Physical Therapy of the Shoulder

FIFTH EDITION

Physical Therapy of the Shoulder

FIFTH EDITION

Edited by

Robert A. Donatelli, PhD, PT, OCS
National Director of Sports Rehabilitation
Physiotherapy Associates
Las Vegas, Nevada

ELSEVIER
CHURCHILL
LIVINGSTONE

ELSEVIER

RELX India Pvt. Ltd.
Registered Office: 818, Indraprakash Building, 8th Floor, 21, Barakhamba Road, New Delhi-110001
Corporate Office: 14th Floor, Building No. 10B, DLF Cyber City, Phase II, Gurgaon-122002, Haryana, India

Physical Therapy of the Shoulder, 5e, Robert A. Donatelli

Original ISBN: 978-1-4377-0740-3

This reprint of **Physical Therapy of the Shoulder, 5e** by Robert A. Donatelli was undertaken by RELX India Pvt. Ltd. and is published by arrangement with Elsevier Ltd.

Indian Reprint ISBN: 978-81-312-5758-6
First Reprinted in India 2019

Printed at EIH Ltd., Unit: Printing Press, IMT Manesar, Gurugram, Haryana.

Dedication

I would like to dedicate this book to my family—my wife Georgi Donatelli, my son, Robby, and my daughters, Briana and Rachel. They have added a new meaning of love, joy and happiness to my life.

Contributors

Randa A. Bascharon, DO, AT
Owner, President, Orthopedic and Sports Medicine Institute Of Las Vegas, Sports Performance Institute of Las Vegas, Las Vegas, Nevada

Mollie Beyers, DPT
Physical Therapist, Biomax Rehabilitation, Effingham, Illinois

Peter Bonutti, MD, FACS, FAAOS, FAANA
Founder and Director, Bonutti Clinic, Founder and Director, Bonutti Technology, Effingham, Illinois, Assistant Clinical Professor, Department of Orthopedic Surgery, University of Arkansas, Fayetteville, Arkansas

Kenji C. Carp, MPT, OCS, ATC
Certified Vestibular Therapist, Director, Owner, Cooperative Performance and Rehabilitation, Eugene, Oregon

Jeff Cooper, MS, ATC
Athletic Training Solutions, Wilmington, Delaware, Consultant, Player Development, Philadelphia Phillies, Philadelphia, Pennsylvania

Donn Dimond, PT, OCS
Director of Clinical Operations, Owner, The KOR Physical Therapy, Portland, Oregon

Jan Dommerholt
President and Physical Therapist, Bethesda Physiocare, Inc/Myopain Seminars, LLC, Bethesda, Maryland

Phillip B. Donley, PT ATC MS
Optimum Physical Therapy, West Chester, Pennsylvania

Xavier A. Duralde, MD
Peachtree Orthopedics Clinic, Assistant Clinical Professor of Orthopedic Surgery, Clinical Instructor, Emory University School of Medicine, Atlanta, Georgia

Richard A. Ekstrom, PT, DSc, MS
Professor, Department of Physical Therapy, University of South Dakota, Vermillion, South Dakota

Todd S. Ellenbecker, DPT, MS, SCS, OCS, CSCS
Clinic Director, Physiotherapy Associates Scottsdale Sports Clinic, National Director of Clinical Research, Physiotherapy Associates, Director of Sports Medicine, ATP World Tour, Scottsdale, Arizona

Robert L. Elvey, BAppSc, Grad. Dip. Manip. Ther.
Senior Lecturer, Curkin University, Physiotherapy Consultant, Southcare Physiotherapy, Perth, Australia

Kathleen Geist, PT, DPT, OCS, COMT
Assistant Professor, Division of Physical Therapy, Department of Rehabilitation Medicine, Emory University School of Medicine, Atlanta, Georgia

John C. Gray, DPT, OCS, FAAOMPT
Lead Clinical Specialist, Department of Physical Therapy, Sharp Rees-Stealy, Clinical Instructor, Ola Grimsby Institute, Credentialed Clinical Instructor, American Physical Therapy Association, Associate Editor, Journal of Manual and Manipulative Therapy, San Diego, California

Bruce H. Greenfield, PT, PhD, OCS
Assistant Professor, Department of Rehabilitation, Center for Ethics, Emory University, Atlanta, Georgia

Ola Grimsby, PT
Chairman of the Board, Ola Grimsby Institute, San Diego, California

Toby M. Hall, PhD, MSc, Post Grad Dip Manip Ther, Assoc in Physiotherapy
Director Manual Concepts, Perth, Australia, Adjunct Senior Teaching Fellow, School of Physiotherapy, Curtin Innovation Health Research Institute, Curtin University of Technology, Bentley, Australia, Senior Teaching Fellow, The University of Western Australia, Perth, Australia, Director Manual Concepts, Perth, Australia

Scot Irwin, DPT, CCS[†]
Formerly, Associate Professor, Department of Physical Therapy, North Georgia College and State University, Dahlonega, Georgia

Robert C. Manske, PT, DPT, SCS, MEd, ATC, CSCSC
Associate Professor, Department of Physical Therapy, Wichita State University, Wichita, Kansas

Johnson McEvoy, PT, BSc, MSc, DPT, MISCP, MCSP
Chartered Physiotherapist in Private Practice, United Physiotherapy Clinic, Limerick, Ireland, Head Physiotherapist, Irish Boxing High Performance Team, Dublin, Ireland, External Lecturer, Sports Science, University of Limerick, Limerick, Ireland

Craig D. Morgan, MD
Clinical Professor, University of Pennsylvania, Department of Orthopaedics, Philadelphia, Pennsylvania, Morgan Kalman Clinic, Wilmington, Delaware

Douglas M. Murray, MD
Surgeon, Peachtree Orthopedic Clinic, Consulting Physician, Shepherd Center, Atlanta, Georgia

Roy W. Osborn, PT, MS, OCS
Associate Professor, Physical Therapist, Physical Therapy Department, Avera McKennan Hospital and University Health System, Sioux Falls, South Dakota

Jaime C. Paz, PT, DPT, MS
Clinical Associate Professor, Division of Physical Therapy, Walsh University, North Canton, Ohio

Scott D. Pennington, MD
Surgeon, Peachtree Orthopedic Clinic, Atlanta, Georgia

Vijay B. Vad, MD
Assistant Professor of Rehabilitation Medicine, Hospital for Special Surgery, New York, New York

Joseph S. Wilkes, MD
Clinical Associate Professor, Orthopedics, Emory University, Active Staff Member, Piedmont Hospital, Specialty Consulting, Crawford Long Hospital, Atlanta, Georgia, Active Staff Member, Fayette Community Hospital, Fayetteville, Georgia

Michael S. Zazzali, DSc, PT, OCS
Co-Director and Partner, Physical Therapy Associates of New York, New York, New York

[†]Deceased.

Preface

The first edition of *Physical Therapy of the Shoulder* was published in 1987, and now we are publishing the fifth edition nearly 25 years later. I would like to thank my readers for their support throughout the years that has made this book successful. The fifth edition has kept up with the tradition of Physical Therapy evidence-based practice. It is amazing how the literature now has developed our profession from and art to a science. Each chapter is a excellent example of how the science of Physical Therapy continues to grow.

The shoulder joint is a complicated structure consisting of three synovial joints, the scapula thoracic articulation, and 17 muscles. The shoulder complex hangs off the rib cage and is connected to the cervical and thoracic spine. The complexity of the shoulder makes many rehabilitation students and clinicians uncertain in assessing shoulder pathomechanics and in establishing treatment approaches for different shoulder pathologies.

In keeping up to date with new and innovative treatment techniques, surgical procedures, and evaluation methods for the shoulder, this fifth edition of *Physical Therapy of the Shoulder* has been updated appropriately. There are 7 new chapters and 8 new authors. The fifth edition is once again divided into five parts; Mechanics of Movement and Evaluation, Neurologic Considerations, Special Considerations, Treatment Approaches, and Surgical Considerations.

In honor of the memory of the late Scot Irwin, Jaime Paz helped to revise the Guide to Physical Therapist Practice. The chapter is an overview of the Guide. Chapter 2 was updated with new anatomic and biomechanical information on how the shoulder moves. Chapter 3 was rewritten by Jeff Cooper with all the new information on the throwing injuries to the shoulder. Jeff has included new research data that he has collected over the past several years on professional baseball pitchers. His approach to evaluation and treatment is state of the art. Chapter 4 is a new chapter by Donn Dimond that finishes the first section with updates on all the new-evidenced-based special tests for the shoulder. The special tests on the shoulder greatly assist the clinician in the development of a differential soft tissue diagnosis. In addition, manual muscle testing to isolate the shoulder muscles is illustrated.

Part 2, Neurologic Considerations, has been updated with new information and references. John C. Gray and Ola Grimsby's chapter, Interrelationship of the Spine, Rib Cage, and Shoulder, along with Neural Tension Testing by Tobby Hall and Bob Elvy have been revised, and Bruce H. Greenfield and Kathleen Geist did a great job updating the chapter on Evaluation and Treatment of Brachial Plexus Lesions. A new chapter, Sensory Integration and Neuromuscular Control of the Shoulder by Kenji Carp has been added to the neurological section. I think you will find that Kenji did an excellent job on defining neuromuscular control in the upper limb. The chapter is an excellent representation of state of the art information that is critical to the rehabilitation of shoulder patients.

Part 3, Special Considerations, was highlighted by the separation of Chapter 10 into two chapters, Impingement Syndrome and Shoulder Instabilities. Bruce Greenfield did an excellent job on describing the mechanisms of impingement and the new chapter, on shoulder instabilities, by Michael Zazzali, focused on the conservative approach to the evaluation and treatment of shoulder instabilities. The Frozen Shoulder chapter was update by Mollie Beyers and Peter Bonutti. This chapter provides an excellent summary of the evidence-based research on treatment of frozen shoulder pathology. John C. Gray's chapter on Visceral Referred Pain to the Shoulder, was rewritten, along with important updates from Todd S. Ellenbecker on rotator cuff pathology.

In the Treatment Approaches Section, Richard A. Ekstrom and Roy W. Osborn did an excellent job on adding addition research on Muscle Length Testing and Electromyographic Evidence for Manual Strength Testing and Exercises for the Shoulder. The Manual Therapy Techniques was updated with additional illustrations of new manual procedures for the shoulder, with a section on evidence-based manual therapy treatment approaches. The treatment section was highlighted by one of two new chapters by Donn Dimond on strength training in the shoulder. As previously noted the shoulder has 17 muscle that allow it to move in multiple planes. Therefore this chapter is long awaited as the strength of the shoulder muscles is critical to the overall function. Finally,

I am honored to have Johnson McEvoy and Jan Dommerholt in the fifth edition with a new chapter on Myofascial Trigger Points of the Shoulder. The chapter is very comprehensive covering evaluation and treatment of trigger points. The treatment approaches described include, Myofascial release techniques using manual therapy, massage techniques, dry needling, spray and stretch, and the use of modalities.

The Surgical Considerations Section includes the addition of a chapter by Dr. Ronda Bascharon and Robert Manske on the Surgical Approach to Shoulder Instabilities. The chapter includes state-of-the-art concepts in evaluation and treatment of the Bankart lesion, S.L.A.P lesions, and rotator cuff interval concepts. Dr. Joseph Wilkes and Dr. Xavier Duralde made important updates in their chapters on Rotator Cuff Repairs and Total Shoulder Replacements, respectively.

I am pleased to include a companion Evolve site with the fifth edition of *Physical Therapy of the Shoulder.* The Evolve site compliments the text and enhances the clinical application with excerpts of an evaluation of a patient using manual therapy treatment techniques of the shoulder. A link to an electronic image collection that features most of the illustrations contained in the book are included on Evolve.

Any rehabilitation professional entrusted with the care and treatment of mechanical and pathologic shoulder dysfunction will benefit from this book. I trust that the fifth edition will meet the reader's expectation of comprehensive, clinically relevant presentations and case studies that are well documented, contemporary, and personally challenging to the student and the experienced specialist alike.

Robert A. Donatelli, PhD, PT, OCS

Contents

CHAPTER

1

Scot Irwin and Jaime C. Paz

The Guide to Practice

In this fifth edition of Donatelli's *Physical Therapy of the Shoulder*, the clinical cases continue to be written in the format of *Guide to Physical Therapist Practice*[1] (the *Guide*) of the American Physical Therapy Association (APTA). This format was developed and has been promoted by the APTA, which is the largest professional representative for physical therapists, physical therapy assistants, and physical therapy students in the United States.

This chapter is designed to orient the reader to the origins, purposes, content, and nature of the *Guide*. In this way, the intent of this chapter is to encourage clinicians and students who use this current book to incorporate the *Guide*'s language and philosophy into the examination, evaluation, diagnosis, prognosis, intervention, and outcome provided for their patients with shoulder dysfunction.

ORIGINS

To speak at any length about the origins of this document would take most of this text. For the abbreviated yet complete review, the reader is encouraged to read the *Guide.*[1] Since Mary McMillan first constructed and presided over the Women's Physiotherapy Association in the early 1920s—and until the first edition of the *Guide* in 1997—the reconstruction aides, general practitioners, and certified clinical specialists all intuitively have known the value and importance of rehabilitation services. Throughout that short but illustrious history, the association members have professed the uniqueness and talent within the physical therapy profession to any who cared to listen. The scientific evidence of this effectiveness, in contrast, remains to be presented. No defined body of knowledge for physical therapists exists. The *Guide* provides a foundation for developing the evidence for the effectiveness of physical therapist interventions. The body of knowledge will be defined from the evidence that proves the value of these interventions.

Physical therapy originated from many facets of health care and health sciences, nursing, physical education, medicine, pathology, and rehabilitation—yet physical therapists claim none alone. For most of the decade of the 1980s and early 1990s, the APTA debated the merits and even the existence of physical therapy diagnoses. The term *diagnosis* is so fraught with interpretations that, within the APTA, confusion and debate have consumed an inordinate amount of the association's governance time. Finally, the APTA House of Delegates came to an agreement that physical therapists did diagnose and that those diagnoses were directed at movement and movement dysfunction.

The basic premise here is that human movement, like digestion, is a system. The movement system has normal behaviors that can become dysfunctional, and a physical therapist can provide remedies for those dysfunctions. Eventually, because of a need to describe the scope of a physical therapist's practice more clearly for many health care agencies and for the physical therapy profession, the APTA undertook the development of the *Guide*. From 1992 through the completion of the current edition, a handful of physical therapists and staff members of the APTA constructed this document. Those who have tried to produce anything by committee can imagine the amount of time and effort required to write the *Guide*. The authors of the *Guide* are too numerous to list, but they are acknowledged within the *Guide* itself, and they deserve the respect and thanks of every physical therapist. All the authors were chosen for their expertise and knowledge in a particular practice pattern arena (musculoskeletal, neuromuscular, cardiovascular/pulmonary, and integumentary). Each of those authors is quick to point out that this document is not written on a stone tablet. Its origins derive from the cataclysmic changes that have occurred in health care delivery and reimbursement in the United States. Those driving forces, along with the dynamic growth and development of the profession of physical therapy, created an environment that required this document's publication and demanded that the *Guide* be in constant evolution. Evidence of this evolution is electronic access to the revised second edition of the *Guide* in compact disk format, which includes a catalog of tests and measures employed by physical therapists. Furthermore, the APTA has provided Internet access to the latest edition of the Guide.[2]

The challenge for future physical therapists is to continue to amend and edit the *Guide* by documenting errors and omissions and by providing new practice patterns for impairments and functional limitations yet to be identified or discovered. A future edition of the *Guide* is likely to include the International Classification of Functioning, Disability, and Health (ICF) developed by the World Health Organization (WHO) to promote human functioning with a standardized framework and language. The APTA House of Delegates endorsed this model in 2008.[3]

PURPOSES

The list of purposes for the *Guide* can be found in the first section, "About the Guide," of the revised second edition.[1] Throughout the document, these purposes are reiterated. Each of the diagnostic patterns described in the *Guide* uses terminology found in the list of purposes. Although many readers find this constant redundancy a distracting feature of the *Guide*, it is used to demonstrate the basic constructs of a physical therapist's approach to patient management. The authors of the *Guide* also used the combined term patient/client throughout the *Guide*. For this chapter, the term *client* is used.

A summary of the purposes is as follows: The *Guide* was developed to assist internal (physical therapists) and external (all others involved in health care delivery and reimbursement) individuals in understanding the scope of a physical therapist's practice. As stated in the *Guide*, this list includes—but is not limited to—practice settings, roles, terminology, tests and measures, and interventions used by physical therapists in the delivery of physical therapy. Perhaps most important, the *Guide* establishes preferred practice patterns based on the Nagi model of disablement.[4] Common themes within the purposes listed in the *Guide* are the promotion of health, wellness, and fitness along with prevention of movement dysfunction and the appropriate use of physical therapy services as provided by physical therapists.

The authors of the *Guide* clearly describe what the *Guide* is not. To quote the authors: "The *Guide* does not provide specific protocols for treatments, nor are the practice patterns contained in the *Guide* intended to serve as clinical guidelines."[1] The authors go on to state that the *Guide* is only an initial step in the development of clinical guidelines. Clinical guideline development requires evidence from peer-reviewed research. The current edition of the *Guide* was not written to provide that level of information.

In this book, the case examples have been "Guideized," including formatting and terminology. It is the intention that the reader should become familiar with this system of patient evaluation and treatment and incorporate it into his or her daily practice. It is also hoped that academic and clinical faculty will use the *Guide* approach when instructing future generations of physical therapists and will thus fulfill the purpose of the *Guide*.

CONTENT

The *Guide* was developed with three key concepts in mind: (1) the Nagi model of disablement[4] (Table 1-1); (2) the variety of work settings for physical therapists; and (3) the provision of services by physical therapists through the continuum of health care.

To understand the *Guide*, a good understanding of the disablement model is required. Articles by Guccione[5] and Jette[6] have provided the background for understanding disablement. The reader can find these articles in the journal *Physical Therapy* from 1991 and 1994, respectively. The Nagi model[4] was selected by the authors of the *Guide* because it provides the best fit for the development of physical therapy practice patterns and diagnoses. As Guccione's diagram (Fig. 1-1) so aptly demonstrates, the Nagi model encompasses the entire spectrum of health care. Pathology and pathophysiology lead to impairment, which can either cause more pathology or lead to functional limitations. These functional limitations may revert back to impairments or progress to disability. The domain of a physical therapist's practice is outlined by the dotted lines in Figure 1-1. The *Guide* was developed to address the delivery of health care services by physical therapists from pathology to impairment to functional limitation and to disability with the greatest emphasis on identification and rectification of impairments and functional limitations. In effect, the *Guide* is saying that physical therapists are the diagnosticians of movement impairments and provide interventions to prevent, improve, or eliminate functional limitations and disability.

The *Guide* goes on to enhance and adapt the Nagi model by expanding it to include the larger arena of quality of life (Fig. 1-2). This enhancement requires that the *Guide* include psychological and social functions, as well as the constructs of the promotion of wellness, prevention, and fitness.

Table 1-1 Nagi Model of Disablement

Active Pathology	Impairment	Functional Limitation	Disability
Interruption or interference with normal processes, and efforts of the organism to regain normal state	Anatomic, physiologic, mental, or emotional abnormalities or loss	Limitation in performance at the level of the whole organism or person	Limitation in performance of socially defined roles and tasks within a sociocultural and physical environment

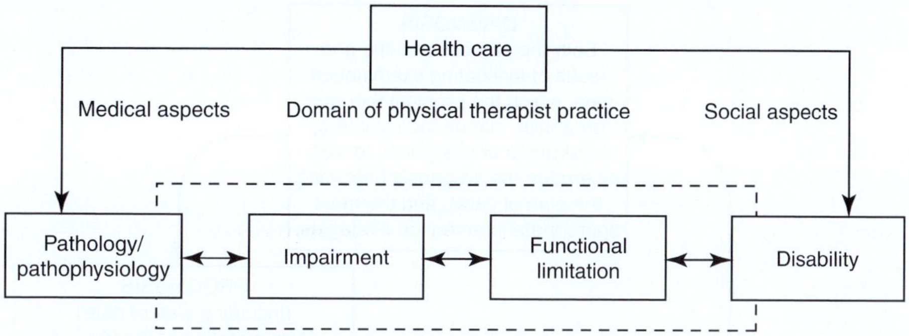

Figure 1-1 Scope of physical therapist practice within the continuum of health care services and the context of the disablement model. (Modified from the American Therapist Association from Guccione AA: Physical therapy diagnosis and the relationship between impairments and function, *Phys Ther* 71:499–504, 1991.)

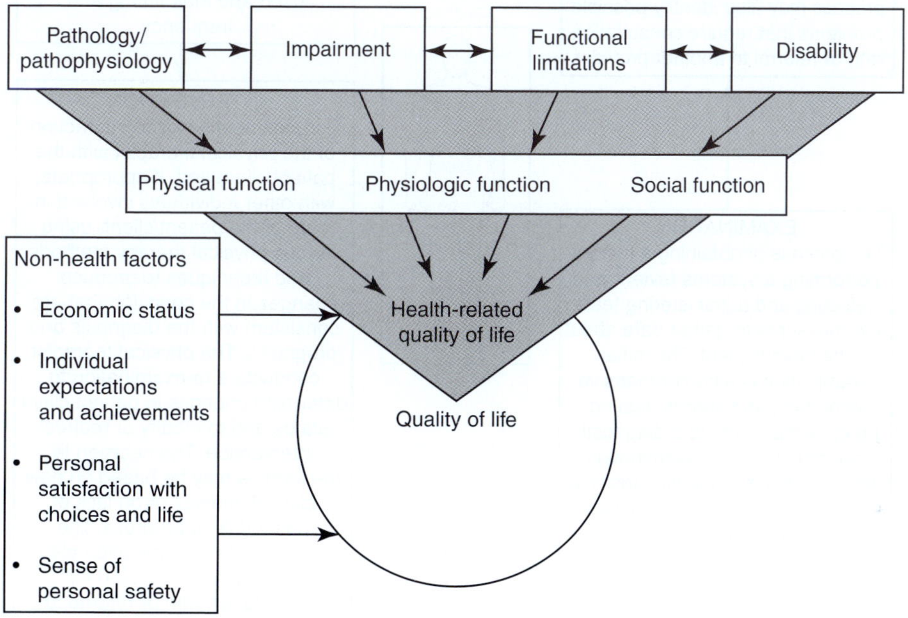

Figure 1-2 Relationship of the disablement model, health-related quality of life, and quality of life.

The actual content of the *Guide* currently includes five major parts. The first part is a description of the *Guide* itself that provides insight into its development, purpose, scope, and content overview. The second part of the *Guide* defines who physical therapists are and describes their approaches to the management of clients. The second part of the *Guide* also provides a description of the tests and measures used by physical therapists as a part of their examination process. In addition, the second part provides definitions and lists of physical therapists' interventions. The third and by far the longest portion of the *Guide* is made up of preferred practice patterns. The fourth part provides expanded access to the catalog of tests and measures. The fifth part provides a document template to facilitate the use of *Guide* terminology and the patient management system in clinical practice. A glossary is included at the end of the *Guide*.

The section that describes physical therapists provides information on the following: the prerequisites required to become a physical therapist; the types of settings in which physical therapists practice; the roles of physical therapists in primary, secondary, tertiary, and preventive care; the components of a physical therapist's episode of care; and the criteria for termination of physical therapy services. In addition, this section describes in greater detail the six elements of patient management: (1) examination, (2) evaluation, (3) diagnosis, (4) prognosis, (5) intervention, and (6) outcomes (Fig. 1-3). Finally, this section gives a broader description of the roles of physical therapists in management, administration, communication, critical inquiry, and education.

The second part of the *Guide* provides the list of the tests and measures used by physical therapists in their examination of clients. If a test or measure is not listed in the *Guide*, this does not preclude physical therapists from using that test or measure. It is the intent of the *Guide*, however, that any test or measure used is valid and reliable and that each follows

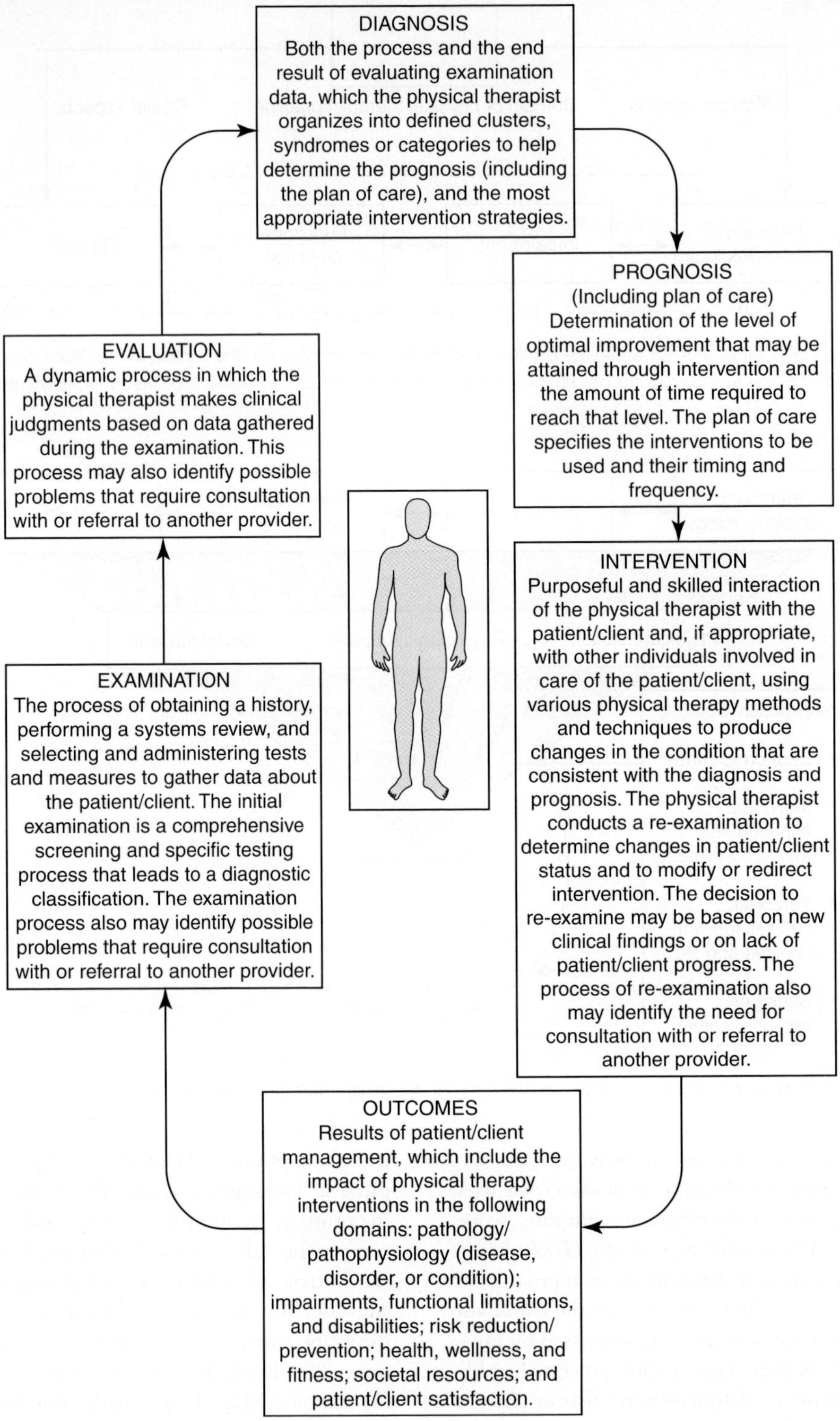

Figure 1-3 The elements of patient management leading to optimal outcomes. (From American Physical Therapy Association: *Guide to Physical Therapist Practice*, ed 2. Baltimore, APTA, 2003.)

the Standards for Tests and Measurements in Physical Therapy Practice as presented in the journal *Physical Therapy* in 1991.[7]

The interventions section is provided primarily for external groups. This section contains definitions and descriptions of all the activities in which physical therapists are trained and required to perform when intervening on behalf of a client. This list includes coordination, communication, administration, client education, and the entire spectrum of the physical therapists' interventions from therapeutic exercise to physical agents and modalities.

The bulk of the *Guide* is dedicated to the practice patterns. The patterns are broken up into four broad classifications: (1) musculoskeletal, (2) neuromuscular, (3) cardiovascular/pulmonary, and (4) integumentary. All the client cases described in this edition of *Physical Therapy of the Shoulder* can be found in the musculoskeletal and neuromuscular practice patterns. Although the physical therapists' evaluations direct them initially to a specific pattern, this does not preclude therapists from changing to an alternative pattern if the examination information leads them to another conclusion. It is also possible for a client to fit into more than one pattern. In this case, the professional opinion of the therapist directs the allocation of resources and time to the pattern of highest priority.

The practice patterns were developed using the Nagi model[4] and the patient management system previously described.[1] This system includes six components. Each component in the patient management system is found in every practice pattern. The purpose of this format is to create a consistent, uniform methodology for patient examination and treatment. As depicted in Figure 1-3, each component of this system has specific supportive parts. Examination includes obtaining a history, review of systems (cardiopulmonary, musculoskeletal, neuromuscular, and integumentary), choice and administration of tests, measurements of appropriate values, and identification of any need for referral to another practitioner.

Figure 1-4 provides an in-depth summary of the data that can be gathered during client history taking. The evaluation is the process of using the information obtained during the examination to determine a diagnosis or need for referral. This process continues throughout the client's contact with the therapist and requires clinical judgment on a regular and routine basis. The diagnosis is a determination of which practice pattern is a "best fit" for the previously gathered examination and evaluation information. This physical therapist diagnosis relates directly to an impairment classification in the Nagi model[4] and should lead the therapist to determine the relative level of functional loss the client is experiencing. This information, in turn, directs the therapist to the appropriate intervention to obtain the optimal outcome for the client.

The next component is the prognosis. This component also includes the plan of care. The prognosis is a natural extension of the diagnosis. Once the diagnosis has been made, the therapist should begin to formulate a realistic prognosis and estimate how much improvement in function can be achieved given the amount of impairment suffered as a result of the disease. The logical progression of these interwoven formulations between the Nagi model and the patient management system has been included in the *Guide* to create a continuum of care that leads to improved function or appropriate referral.

The plan of care is the culmination of all the steps previously listed and includes the client's goals, the short- and long-term goals of the therapist, specific interventions, and the projected outcomes of those interventions. Included within the interventions and outcomes should be some projection of the frequency and duration of treatment required and plans for discharge from therapy.

Perhaps the most important contribution of the *Guide* to the clinician is in the intervention segments of each practice pattern. These *suggested* interventions are not cookbooks for care, but rather are listed specifically as *possible* physical therapist approaches to achievement of the desired outcomes for the client. In all cases, education of the client or of supportive personnel is included as part of the interventions listed regardless of the selected practice pattern. Alternative interventions listed under a particular pattern should not be interpreted by the therapist as an indication to try one or two interventions and then move on to the next practice pattern if the interventions do not work. Each intervention should be applied as appropriate to the client's responses, goals, needs, and projected outcomes. Nowhere in the *Guide* is it suggested that the interventions listed are the only ones appropriate to a particular practice pattern. As the reader will learn later in this book, however, application of the correct intervention to the client with shoulder dysfunction has been found to improve the client's functional level and to reduce his or her overall impairment.

In few, if any, cases are the interventions of the physical therapist directed solely toward the pathologic or pathophysiologic features of the client's medical condition. The *Guide* is a textbook for providing direction for physical therapists to intervene at the level of impairment and functional limitation without the use of medication for the most part or surgical interventions. Intervention also includes the need for the therapist to interact with the rest of the medical community involved in the client's care. This interaction requires coordination and communication with, and documentation of, all the physical therapist's clients.

Inherent in the system of patient management is that at any point during the client's treatment, the therapist is mandated to provide re-examination. The re-examination should be performed periodically during an episode of care, to ensure that the client is progressing according to his or her prognosis and that short- and long-term goals are being achieved. During re-examination, the patient management system steps are repeated as in the original examination process.

SUMMARY

Why is the *Guide* entitled *Guide to Physical Therapist Practice* and not *Guide to Physical Therapy Practice*? That is the nature of the document. It is intended to describe the scope, role, and spectrum of the physical therapist's activity. Why not physical therapy? Because many other practitioners who are not physical therapists are legally allowed to provide and be reimbursed for physical therapy. The APTA believes that physical therapy per se is well described within the *Guide,* but physical therapy is really performed only by physical therapists. Therefore, the *Guide* correctly describes the physical therapists' diagnoses (practice patterns), tests and measures, interventions, and responsibilities within the context of the Nagi model.[4]

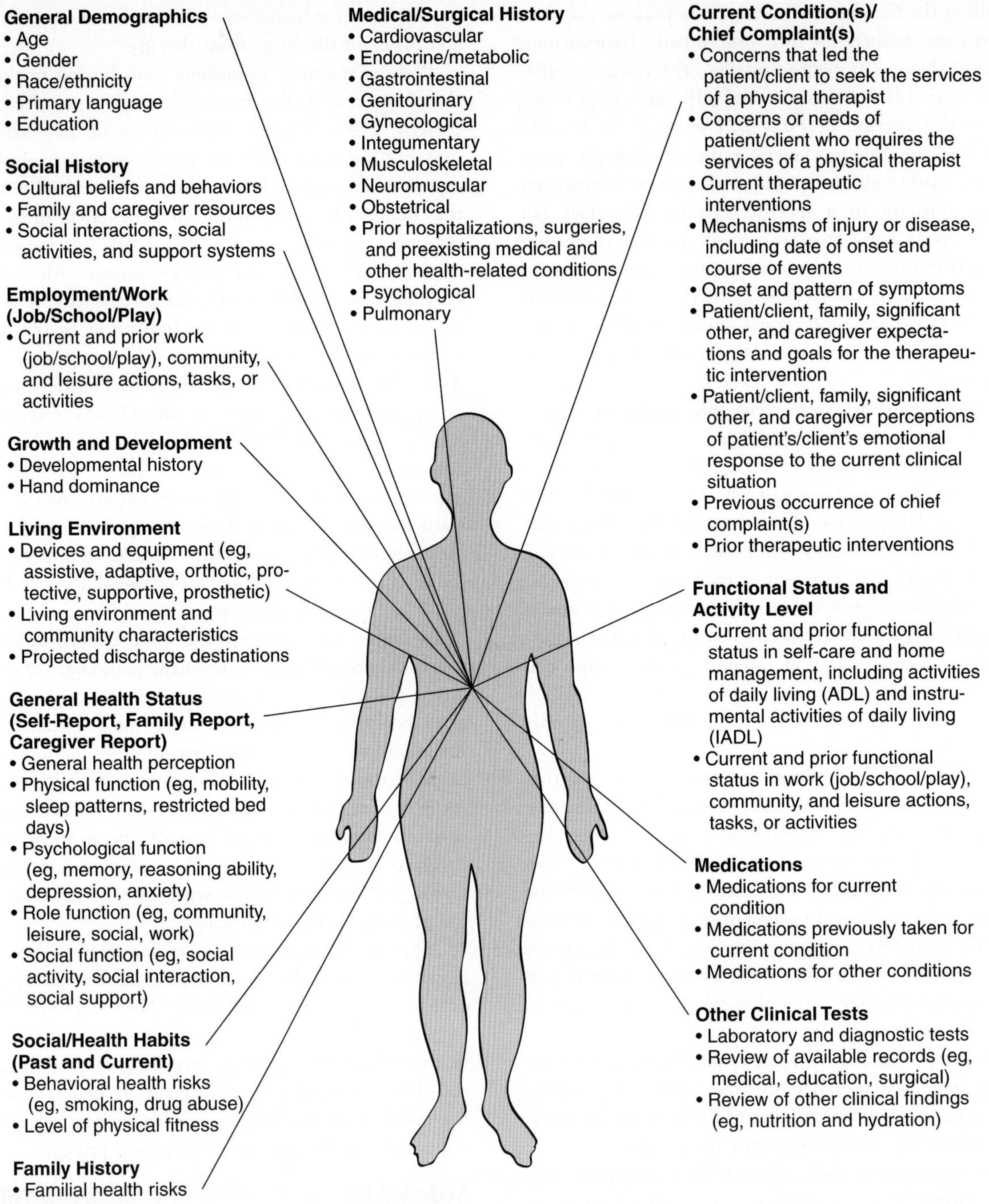

Figure 1-4 Types of data that may be generated from a client history. (From American Physical Therapy Association: *Guide to Physical Therapist Practice*, ed 2. Baltimore, 2003, APTA.)

The template for defining the body of knowledge of physical therapy has been produced in the *Guide*. The physical therapist community has been challenged to provide the evidence to prove or disprove the usefulness of the interventions provided within each practice pattern. The *Guide* has provided all physical therapists with a common language, a patient management system, and an opportunity to develop definitive and reproducible methods of optimally improving impairments and functional limitations of a physical therapist's clients. The *Guide to Physical Therapist Practice* is indeed a truly epic document.

REFERENCES

1. American Physical Therapy Association: *Guide to physical therapist practice*, ed 2 rev, Alexandria, Va, 2003, American Physical Therapy Association.
2. American Physical Therapy Association: *Guide to physical therapist practice* (website). http://guidetoptpractice.apta.org/. Accessed May 17, 2010.
3. American Physical Therapy Association: *House of Delegates Policies 2009, Page 32, line 8.* http://www.apta.org/AM/Template.cfm?Section=Policies_and_Bylaws1&TEMPLATE=/CM/ContentDisplay.cfm&CONTENTID=67833. Accessed October 28, 2010.

4. Nagi S: *Disability and rehabilitation*, Columbus, Ohio, 1969, Ohio State University Press.
5. Guccione AA: Physical therapy diagnosis and the relationship between impairments and function, *Phys Ther* 71:499–504, 1991.
6. Jette AM: Physical disablement concepts for physical therapy research and practice, *Phys Ther* 74:381, 1994.
7. American Physical Therapy Association: Standards for tests and measurements in physical therapy practice, *Phys Ther* 71:589–622, 1991.

PART 1
MECHANICS OF MOVEMENT AND EVALUATION

CHAPTER 2

Robert A. Donatelli

Functional Anatomy and Mechanics

One of the most common peripheral joints to be treated in a physical therapy clinic is the shoulder joint. The physical therapist must have an in-depth understanding of the anatomy and mechanics of this joint to evaluate and design a treatment program most effectively for the patient with shoulder dysfunction. This chapter describes the pertinent functional anatomy of the shoulder complex and relates this anatomy to functional movements, stability, muscle activity, and clinical application.

The shoulder joint is better called the shoulder complex, because a series of articulations are necessary to position the humerus in space (Fig. 2-1). Most authors, when describing the shoulder joint, discuss the acromioclavicular (AC) joint, the sternoclavicular joint (SC), the scapulothoracic articulation, and the glenohumeral joint.[1-4] Dempster[5] related all these areas by using a concept of links. The integrated and harmonious roles of all the links are necessary for full normal mobility.[5]

The glenohumeral joint sacrifices stability for mobility. This joint is characterized by its large range of motion. The shoulder is capable of moving in more than 16,000 positions, which can be differentiated by 1° in a normal person.[6] The mobility of the shoulder relies on the congruent articulating surfaces and the surrounding soft tissue envelope for static and dynamic stability. The position of the humerus and scapula must change throughout each movement to maintain stability.[6]

OSTEOKINEMATIC AND ARTHROKINEMATIC MOVEMENT

Analysis of shoulder movement emphasizes the synchronized movement of four joints: the glenohumeral, scapulothoracic, SC, and AC joints.[2,4,7,8] As the humerus moves into elevation, movement must occur at all four joints. Elevation of the arm can be observed in three planes: the frontal plane (abduction), the sagittal plane (flexion), and the plane of the scapula (POS; scaption).[8,9] Movement of the long bones of the arm into elevation is referred to as *osteokinematics.* The term *arthrokinematics* describes the intricate movement of joint surfaces: rolling, spinning, and sliding.[10]

Osteokinematic Movement

Scaption-Abduction: Plane of the Scapula

Abduction of the shoulder in the frontal or coronal plane has been extensively researched.[4,8,11-17] Poppen and Walker[15] and Johnston[8] suggested that the true plane of movement in the shoulder joint occurs in the POS. The term *plane of the scapula* is defined as elevation of the shoulder in a range between 30° and 45° anterior to the frontal plane (Figs. 2-2 and 2-3).[15]

Kondo et al[18] devised a method for taking radiographs to define scaption during elevation. The medial tilting angle was used to describe scaption. The *medial tilting angle* refers to the tilting of the scapula toward the sagittal plane. As the medial tilting angle increases, movement of the scapula around the thoracic cage occurs. Kondo et al[18] demonstrated that the medial tilting angle was constant at 40° anterior to the frontal plane throughout a range of 150° of elevation.

Several authors believe that the POS is clinically significant because the length-tension relationship of the shoulder abductors and rotators is optimum in this plane of elevation.[8,15] Research has demonstrated that the length of the muscle determines the amount of stretch applied to the individual sarcomeres, thus enabling them to exert maximum tension.[19] The length-tension curves obtained from normal muscles show that maximum tension develops when the muscle length is approximately 90% of its maximum length.[19] Conversely, when the muscle is fully shortened, the tension developed is minimal.[20,21] Therefore, the optimal lengthened position of the muscle tendon facilitates optimal muscle contraction.[22]

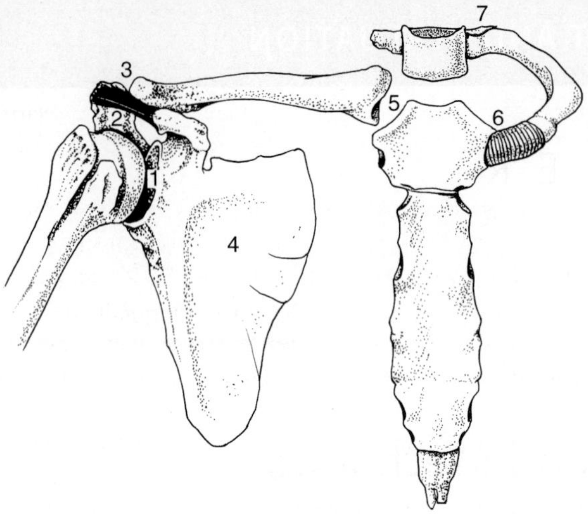

Figure 2-1 The components of the shoulder joint complex: 1, glenohumeral joint; 2, subdeltoid joint; 3, acromioclavicular joint; 4, scapulothoracic joint; 5, sternoclavicular joint; 6, first costosternal joint; 7, first costovertebral joint.

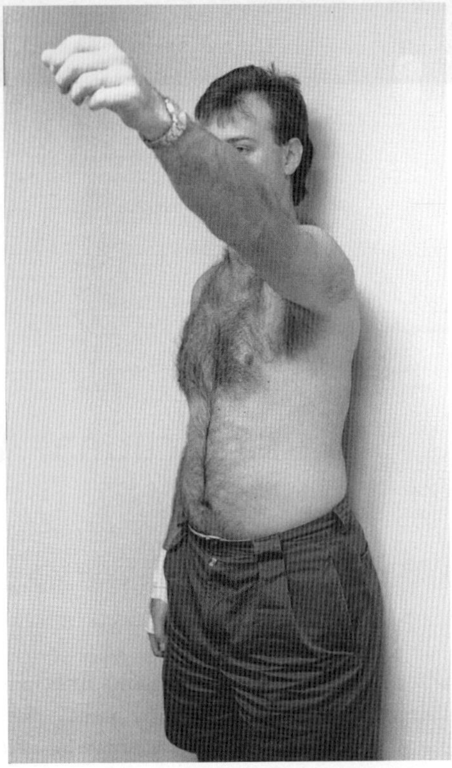

Figure 2-2 Elevation in the plane of the scapula.

Several studies have compared the torque production of different shoulder muscle groups when tested in scaption versus other body planes.[23-27] Soderberg and Blaschak[23] and Hellwig and Perrin[24] demonstrated no significant differences in the peak torque of the glenohumeral rotators between scaption and other body planes. These studies used 45° and 40° anterior to the frontal plane, respectively, for the scaption test position. Greenfield et al[25] reported greater torque in the external rotators when tested in scaption versus the coronal plane. Furthermore, Tata et al[26] reported higher ratios of abduction to adduction and external to internal torque when tested in the scapular plane at 30° and 35° anterior to the frontal plane, respectively. Whitcomb et al[27] found no significant difference in torque produced by the shoulder abductors in the coronal and scapular planes when a scaption position 35° anterior to the frontal plane was used.

The studies cited indicate that the external rotators are the only muscle group that demonstrate a significant increase in torque in the scaption plane 30° anterior to the frontal plane. The pectoralis major and the latissimus muscle groups are not attached to the scapula. Therefore, it would seem reasonable that when the torque output of the internal rotators is compared, the change in position of the scapula should not influence the optimal length-tension relationship. The internal rotators exhibit no change in torque when they are tested in different planes of movement.

In addition to optimal muscle length-tension relationship in the POS, the capsular fibers of the glenohumeral joint are relaxed.[8] Because the capsule is untwisted in the POS, mobilization and stretching in this plane may be tolerated better than in other planes, where the capsule is starting in a twisted position.

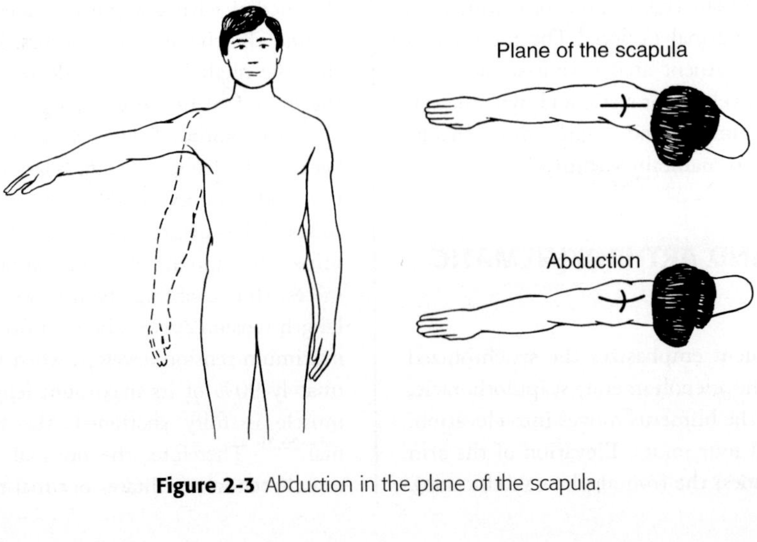

Figure 2-3 Abduction in the plane of the scapula.

Poppen and Walker[14] demonstrated that an increase in joint congruity occurs in scaption that allows for greater joint stability. Therefore, for reasons of glenohumeral stability, minimal scapular torsion, avoidance of impingement, and balance of muscle action, scaption may be the plane in which shoulder trauma is minimal and may thus be the most advantageous plane for mobilization, stretching, testing, and strengthening of the glenohumeral rotators.

Flexion

The movement of flexion has been investigated less thoroughly. *Flexion* is movement in the sagittal plane. Full flexion from 162° to 180° is possible only with synchronous motion in the glenohumeral, AC, SC, and scapulothoracic joints.[14] The movement is similar to that of abduction.

Arthrokinematic Movement

The motion occurring at joint surfaces is *arthrokinematic motion,* the three types of which are rolling, gliding, and rotation (Fig. 2-4). *Rolling* occurs when various points on a moving surface contact various points on a stationary surface. *Gliding* occurs when one point on a moving surface contacts multiple points on a stationary surface. During rolling or gliding, a significant change occurs in the contact area between the two joint surfaces. The third type of arthrokinematic movement, *rotation,* occurs when one or more points on a moving surface contact one point on a stationary surface. Displacement between the two joint surfaces in rotation is minimal.

All three arthrokinematic movements can occur at the glenohumeral joint, but not in equal proportions. These motions are necessary for the large humeral head to take advantage of the small glenoid articulating surface.[16] Saha[16] investigated the contact area between the head of the humerus and the glenoid with abduction in the POS and found that the contact area on the head of the humerus shifted upward and forward, whereas the contact area on the glenoid remained relatively constant, a finding indicating a rotation movement. Poppen and Walker[15] measured the instant centers of rotation for the same movement. These investigators found in the first 30°, and often between 30° and 60°, that the head of the humerus moved superiorly in the glenoid by 3 mm, a finding indicating rolling or gliding. At more than 60°, movement of the humerus was minimal, a sign of almost pure rotation.[15]

Effective arthrokinematic movements are achieved by complex interaction between the various articular and soft tissue restraints in addition to the dynamic action of the rotator cuff muscles. For example, the rotator cuff muscles center the humeral head in the congruent glenoid fossa during the midrange of motion when the capsuloligamentous structures are lax.[28] Dysfunction of this complex mechanism occurs with tightening of the capsule anteriorly, a situation that results in anterior restriction and causes an associated posterior shift in contact of the humerus on the glenoid. The posterior migration of the humeral head center and glenohumeral contact are pronounced in shoulder joints with poor congruence.[28] To re-establish harmonious movement within the shoulder complex, the therapist must rehabilitate the connective tissue by restoring its extensibility and the normal balance of muscles.

ROTATIONS OF THE HUMERUS

Rotations of the humerus are important for elevation. Concomitant external rotation of the humerus is necessary for abduction in the coronal plane.[4,8,10,14,17] Some investigators have postulated that this motion is necessary for the greater

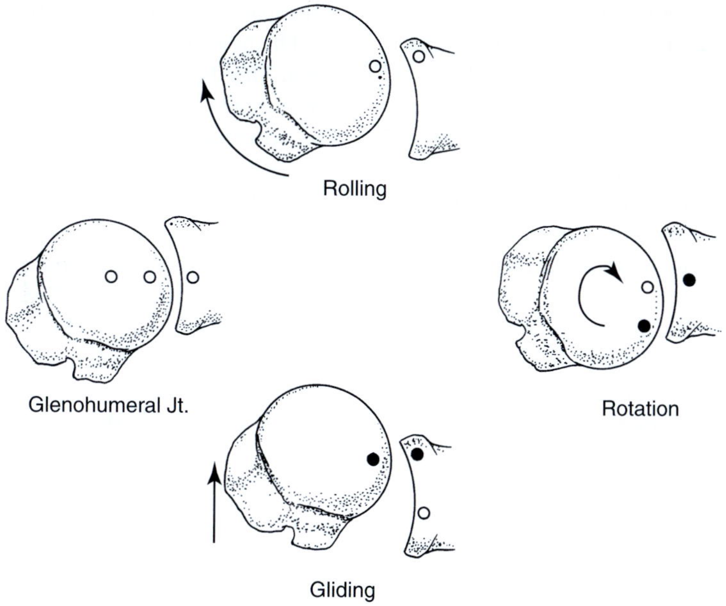

Figure 2-4 Arthrokinematic motion occurring at the glenohumeral joint: rolling, rotation, and gliding.

tuberosity to clear the acromion and the coracoacromial ligament.[1,2,17] Saha[16] reported sufficient room between the greater tuberosity and the acromion to prevent bone impingement. External rotation also remains necessary for full coronal abduction even after surgical removal of the acromion and the coracoacromial ligament. Saha[16] reasoned that external rotation is necessary to prevent the humeral head from impinging on the glenoid rim.

Using cadaveric glenohumeral joints, Rajendran[29] demonstrated that automatic external rotation of the humerus is an essential component of active and passive elevation of the arm through abduction. Even in the absence of extra-articular influences, such as the coracoacromial arch and glenohumeral muscles, external rotation of the humerus was spontaneous. An et al[30] used a magnetic tracking system to monitor the three-dimensional orientation of the humerus with respect to the scapula. Appropriate coordinate transformations were then performed for the calculation of glenohumeral joint rotation. Maximum elevation in all planes anterior to the scapular plane required external axial rotation of the humerus. Browne et al,[31] using three-dimensional magnetic field tracking, demonstrated that elevation in any plane anterior to the scapula required external humeral rotation. Furthermore, maximum elevation was associated with approximately 35° of external humeral rotation. Conversely, internal rotation was necessary for increased elevation posterior to the POS.

Otis et al[32] demonstrated that external rotation of the humerus allows the insertion of the subscapularis tendon to move laterally, with a resulting increase in the distance from the axis of elevation in the scapular plane. An increase in the moment arm enhances the ability of the superior fibers of the subscapularis to participate in scaption. Conversely, internal rotation of the humerus increases the moment arm of the superior fibers of the infraspinatus and increases the ability of the muscle to participate in scaption. Flatow et al[33] reported that acromial undersurface and rotator cuff tendons are in closest proximity between 60° and 120° of elevation.

Conditions limiting external rotation or elevation may increase rotator cuff compression. Rajendran and Kwek[34] described how the course of the long head of the biceps (LHB) would influence external rotation of the humerus, which, in turn, prevents tendon impingement between the greater tuberosity and the glenoid labrum and allows glenohumeral elevation to move to completion. Brems[35] reported that external rotation is possibly the most important functional motion that the shoulder complex allows. Loss of external rotation can result in significant functional disability. Walker[36] described external rotation of the humerus as necessary for the greater tuberosity to clear the glenoid, thus providing more articular cartilage motion to produce elevation of the arm. Abboud and Soslowsky[37] reported that loss of rotational range of motion is deleterious because of its effect on activities of daily living and sports and its likely relation to the development of osteoarthritis.

External rotation is an important component for active abduction in POS elevation. In a pilot study, Donatelli[38] demonstrated a direct correlation between passive external rotation, measured in the adducted position, and active abduction in the POS.

When treating patients with limited active elevation, the practitioner should avoid pushing the joint into painful elevation activities. Restoring passive external rotation in the adducted position is a safe and effective way of restoring extensibility to the capsule and enhancing active abduction in the POS.

STATIC STABILIZERS OF THE GLENOHUMERAL JOINT

The stability of the glenohumeral joint depends on the integrity of soft tissue and bony structures such as the labrum, glenohumeral ligaments, capsular ligaments, and bony glenoid.[39] The glenohumeral joint contributes the greatest amount of motion to the shoulder because of its ball and socket configuration. Saha[40] confirmed the ball and socket joint of the glenohumeral articulation in 70% of his subjects. In the remaining 30%, the radius of curvature of the humeral head was greater than the radius of curvature of the glenoid. Thus, the joint was not a true enarthrosis.[16] Saha[16] further described the joint surfaces, especially on the head of the humerus, to be very irregular and to demonstrate a great amount of individual variation.

The head of the humerus is a hemispherical convex articular surface that faces superiorly, medially, and posteriorly. This articular surface is inclined 130° to 150° to the shaft of the humerus and is retroverted 20° to 30°.[3] The retroversion and the posterior tilt of the head of the humerus and the glenoid cultivate joint stability (Fig. 2-5). This retroversion of the head of the humerus corresponds to the forward inclination of the scapula, so that free pendulum movements of the arm do not occur in a straight sagittal plane but at an angle of 30° across the body.[41] Retroversion of the humeral head corresponds to the natural arm swing evident in ambulation.

The head of the humerus is large in relation to the glenoid fossa. Therefore, only one third of the humeral head can contact the glenoid fossa at a given time.[1,41] The glenoid fossa is a shallow structure deepened by the glenoid labrum. The labrum is wedge shaped when the glenohumeral joint is in a resting position and changes shape with various movements.[42] The glenoid and the labrum combine to form a socket with a depth up to 9 mm in the superior-inferior direction and 5 mm in the anterior-posterior direction.[43] The functional significance of the labrum is questionable. Most authors agree that the labrum is a weak supporting structure.[42,44] The function of the labrum has also been described as a "chock block" preventing humeral head translation.[45] Moseley and Overgaard[42] considered the labrum a redundant fold of the capsule composed of dense fibrous connective tissue but generally devoid of cartilage except in a small zone near its osseous attachment.

The glenohumeral joint was described by Matsen et al[46] as a suction cup because of the seal of the labrum and glenoid to the humeral head. This phenomenon is caused by the graduated flexibility of the glenoid surface, which permits

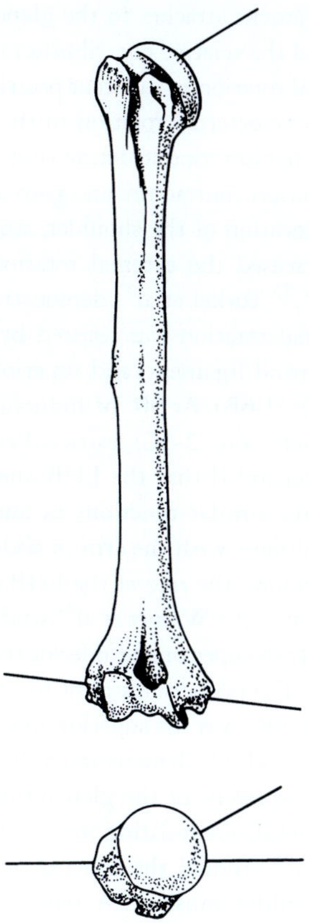

Figure 2-5 A, Humerus with marker through the head-neck and a second marker through the epicondyles. **B,** Retroversion of the humerus as seen from above.

the glenoid to conform and seal to the humeral head. Compression of the head into the socket expels the synovial fluid to create suction that resists distraction. Negative intra-articular joint pressure is produced by the limited joint volume.[47] Matsen et al[46] illustrated the importance of an intact glenoid labrum in establishing concavity compression stabilization. The compressive load is provided by dynamic muscle contraction. In addition, Matsen et al[46] discussed the importance of the central position of the humerus on the glenoid, to optimize the mechanical advantage of the rotator cuff muscles.

The glenoid fossa faces laterally. Freedman and Munro[48] found that the glenoid faced downward in 80.8% of the shoulders they studied radiographically. Saha[40] found a 7.4° retrotilt of the glenoid in 73.5% of normal subjects. The retrotilt is a stabilizing factor in the glenohumeral joint. Both the humeral and glenoid articular surfaces are lined with articular cartilage. The cartilage is the thickest at the periphery on the glenoid fossa and at the center of the humeral head.[16]

Central Position of the Humerus on the Glenoid

Because the shoulder is not inherently stable, the orientation and location of the joint reaction force with respect to the glenoid surface are important considerations in joint stability and function. The central location of the humeral head is maintained by a balance of muscle forces and connective tissue extensibility. Off-center joint force has more potential for subluxation and dislocation.[49]

If the head of the humerus is not in a central position, it will reduce the compressive forces of the rotator cuff muscles, thereby decreasing dynamic stability by altering the length tension of the rotator cuff muscles. A reduction in rotator cuff strength promotes destabilizing forces and poor joint arthrokinematics.

Clinical Evaluation of Humeral Head Central Position

- Evaluation of scapula posture
- Assessment of glenohumeral capsular extensibility by tests of external and internal rotation in various positions
- Assessment of strength of the rotator cuff muscles
- Assessment of strength of the scapula rotators

A centrally located humeral head on the glenoid enhances the dynamic stability of the glenohumeral joint. Joint forces associated with the rotator cuff muscles are stabilizing to the glenohumeral joint, whereas the forces produced by the deltoid muscles deviate from the surface of the glenoid joint during elevation of the arm. At 60° of glenohumeral abduction the shearing force is the greatest. The line of pull of the deltoid is oriented superiorly and parallel to the glenoid surface; this can be described as a shearing force. This parallel and superior action of the deltoid muscle may therefore result in a more off-center joint reaction force at the glenoid surface. This off-centered joint force could be the cause of several mechanic dysfunctions of the shoulder, including impingement and rotator cuff tears. Ideally, the best strategy for a glenohumeral elevation would be the combination of a strong deltoid muscle and the rotator cuff muscles to stabilize the joint by directing the joint force toward the a stable compressive force that is the center of the joint surface.

Anatomy of the Glenohumeral Ligaments

The coracohumeral ligament is the strongest supporting ligament of the glenohumeral joint. Fibers of the capsule and coracohumeral ligament blend together and insert into the borders of the supraspinatus and subscapularis.[50] Portions of the coracohumeral ligament form a tunnel for the biceps tendon on the anterior side of the joint. The *rotator cuff interval,* the region of the capsule between the anterior border of the supraspinatus and the superior border of the subscapularis muscle, is reinforced by the coracohumeral ligament.[45] The superior glenohumeral ligament and the coracohumeral ligament limit external rotation and abduction of the humerus and are important stabilizers in the inferior direction from 0° to 50° of abduction.[45,51]

The superior glenohumeral ligament forms an anterior cover around the LHB tendon and is also part of the rotator cuff interval.[45] The coracohumeral ligament blends with the superior glenohumeral ligament. The anatomy of the middle glenohumeral ligament is similar to that of the superior glenohumeral ligament. The middle glenohumeral ligament blends with portions of the subscapularis tendon medial to its insertion on the lesser tuberosity. The middle glenohumeral ligament has been shown to become taut at 45° of abduction, and at 10° of extension and external rotation, and it provides anterior stability between 45° and 60° of abduction.

The inferior glenohumeral ligament complex is a hammock-like structure with attachments on the anterior and posterior sides of the glenoid. The anterior band of the inferior glenohumeral ligament is attached to the anterior labrum. At the neutral position (0° of abduction and 30° of horizontal extension), the anterior band of the inferior glenohumeral ligament becomes the primary stabilizer. The inferior glenohumeral ligament complex was found to be the most important stabilizer against anterior-inferior shoulder dislocation.[45,52]

The capsule and ligaments reinforce the glenohumeral joint. The capsule attaches around the glenoid rim and forms a sleeve around the head of the humerus, by attaching on the anatomic neck. A functional interplay or interdependence exists between the anterior and posterior and superior and inferior capsuloligamentous system. This concept is referred to as the *circle theory,* a term implying that excessive translation in one direction may damage the capsule on the same and opposite sides of the joint.[37] The capsule is a lax structure. The head of the humerus can be distracted one-half inch when the shoulder is in a relaxed position.[51] The anterior capsule is reinforced by the glenohumeral ligaments noted earlier. The support these ligaments lend to the capsule is insignificant.[53]

Turkel et al[54] described the inferior glenohumeral ligament as the thickest and most consistent structure. The inferior glenohumeral ligament attaches to the glenoid labrum. Turkel et al[54] determined the relative contribution to anterior stability by testing external rotation in different positions. The subscapularis resisted passive external rotation in the adducted position more than any other anterior structure (Fig. 2-6A). In patients with internal rotation contracture and pain after anterior repair for recurrent dislocation of the shoulder, surgical release of the subscapularis increased the external rotation range of motion an average of 27°.[55] Turkel et al[54] demonstrated that, at 45° of abduction, external rotation was resisted by the subscapularis, middle glenohumeral ligament, and superior fibers of the inferior ligament (Fig. 2-6B). At 90° of abduction, the inferior glenohumeral ligament (Fig. 2-6C) restricted external rotation.

Itoi et al[56] concluded that the LHB and short head of the biceps (SHB) have similar functions as anterior stabilizers of the glenohumeral joint with the arm in abduction and external rotation. Furthermore, the role of the LHB and SHB increased with shoulder instability. Warner et al[57] studied the capsuloligamentous restraints to superior and inferior translation of the glenohumeral joint. The primary restraint to inferior translation of the adducted shoulder was the superior glenohumeral ligament. Abduction to 45° and 90° demonstrated the anterior and posterior portions, respectively, of the glenohumeral ligament to be the main static stabilizers resisting inferior translation.

Guanche et al[58] studied the synergistic action of the capsule and the shoulder muscles. A reflex arch was identified from mechanoreceptors within the glenohumeral capsule to muscles crossing the joint. Stimulation of the anterior and inferior axillary articular nerves elicited electromyographic (EMG) activity in the biceps, subscapularis, supraspinatus, and infraspinatus muscles. Stimulation of the posterior

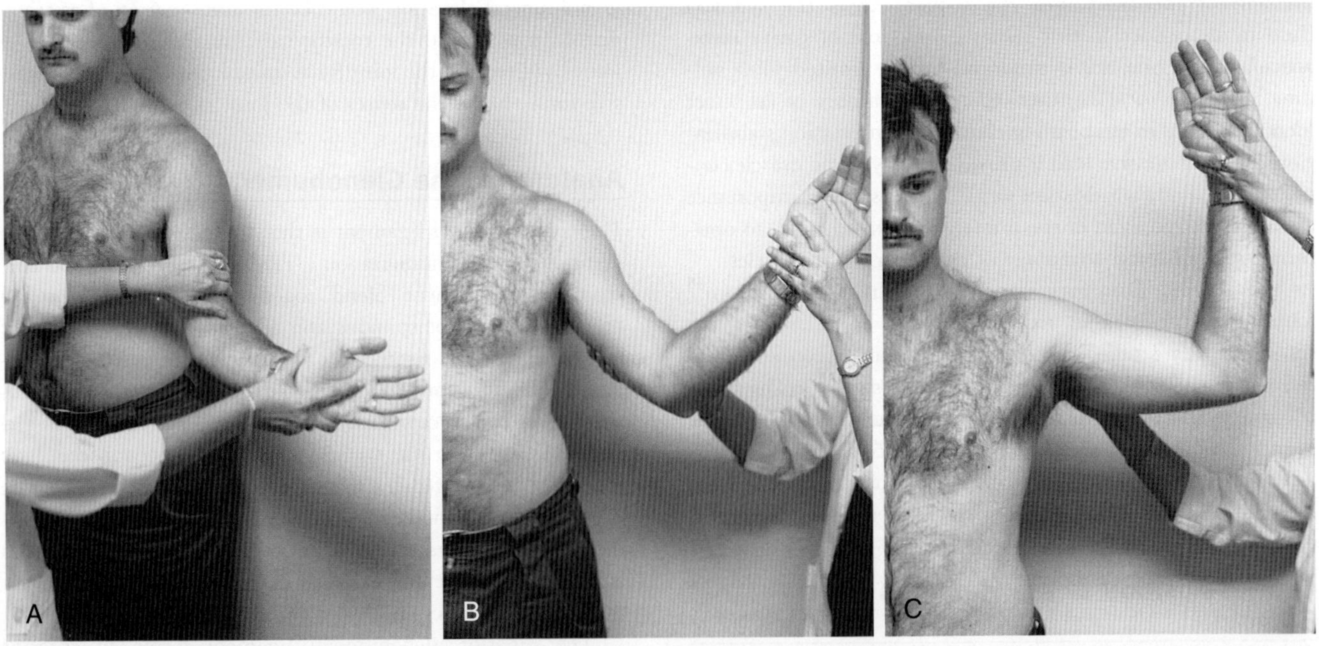

Figure 2-6 External rotation of the humerus. **A,** In the adducted position. The most stabilizing structure to this movement is the subscapularis muscle. **B,** At 45° of abduction. The most stabilizing structures for this movement are the middle and inferior ligaments and the subscapularis muscle. **C,** At 90° of abduction. The most stabilizing structure for this movement is the inferior ligament.

axillary articular nerve elicited EMG activity in the acromiodeltoid muscle.

Between the supporting ligaments and muscles lie synovial bursae or recesses. Anteriorly, three distinct recesses are present.[59] The superior recess is the subscapular bursa, which normally communicates with the shoulder joint. The inferior recess is referred to as the axillary pouch, and the middle synovial recess lies posterior to the subscapularis tendon. Arthrograms of frozen shoulders in relatively early stages, before glenohumeral abduction is completely restricted, show obliteration of the anterior glenoid bursa.[60]

DYNAMIC STABILIZERS OF THE GLENOHUMERAL JOINT

The major muscles that act on the glenohumeral and scapulothoracic joints may be grouped into the scapulohumeral, axiohumeral, and axioscapular muscles. The muscles of the scapulohumeral group, which include the rotator cuff muscles, originate on the scapula and insert on the humerus. The rotator cuff muscles insert on the tuberosities and along the upper two thirds of the humeral anatomic neck.[10] The contribution of the shoulder musculature to joint stability may be caused by the following mechanisms: muscle bulk acting as a passive muscle tension, contraction of the rotator cuff muscles primarily causing compression of the articular surfaces, joint motion that secondarily tightens the ligamentous constraints, barrier or restraint effects of the contracted muscle, and redirection of the joint force to the center of the glenoid surface by coordination of muscle forces.[37]

The infraspinatus and teres minor control external rotation of the humerus and reduce anterior-inferior capsuloligamentous strain. The subscapularis muscle is the strongest stabilizer of the rotator cuff muscles. It has the largest amount of muscle mass of the four rotator cuff muscles.[4] Combined contraction of the subscapularis and the infraspinatus forms a force couple, providing stability throughout the midrange of elevation, which is from 60° to 150° of abduction.[52]

Researchers showed that during late cocking by baseball pitchers, the glenohumeral joint reaches extreme external rotation. The subscapularis is the strongest activity stabilizer, followed by the infraspinatus and teres minor. The supraspinatus has the least stabilizing activity.[37] In addition, the subscapularis of a professional baseball pitcher is more active in the propulsive phase than any other internal rotator.[37]

Travell and Simons[60] believed that a trigger point within the subscapularis may spur the other shoulder girdle musculature into developing secondary and satellite trigger points. These points would lead to major restrictions in glenohumeral joint motion and cause adhesive capsulitis.

The rotator cuff muscles have been described as steering mechanisms for the head of the humerus on the glenoid.[16] The subscapularis, latissimus dorsi, teres major, and teres minor act as humeral depressors.[16,61] The arthrokinematics (rolling, spinning, and sliding) of the glenohumeral joint result from the action of the steering mechanisms and the depressors of the humeral head. Translation of the humeral head is of clinical interest in most shoulder disorders. At the glenohumeral joint, the amount and direction of translation define the type of instability. Wuelker et al[62] demonstrated that translation of the humeral head during elevation of the glenohumeral joint between 20° and 90° averaged 9 mm superiorly and 4.4 mm anteriorly. Translation of the humeral head during active elevation may be diminished by the coordinated activity of the rotator cuff muscles. This active control of translation forces provides dynamic stability to the glenohumeral joint. Perry[63] described 17 muscle groups that provide dynamic interactive stabilization of the composite movement of the thoracoscapular humeral articulation.

The deltoid muscle makes up 41% of the scapulohumeral muscle mass.[4] This muscle, in addition to its proximal attachment on the acromion process and the spine of the scapula, also stems from the clavicle. The distal insertion is on the shaft of the humerus at the deltoid tubercle. The mechanical advantage of the deltoid is enhanced by the distal insertion and the evolution of a larger acromion process.[4] The deltoid is a multipennate and fatigue-resistant muscle. These characteristics may explain the rare involvement of this muscle in pathologic shoulder conditions.[64] The deltoid and the clavicular head of the pectoralis major muscles have been described as prime movers of the glenohumeral joint because of their large mechanical advantage.[4] Michiels and Bodem[65] demonstrated that deltoid muscle action is not restricted to the generation of abduction in the shoulder joint.

The deltoid provides dynamic stability with the arm in the scapular plane and decreases stability with the arm in the coronal plane. The middle and posterior heads of the deltoid provide more stability by generating more compressive forces and lower shearing forces than the anterior head. Therefore, the middle and posterior heads of the deltoid should strengthen vigorously in anterior shoulder instability.[66]

Itoi et al[56] reported that the biceps muscle group becomes more important than the rotator cuff muscles as stability from the capsuloligamentous structure decreases. The anterior displacement of the humeral head under a 1.5-kg force was significantly decreased by both LHB and SHB loading in all capsular conditions when the arm was in 60° or 90° of external rotation and abduction. Abboud and Soslowsky[37] demonstrated that the LHB in the shoulder neutral position is anterior to the joint. Internal rotation of the humerus positions the tendon of the biceps further anterior to the joint, and external rotation positions the biceps tendon posterior to the joint. The forces generated by the LHB help to stabilize the glenohumeral joint and assist in restricting the translations of the humeral head. The restrictions in translation of the humeral head result from internal and external rotation of the humerus that allow the forces generated by the tendon to change to compressive with a posterior-directed force and compressive with an anterior-directed force, respectively (Fig. 2-7).

The deltoid and the rotator cuff muscles produce shearing and compressive forces in the glenohumeral joint. These forces vary as the alignment of the muscles changes.[67] The compressive forces produced by those muscles acting parallel to the

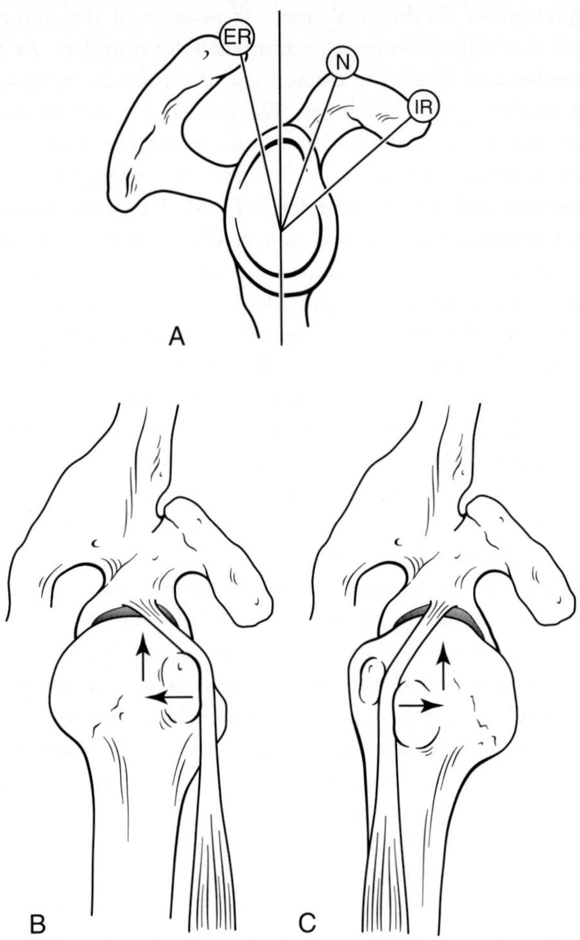

Figure 2-7 Forces produced by the long head of the biceps tendon in conjunction with internal rotation (IR) and external rotation (ER) of the humerus. **A,** Tendon position neutral and anterior to joint, ER posterior to joint, IR anterior to joint. **B,** Forces are compressive and posterior with IR. **C,** Forces are compressive and anterior with ER. (Modified from Pagnani MJ, Xiang-Hua D, Warren RF, et al: Role of the long head of the biceps brachii in glenohumeral stability: a biomechanical study in cadavers, *J Shoulder Elbow Surg* 5:225–262, 1996.)

glenoid fossa stabilize the humeral head. Muscles acting more perpendicular to the glenoid produce a translational shear. A larger superior shear produces impingement, whereas a larger compressive force centers the humeral head in the glenoid and reduces impingement of the rotator cuff under the acromion.[67] The central position of the humeral head on the glenoid helps to stabilize the glenohumeral joint.

Payne et al[67] simulated rotator cuff, deltoid, and biceps muscle forces on 10 human cadaver shoulders using transducers within the acromial arch. The muscle forces that reduced acromial pressure included the biceps, which decreased acromial pressure by 10% in all the shoulders and 34% in 6 of the shoulders. Rotator cuff muscle force, without simulating supraspinatus, was very effective in reducing the acromial pressure. With simulation of the subscapularis, infraspinatus, and teres minor, these investigators noted a 52% decrease in the anterior-lateral acromion pressure in neutral shoulders with type III acromion. Without the rotator cuff force, the amount of deltoid force required to abduct the arm increased by 17%. According to the study by Payne et al,[67] the action of the deltoid muscle increased the pressures under the acromion by 1240%.

One study described the lines of action of 18 major muscles spanning the shoulder joint during abduction and flexion and their potential contributions to glenohumeral joint stability.[68] The superior pectoralis major and inferior latissimus dorsi were the chief scapular plane destabilizers, with a demonstrated ability to provide superior and inferior shear to the glenohumeral joint, respectively. Evaluation of the middle and anterior deltoid during flexion and abduction demonstrated a potential contribution to superior shear, by opposing the combined destabilizing inferior shear potential of the latissimus dorsi and inferior subscapularis. The rotator cuff muscles were more aligned to stabilize the glenohumeral joint in the transverse plane than in the scapular plane. Overall, the anterior supraspinatus was most favorably oriented to apply glenohumeral joint compression. The study identified the posterior deltoid and subscapularis as potential stabilizers because they had posteriorly directed muscle lines of action, whereas the teres minor and infraspinatus had anteriorly directed lines of action.

The foregoing study helps the clinician identify the dynamic action of muscles surrounding the shoulder. A coordinated activation of the destabilizers and stabilizer muscles results in movement patterns that are not destructive to the shoulder. However, muscle imbalances around the shoulder may be the underlying cause of abnormal movement patterns and the resultant pathologic process. Knowledge of the stabilizing potential of shoulder musculature may assist clinicians in identifying muscle-related instabilities and may aid in the development of rehabilitation programs to improve joint stability and prevention programs.

STERNOCLAVICULAR JOINT

The SC joint is the only articulation that binds the shoulder girdle to the axial skeleton (Fig. 2-8). This is a sellar joint, with the sternal articulating surface greater than the clavicular surface, thus providing stability to the joint.[10] The joint is also stabilized by its articular disk, joint capsule, ligaments, and reinforcing muscles.[5,69] The disk binds the joint together

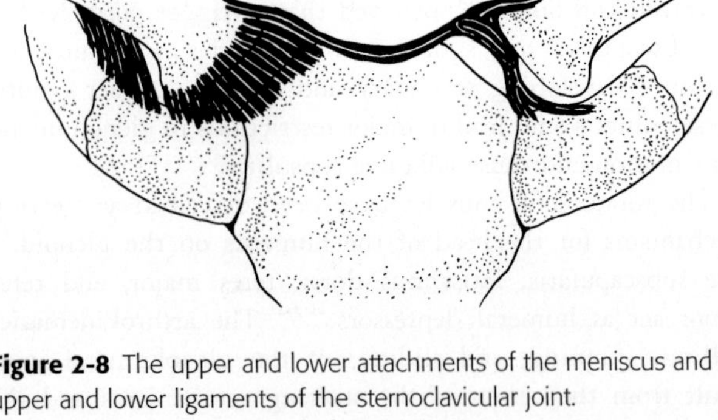

Figure 2-8 The upper and lower attachments of the meniscus and the upper and lower ligaments of the sternoclavicular joint.

and divides the joint into two cavities. The capsule surrounds the joint and is thickest on the anterior and posterior aspects. The section of the capsule from the disk to the clavicle is more lax and allows more mobility than among the disk, sternum, and first rib.[10] The interclavicular ligament anteriorly and inferiorly reinforces the capsule. The costoclavicular ligament connects the clavicle to the first rib.[10] The SC joint gains increased stability from muscles, especially the sternocleidomastoid, sternohyoid, and sternothyroid.[69]

ACROMIOCLAVICULAR JOINT

At the other end of the clavicle is the AC joint. This articulation is characterized by variability in size and shape of the clavicular facets and the presence of an intra-articular meniscus.[66] The AC joint capsule is more lax than the SC joint, and thus a greater degree of movement occurs at the AC joint that contributes to the increased incidence of dislocations.[69] The AC joint has three major supporting ligaments. The conoid and trapezoid ligaments are collectively called the *coracoclavicular ligament* and the *AC ligament*. It is through the conoid and trapezoid ligaments that scapula motion is translated to the clavicle.[5]

Rotation of the clavicle is the major movement at the AC joint. Steindler[70] described AC joint rotation occurring around three axes. Longitudinal axial rotation, vertical axis for protraction and retraction, and horizontal axis for elevation and depression are all controlled and facilitated by the conoid, trapezoid, and AC ligaments (Fig. 2-9).

Scapulothoracic Joint

The scapulothoracic joint is not an anatomic joint, but it is an important physiologic joint that adds considerably to motion of the shoulder girdle. The scapula is concave, articulating with a convex girdle.[1,63] The scapula is without bony or ligamentous connections to the thorax, except for its attachments at the AC joint and coracoacromial ligament. The scapula is primarily stabilized by muscles. The importance of the scapula rotators has been established as an essential ingredient of glenohumeral mobility and stability (Fig. 2-10). The stable base and therefore the mobility of the glenohumeral joint largely depend on the relationship of the scapula and the humerus. The scapula and humerus must accommodate to ever-changing positions during shoulder movement to maintain stability.[6] Figure 2-11 demonstrates the force couple of the scapula rotators.

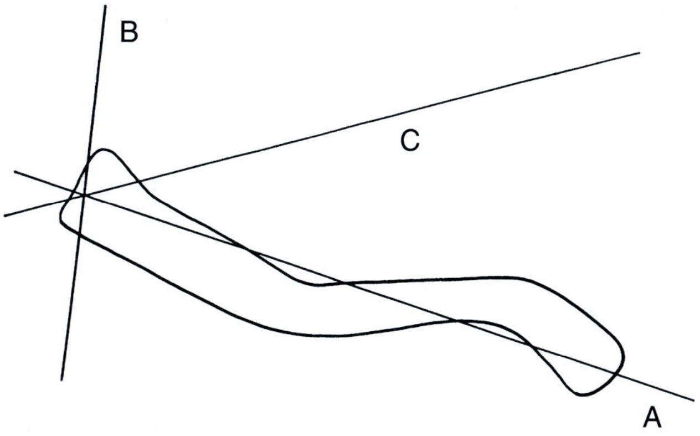

Figure 2-9 Axes of motion of the clavicle. **A,** Longitudinal axis of rotation. **B,** Vertical axis for protraction and retraction. **C,** Horizontal axis for elevation and depression. The sternal end of the scapula is on the *left*. (From Schenkman M, Rugo de Cartaya V: Kinesiology of the shoulder complex, *J Orthop Sports Phys Ther* 8:438, 1987, with permission of the Orthopaedic and Sports Physical Therapy Sections of the American Physical Therapy Association).

Scapulothoracic kinematics involve combined SC and AC joint motions.[71,72] Three-dimensional motion occurs at both the SC and AC joints during arm elevation in healthy subjects.[71,72] The clavicle demonstrates a pattern of slight elevation and increasing retraction as arm elevation progresses overhead.[72]

Teece et al[71] described that the scapula is simultaneously upwardly rotating, internally rotating, and posteriorly tilting relative to the clavicle at the AC joint (Fig. 2-12). In addition, scapulothoracic "translations" of elevation and depression and abduction and adduction were observed by the Teece et al.[71] These scapula movements actually derive from clavicular motions at the SC joint. Scapulothoracic elevation is a result of SC elevation, and abduction and adduction result from SC protraction and retraction.[72,73]

FUNCTIONAL BIOMECHANICS

As previously noted, *shoulder elevation* is defined as the movement of the humerus away from the side. It can occur in a seemingly infinite number of body planes.[47]

Shoulder elevation can be divided into three phases. The initial phase of elevation is 0° to 60°. The middle or "critical" phase is 60° to 140°. The final phase of elevation is 140° to 180°. Specific to each phase of movement, precise muscle function and joint kinematics allow normal, pain-free motion. Analysis of the precise components critical for each phase of shoulder elevation determines the success of clinical management of shoulder dysfunction.

Initial Phase of Elevation: 0° to 60°

All three arthrokinematic movements occur at the glenohumeral joint, but they do not occur in equal proportions. These movements—roll, spin, and glide—are necessary for the large humeral head to take advantage of the small glenoid articulating surface.[16] Saha[74] and Sharkey and Marder[75] investigated the contact area between the head of the humerus and the glenoid with elevation in abduction and in scaption. The studies found that the contact area on the head of the humerus was centered at 30° and was superiorly shifted 1.5 mm by 120°. Poppen and Walker[14] also studied the instant centers of rotation for abduction. These investigators reported that in the first 30° and often between 30° and 60° of abduction, the

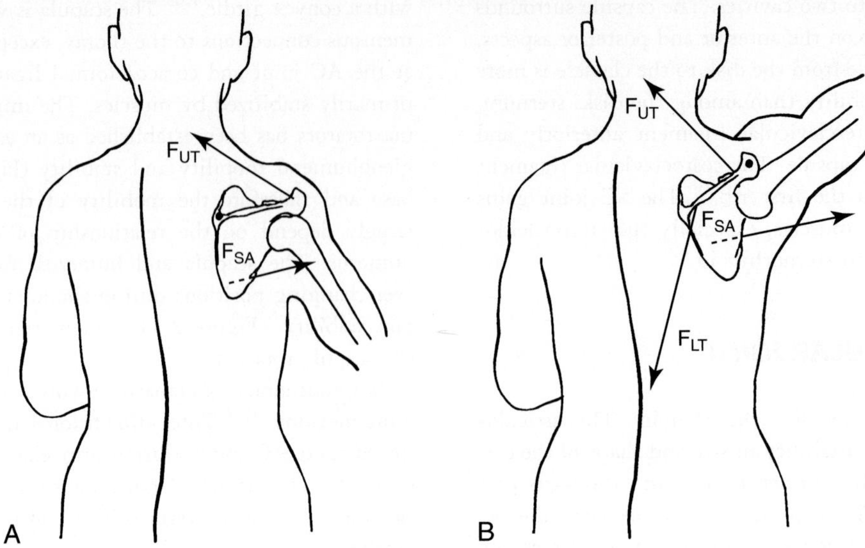

Figure 2-10 Force couple of muscles acting at scapula. **A,** Axis of scapular rotation from 0° to 30°. **B,** Axis of scapular rotation from 30° to 60°. FLT, force of lower trapezius; FSA, force of serratus anterior; FUT, Force of upper trapezius. (Modified from Schenkman M, Rugo de Cartaya V: Kinesiology of the shoulder complex, *J Orthop Sports Phys Ther* 8:438, 1987, with permission of the Orthopaedic and Sports Physical Therapy Sections of the American Physical Therapy Association.)

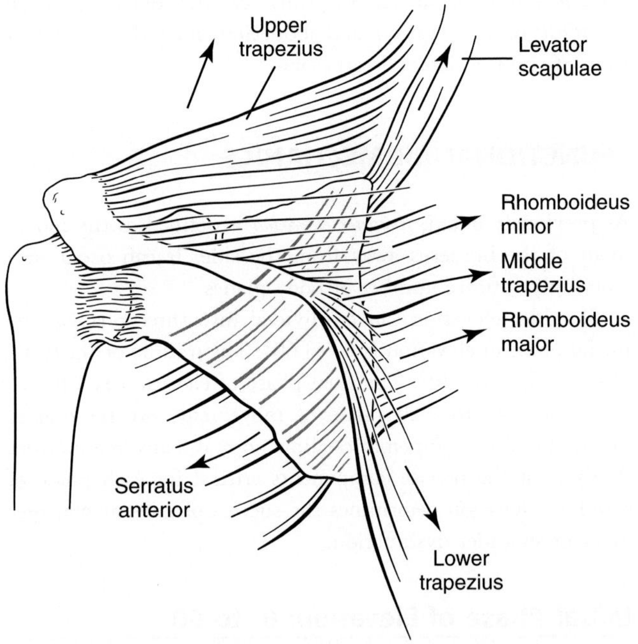

Figure 2-11 Force couple of the scapula rotators.

head of the humerus moved superiorly in the glenoid by 3 mm, a finding that indicates the occurrence of rolling or gliding of the head. The EMG activity of the supraspinatus muscle indicates an early rise in tension that produces a compressive force on the glenohumeral joint surface.

The deltoid muscle also demonstrates EMG activity in the initial phase of elevation. The subscapularis, infraspinatus, and teres minor muscles are important stabilizers of the humerus in the initial phase of elevation.[3] Kadaba et al[61] reported EMG activity of the upper and lower portions of the subscapularis muscle recorded by intramuscular wire electrodes. During the initial phase of elevation, EMG activity of the upper subscapularis was greater at the beginning of the range, whereas the lower subscapularis increased as the elevation reached 90°.[54] A significant amount of force is generated at the glenohumeral joint during abduction.[4,15] In the early stages of abduction, the loading vector is beyond the upper edge of the glenoid.[76]

During the initial stage of elevation, the pull of the deltoid muscle produces an upward shear of the humeral head.[3] This shearing peaks at 60° of abduction and is counteracted by the transverse compressive forces of the rotator cuff muscles.[3,15] The primary function of the subscapularis muscle is to depress the humeral head, thus counteracting the superior migrating force of the deltoid.[61] At 60° (abduction), the downward (short rotator) force is maximal at 9.6 times the limb weight or 0.42 times the body weight.[2,15] The subscapularis, infraspinatus, and latissimus dorsi muscle have small lever arms that form 90° angles to the glenoid face, thereby producing compressive forces to the joint.

Movement of the AC and SC joints permits movement of the scapula. Shoulder abduction is accompanied by clavicular elevation. SC elevation is most evident during the initial phase of arm elevation. A 4° SC movement occurs for each 10° of shoulder abduction.[4] The AC joint moves primarily before 30° and after 135°.[4]

The instantaneous center of rotation (ICR) of the scapula during the initial phase of elevation is located at or near the root of the scapula spine in line with the SC joint.[77] The initial phase of arm elevation was referred to by Poppen and Walker[15] as the *setting phase;* scapula rotation occurs

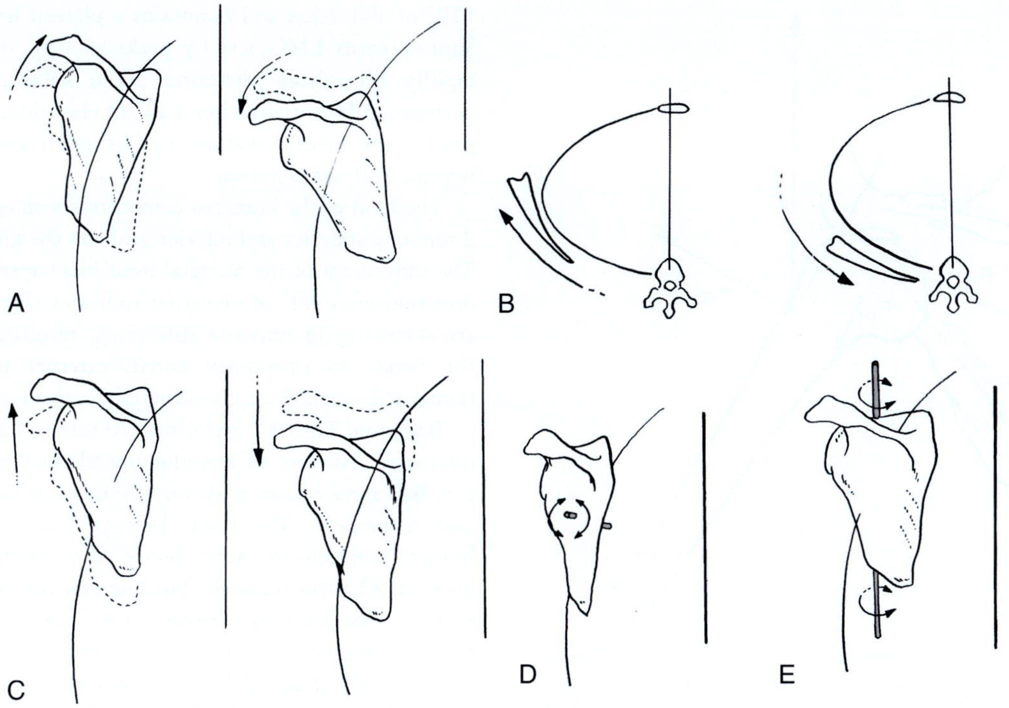

Figure 2-12 It is important to understand the various motions of the scapula relative to the thorax: **A,** upward and downward rotation; **B,** protraction and retraction; **C,** elevation and depression; **D,** tilting about a frontal axis; and **E,** tilting about a vertical axis. (Porterfield, James A. Mechanical Shoulder Disorders: Perspectives in Functional Anatomy. W.B. Saunders Company, 102003.)

about the lower midportion. The relative contribution from scapular rotation during the initial phase of elevation is considerably less than from glenohumeral motion. Bagg and Forest[77] estimated a 3.29:1 ratio of glenohumeral to scapulothoracic mobility during the initial phase of elevation. The upper trapezius and lower serratus anterior muscles provide the necessary rotatory force couple to produce upward scapular rotation during the early phase of arm abduction.[78]

Middle or Critical Phase of Elevation: 60° to 100°

The middle or critical phase of elevation is initiated by excessive force at the glenohumeral joint. As previously noted, the shearing of the deltoid muscle is maximal at 60° elevation (Fig. 2-13). Wuelker et al[62] simulated muscle forces under the coracoacromial vault. The forces at the glenohumeral joint were recorded and applied to the shoulder muscles at a constant ratio approximating physiologic conditions of shoulder elevation: deltoid, 43%; supraspinatus, 9%; subscapularis, 26%; and infraspinatus/teres minor, 22% (Fig. 2-14). Peak forces under the coracoacromial vault occurred between 51° and 82° of glenohumeral joint elevation. These force values may represent the pathomechanics of shoulder impingement. Figure 2-15 demonstrates the compressive and depressive forces generated by the muscles that provide a parallel force to the glenohumeral joint to counteract the shearing of the deltoid muscle group, which is perpendicular to the glenohumeral joint.

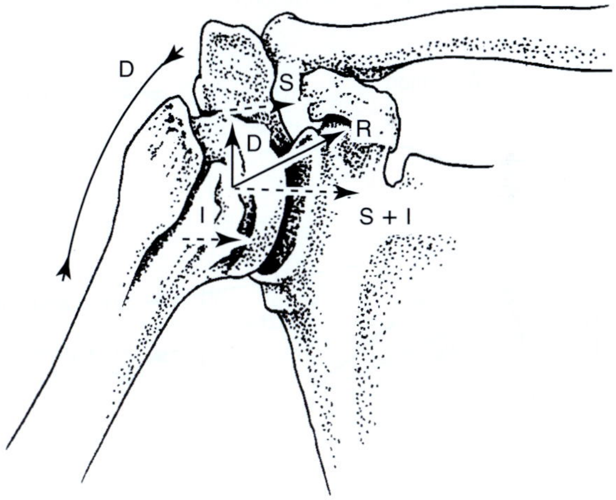

Figure 2-13 In the early stages of glenohumeral abduction, the deltoid reactive force (D) is located outside the glenoid fossa. The transverse compressive forces of the supraspinatus (S) and infraspinatus (I) muscles are counteracted by this force. The resultant reactive force (R) is therefore more favorably placed within the glenoid fossa for joint stability.

The resultant acting forces, which help to stabilize the joint, are maximal at 90° of elevation,[3] with shear and compressive forces equal.[78] As the arm reaches the end of the critical phase, the resultant and shearing forces of the deltoid are almost zero.[3,15]

The balance of shearing and compressive force establishes dynamic stability of the glenohumeral joint. In the early part

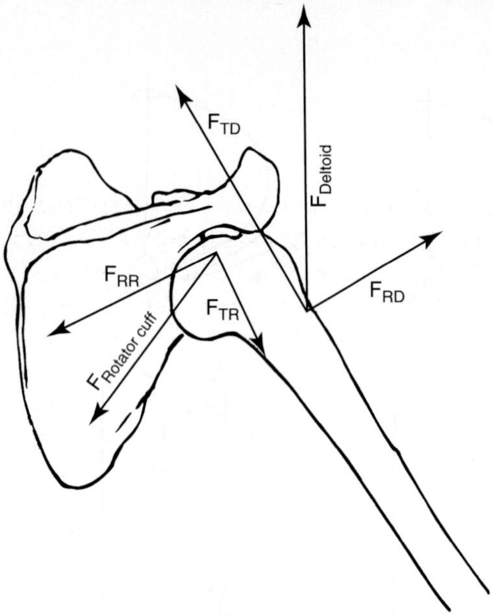

Figure 2-14 Force couple of deltoid and rotator cuff muscles. Rotatory forces, acting on opposite sides of the axis of motion, combine to produce upward rotation. Translatory forces cancel each other out. FRD, rotatory force of deltoid; FRR, Rotatory force of rotator cuff; FTD, translatory force of deltoid; FTR, translatory force of rotator cuff. (Modified from Schenkman M, Rugo de Cartaya V: Kinesiology of the shoulder complex, *J Orthop Sports Phys Ther* 8:438, 1987, with permission of the Orthopaedic and Sports Physical Therapy Sections of the American Physical Therapy Association.)

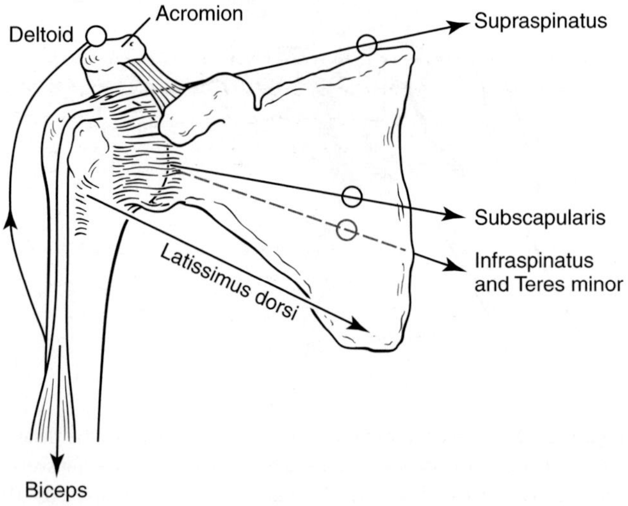

Figure 2-15 Forces provided to the muscles that are parallel to the glenohumeral joint. These muscles produce compressive and depressive forces to help stabilize the glenohumeral joint. The deltoid muscle is perpendicular to the glenohumeral joint.

of the critical phase, dynamic stability must be initiated before further progression of pain-free movement can occur. As previously noted, the lower fibers of the subscapularis muscle showed more activity at 90° of abduction.[61] The deltoid muscle reaches maximum EMG activity at approximately 110° of abduction and maintains a plateau level of activity.[3] Supraspinatus EMG activity peaks at 100° of elevation and rapidly diminishes thereafter.[3] The subscapularis activity decreases substantially after 130° of elevation, a finding supporting the concept that anterior ligament stability is critical beyond 130° of elevation.[3]

The head of the humerus demonstrates an excursion of 1 to 2 mm of a superior and inferior glide on the glenoid surface.[14] The movement of the humeral head in a superior and inferior direction after 60° of elevation indicates that roll and glide are occurring in opposite directions, resulting in a spin of the bone. As previously noted, external rotation of the humerus is critical for elevation (abduction) of the arm.

Bagg and Forrest[77] examined 20 subjects and found three distinctive patterns of scapulohumeral movement. Each pattern had three phases with varying ratios of humeral to scapular movement. The most common pattern had 3.29° of humeral motion to every degree of scapular motion from 20.8° to 81.8° of scaption. The humeral component decreased to 0.71° for scaption between 81.8° and 139.1°. Therefore, the greatest relative amount of scapular rotation occurs between 80° and 140° of arm abduction.[77] The ratio of glenohumeral to scapulothoracic motion has been calculated to be 0.71:1 during the middle phase of elevation.[78] Doody et al,[12] along with Freedman and Munro,[48] proposed that the significant role of the scapular rotators during the critical phase of elevation is secondary to the relatively long moment arms of the upper trapezius, lower trapezius, and lower serratus anterior muscles. Therefore, during the middle phase of elevation, the scapular rotators provide an important contribution to elevation of the humerus in the POS.

Movement of the AC and SC joints permits movement of the scapula. The relative contribution of these two joints changes throughout the range of motion, depending on where the ICR lies.[77] During the middle phase of abduction, the ICR of the scapula begins to migrate toward the AC joint. Clavicular elevation about the SC joint, coupled with scapular rotation about the AC joint, facilitates normal scapula mobility. Motion can occur at the AC joint, with less movement occurring at the SC joint because of the clavicular rotation around its long axis.[4] The double-curved clavicle acts like a crankshaft, to permit elevation and rotation at the AC end. The rotation of the scapula about the AC joint is initiated between 60° and 90° of elevation.[78] Clavicular elevation is completed between 120° and 150° of humeral abduction.[77] Clavicular elevation at the AC joint permits maximum scapular rotation. At approximately 150° of elevation, the ICR of the scapula is in line with the AC joint.[77]

Final Phase of Elevation: 140° to 180°

During the final phase of elevation, the ratio of glenohumeral to scapulothoracic motion is 3.49:1, a finding indicating relatively more glenohumeral motion.[77] The ICR of the scapula has relocated upward and laterally. The rotatory force arm of the upper trapezius muscle has reduced in length, and the role of this muscle is now supportive of the scapula.[78] The new location of the ICR of the scapula allows the middle trapezius to become a prime mover for downward scapular rotation.[78] The lower trapezius and the serratus anterior muscles continue to increase in activity during the final phase of elevation, and they act as an upward rotator and oppose the forces of the upper and middle trapezius.[77]

As the humerus elevates toward the end of the elevation range of motion, it must disengage itself from the scapula. As previously noted, the ratio of glenohumeral to scapulothoracic motion is 3.49:1. Good extensibility of the teres major and the subscapularis muscles is important, to allow the humerus to disassociate itself from the scapula. Often, with passive humeral elevation, a bulge of the scapula is noted laterally. The bulge is usually the inferior angle that is secondary to increased protraction of the scapula. Lack of elongation of these muscles prevents the normally dominant movement of the humerus at the end of the elevation range. Tightness of the subscapularis muscle, teres major muscle, or both, is often observed.

Furthermore, observation of limited passive humeral elevation may exhibit elevation of the chest cavity. If muscles connecting the humerus and rib cage are not flexible enough, movement will occur at both ends. The latissimus and pectoralis major muscles connect the humerus to the rib cage. Lack of dissociation of the rib cage from the humerus results in excessive rib cage mobility in passive terminal elevation.

Summary of Shoulder Phases of Movement

The initial phase of elevation occurs predominantly at the glenohumeral joint. A 3-mm superior glide of the humeral head has been observed in the initial phase of elevation. The activity of the deltoid muscle produces this superior shearing at the glenohumeral joint. The activity of the supraspinatus, infraspinatus, teres minor, and subscapularis muscles counteracts the forces of the deltoid muscle and creates a resultant force that helps to stabilize the joint and is necessary for full pain-free movement to continue. The resultant force in the normal glenohumeral joint is maximal at 90° of elevation. The early phase of scapula movement is described as the setting phase, with the majority of movement occurring at the glenohumeral joint.

The middle phase of elevation is referred to as the critical phase. At the beginning of the critical phase, maximum shearing forces of the deltoid muscle occur. The ratio of glenohumeral to scapulothoracic movement shifts and emphasizes scapulothoracic movement. The increased scapula movement is established by the activity of the upper and lower trapezius and lower anterior serratus muscles. The arthrokinematic movement of the head of the humerus on the glenoid has been observed as an inferior and superior glide of 1.5 mm.

During the final phase of elevation, the glenohumeral joint once again dominates the movement. Good extensibility of the latissimus, pectoralis major, teres major, teres minor, and subscapularis muscles is necessary to allow the increased and unconstrained movement of the humerus away from the scapula.

SUMMARY

Patients with shoulder dysfunction are routinely treated in the physical therapy clinic. An understanding of the anatomy and biomechanics of this joint can help to provide the physical therapist with a rationale for evaluation and treatment. Most studies involving shoulder anatomy and biomechanics reveal a common pattern, along with a wide variation among subjects. The physical therapist should keep this variation in mind when treating an individual patient.

Treatment may be directed toward restoring mobility, providing stability, or a combination of the two. The shoulder is an inherently mobile complex, with various joint surfaces adding to the freedom of movement. The shallow glenoid, with its flexible labrum and large humeral head, provides mobility. At times, this vast mobility occurs at the expense of stability. The shoulder relies on various stabilizing mechanisms, including shapes of joint surfaces, ligaments, and muscles to prevent excessive motion. Almost 20 muscles act on this joint complex in some manner, and at different times these muscles can be both prime movers and stabilizers. Harmonious actions of these muscles are necessary for the full function of this joint.

REFERENCES

1. Kent BE: Functional anatomy of the shoulder complex: a review, *Phys Ther* 51:867, 1971.
2. Lucas D: Biomechanics of the shoulder joint, *Arch Surg* 107:425, 1973.
3. Sarrafian SK: Gross and functional anatomy of the shoulder, *Clin Orthop Relat Res* 173:11, 1983.
4. Inman VT, Saunders M, Abbott LC: Observations on the function of the shoulder joint, *J Bone Joint Surg Am* 26:1, 1944.
5. Dempster WT: Mechanism of shoulder movement, *Arch Phys Med Rehabil* 46A:49, 1965.
6. Moseley JB Jr, Jobe FW, Pink M, et al: EMG analysis of the scapular muscles during a shoulder rehabilitation program, *Am J Sports Med* 20:128, 1992.
7. Bechtol C: Biomechanics of the shoulder, *Clin Orthop Relat Res* 146:37, 1980.
8. Johnston TB: Movements of the shoulder joint: plea for use of "plane of the scapula" as plane of reference for movements occurring at humero-scapular joint, *Br J Surg* 25:252, 1937.
9. Townsend H, Jobe F, Pink M, et al: Electromyographic analysis of the glenohumeral muscles during a baseball rehabilitation program, *Am J Sports Med* 19:264, 1991.
10. Warwick R, Williams P, editors: *Gray's anatomy*, British ed 35, Philadelphia, 1973, Saunders.
11. Calliet R: *Shoulder pain*, Philadelphia, 1966, Davis.
12. Doody SG, Freedman L, Waterland JC: Shoulder movements during abduction in the scapular plane, *Arch Phys Med Rehabil* 51:595, 1970.
13. Saha AK: Mechanics of elevation of glenohumeral joint, *Acta Orthop Scand* 44:668–678, 1973.
14. Poppen NK, Walker PS: Forces at the glenohumeral joint in abduction, *Clin Orthop Relat Res* 135:165, 1978.
15. Poppen NK, Walker PS: Normal and abnormal motion of the shoulder, *J Bone Joint Surg Am* 58:195, 1976.
16. Saha AK: *Theory of shoulder mechanism: descriptive and applied*, Springfield, Ill, 1961, Charles C Thomas.

17. Codman EA: *The shoulder*, Boston, 1934, Thomas Dodd.
18. Kondo M, Tazoe S, Yamada M: Changes of the tilting angle of the scapula following elevation of the arm. In Gateman JE, Welsh RP, editors: *Surgery of the shoulder*, Philadelphia, 1984, Mosby.
19. Williams PE, Goldspink G: Changes in sarcomere length and physiological properties in immobilized muscle, *J Anat* 127:459, 1978.
20. Tabury JC, Tabary C, Tardieu C, et al: Physiological and structural changes in the cat's soleus muscle due to immobilization at different lengths by plaster casts, *J Physiol* 224:231, 1972.
21. Tardieu C, Huet E, Bret MD, et al: Muscle hypoextensibility in children with cerebral palsy: clinical and experimental observations, *Arch Phys Med Rehabil* 63:97, 1982.
22. Lucas D: Biomechanics of the shoulder joint, *Arch Surg* 107:425, 1973.
23. Soderberg GJ, Blaschak MJ: Shoulder internal and external rotation peak torque production through a velocity spectrum in differing positions, *J Orthop Sports Phys Ther* 8:518, 1987.
24. Hellwig EV, Perrin DH: A comparison of two positions for assessing shoulder rotator peak torque: the traditional frontal plane versus the plane of the scapula, *Isokinet Exerc Sci* 1:202, 1991.
25. Greenfield BH, Donatelli R, Wooden MJ, et al: Isokinetic evaluation of shoulder rotational strength between the plane of the scapula and the frontal plane, *Am J Sports Med* 18:124, 1990.
26. Tata EG, Ng L, Kramer JF: Shoulder antagonistic strength ratios during concentric and eccentric muscle actions in the scapular plane, *J Orthop Sports Phys Ther* 18:654, 1993.
27. Whitcomb LJ, Kelley MJ, Leiper CI: A comparison of torque production during dynamic strength testing of shoulder abduction in the coronal plane and the plane of the scapula, *J Orthop Sports Phys Ther* 21:227, 1995.
28. Bigliani L, Kelkar R, Faltow E, et al: Glenohumeral stability: biomechanical properties of passive and active stabilizers, *Clin Orthop Relat Res* 330:13–30, 1996.
29. Rajendran K: The rotary influence of articular contours during passive glenohumeral abduction, *Singapore Med J* 33:493, 1992.
30. An KN, Browne AO, Korinek S, et al: Three-dimensional kinematics of glenohumeral elevation, *J Orthop Res* 9:143, 1991.
31. Browne A, Hoffmeyer P, Tanka S, et al: Glenohumeral elevation studied in three dimensions, *J Bone Joint Surg Br* 72:843–845, 1990.
32. Otis JC, Jiang CC, Wickiewicz TL, et al: Changes in the moment arms of the rotator cuff and deltoid muscles with abduction and rotation, *J Bone Joint Surg Am* 76:667, 1994.
33. Flatow EL, Soslowsky LJ, Ticker JB: Excursion of the rotator cuff under the acromion: patterns of subacromial contact, *Am J Sports Med* 22:779, 1994.
34. Rajendran K, Kwek BH: Glenohumeral abduction and the long head of the biceps, *Singapore Med J* 32:242, 1991.
35. Brems JJ: Rehabilitation following total shoulder arthroplasty, *Clin Orthop Relat Res* 307:70, 1994.
36. Walker PS: *Human joints and their artificial replacement*, Springfield, Ill, 1977, Charles C Thomas.
37. Abboud J, Soslowsky L: Interplay of the static and dynamic restraints in glenohumeral instability, *Clin Orthop Relat Res* 1:48–57, 2002.
38. Donatelli R, Wilkes J, Hall W, Cole S: Frozen shoulder encapsulates therapy challenges, *Biomech* 2:31–42, 2006.
39. Terry GC, Hammon D, France P, et al: The stabilizing function of passive shoulder restraints, *Am J Sports Med* 19:26–34, 1991.
40. Saha AK: Dynamic stability of the glenohumeral joint, *Acta Orthop Scand* 42:491, 1971.
41. Kessell L: *Clinical disorders of the shoulder*, ed 2, Edinburgh, 1986, Churchill Livingstone.
42. Moseley HP, Overgaard B: The anterior capsular mechanism in recurrent anterior dislocations of the shoulder: morphological and clinical studies with special reference to the glenoid labrum and glenohumeral ligaments, *J Bone Joint Surg Br* 44:913, 1962.
43. Bowen MK, Russell FW: Ligamentous control of shoulder stability based on selective cutting and static translation experiments, *Clin Sports Med* 10:757, 1991.
44. Reeves B: Experiments in the tensile strength of the anterior capsular structures of the shoulder in man, *J Bone Joint Surg Br* 50:858, 1968.
45. Burkart A, Debski R: Anatomy and function of the glenohumeral ligaments in anterior shoulder instability, *Clin Orthop Relat Res* 1:32–39, 2002.
46. Matsen FA, Lippitt SB, Slidles JA, et al: Stability. In Matson FA, Lippitt SB, Slides JA, et al, editors: *Practical evaluation and management of the shoulder*, Philadelphia, 1993, Saunders.
47. Pagnani MJ, Galinat BJ, Warren RF: Glenohumeral instability. In DeLee JC, Drez D, editors: *Orthopaedic sports medicine: principles and practice*, Philadelphia, 1993, Saunders.
48. Freedman L, Munro RH: Abduction of the arm in the scapular plane: scapular and glenohumeral movements: a roentgenographic study, *J Bone Joint Surg Am* 48:1503, 1966.
49. An KN, Himeno S, Tsumura H, et al: Pressure distribution on articular surfaces: application to joint stability evaluation, *J Biomech* 23:1013–1020, 1990.
50. Harryman DT, Sidles JA, Harris SL, et al: The role of rotator interval capsule in passive motion and stability of the shoulder, *J Bone Joint Surg Am* 74:53, 1992.
51. Kapanji IA: *The physiology of the joints and upper limb*, New York, 1970, Churchill Livingstone.
52. Eberly V, McMahon P, Lee T: Variation in the glenoid origin of the anteroinferior glenohumeral capsulolabrum, *Clin Orthop Relat Res* 1:26–31, 2002.
53. Basmajian J: The surgical anatomy and function of the arm-trunk mechanism, *Surg Clin North Am* 43:1475, 1963.
54. Turkel SJ, Panio MW, Marshall JL, et al: Stabilizing mechanisms preventing anterior dislocation of the glenohumeral joint, *J Bone Joint Surg Am* 63:1208, 1981.
55. MacDonald PB, Hawkins RJ, Fowler PJ, et al: Release of the subscapularis for internal rotation contracture and pain after anterior repair for recurrent anterior dislocation of the shoulder, *J Bone Joint Surg Am* 74:734, 1992.
56. Itoi E, Kuechle DK, Newman SR, et al: Stabilizing function of the biceps in stable and unstable shoulders, *J Bone Joint Surg Br* 75:546, 1993.
57. Warner JJ, Deng XH, Warren RF, et al: Static capsuloligamentous restraints to superior inferior translation of the glenohumeral joint, *Am J Sports Med* 20:675, 1992.
58. Guanche C, Knatt T, Solomonow M, et al: The synergistic action of the capsule and the shoulder muscles, *Am J Sports Med* 23:78–89, 1995.
59. Kummell BM: Spectrum of lesions of the anterior capsular mechanism of the shoulder, *Am J Sports Med* 7:111, 1979.
60. Travell J, Simons D: *Myofascial pain and dysfunction: the trigger point manual*, Baltimore, 1993, Williams & Wilkins.
61. Kadaba MP, Cole MF, Wooten P, et al: Intramuscular wire electromyography of the subscapularis, *J Orthop Res* 10:394, 1992.
62. Wuelker N, Schmotzer H, Thren K, et al: Translation of the glenohumeral joint with simulated active elevation, *Clin Orthop Relat Res* 309:193, 1994.

63. Perry J: Muscle control of the shoulder. In Rowe CR, editor: *The shoulder*, New York, 1988, Churchill Livingstone.
64. Hagberg M: Electromyographic signs of shoulder muscular fatigue in two elevated arm positions, *Am J Phys Med* 60:111, 1981.
65. Michiels I, Bodem F: The deltoid muscle: an electromyographical analysis of its activity in arm abduction in various body postures, *Int Orthop* 16:268, 1992.
66. Lee S, An K: Dynamic glenohumeral stability provided by three heads of the deltoid muscle, *Clin Orthop Relat Res* 1:40–47, 2002.
67. Payne L, Xiang-Hua D, Edward C, et al: The combined dynamic and static contributions to subacromial impingement: a biomechanical analysis, *Am J Sports Med* 25:801–808, 1997.
68. Ackland DC, Pandy MG: Lines of action and stabilizing potential of the shoulder musculature, *J Anat* 215:184–197, 2009.
69. Moseley HF: The clavicle: its anatomy and function, *Clin Orthop Relat Res* 58:17, 1968.
70. Steindler A: *Kinesiology of the human body under normal and pathological conditions*, Springfield, Ill, 1955, Charles C Thomas.
71. Teece R, Lunden J, Lloyd A, et al: Three-dimensional acromioclavicular joint motions during elevation of the arm, *J Orthop Sports Phys Ther* 38:181–190, 2008.
72. Ludewig PM, Behrens SA, Meyer SM, et al: Three-dimensional clavicular motion during arm elevation: reliability and descriptive data, *J Orthop Sports Phys Ther* 34:140–149, 2004.
73. Ludewig PL, Reynolds J: The association of scapular kinematics and glenohumeral joint pathologies, *J Orthop Sports Phys Ther* 39:90–104, 2009.
74. Saha AK: Mechanism of shoulder movements and a plea for the recognition of "zero position" of glenohumeral joint, *Clin Orthop Relat Res* 173:3, 1983.
75. Sharkey NA, Marder RA: The rotator cuff opposes superior translation of the humeral head, *Am J Sports Med* 23:270, 1995.
76. Himeno S, Tsumura H: The role of the rotator cuff as a stabilizing mechanism of the shoulder. In Bateman S, Welch P, editors: *Surgery of the shoulder*, St. Louis, 1984, Mosby.
77. Bagg DS, Forrest WJ: A biomechanical analysis of scapular rotation during arm abduction in the scapular plane, *Am J Phys Med Rehabil* 67:238, 1988.
78. Bagg DS, Forrest WJ: Electromyographic study of the scapular rotators during arm abduction in the scapular plane, *Am J Phys Med* 65:111, 1986.

CHAPTER

3

Jeff Cooper, Phillip B. Donley
and Craig D. Morgan

Throwing Injuries

To throw a baseball with high velocity and with great accuracy is a skill that escapes the majority of the population. Those who have accomplished this skill often demonstrate a heightened neuromuscular system and have invested thousands of hours of sport-specific training. This unique athletic act has produced a wide array of disabilities that have been reported in the literature. These disabilities include neurologic entrapments, arterial and venous thrombosis, acromioclavicular joint degeneration, primary impingement, secondary impingement, glenohumeral instabilities, labral lesions, subdeltoid bursitis, biceps tendinitis, subluxing bicipital tendon, undersurface tears of the rotator cuff, full-thickness tears of the rotator cuff, lesions of the humeral head, fracture of the humerus, fracture of the lateral border of the scapula, fracture of the coracoid, rib fractures, posterior capsular syndrome, and muscle imbalances, among others.[1-19]

During the years 1995 to 2006, an estimated 1,595,000 baseball-related injuries were treated in US hospital emergency facilities. Upper extremity injuries were second (32.4%) only to injuries of the face (33.5%).[20] An estimated 131,555 high school baseball injuries occurred during the school years 2005 to 2007. The shoulder was involved in 17.6% of the reported injuries.[21] Nationally, the estimated number of injuries in high school baseball players during the 2007 to 2008 school year was 44,760, occurring at a rate of 0.93 per exposure. The injury rate during competition (1.37) was twice as high as reported during practices (0.68). The number of injuries increased from the freshman player (16.6%) to the senior players (33.0%). Shoulder injuries were reported to be 16% of all injuries, second only to reported hand and wrist injuries (17.9%). Eighteen percent of all injuries occurred in the pitcher, and 15.7% of these injuries were specific to pitching. An additional 7.4% of all injuries were related to nonpitching throwing.[22] From 2005 to 2007, an estimated 19,988 baseball injuries in high school athletes were considered severe, defined as causing a loss of more than 21 days. Severe shoulder injuries accounted for 21.5% of the total.[23]

A study of collegiate baseball injuries over a 3-year period revealed that upper extremity injuries accounted for 58% of the total, and those injuries accounted for 75% of time loss. Pitchers sustained 69% of the reported shoulder injuries.[24] Collegiate players, like high school players, are more likely to be injured during games than practices. A study conducted over 16 years calculated the injury rate to be 5.78 versus 1.85 per 100 athlete exposures, competition versus practice. The chance of an athlete's sustaining a shoulder strain was twice as high in a game as in practice (0.37 versus 0.18 per athlete exposures). Shoulder injuries accounted for 23.4% of all game injuries and for 16% of all practice injuries. Throwing accounted for 59.5% shoulder injuries, and pitching accounted for 73%.[25]

In an attempt to identify causal factors in injury in youth baseball, a prospective injury study was conducted of 298 youth pitchers over the course of two seasons. The reported frequency of shoulder pain was 32%, and that of elbow pain was 26%. The following were identified as risk factors related to shoulder pain: decreased self-satisfaction, arm fatigue during one game pitched, throwing more than 75 pitches in one game, and throwing fewer than 300 pitches in a season. Risk factors for reported elbow pain were increased age, increased weight, decreased height, lifting weights during the season, playing baseball outside the league, decreased self-satisfaction, throwing more than 75 pitches in one game, and throwing fewer than 300 pitches or more than 600 pitches during the season.[26]

A follow-up study by the same authors reported an increased injury risk associated with youth baseball pitchers who threw breaking balls. Of the 476 youth baseball pitchers participating in the study, half of the players reported either shoulder pain or elbow pain during the competitive season. The investigators determined that the throwing of a curve ball was associated with an increased the risk of shoulder pain by 52%, and the throwing of a slider was associated with an increased the risk of elbow pain by 86%. Whether the primary offender is the specific mechanics of the breaking pitch or the increased load placed on the youth baseball pitcher trying to learn a new pitch, it is prudent to develop the breaking ball as an older teenager.[27]

In a retrospective cohort study of adolescent pitchers 14 to 20 years old, 95 injured pitchers who required either shoulder or elbow surgery were matched with 45 uninjured pitchers. The 29 injured pitchers who required shoulder surgery were more frequently used as starting pitchers. They threw at higher velocities and pitched significantly more months of the year, more innings per game, and thus more pitches per game. These pitchers reported using more warm-up pitches before their starts, pitching when fatigued, and using more anti-inflammatory medication. Almost 60% of these injured pitchers reported playing another position when not pitching.[28]

An examination of the 3282 disabled players in Major League Baseball between 1989 and 1999 showed revealed that 48.4% of all injuries occurred in pitchers. A team's pitching staff comprises 40% to 46% of the club roster; however, not all pitchers are active on a game-to-game basis. In the 5-year period from 1995 to 1999, 27.8% of all disabled Major League players had shoulder injuries. Elbow injuries accounted for an additional 22% of the disablement days. Thus, upper extremity injuries in this period constituted half of all the Major League Baseball injuries that required removal of an athlete from the active roster for a minimum of 15 days. In days lost, this figure converts to an average loss to Major League Baseball of 5619 days per year for shoulder injuries and an additional 4452 days per year for elbow injuries. On average, each club lost 336 days or 1.84 years of service time (182 days constitutes a service year) to upper extremity injuries.[29]

Injury to the shoulder complex precipitated by overhand throwing is most often the result of a failure in the kinetic chain manifesting itself in the weakest link. This weakest link is usually the glenohumeral joint. Macrotrauma injuries, such as a fracture of the humerus, can often be related to this proximal kinetic chain failure, which imposes higher demands on distal structures. Injury to the elbow is often precipitated by a dysfunction of the shoulder complex.[30,31] This chapter focuses on the underlying causes of most shoulder injuries and a preventive conditioning program that can be applied to the treatment of these injuries in the overhand throwing athlete.

OVERHAND THROWING

The biomechanical and electromyographic activity of overhand throwing has been investigated to give a relative model of function in a controlled environment.[32-40] Electromyographic sequence activity appears fairly consistent regardless of generated velocities and is discussed here. Whiteley[41] presented an excellent review of biomechanical investigations on this topic.

The overhand throw as it relates to pitching has been divided, depending on the investigator, into three, four, five, or six phases. This discussion explores a five-phase model consisting of (1) windup, (2) early cocking, (3) late cocking, (4) acceleration, and (5) follow-through.

Windup

The *windup* is an activity that is highly individualized. Its purpose is to organize the body beneath the arm to form a stable platform. As with all overarm activities, it is vital that the body perform in sequential links to enable the hand to be in the correct position in space to complete the assigned task. The hand can be placed in an infinite number of localities, and it is essential that the scapula humeral rhythm place it in an optimum setting for the task of propulsion. The drawing of the humerus into the moment center of the glenoid fossa is accomplished during the first 30° of elevation as the arm is brought upward by the deltoid and supraspinatus. Because of these many individual styles, no consistent pattern of muscle activity occurs during the windup phase.

Early Cocking

Early cocking is the period when the dominant hand is separated from the gloved hand, and it ends when the forward foot makes contact with the mound. The scapula is retracted and maintained against the chest wall by the serratus anterior. The humerus is brought into 90° of abduction and horizontal extension, with a minimal external rotation of approximately 50°. This position is accomplished by activation of the anterior, middle, and posterior deltoid. The external rotators of the cuff are activated toward the end of early cocking, with the supraspinatus more active than the infraspinatus and the teres minor as it steers the humeral head in the glenoid. The biceps brachii and brachialis act on the forearm to develop the necessary angle of the elbow.

As the body moves forward, the humerus is supported by the anterior and middle deltoid as the posterior deltoid pulls the arm into approximately 30° of horizontal extension. At this time, the static stability of the humeral head becomes dependent on the anterior margin of the glenoid, notably the inferior glenohumeral ligament and the inferior portion of the glenoid labrum.

Late Cocking

Late cocking is the interval in the throwing motion when the lead foot makes contact with the mound, and it ends when the humerus begins internal rotation. The lead foot applies an anterior shear force to slow the lower extremity and to transfer energy. The foot serves as an anchor; the forward and vertical momentum is transformed into rotational components. During this time, the humerus is moved into a position more forward in relation to the trunk and begins to come into alignment with the upper body. The extreme of external rotation, an additional 125°, is achieved to provide positioning for the power phase or acceleration. This is the first of two critical instants.[40]

The supraspinatus, infraspinatus, and teres minor are active in this phase but become quiet once external rotation is achieved. Deceleration of the externally rotating humerus is accomplished by the contraction of the subscapularis. It remains active until the completion of late cocking. The serratus anterior and the clavicular head of the pectoralis major have their greatest activity during deceleration. The biceps brachii aids in maintaining the humerus in the glenoid by producing compressive axial load. At the end of this phase, the triceps begins activity by providing compressive axial loading to replace the force of the biceps. The capsule becomes wound tight in preparation for acceleration.

Acceleration

Acceleration is a ballistic action lasting less than one tenth of a second. The ball is accelerated from 4 miles per hour to a speed of more than 90 miles per hour.[39] The scapula is protracted and rotated downward and held to the chest wall by the serratus anterior. The arm continues into forward flexion and is marked by a maximum internal rotation of the humerus. The humerus travels forward in 100° of abduction but adducts approximately 5° just before release. The latissimus dorsi and pectoralis major provide power to the forward moving shoulder. Subscapularis activity is at maximum levels as the humerus travels into medial rotation. The triceps develops strong action in accelerating the extension of the elbow.

The forces developed in this instant reflect the body's amazing ability to develop power and encase itself in a protective mechanism. This acceleration produces angular velocities that have been reported in excess of 10,000°/second.[41] Gainor et al[1] reported 14,000 inch pounds of rotatory torque produced at the shoulder. This torque develops 27,000 inch pounds of kinetic energy in the humerus. Control of the ball is lost approximately midway through the acceleration phase, when the humerus is positioned slightly behind the forward-flexing trunk and at an angle of approximately 110° of external rotation. The hand follows the ball after release and is unable to apply further force.

Follow-through

Follow-through begins with the release of the ball. Within the first tenth of a second, the humerus travels across the midline of the body and develops a slight external rotation before finishing in internal rotation. The second critical instant occurs during this segment.[18] This is a very active phase for all glenohumeral muscles as the arm is decelerated. The deltoid and upper trapezius have strong activity, as does the latissimus dorsi. The infraspinatus, teres minor, supraspinatus, and subscapularis are all active as eccentric loads are produced. The biceps develops peak activity in decelerating the forearm and imposes a traction force within the glenohumeral joint.

The task of documenting the sequence of muscle activity during the act of pitching has allowed the musculature acting on the glenohumeral joint to be divided into two groups.[19] The first group of muscles contains those that are most active during the second and third phases of throwing: early and late cocking. These muscles are least active during the acceleration phase. The deltoid, trapezius, external rotators, supraspinatus, infraspinatus, teres minor, and biceps brachii comprise this first group.

The second group of muscles contains those used primarily for the fourth phase of throwing: acceleration. These muscles are necessary to protract the scapula, horizontally forward flex and internally rotate the humerus, and extend the elbow. This group consists of the subscapularis, serratus anterior, pectoralis major, latissimus dorsi, and triceps brachii. The first phase of throwing is not included in either group because of the nonspecific generalized activity.

Professional versus Amateur Pitchers

Gowan et al[36] conducted a study to determine whether the muscle firing sequence of professional pitchers was significantly different from that of amateur pitchers. No significant differences were noted in the first three phases of the pitch: the windup and early and late cocking. No significant differences were noted in the follow-through, in which muscle activity was described as general.

During the acceleration phase, professional pitchers recorded increased activity of the pectoralis major and latissimus dorsi. They also had increased activity in the serratus anterior muscle. The professional pitchers had decreased activity in the supraspinatus, infraspinatus, and teres minor during acceleration. The professional pitchers used the subscapularis predominantly during acceleration and internal rotation. Activity in the biceps brachii was also lower in the professional than in the amateur pitchers.

Electromyographic Activity in the Injured Thrower

Athletes who were diagnosed as having subacromial impingement demonstrated differences in their electromyographic studies compared with uninjured throwers.[37] During the second phase of throwing, early cocking, the injured athletes had continued deltoid activity, whereas the healthy athletes had decreased deltoid activity. A lower level of supraspinatus activity was also noted during this period. During early cocking and late cocking, the internal rotators, subscapularis, pectoralis major, and latissimus dorsi had decreased activity. The serratus anterior followed this pattern and was less effective. Investigators theorized that the combination of these differences may lead to increased external rotation, superior humeral migration, and impaired scapular rotation. All or some of these factors may be the underlying cause of the initial problem or a factor in the continuum of the syndrome.

Throwing athletes who have been hampered by glenohumeral instabilities were compared with healthy athletes in a similar fashion.[38] This series tested the activity of the biceps, middle deltoid, supraspinatus, infraspinatus, pectoralis major, subscapularis, latissimus dorsi, and serratus anterior. Noted were differences in every muscle except the middle deltoid. These investigators suggested that the mildly increased activity of the biceps and supraspinatus may be compensatory for the laxity present in the anterior capsule. The infraspinatus developed a pattern of activity during early cocking, reduced activity during late cocking, and again increased activity in follow-through. As noted with the impingement group, the internal rotators, consisting of the subscapularis, pectoralis major, and latissimus dorsi, had decreased activity, which was marked in the early cocking phase. The serratus anterior showed decreased activity as well.

These investigators concluded that these changes in muscle activity allowed decreased internal rotation force needed in both late cocking and acceleration.[38] Reduced activity demonstrated in controlling the scapula by the serratus anterior allowed the glenoid to be placed in a compromising position during late cocking and increased the stress on the labrum and capsule. Microtraumas can be associated with deficiencies in a muscle or muscle group that fails to aid in stabilizing the glenohumeral joint or fails to become active in the proper sequence during the distinct phases of throwing. Lack of flexibility can be a factor leading to disability, particularly in the deceleration phase, when tremendous eccentric forces develop.

CAPSULE

A more detailed description of the function of the capsule of the glenohumeral joint and its ligaments can be found in Chapter 2. Here, it is necessary to describe some works in regard to the capsule in the cocked position in the overhand-throwing athlete. Harryman et al[42] indicated that oblique glenohumeral translations are not the result of ligament insufficiency or laxity, but rather translation results when the capsule is asymmetrically tight. He surgically tightened fresh cadaver posterior capsules and found increased anterior humeral head translation during cross-body movement, flexion, and internal rotation and increased superior translation with flexion.

O'Brien et al[43] demonstrated that the posterior band of the inferior glenohumeral ligament complex, which is a thickening of the posterior capsule, is the primary restraint to any posterior force when the arm is positioned at 90° of abduction and is internally rotated. Tightening of the posterior or posterior-inferior capsule causes a posterior-superior shift of the glenohumeral fulcrum, which allows contact of the labrum in the posterior-superior glenoid.

Collagen fiber bundle patterns of the capsule were reported by Gohlke et al.[44] These investigators described both the radial and circular components of this structure. The nature of these patterns predisposes the capsule to dual action during glenohumeral rotation. During rotation, the capsule becomes shortened and produces both a compressive force and a centering of the humerus on the glenoid. The role of the glenohumeral ligaments depends on humeral position. When the humerus is abducted to 90° and the motion of external rotation is introduced, the anterior band of the inferior glenohumeral ligament becomes the supporting structure to resist anterior displacement of the humeral head. The posterior band of the glenohumeral ligament is now positioned under the humeral head and resists inferior displacement. As the humerus is rotated medially into internal rotation with the elevated humerus, the posterior band of the inferior glenohumeral ligament becomes the structure to prevent posterior translation and the anterior portion of the ligament then has the inferior position.

Branch et al[45] investigated the function of the capsule in its relation to anterior and posterior translation of the humerus during internal and external rotation. An artificially constructed lengthening of the capsule tissue and its relation to the changes in anterior-posterior translation were also investigated. Measurements were made at intervals of 20° of internal and external rotation. The investigations concluded with an intact capsuloligamentous complex with the humerus translated maximally in the glenoid when the humerus was between 40° and 100° of external rotation. When the glenohumeral capsuloligamentous complex was increased in length, translation increased. During internal rotation, the length of the posterior capsule had a greater influence on anterior-posterior translation, and the anterior capsule length had a greater effect on external rotation.

Anterior translation and inferior glenohumeral ligament strain in simulated scapular protraction were investigated by Weiser et al.[46] This cadaver study was conducted with the specimens placed in the position of apprehension and simulated protraction. With anteriorly directed loads, the investigators reported increasing strain in the anterior band of the inferior glenohumeral ligament with increased scapular protraction.

Novotny et al[47] used an analytical model to predict glenohumeral kinematics and to view the way in which the glenohumeral capsule and bony contact stabilize the joint. The simulation was conducted in the cocking phase of throwing with an abducted extended external rotated humerus. In this position, the center of the humeral head translated posteriorly and superiorly during external rotation. The anterior band of the inferior glenohumeral ligament increased in tension with external rotation. The axillary pouch and posterior band decreased in tension. The contact area, stress, and force increased with external rotation. The contact area moved posteriorly and inferiorly on the area of the glenoid.

In a cadaver study by Kuhn et al,[48] the ligamentous restraints of the glenoid capsuloligamentous complex were investigated in the late cocking phase of throwing. This study involved cutting selected structures and measuring the increase in external rotation. The release of the entire inferior glenohumeral ligament allowed the greatest increase in external rotation. Isolating the loss of the anterior band of the inferior glenohumeral produced the greatest external rotation when compared with the loss of either the superior or middle glenohumeral ligaments.

Pollock et al[49] examined the mechanical response of the inferior glenohumeral ligament of cadaver shoulders that were exposed to different levels of subfatigue cycle strains. Three groups of specimens received increased loads and frequency of subfatigue strains. The repeated loading of the inferior glenohumeral ligament induced laxity. The mechanical response reflected the magnitude of the cycles, strain, and frequency of the loading. A ligament length increase noted in all specimens led the investigators to believe that this could be a mechanism for acquired glenohumeral instability.

A three-dimensional kinematic study was designed by Baeyens et al[50] to determine the rotation and shift of the humeral head in the glenoid cavity and the migration of contact of the articular surfaces. Helical axis parameters of rotation, shift, and direction were compared between the glenoid and the articulation surface of the humerus. Calculations were made from the beginning position of 90° of abduction and 90° of external rotation to full cocking (full external rotation and horizontal extension). The humeral head in normal shoulders did not externally or internally rotate on the glenoid. In shoulders deemed clinically as having minor anterior glenohumeral instability, a larger external rotational component was found. Thus, the humeral head of the normal shoulder translated into the posterior portion of the glenoid, and the shoulder with minor anterior instability translated centrally in the glenoid. When the anterior part of the inferior glenohumeral ligament limits anterior translation and external rotation, minor anterior instability is the result of dysfunction of the anterior part of the inferior glenohumeral ligament.

Grossman et al[51] conducted a cadaveric study in which the anterior capsule was stretched and the posterior capsule was tightened. Stretching the anterior capsule alone produced a significant increase in total range of motion, with the primary gains in external rotation. When the posterior capsule was tightened, a significant decrease in total motion was noted when compared with the stretched anterior capsule. When both alterations were applied, the stretched anterior capsule and the contracted posterior capsule, a significant increase in external rotation and a significant decrease in internal rotation occurred.

This study also examined the position of the humeral head on the glenoid with each capsule alteration. Normally, the humeral head settles in a posterior-inferior position during maximum external rotation. When the anterior capsule was stretched, the externally rotation humeral head settled into a position that was more inferior but less posterior. When the condition of a posterior capsule contracture was added, the externally rotating humeral head settled more posteriorly and less inferiorly. Although these humeral head positional changes on the glenoid were not significant, the investigators suggested that posterior capsular tightness, as opposed to anterior capsular laxity, may be a causative factor in posterior-superior glenoid internal impingement.

In yet another cadaveric study,[52] with similarly simulated conditions of a stretched anterior capsule and a contracted posterior-inferior capsule, an attempt was made to measure the glenohumeral articulation throughout the rotational range of motion, not just maximum external rotation. This study incorporated twice the compression forces (44 N) and equal translation forces (20 N) and incorporated a three-dimensional digitized system to record the apex of the humeral head throughout the test range of motion. Measurements were recorded at 15° intervals. When the range of motion measurements of the altered specimens were compared with their previous state, the investigators noted a significant increase in external rotation. The changes in internal rotation were deemed not statistically significant. In maximum external rotation, the humeral head apex was posteriorly displaced an average 7.5 mm with the combined condition. No significant difference was noted between the individual conditions. This shift began occurring at 120° of external rotation to the maximum at the tested end range of 150°. Maximum internal rotation of the humeral head apex had an anterior shift of 3.5 mm and an inferior shift of 2.8 mm. The changes were most evident at 15° to terminal internal rotation. These changes were considered significant.

This study[52] suggested that posterior-inferior capsule contracture not only changes the humeral head apex in extremes of external rotation but also significantly alters the course of the articulation at the end ranges of internal rotation. The investigators suggested that this occurrence may be more relevant to traction injury than to internal impingement.

BICEPS TENDON–SUPERIOR LABRAL COMPLEX: SLAP LESIONS

The role of the long head of the biceps tendon within the glenohumeral mechanism has long been overlooked. Often dismissed as only a minor player at the shoulder as a humeral head depressor, long head of the biceps tendon was recognized for its role as an elbow stabilizer and decelerator. Since the advent of shoulder investigation by arthroscopy, the role of this structure has been better appreciated. The data of Snyder et al[53] suggested that the superior labrum anterior to posterior (SLAP) lesion occurs in a very limited number of cases among the general population, and the mechanism of trauma is varied. Maffet et al,[54] in a review of 712 surgical shoulders with significant biceps tendon and superior labral abnormalities, suggested that these separations are indeed caused by various events. In the general population, injury to the biceps tendon–labral complex is mostly a traumatic event. Two injury mechanisms for a disabling injury to this structure in the overhand-throwing athlete have been put forth: maximum forces occurring at deceleration and the peel back mechanism during terminal external rotation.

Andrews et al[2] examined a population of 73 throwing athletes and observed that 60% of this group had tears in the anterior-superior labrum, and another 23% had tears in both the anterior-superior and posterior-superior portion. In a subgroup of baseball pitchers, this lesion was associated with a partial tear of the supraspinatus in 73% of the athletes. A smaller group of 7% demonstrated a partial tear of the long head of the biceps. The investigators hypothesized that the incident of injury to this region of the glenoid labrum was the result of the tremendous eccentric stresses placed on the biceps in an attempt to decelerate the arm during the follow-through phase of the overhand throw.

A correlation with patient history revealed that 95% of the patients reported pain during the overhand throw, and 45% of the population reported a popping or catching sensation. On physical examination, the popping was evident in the position of full abduction and full flexion as the upper arm was aligned with the ear in 79% of the athletes. None of the population demonstrated a significant weakness of either the rotator cuff or biceps tendon. This lesion gave the athlete a sensation of instability.

In a retrospective totaling 2375 arthroscopically evaluated shoulders, Snyder et al[53] reported 140 cases with superior glenoid labrum injuries. These cases represented only 6% of the sample population. The involvement of the dominant shoulder versus the nondominant shoulder was greater than 2 to 1.

No radiographic findings could be correlated with the disorder. At the time, no clinical examination was considered specific for the superior labrum. Approximately half of the patients described a painful catching or popping, a finding consistent with the previous study. Only approximately one third demonstrated a positive biceps tension test. Fifty-five percent of these shoulders were categorized as having a type II SLAP lesion consisting of detachment of the superior labrum and biceps tendon from the glenoid rim. Of these shoulders, only 28% were isolated from a rotator cuff injury or other labral problems.

Rodosky et al[55] investigated the role of the long head of the biceps and its attachment to the superior labrum in a laboratory model of the glenohumeral joint positioned in abduction and external rotation as experienced by the overhand thrower. The investigators hypothesized that the presence of the long head of the biceps acted to help limit the external rotating shoulder. The biceps compressed the humeral head against the glenoid resisting the rotation. The long head of the biceps withstood higher external rotational forces without the inferior glenohumeral ligament's experiencing a greater strain. This finding suggested that the biceps has a role in the provision of anterior stability. The glenohumeral joint demonstrated heightened torsional stiffness as force was increased through the long head of the biceps.

When a surgical SLAP lesion was created, torsional rigidity decreased 26%, and the strain on the inferior glenohumeral ligament was increased by 33%. This model suggested that the shoulder thus depends on the long head of the biceps to provide dynamic stability to the glenohumeral joint in the cocking, acceleration, and follow-through phases. This dynamic stability ensures a consistent stress on the inferior glenohumeral ligament. The long head of the biceps acts as a continuum provider of axial tension as a protective mechanism for the humerus and the inferior glenohumeral ligament.

A cadaveric study measuring strain to the superior labrum and biceps anchor through the phases of throwing reported increased labral strain during the late cocking phase of throwing.[56] In another cadaveric study that compared the late cocking and a simulated deceleration phase of throwing (in-line loading), the biceps anchor was loaded to failure.[57] Anchor failure in the late cocking position resulted in a type II SLAP lesion. Most deceleration failures resulted in midsubstance tears of the tendon itself. This study reported significantly higher structure strength with the in-line loading–deceleration phase.

In a study incorporating a three-dimensional finite element model, the superior labrum was stressed through the long head of the biceps tendon in four phases of throwing.[58] In addition to the throwing phases, three types of insertions were analyzed: a mostly posterior origin, an equal anterior and posterior origin, and a mostly anterior origin. The deceleration phase provided the highest labrum stress in all orientation types, and the highest stress orientation was in the mostly anterior model.

Investigators have suggested that lesions that produce small increases in external rotation and glenohumeral translation and lack involvement of superior glenohumeral ligament and middle glenohumeral ligament may allow overhand-throwing athletes to continue to function in the absence of mechanical symptoms or pain.[59] However, once the integrity of the glenohumeral joint is reduced by superior labrum dissociation, the shoulder sacrifices stability. Shoulder instability clearly coexists with a SLAP lesion.[37] A SLAP lesion must be among the suspected diagnoses in the overhand-throwing athlete who complains of instability or a sense of instability of the shoulder.

Morgan et al[60] suggested that the mechanism of injury extending or potentially producing a type II SLAP lesion is a torsional force that "peels back" the biceps and posterior labrum from the neck of the glenoid. The investigators suggested that when the shoulder is placed in extreme abduction and external rotation, torsion is applied to the biceps tendon. Placing the upper extremity in this position of cocking the biceps creates a more vertical and posterior angle. When a force is applied, a twist is produced at the base of the biceps, and this transmits a torsional force to the posterior-superior labrum.

Morgan et al[60] reviewed a group of 102 patients with type II SLAP lesions. Of this group, 53 were overhand-throwing athletes, 44 of whom were baseball pitchers. A common history for these individuals included the development of pain in the cocking phase of throwing, pain arising either anteriorly or posteriorly, and decreased performance or decreased velocity. These symptoms were often described as a "dead arm." The clinical examination included the following tests: (1) bicipital groove tenderness, (2) Speed's test, (3) O'Brien's cross-arm test (active compression test),[61] and (4) Jobe's relocation test[62] in which pain and apprehension posteriorly and superiorly are relieved by a force directed posteriorly to the humeral head. These clinical findings were then correlated to a further classification of type II SLAP lesion. In the overhand throwing athletes, 19% had anterior-superior lesions, 47% had posterior-superior lesions, and 34% had a combined anterior-posterior lesion. Thus, 81% of the SLAP lesions in the throwing group had a posterior component.

When compared with the entire group of 102 patients, the posterior type II SLAP lesion was three times more common in the overhead-throwing athletes, and the anterior type II SLAP was three times more common in the nonthrowing group who had sustained trauma. When the clinical examination was correlated with the arthroscopic findings, the investigators generally determined that Speed's test and O'Brien's test were useful in predicting anterior-superior lesions, and Jobe's relocation test was useful in predicting posterior-superior lesions.[60]

Of the 53 overhand-throwing athletes, 10 presented with a partial-thickness undersurface tear of the rotator cuff, and 1 presented with a complete tear. Eighty-seven percent of the overhand throwers reported an excellent result with internal fixation of their SLAP lesion. The other 13% reported a good result. Eighty-four percent returned to their preinjury level of sports participation. Sixteen percent reported decreased velocity and control. Those 7 athletes all had associated rotator cuff disorders.[60]

All overhead-throwing athletes in this study were measured for internal and external rotation at 90° of abduction in the plane of the scapula. A noted lack of internal rotation in the surgical shoulder was present. On average, a loss of 45° of internal rotation (range, –35° to –60°) occurred. External rotation in the plane of the scapula had an average gain of 40° (range, +20° to +45°).[60]

The final observation in this investigation is the relationship of the posterior-superior SLAP and rotator cuff disease. Thirty-one percent of those patients with chronic SLAP had associated undersurface rotator cuff involvement. The investigators postulated that the humeral head acquired the ability to translate superiorly or to sublux because of the lack of a fixed biceps labrum. This combination of superior translation and repetitive twisting of the rotator cuff in the cocking phase of throwing results in fiber fatigue and failure of the cuff.[60]

The foregoing group of investigators[63] reinforced their position on the mechanism of injury of the biceps tendon–superior labral complex in the overhead throwing athlete. Their model encompassed the following:

1. A type II posterior-superior glenoid labrum tear. This tear causes anterior pseudolaxity and a positive arthroscopic drive-through sign.
2. The upper extremity positioned in abduction and external rotation with a type II posterior-superior glenoid labrum tear and unstable biceps anchor will cause the biceps–superior labral complex to "peel back" over the posterior-superior corner of the labrum.
3. A contracted posterior-inferior capsule resulted in a reduction of internal rotation in abduction. This clinical finding is present in all overhand-throwing athletes who develop posterior-superior SLAP lesions.

The mechanism is as follows: When an overhand-throwing athlete with an acquired tight posterior capsule places the shoulder in the cocking position of abduction and external rotation, the posterior capsule inhibits normal full external rotation. This situation causes a posterior-superior shift of the moment center of the glenohumeral joint. This new center of rotation places the humeral head in increased contact with the internal impingement zone and thus causes increased forces to the biceps tendon–superior labrum complex through external rotation. This mechanism produces the SLAP lesion, and the creation of the SLAP lesion contributes to a posterior-superior shift and instability.

Given that deceleration produces the greatest force through the phases of overhand throwing, the biceps-labrum complex also exhibits its greatest strength in this in-line position. Deceleration does play a role in the creation of a SLAP lesion, probably by being the force that generates the adaption of the posterior capsule. A restricted posterior capsule intensifies the superior shear force in terminal external rotation and becomes a component of this disabling injury.

ASYMMETRICAL SCAPULAR MALPOSITION

Five roles of the scapula have been described[64]:

- Being a stable part of the glenohumeral articulation
- Retraction and protraction along the thoracic wall
- Elevation of the acromion
- Being a base for muscle attachment
- Serving as a link in the proximal to distal sequence energy delivery

A dysfunction in one role or a combination of dysfunctions in other scapular roles puts the throwing athlete at risk.

Normal scapular kinematics is necessary for optimum upper extremity motion. The glenoid must be continually repositioned to correlate with the moving humerus to maintain the stable glenohumeral joint. A malpositioned scapula has been demonstrated to place greater demands on the anterior capsule.[46] The ability of the scapula to retract places the upper extremity in the "full tank of energy" position for throwing, and the ability to protract through the delivery is necessary for the scapula to follow the moving humerus while providing a stable platform. Elevation of the acromion increases the subacromial space to prevent impingement of the rotator cuff. Certain muscular force couples are necessary to move the scapula through its three axes of motion. In the active scapular plane, upward rotation has been reported to be 50° (–SD 4.8°), posterior tilting on a medial to lateral axes is 30° (–SD 13°), and external rotation around a vertical axis is 24° (–SD 12.8°).[65] Scapular positioning has also been reported in nondominant movement patterns of abduction and horizontal adduction, as well as in the tasks of reaching and hand-behind-the-back maneuvering.[66]

An adaptive change of greater upward rotation of the scapula in the overhand-throwing athlete has been recognized at an early age and can be a consistent finding in the professional athlete.[67,68] Myers et al[69] investigated this adaptation in throwing athletes as compared with a control group. The motion of humeral elevation in the scapular plane demonstrated significant increased upward rotation at 0° to 30°, 60° to 90°, and 120°. In addition, the throwing athlete demonstrated significant increases of retraction at both 90°and 120° of humeral elevation in the scapular plane. No significant differences were in anterior and posterior scapular tipping or in scapular elevation and depression. However, increased scapular internal rotation in the throwing group was present in all test positions.

In a study comparing scapular upward rotation in high school and collegiate baseball players, a significant decrease of motion was determined in the older group at both 90° and 120° in abduction. Collegiate players also demonstrated more scapular protraction when they were assessed in the hands-on-hips and 90° abduction with internal rotation positions.[70] A comparison of upward scapular rotation during humeral elevation in the plane of the scapula of dominant shoulders of professional position players and professional pitchers revealed decreased motion at the four static test positions: rest, 60°, 90°, and 120°. A significant difference was seen between the groups at both 60° and 90°.[71]

Oyama et al,[72] in a three-dimensional study, investigated the scapular resting position bilaterally in three male overhand athlete groups: baseball pitchers, volleyball players, and tennis players. The dominant scapula in all groups was more internally rotated and anteriorly tilted. Tennis players had a more protracted scapula. The investigators suggested that these changes in scapular position could be defined as normal for these populations because all subjects were asymptomatic. Decreased scapular upward rotation was not present in these subjects, and this finding could suggest that this component may be associated with the injured athlete.

More often than not, the disabled overhand-throwing athlete clinically presents with a markedly asymmetrical, malpositioned scapula. This malpositioned scapula is referred to by the acronym *SICK scapula*[73]: (1) *s*capula, (2) *i*nfera, (3) *c*oracoid, and (4) dys*k*inesis. A SICK scapula is a muscular overuse fatigue syndrome that manifests clinically with three major components. First, the scapula drops or is lower when compared with the nondominant scapula. Second, the scapula is protracted or lies farther laterally from the spine when compared with the nondominant scapula. Third, the scapula has increased abduction or a greater angle from the spine to the medial scapula border when compared with the nondominant scapula. One, any combination, or all of these components can be present at the time of examination.

An athlete often presents with one or more of the following symptoms in association with a SICK scapula:

1. Pain located on the medial aspect of the coracoid
2. Pain located at the superior-medial aspect of the scapula
3. Painful subacromial space
4. Painful acromioclavicular joint
5. Thoracic outlet symptoms or radicular pain

The onset of these symptoms is usually insidious and occurs when the athlete passes a pathologic threshold. A careful medical history does not reveal a single event or rapid progression to disability.

Because of the components of a malpositioned scapula, which is located inferiorly, protected, and abducted, increased tension is placed on the coracoid by virtue of a shortened pectoralis minor tendon and conjoined tendon. With repetitive overhand motions, the restrictive nature of these shortened tendon structures encourages tendinopathy that results in a painful medial coracoid.

Pain located at the superior-medial aspect of the scapula is present in the malpositioned scapula at the insertion of the levator scapulae, upper rhomboids, and upper trapezius. Because these scapular control muscles originate from the essentially fixed spine, they are required to function in an overtensioned pattern of pain referral into the muscle belly. Most often, the key indicator in this sequence is posterior neck pain on the dominant side. Dyskinesis of the scapula is the primary offender, and a treatment protocol should be designed to rectify the malposition of the scapula to resolve the posterior neck symptoms. Any attempt to stretch the offended musculature will add insult to the present injury.

Subacromial pain often results from the infera component of the SICK scapula, which reduces the subacromial space by essentially lowering the acromion (Fig. 3-1). This reduction of space hinders the function of the rotator cuff in all phases of the overhand throw. The coinciding lack of posterior tilting of the scapula with elevation increases the impingement symptoms.[74,75] A scapular relocation test that relieves these symptoms also increases the athlete's ability to forward flex, which is often restricted and painful.

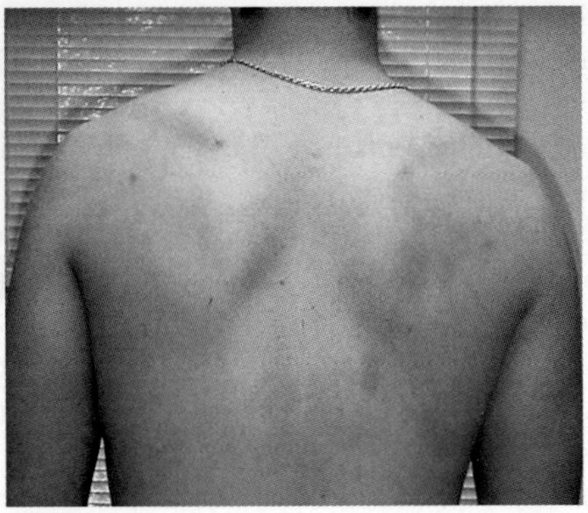

Figure 3-1 SICK scapula: right scapula is lower, protracted, and abducted.

The acromioclavicular joint becomes symptomatic as a result of the altered kinematics of the malpositioned scapula. Because the clavicle is more rigidly secured at the sternum, stresses from the infera and from protraction and abduction of the scapula are imposed on the distal clavicle articulation. Thoracic outlet symptoms are present in a few athletes because of the pressure on the neurovascular structures by the unsupported scapula and clavicle.

The challenge for the clinician is to recognize the subtle changes in the position of the scapula and the way in which those subtle changes put the glenohumeral joint at risk. The task of repositioning the scapula by stretching the contracted structures and strengthening the supporting musculature in the corrected position is paramount in the sequence of rehabilitation of the overhand-throwing athlete.

POSTERIOR SHOULDER TIGHTNESS: GLENOHUMERAL INTERNAL ROTATION DEFICIT

Adaptive range-of-motion changes in overhand-throwing athletes have been observed for some time.[76,77] Common adaptations occur in horizontal adduction and in external and internal rotation of the glenohumeral joint at 90° of abduction. Asymptomatic pitchers have been reported to manifest an increase of up to 30° of glenohumeral external rotation in both the frontal and scapular plane when compared with their nondominant shoulders.[1] Glenohumeral internal rotation deficits of 15° to 20° have also been associated with asymptomatic pitchers,[46,48-51] whereas symptomatic pitchers have reported deficits as high as 45°.[38] These changes have been attributed to numerous factors including a posterior-inferior capsular restriction, muscular inflexibility of the external rotators, eccentric loading of the external rotators, and osseous adaptations of humeral head or glenoid.[52-54,78]

Since the late 1990s, numerous studies have determined the passive range of motion of the overhand-throwing athlete.[78-94] Some of these studies have addressed the issue of humeral retroversion.[83,87] The study of humeral retroversion may be relatively new in the sports medicine world; however, it was described as far back as 1881 in the anthropology literature.[95] The relationship of the distal humerus with the proximal humerus changes through the skeletal maturation process. Adults have humeral retroversion in the range of 25° and 35°. Fetal skeletons ($N = 50$) have been measured with a mean retroversion angle of 78°.[96] By the age of 8 years, most of the derotation occurs, and in the following 8 years, the process is complete.[97]

During overhand throwing, humeral torque is developed as the distal portion of the humerus is externally rotated at a rate greater than the proximal end, in an attempt to achieve maximum glenohumeral rotation. Humeral peak torque peaks immediately before maximum external rotation.[98] It appears that the stress endured by the maturing proximal humerus during the overhand throw slows the derotation in the dominant arm.[99,100]

In a cross-sectional study of 294 Little League and adolescent baseball players between 8 and 16 years old, peak changes in elevation, external rotation, and internal rotation occurred between the ages of 11 and 13 years. Significant changes in internal rotation of the dominant shoulder occurred between the 12- and 13-year-old groups. Changes in internal rotation of the nondominant shoulder was seen between the 14- and 15-year-old groups.

When the youngest group of baseball players was compared with the oldest group, the differences in internal rotation, external rotation, and total range of motion were significant. Internal rotation in the dominant shoulder decreased by an average of 17.7°, and it decreased by 9.1° in the nondominant shoulder. External rotation in the dominant shoulder decreased by an average of 20.5°, and this value decreased by 23.5° in the nondominant shoulder. Thus, the total range of motion decreased by 38.2° in the dominant shoulder as compared with 32.5° in the nondominant shoulder.[101]

Pappas et al[102] reported a significant limitation of glenohumeral internal rotation range of motion and posterior shoulder tightness as measured by horizontal abduction with scapula stabilization in patients diagnosed as having subacromial impingement. Brown et al[80] recorded the range of motion for multiple upper extremity movements in two separate groups consisting of professional pitchers and position players. The pitchers had significant increases of 9° of external rotation in 90° abduction. The pitchers had significant decreases of 5° shoulder flexion and 15° internal rotation in 90° of abduction when compared with their nondominant side. Position players had a significant increase of 8° external rotation in 90° of abduction.

Verna et al[103] measured 137 professional baseball players bilaterally for internal rotation by fixing the scapula and medially rotating the humerus while in 90° of abduction in the supine position. Correlating the internal rotation deficits of the dominant shoulder with injury history revealed that those pitchers who reported a shoulder or an elbow problem averaged an internal rotation deficit of 41%. Position players reporting a shoulder or an elbow problem averaged a deficit of 43%. Uninjured athletes, whether pitchers or position players, averaged an internal rotation deficit of only 24%.

Warner et al[104] demonstrated a significant limitation of internal rotation range of motion and posterior shoulder tightness, as measured in horizontal abduction, in a group of patients with impingement compared with patients with shoulder instability and control patients. Kugler et al[105] attempted to identify features that could correlate with shoulder injuries in highly skilled volleyball attackers, an overhand activity. To measure posterior shoulder tightness, the researchers measured the distance from the lateral epicondyle to the acromion of the opposite shoulder during maximal horizontal adduction. The researchers did not report whether the scapula was stabilized. They found that the dominant posterior shoulder was significantly tighter in attackers with shoulder pain compared with attackers without shoulder pain or compared with a control group. Attackers without shoulder pain had significantly tighter shoulders than did the control group. Both groups of volleyball players had an increase in tightness in their dominant shoulder compared with their nondominant shoulder.

Bigliani et al[79] examined upper extremity range of motion and glenohumeral joint laxity in a study of 148 healthy professional baseball players, 72 pitchers and 76 position players. Glenohumeral internal rotation was recorded as the highest vertebral level reached by the thumb up the spine.[106] This recording was converted to a number value according to the American Shoulder and Elbow Surgeons' standards, to permit statistical comparisons. Shoulder external rotation with the humerus at 90° of abduction in the frontal plane and internal rotation, measured as previously described, both demonstrated statistically significant differences between dominant and nondominant shoulders.

For pitchers, the dominant glenohumeral external rotation range of motion averaged 118° (range, 95° to 145°), and the nondominant glenohumeral external rotation range of motion averaged 102° (range, 85° to 130°). The difference was 15.2° or a 13% increase in external rotation in the dominant extremity. Pitchers' dominant glenohumeral internal rotation range of motion averaged 15.5° (T6-7) (range, L3-T2); the nondominant glenohumeral internal rotation range of motion averaged 17.6° (T4-5) (range, T8-T2) or a loss of 14%. Positional players measured in similar fashion had an average dominant glenohumeral external rotation range of 109.3° (range, 80° to 150°) and a nondominant glenohumeral external rotation range of motion averaging 97.1° (range, 80° to 120°). Positional players recorded a loss of two levels of vertebrae calculated to 12.2° or 11% of their internal rotation in their dominant shoulder.

In a similar study,[107] 152 right-handed professional baseball pitchers were measured for glenohumeral internal rotation with three different protocols: vertebrae level/thumb up spine, glenohumeral internal rotation in the frontal plane at 90° of abduction with a stabilized scapula, and glenohumeral internal rotation in the scapular plane at 90° of abduction with a stabilized scapula. Correlation between the vertebrae level/thumb up spine (average loss of 7.8 ± 4.8 cm in the dominant arm) and glenohumeral internal rotation in the frontal plane ($r = 0.176$; $P \leq .03$) or glenohumeral internal rotation in the scapular plane ($r = 0.226$; $P \leq .005$) was poor.

The indirect behind-the-back measurement for internal rotation has been studied by others, and this method has been suggested as problematic.[108,109] It involves shoulder extension, scapular retraction and downward rotation, elbow flexion, and mobility of the forearm, wrist, and thumb. Mallon et al,[110] in a radiographic study, estimated that 35% of the motion in this test occurred at the scapulothoracic articulation. The vertebrae level/thumb up spine may be a test of functionality, but it is not a valid measure of glenohumeral internal rotation in the overhand-throwing athlete because of the inability to stabilize the scapula.

Tyler et al,[82] while describing a proposed alternate method for measuring posterior shoulder tightness, recorded bilateral external and internal rotation of the glenohumeral joint with 90° of humeral abduction in 22 collegiate baseball pitchers. The scapula was stabilized only by the weight of the subject. The baseball pitchers recorded significantly more external rotation bilaterally than did the control group. The pitchers' dominant shoulders recorded an average range of external rotation of 109.7° ± 2.4° compared with the control 95.9° ± 1.6°. The nondominant shoulders of the baseball pitchers recorded 98.9° ±1.6° of external rotation, and the controls recorded 95.2° ± 1.6°. The dominant shoulders of the baseball pitchers averaged 50.0° ± 2.0° of internal rotation compared with 46.4° ± 1.3° in the control group. Internal rotation of the baseball pitchers' nondominant shoulders averaged 69.5° ± 2.5° compared with 50.2° ± 1.4° in the control group.

When one examines these data further, the pitchers in this study experienced an average glenohumeral external rotation gain of 10.8° or 10.9% in the dominant shoulder as compared with the nondominant shoulder. The average loss of glenohumeral internal rotation was 19.5° or 28% of the dominant shoulder as opposed to the nondominant shoulder. The control group had essentially no gain in glenohumeral external rotation in the dominant shoulder and an average loss of only 3.8° or 7.5% of internal rotation.

The larger purpose of the study by Tyler et al[82] was to introduce an alternative for measuring posterior shoulder tightness to that method reported by previous investigators.[104,105] This alternate method involved a side-lying position in which the scapula was manually stabilized and the humerus was horizontally adducted without rotation to a firm end feel. The distance from the medial epicondyle to the surface of the examination table was measured in centimeters. Essentially, the supine test position was rotated 90°, and a linear measure, such as Kugler's, was used instead of a goniometric measure. When Tyler et al[82] compared these linear measure data with their internal rotation data, they reported that every centimeter of horizontal adduction lost corresponded to 4° of internal rotation lost in the baseball pitcher.

In a group of 372 professional baseball pitchers, Wilk et al[111] reported an average total shoulder range of motion of 129.9° ± 10° of external rotation and 62.6° ± 9° of internal rotation when it was passively measured at 90° of abduction. These measurements represent an unstabilized glenohumeral joint. When the dominant shoulder was compared with the nondominant shoulder, a 7° increase in external rotation and a 7° decrease in internal rotation in the dominant shoulder were noted. This finding was coined the "total motion concept" in which total shoulder rotation is equal to the sum of external rotation and internal rotation.

The previous discussion on the biceps tendon–superior labral complex demonstrated a strong relationship between glenohumeral internal rotation deficits in the overhand-throwing athlete and a surgical shoulder. Burkhart et al[81] reported that 53 overhand throwers with SLAP lesions had an average internal rotation deficit at 90° of abduction of −45° preoperatively. One year postoperatively, internal rotation deficits were only −15°. These investigators emphasized that the required rehabilitation protocol was an aggressive stretching program for a tight posterior-inferior capsule, which had been thought to initially cause the SLAP lesion.

Morgan[112] introduced the *rotational unity rule* stating that an overhand-throwing athlete will maintain normal glenohumeral mechanics if the internal rotational deficit is less than or equal to the external rotational gain. A humeral posterior-superior shift will occur if the internal rotation deficit is greater than the external glenohumeral gain. Morgan supported this theory with a series of 124 baseball pitchers surgically treated for SLAP lesions. This group was equally divided by thirds into professional athletes, college athletes, and high school or recreational athletes. Preoperatively, the group, as measured in 90° of abduction with a stabilized scapula, averaged a glenohumeral internal rotation deficit of 53° (range, 26° to 80°). The external rotation gain, similarly measured, in this group was 33° (range, 22° to 45°). Thus, a larger glenohumeral internal rotation deficit was present compared with the external rotational gain in these 124 surgical patients.

The rotational unity rule was supported by a study of 67 college-aged baseball players who were grouped by reported shoulder pain.[113] Thirty-seven (55%) reported no shoulder pain. Ten (15%) reported mild pain with no loss in strength or performance. Twelve (18%) reported moderate pain with a performance drop but no time loss. Eight (12%) reported severe pain requiring time off or rest. All players were measured for both internal and external glenohumeral rotation in 90° of abduction while in a seated position. The scapula was stabilized by the examiner. When total arc was examined in the asymptomatic group, the dominant and nondominant sides were essentially equal. The dominant side exhibited 8.8° more external rotation, offset by an 8.9-degree loss in internal rotation. Players who reported pain affecting performance had a total arc reduction in their dominant shoulders by an average of 10.4°. The average external rotation gain was 4.4 degrees, as compared with a significant internal rotation loss of 13.7°.

Myers et al[114] employed the side-lying method to measure posterior shoulder tightness and the supine 90/90 method to measure glenohumeral external and internal rotation in a group of overhand-throwing athletes with pathologic internal impingement. Compared with a control group, the injured athletes demonstrated significantly increased posterior tightness and loss of internal rotation. No significant external rotation gains were reported between the groups.

Glenohumeral joint horizontal adduction assessment for posterior shoulder tightness has been used in many of these and other studies. Laudner et al[115] conducted a study to determine the reliability and validity of this test. Twelve controls and 23 professional baseball players were involved. All subjects were tested from the supine position with a fixed scapula. The lateral border of the scapula was pressed posteriorly to the examination table before any humeral movement. Once terminal horizontal adduction was achieved, the angle was recorded with a digital inclinometer. In this study, both intratester and intertester reliability were 0.91. This study also measured the external and internal glenohumeral range of motion in 20 of the subjects. Repeat measurements were made in approximately 24 hours. The Intraclass Correlation Coefficient was reported as 0.95 for external rotation and 0.98 for internal rotation.

Myers et al[116] investigated the reliability, precision, accuracy, and validity of both side-lying and supine horizontal humeral adduction assessments for posterior shoulder tightness. With the aid of an electronic tracking device, four groups were tested: 15 controls, 15 non–overhead-throwing athletes, 15 baseball players, and 13 tennis players. The scapula was fixed in maximum retraction by the examiner before movement of the humerus into adduction. External range of motion and internal range of motion were also recorded.

Both methods for measuring posterior shoulder tightness resulted in low clinical error with good precision. Scapular stabilization was held within tolerable limits by both methods. The supine method proved to be more reliable between both testing sessions and testers. When both methods were compared with glenohumeral internal rotation measurements, the supine method was able to determine the differences between the control group and the overhand athletes.

The "posterior syndrome" was described as an enigma in the late 1970s.[77] Factors limiting horizontal adduction and internal rotation at 90° of abduction may include posterior-inferior capsular restrictions, muscular inflexibility of the external rotators, and osseous adaptations of humeral head or glenoid. Significant loss of motion in either plane may suggest the diagnosis of posterior capsular contracture. Clinical measurements that have been studied as reliable should be incorporated into a proactive preventive protocol.

ESSENTIAL-ESSENTIAL LESION

In this chapter, the relationship between a glenohumeral internal rotation deficit resulting from a posterior-inferior capsule contraction and the injured overhand-throwing athlete has been suggested. The posterior-inferior capsule often becomes thickened and contracted as a reaction to the tremendous distraction forces placed on the glenohumeral joint during deceleration. As this slow and insidious adaptive change occurs, it dictates altered dynamics of the glenohumeral joint by the shifting the humeral head during the cocking phase of throwing from its true moment center to a more posterior-superior position.

Previous studies indicated an anterior-superior migration of the humeral head in relation to a posteriorly and inferiorly contracted capsule; however, these investigations were focused on the motion of forward flexion.[18] With the introduction of external rotation at 90° of abduction, the posterior-inferior capsule is positioned inferiorly and becomes the supporting structure of the humeral head. Once this structure becomes shortened, the tethered posterior cable and cam effect[117] puts the overhand-throwing athlete's shoulder at risk by altering the mechanics of the glenohumeral joint to begin the potential crescendo of internal impingement, labral lesions, and undersurface rotator cuff disease.

Additionally, a contracted posterior-inferior capsule becomes the steering mechanism for the upper quadrant during the follow-through phase. The rapidly moving humerus begins to dictate the position of the scapula. When the posterior-inferior capsule is contracted, the scapula's position on the thorax often becomes altered. Upward rotation is decreased, and anterior tilt and protraction is increased.[118,119] Over time, in an adaptive attempt to normalize its position, the scapula settles into a depressed position or one previously described as infera.[64] This combination of a glenohumeral internal rotation deficit and asymmetrical scapular malposition has the greatest potential of producing a significant injury in the upper extremity in the overhand-throwing athlete.

PREVENTIVE PROTOCOL

The knowledge gained since the late 1990s in the rehabilitation of the overhand-throwing athlete has allowed improved preventive protocols to be designed. These protocols not only have made a significant impact in the prevention of disabilities but also have played an important role in the reduction of severity and playing time loss by the athlete. As the surgeon's knowledge expands and is supported by the technical tools necessary to repair previously undiagnosed lesions, a whole generation of athletes has been given a second opportunity. Overhand-throwing athletes who were previously cast aside because of interarticular structural damage can now entertain surgical options once a period of conservative care has proven fruitless. Athletes must understand that a return to play demands that rehabilitation will be a continuing process. At no time should these athletes think that they have obtained a cure. If athletes abandon the rehabilitation process, they will revert to the previous stress cycle and will predispose themselves to reinjury.

For an overhand-throwing athlete to be most efficient, he or she must obtain congruent glenohumeral stability throughout the full range of motion.[63] Because the scapula must continually reposition itself to maintain this stability, it is necessary to ensure unrestricted range of motion and some balanced force couples. Kibler[120] identified three scapular patterns related to shoulder injuries:

1. The lack of retraction, resulting in the loss of the ability to place the scapula in the position of full cocking and hence the loss of acceleration
2. The lack of protraction, resulting in increased deceleration forces on the shoulder and an altered safe zone for the glenohumeral joint in acceleration
3. Excessive protraction, resulting in a scapula that is rotated downward and forward

Therefore, the first objective in the preventive protocol is to attempt to maintain an anatomically correct position of the scapula or to reposition the asymmetrical scapula. This is accomplished by mobilizing the restrictive structures that have permitted the humerus and a tethered coracoid to dictate the position of the scapula. These structures are a contracted posterior capsule and a contracted pectoralis minor and conjoined tendon.

Exercises are then introduced for scapular elevation and depression, protraction and retraction, and upward and downward rotation, to restore a normal range of motion. These exercises can be accomplished in a closed-chain manner for glenohumeral joint protection.[121] Muscle strengthening should begin with the scapular pivoters and glenohumeral protectors.[122] Special attention should be paid to the serratus anterior and the lower trapezius, for this force couple is responsible for the elevation of the acromion.

The training or retaining of the humeral positioners and rotators is begun with closed-chain exercises in 60° of humeral abduction, a safe zone for the rotator cuff. The exercises are progressively elevated to 90° of humeral abduction. Once the scapula can be adequately positioned and stabilized, the humeral positioners and humeral rotators can be exercised in an open chain.

Contained within the following base exercise protocol are five movements identified as core exercises. These exercises, commonly used by many throwing athletes, have been popularized by two studies from the Kerlan-Jobe Clinic.[123,124] Because the experimental models used small weights at low intensities, the full benefit of these exercises may not be apparent from these data. First, some of these exercises are not performed in the arc of greatest benefit if one limits the exercises to what is commonly referred to as *below the plane*. Most of the tested exercises qualify at the extreme of the available range of motion. Second, less than adequate resistance may have been employed to elicit the desired muscle response. Third, the inclusion of a high-repetition program was not explored using these tested exercises. Fourth, the exercises lend themselves easily to an eccentric, or deceleration, program. When the concentric component of the exercise is provided for the athlete, the resistance of the eccentric component can be significantly increased. It is paramount that a negative exercise base be established before the introduction of stretch-shortening exercises.

The mass movement patterns contained with the following protocol are used to choreograph functional activity so the scapula is placed in the optimum position for the desired activity at the distal segment. Global pattern exercises are incorporated not only for their specific core and shoulder strength training but also to elicit a crossover of upper extremity synchrony. The combination of these exercises moves the athlete closer to a return to activity.

The final step in conditioning or rehabilitating an overhand-throwing athlete is to train the accelerators. This is done through a throwing program that builds on and emphasizes long throwing. The act of long throwing enhances acceleration and builds upper extremity strength in the required rotational pattern. It provides a step-by-step form to evaluate the coexistent stretching and strengthening protocol. Long throwing also provides an excellent base for protective deceleration conditioning. As the neuromuscular system is trained or retrained to provide synchrony of movement, the capsule must be conditioned to withstand the tremendous traction forces it is exposed to during deceleration.

As previously stated, injury to the shoulder complex precipitated by overhand throwing is most often the result of a failure in the kinetic chain manifesting itself in the weakest link, the glenohumeral joint. Because the lower body and trunk develop 46.7% of the velocity for the throwing arm,[125] it is important to focus on proximal joint contractures and muscular imbalances in the conditioning of these segments as part of the entire rehabilitation process. If one maintains a glenohumeral vision in the design of preventive or rehabilitation protocols for the overhand-throwing athlete, the process will be guaranteed to fail.

MEASUREMENTS

Previously, two reliable methods were presented to measure posterior capsular restriction in the overhand-throwing athlete: horizontal adduction and internal rotation at 90°. One author attempted to find a correlation among the two methods.[126] The following are a few suggested ways of measuring both these motions and external rotation in 90° of abduction. Because the act of overhand throwing is rotational, the measurements made with the capsule in a state of rotation are extremely important. All measurements are made bilaterally, and a deficit of internal rotation greater than 20% in the dominant shoulder is cause for concern.

$$([ND - D]/ND) \times 100$$

The measurement of external rotation in 90° of abduction is necessary to establish an individual's total motion or rotational unity. However, the arc is critical. If the total rotational range of motion at 90° of abduction is within bounds bilaterally, a limit of 120° of external rotation should be considered the maximum in most athletes unless this value is noted in the nondominant glenohumeral joint. In a proactive preventive protocol, these measurements should be obtained often during a competitive sports season to ensure the necessary posterior muscle and capsule flexibility.

Horizontal Adduction: Supine

The athlete is positioned supine, and the lateral border of the scapula is stabilized against the chest wall with one hand (Fig. 3-2). The humerus is then horizontally adducted in neutral rotation until a firm end feel is obtained or scapular movement is detected. A measurement is then made using a goniometer with an attached level or digital inclinometer for greater accuracy.

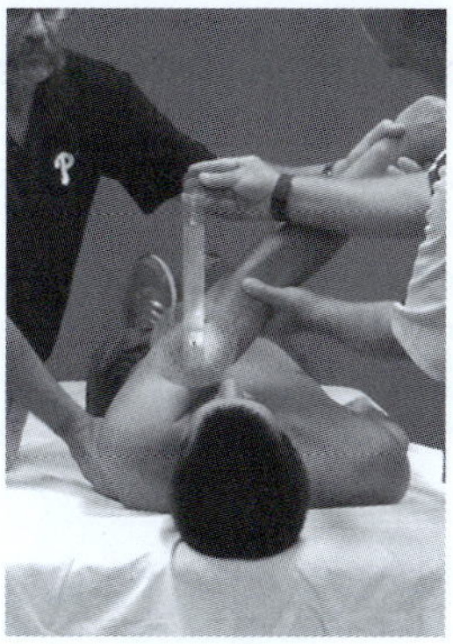

Figure 3-2

Glenohumeral Internal Rotation in 90° of Abduction Frontal Plane: Supine

The athlete is positioned supine and the humerus is abducted to 90° (Fig. 3-3). The scapula is stabilized with a downward force on the coracoid process with one hand while the humerus is medially rotated until an end feel is obtained or scapular movement is detected. A measurement is then made using a goniometer with an attached level or digital inclinometer for greater accuracy.

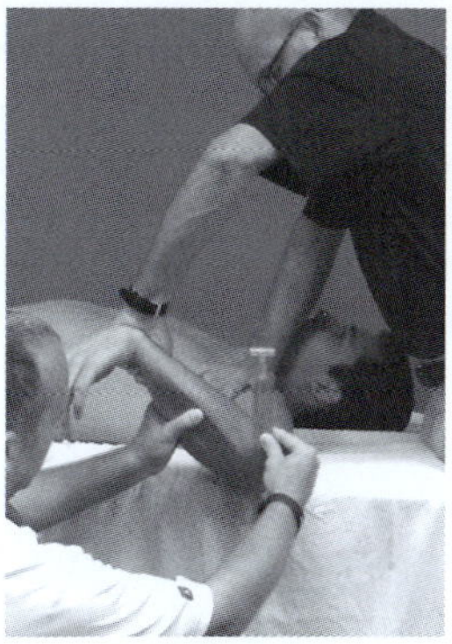

Figure 3-3

Glenohumeral External Rotation in 90° of Abduction Frontal Plane: Supine

The athlete is positioned supine and the humerus is abducted to 90° (Fig. 3-4). The scapula is stabilized with a downward force on the coracoid process with one hand while the humerus is laterally rotated until an end feel is obtained or scapular movement is detected. A measurement is then made using a goniometer with an attached level or digital inclinometer for greater accuracy.

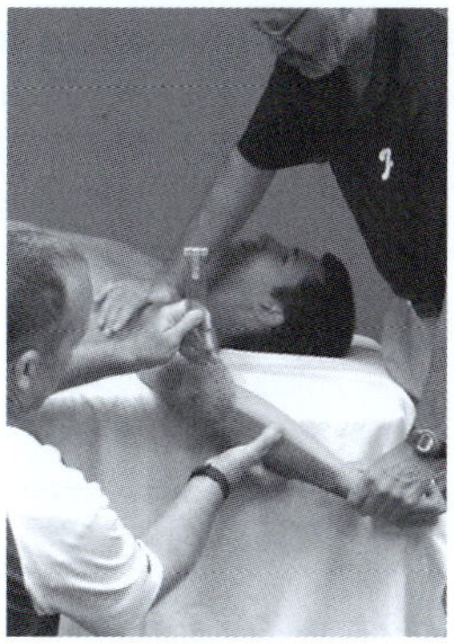

Figure 3-4

Glenohumeral Internal Rotation in 90° of Abduction Scapular Plane: Supine

The athlete is positioned supine and the humerus is abducted to 90° and horizontally adducted 30° with a wedge (Fig. 3-5). The scapula is stabilized with a downward force with one hand on the coracoid process while the humerus is medially rotated until an end feel is obtained or scapular movement is detected. A measurement is then made using a goniometer with an attached level or digital inclinometer for greater accuracy

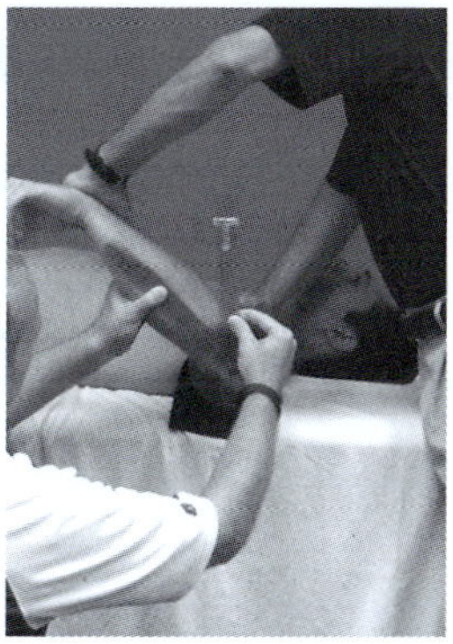

Figure 3-5

Glenohumeral External Rotation in 90° of Abduction Scapular Plane: Supine

The athlete is positioned supine and the humerus is abducted to 90° and horizontally adducted 30° with a wedge (Fig. 3-6). The scapula is stabilized with a downward force with one hand on the coracoid process while the humerus is laterally rotated until an end feel is obtained or scapular movement is detected. A measurement is then made using a goniometer with an attached level or digital inclinometer for greater accuracy.

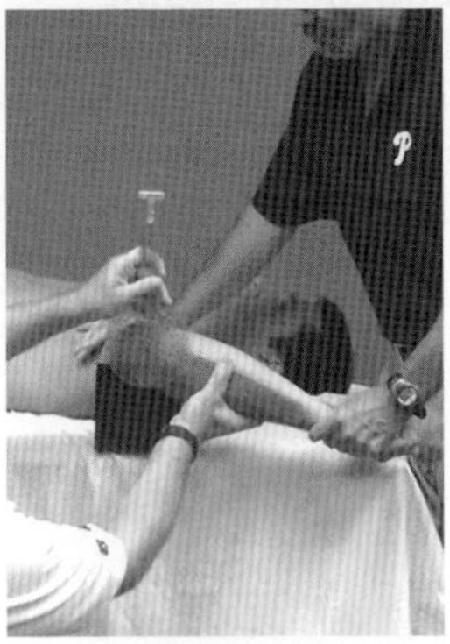

Figure 3-6

Glenohumeral Internal Rotation in 90° of Forward Flexion: Side Lying

The athlete is positioned in a side-lying position, and the humerus is forward flexed 90° (Fig. 3-7). The scapula is stabilized by the athlete's body weight and is monitored for movement with one hand. The humerus is medially rotated until an end feel is obtained or scapular movement is detected. A measurement is then made using a goniometer with an attached level or digital inclinometer for greater accuracy.

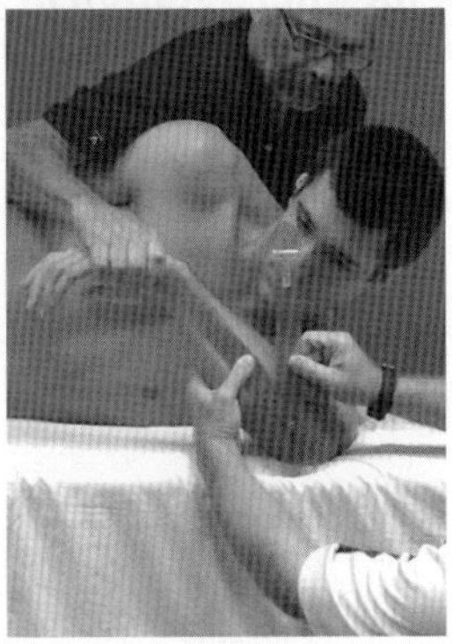

Figure 3-7

Glenohumeral External Rotation in 90° of Forward Flexion: Side Lying

The athlete is positioned in a side-lying position, and the humerus is forward flexed 90° (Fig. 3-8). The scapula is stabilized by the athlete's body weight and is monitored for movement with one hand. The humerus is laterally rotated until an end feel is obtained or scapular movement is detected. A measurement is then made using a goniometer with an attached level or digital inclinometer for greater accuracy.

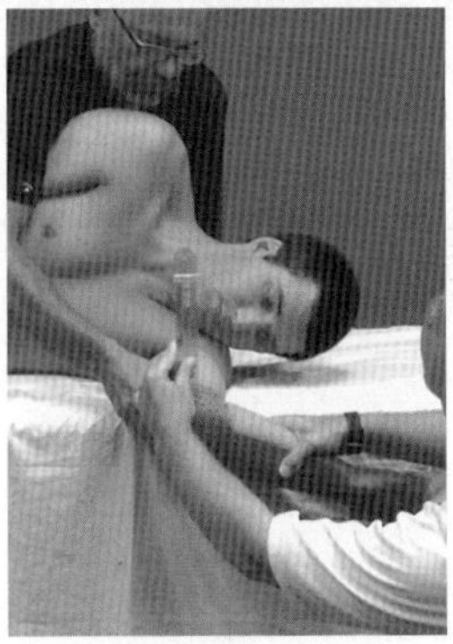

Figure 3-8

MOBILIZATION OF THE SCAPULA

Pectoralis Minor/Conjoined Tendon Stretch: Supine

The athlete is positioned supine with a rigid bolster place in line with the medial border of the scapula to elevate the shoulder girdle (Fig. 3-9A). In a crossed-hand fashion, one hand is placed on inferiorly and medial to the coracoids. The heel of the other hand is placed on the coracoid (Fig. 3-9B). A downward motion while separating the hands accomplishes the stretch.

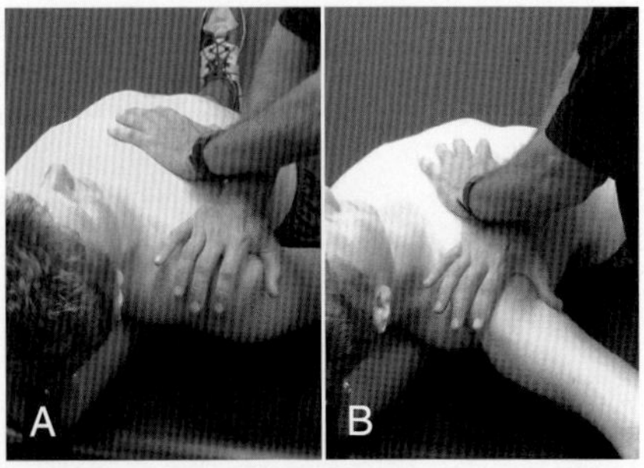

Figure 3-9

Pectoralis Minor/Conjoined Tendon Self Stretch

The athlete stands with the humerus abducted to 90° with the elbow flexed to 90° (Fig. 3-10A). The palm and forearm are placed against a vertical structure such as a doorway, and the trunk is rotated away from the arm to accomplish the desired stretch (Fig. 3-10B).[127]

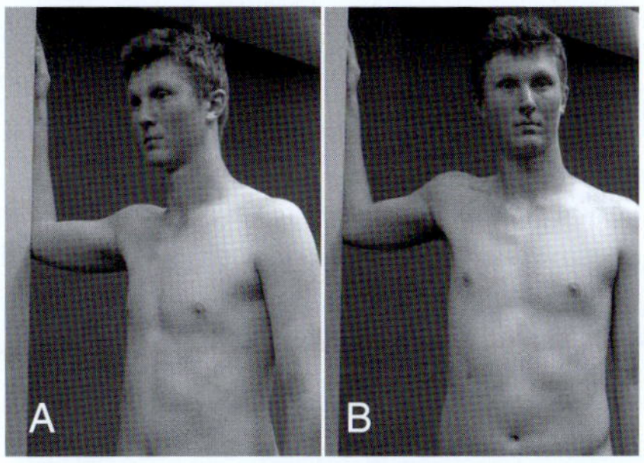

Figure 3-10

Protraction/Retraction Stretch: Side Lying

The athlete is placed in a side-lying position. By grasping the medial border of the scapula, it is protracted by moving it laterally against the chest wall (Fig. 3-11A). By placing the heels of the hands on the lateral border of the scapula, the scapula is moved into retraction by moving it medially against the chest wall (Fig. 3-11B).

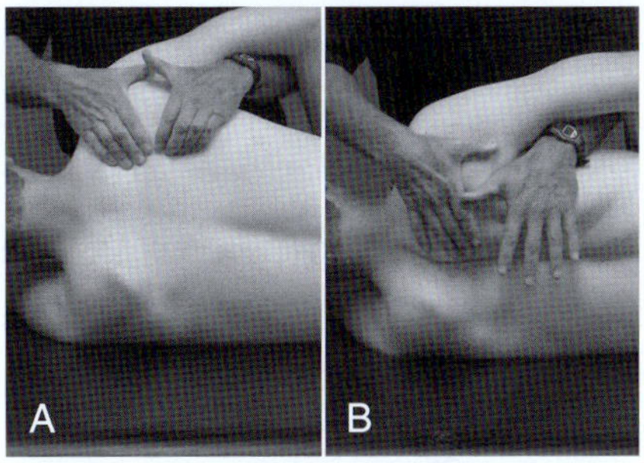

Figure 3-11

Upward/Downward Rotation Stretch: Side Lying

The athlete is placed in a side-lying position. By grasping the inferior medial border of the scapula with one hand and the lateral border with the heel of the other hand, upward rotation along the chest wall is achieved (Fig. 3-12A). Downward rotation can be achieved by reversing the hands, grasping the superior-medial border of the scapula with one hand, and placing the heel of the other hand on the inferior-lateral border (Fig. 3-12B).

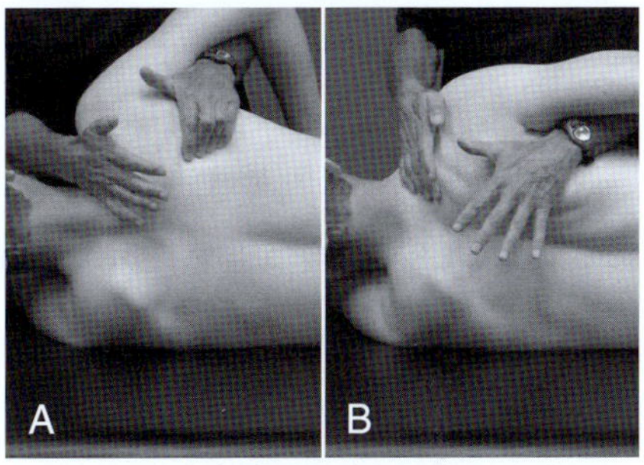

Figure 3-12

Posterior Tilting Stretch: Side Lying

The athlete is placed in a side-lying position. One hand is placed on the inferior angle of the scapula, and the heel of the other hand is placed on the coracoid (Fig. 3-13A). The scapula is then elevated from the inferior angle and then pressed against the chest wall. Once full elevation is achieved, the scapula is posteriorly tilted by pressure against the coracoid (Fig. 3-13B).

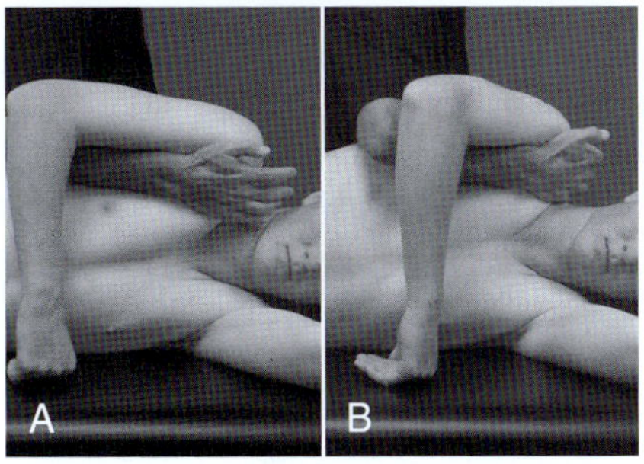

Figure 3-13

Posterior Tilting Stretch: Prone

The athlete is placed in a prone position with the shoulder abducted to 90° and the elbow flexed 90°. One hand is placed on the inferior angle of the scapula, and the fingers of the other hand reach under the chest to locate the coracoid (Fig. 3-14A). The scapula is then elevated from the inferior angle and then pressed against the chest wall. Once full elevation is achieved, lifting the coracoid posteriorly tilts the scapula (Fig. 3-14B).

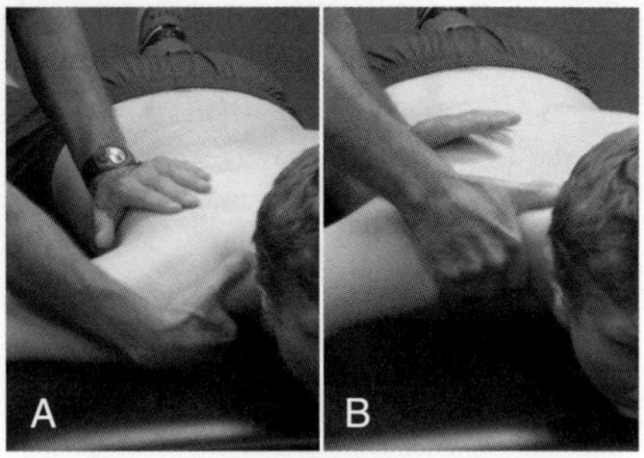

Figure 3-14

POSTERIOR-INFERIOR CAPSULE STRETCHING

Horizontal Adduction: Supine

The athlete is positioned supine on the table close enough to the edge to expose the lateral border of the scapula. The scapula is stabilized with the hip, and the humerus is moved into horizontal adduction (Fig. 3-15).

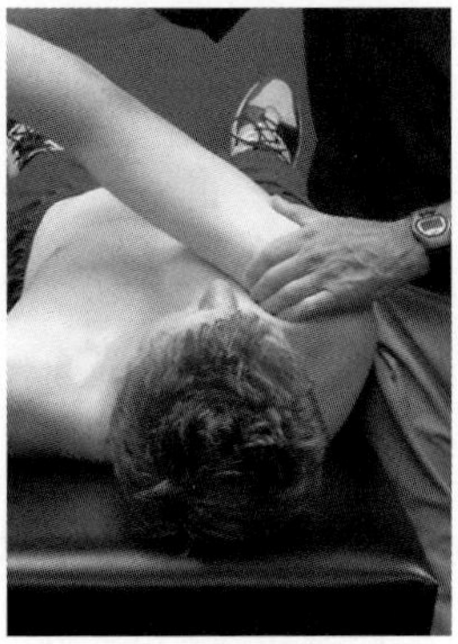

Figure 3-15

Abduction 90°/Scapular Plane Internal Rotation: Supine

The athlete is positioned supine on the table close enough to the edge to expose the lateral border of the scapula. The humerus is abducted to 90° and is horizontally adducted into the plane of the scapula. The elbow is flexed 90°. One hand is passed under the ulna and is placed on the anterior aspect of the shoulder. This hand applies a downward pressure to stabilize the scapula. Applying downward pressure at the distal end of the ulna with the other hand medially rotates the humerus (Fig. 3-16).

Forward Flexion with Internal Rotation: Supine

The athlete is positioned supine on the table close enough to the edge to expose the lateral border of the scapula. The humerus is forward flexed approximately 60°, and the elbow is flexed 90°. The scapula is stabilized with the hip. One hand is passed under the humerus and is placed on the anterior aspect of the shoulder. This hand applies a downward pressure to stabilize the scapula. Applying downward pressure at the distal end of the ulna with the other hand medially rotates the humerus.

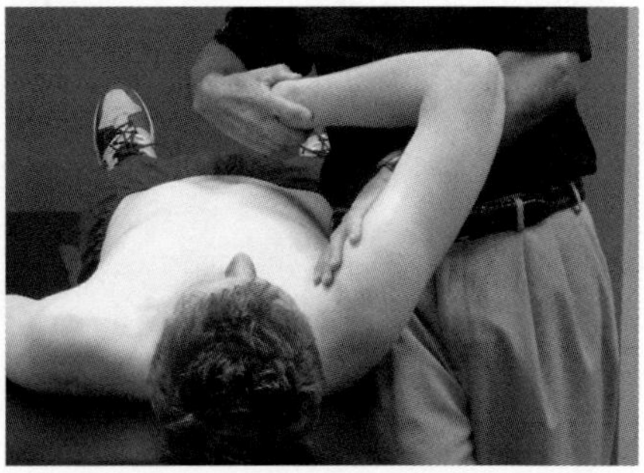

Figure 3-16

Diagonal with Internal Rotation: Supine

The athlete is positioned supine on the table close enough to the edge to expose the lateral border of the scapula. The scapula is stabilized with the hip. The humerus is forward flexed 45° and is maximally internally rotated. The elbow is flexed 90°. One hand is placed on the posterior aspect of the humerus, and the other hand grasps the distal end of the ulna. Pressure is applied to the posterior humerus to move it in the direction of the opposite hip. The elbow is extended to enhance the stretch.

Abduction 90°/Supported Frontal Plane Internal Rotation: Supine

The athlete is positioned supine on the table so the majority of the humerus is supported in 90° of abduction in the frontal plane. The scapula is stabilized by a downward pressure on the coracoid with one hand as the other hand, grasping the distal end of the ulna, internally rotates the humerus (Fig. 3-17).

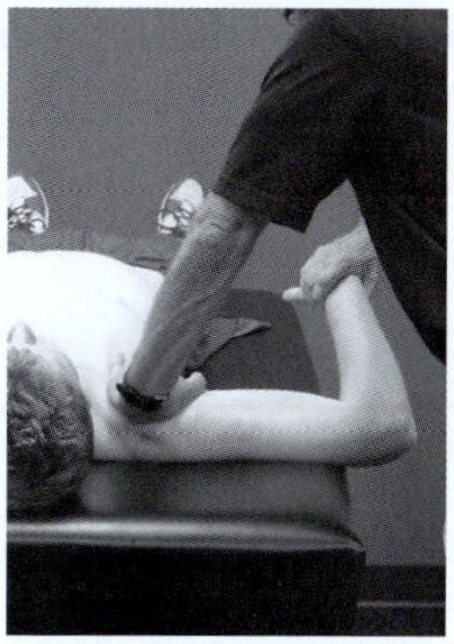

Figure 3-17

Abduction 90°/Supported Scapular Plane Internal Rotation: Supine

The athlete is positioned supine on the table so the majority of the humerus is supported at 90° of abduction on a 30° wedge. The scapula is stabilized by a downward pressure on the coracoid with one hand as the other hand, grasping the distal end of the ulna, internally rotates the humerus (Fig. 3-18).

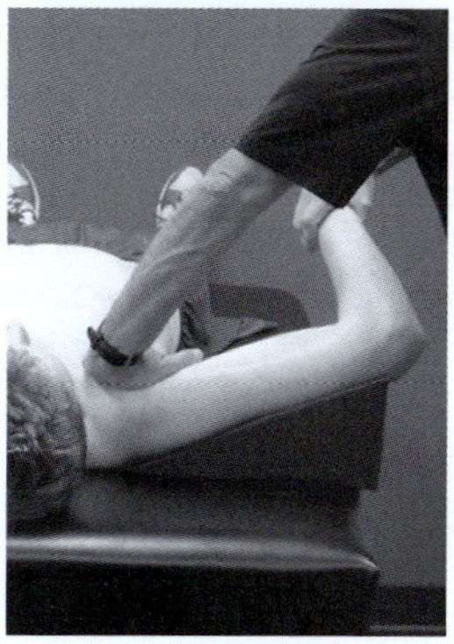

Figure 3-18

Forward Flexion 70° with Internal Rotation: Side Lying

The athlete is positioned in a side-lying position with the humerus forward flexed 70°. The elbow is flexed 90°. One hand is placed on the proximal humerus to assist the body weight in stabilizing the scapula. The other hand is placed on the posterior aspect of the distal ulna. A downward motion at the distal ulna medially rotates the humerus (Fig. 3-19). (Should be included in a self-stretch protocol.)

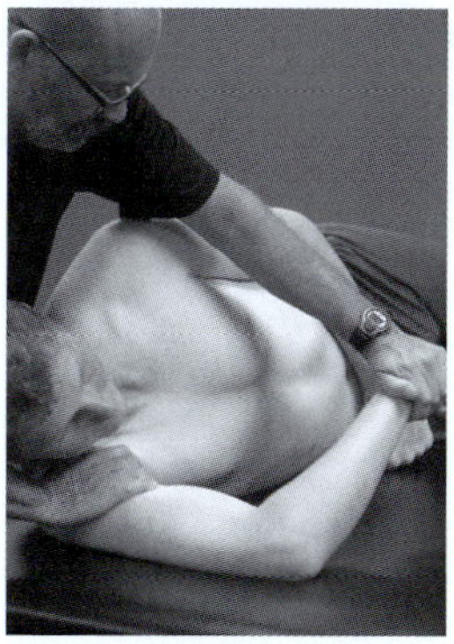

Figure 3-19

Forward Flexion 90° with Internal Rotation: Side Lying

The athlete is positioned in a side-lying position with the humerus forward flexed 90°. The elbow is also flexed 90°. One hand is placed on the proximal humerus to assist the body weight in stabilizing the scapula. The other hand is placed on the posterior aspect of the distal ulna. A downward motion at the distal ulna medially rotates the humerus (Fig. 3-20). (Should be included in a self-stretch protocol.)

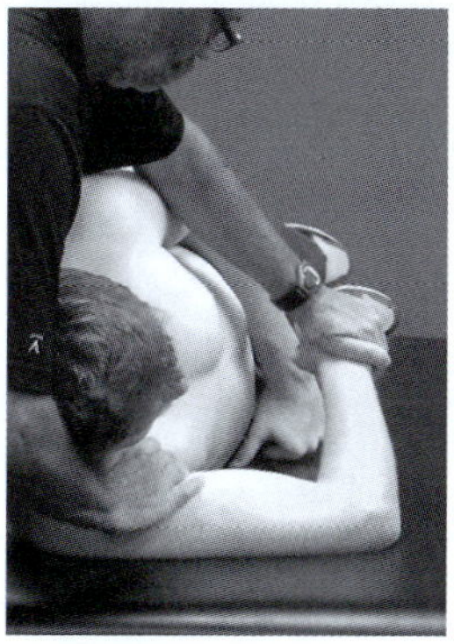

Figure 3-20

Forward Flexion 110° with Internal Rotation: Side Lying

The athlete is positioned in a side-lying position with the humerus forward flexed 100°. The elbow is flexed 90°. One hand is placed on the proximal humerus to assist the body weight in stabilizing the scapula. The other hand is placed on the posterior aspect of the distal ulna. A downward motion at the distal ulna medially rotates the humerus (Fig. 3-21). (Should be included in a self-stretch protocol.)

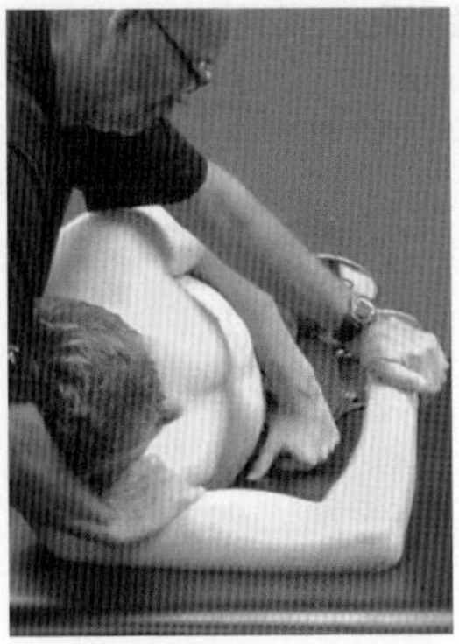

Figure 3-21

Forward Flexion 90° with Internal Rotation: Side Lying and Roll Over

The athlete is positioned in a side-lying position with the humerus forward flexed 90°. The elbow is also flexed 90°. One hand is placed on the uninvolved shoulder. The other hand is placed on the posterior aspect of the distal ulna. A downward motion at the distal ulna medially rotates the humerus. At the completion of medial rotation, the torso is rotated toward the humerus to enhance the stretch (Fig. 3-22). (Should be included in a self-stretch protocol.)

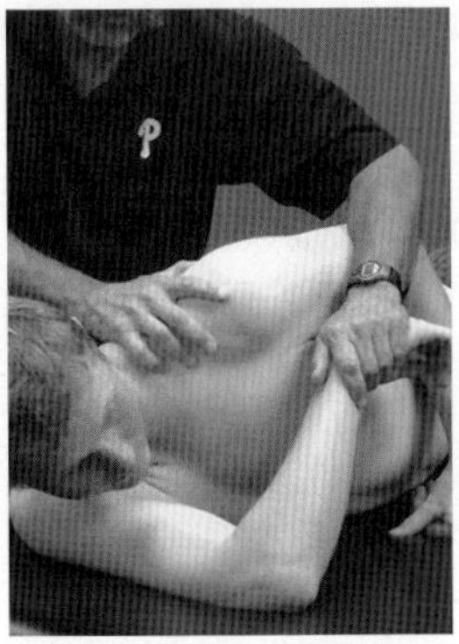

Figure 3-22

Abduction 90°/Frontal Plane Internal Rotation: Prone

The athlete is positioned prone on the table so the entire length of the humerus is supported when abducted to 90°. The elbow is flexed 90°, and the back of the hand is supported on the table. In a crossed-hand fashion, one hand stabilizes the scapula against the chest wall, and the other hand is positioned at the distal end of the humerus. A downward motion while separating the hands accomplishes the stretch (Fig. 3-23). Note: In the case of a severe posterior-inferior capsule contracture, this stretch may have to accomplished in less humeral abduction.[128]

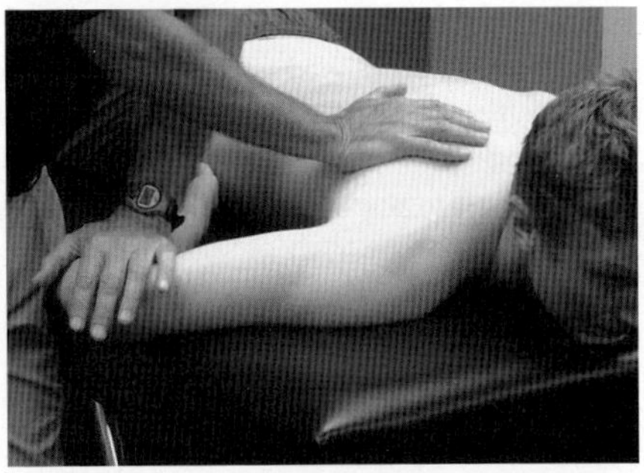

Figure 3-23

Scapular Elevation and Internal Rotation: Prone

The athlete is positioned prone on the table so the entire length of the humerus is supported when abducted to 90°. The elbow is flexed 90° and is unsupported. One hand is placed at the inferior angle of the scapula, and the other hand grasps the distal end of the ulna (Fig. 3-24A). The scapula is elevated with a superior motion, and lifting the distal ulna medially rotates the humerus (Fig. 3-24B).

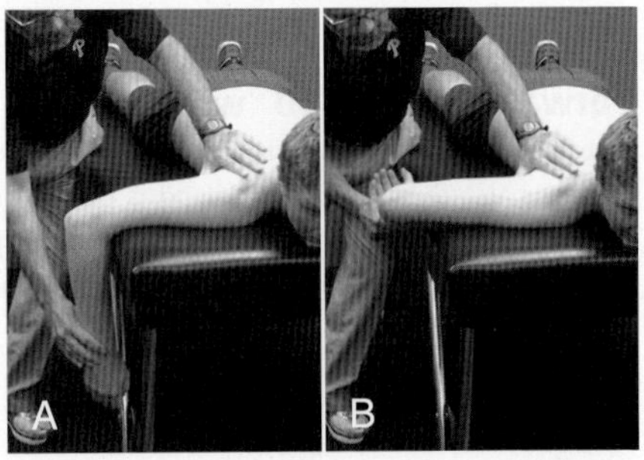

Figure 3-24

EXERCISE PROTOCOL

Table-Top Exercises

Weight Shift with Scapular Movement

Support your body weight on the edge of a table in a forward leaning position with the shoulders forward flexed and the hands wider than the shoulder width (Fig. 3-25A). Shift your body weight over your right shoulder by moving your body towards right side (Fig. 3-25B). The right scapula retracts as the left scapula protracts. Shift body weight over your left shoulder by moving your body toward the left side (Fig. 3-25C). The left scapula retracts, and the right scapula protracts.

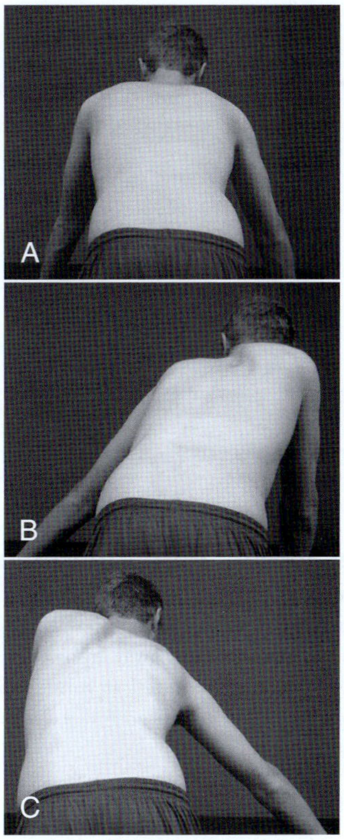

Figure 3-25

Seated: Scapular Protraction/Retraction

Sit with your shoulder abducted with a towel placed between your hand and the table. Place your opposite hand behind your head to maintain your posture. Fully protract your scapula by advancing your hand forward (Fig. 3-26A). Fully retract the scapula by drawing your hand backward (Fig. 3-26B). Be careful not to elevate the shoulder during this exercise.

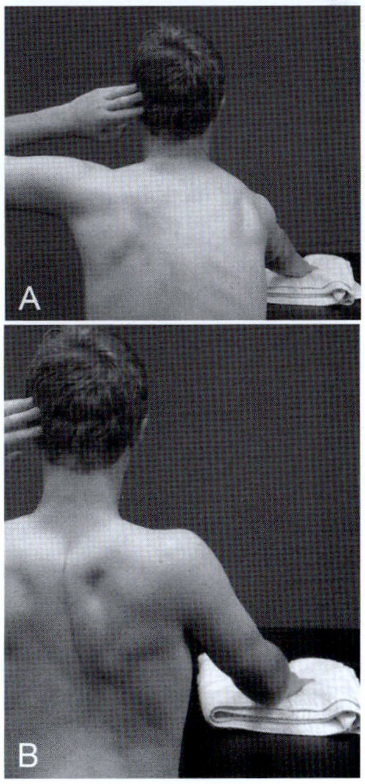

Figure 3-26

Seated: Scapular Depression/Elevation

Sit with the shoulder abducted with a towel placed between your hand and the table. Place your opposite hand behind your head to maintain your posture. Fully depress your scapula by advancing your arm forward. Fully elevate your scapula by drawing your hand backward (Fig. 3-27).

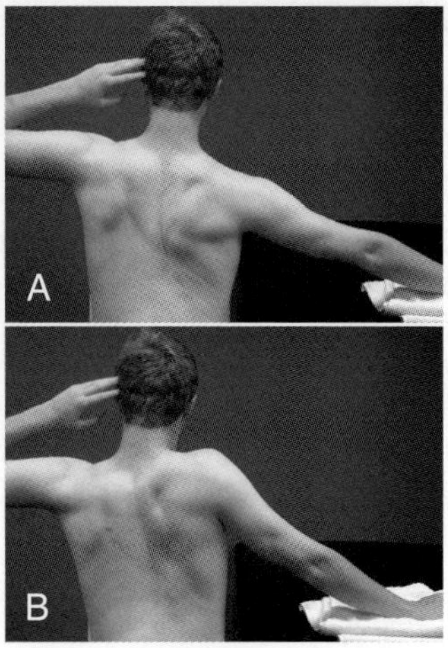

Figure 3-27

Wall Exercises

Shoulder Flexion: Protraction/Retraction

Stand with your shoulder in 90° of forward flexion with your hand placed against the wall. Allow your body to lean toward the wall. Place your opposite hand behind your head to maintain your posture. Push away from wall at your shoulder by fully protracting the scapula (Fig. 3-28A). Lean into the wall at your shoulder by retracting your scapula (Fig. 3-28B). Be certain to pinch your scapulae on full retraction. Be careful not to elevate your shoulder during this exercise.[64]

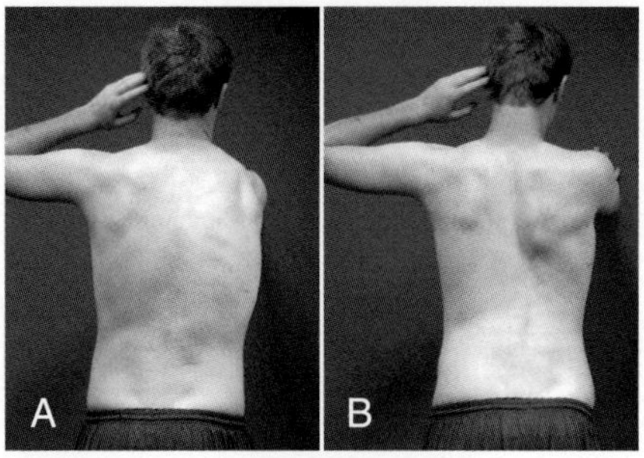

Figure 3-28

Shoulder Abduction: Protraction/Retraction

Stand with your shoulder in 90° of abduction with your hand placed against the wall. Allow your body to lean toward the wall. Place your opposite hand behind your head to maintain your posture. Push away from wall at your shoulder by fully protracting the scapula (Fig. 3-29A). Lean into the wall at your shoulder by retracting your scapula (Fig. 3-29B). Be certain to pinch your scapulae on full retraction. Be careful not to elevate your shoulder during this exercise.

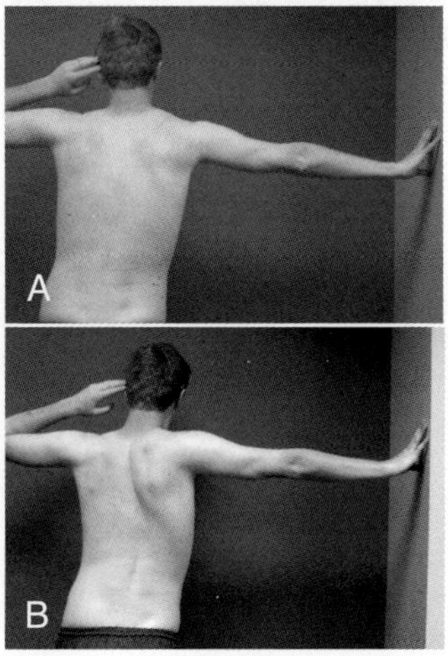

Figure 3-29

Shoulder Flexion: Elevation/Depression

Stand with your shoulder in 90° of flexion with your hand placed against the wall. Allow your body to lean toward the wall. Place your opposite hand behind your head to maintain your posture. Completely elevate your scapula (Fig. 3-30A). Completely depress your scapula. While in full depression, squeeze your scapulae together (Fig. 3-30B).

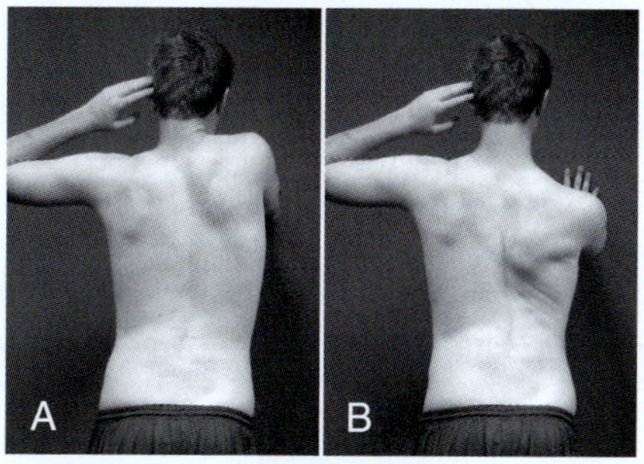

Figure 3-30

Shoulder Abduction: Elevation/Depression

Stand with your shoulder in 90° of abduction with your hand placed against the wall. Allow your body to lean toward the wall. Place your opposite hand behind your head to maintain your posture. Completely elevate your scapula (Fig. 3-31A). Completely depress your scapula. While in full depression, squeeze your scapulae together (Fig. 3-31B).

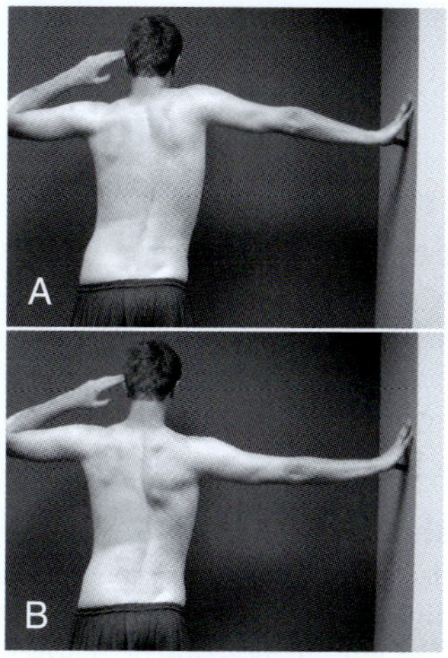

Figure 3-31

Shoulder Rotation: Flexion

Stand with your shoulder in 90° of flexion with your thumb placed against the wall. Allow your body to lean slightly toward the wall. Place your opposite hand behind your head to maintain your posture. Completely internally rotate your arm by using your thumb as a fulcrum. Obtain full upward rotation of your scapula (Fig. 3-32A). Completely externally rotate your arm by using your thumb as a fulcrum (Fig. 3-32B). Obtain full downward rotation of your scapula. When your scapula is in the full downward rotational position, squeeze your scapulae together.

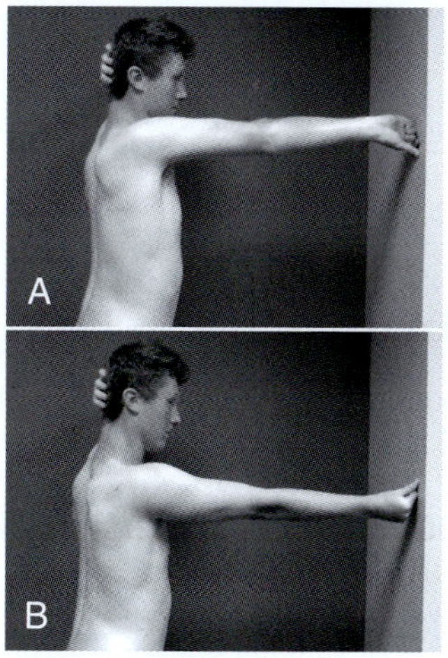

Figure 3-32

Shoulder Rotation: Abduction

Stand with your shoulder in 90° of abduction with your thumb placed against the wall. Allow your body to lean slightly toward the wall. Place your opposite hand behind your head to maintain your posture. Completely internally rotate your arm by using your thumb as a fulcrum (Fig. 3-33A). Obtain full upward rotation of your scapula. Completely externally rotate your arm by using your thumb as a fulcrum (Fig. 3-33B). Obtain full downward rotation of your scapula. When your scapula is in the full downward rotational position, squeeze your scapulae together.

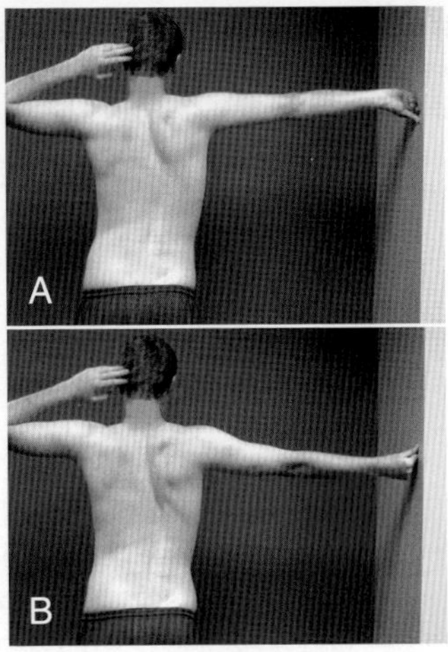

Figure 3-33

Wall Slide

Stand facing the wall with one foot against the wall and the other staggered behind, a shoulder's width apart. The forearms are supinated and placed on the wall so the shoulders are forward flexed 90° and the elbows are flexed 90°. Elevate your forearms in a scapular plane by transforming your body weight forward until terminal extension is achieved.[129]

Wall Push

Sit facing the wall and place your fingertips on the wall at shoulder height and shoulder width. Press your fingertips into the wall (Fig. 3-34A). Slowly continue to push your fingers and then hands into the wall for an isometric contraction (Fig. 3-34B).

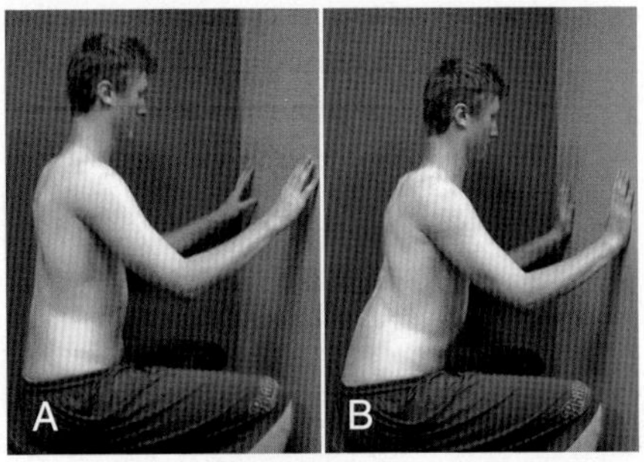

Figure 3-34

Prone Exercises: The Six Backs

These exercises can be accomplished on a stability ball for an additional core challenge.[130]

Prone: 90° Shoulder Abduction with Thumbs Forward (Neutral Rotation)

Lie prone with your shoulders abducted to 90° with your thumbs forward. Fully horizontally abduct your arms with full scapular retraction. Squeeze your scapulae together, and hold this position for 6 seconds (Fig. 3-35).

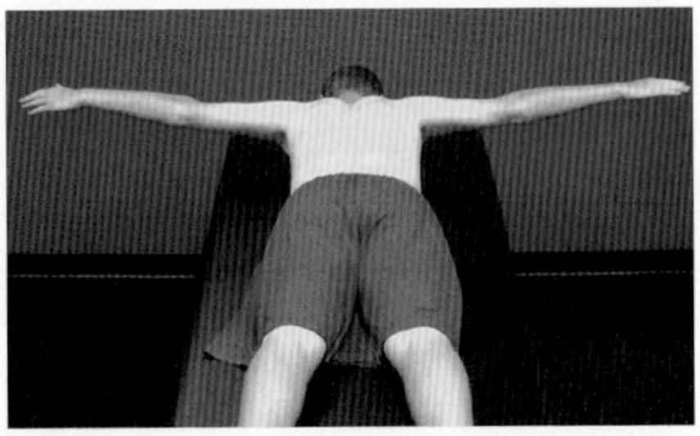

Figure 3-35

Prone: 90° Shoulder Abduction with Thumbs Up (External Rotation)

Lie prone with your shoulders abducted to 90° with your thumbs up. Fully horizontally abduct your arms with full scapular retraction. Squeeze your scapulae together, and hold this position for 6 seconds (Fig. 3-36).

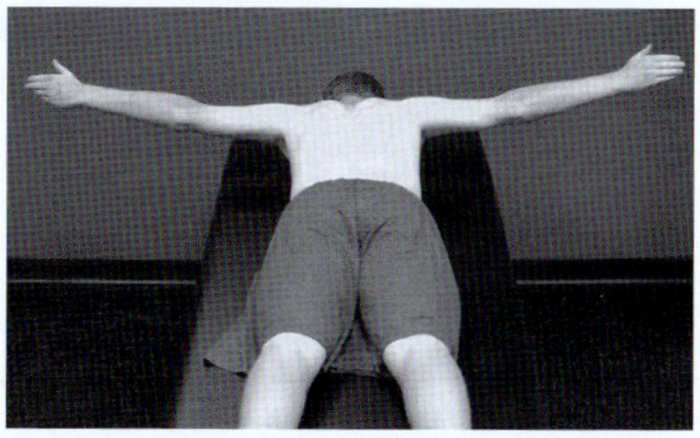

Figure 3-36

Prone: 100° Shoulder Abduction with Thumbs Forward (Neutral Rotation)

Lie prone with your shoulders abducted to 100° with your thumbs forward. Fully horizontally abduct your arms with full scapular retraction. Squeeze your scapulae together, and hold this position for 6 seconds (Fig. 3-37).

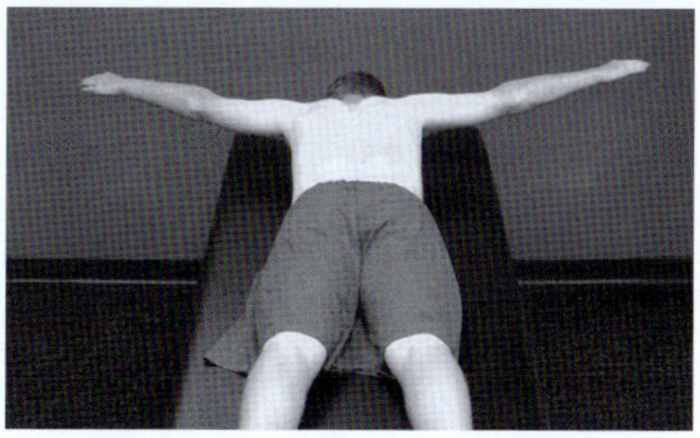

Figure 3-37

Prone: 100° Shoulder Abduction with Thumbs Up (External Rotation)

Lie prone with your shoulder abducted to 100° with your thumbs up. Fully abduct your arms horizontally with full scapular retraction. Squeeze your scapulae together, and hold this position for 6 seconds (Fig. 3-38).

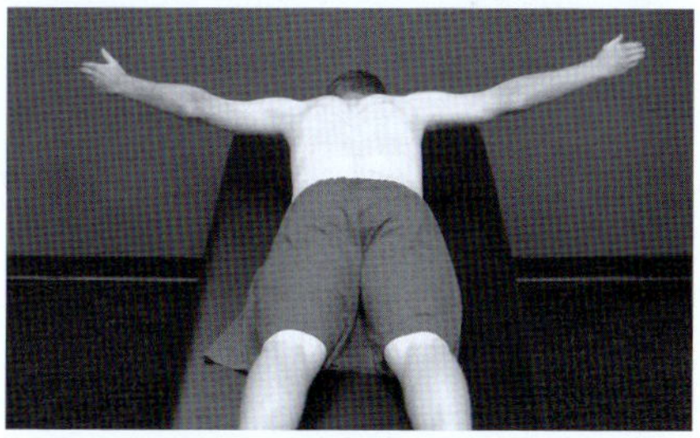

Figure 3-38

Prone: 90° Shoulder Abduction with 90° Elbow Flexion (90/90 position)

Lie prone with your shoulders abducted and your elbows flexed to 90°, thumbs up. Fully abduct your arms horizontally with full scapular retraction. Squeeze your scapulae together, and hold this position for 6 seconds (Fig. 3-39).

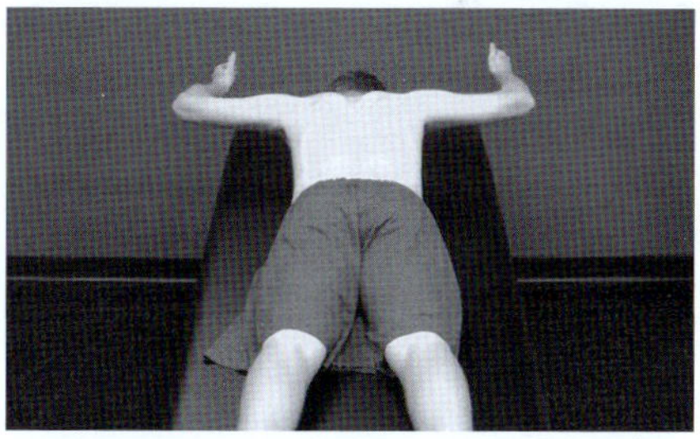

Figure 3-39

Prone: Shoulder Extension

Lie prone with your arms at sides and your palms facing down. Lift your hands away from the table to produce full shoulder extension. Squeeze your scapulae together, and hold this position for 6 seconds (Fig. 3-40).

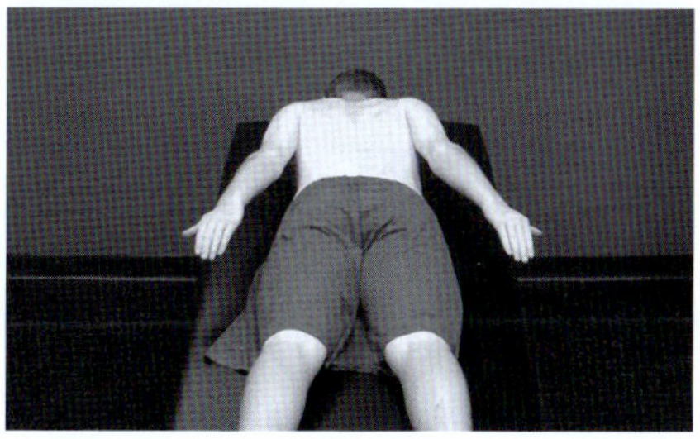

Figure 3-40

Quadriped 120° Extension with External Rotation

Begin in a quadruped position and then flex your hips and knees to assume a position over the contralateral lower leg. Position your arm in 120° of abduction and external rotation (Fig. 3-41A). The arm is lifted into extension by moving the scapula into retraction and depression (Fig. 3-41B).

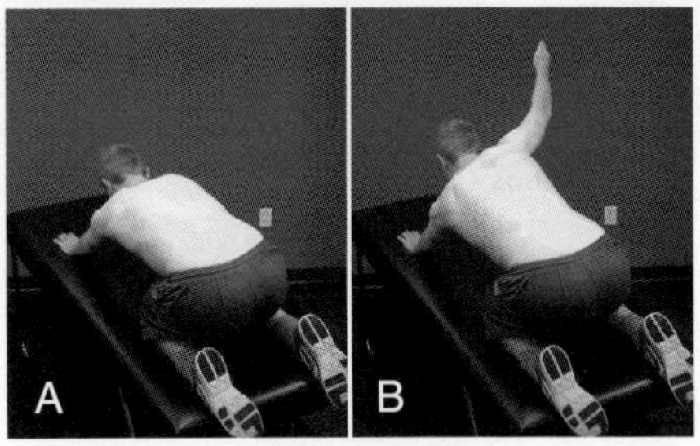

Figure 3-41

Base Exercises

Pillow Squeezes

Place small pillows under arms. Your elbows should be flexed to 90° (Fig. 3-42A). Squeeze pillows to your sides by retracting your scapulae and externally rotating your shoulders (Fig. 3-42B).

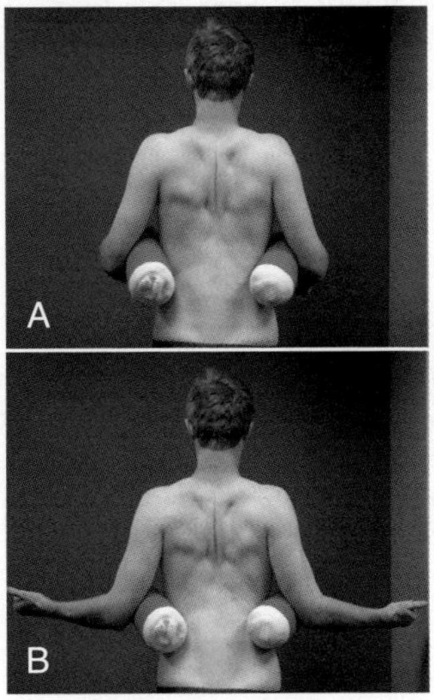

Figure 3-42

Low Row

Stand at the end of the table, and place a pronated hand on its edge. Extend your trunk. Press your hand maximally in an isometric contraction to create shoulder extension (Fig. 3-43). Retract and depress your scapula.[131]

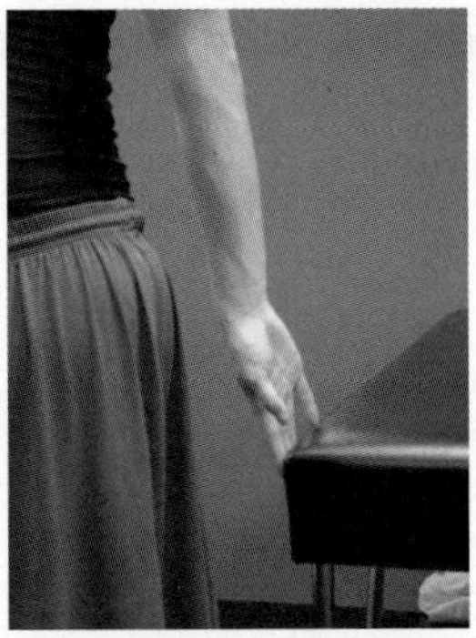

Figure 3-43

Shoulder Shrugs

Stand with your arms at your sides. Fully retract your scapulae (Fig. 3-44A). Perform a shoulder shrug by elevating your scapulae toward the back of your neck. Maintain good posture by avoiding forward tilting of the head (Fig. 3-44B). Make certain to keep your scapulae fully retracted throughout movement.

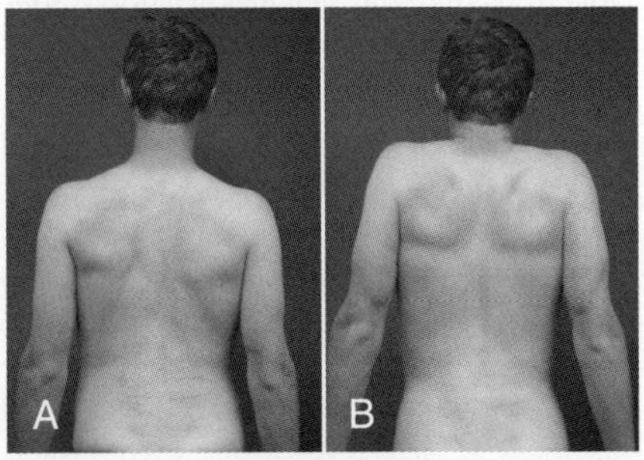

Figure 3-44

Scapula Circles

Stand with your arms at your sides. This is a four-count exercise. Elevate your scapulae (Fig. 3-45A). Fully retract your scapulae (Fig. 3-45B). Fully depress your scapulae (Fig. 3-45C). Protract your scapulae to the starting position (Fig. 3-45D). Do not protract your scapulae beyond the neutral starting position.

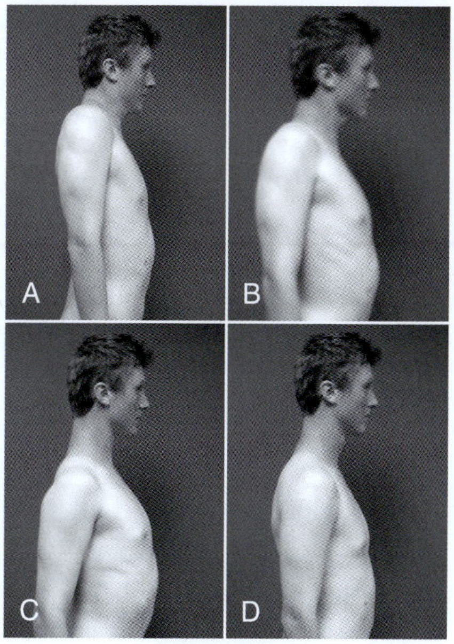

Figure 3-45

Scaption: External Rotation (Core 1)

Stand with your arms at your sides. Externally rotate your humerus, and move your hands forward into the plane of the scapula (Fig. 3-46A and B). Elevate your arms in scapular plane until the arc is completed (Fig. 3-46C). Return to starting position in same manner. Perform scapular retraction at the end of each repetition.[132]

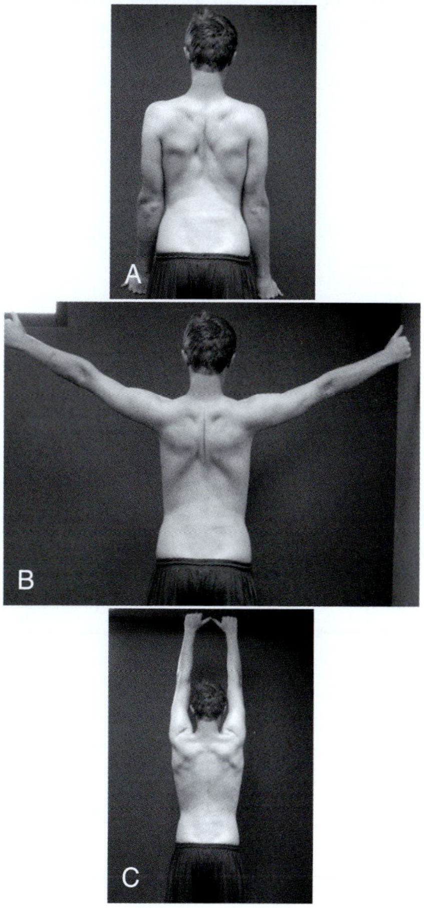

Figure 3-46

Horizontal Abduction and External Rotation (Core 2)

Standing, bend forward at the waist until your torso is parallel to the floor. Bend your knees for balance. You may place your forehead on an appropriate height table for support. Externally rotate your humerus, and contract your abdominal muscles. Horizontally abduct your arms until they are parallel to the floor (Fig. 3-47A). Squeeze your scapulae into complete retraction at end of movement (Fig. 3-47B). Return your arms to the starting position.

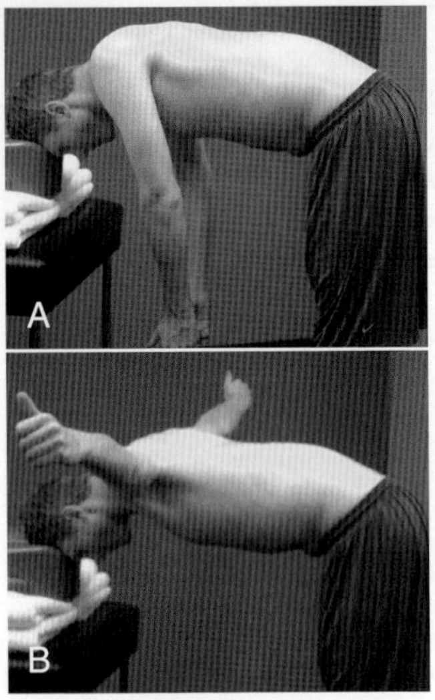

Figure 3-47

Prone Scapular Rowing

Lie prone on a table with your shoulder forward flexed to 90° and your elbow fully extended. Your shoulder should be far enough off the table to allow complete freedom of scapular motion. Fully retract your scapula while maintaining full elbow extension (Fig. 3-48A). Return to the starting position by protracting your scapula (Fig. 3-48B).

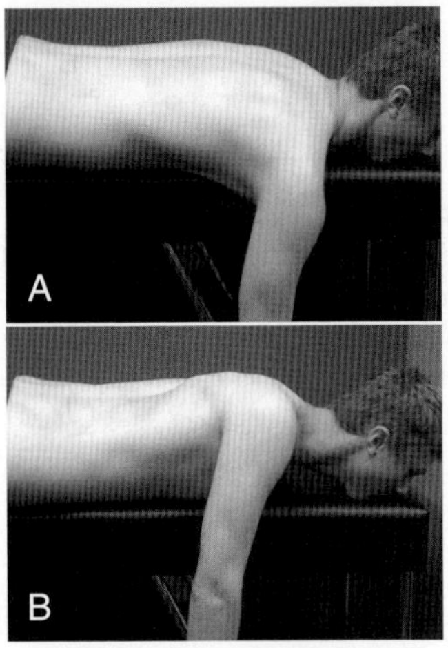

Figure 3-48

Prone Rowing (Core 3)

Lie prone on a table with your shoulder forward flexed to 90° and your elbow fully extended. Your shoulder should be far enough off the table to allow complete freedom of scapular motion. Fully retract scapula while maintaining full elbow extension (Fig. 3-49A). Once your scapula is in full retraction, extend the shoulder and flex the elbow in a rowing motion (Fig. 3-49B). Return to the starting position by extending the elbow and forward flexing the shoulder. Protract the scapula at the completion of arm movement (Fig. 3-49C).

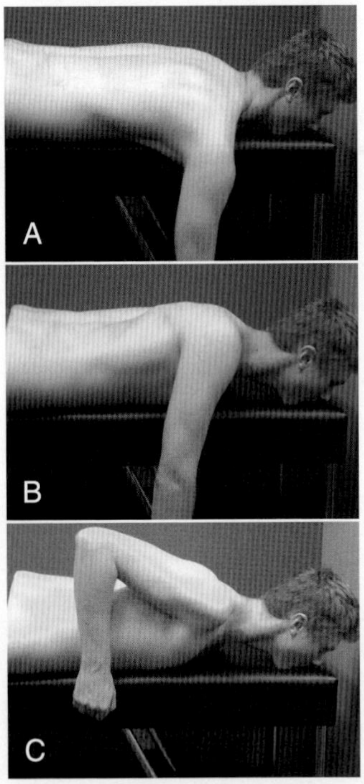

Figure 3-49

Bench Press Plus

Lie supine on a table with your shoulder fully extended and your elbow fully flexed. Your shoulder should be far enough off the table to allow complete freedom of scapular motion. Extend your elbow while forward flexing your shoulder until full elbow extension and 90° of shoulder forward flexion is achieved (Fig. 3-50A). Fully protract the scapula (Fig. 3-50B). Fully retract the scapula (Fig. 3-50C). Lower your arm by elbow flexion and shoulder extension to the starting position.

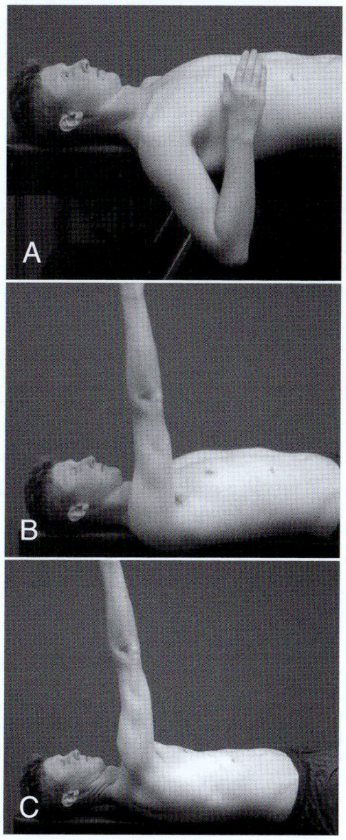

Figure 3-50

Push-up Plus (Core 5)

Begin in a forward leaning position supported by a table. Lower your chest between your hands by extending your shoulders and flexing your elbows (Fig. 3-51A). Perform a push-up by extending your elbows and forward flexing your shoulders (Fig. 3-51B). At the end of this motion, fully protract the scapulae by pushing the torso further away from the table. Progress this exercise to the tabletop or floor (Fig. 3-51C).

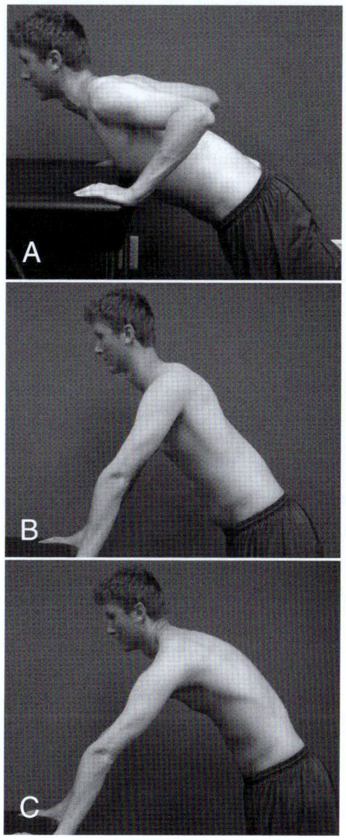

Figure 3-51

Press-Ups: Seated Dips (Core 5)

Position your hands on supports to allow your shoulders to support some of your body weight (Fig. 3-52A). Extend your elbows and depress your arms to lift your body weight. Push yourself higher by depressing your scapulae into a plus position (Fig. 3-52B).

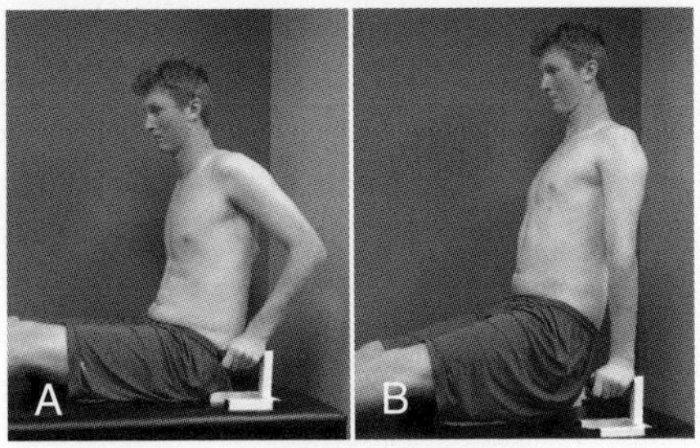

Figure 3-52

Side-Lying External Rotation

Lie on the table on your uninvolved side with a bolster between the distal end of your humerus and your side. The elbow is flexed to 90°, and the forearm is supinated (Fig. 3-53A). Retract your scapula. Laterally rotate your humerus (Fig. 3-53B).

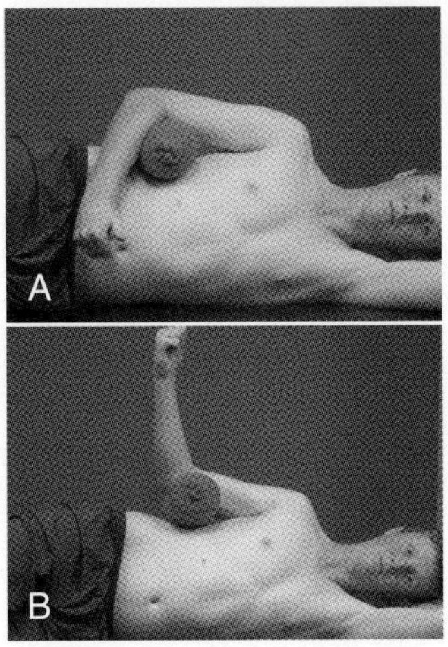

Figure 3-53

Scapula Depression: Unilateral

Stand with your arms at your sides. Fully retract your scapulae, and place your nonexercise hand behind your head to maintain your posture (Fig. 3-54A). Using a pulley, tubing, or manual resistance, depress the scapula (Fig. 3-54B). Return to the starting position. Be certain to keep the scapulae fully retracted throughout the movement.

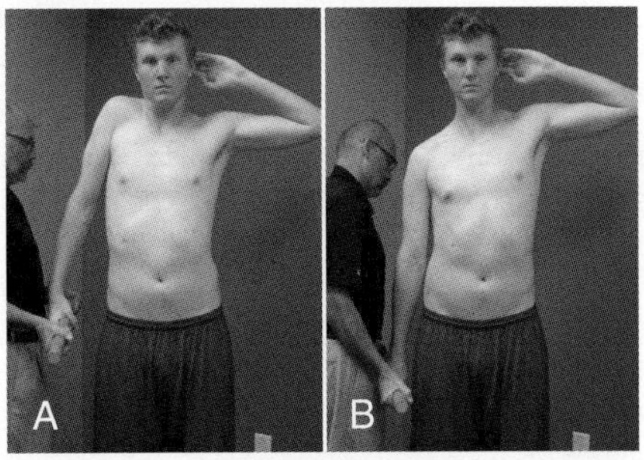

Figure 3-54

Scapular Elevation: Unilateral

Stand with your arms at your sides. Fully retract your scapulae, and place your nonexercise hand behind your head to maintain your posture (Fig. 3-55A). Using a pulley, tubing, or manual resistance, elevate the scapula (Fig. 3-55B). Return to the starting position. Be certain to keep the scapula fully retracted throughout the movement.

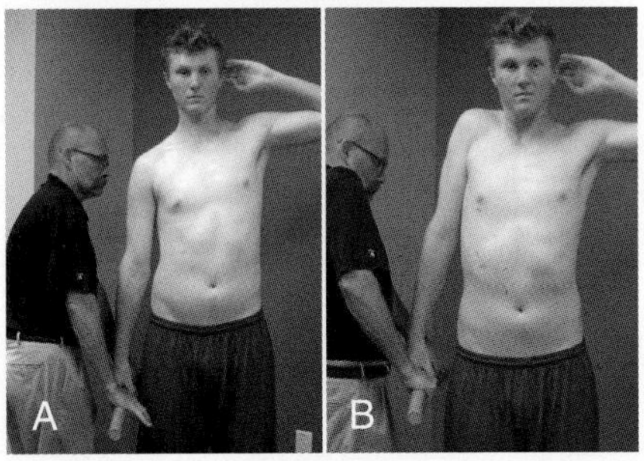

Figure 3-55

Scapula Depression: Bilateral

Place yourself in a position so resistance can be provided from an area forward and above your shoulders. Your shoulders are forward flexed approximately 120°, and your elbows are fully extended (Fig. 3-56A). Retract and depress the scapulae in one motion (Fig. 3-56B). Return to the starting position using scapulae control.

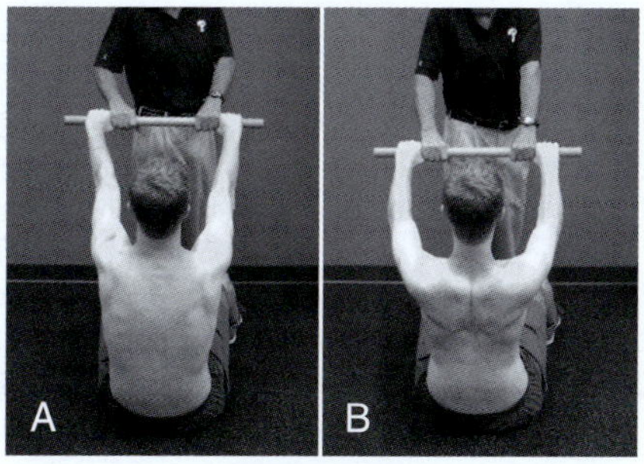

Figure 3-56

Mass Movement Patterns

Lateral Lunge

Stand with both hands placed on your chest with your knees slightly bent, feet apart. Begin the movement by stepping laterally with your right foot while moving the right hand, in a sweeping motion, down from chest into a finished laterally elevated position (Fig. 3-57A). This motion should occur in the plane of the scapula. The exercise concentration should be on the movement of the scapula. Return to your starting position by reversing the sequence of movements, sweeping your right hand down, and drawing it to your chest while steeping back to your original position (Fig. 3-57B). Perform scapular retraction at the midpoint of this exercise. Complete the exercise by performing the movement to your left (Fig. 3-57C).

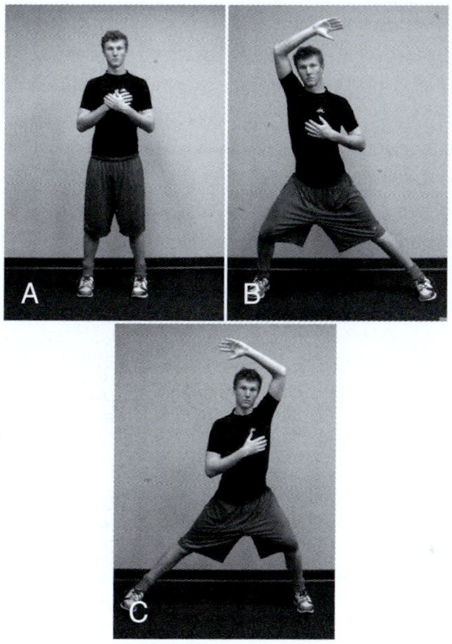

Figure 3-57

Forward Lunge

Stand with right shoulder in 90° to 100° of abducted and full horizontal extension. Retract the scapula. The elbow should be flexed to 90°. Place your left hand on your chest, and step backward with your left foot (Fig. 3-58A). Step forward with your left foot while moving your right arm in a fully extended position with full scapular protraction. Internally rotate the humerus toward the end of the movement (Fig. 3-58B). Reverse the movement by stepping backward with your left foot to its beginning position. Draw the right arm back into horizontal extension and full scapula retraction. The elbow returns to its flexed position. Perform scapular retraction at the midpoint and end of each repetition. At the completion of the assigned number of repetitions, the exercise is then performed using the left shoulder and right foot.

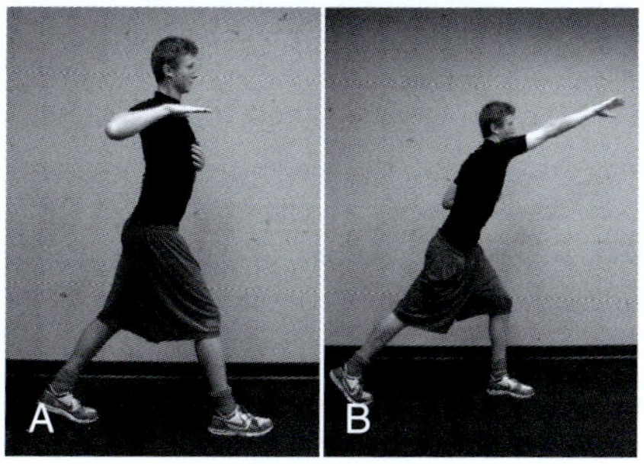

Figure 3-58

Diagonal Pull

Stand with right shoulder abducted to 90° to 100°. Your elbow should be in full flexion. Place your left hand on your chest. Your feet should be placed a shoulder width apart (Fig. 3-59A). Squat to approximately 45° while moving your hand down and across your body toward the outside of left knee in a diagonal movement pattern. Internally rotate your humerus toward the end of the movement (Fig. 3-59B). Return to the starting position by extending your knees and drawing your hand back across your chest. Perform scapular retraction at the end of each repetition. At the completion of the assigned number of repetitions, the exercise is then performed using the left shoulder.

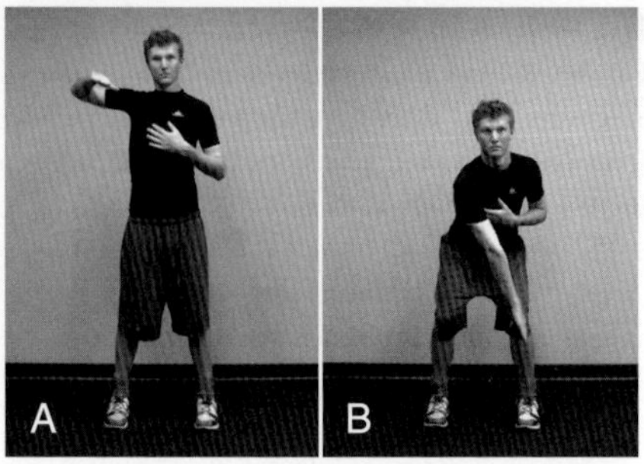

Figure 3-59

Same Side Pull

Stand with right arm at side. Place your left hand on your chest. Your feet should be placed shoulder width apart. Squat to approximately 45° while fully depressing the scapula (Fig. 3-60A). Extend your knee to a full standing position while elevating your scapula. Simultaneously move the humerus into an abducted position of 90° to 100° with elbow flexion. Fully retract the scapula (Fig. 3-60B). Change the motion of the upper extremity by moving your hand across your midline and bringing the shoulder into horizontal adduction and full elbow extension. Internally rotate the humerus toward the end of this movement (Fig. 3-60C). Return to the starting position by retracting your movements. Be certain to include full scapular retraction before lowering the hand to the starting position. At the completion of the assigned number of repetitions, the exercise is then performed using the left shoulder.

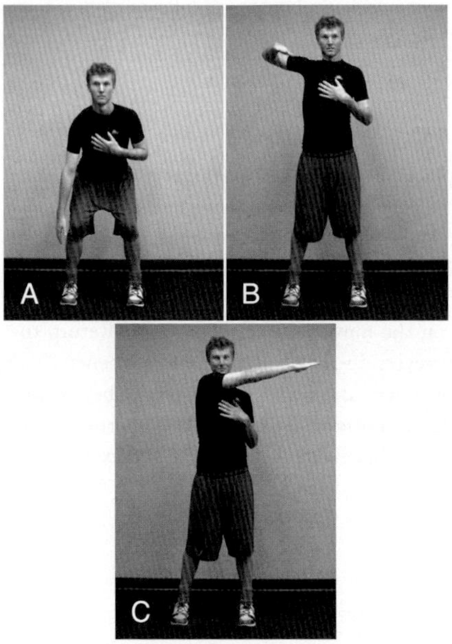

Figure 3-60

Bilateral Lunge

Stand with both shoulders in extension with elbows flexed. Retract your scapulae. Step backward with your nondominant foot to establish the beginning position. Step forward with the nondominant foot while moving your shoulders into a forward flexed position of approximately 150°. Your elbows should be fully extended (Fig. 3-61A). The final forward movements should be full scapular protraction and humeral internal rotation (Fig. 3-61B). Complete the exercise by stepping back with the nondominant foot and moving the shoulders back into the position of extension with elbow flexion. Retract the scapulae at the end of the repetition. Nondominant hip stability can be enhanced by the use of a step-up.

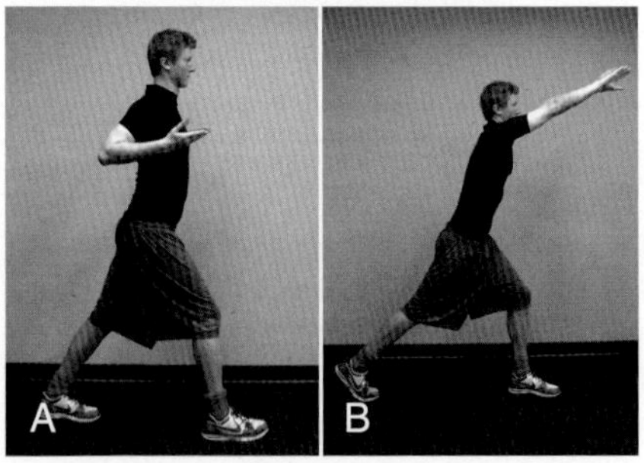

Figure 3-61

Global Supine Incline: Abduction and Adduction

Position yourself on a stability ball supine with your hips lower than your shoulders. Your hands should be resting on your anterior thighs. Sweep your hands away from your midline in the plane of the scapula until the arc is completed (Fig. 3-62). Move your hands back to the starting position by adducting along your midline. Perform a scapular retraction at the end of each repetition.

Additional exercises can be preformed on the exercise ball in the supine incline position adduction can be performed by reversing the abduction pattern.

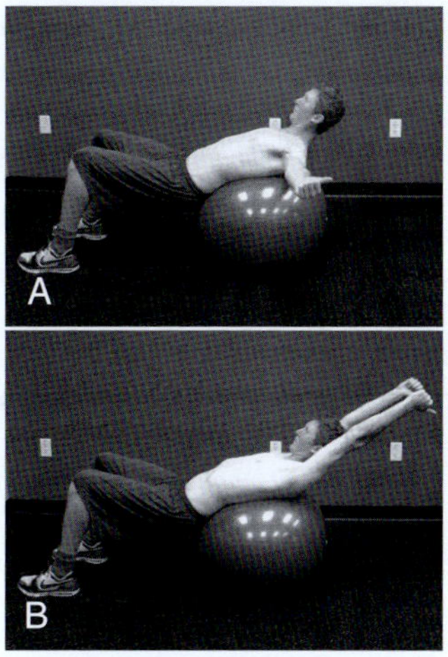

Figure 3-62

Global Supine Decline and Level: Abduction and Adduction

The position on the exercise ball can be changed to a level position and with the ball and a decline position with the ball. In the supine level position the hips and shoulders are at the same height. In the decline position the shoulders are lower than your hips. Abduction and adduction movements can be performed in the same manner as described above.

Global Prone Incline: Abduction & Adduction

Position yourself on a stability ball prone with your shoulders elevated higher than your hips. Your hands should be resting at your lateral thighs. Retract your scapulae (Fig. 3-63A). Sweep your hands away from your midline in the plane of the scapula (Fig. 3-63B) until the arc is completed (Fig. 3-63C). Move your hands back to the starting position by adducting along your midline (Fig. 3-63D). (Elbow flexion will be necessary to clear your hands.)

Reverse of the abduction pattern for adduction.

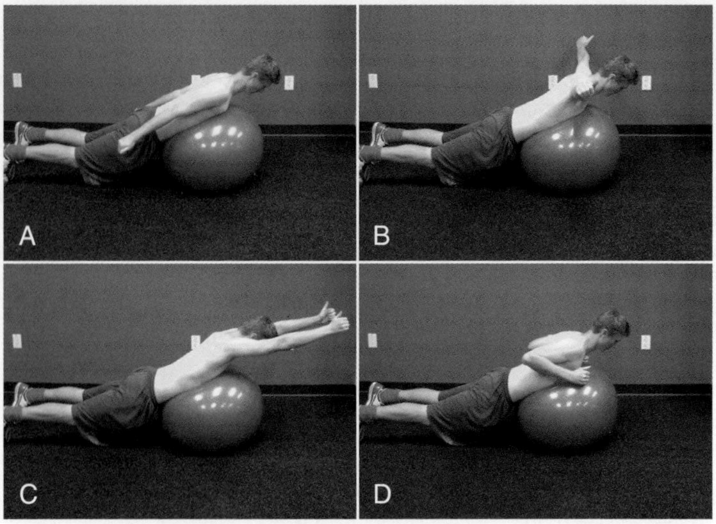

Figure 3-63

Global Prone Decline and Level: Abduction and Adduction

In the supine level position the hips and shoulders are at the same height. In the decline position the shoulders are lower than your hips. Abduction and adduction movements can be performed in the same manner as described above.

Stability Ball: Horizontal Abduction with 90/90

Position yourself on a stability ball prone with your shoulders horizontally extended, elbows flexed to 90° and thumbs up (Fig. 3-64A). Horizontally abduct your shoulders and retract your scapulae (Fig. 3-64B). Externally rotate your humerus.

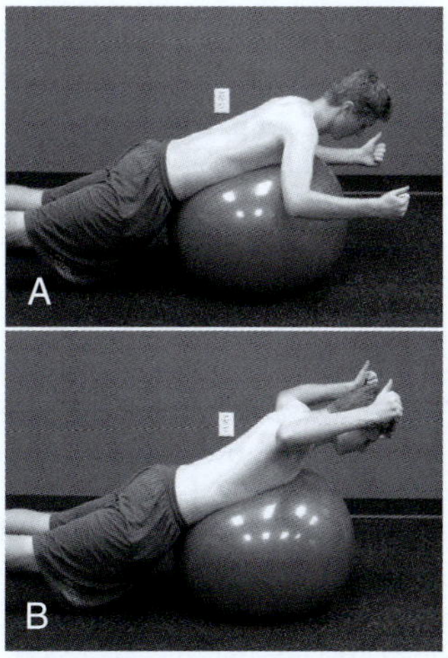

Figure 3-64

Stability Ball: Dynamic Hug

Position yourself on a stability ball supine with your shoulders horizontally extended and your elbow flexed to 90° (Fig. 3-65A). Move your hands toward your midline in the same plane without changing the angle of your elbows (Fig. 3-65B).[133]

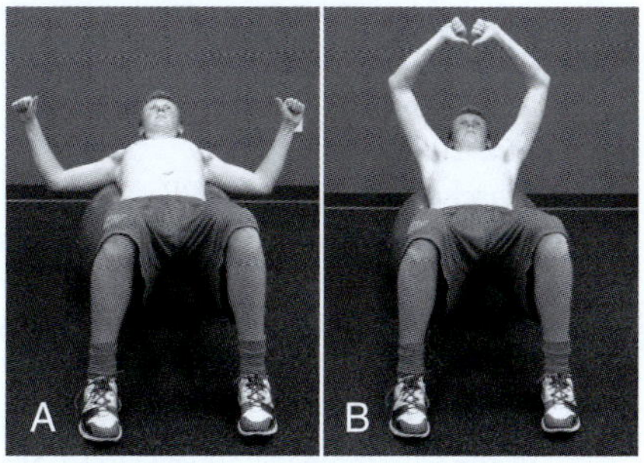

Figure 3-65

REFERENCES

1. Gainor BJ, Piotrowski G, Puhl J, et al: The throw: biomechanics and acute injury, *Am J Sports Med* 8:114, 1980.
2. Andrews JR, Carson WG Jr, McLeod WD: Glenoid labrum tears related to the long head of the biceps, *Am J Sports Med* 13:337, 1985.
3. Garth WP, Allman FL, Armstrong WS: Occult anterior subluxations of the shoulder in noncontact sports, *Am J Sports Med* 15:579, 1987.
4. Jobe FW, Kvitne RS: Shoulder pain in the overhand or throwing athlete, *Othop Rev* 18:963, 1989.
5. Simon ER, Hill JA: Rotator cuff injuries: an update, *J Orthop Sports Phys Ther* 10:394, 1989.
6. Ringel SP, Treihaft M, Carry M, et al: Suprascapular neuropathy in pitchers, *Am J Sports Med* 18:80, 1990.
7. Black KP, Lombardo JA: Suprascapular nerve injuries with isolated paralysis of the infraspinatus, *Am J Sports Med* 18:225, 1990.
8. Branch T, Partin C, Chamberland P, et al: Spontaneous fractures of the humerus during pitching: a series of 12 cases, *Am J Sports Med* 20:468, 1992.
9. Altchek DW, Warren RF, Wickiewicz TL, et al: Arthroscopic labral debridement: a three-year follow-up study, *Am J Sports Med* 20:702, 1992.
10. Schachter CL, Canham PB, Mottola MF: Biomechanical factors affecting Dave Dravecky's return to competitive pitching: a case study, *J Orthop Sports Phys Ther* 16:2, 1992.
11. Carson WG, Gasser SI: Little League shoulder: a report of 23 cases, *Am J Sports Med* 26:575, 1998.
12. DiFelice GS, Paletta GA, Phillips BB, et al: Effort thrombosis in the elite throwing athlete, *Am J Sports Med* 30:708, 2002.
13. Soeda T, Nakagawa Y, Suzuki T, et al: Recurrent throwing fracture of the humerus in a baseball player: case report and review of the literature, *Am J Sports Med* 30:900, 2002.
14. Yoshikawa GI, Hori K, Kaneko H, et al: Acute subscapularis tendon rupture caused by throwing: a case report, *J Shoulder Elbow Surg* 14:218, 2005.
15. Coris EE, Higgins HW: First rib fractures in throwing athletes, *Am J Sports Med* 33:1400, 2005.
16. Baumgarten KM, Dines JS, Winchester PA, et al: Axillary artery aneurysm with distal embolization in a major league pitcher, *Am J Sports Med* 35:650, 2007.
17. Noonan TJ, Sakryd G, Espinoza LM, et al: Posterior rib stress fracture in professional baseball pitchers, *Am J Sports Med* 35:654, 2007.
18. Hsu JC, Paletta GA, Gambardella RA, et al: Musculocutaneus nerve injury in Major League Baseball pitchers: a report of two cases, *Am J Sports Med* 35:1003, 2007.
19. Herickhoff PK, Keyurapan E, Fayad LM, et al: Scapular stress fracture in a professional baseball player: a case report and review of literature, *Am J Sports Med* 35:1193, 2007.
20. Radelet MA, Lephart SM, Rubinstein EN, et al: Survey of the injury rate for children in community sports, *Pediatrics* 3:110, 2002.
21. Centers for Disease Control and Prevention: Physical activity levels among children aged 9–13 years: United States, 2002, *Morb Mortal Wkly Rep* 52:785, 2003.
22. Pray WS, Pray JJ: Sports injuries in children. Medscape Today Nov 2004.
23. Centers for Disease Control and Prevention: Sports-related injuries among high school athlete: United States, 2005–06 school year, *Morb Mortal Wkly Rep* 55:1037, 2006.
24. McFarland EG, Wasik M: Epidemiology of college baseball injuries, *Clin J Sports Med* 8:10, 1998.
25. Dick R, Sauners E, Agle J, et al: Descriptive epidemiology of collegiate men's baseball injuries: National Collegiate Athletic Association injury surveillance system, 1988–1989 through 2003–2004, *J Athl Train* 42:183, 2007.
26. Lyman S, Fleisig GS, Waterbor JW, et al: Longitudinal study of elbow and shoulder pain in youth baseball pitchers, *Med Sci Sports Exerc* 33:1803, 2001.
27. Lyman S, Fleisig GS, Andrews JR, et al: Effect of pitch type, pitch count, and pitching mechanics on risk of elbow and shoulder pain in youth baseball pitchers, *Am J Sports Med* 30:463, 2002.
28. Olsen S, Fleisig G, Dun S, et al: Risk factors for shoulder and elbow injuries in adolescent baseball pitchers, *Am J Sports Med* 34:905, 2006.
29. Conte S, Requa R, Garrick JG: Disability days in Major League Baseball, *Am J Sports Med* 29:431, 2001.
30. Morgan CD: Glenohumeral internal rotation deficit and its relationship to ulnar collateral ligament injury in throwing athletes. In *Shoulder and elbow injuries in baseball, Little League to Major Leagues: southern orthopedics lecture symposium*, Cooperstown, NY, 2002, Baseball Hall of Fame.
31. Dines JS, Frank JB, Akerman M, et al: Glenohumeral internal rotational deficits in baseball players with ulnar collateral ligament insufficiency, *Am J Sports Med* 37:566, 2009.
32. Jobe FW, Tibone JE, Perry J, et al: An EMG analysis of the shoulder in throwing and pitching: a preliminary report, *Am J Sports Med* 11:3, 1983.
33. Jobe FW, Moynes DR, Tibone JE, et al: An EMG analysis of the shoulder in pitching: a second report, *Am J Sports Med* 12:218, 1984.
34. Pappas AM, Zawacki RM, Sullivan TJ: Biomechanics of baseball pitching: a preliminary report, *Am J Sports Med* 14:216, 1985.
35. Moynes DR, Perry J, Antonelli DJ, et al: Electromyographic and motion of the upper extremity in sports, *Phys Ther* 66:1905, 1986.
36. Gowan ID, Jobe FW, Tibone JE, et al: A comparative electromyographic analysis of the shoulder during pitching, *Am J Sports Med* 15:586, 1987.
37. Nicholas J, Hershman E, editors: *The upper extremity in sports medicine*, St. Louis, 1990, Mosby, p 741.
38. Glousman R, Jobe F, Tibone J, et al: Dynamic electromyographic analysis of the throwing shoulder with glenohumeral instability, *J Bone Joint Surg Am* 70:220, 1988.
39. Dillman CJ, Fleisig GS, Andrews JR: Biomechanics of pitching with emphasis upon shoulder kinematics, *J Orthop Sports Phys Ther* 18:402, 1993.
40. Fleisig GS, Andrews JR, Dillman CJ, et al: Kinetics of baseball pitching with implications about injury mechanisms, *Am J Sports Med* 23:233, 1995.
41. Whiteley R: Baseball throwing mechanics as they relate to pathology and performance - A review, J Sport Science & Med 6:1, 2007.

41a. Werner SL, Gill TJ, Cook TD, et al: Relationships between throwing mechanics and shoulder distraction in professional baseball pitchers, *Am J Sports Med* 29:354, 2001.

42. Harryman DT, Sidles JA, Clark JM, et al: Translation of the humerus on the glenoid with passive glenohumeral motion, *J Bone Joint Surg Am* 72:1334, 1990.

43. O'Brien SJ, Neves MC, Arnoczky SP, et al: The anatomy and histology of the inferior glenohumeral complex of the shoulder, *Am J Sports Med* 18:449, 1990.
44. Gohlke F, Essigkrug B, Schnitz F: The pattern of the collagen fiber bundles of the capsule of the glenohumeral joint, *J Shoulder Elbow Surg* 3:111–128, 1994.
45. Branch TP, Avilla O, London L, et al: Correlation of medial/lateral rotation of the humerus with glenohumeral translation, *Br J Sports Med* 33:347, 1999.
46. Weiser WM, Lee TQ, McMaster WC, et al: Effects of simulated scapular protraction on anterior glenohumeral stability, *Am J Sports Med* 27:801, 1999.
47. Novotny JE, Beynnon BD, Nichols CE: Modeling the stability of the human glenohumeral joint during external rotation, *J Biomech* 33:345, 2000.
48. Kuhn JE, Bey MJ, Huston LJ, et al: Ligamentous restraints to external rotation in the humerus in the late-cocking phase of throwing: a cadaveric biomechanical investigation, *Am J Sports Med* 28:200, 2000.
49. Pollock RG, Wang VM, Bucchieri JS, et al: Effects of repetitive subfailure on the mechanical behavior of the inferior glenohumeral ligament, *J Shoulder Elbow Surg* 9:427, 2000.
50. Baeyens JP, Van Roy P, De Schepper A, et al: Glenohumeral joint kinematics related to minor anterior instability at the end of the late preparatory phase of throwing, *Clin Biomech* 16:752, 2001.
51. Grossman MG, Tibone JE, McGarry MH, et al: A cadaveric model of the throwing shoulder: a possible etiology of superior labrum anterior to posterior lesions, *J Bone Joint Surg Am* 87:824, 2005.
52. Hufman GR, Tibone JE, McGarry MH, et al: Path of glenohumeral articulation throughout the rotational range of motion in a thrower's shoulder model, *Am J Sports Med* 34:1662, 2006.
53. Snyder SJ, Banas MP, Karzel RP: An analysis of 140 injuries to the superior labrum, *J Shoulder Elbow Surg* 4:243, 1995.
54. Maffet MW, Gartsman GM, Moseley B: Superior labrum–biceps tendon complex lesions of the shoulder, *Am J Sports Med* 23:93, 1995.
55. Rodosky MW, Harner CD, Fu FH: The role of the long head of the biceps muscle and superior glenoid labrum in anterior stability of the shoulder, *Am J Sports Med* 22:121, 1994.
56. Pradhan RL, Itol E, Hatakeyama Y, et al: Superior labral strain during the throwing motion: a cadaveric study, *Am J Sports Med* 29:488, 2001.
57. Sheppard MF, Dugas JR, Zeng N, et al: Differences in the ultimate strength of the biceps anchor and the generation of type II superior labral anterior posterior lesions in a cadaveric model, *Am J Sports Med* 32:1197, 2004.
58. Yeh M, Litner D, Luo Z: Stress distribution in the superior labrum during throwing motion, *Am J Sports Med* 33:395, 2005.
59. Youm T, Tibone JE, ElAttrache NS: Simulated type II superior labral anterior posterior lesions do not alter the path of glenohumeral articulation: a cadaveric biomechanical study, *Am J Sports Med* 36:767, 2008.
60. Morgan CD, Burkhart SS, Palmeri M, et al: Type II SLAP lesions: three subtypes and their relationships to superior instability and rotator cuff tears, *Arthroscopy* 14:553, 1998.
61. O'Brien SJ, Pagnani MJ, Fealy S, et al: The active compression test: a new and effective test for diagnosing labral tears and acromioclavicular joint abnormality, *Am J Sports Med* 26:610, 1998.
62. Jobe CW, Pink MM, Jobe FW, et al: Anterior shoulder instability, impingement, and rotator cuff tear: theories and concepts. In Jobe FW, editor: *Operative techniques in upper extremity sports injuries*, St. Louis, 1996, Mosby Year-Book, pp 164–176.
63. Barber FA, Morgan CD, Burkhart SS, et al: Labrum/biceps/cuff dysfunction in the throwing athlete, *Arthroscopy* 15:852, 1999.
64. Kibler WB: The role of the scapula in athletic shoulder function, *Am J Sports Med* 26:325, 1998.
65. McClure PW, Michener LA, Sennett BJ, et al: Direct 3-dimensional measurement of scapular kinematics during dynamic movements in vivo, *J Shoulder Elbow Surg* 10:269, 2001.
66. Bourne DA, Choo AMT, Regan WD, et al: Three-dimensional rotation of the scapula during functional movements: an in vivo study in healthy volunteers, *J Shoulder Elbow Surg* 16:150, 2007.
67. Downar JM, Sauers EL: Clinical measures of shoulder mobility in the professional baseball player, *J Athl Train* 40:23, 2005.
68. Mourtacos SL, Sauers EL, Downar JM: Adolescent baseball players exhibit differences in shoulder mobility between the throwing and non-throwing shoulder and between divisions of play, *J Athl Train* 38:S72, 2003.
69. Myers JB, Laudner KG, Pasquale MR, et al: Scapular position and orientation in throwing athletes, *Am J Sports Med* 33:263, 2005.
70. Thomas SJ, Swanik KA, Swanik CB, et al: Internal rotation and scapular differences: a comparison of collegiate and high school baseball players, *J Athl Train* 45:44, 2010.
71. Laudner KG, Stanek JM, Meister K: Differences in scapular upward rotation between baseball pitchers and position players, *Am J Sports Med* 35:2091, 2007.
72. Oyama S, Myers JB, Wassinger CA, et al: Asymmetric resting scapular posture in healthy overhead athletes, *J Athl Train* 43:565, 2008.
73. Morgan CD: The S.I.C.K. scapula syndrome in overhead/throwing athletes. In *Shoulder and elbow injuries in baseball, Little League to Major Leagues: southern orthopedics lecture symposium*, Cooperstown, NY, 2002, Baseball Hall of Fame.
74. Lukasiewicz AC, McClure P, Michener L, et al: Comparison of 3-dimensional scapular position and orientation between subjects with and without shoulder impingement, *J Orthop Sports Phys Ther* 29:574, 1999.
75. Ludewig PM, Cook TM: Alterations in shoulder kinematics and associated muscle activity in people with symptoms of shoulder impingement, *Phys Ther* 80:276, 2000.
76. King JW, Brelsford HJ, Tullos HS: Analysis of the pitching arm of the professional baseball pitcher, *Clin Orthop Relat Res* 67:116, 1969.
77. Barnes DA, Tullos HS: An analysis of 100 symptomatic baseball players, *Am J Sports Med* 6:62, 1978.
78. Reinold MM, Wilk KE, Macrina LC, et al: Changes in shoulder and elbow passive range of motion after pitching in professional baseball players, *Am J Sports Med* 36:523, 2008.
79. Bigliani LU, Codd TP, Connor PM, et al: Shoulder motion and laxity in the professional baseball player, *Am J Sports Med* 25:609, 1997.
80. Brown LP, Niehues SL, Harrah A, et al: Upper extremity range of motion and isokinetic strength of the internal and external shoulder rotators in Major League Baseball players, *Am J Sports Med* 16:577, 1988.
81. Burkhart SS, Morgan CD, Kibler WB: Shoulder injuries in overhead athletes: the "dead arm" revisited, *Clin Sports Med* 19:125, 2000.

82. Tyler TF, Roy T, Nicholas SJ, et al: Reliability and validity of a new method of measuring posterior shoulder tightness, *J Orthop Sports Phys Ther* 29:262, 1999.
83. Crockett HC, Gross LB, Wilk KE, et al: Osseous adaptation and range of motion at the glenohumeral joint in professional baseball pitchers, *Am J Sports Med* 30:20, 2002.
84. Osbahr DC, Cannon DL, Speer KP: Retroversion of the humerus in the throwing shoulder of college baseball pitchers, *Am J Sports Med* 30:347, 2002.
85. Reagan KM, Meister K, Horodyski MB, et al: Humeral retroversion and its relationship to glenohumeral rotation in the shoulder of college baseball players, *Am J Sports Med* 30:354, 2002.
86. Chant C, Litchfield R, Griffin S, et al: Humeral head retroversion in competitive baseball players and its relationship to glenohumeral rotation range of motion, *J Orthop Sports Phys Ther* 39:514, 2007.
87. Whiteley RJ, Ginn K, Nicholson LL, et al: Sports participation and humeral torsion, *J Orthop Sports Phys Ther* 39:256, 2009.
88. Donatelli R, Ellenbecker T, Ekedahl SR, et al: Assessment of shoulder strength in professional baseball pitchers, *J Orthop Sports Phys Ther* 30:544, 2000.
89. Baltaci G, Johnson R, Kohl H: Shoulder range of motion characteristics in college baseball players, *J Sports Med Phys Fitness* 41:236, 2001.
90. Ellenbecker T, Roetert EP, Bailie DS, et al: Glenohumeral joint total rotation range of motion in elite tennis players, *Med Sci Sports Exerc* 34:2052, 2002.
91. Sethi PM, Tibone JE, Lee TQ: Quantitative assessment of glenohumeral translation in baseball players: a comparison of pitchers verus nonpitching athletes, *Am J Sports Med* 32:1711, 2004.
92. Myers JB, Laudner KG, Pasquale MR, et al: Glenohumeral range of motion deficits and posterior shoulder tightness in throwers with pathologic internal impingement, *Am J Sports Med* 34:385, 2006.
93. Ruotolo C, Price E, Panchal A: Loss of motion in collegiate baseball players, *J Shoulder Elbow Surg* 15:67, 2006.
94. Borsa PA, Dover GC, Wilk KE, et al: Glenohumeral range of motion and stiffness in professional baseball players, *Med Sci Sport Exerc* 34:21, 2006.
95. Broca P: La torsion de l'humerus et le tropometer, *Rev Anthrop* 4:193–210, 1881 385–425, 577–592.
96. Edelson G: Variations in the retroversion of the humeral head, *J Shoulder Elbow Surg* 8:142, 1998.
97. Edelson G: The development of humeral head retroversion, *J Shoulder Elbow Surg* 9:316, 1999.
98. Sabick MD, Torry MR, Young-Kyu K, et al: Humeral torque in professional baseball pitchers, *Am J Sports Med* 32:892, 2004.
99. Yamamoto N, Minagawa H: Why is the humeral retroversion of throwing athletes greater in dominate shoulders than in nondominant shoulders? *J Shoulder Elbow Surg* 15:5, 2006.
100. Sabick MB, Young-Kyu K, Torry MR, et al: Biomechanics of the shoulder in youth baseball pitchers: implications for the development of proximal humeral epiphysiolysis and humeral retrotorsion, *Am J Sports Med* 33:1716, 2005.
101. Meisner K, Day T, Horodyski M, et al: Rotational motion changes in the glenohumeral joint of the adolescent/Little League baseball player, *Am J Sports Med* 33:693, 2005.
102. Pappas AM, Zawacki RM, McCarthy CF: Rehabilitation of the pitching shoulder, *Am J Sports Med* 13:223, 1985.
103. Verna C: Analysis of the relationship of shoulder rotation deficit to shoulder, elbow and low back problems in professional baseball players. In *PBATS sports medicine symposium*, Phoenix, 1991, Professional Baseball Athletic Trainers Society.
104. Warner JJ, Micheli LJ, Arslanian LE, et al: Patterns of flexibility, laxity, and strength in normal shoulders and shoulders with instability and impingement, *Am J Sports Med* 18:366, 1990.
105. Kugler A, Kruger-Franke M, Reininger S, et al: Muscular imbalance and shoulder pain in volleyball attackers, *Br J Sports Med* 30:256, 1996.
106. Green WB, Heckman JD, editors: *The clinical measurement of joint motion*, Rosemont, Illinois, 1994, American Academy of Orthopaedic Surgeons, pp 24–25.
107. Cooper JS, Donley P: Unpublished data, 2000.
108. Ginn KA, Cohen ML, Herbert RD: Does hand-behind-back of motion accurately reflect shoulder internal rotation? *J Shoulder Elbow Surg* 15:311, 2006.
109. Wakabayashi I, Itol E, Minagawa H, et al: Does reaching the back reflect the actual rotation of the shoulder? *J Shoulder Elbow Surg* 15:306, 2006.
110. Mallon W, Herring C, Sallay P, et al: Use of vertebral levels to measure presumed internal rotation at the shoulder: a radiological analysis, *J Shoulder Elbow Surg* 5:299, 1996.
111. Wilk KE, Meister K, Andrews JR: Current concepts in the rehabilitation of the overhead throwing athlete, *Am J Sports Med* 30:136, 2002.
112. Morgan CD: The throwers shoulder: spectrum of pathology. In *Shoulder and elbow injuries in baseball, Little League to Major Leagues: southern orthopedics lecture symposium*, Cooperstown, NY, 2002, Baseball Hall of Fame.
113. Ruotolo C, Price E, Panchal A: Loss of total arc of motion in collegiate baseball players, *J Shoulder Elbow Surg* 15:67, 2006.
114. Myers JB, Lauder KG, Pasquale MR, et al: glenohumeral range of motion deficits and posterior shoulder tightness in throwers with pathologic internal impingement, *Am J Sports Med* 34:385, 2006.
115. Laudner KG, Stanek JM, Meister K: Assessing posterior shoulder contracture: the reliability and validity of measuring glenohumeral joint horizontal adduction, *J Athl Train* 41:375, 2006.
116. Myers JB, Oyama S, Wassinger CA, et al: Reliability, precision, accuracy, and validity of posterior shoulder tightness in overhead athletes, *Am J Sports Med* 35:1922, 2007.
117. Burkhart SS, Morgan CD, Kibler WB: The disabled throwing shoulder: spectrum of pathology. Part I. Pathoanatomy and biomechanics, *Arthroscopy* 19:404, 2003.
118. Borich MR, Bright JM, Lorello DJ, et al: Scapular angular position at end range internal rotation in cases of glenohumeral internal rotation deficit, *J Orthop Sports Phys Ther* 36:926, 2006.
119. Thomas SJ, Swanik KA, Swanik CB, et al: Internal rotation and scapular differences: a comparison of collegiate and high school baseball players, *J Athl Train* 45:44, 2010.
120. Kibler WB: Role of the scapula in the overhand throwing motion, *Contemp Orthop* 22:525, 1991.
121. Kibler WB: Shoulder rehabilitation: principles and practice, *Med Sci Sports Exerc* 30:S40, 1998.
122. Jobe FW, Pink M: Classification and treatment of shoulder dysfunction in the overhead athlete, *J Orthop Sports Phys Ther* 18:427, 1993.
123. Townsend H, Jobe F, Pink M, et al: Electromyographic analysis of the glenohumeral muscles during a baseball rehabilitation program, *Am J Sports Med* 19:264, 1991.
124. Moseley J, Jobe F, Pink M, et al: EMG analysis of the scapular muscles during a shoulder rehabilitation program, *Am J Sports Med* 20:128, 1992.

125. Toyoshima S, Hoshikawa T, Miryashita M, et al: Contribution of the body parts to throwing performance. In Nelson RC, Morehouse CA, editors: *Biomechanics* 4:Baltimore, 1974, University Park Press, p 169.
126. Tyler TF, Nicholas SJ, Roy T, et al: Quantification of posterior capsule tightness and motion loss in patients with shoulder impingement, *Am J Sports Med* 28:668, 2000.
127. Borstad JD, Ludewig PM: Comparison of three stretches for the pectoralis minor muscle, *J Shoulder Elbow Surg* 15:324, 2006.
128. Johansen RL, Callis M, Potts J, et al: A modified internal rotation stretching technique for overhand and throwing athletes, *J Orthop Sports Phys Ther* 21:216, 1995.
129. Hardwick DH, Beebe JA, McDonnell MK, et al: A comparison of serratus anterior muscle activation during a wall slide exercise and other traditional exercises, *J Orthop Sports Phys Ther* 36:903, 2006.
130. Blackburn TA, McLeod WD, White B, et al: EMG analysis of posterior rotator cuff exercises, *Athl Train* 25:40, 1990.
131. Kibler WB, Sciascia AD, Uhl TL, et al: Electromyographic analysis of specific exercises for scapular control in early phases of shoulder rehabilitation, *Am J Sports Med* 36:1789, 2008.
132. Thigpen CA, Padua DA, Morgan N, et al: Scapular kinematics during supraspinatus rehabilitation exercise: a comparison of full-can versus empty-can techniques, *Am J Sports Med* 34:644, 2006.
133. Decker MJ, Hintermeister RA, Faber KJ, et al: Serratus anterior muscle activity during selected rehabilitation exercise, *Am J Sports Med* 27:784, 1999.

APPENDIX 3-1 GUIDELINES FOR OFF-SEASON UPPER EXTREMITY CONDITIONING PROTOCOL

This conditioning protocol has been designed for three 5-week blocks. The first block relies on a three-day workout to re-establish the upper extremity exercises you have used this past season. This is your active rest period. The second block is a strength-building period with workouts three times a week using a five repetition–five set format with controlled 3-minute rest periods. The third block, beginning after a week of rest, moves to a 4 day a week format with increasing repetitions.

You determine the weight that you begin with and when to increase that weight. Generally, you begin with half the weight you were using at the conclusion of the season and begin the second and third blocks with half the weight you were using at the conclusion of the previous block.

At the conclusion of the third block is a week of modified activity followed by a week of activity, which mimics your spring training protocol. A suggested throwing protocol is included.

BLOCK ONE: WEEKS 1 TO 5

- Progress through this period beginning with 16 repetitions and ending with 20.
- Six backs begin with 1 set of 3 repetitions and progress to 1 set of 6 repetitions.
- Global patterns begin with 3 repetitions per position per direction. Three supine positions (incline, level, and decline) are used, for a total of 18 repetitions. Three prone positions (incline, level, are decline) are used, for a total of 18 repetitions.
- The dynamic hug and reverse fly are included in the global patterns because of the use of the stability ball. Repetitions should follow the 16-to-20 formats.
- Add weight as necessary to ensure maximum benefit.

BLOCK TWO: WEEKS 6 TO 10

- Range-of-motion (ROM) exercises are done in 1 set of 25 repetitions.
- Core, base, and movement patterns are done in a 5 repetition–5 set sequence.
- Once the first exercise is completed in a group, a clock is started for 3 minutes.
- The remaining exercises are completed to finish the first set. The second set is not begun until the 3-minute period has elapsed.
- The timing continues through each of the 5 sets.
- The dynamic hug and reverse fly are accomplished in 1 set of 25.

RECOVERY WEEK 11

- Recovery week: ROM exercises.

BLOCK THREE: WEEKS 12 TO 16

- ROM, core, and base exercises return to a 1 set of 20 format.
- Six backs and global exercises remain at 1 set of 6.
- The dynamic hug and reverse fly are 1 set of 20.
- Movement patterns break into 2 sets. One set is to be performed after the range-of-motion exercises and before the other exercises. The second movement pattern set is performed at the conclusion of the workout.

WEEK 17

- ROM exercises remain at 1 set of 20.
- Core and base exercises are eliminated.
- One set of 25 movement patterns precedes global patterns.
- One set of 25 movement patterns follows global patterns.

WEEK 18

- Return to Block Three format.
- Movement patterns remain at 2 sets of 25 as in Block Three.

Table A-1 Block One: Weeks 1 to 5

Week 1: Day 1	Week 1: Day 2	Week 1: Day 3
ROM exercises 1 × 16	ROM exercises 1 × 16	ROM exercises 1 × 16
Six backs 1 × 4	Six backs 1 × 4	Six backs 1 × 4
Core exercises 1 × 16	Core exercises 1 × 16	Core exercises 1 × 16
Base exercises 1 × 16	Base exercises 1 × 16	Base exercises 1 × 16
Movement patterns 1 × 16	Movement patterns 1 × 16	Movement patterns 1 × 16
Global patterns 3 per position	Global patterns 3 per position	Global patterns 3 per position
Week 2: Day 1	**Week 2: Day 2**	**Week 2: Day 3**
ROM exercises 1 × 17	ROM exercises 1 × 17	ROM exercises 1 × 17
Six backs 1 × 5	Six backs 1 × 5	Six backs 1 × 5
Core exercises 1 × 17	Core exercises 1 × 17	Core exercises 1 × 17
Base exercises 1 × 17	Base exercises 1 × 17	Base exercises 1 × 17
Movement patterns 1 × 17	Movement patterns 1 × 17	Movement patterns 1 × 17
Global patterns 3 per position	Global patterns 3 per position	Global pattern 3 per positions
Week 3: Day 1	**Week 3: Day 2**	**Week 3: Day 3**
ROM exercises 1 × 18	ROM exercises 1 × 18	ROM exercises 1 × 18
Six backs 1 × 6	Six backs 1 × 6	Six backs 1 × 6
Core exercises 1 × 18	Core exercises 1 × 18	Core exercises 1 × 18
Base exercises 1 × 18	Base exercises 1 × 18	Base exercises 1 × 18
Movement patterns 1 × 18	Movement patterns 1 × 18	Movement patterns 1 × 18
Global patterns 4 per position	Global patterns 4 per position	Global patterns 4 per position
Week 4: Day 1	**Week 4: Day 2**	**Week 4: Day 3**
ROM exercises 1 × 19	ROM exercises 1 × 19	ROM exercises 1 × 19
Six backs 1 × 6	Six backs 1 × 6	Six backs 1 × 6
Core exercises 1 × 19	Core exercises 1 × 19	Core exercises 1 × 19
Base exercises 1 × 19	Base exercises 1 × 19	Base exercises 1 × 19
Movement patterns 1 × 19	Movement patterns 1 × 19	Movement patterns 1 × 19
Global patterns 4 per position	Global patterns 4 per position	Global patterns 4 per position
Week 5: Day 1	**Week 5: Day 2**	**Week 5: Day 3**
ROM exercises 1 × 20	ROM exercises 1 × 20	ROM exercises 1 × 20
Six backs 1 × 6	Six backs 1 × 6	Six backs 1 × 6
Core exercises 1 × 20	Core exercises 1 × 20	Core exercises 1 × 20
Base exercises 1 × 20	Base exercises 1 × 20	Base exercises 1 × 20
Movement patterns 1 × 20	Movement patterns 1 × 20	Movement patterns 1 × 20
Global patterns 5 per position	Global patterns 5 per position	Global patterns 5 per position

ROM, range-of-motion.

Table A-2 Block Two: Weeks 6 to 10

Week 6: Day 1	Week 6: Day 2	Week 6: Day 3
ROM exercises 1 × 25	ROM exercises 1 × 25	ROM exercises 1 × 25
Six backs 1 × 6	Six backs 1 × 6	Six backs 1 × 6
Core exercises 5 × 5	Core exercises 5 × 5	Core exercises 5 × 5
Base exercises 5 × 5	Base exercises 5 × 5	Base exercises 5 × 5
Movement patterns 5 × 5	Movement patterns 5 × 5	Movement patterns 5 × 5
Global patterns 5 per position	Global patterns 5 per position	Global patterns 5 per position
50 throws at 60 feet	50 throws at 60 feet	50 throws at 60 feet

Table A-2 Block Two: Weeks 6 to 10—cont'd

Week 7: Day 1	Week 7: Day 2	Week 7: Day 3
ROM exercises 1 × 25	ROM exercises 1 × 25	ROM exercises 1 × 25
Six backs 1 × 6	Six backs 1 × 6	Six backs 1 × 6
Core exercises 5 × 5	Core exercises 5 × 5	Core exercises 5 × 5
Base exercises 5 × 5	Base exercises 5 × 5	Base exercises 5 × 5
Movement patterns 5 × 5	Movement patterns 5 × 5	Movement patterns 5 × 5
Global patterns 6 per position	Global patterns 6 per position	Global patterns 6 per position
60 throws at 60 feet	60 throws at 60 feet	60 throws at 60 feet
Week 8: Day 1	**Week 8: Day 2**	**Week 8: Day 3**
ROM exercises 1 × 25	ROM exercises 1 × 25	ROM exercises 1 × 25
Six backs 1 × 6	Six backs 1 × 6	Six backs 1 × 6
Core exercises 5 × 5	Core exercises 5 × 5	Core exercises 5 × 5
Base exercises 5 × 5	Base exercises 5 × 5	Base exercises 5 × 5
Movement patterns 5 × 5	Movement patterns 5 × 5	Movement patterns 5 × 5
Global patterns 6 per position	Global patterns 6 per position	Global patterns 6 per position
70 throws at 60 feet	70 throws at 60 feet	70 throws at 60 feet
Week 9: Day 1	**Week 9: Day 2**	**Week 9: Day 3**
ROM exercises 1 × 25	ROM exercises 1 × 25	ROM exercises 1 × 25
Six backs 1 × 6	Six backs 1 × 6	Six backs 1 × 6
Core exercises 5 × 5	Core exercises 5 × 5	Core exercises 5 × 5
Base exercises 5 × 5	Base exercises 5 × 5	Base exercises 5 × 5
Movement patterns 5 × 5	Movement patterns 5 × 5	Movement patterns 5 × 5
Global patterns 6 per position	Global patterns 6 per position	Global patterns 6 per position
80 throws at 60 feet	80 throws at 60 feet	80 throws at 60 feet
Week 10: Day 1	**Week 10: Day 2**	**Week 10: Day 3**
ROM exercises 1 × 25	ROM exercises 1 × 25	ROM exercises 1 × 25
Six backs 1 × 6	Six backs 1 × 6	Six backs 1 × 6
Core exercises 5 × 5	Core exercises 5 × 5	Core exercises 5 × 5
Base exercises 5 × 5	Base exercises 5 × 5	Base exercises 5 × 5
Movement patterns 5 × 5	Movement patterns 5 × 5	Movement patterns 5 × 5
Global patterns 6 per position	Global patterns 6 per position	Global patterns 6 per position
90 throws at 60 feet	90 throws at 60 feet	90 throws at 60 feet

ROM, range-of-motion.

Table A-3 Recovery Week 11

Week 11: Day 1	Week 11: Day 2	Week 11: Day 3
ROM exercises 1 × 25	ROM exercises 1 × 25	ROM exercises 1 × 25
100 throws at 60 feet	100 throws at 60 feet	100 throws at 60 feet

ROM, range-of-motion.

Table A-4 Block Three: Weeks 12 to 16

Week 12: Day 1	Week 12: Day 2	Week 12: Day 3	Week 12: Day 4
ROM exercises 1 × 20	ROM exercises 1 × 20	ROM exercises 1 × 20	ROM exercises 1 × 20
Six backs 1 × 6	Six backs 1 × 6	Six backs 1 × 6	Six backs 1 × 6
Core exercises 1 × 20	Core exercises 1 × 20	Core exercises 1 × 20	Core exercises 1 × 20
Base exercises 1 × 20	Base exercises 1 × 20	Base exercises 1 × 20	Base exercises 1 × 20
Movement patterns 2 × 12	Movement patterns 2 × 12	Movement patterns 2 × 12	Movement patterns 2 × 12
Global patterns 1 × 6	Global patterns 1 × 6	Global patterns 1 × 6	Global patterns 1 × 6
75 throws at 60 feet	75 throws at 60 feet	75 throws at 60 feet	75 throws at 60 feet
25 throws at 90 feet	25 throws at 90 feet	25 throws at 90 feet	25 throws at 90 feet

Week 13: Day 1	Week 13: Day 2	Week 13: Day 3	Week 13: Day 4
ROM exercises 1 × 20	ROM exercises 1 × 20	ROM exercises 1 × 20	ROM exercises 1 × 20
Six backs 1 × 6	Six backs 1 × 6	Six backs 1 × 6	Six backs 1 × 6
Core exercises 1 × 20	Core exercises 1 × 20	Core exercises 1 × 20	Core exercises 1 × 20
Base exercises 1 × 20	Base exercises 1 × 20	Base exercises 1 × 20	Base exercises 1 × 20
Movement patterns 2 × 14	Movement patterns 2 × 14	Movement patterns 2 × 14	Movement patterns 2 × 14
Global patterns 1 × 6	Global patterns 1 × 6	Global patterns 1 × 6	Global patterns 1 × 6
75 throws at 60 feet	75 throws at 60 feet	75 throws at 60 feet	75 throws at 60 feet
25 throws at 120 feet	25 throws at 120 feet	25 throws at 120 feet	25 throws at 120 feet

Week 14: Day 1	Week 14: Day 2	Week 14: Day 3	Week 14: Day 4
ROM exercises 1 × 20	ROM exercises 1 × 20	ROM exercises 1 × 20	ROM exercises 1 × 20
Six backs 1 × 6	Six backs 1 × 6	Six backs 1 × 6	Six backs 1 × 6
Core exercises 1 × 20	Core exercises 1 × 20	Core exercises 1 × 20	Core exercises 1 × 20
Base exercises 1 × 20	Base exercises 1 × 20	Base exercises 1 × 20	Base exercises 1 × 20
Movement patterns 2 × 16	Movement patterns 2 × 16	Movement patterns 2 × 16	Movement patterns 2 × 16
Global patterns 1 × 6	Global patterns 1 × 6	Global patterns 1 × 6	Global patterns 1 × 6
75 throws at 60 feet	75 throws at 60 feet	75 throws at 60 feet	75 throws at 60 feet
25 throws at 150 feet	25 throws at 150 feet	25 throws at 150 feet	25 throws at 150 feet

Week 15: Day 1	Week 15: Day 2	Week 15: Day 3	Week 15: Day 4
ROM exercises 1 × 20	ROM exercises 1 × 20	ROM exercises 1 × 20	ROM exercises 1 × 20
Six backs 1 × 6	Six backs 1 × 6	Six backs 1 × 6	Six backs 1 × 6
Core exercises 1 × 20	Core exercises 1 × 20	Core exercises 1 × 20	Core exercises 1 × 20
Base exercises 1 × 20	Base exercises 1 × 20	Base exercises 1 × 20	Base exercises 1 × 20
Movement patterns 2 × 18	Movement patterns 2 × 18	Movement patterns 2 × 18	Movement patterns 2 × 18
Global patterns 1 × 6	Global patterns 1 × 6	Global patterns 1 × 6	Global patterns 1 × 6
75 throws at 60 feet	75 throws at 60 feet	75 throws at 60 feet	75 throws at 60 feet
25 throws at 180 feet	25 throws at 180 feet	25 throws at 180 feet	25 throws at 180 feet

Week 16: Day 1	Week 16: Day 2	Week 16: Day 3	Week 16: Day 4
ROM exercises 1 × 20	ROM exercises 1 × 20	ROM exercises 1 × 20	ROM exercises 1 × 20
Six backs 1 × 6	Six backs 1 × 6	Six backs 1 × 6	Six backs 1 × 6
Core exercises 1 × 20	Core exercises 1 × 20	Core exercises 1 × 20	Core exercises 1 × 20
Base exercises 1 × 20	Base exercises 1 × 20	Base exercises 1 × 20	Base exercises 1 × 20
Movement patterns 2 × 20	Movement patterns 2 × 20	Movement patterns 2 × 20	Movement patterns 2 × 20
Global patterns 1 × 6	Global patterns 1 × 6	Global patterns 1 × 6	Global patterns 1 × 6
75 throws at 60 feet	75 throws at 60 feet	75 throws at 60 feet	75 throws at 60 feet
25 throws at 210 feet	25 throws at 210 feet	25 throws at 210 feet	25 throws at 210 feet

ROM, range-of-motion.

Table A-5 Week 17

Week 17: Day 1	Week 17: Day 2	Week 17: Day 3	Week 17: Day 4
ROM exercises 1 × 20	ROM exercises 1 × 20	ROM exercises 1 × 20	ROM exercises 1 × 20
Movement patterns 2 × 25	Movement patterns 2 × 25	Movement patterns 2 × 25	Movement patterns 2 × 25
Global patterns 1 × 3	Global patterns 1 × 3	Global patterns 1 × 3	Global patterns 1 × 3
75 throws at 60 feet	75 throws at 60 feet	75 throws at 60 feet	75 throws at 60 feet
25 throws at 240 feet	25 throws at 240 feet	25 throws at 240 feet	25 throws at 240 feet

ROM, range-of-motion.

Table A-6 Week 18

Week 18: Day 1	Week 18: Day 2	Week 18: Day 3	Week 18: Day 4
ROM exercises 1 × 20	ROM exercises 1 × 20	ROM exercises 1 × 20	ROM exercises 1 × 20
Six backs 1 × 6	Six backs 1 × 6	Six backs 1 × 6	Six backs 1 × 6
Core exercises 1 × 20	Core exercises 1 × 20	Core exercises 1 × 20	Core exercises 1 × 20
Base exercises 1 × 20	Base exercises 1 × 20	Base exercises 1 × 20	Base exercises 1 × 20
Movement patterns 2 × 25	Movement patterns 2 × 25	Movement patterns 2 × 25	Movement patterns 2 × 25
Global patterns 1 × 6	Global patterns 1 × 6	Global patterns 1 × 6	Global patterns 1 × 6
Begin mound work			

ROM, range-of-motion.

APPENDIX 3-2 NINE-LEVEL REHABILITATION THROWING PROGRAM

This program is designed for athletes to work at their own pace to develop the necessary arm strength to begin throwing from a mound. The athlete is to throw 2 days in a row and then rest for 1 day. Progressing to the next throwing level with each outing is not important. It is preferred that several outings at the same level be completed before progressing. It is important to throw with comfort, which may necessitate moving back a level on occasion.

Table B-1

Level	Throws	Feet	Throws	Feet	Throws	Feet
One	25	25	25	60		
Two	25	25	50	60		
Three	25	25	75	60		
Four	25	25	50	60	25	90
Five	25	25	50	60	25	120
Six	25	25	50	60	25	150
Seven	25	25	50	60	25	180
Eight	25	25	50	60	25	210
Nine	25	25	50	60	25	240

APPENDIX 3-3 REHABILITATION PROTOCOL

Craig Morgan and Phillip B. Donley

ARTHROSCOPIC REPAIR OF A SLAP LESION IN A THROWING ATHLETE

Under optimal conditions, early healing of a superior labrum anterior to posterior (SLAP) lesion occurs at 3 weeks and progresses to a soft union at 6 weeks. Remodeling and continued strengthening of the repair continue for 8 to 12 months in most cases. Fine-tuned athletic performance may take up to 18 months. Upper quadrant strength, flexibility, and sound body mechanics are critical to prevent a recurrence.

WEEK 1: ACUTE STAGE

- Objectives: Avoid causing compression, traction, or shearing forces on the repaired labrum. Avoid stress to the biceps. Allow nonpainful limited range of motion (ROM). Full passive shoulder flexion should be achieved by the end of week 3.
- The patient should use a sling until first postoperative visit.

- Pendulum exercise 3 to 4 times per day in flexion, extension, abduction, and adduction.
- Passive ROM (PROM) in the pain-free range followed by ice and transcutaneous elecrical nerve stimulation (TENS).
- Sets and repetitions are completed to the patient's tolerance.
- The patient may perform very light pendulum exercises in flexion, extension, abduction, and adduction.

WEEKS 2 TO 3: STITCHES REMOVED

- The patient should use a sling for sleeping and as needed during the day. The elbow may be flexed and extended for light activities of daily living (ADLs).
- Full elbow, wrist, and hand motion may be used for ADLs.
- Use a rope and pulley for ROM exercises with elbow in 90° to 45° of flexion and 90° of abduction with no external rotation. Also include pendulum exercises.
- Increase ROM so that by the end of 3 weeks, the patient has full flexion.
- The patient should perform shoulder shrugs and circular rotation.
- Hand and wrist isometrics and isotonics are performed in the sling.
- Use ice as needed.

Goals

- Full flexion, 45° of external rotation, and 15° of horizontal adduction will be achieved after 3 weeks.

Clinical Protocol

- In scaption, perform PROM stretching with gentle contraction and relaxation techniques in the painful arc.
- Week 3: Isometrics with 0° of abduction and adduction, extension, and internal and external rotation are used.
- Week 3: Active assistive ROM is used for abduction and flexion to 90°.
- Scapular isotonics are used in four directions, with no load on the arm.
- Passive capsular ligament stretch is used.
- The emphasis is on posterior rotator cuff mobilization.
- Myofascial stretching is performed for superficial structures of the anterior and posterior shoulder.

WEEKS 4 TO 6: SUBACUTE PHASE: DISCONTINUE SLING

- Continue the ROM pulley and pendulum exercises if the patient does not have full passive flexion.
- Protraction and retraction exercises are performed.
- Continue overall fitness for the uninvolved arm and lower extremities.
- Do *not* load the elbow.
- Stretch the posterior rotator cuff in horizontal adduction with the shoulder in 45° to 90° of flexion. Hold only 30 seconds.
- Wrist and hand isotonics and isometrics are performed. Avoid loading the biceps by keeping the elbow in flexion. Use wrist curls, forward and reverse.

Goals

- The patient will have full ROM with the patient in the supine position.
- Focus on posterior rotator cuff stretching because this may be a causative effect of labral disease.

Clinical Protocol

- Perform wrist and hand strengthening without loading the biceps.
- Continue scapular isometrics in 60° to 90° of flexion and abduction.
- Perform full antigravity ROM with no external loads.
- Isometrics: Emphasize adduction and extension in pain-free positions.
- Provide posture and gait training, cervical and thoracic.
- Perform closed-chain rotator cuff exercises by week 6.
- Perform pelvic and trunk stabilization exercises.
- Perform isotonics of the lower extremities.
- Build endurance with stationary equipment, bicycle.

WEEKS 6 TO 12: INTERMEDIATE PROGRAM

- Begin upper quadrant progressive strengthening exercises with pain free light loads.
- Continue the progression of flexibility of the posterior rotator cuff and scapula motions.
- Protect the labrum with low-velocity motions.
- *No* throwing or racquet use is allowed.

Goals

- Throwers will have 90° of external rotation in 90° of abduction.
- At end of week 12: The patient should be jogging off the treadmill.
- Overall body conditioning should include scapula/thoracic, wrist/hand, cervical/thoracic, lower extremities, and uninvolved extremity conditioning.
- The patient will have full ROM.

Clinical Protocol

- Isotonic strengthening is performed in all planes using free weights and tubing. Emphasize high repetitions with low weight when the patient has achieved full ROM.
- Continue to emphasize stretching of the posterior rotator cuff and increasing scapular motion.

- Begin treadmill jogging.
- Proprioceptive neuromuscular facilitation (PNF) patterns (D1 and D2) should be used at week 10.
- Stretch with contraction and relaxation in both scaption and neutral positions.
- The upper body ergometer (UBE) is used with progressive endurance loads.
- Start biceps loading.
- Increase loads and repetitions with all activities.
- Promote lower extremity agility and functional activities.
- Internal and external rotation: Use multiple sets and varying degrees of abduction.
- Emphasize proprioceptive activities for the shoulder.
- Promote pelvic and trunk stabilization.

WEEKS 13 TO 18: STRENGTHENING PHASE

- At 16 weeks: Begin tossing a ball.
- Eliminate any mechanical flaws in throwing: promote coordination and timing for the entire body.

Goals

- The patient will have full nonpainful ROM.
- The strength of the involved side will be equal to 80% of that of the uninvolved side.

Clinical Protocol

- The pool is used, with no overhand strokes: Shoulder press or punch, paddles or gloves, and breast stroke.
- At 16 weeks: Begin plyoball activities (with a shoulder rebounder if available).
- Isokinetics are used (at 45° of abduction of internal and external rotation) at no less than 90° per second.
- Increase free weights with machines for all planes of the shoulder, with high repetitions.
- Rubber tube exercises include diagonal planes with all on a physioball.
- UBE is used in both directions with the shoulder arc at 90° to 110° of flexion.
- Begin plyoball exercises: One hand on wall dribble, two-hand push pass, overhead pass, and lateral pass.
- Begin the impulse machine at 14 weeks.

WEEKS 18 TO 24

Goals

- The patient will return to full activity with no restrictions.
- The strength of the involved side will be 80% to 90% of that of the uninjured side.

Clinical Protocol

- Begin a rehabilitation throwing program when 75 throws can be successfully completed.
- Initiate sports-specific simulation activities, including plyometrics.
- Initiate isokinetic testing.
- *Remember*: A tight posterior capsule is a primary cause of a SLAP lesion. Maintain posterior capsule flexibility.

WEEKS 24 PLUS

- The patient should have a full return to presurgical activities, per physician's orders.
- A preventive maintenance program should be followed.
- A regular posterior capsule stretching program should be followed as long as overhead motions are continued.
- **It is *very* important to maintain posterior cuff and posterior capsule stretching while continuing to perform overhead activities.**

CHAPTER

4

Donn Dimond
and Robert A. Donatelli

Examinations and Evaluation of the Shoulder

Patients with cervical and shoulder symptoms make up a large portion of the patient mix of an orthopedic physical therapist (PT). In fact, 8.5% of adults at any given time will have had a complaint of shoulder pain within the last 30 days.[1] An efficient and effective examination is needed to treat appropriately the cause of the patient's functional limitation as opposed to just treating their symptoms. Otherwise, the PT is not much better than pain medication. This chapter first describes the symptom investigation and examination of the shoulder. This discussion includes the history of the symptoms, the screening process of the cervical spine and related upper quarter structures, the examination of the glenohumeral, sternoclavicular, acromioclavicular, and scapulothoracic joints, and special tests.

Next, the chapter discusses the evaluation process and the examination results as they relate to the importance of the central position of the humeral head on the glenoid. The operating premise is that most shoulder pain and dysfunction are secondary to this lack of central position of the humerus.

HISTORY

Shoulder Pain and Disability Index

Because the need for PTs to use standardized outcome measures has been recognized at the national level in the United States, it is appropriate to include use of one with patients with complaints encompassing the shoulder.[2] The Shoulder Pain and Disability Index (SPADI) measures the pain and disability associated with shoulder disease and has been shown to be valid and reliable.[3] The patient should fill out this questionnaire before meeting with the PT.

The SPADI gives the clinician a score for pain and a score for disability, as well as an overall score. The maximum score is 100% in each section and overall. This score gives the clinician a general idea of what the patient is feeling even before asking the patient a single question. Although the SPADI was not designed to compare scores among patients, it was designed to look at scores between patient visits. The minimal detectable change (90% confidence) is 13 points.[2] Change less than this may be attributable to measurement error.

Chief Complaint

The clinician must first establish the patient's chief complaint. This is best accomplished by having the patient describe which side is affected and which complaints are the main reasons for seeking care. Such complaints may include difficulty with daily activities, fatigue or poor endurance, headache, impaired sensation, joint stiffness, joint swelling, muscle tenderness, muscle weakness, problems with breathing or shortness of breath, and tingling or numbness. The PT must also ascertain from the patient which joints are involved. Joint complaints may include hand pain, neck pain, rib pain, shoulder pain, upper extremity or arm pain, and wrist pain. By asking these questions first, before the history of the chief complaint, the PT can better identify the true complaints and also become aware of other possible pain generators. The PT also needs to perform a medical screening at this point.

The PT should ask the patient whether or she has experienced any of these symptoms in the past year: abdominal pain; bowel problems; chest pain; constant pain in body; coordination problems; cough; difficulty sleeping; difficulty or changes in swallowing; difficulty walking; dizziness or blackouts; excessive thirst; fainting spells; feeling downhearted or blue; fever, chills, or sweats; foot pain or discoloration; frequent or severe headaches; frequent heartburn or indigestion; hearing impairment or hearing problems; heart palpitations; hoarseness or changes in speech; insomnia; joint pain, swelling, or redness; loss of appetite; loss of balance or falling; loss of pleasure in things usually enjoyed; nausea or vomiting; numbness or changes in sensation, especially in more than one extremity; pain at night; and pain or cramping in the lower leg (calf). If the patient answers yes to any of these questions, then the PT should at least ask whether the patient's primary care physician is aware of any of these symptoms. If not, the patient should be advised to contact his or her physician.

Once the chief complaint is established, it is important for the clinician to review the history of the patient's complaint. This review includes the date the current problems started, the date the injury took place, whether it came on during a onetime event (macrotrauma) or over a period of time (microtrauma), the activity the patient was engaged in when the complaints started, the action the patient is taking now to help take care of the current problem, and whether the patient is currently seeing anybody else for the current problem. The PT must also know whether the patient had surgery for the current complaint, and, if so, the therapist should obtain a copy of the operative report and any precautions that the surgeon may have for the patient. The PT must also ascertain whether the patient had this complaint before and, if so, whether the patient sought treatment. If the patient did seek treatment before, from whom did the patient seek treatment, and did it help? What was the duration of previous care, and did that help? What did the patient do initially to help alleviate the complaint? Finally, the PT must know whether the patient has had any recent hospitalizations and, if so, for how long and for what condition.

Pain Scale

The PT must also know what the patient's complaint of pain has been. A numeric rating schedule (NRS) to determine the pain rating is indicated in all settings for adults and children who are more than 9 years old.[4] The scale consists of a straight horizontal line numbered at equal intervals from 0 to 10 with anchor words of "no pain" for 0, "moderate pain" for 5, and "worst pain" for 10.[4] The therapist should also ask the patient about the following: activities that make the pain worse and activities that make the pain better; any difficulties at work; any difficulties with activities of daily living or difficulties with recreational activities; whether sleep is disturbed and, if so, the preferred sleep position; how the patient feels in the morning, whether it feels better once the patient moves about, and what it feels like at the end of the day. The therapist should also ask whether the patient has headaches and, if so, their location, duration, and frequency.

Environmental Factors

The PT should also be aware of any environmental factors that may affect the patient's current condition for better or for worse. Effects can include but are not limited to carrying, crawling, fatigue, lifting, lying down, pulling, pushing, reaching, repetitions, and resting.

Supplemental Questions

When dealing with the shoulder, it is important to screen the patient for other possible disorders. At the very least, the therapist should ask whether the pain causes the patient to wake from sleep and whether the pain or symptoms extend below the elbow. If the pain does wake the patient from sleep, the therapist should note whether the night pain is the patient's worst pain during a 24-hour period and whether it takes more than a minimal effort for the patient to fall back asleep. If so, then the patient should be directed to discuss this problem with his or her physician. If the pain radiates past the elbow, then a strong potential exists that more than just the shoulder joint is involved.

EXAMINATION FOR POSTURE

The examination starts with a look at the patient's posture. Most commonly, patients present with a forward head and rounded shoulders, and this can be a source of neck and shoulder pain. Kebaetse et al[5] found that thoracic posture affects the position of the scapula and glenohumeral joint. Posture should be viewed from the anterior, lateral, and posterior views. The PT should take note of head position, both in frontal and transverse planes, shoulder height, scapular position (superior, inferior, abducted), inferior angle position, and thoracic spine position.

MOBILITY

Active Range of Motion

Once the posture examination is complete, the PT can look at the active range of motion of the patient's shoulder, cervical spine, and thoracic and lumbar spine.

Shoulder Elevation

With the patient standing, the patient is asked to raise his or her arm up as high as possible in the plane of the scapula (scaption; POS), 30° to 45° anterior to the frontal plane (Fig. 4-1). The more kyphotic a patient is, the more anterior to the frontal plane the POS will be. The physical therapist should also take note of how well the humerus "dissociates" from the scapula in the last phase of elevation (140° to 180°).

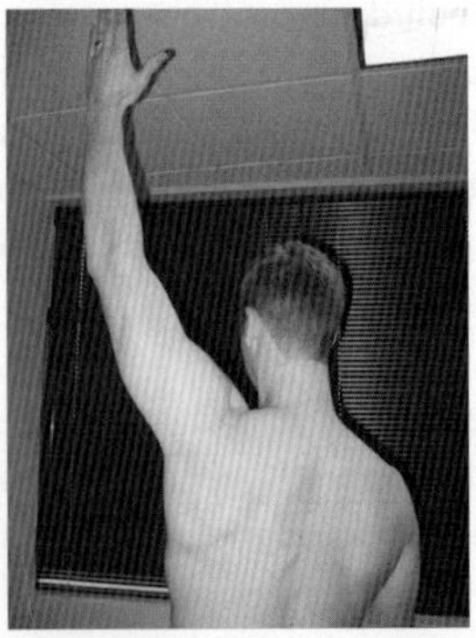

Figure 4-1 Shoulder elevation.

Cervical Motion

The PT measures the amount of cervical rotation, side bending, flexion, and extension. At this point, the PT should perform Spurling's test to see whether any of the shoulder symptoms originate from the cervical spine. The test is performed by extending the patient's neck, rotating the head, and then applying downward pressure on the head. The test result is considered positive if pain radiates into the limb ipsilateral to the side to which the head is rotated. The PT should also perform the cervical distraction spine distraction test. This test is done with the patient seated. The PT grasps the patient's head around the jaw and the back of the head and applies a superior distraction force. If the patient's pain is alleviated by the distraction force, then some or all of the pain may be diskogenic.

Thoracic and Lumbar Motion

With the patient sitting, the PT asks the patient to cross his or her arms across the chest and rotate to the right as far as possible. The PT then measures the amount of right rotation and then repeats the measurement with the patient rotating to the left.

Passive Range of Motion

External Rotation at 0° of Abduction (Subscapularis Length)

While the patient is supine, the PT holds the patient's arm with one hand in midline (Fig. 4-2). The other hand holds a goniometer to the patient's radius and rotates the radius away from the patient's body until the PT feels the slack being taken up. The PT measures the amount of rotation.[6]

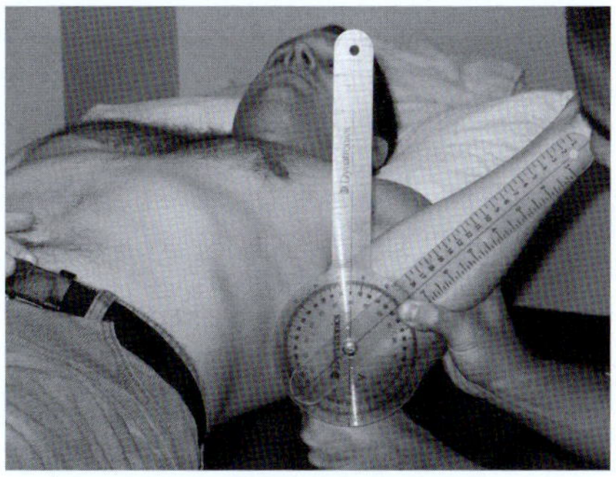

Figure 4-2

External Rotation at 45° of Abduction (Superior and Middle Glenohumeral Ligament and Coracohumeral Ligament Length)

With the patient supine, the PT moves the patient's arm up to 50° of abduction (Fig. 4-3). The PT then externally rotates the patient's arm out until the PT feels that the slack is taken up. Please refer to reference 6 for more information

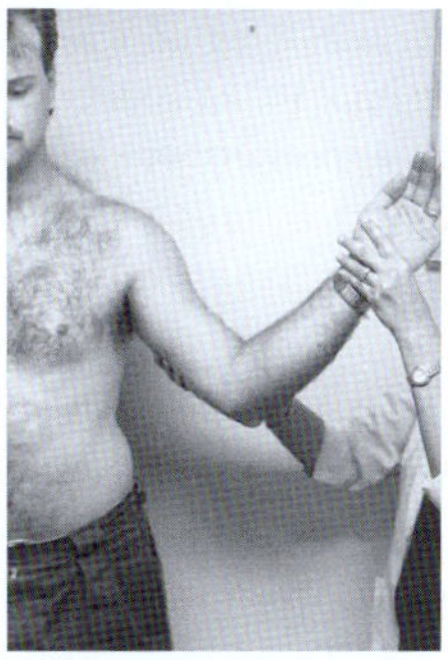

Figure 4-3

External Rotation at 90° of Abduction (Inferior Glenohumeral Ligament Complex)

With the patient supine, the PT moves the patient's arm up to 90° of abduction (Fig. 4-4). The PT then externally rotates the patient's arm back until the PT feels that the slack is taken up. Please refer to reference 6 for more information

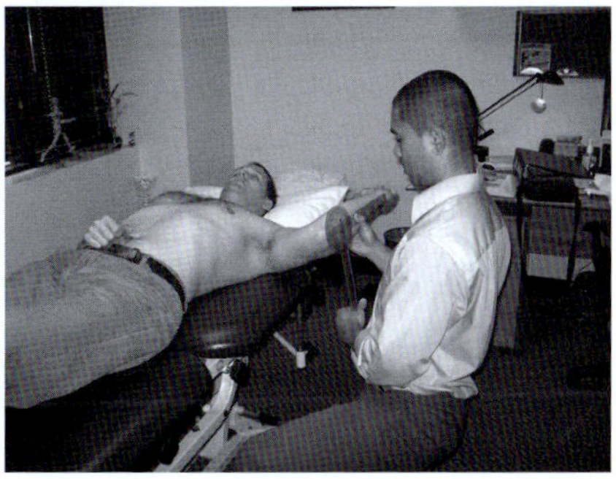

Figure 4-4

General Internal Rotation (Posterior Capsule in General)

With the patient in the side-lying position, the arm is placed in 90° of flexion in the sagittal plane with the elbow bent at 90° (Fig. 4-5). The PT rotates the patient's arm toward the patient's hips until the slack is taken up in the patient's shoulder. The PT then measures the angle of rotation.[7]

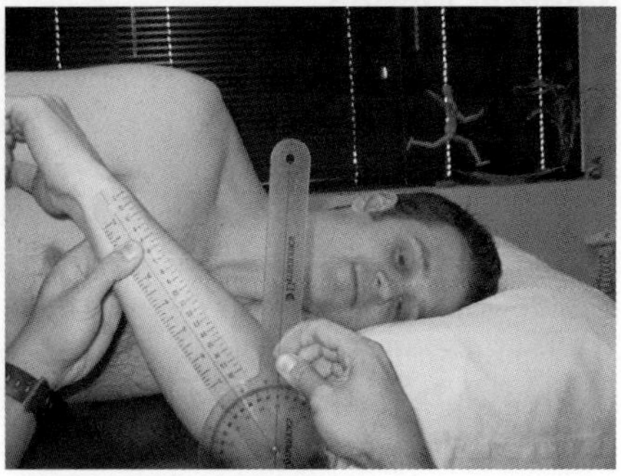

Figure 4-5

30° of Extension and Internal Rotation (Lower Fibers of the Posterior Capsule)

With the patient prone, the PT moves the patients arm back into 30° of shoulder extension (Fig. 4-6). While the hand is resting on the patient's waist, the PT pushes the patient's scapula against the patient's rib cage. The distance from the patient's elbow to the plinth is noted and compared with the contralateral arm.[7]

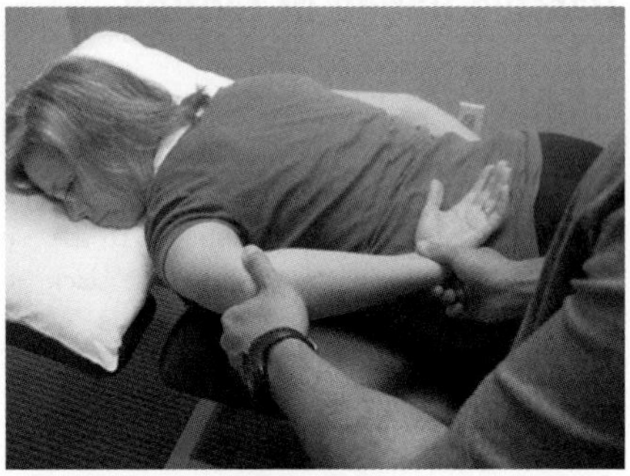

Figure 4-6

Internal Rotation in 30° of Abduction in the Plane of the Scapula (30° Anterior to the Frontal Plane) (Superior and Middle Fibers of the Posterior Capsule)

With the patient in the side-lying position, enough to place the patient's shoulder in the POS, the PT moves the arm into 30° of abduction (Fig. 4-7). The PT then internally rotates the patient's arm and takes a measurement with the goniometer.[7]

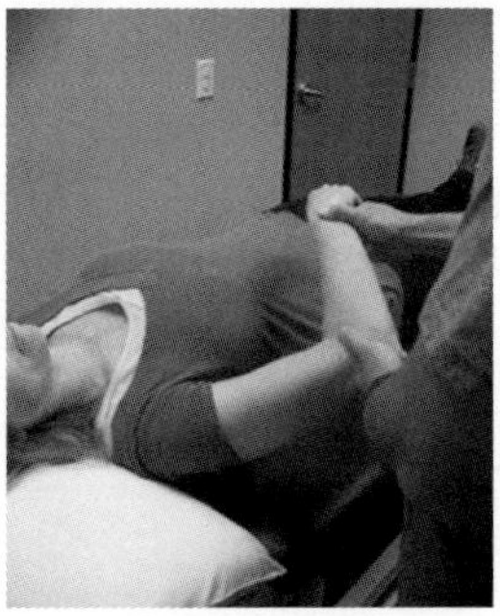

Figure 4-7

60° of Abduction in the Frontal Plane and Internal Rotation (Posterior Capsule)

With the patient supine, the PT brings the patient's out to 60° of abduction (Fig. 4-8). The PT then rotates the arm internally until the slack is taken up while making sure not to allow the scapula to come off the plinth.[7]

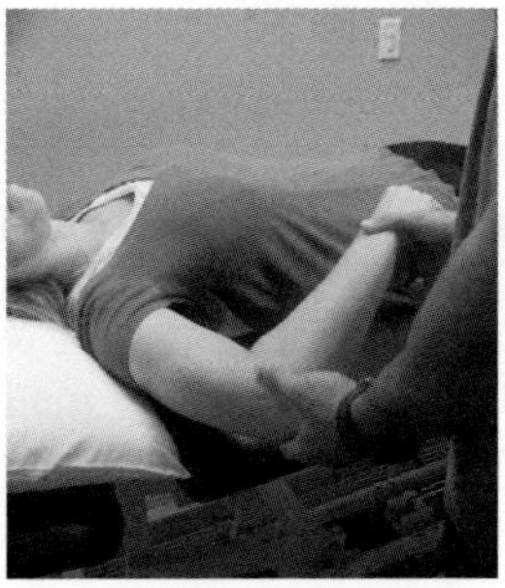

Figure 4-8

STRENGTH

The order of the manual muscle tests minimizes the patient's having to get onto and off the plinth.

Middle Trapezius (Scapular Rotator)

With the patient prone, the shoulder is placed in 90° of abduction and lateral rotation of the humerus (Fig. 4-9). The patient is instructed to resist downward pressure provided by the examiner toward horizontal adduction. Lateral rotation minimizes contribution from the elbow extensors.[8]

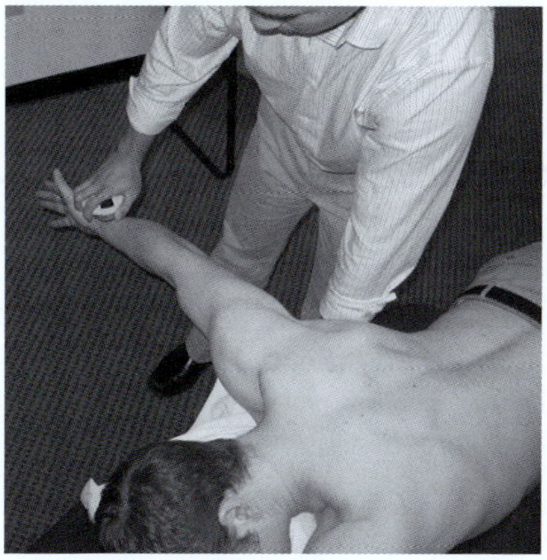

Figure 4-9

Lower Trapezius (Scapular Rotator)

With the patient prone, the shoulder is placed in 90° abduction, 90° of lateral rotation, and 90° of elbow flexion (Fig. 4-10). The patient is instructed to resist the examiner's downward pressure to the lateral elbow directed toward the table. Ekstrom et al[8] reported that this movement was the most effective at isolating the lower trapezius from the upper and middle trapezius.

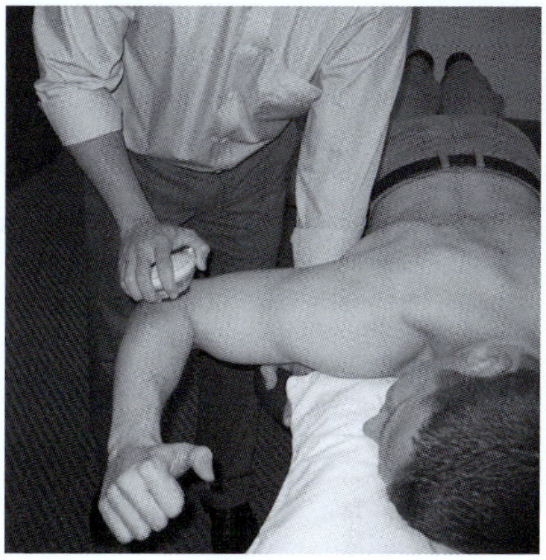

Figure 4-10

Teres Major (Glenohumeral Rotator)

With the patient prone, the shoulder is placed in medial rotation with the hand resting on the posterior iliac crest (Fig. 4-11). The patient resists as the examiner applies a force above the elbow in the direction of abduction and flexion.[9]

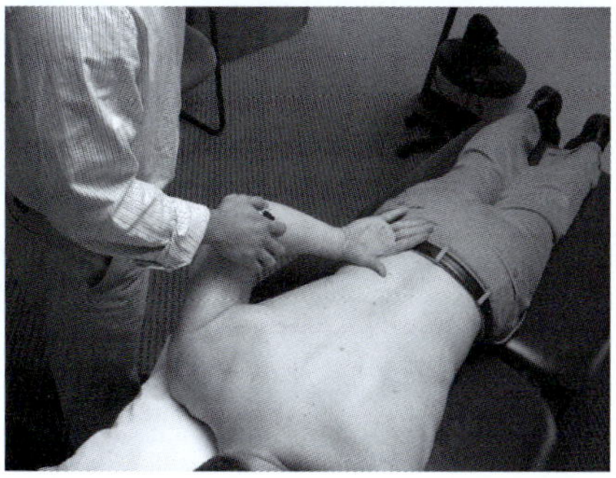

Figure 4-11

Latissimus Dorsi (Glenohumeral Rotator)

With the patient prone, the shoulder is placed in extension, adduction, and medial rotation (Fig. 4-12). The patient resists as the examiner applies a force against the forearm in the direction of abduction and slight flexion.[9]

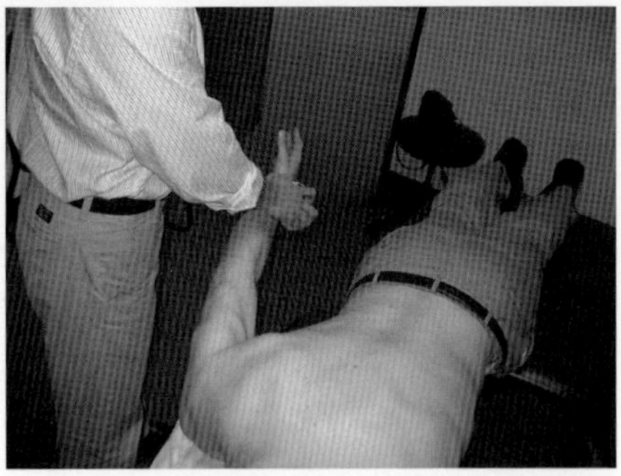

Figure 4-12

Rhomboids (Scapular Rotator)

With the patient prone and arm resting at the side, the patient resists as the examiner attempts to pull the lateral border of the scapula away from the spine into abduction (Fig. 4-13).[9]

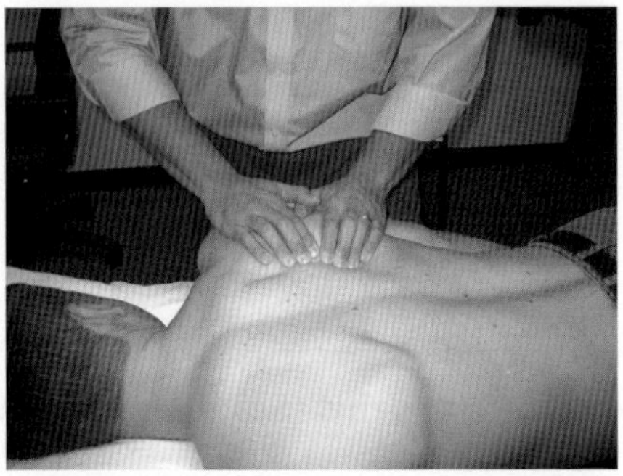

Figure 4-13

Teres Minor (Glenohumeral Rotator)

With the patient prone, the shoulder is placed in 90° of abduction and 90° of external rotation, with the elbow bent to 90° (Fig. 4-14).The examiner places one hand under the elbow to ensure pure rotation through the humerus. Using the forearm as a lever, pressure is applied in the direction of medial rotation as the patient resists.[9]

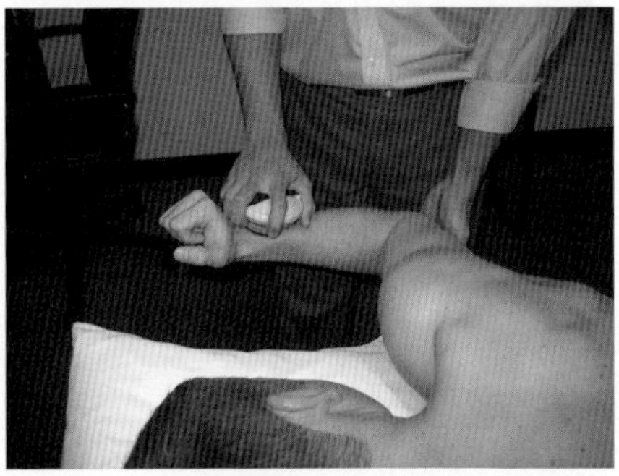

Figure 4-14

Infraspinatus (Glenohumeral Rotator)

The patient stands with the arm at the side with the elbow at 90° and the humerus medially rotated to 45° (Fig. 4-15). The examiner then applies a medial rotation force that the patient resists. Counterpressure is applied by the examiner against the inner aspect of the distal end of the humerus to ensure a rotation movement.[10,11]

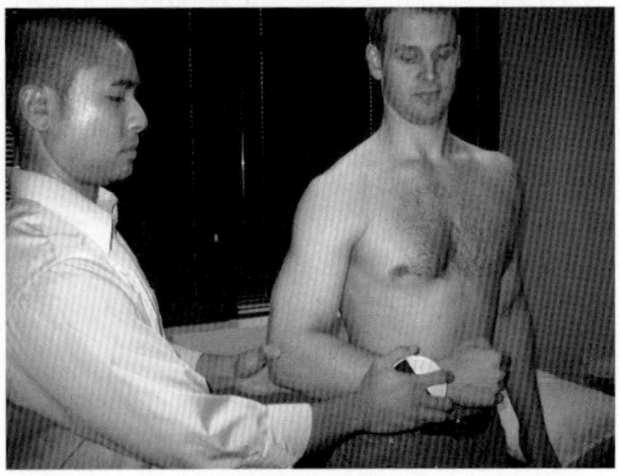

Figure 4-15

Supraspinatus (Glenohumeral Rotator)

The patient elevates the arm to 90° in the scapular plane in the "full can" position with the thumb pointing upward (Fig. 4-16). The patient is asked to resist as the examiner applies a downward force to the distal forearm. Kelly et al[10] found no significant difference in supraspinatus muscle activation when comparing the "full can" and "empty can" positions. Furthermore, the "full can" activates the infraspinatus muscle significantly less and avoids the positional pain provocation associated with the "empty can" position.[10,11]

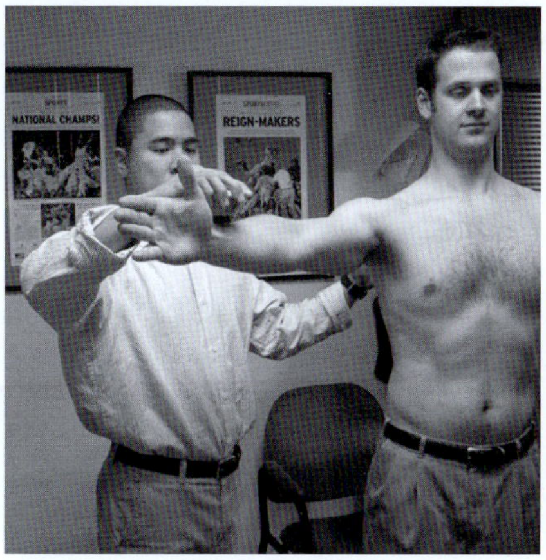

Figure 4-16

Subscapularis (Glenohumeral Rotator)

The patient places the dorsum of the hand against the midlumbar spine (Fig. 4-17). The patient is instructed to take the hand away from the back, and the examiner applies a load pushing the hand toward the back. This test maximizes subscapularis muscle activation and minimizes the activation from the pectoralis and latissimus muscles.[12,13]

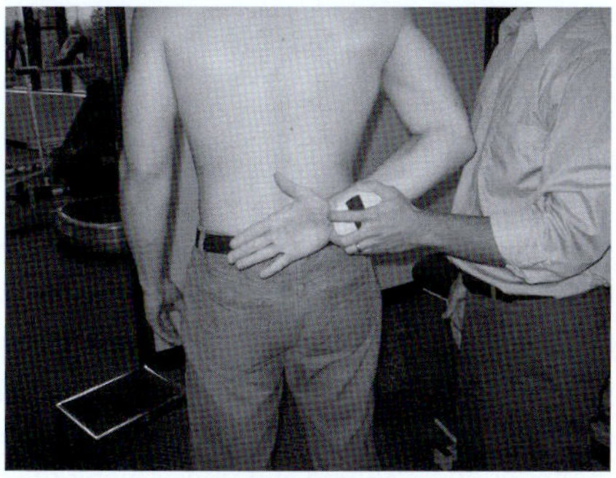

Figure 4-17

Serratus Anterior (Scapular Rotator)

The patient's arm is elevated to 125° in the scapular plane with the thumb pointing upward (Fig. 4-18). The patient is instructed to resist as the examiner applies downward pressure to the distal forearm. Ekstrom et al[8] demonstrated high serratus anterior electromyographic activity as the scapula upwardly rotates above 120° of shoulder elevation.

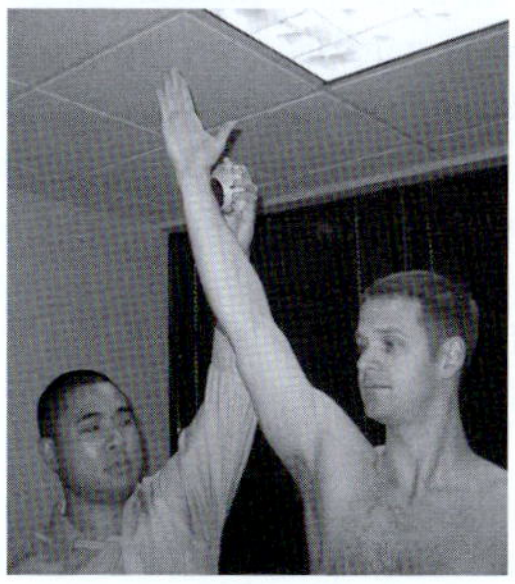

Figure 4-18

SPECIAL TESTS

Instability Tests

Sulcus Sign

The patient sits with arm by the side and shoulder muscles relaxed (Fig. 4-19). The examiner grasps the patient's forearm below the elbow and pulls the arm distally while palpating the inferior margin of the acromion for inferior translation of the humeral head. The presence of a sulcus is considered a positive test result and may indicate inferior instability or inferior glenohumeral ligament laxity.[11]

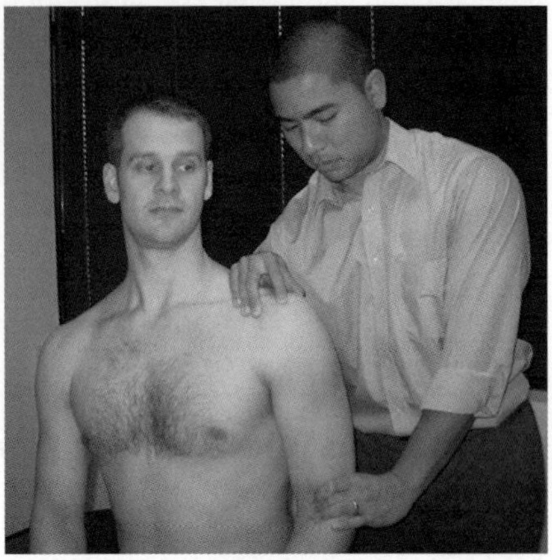

Figure 4-19

Load and Shift Test

The patient sits in upright posture with arm at the side and shoulder muscles relaxed (Fig. 4-20). The examiner stabilizes the shoulder with one hand over the clavicle and scapula. With the other hand, the examiner grasps the head of the humerus with the thumb over the posterior humeral head and fingers along the anterior humerus. The examiner assesses the initial position of the humeral head relative to the glenoid. The humerus is then gently pushed anteriorly or posteriorly to "seat" it into a centered position relative to the glenoid. This is the "load portion" of the test. The examiner then pushes the humeral head anteriorly or posteriorly noting the amount of translation and end feel. This is the "shift" portion of the test. Translation of 25% or less, of the humeral head diameter anteriorly, is considered normal, although variability occurs among patients. Hawkins and Mohtadi[14] advocated a three-grade system for anterior translation: grade I, the humeral head translates up to 50% riding up to the glenoid rim; grade II, the humeral head translates more than 50% over the glenoid rim, but spontaneously reduces; and grade III, the humeral head rides over the glenoid rim and does not spontaneously reduce and remains dislocated.[11]

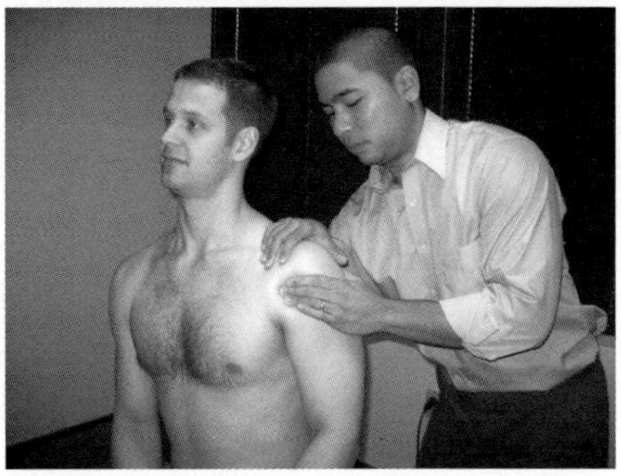

Figure 4-20

Apprehension and Relocation Tests

The examiner abducts the arm to 90° and laterally rotates the patient's shoulder slowly (Fig. 4-21). A positive test result is indicated by a look or feeling of apprehension or alarm on the patient's face and the patient's resistance to further motion. If the apprehension test result is positive, the examiner then applies a posterior translation stress to the head of the humerus (relocation test). The test result is considered positive if the patient loses the apprehension, pain decreases, and further lateral rotation is possible before the apprehension or pain returns. These tests are primarily designed to test for traumatic instability problems causing gross or anatomic instability of the shoulder.[11,14]

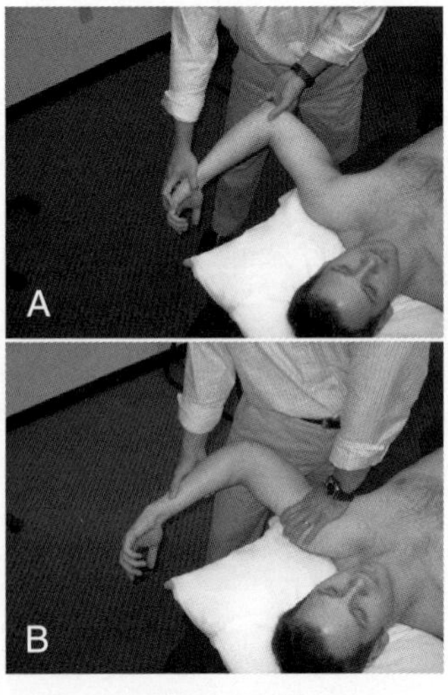

Figure 4-21

Labral Tests

Active Compression Test of O'Brien

The patient is placed in the standing position with the arm forward flexed to 90° and the elbow in full extension (Fig. 4-22). The arm is then horizontally adducted 10° to 15° and is medially rotated so the thumb faces downward. The examiner stands behind the patient and applies a downward force to the distal arm. With the arm in the same position, the palm is fully supinated and the downward force is repeated. The test result is considered positive for labral abnormality if pain or clicking is produced "inside" the shoulder with the first maneuver and reduced or eliminated with the second maneuver. Pain localized to the acromioclavicular joint or on top of the shoulder is diagnostic of acromioclavicular joint abnormality.[11,15]

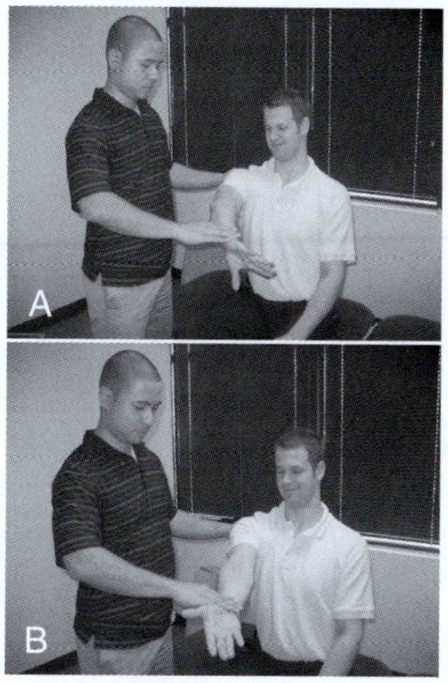

Figure 4-22

Biceps Load Test and Biceps Load II

The arm to be examined is elevated to 90° (biceps load) and 120° (biceps load II) and is laterally rotated to its maximal point with the elbow in 90° flexion and the forearm in the supinated position (Fig. 4-23). The patient is asked to flex the elbow while resisting the examiner's resistance at the wrist. The test result is considered positive if the patient complains of increased pain during the resisted elbow flexion. The test result is negative if pain is not elicited by the resisted elbow flexion or if the preexisting pain during the elevation and external rotation of the arm is unchanged or diminished by the resisted elbow flexion.[11,16]

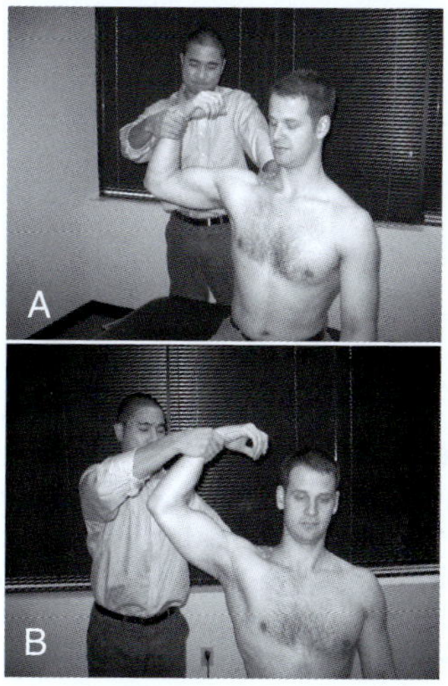

Figure 4-23

New Pain Provocation Test

The patient is seated, the arm is abducted to between 90° and 100°, and the arm is laterally rotated by the examiner by holding the wrist (Fig. 4-24). The forearm is taken into maximum supination and then maximum pronation. If pain is provoked only in the pronated position, the test is considered positive for a superior labrum anterior posterior (SLAP) tear. In this position, forearm pronation produces additional stretch to the biceps tendon.[11,17]

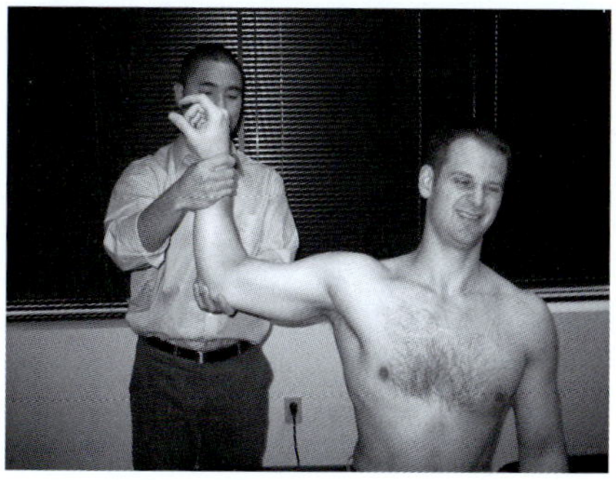

Figure 4-24

Speed's Test

The patient resists downward force with shoulder flexed to 90° and elbow fully extended (Fig. 4-25). A positive test result elicits increased tenderness in the bicipital groove and indicates a SLAP lesion or bicipital tendinosis.[11,18]

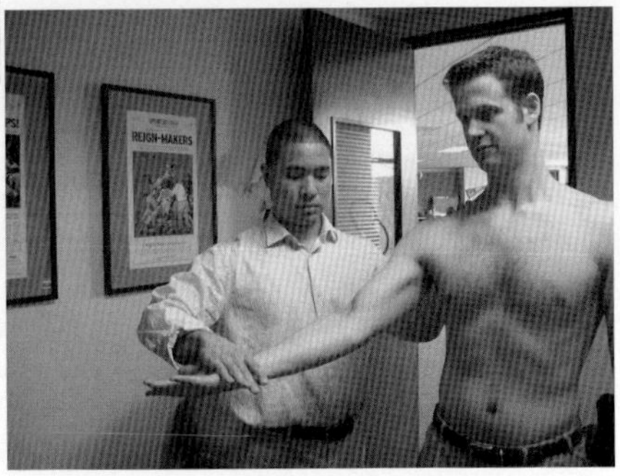

Figure 4-25

Dynamic Speed's Test

The examiner provides resistance against both shoulder elevation and elbow flexion (Fig. 4-26) simultaneously as the patient elevates the arm overhead. Deep pain within the shoulder during shoulder elevation is positive for labral disease.[11,18]

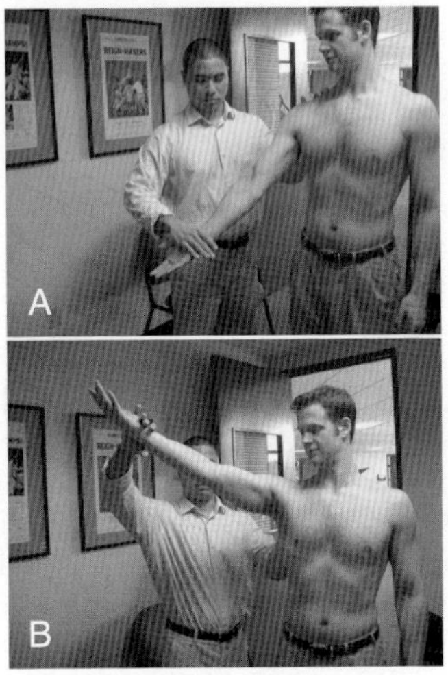

Figure 4-26

Crank Test

The patient is in the supine lying or sitting position (Fig. 4-27). The examiner elevates the arm to 160° in the scapular plane. In this position, an axial load is applied to the humerus with one hand of the examiner while the other hand rotates the humerus medially and laterally.
A positive test result is indicated by pain on rotation. Symptomatic clicking or grinding may also be present during this maneuver.[11,18]

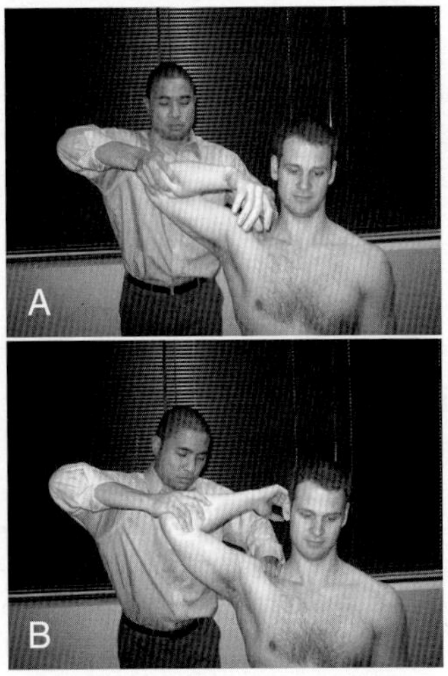

Figure 4-27

Acromioclavicular Tests

Acromioclavicular Shear Test

With the patient in the sitting position, the examiner cups his or her hands over the deltoid muscle, with one hand on the clavicle and one hand on the spine of the scapula (Fig. 4-28). The examiner then squeezes the heels of the hands together. A positive test result is indicated by pain or abnormal movement at the acromioclavicular joint and represents of acromioclavicular joint disease.[11]

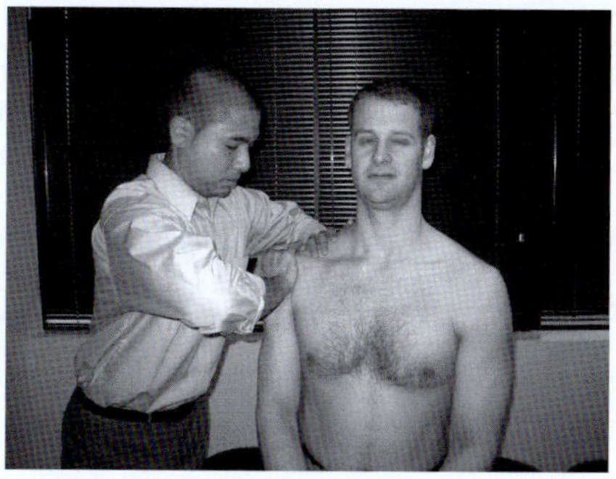

Figure 4-28

Impingement Tests

Neer's Impingement Test

The patient's arm is passively and forcibly fully elevated in the scapular plane with the arm medially rotated by the examiner (Fig. 4-29). A positive Neer impingement sign is present if pain is produced when the arm is forcibly flexed, jamming the greater tuberosity against the anteroinferior border of the acromion.[11]

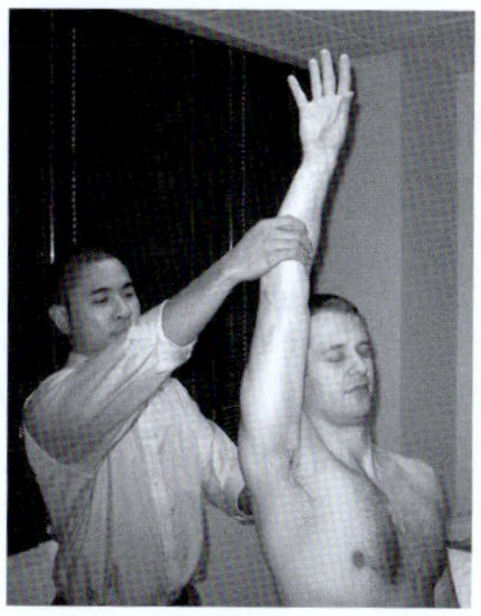

Figure 4-29

Hawkins-Kennedy Impingement Test

The examiner forward flexes the arm to 90° and then forcibly medially rotates the shoulder (Fig. 4-30). This movement pushes the supraspinatus tendon against the anterior surface of the coracoacromial ligament and coracoid process. Pain indicates a positive test result for supraspinatus tendinosis or secondary impingement.[11]

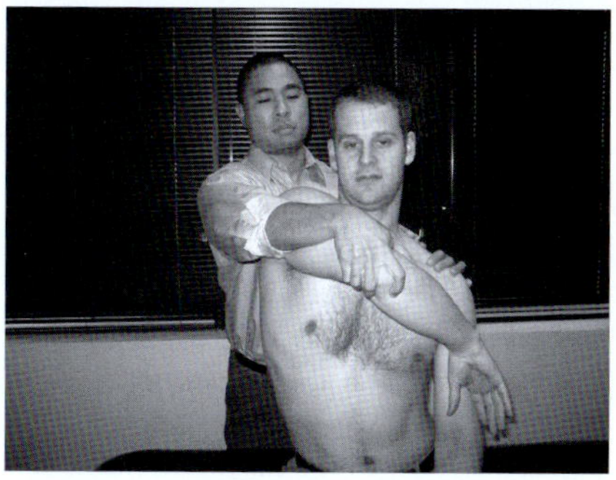

Figure 4-30

Yocum's Test

The patient's hand is placed on the opposite shoulder, and the elbow is actively elevated by the patient with some overpressure by the examiner (Fig. 4-31). Pain indicates a positive test result for supraspinatus tendinosis or secondary impingement.[11]

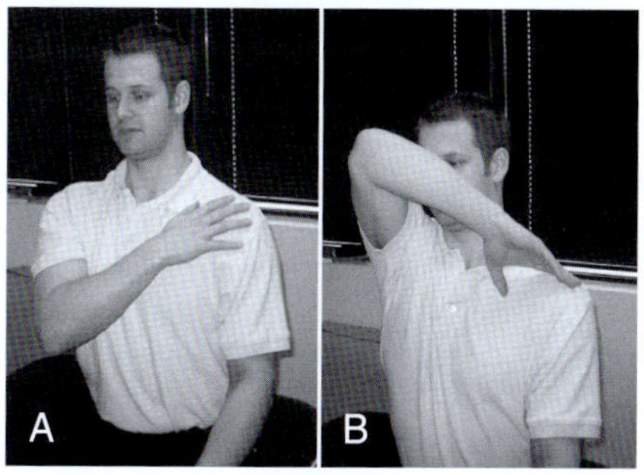

Figure 4-31

Rotator Cuff Disease Tests

Internal Rotation Lag Sign

The patient's hand is passively medially rotated and brought behind the back as far as possible (Fig. 4-32). The elbow is flexed at 90°, and the shoulder is held at 20° of elevation and 20° of extension. The patient is then asked to hold the position as the examiner releases the wrist while maintaining support at the elbow. The sign is considered positive when a lag occurs and the patient is unable to maintain maximum internal rotation and the hand moves toward the back. Inability to hold the position because of weakness or pain may indicate a lesion of the subscapularis muscle or tendon.[11,19]

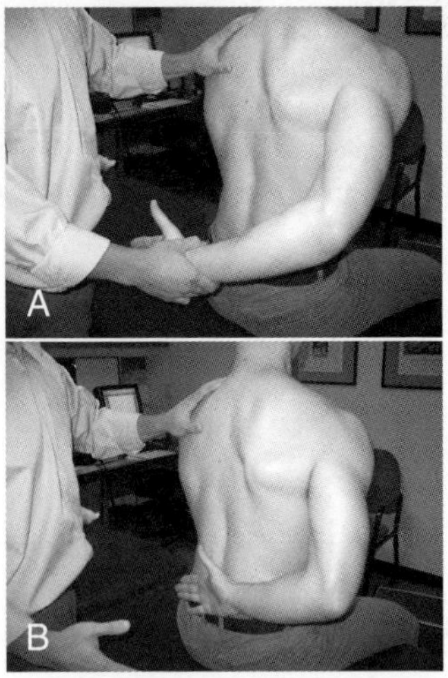

Figure 4-32

External Rotation Lag Sign

The patient's elbow is passively flexed to 90°, and the shoulder is held at 20° of elevation in the scapular plane (Fig. 4-33). The examiner then takes the patient's arm into maximum lateral rotation and asks the patient to hold the position as he or she releases the wrist while maintaining support at the elbow. If the supraspinatus and infraspinatus tendons are torn, the arm will medially rotate and spring back anteriorly, indicating a positive test result.[11,19]

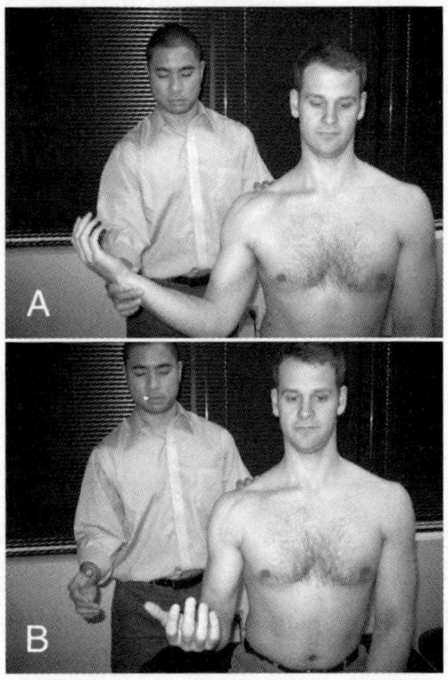

Figure 4-33

External Rotation Lag Sign at 90°

The examiner holds the affected arm at 90° of elevation in the scapular plane at maximal external rotation with the elbow flexed at 90° (Fig. 4-34). The patient is asked to maintain this position actively as the examiner releases the wrist while supporting the elbow. If the patient's hand springs forward and "drops" back to neutral rotation, the test result is considered positive for a lesion of the infraspinatus.[11,19]

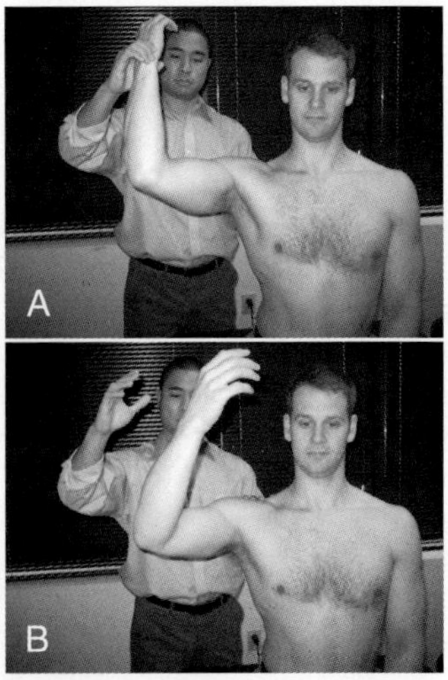

Figure 4-34

Bear Hug Test

The patient's fist is placed on their opposite shoulder, and the PT tries to lift the patient's wrist off the opposite shoulder while the patient resists (Fig. 4-35). Inability to hold the position because of weakness or pain may indicate a lesion of the subscapularis muscle or tendon.[20]

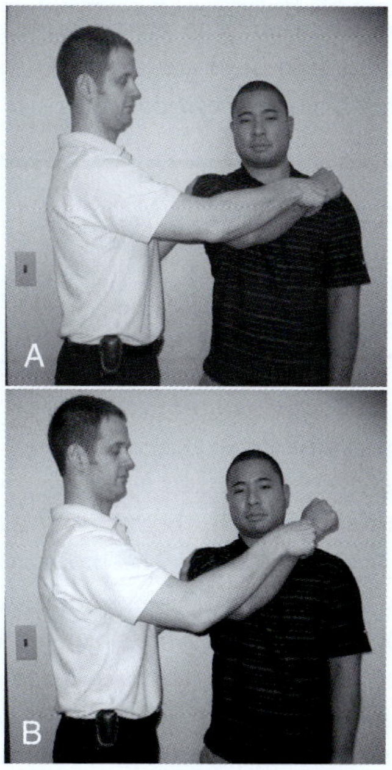

Figure 4-35

EVALUATION

Whereas the *examination* is the process of obtaining a history, performing a systems review, and selecting and administering tests and measures to gather data about a patient, the *evaluation* is the dynamic process in which the PT makes clinical judgments based on data gathered during the examination. Once the examination is complete, the PT must start the evaluation process.

The first objectives of the examination that must be answered are whether (1) PT intervention is appropriate; (2) consultation with another health care provider is appropriate; and (3) PT intervention is not indicated, and the patient should be managed by another provider.

The main purpose of the preceding examination is to determine a differential soft tissue diagnosis. The differential soft tissue diagnosis allows the PT to determine the specificity of the treatment approach. The foregoing assessment helps to determine the soft tissue barriers that limit mobility of the joint, specific muscle deficits and muscle restrictions, and the postural asymmetries of the scapula and glenohumeral joints.

The specificity of manual therapy depends on determining the direction of the restrictions in the soft tissue structures. As noted earlier, by assessing passive rotation of the glenohumeral joint, the PT can determine specific parts of the capsule that are restricted. The manual therapy techniques discussed in Chapter 13 are directed at the specific barriers in the soft tissue.

The manual muscle testing note just mentioned will help to determine the specific muscle deficits. The combination of passive testing, to determine the length of the tissue, and muscle testing, to determine strength, helps the PT to identify muscle imbalances. Muscle imbalances are identified by tightness in dysfunction of some muscles and soft tissue and weakness in some muscles, with increased extensibility of soft tissue structures. Based on the foregoing potential changes in the soft tissue structures, a change in posture of the scapula and glenohumeral joint can occur.

It is very important in the shoulder to maintain a central position of the humeral head on the glenoid. The large discrepancy between the size of the humeral head and the glenoid surface reinforces the importance of the central position. This issue is discussed further in Chapter 2. Tightness of the soft tissue structures and muscle imbalances change the position of the scapula. As the scapula changes position, it affects the central position of the humeral head on the glenoid.

Therefore, to assess the central position of the humerus on the glenoid and the ability of the glenohumeral and scapular rotators to maintain this position with movement, the PT needs to evaluate the following, as described earlier:

1. Scapula posture
2. Glenohumeral soft tissue extensibility
3. Strength of the rotator cuff muscles
4. Strength of the scapula rotators

Because few valid reported norms for shoulder mobility exist in the POS, the PT must compare the affected side with the unaffected side. A difference greater than 20% is considered an impairment. The more impairments a patient has, the greater the potential will be for a humeral head that is not in the central position.

While evaluating the strength of the glenohumeral and scapular rotators, the PT must understand that no reported studies of "normal strength" in any of these muscle groups exist. Again, a significant difference between the sides would warrant intervention. The greater number of muscle impairments would also indicate a greater potential for lack of humeral head central position.

The most successful treatment approach is to use manual therapy techniques to reduce the soft tissue restrictions and specific strengthening exercises to increase the strength deficits noted.

CASE STUDY 4.1

Examination Results

Chief Complaint

Ms. Smith is a 22-year-old female patient. She has a chief complaint comprising joint stiffness, joint swelling, muscle tenderness, muscle weakness, shoulder pain, and tingling.

History of Present Illness or Injury

The current problems began on 7/23/2009. The date of injury was 11/27/2006. The problems affect the left side. She is a swimmer of 15 years. Approximately 4 years ago, her shoulder started to hurt badly and was written off as shoulder tendinitis. It has become worse every year. These complaints are exacerbated by carrying, crawling, lifting, lying down, pulling, pushing, reaching, and running and sitting. The patient has the need for and interest in education, exercise, fitness, and prevention. The patient states that the pain at its best is 5 out of a rating scale of 10. The pain at its worst is 10 out of 10. The pain at present is 6 out of 10. According to the patient, the activities that make the symptoms worse are swimming, lifting, stretching, and any rotation of her arm. The activities that make the symptoms better are holding her arm closer to her body and supporting it. The patient's sleep is disturbed by this pain. The patient sleeps in the left side position. The patient has the following difficulties at school: pain. The patient has the following difficulties with recreational activities: cannot do anything with her left arm without pain afterward. The patient feels sore in the morning. The patient feels worse after moving about. The patient feels worse at the end of the day.

The patient is taking care of the problems through ice, naproxen (Aleve), and some exercises such as pendulums. The patient is under the care of an athletic trainer and orthopedist for these complaints.

Patient History

The patient has not experienced any recent weight change.

Examination Findings

Ms. Smith was seen at ABC PT for an evaluation on 12/17/2009. The examination findings are as follows:

Observation/Posture

Head forward: Yes
Shoulder forward: Left
Shoulder low: Left
Scapula abducted: Left
Scapula winging: Bilateral

Special Tests: Cervical Spine

Spurling's: Negative
Distraction: Negative

Supplemental Questions: Shoulder

Pain wakes from sleep: Yes
Pain/symptoms below elbow: No

Range of Motion: Shoulder

Shoulder Girdle Range of Motion (Active)

Right ROM		Left ROM
180	Elevation in scapular plane	150
90	External rotation in adducted position	35
120	External rotation in 90°/POS	110
45	Internal rotation in sleeper position	40

Manual Muscle Testing: Muscle Examination of the Shoulder

Shoulder Muscle Test

Right Dynamometer		Left Dynamometer
11	Supraspinatus	10
22	Infraspinatus	8
9	Subscapularis	9
9	Latissimus dorsi	8

Scapula Muscle Test

Right Dynamometer		Left Dynamometer
9	Serratus	6
9	Middle trapezius	5
13	Lower trapezius	9

Special Tests: Shoulder

Laxity and Instability Tests

Right Findings		Left Findings
Positive	Load and shift test	Positive
Negative	Sulcus sign test at 0°	Negative
Negative	Anterior apprehension test	Negative
Negative	Relocation test	Negative

Rotator Cuff Impingement Tests

Right Findings		Left Findings
Negative	Neer's impingement test	Positive
Negative	Hawkins-Kennedy test	Positive
Negative	Speed's test	Negative
Negative	Yocum's test	Negative

CASE STUDY 4.1—cont'd

Biceps and Labral Tests

Right Findings		Left Findings
Negative	O'Brien's test	Negative
Negative	Crank test	Negative
Negative	New pain provocation	Negative
Negative	Biceps load	Negative

Scores for the Patient

The SPADI total score is 104.00.

Score Category	Score
Pain score	39.00
Disability score	65.00
Total score	104.00
Pain score (%)	78.00
Disability score (%)	81.25
Total score (%)	80.00

Evaluation

- *Problem list/impairment*: Joint mobility, muscle strength, and pain.
- *Functional limitation*: Performance in leisure activities and performance in sport activities.
- *Clinical impression*: The patient presents with a significant decrease in scapular and glenohumeral rotator strength and decreased subscapularis mobility that are limiting her ability to perform her needed activities pain free.

Plan of Care

Short-Term Goals

All goals are short term secondary to the patient's returning to school in 3 weeks:

1. The patient's left external rotation in adduction will be greater than 60° in 3 weeks.
2. The patient's left shoulder strength will increase by 30% in 3 weeks.
3. The patient will be independent with a home exercise program in 3 weeks (frequency and duration: twice/week × 3 weeks).

Evaluation Process

The glenohumeral joint is a unique articulation that, under normal circumstances, maintains a balance between its large degree of mobility and its lack of inherent stability. For normal articular motion to occur, the joint depends heavily on the synergistic relationship between the dynamic and static stabilizers.[21] When this relationship is interrupted by injury or muscle imbalances about the shoulder, impingement of the glenohumeral joint may result. *Shoulder impingement* has been defined as compression and mechanical abrasion of the rotator cuff components as they pass beneath the coracoacromial arch during elevation of the arm.[22-25]

When exploring the relationship among clinical findings of limited passive external rotation in the adducted position, limited active elevation in the POS, and scapular asymmetry, positive impingement tests may be helpful in gaining an understanding of shoulder function and injury treatment. For the purpose of this chapter, *subscapularis syndrome* is defined as a constellation of signs and symptoms associated with the subscapularis muscle, glenohumeral joint dysfunction, and subacromial impingement.

Patients suffering from shoulder pain and stiffness often demonstrate common clinical signs such as limited passive glenohumeral external rotation in the adducted position, pain on palpation of trigger points that may be scar tissue within the subscapularis muscle belly or tendon, asymmetrical positioning of the scapula, muscle pain and weakness during the lift-off test for subscapularis syndrome, and positive impingement test results. All the foregoing signs may be associated with dysfunction of the subscapularis muscle and the glenohumeral joint.

An "obligatory" axial external rotation of the humerus is necessary to clear the greater tuberosity from the acromial arch and to accommodate the retroverted articular surface of the humerus, to gain an optimum position for glenoid contact and stability. Brems[26] reported that external rotation at the glenohumeral joint is possibly the most important functional motion that the shoulder complex allows. Most patients need a minimum of 45° of external rotation to maintain functional overhead movements and avoid subacromial impingement.

Many studies have focused on the supraspinatus and infraspinatus as the rotator cuff tendons most likely to be the sources of pain in subacromial impingement.[27,28] The subscapularis is often overlooked.[29] Although anatomically the subscapularis does not pass under the subacromial region, it has been shown to limit glenohumeral external rotation in the adducted position.[30] Turkel et al[6] reported that, during passive external rotation of the glenohumeral joint in 0° of abduction, the subscapularis muscle was the most important stabilizer.

The subscapularis is the largest of the four rotator cuff muscles, and it has a physiologic cross-sectional area two to three times the size of the remaining rotator cuff muscles.[12,13] The subscapularis originates in the subscapular fossa on the costal face of the scapula. The muscle arises from an anterior position on the scapular body and converges laterally to insert anteriorly into the lesser tuberosity of the humerus. One of the main functions of the subscapularis muscle is as a humeral depressor to counteract the superiorly directed shearing forces of the deltoid.[12] The subscapularis is an internal rotator of the shoulder and also an important stabilizer of the glenohumeral joint.

Weakness in the rotator cuff muscles induces loss of the force couple at the glenohumeral joint. This costs the rotator cuff muscles the ability to control the superior shear force of the humeral head effectively by contraction of the deltoid muscle during humeral elevation.[31] The consequence may be repetitive subacromial impingement of the humeral head. Another factor found to augment the superior shear force of the deltoid is elevation with the arm in internal rotation.[32] The internal rotation of the humerus was found to decrease the lever arm of the anterior and medial deltoid with a concomitant increase in its superior shear force with abduction.[32]

Many times, trigger points develop within the subscapularis muscle belly secondary to trauma or microtrauma and result in restrictions in external rotation in the neutral position and limited elevation at the glenohumeral joint. Travell and Simons[33] proposed that a trigger point within the subscapularis muscle may sensitize the other muscles of the shoulder girdle into developing secondary and satellite trigger points, leading to major restrictions in motion at the glenohumeral joint. Therefore, fibrosis or tears of the subscapularis may alter the resultant moment of adjacent muscles, as well as limit external rotation in the adducted position. Subscapularis fibrosis or tears should therefore be considered in the etiology of shoulder impingement. One study demonstrated a positive correlation between soft tissue mobilization with proprioceptive neuromuscular facilitation to the subscapularis muscle belly and an increase in external rotation and overhead reach.[34]

Clinically, over the past 5 to 10 years we have been observing a relationship between a loss of external rotation in the adducted position, scapula asymmetry, rotator cuff weakness, and signs and symptoms consistent with subacromial impingement have become apparent. Furthermore, concurrent patients have demonstrated nearly full external rotation in 90° of abduction, a finding implicating the subscapularis as the restricting tissue.

REFERENCES

1. Centers for Disease Control and Prevention National Center for Health Statistics: *Health, United States, 2007: with chartbook on trends in the health of Americans*, Hyattsville, Md, 2007, National Center for Health Statistics.
2. Jette D, Halbert J, Iverson C, et al: Use of standardized outcome measures in physical therapist practice: perceptions and applications, *Phys Ther* 89(2):125–135, 2009.
3. Roach KE, Budiman-Mak E, Songsiridej N, et al: Development of a shoulder pain and disability index, *Arthritis Care Res* 4 (4):143–149, 1991.
4. Agency for Healthcare Research and Quality: *Acute pain management guideline panel*, Rockville, Md, 1994, Agency for Healthcare Research and Quality.
5. Kebaetse M, McClure P, Pratt NA: Thoracic position effect on shoulder range of motion, strength, and three-dimensional scapular kinematics, *Arch Phys Med Rehabil* 80(8):945–950, 1999.
6. Turkel SJ, Panio MW, Marshall JL, et al: Stabilizing mechanisms preventing anterior dislocation of the glenohumeral joint, *J Bone Joint Surg Am* 63(8):1208–1217, 1981.
7. Izumi T, Aoki M, Muraki T, et al: Stretching positions for the posterior capsule of the glenohumeral joint: strain measurement using cadaver specimens, *Am J Sports Med* 36(10):2014–2022, 2008.
8. Ekstrom RA, Donatelli RA, Soderberg GL: Surface electromyographic analysis of exercises for the trapezius and serratus anterior muscles, *J Orthop Sports Phys Ther* 33:247–258, 2008.
9. Kendall FP, McCreary EK, Provance PG: *Muscles: testing and function*, Baltimore, 1993, Williams & Wilkins.
10. Kelly BT, Kadrmas WR, Speer KP: The manual muscle examination for rotator cuff strength: an electromyographic investigation, *Am J Sports Med* 24:581–588, 1996.
11. Magee DJ: *Orthopedic physical assessment*, ed 4, Philadelphia, 2002, Saunders.
12. Gerber C, Hersche O, Farron A: Isolated rupture of the subscapularis tendon, *J Bone Joint Surg Am* 78:1015–1023, 1996.
13. Greis PE, Kuhn JE, Schultheis J, et al: Validation of the lift-off test and analysis of subscapularis activity during maximal internal rotation, *Am J Sports Med* 24:589–593, 1996.
14. Hawkins RJ, Mohtadi NG: Clinical evaluation of shoulder instability, *Clin J Sports Med* 1:59–64, 1991.
15. O'Brien SJ, Pagnani MJ, Fealy S, et al: The active compression test: a new and effective test for diagnosing labral tears and acromioclavicular joint abnormality, *Am J Sports Med* 26:610–613, 1998.
16. Kim SH, Ha KI, Han KY: Biceps load test: a clinical test for superior labrum anterior and posterior lesions in shoulder with recurrent anterior dislocations, *Am J Sports Med* 27:300–303, 1999.
17. Mimori K, Menta T, Nakagawa T, et al: A new pain provocation test for superior labral tears of the shoulder, *Am J Sports Med* 27(2):137–142, 1999.
18. Wilk KE, Reinold MM, Dugas JR, et al: Current concepts in the recognition and treatment of superior labral (SLAP) lesions, *J Orthop Sports Physical Ther* 35(5):273–291, 2005.
19. Tennent TD, Beach WR, Meyers J: Clinical sports medicine update. a review of the special tests associated with shoulder examination. Part I. The rotator cuff tests, *Am J Sports Med* 31:154–160, 2003.
20. Barth JR, Burkhart SS, De Beer JF: The bear hug test: a new and sensitive test for diagnosing a subscapularis tear, *Arthroscopy* 22(10):1076–1084, 2006.
21. Matsen FA 3rd, Harryman DT 2nd, Sidles JA: Mechanics of glenohumeral instability, *Clin Sports Med* 10(4):783–788, 1991.
22. Hannafin J, Griffin L, Garrick J: Adhesive capsulitis: a treatment approach, *Clin Orthop Relat Res* 372:95–109, 2000.
23. Hawkins RJ, Kennedy JC: Impingement syndrome in athletes, *Am J Sports Med* 8(3):151–157, 1980.
24. Matsen FA 3rd: Stabilization of the glenohumeral joint: overview and directions for future research. In Matsen FA 3rd, Fu FH, Hawkins RJ, editors: *The shoulder: a balance of mobility and stability*, Rosemont, Ill, 1993, American Academy of Orthopaedic Surgeons, pp 3–5.
25. Neer CS 2nd: Impingement lesions, *Clin Orthop Relat Res* 173:70–77, 1983.
26. Brems JJ: Rehabilitation following total shoulder arthroplasty, *Clin Orthop Relat Res* 307:70–85, 1994.

27. Budoff J, Nirschl R, Guidi EJ: Debridement of partial-thickness tears of the rotator cuff without acromioplasty: long-term follow-up and review of the literature, *J Bone Joint Surg Am* 80 (5):733–748, 1998.
28. Codman EA: *The shoulder: rupture of the supraspinatus tendon and lesions in or about the subacromial bursa*, Boston, 1934, Thomas Todd, pp 262–312.
29. Inman VT, Saunders JB, Abbott LC: Observations on the function of the shoulder joint: 1944, *Clin Orthop Relat Res* 330:3–12, 1996.
30. Neer CS 2nd: Anterior acromioplasty for the chronic impingement syndrome in the shoulder: a preliminary report, *J Bone Joint Surg Am* 54(1):41–55, 1972.
31. Kamkar A, Irrgang JJ, Whitney SL: Nonoperative management of secondary shoulder impingement syndrome, *J Orthop Sport Phys Ther* 17(5):212–224, 1993.
32. Saha AK: Dynamic stability of the glenohumeral joint, *Acta Orthop Scand* 42(6):491–505, 1971.
33. Travell J, Simons DG: *Myofascial pain and dysfunction: the trigger point manual*, Baltimore, 1993, Williams & Wilkins, pp 410–424.
34. Godges J, Mattson-Bell M, Thorpe D, et al: The immediate effects of soft tissue mobilization with proprioceptive neuromuscular facilitation on glenohumeral external rotation and overhead reach, *J Orthop Sports Phys Ther* 33(12):713–718, 2003.

PART 2
NEUROLOGIC CONSIDERATIONS

CHAPTER

5

John C. Gray and Ola Grimsby

Interrelationship of the Spine, Rib Cage, and Shoulder

One of the most difficult and challenging aspects of the orthopedic physical therapist's work is to determine the primary tissue responsible for a patient's complaints of pain, or the nociceptive generator. This is particularly true when evaluating the shoulder. Pain and dysfunction in the shoulder may arise from intrinsic pathologic conditions in the shoulder or extrinsic pathologic conditions in the spine, rib cage, or viscera. The clinician needs to recognize that pain may be referred directly to the shoulder from cervical, thoracic, or rib injuries, and that dysfunctions anywhere in the spine or rib cage can precipitate and exacerbate shoulder dysfunction. For these reasons, an understanding of the interrelationships among the spine, ribs, and shoulder is important. Central sensitization also plays an important role in the maintenance of chronic shoulder pain and dysfunction. This chapter reviews the musculoskeletal, biomechanical, postural, occupational, and neurologic relationships among the spine, ribs, and shoulder. It also briefly reviews musculoskeletal syndromes that contribute to pain and dysfunction in the shoulder. In addition, the chapter reviews spine and rib injuries that can cause shoulder pain and dysfunction. Finally, this chapter closes with a case study to illustrate the important preceding concepts.

MUSCULOSKELETAL RELATIONSHIP

One of the most direct relationships between the spine and the shoulder girdle is through muscle, tendon, and fascial attachments. Seven muscles of the shoulder, the rotator cuff group in addition to the deltoid, teres major, and latissimus dorsi, are thought to be related morphologically to the spine. They appear to originate from cervical myotomes.[1]

Shoulder Muscles and Fascia with a Direct Relationship with the Spine

The trapezius muscle originates from the medial third of the superior nuchal line and the external protuberance of the occipital bone. The muscle also extends from the ligamentum nuchae, the spinous processes of the seventh cervical vertebra and all the thoracic vertebrae, and the intervening supraspinal ligament (Fig. 5-1).[2,3] This muscle inserts on the lateral third of the clavicle, the medial border of the acromion, and the upper border of the crest of the spine of the scapula.[2,3] The trapezius assists in suspension of the shoulder girdle, in pulling or extension movements of the arm, in abduction of the arm, and in upward rotation of the scapula.[2,3] With the shoulder fixed, the trapezius may bend the head and neck posteriorly and laterally.[2,3]

The latissimus dorsi muscle originates medially from tendinous fibers that attach to the lower six thoracic spines. The muscle also originates from the thoracolumbar fascia, which has attachments to the lumbar and sacral spines, the supraspinous ligaments, and the posterior portion of the iliac crest (see Fig. 5-1).[2,3] It also originates, by muscular attachments, from the outer lip of the iliac crest, the lower three or four ribs, and the inferior angle of the scapula.[2,3] This broad muscle subsequently inserts into the floor of the intertubercular groove of the humerus.[2,3] The latissimus dorsi muscle is active in adduction, extension, and medial rotation of the humerus.[2,3] It helps to support the weight of the body during ambulation on crutches and is typically active during swimming, pulling movements, coughing, sneezing, and deep inspiration.[2,3]

The levator scapulae muscle originates by four separate tendons from the transverse processes of the first three or four cervical vertebrae.[2,3] The origin of this muscle often has various accessory attachments that may include the mastoid process, occipital bone, first or second rib, scaleni, trapezius, and serrate muscles.[3] It inserts into the medial border of the scapula from the superior angle to the spine.[2,3] The levator scapulae works with the rhomboids to control scapula motion and to stabilize the position of the scapula. The levator scapulae, working with the rhomboids and pectoralis minor muscles, assists in the downward rotation and depression of the scapula. It works with the trapezius and assists in elevation of the scapula.[3] With the distal attachments to the scapula fixed, the levator scapulae produces ipsilateral side bending of the cervical spine.[3]

The rhomboideus minor muscle originates from the lower part of the ligamentum nuchae, the spinous process of the last cervical and first thoracic vertebrae, and the associated segment of the supraspinal ligament.[2,3] It inserts into the medial border of the scapula at the root of the scapular spine.[2,3] The rhomboideus major muscle originates from the spinous processes of the second to the fifth thoracic vertebrae and the corresponding segment of the supraspinous ligament.[2,3] It inserts into the medial border of the scapula below its spine.[2,3] The rhomboideus minor and major muscles work together with the serratus anterior muscle to hold the scapula firmly to the chest wall.[2,3] The trapezius and rhomboid muscles are the primary movers for scapula retraction.[2,3] Rotating and depressing the scapula require the coordinated efforts of the rhomboids, levator scapulae, and pectoralis minor muscles.[2,3]

The deep cervical fascia, internal to platysma, is fibroareolar tissue between muscles, viscera, and vessels.[3] Its superficial layer is continuous with the ligamentum nuchae and the periosteum of the seventh cervical spine.[3] It covers the trapezius and sternocleidomastoid (SCM) muscles and adheres to the symphysis menti and the body of the hyoid bone.[3] The deep fascia is attached to the acromion, clavicle, and manubrium sterni, and it fuses with their periostea (Fig. 5-2).[3]

Shoulder Muscles with a Direct Relationship with the Rib Cage

The SCM muscle originates from the lateral aspect of the mastoid process and, by a thin aponeurosis, the lateral half of the superior nuchal line (Fig. 5-3).[3] It inserts into the upper anterior surface of the manubrium sterni and the medial third of the clavicle.[3] The SCM muscle side bends the head

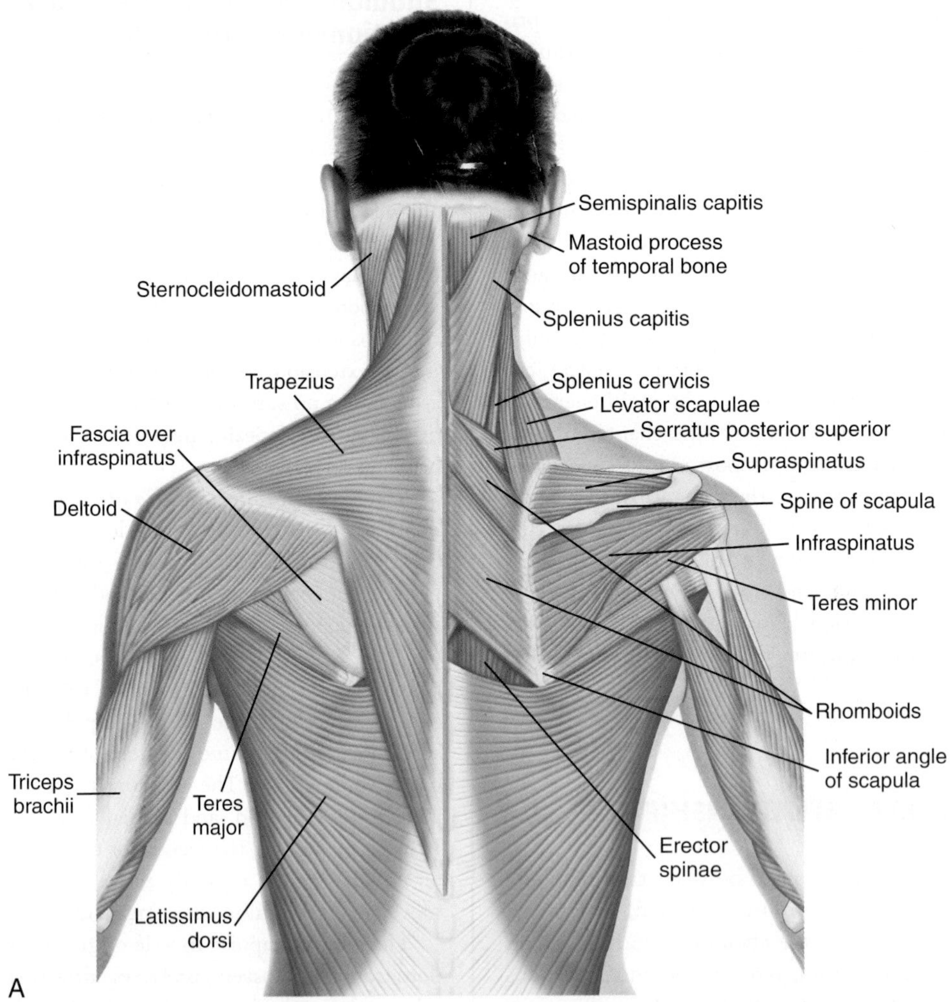

Figure 5-1 Views of the shoulder girdle region. **A,** Posterior view. The left side is superficial; the right side is deep (the deltoid, trapezius, sternocleidomastoid, and infraspinatus fascia have been removed).

Continued

ipsilaterally and rotates it contralaterally.[3] It also assists in flexion of the cervical spine.[3] With the head fixed, the muscles work together to aid thoracic elevation and inspiration.[3]

The suprahyoid muscles (i.e., digastric, stylohyoid, mylohyoid, and geniohyoid) are important in that they work in coordination with the infrahyoid muscles (i.e., sternohyoid, sternothyroid, thyrohyoid, and omohyoid), which have direct attachments to the shoulder girdle (see Fig. 5-3).[3] The suprahyoid muscles are active in mandibular depression, hyoid elevation, swallowing, and chewing.[3] The infrahyoid muscles are active in hyoid depression, elevation and depression of the larynx, speech, and mastication.[3] The omohyoid, one of the infrahyoid muscles, has two bellies that meet at an angle as an intermediate tendon (see Figs. 5-1 to 5-3). The superior belly originates from the lower border of the hyoid bone and descends into the intermediate tendon.[3] This tendon is ensheathed by a band of deep cervical fascia that descends to the clavicle and first rib.[3] The inferior belly descends from this tendon to attach to the upper scapular border, near the scapular notch, and occasionally to the superior transverse scapular ligament.[3] Its actions include hyoid depression during prolonged inspiratory efforts and tensing of the lower deep cervical fascia.[3]

The pectoralis major muscle originates from the sternal half of the clavicle, a region approximating the first through seventh ribs along half of the anterior sternum and costal cartilages, and the aponeurosis of the abdominal external oblique (see Fig. 5-1).[2-4] Variations include a slip of muscle that blends in with the SCM. The insertion site for this muscle is the lateral lip of the intertubercular sulcus along the upper anterior portion of the humerus.[2-4] The pectoralis major muscle primarily adducts and internally rotates the humerus. It can also assist in flexion of the shoulder, in deep inspiration, and in supporting the weight of the body during ambulation on crutches.[2-4]

The pectoralis minor muscle originates from the superior margins and outer surfaces of ribs three to five (sometimes ribs two to four) near the cartilage and from the fascia overlying the respective intercostal muscles (see Fig. 5-1).[2-4] The insertion sites for this muscle are the medial border and superior surface of the coracoid process of the scapula.[2-4] Variations include insertion extending along the coracoacromial ligament or along the coracohumeral ligament to the humerus. The pectoralis minor muscle primarily tilts the scapula anteriorly and assists the serratus anterior in bringing the scapula forward around the thorax. Along with the levator scapulae and the rhomboids, the pectoralis minor assists in rotating the scapula and depressing the shoulder.[2-4] The pectoralis minor muscle may also assist in extreme inspiration.

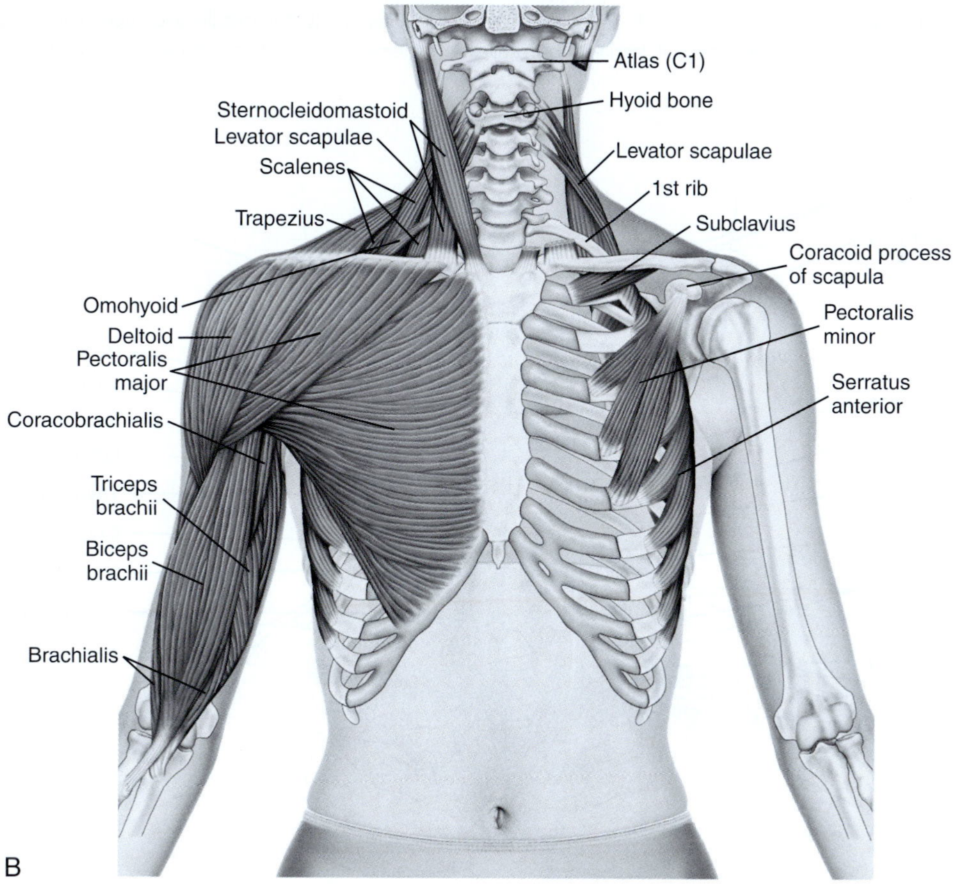

Figure 5-1 Cont'd B, Anterior view. The right side is superficial. The left side is deep (the deltoid, pectoralis major, trapezius, scalenes, omohyoid, and muscles of the arm have been removed; the sternocleidomastoid has been cut). (From Muscolino JE: *The muscle and bone palpation manual: with trigger points, referral patterns, and stretching,* St. Louis, 2009, Mosby Elsevier.)

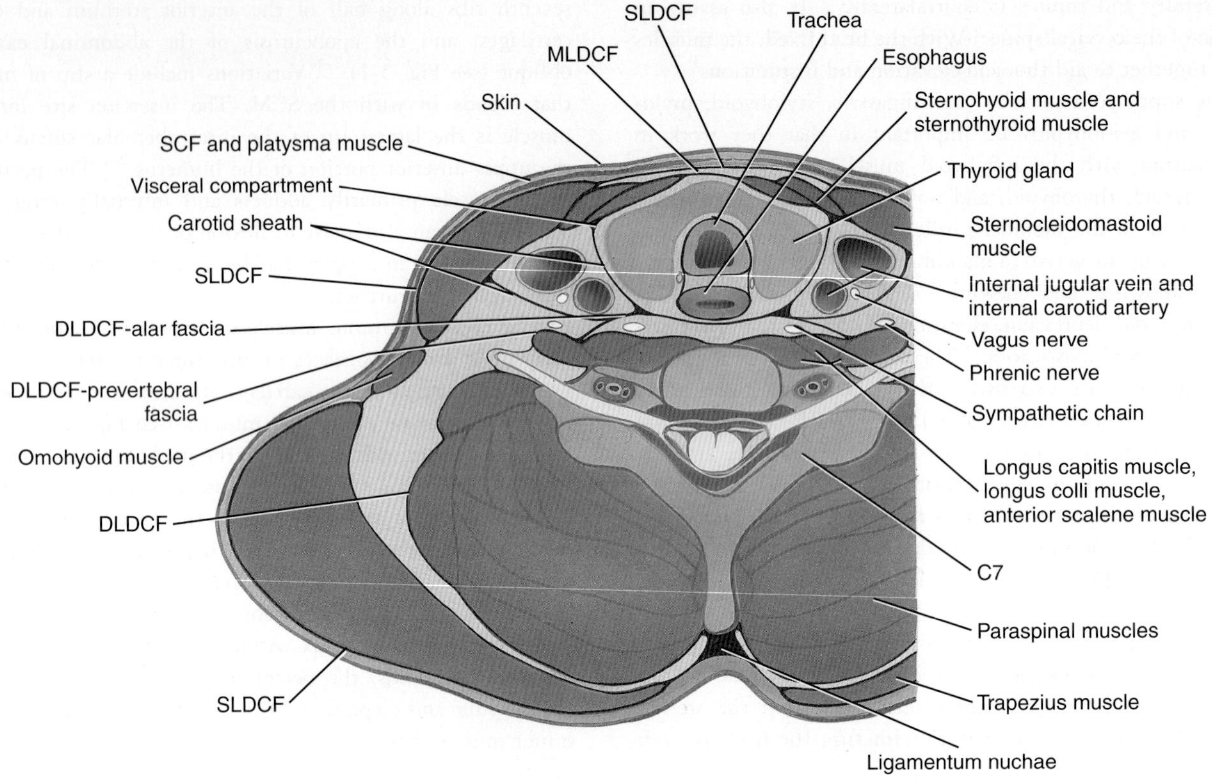

Figure 5-2 Axial view of neck at the level of C7. DLDCF, deep layer, deep cervical fascia; MLDCF, middle layer, deep cervical fascia; SCF, superficial cervical fascia; SLDCF, superficial layer, deep cervical fascia. (From Kelley L, Petersen CM: *Sectional anatomy for imaging professionals,* ed 2, St. Louis, 2007, Mosby Elsevier.)

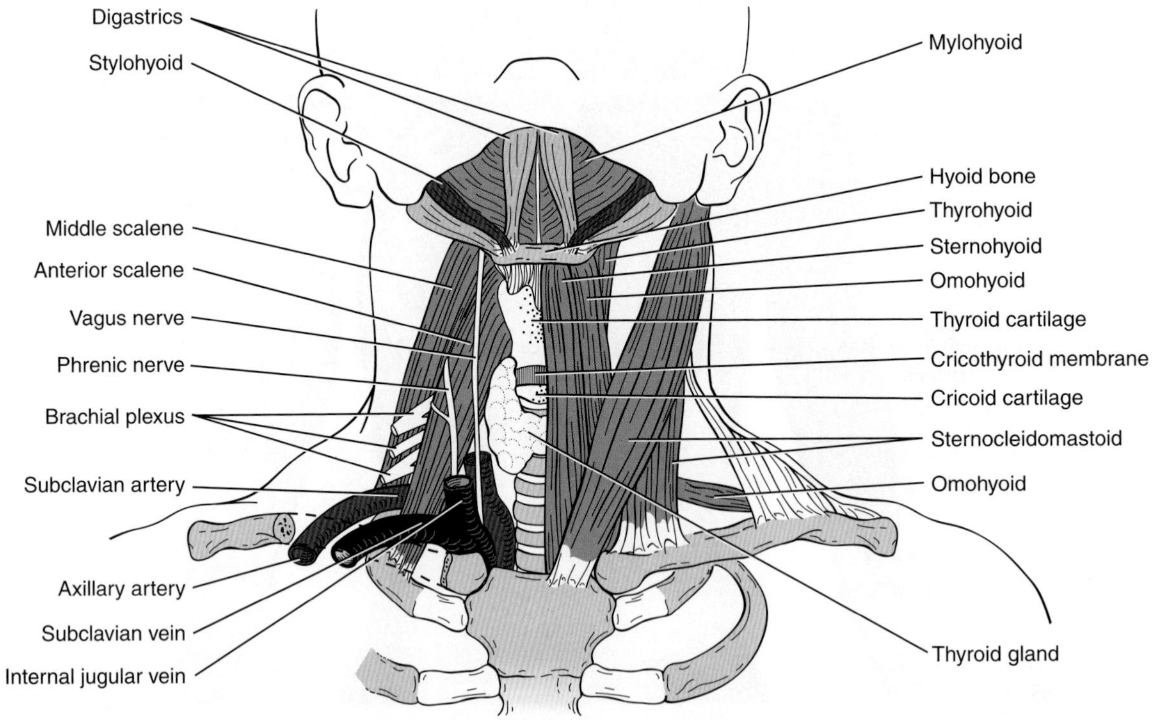

Figure 5-3 Anterior view of the neck. Superficial muscles and the clavicle are omitted on the right side of the illustration to reveal deeper structures. Branches of the subclavian and axillary arteries are not illustrated. (From Jenkins DB: *Hollinshead's functional anatomy of the limbs and back,* ed 9, St. Louis, 2009, Saunders Elsevier.)

The subclavius muscle originates from the junction of the first rib and its cartilage, anterior to the costoclavicular ligament, and inserts on the inferior surface of the middle third of the clavicle (see Fig. 5-1).[2,3] Variations include insertion extending to the coracoid process. The subclavius muscle may participate in pulling the shoulder down and forward. It may also be active in stabilizing the clavicle against the sternoclavicular disk.[2,3]

The serratus anterior muscle originates from the outer surfaces and superior borders of the upper 8 to 10 ribs (see Fig. 5-1).[2-4] Variations include a blended origin with the external intercostals or the abdominal external oblique muscle. A blended insertion with the levator scapulae muscle has also been noted. The insertion site for this muscle is the costal surface of the medial border of the scapula.[2-4] The serratus anterior muscle primarily abducts and rotates the scapula so that the glenoid fossa faces superiorly. This muscle also assists in elevation or depression, is able to move the thorax posteriorly when the humerus is fixed (push-up), and may assist in forced inspiration.[2-4]

The platysma is a broad muscular sheet that spreads from its fascial attachments over the upper parts of the pectoralis major and deltoid muscles and ascends medially across the clavicle to the side of the neck.[3] Attachment sites include the symphysis menti, the lower border of the mandibular body, the lateral half of the lower lip, and muscles at the modiolus near the buccal angle.[3] The platysma wrinkles the nuchal skin obliquely. It also may assist in mandibular depression, helps to express horror and surprise, is active in sudden deep inspiration, and is notably contracted in sudden and violent efforts.[3]

Fascia of the Shoulder with a Direct Relationship with the Rib Cage

The clavipectoral fascia, underneath the clavicular portion of the pectoralis major, fills in the gap between the pectoralis minor and subclavius muscles.[2,3] The fascial attachments include the following: the clavicle, by surrounding the subclavius muscle and blending with the deep cervical fascia that connects the omohyoid to the clavicle; the first rib and the fascia over the first two intercostal spaces; the coracoid process; and the axillary fascia.[2,3] Special features of this fascia include the following: the costocoracoid membrane, which lies superior and medial to the pectoralis minor muscle; the costocoracoid ligament, with attachments from the coracoid process to the first rib; and the suspensory ligament of the axilla, which lies inferior and lateral to the pectoralis minor muscle.[2,3] The axillary fascia blends with the fascia of the serratus anterior muscle and the brachial fascia.[2] This fascia blends anteriorly with the pectoral and clavipectoral fascia; it blends posteriorly with the fascia of the scapula muscles.[2]

Bones of the Shoulder with a Direct Relationship with the Rib Cage

Clavicle

The clavicle is attached to the rib cage by fascia (as noted earlier), the sternoclavicular joint capsule, and associated ligaments (Fig. 5-4).[5] The sternoclavicular joint is sellar and contains a fibrocartilaginous disk. Ligamentous attachments

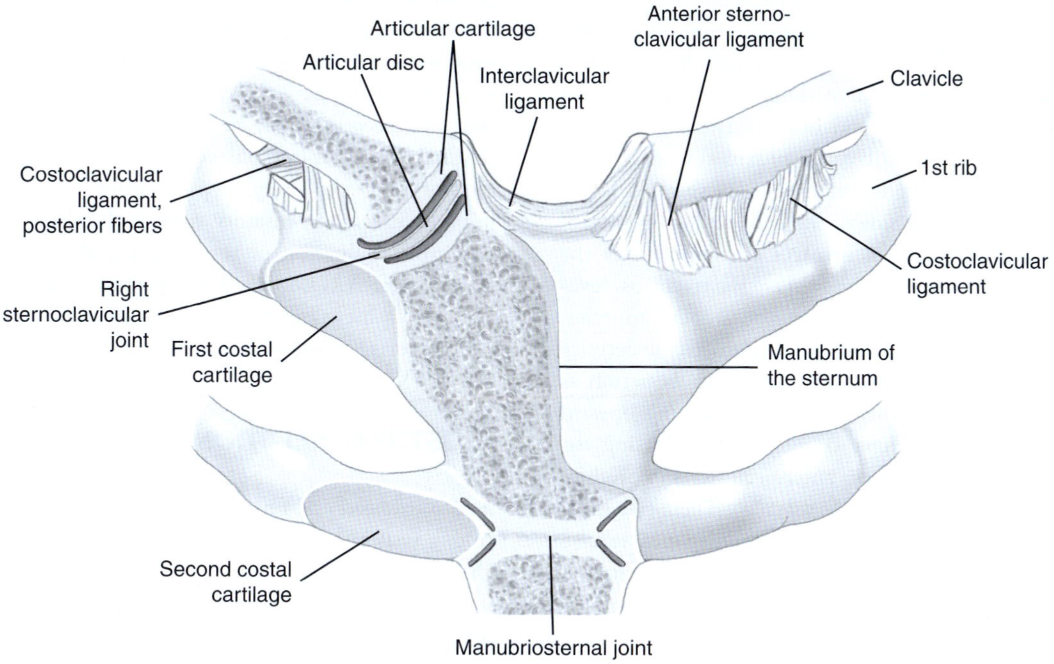

Figure 5-4 Anterior view of the sternoclavicular (SC) joints. The right joint is shown in a frontal (i.e., coronal) section; the left joint is left intact. The SC joint is stabilized by its fibrous capsule, the anterior and posterior SC ligaments, the interclavicular ligament, and the costoclavicular ligament. (From Muscolino JE: Kinesiology: *The skeletal system and muscle function*, 2nd edition, St. Louis, 2011, Mosby.)

of the clavicle to the sternum and first rib include the following: the anterior and posterior sternoclavicular ligaments; the interclavicular ligament, which is continuous with the deep cervical fascia; and the costoclavicular ligament, which attaches to the first rib and its costal cartilage.[5]

Scapula

The scapulothoracic articulation, although not a true joint, has been described as a functional joint because of its close interaction with the rib cage.[6] The main components between the scapula and the ribs (ribs two to seven in the resting position) are the scapulothoracic bursa, the serratus anterior muscle, and the subscapularis muscle.[6] The scapula does, however, have direct fascial and ligamentous connections to the rib cage: the costocoracoid membrane and the costocoracoid ligament (see Fig. 5-4).

BIOMECHANICAL RELATIONSHIP

The shoulder is designed to be extremely mobile. One of its primary functions is to allow the hands to be used to their greatest advantage. All movements of the shoulder involve the direct or indirect participation of the cervical, thoracic, and lumbar spine, and ribs. Most of the movement of the shoulder occurs between the head of the humerus and the glenoid fossa, with notable and important contributions from the sternoclavicular, acromioclavicular, and scapulothoracic joints. What is often less appreciated is the motion that must occur throughout the spine and rib cage to allow the shoulder and upper extremity to attain the maximum amount of reach possible. Clinicians must realize that the spine (cervical to lumbar) and ribs are not held completely rigid during active flexion or abduction of the arm. Although it is well known that distal mobility (shoulder and upper extremity) requires proximal stability (spine and rib cage), proximal stability does not preclude carefully controlled motion of the spine and ribs.

Lifting the arm from the side of the body and up overhead, *abduction* (normal range, 180°), involves all the joints of the shoulder. The primary muscles involved are the trapezius, levator scapulae, serratus anterior, deltoid, and rotator cuff muscles. The rhomboid major and minor muscles simulate the activity of the middle trapezius and are most active in abduction as stabilizing synergists by eccentric contraction during upward rotation of the scapula.[7] A force couple is formed using the upper trapezius and upper serratus anterior muscles to produce upward rotation and elevation of the scapula.[7] These two muscle segments, in concert with the levator scapulae muscle, also support the shoulder against the downward pull of gravity.[7] A second force couple, active in the same task, uses the lower trapezius and lower serratus anterior muscles.[7]

Besides the activity of muscles originating from the spine, direct involvement of the joints of the spine occurs with end-range (usually greater than 150°) abduction. As the shoulder and arm are abducted beyond approximately 150°, one sees a component motion of contralateral side bending (usually coupled with rotation in the opposite direction) and extension of the thoracic spine.[8] When both arms are abducted, a necessary increase in the lumbar lordosis occurs through activity of the lumbar erector spinae muscles.[8] Lumbar lordosis may also be increased secondary to a tight latissimus dorsi muscle. Full flexion of the shoulder is usually achieved in concert with extension of the thoracic and lumbar spine and with some degree of elevation and expansion of the ribs toward the end of range of motion (ROM). Persons with adhesive capsulitis, or other chronic conditions that limit shoulder mobility, necessarily put more stress on regions of their spine (cervical, thoracic, and lumbar) and ribs to achieve the ROM they need for a particular task. When any particular task is repeated over and over in this manner, hypermobilities or overuse injuries may occur in the spine or ribs. The thoracolumbar junction, especially during repeated overhead activities, is particularly vulnerable to overuse stress in this manner. During functional activities of daily living (ADLs), the mobility of the spine and ribs is as important as mobility of the shoulder for a particular task or activity to be successful. If normal mobility is not present in the spine and ribs, then more stress may be directed at the shoulder to complete the task. Again, if any particular task is repeated over and over in this manner, hypermobilities, impingement, or overuse injuries (bicipital or rotator cuff tendinosis) may occur in the shoulder.

To ensure full functional recovery of the shoulder and to prevent future overuse or overstrain injuries, the clinician must treat all relevant spine and rib dysfunctions that may be placing excessive stress and strain on the tissues of the shoulder. It is not enough simply to measure the gross osteokinematic motion of the shoulder. One must also know how the shoulder achieves its end ROM. The clinician also needs to know what is happening arthrokinematically in the relevant joints of the spine and ribs. Even though the patient may appear to have normal active ROM (AROM) at the shoulder, he or she may have thoracic and rib hypomobilities that have resulted in the development of glenohumeral hypermobility or, conversely, hypomobility in the glenohumeral joint with compensatory thoracolumbar hypermobility. A simple evaluation of the patient's ability to achieve full goniometric AROM in a static posture is not sufficient. The ability to achieve full functional ROM during repeated ADLs, work, sports, and hobbies should also be of great concern.

POSTURAL RELATIONSHIP

A forward head and rounded shoulder posture can be common among healthy persons who do not have physical complaints.[9] Unfortunately, poor posture can also be a source of neck and shoulder pain.[9-13] Normal postural alignment, starting at the external auditory meatus of the skull, allows a line of gravity to pass through the odontoid process, anterior to the axis of motion for flexion and extension of the occiput, posterior to the midcervical spine, through the glenohumeral joint, anterior to the thoracic spine, and posterior to the lumbar spine (Fig. 5-5).[14]

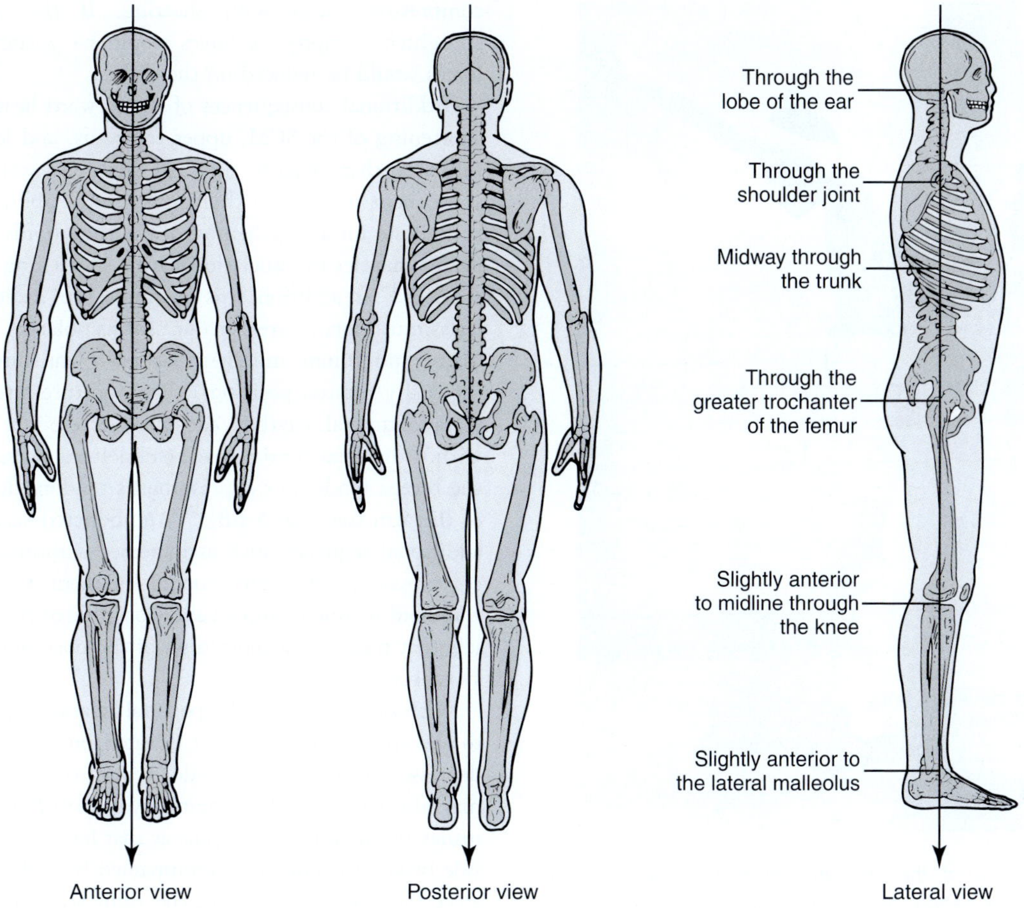

Figure 5-5 Ideal standing posture. Anterior, posterior, and lateral views. (From Cameron MH, Monroe LG: *Physical rehabilitation: evidence-based examination, evaluation, and intervention,* St. Louis, 2008, Saunders Elsevier.)

In a person with good postural alignment, elevation of the arm is free to proceed through a full 160° to 180° of motion without impingement of soft tissues in the subacromial space (Fig. 5-6A). In the patient with the classic forward head, rounded shoulders, and increased thoracic kyphosis, the scapula rotates forward and downward, thus depressing the acromion process and changing the direction of the glenoid fossa. As that patient attempts to elevate the arm, the supraspinatus tendon or the subdeltoid bursa may become impinged against the anterior portion of the acromion process (see Fig. 5-6B). Repeated motions of this nature may accelerate overuse injuries or cumulative trauma disorders (CTDs) and may lead to early changes consistent with tendinosis or bursitis.[15] At least one study found a significant relationship between severe thoracic kyphosis and interscapular pain, between forward head and interscapular pain, and between rounded shoulders and interscapular pain.[9]

Sitting postures with the whole spine flexed result in high levels of electromyographic (EMG) activity in the neck and shoulder muscles. Neck and shoulder muscle activity is lowest in a sitting posture of slight thoracolumbar extension with a vertical cervical spine (Fig. 5-7A and B).[16] Standing postures associated with a forward head demonstrate an increase in cervical and lumbar lordosis and an increase in thoracic kyphosis. In addition, the forward head posture forces the midcervical spine into hyperextension, with subsequent narrowing of the intervertebral foramina and increased weight bearing of the facet joints, especially at the C4-5 and C5-6 segments (Fig. 5-7C).[11,17] This situation may lead to irritation of the C5 and C6 spinal nerve roots, respectively.[11,17,18] It may also lead to irritation of the dorsal root of C1, vertebral artery symptoms, or entrapment of the suprascapular and dorsal scapular nerves.[19] Headaches are a common sequela of chronic poor posture. One source of these headaches is the increased stress on the C2-3 facet joints and the associated intervertebral foramen. Headaches originating from the C2-3 facet joints or the C3 dorsal ramus are fairly common in patients with chronic neck pain and headaches.[20,21]

The cervical facet joints are at risk because of the increased weight-bearing stress encountered in the forward head posture. The articular cartilage, synovial capsule, and meniscoid of the facet joint are exposed to persistent and recurrent trauma.[22] This trauma may lead to arthritic changes and restrictions within the involved joints.[22] Any injury or irritation to these facet joints contributes, through type I mechanoreceptor damage, to disorders involving the static postural reflexes of the spine and upper extremities.[23,24] Finally, the intervertebral disks are put at risk because of the increase in shearing as a result of increased cervical lordosis (see Fig. 5-7C). The normal lordosis in the cervical spine allows for an adequate balance of

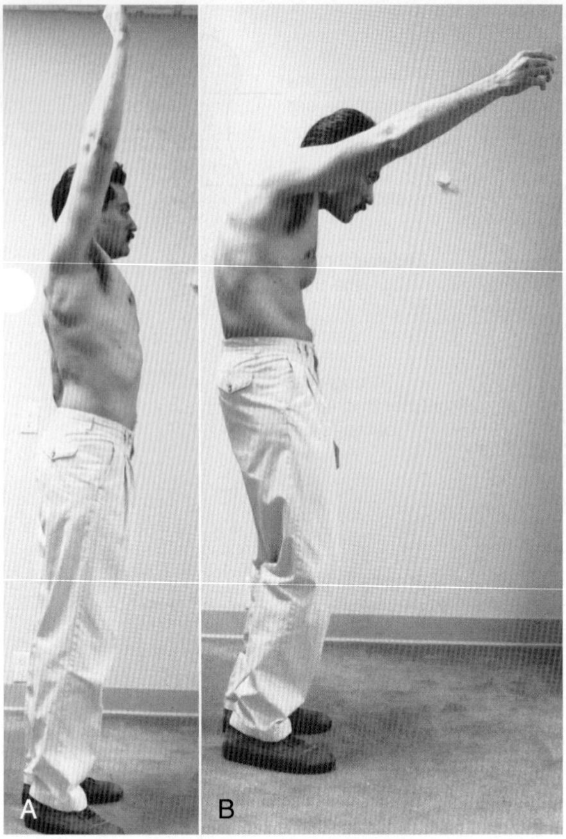

Figure 5-6 Elevation of the arm. **A,** Person with good postural alignment. **B,** Same person, now demonstrating the effect of poor posture on elevation of the arm.

compressive forces with shearing. If the spine were to straighten, compressive forces would be greater and shearing forces would be reduced on the disks.

Additional consequences of the forward head posture are a shortening of the SCM, upper trapezius, and levator scapulae muscles that results in an elevated scapula.[19,25] The subsequent increase in thoracic kyphosis abducts the scapula and allows for a lengthening of the rhomboids and lower trapezius muscles in association with a shortening of the serratus anterior.[19] In addition, this posture causes a shortening of the latissimus dorsi, teres major, subscapularis, and pectoralis major and minor muscles that pulls the humerus into an internally rotated position.[19] This posture alters the normal scapulohumeral rhythm and may precipitate impingement within the subacromial space (subdeltoid bursa, long head of the biceps tendon, or supraspinatus tendon) during elevation of the arm (see Fig. 5-6B).[19] An abducted scapula may have additional sequelae, such as increased acromioclavicular joint compression, a shortened conoid ligament with a lengthened trapezoid ligament, and an anterior glide of the proximal clavicle that results in a shortening of the posterior capsule of the sternoclavicular joint.[19]

Scoliosis also affects the postural relationship of the scapula to the spine. The scapula is elevated on the convex side and depressed on the concave side of the scoliosis.[14] The patient may also have a slight winging over a rib hump secondary to ipsilateral rotation of the spine at that level.[14] For example, left side bending is normally accompanied by right rotation in the erect thoracic spine, so that the right scapula is elevated and winged slightly.

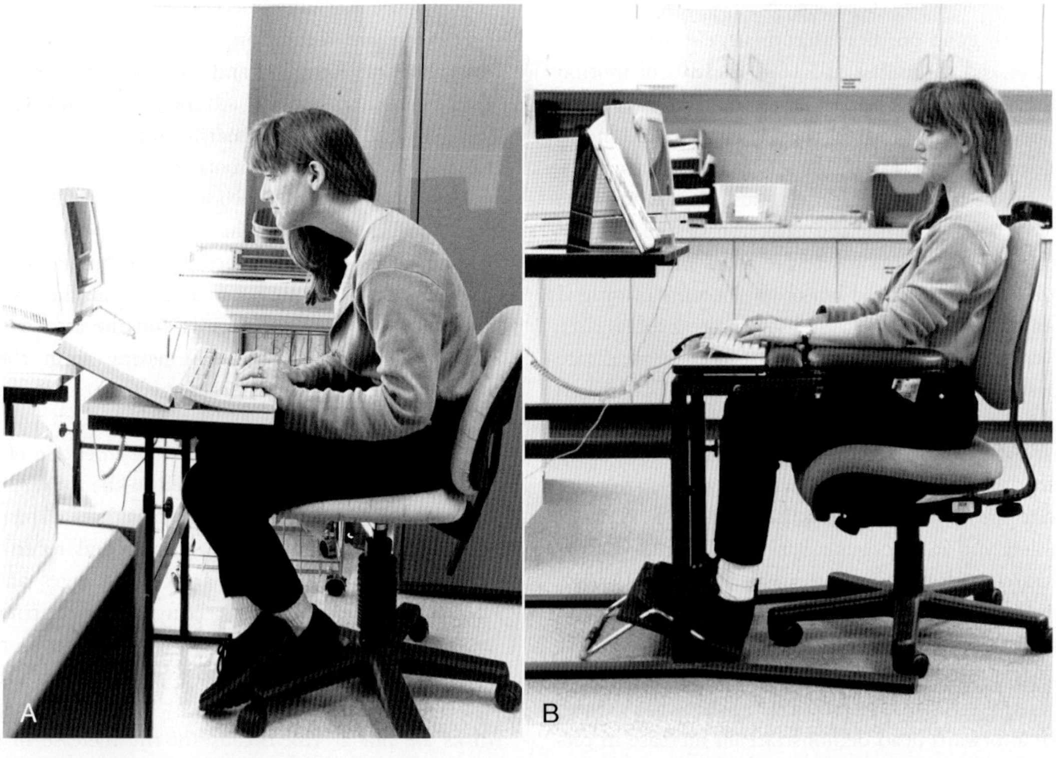

Figure 5-7 Sitting postures. **A,** Poor sitting posture at a workstation. **B,** Good postural alignment with the appropriate use of ergonomic design for a person seated at a visual display terminal.

Continued

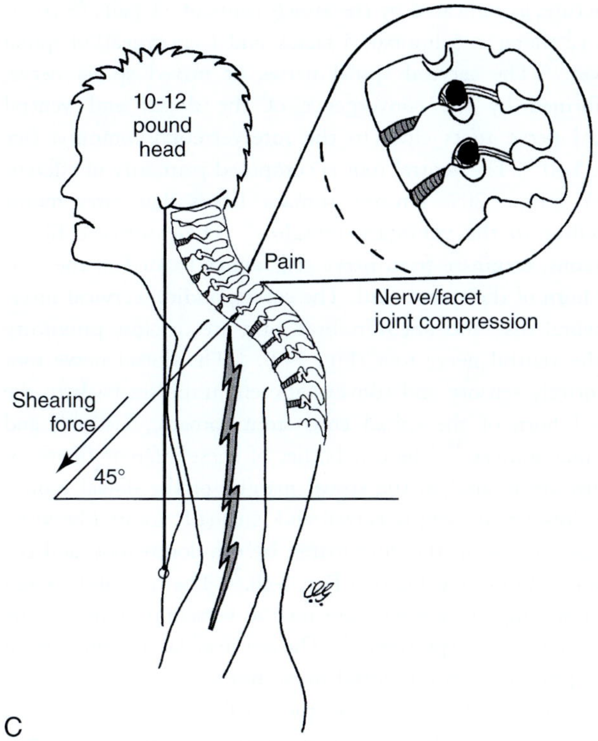

Figure 5-7 Cont'd C, Schematic of a forward head posture resulting in nerve and facet joint compression with increased shearing at the disks.

OCCUPATIONAL RELATIONSHIP

The spine and the shoulder are inseparable with regard to their coordinated functions in job-related tasks. Holding a prolonged and abnormal posture of the neck and shoulder is a major cause of CTD.[26,27] The term *cumulative trauma disorder* represents repetitive microtrauma to specific musculoskeletal tissues over a period of time at a rate faster than that at which the body can heal itself.[26] If the damage continues to exceed the repair process, then it will eventually lead to pain, decreased work performance, and loss of function.[26] Jobs that require sustained elevation of the arms may cause supraspinatus tendinosis because of the compression of the humeral head against the coracoacromial arch as the head of the humerus migrates cranially from rotator cuff fatigue and because of sustained tension in the muscle that can inhibit venous circulation.[28] Bicipital tendinosis can result from similar working postures because of repeated friction between the synovial sheath of the tendon (long head) and the lesser tuberosity of the humerus.[28] The physical work demands that lead to CTD are repetitive motion and holding of a sustained posture (e.g., jobs that require sitting while typing on a computer, carpenters, electricians, mechanics, and musicians).[26,27] Forward head posture is a major risk factor in CTD.[26] The shifting forward of the weight of the head makes the neck and upper back muscles work harder.[26] This stressful posture can upset nerve control and circulation to the arms.[26] Poor posture is as much a problem in CTD as is repetitive motion.[26] Jobs requiring repetitive motion are often carried out in prolonged sitting or standing positions.[26,27] The posture assumed by the neck and shoulder determines how well the arm, wrist, and hand will tolerate the demands of work.[27]

The neck and shoulder are dynamic structures that are mobile by design.[26] The neck and shoulder, however, are often required to perform static work as the hands perform a skilled task.[26,27,29] Maintaining a sustained work posture of the neck, in association with repetitive movements of an elevated shoulder, can restrict circulation to the working tissues of the arm and hand.[29] This situation can be a major hurdle for persons trying to return to work following a musculoskeletal injury. Patients with chronic neck and shoulder pain, following a whiplash injury in a motor vehicle accident, for example, have shown a decreased ability to achieve a normal increase in blood flow to the upper trapezius muscle during progressive workloads.[30] Myofascial disorders of the trapezius, SCM, or infraspinatus muscles can cause referred autonomic phenomena, including vasoconstriction.[31] Jobs that require holding a sustained posture for a prolonged period of time can restrict circulation to working tissues, with resulting early fatigue and a slower rate of repair of microtraumas to the musculoskeletal system.[26]

Occupational neck and shoulder disorders are usually the result of prolonged flexion or abduction of the shoulders, repetitive arm work, high-speed work, poor head posture, and a maintained static muscle load.[12,18,27,28,32-34] A high level of static muscle activity is one reason for the high incidence of neck and shoulder disorders in persons working with cash registers or computer keyboards.[12,27,33,34] Working in a posture with the shoulder flexed or abducted will increase the EMG activity levels in the upper trapezius, cervical, and thoracic erector spinae muscles.[16,27,32] One solution is to have the cashier stand rather than sit, which puts less stress on the trapezius, infraspinatus, and thoracic erector spinae muscles.[27] When someone is seated at a desk or table, the forward head posture may be secondary to one or more of the following: a seat height that is too high, a table or visual display terminal height that is too low, or a seat that is too far away from the table (see Fig. 5-7A).[32] For computer keyboard operators, ergonomically designed chairs with foot and arm rests are available (see Fig. 5-7B). The top portion of the visual display terminal should be at eye level.

Ergonomic solutions to CTD include the following: correction of both sitting and standing posture (see Fig. 5-5); adjustments to seat, table, and visual display terminal heights, to allow for supportive posture (see Fig. 5-7B); brief but frequent rest periods throughout the workday; light exercise during breaks to keep the blood flowing freely to all tissues; creation of a balance between repetitive motions of ADLs or sports that simulate job duties and appropriate periods of rest; and training of the worker's body to become fit—like an athlete—through exercise, nutrition, and rest, to withstand the daily stress on the job.

NEUROLOGIC RELATIONSHIP

The shoulder is tied to the spine neurologically by sensory, motor, and sympathetic relationships. Each of these relationships is evaluated in greater detail throughout this section and the rest of the chapter.

The spinal cord is surrounded by meninges (dura mater, arachnoid mater, and pia mater), which, at the level of the foramen magnum, are directly continuous with those covering the brain (Fig. 5-8).[35] The spinal cord is a segmented structure, as indicated by the attachments of 31 pairs (8 cervical, 12 thoracic, 5 lumbar, 5 sacral, and 1 coccygeal) of spinal nerves.[35] The cervical spinal nerve, or mixed spinal nerve, is formed by the convergence of the dorsal and ventral spinal nerve roots close to the intervertebral foramina (see Fig. 5-8).[35] The ventral root is composed primarily of efferent (80% motor, 20% sensory) somatic fibers that carry motor impulses to the voluntary muscles.[35] These somatic fibers, or axons, originate from nerve cell bodies located in the ventral horn of the spinal cord. The corresponding cervical intervertebral disk and uncovertebral joint are in close proximity to the ventral nerve root (Fig. 5-9).[35] The dorsal nerve root is entirely sensory and conveys afferent impulses back to the dorsal horn of the spinal cord from somatic, visceral, and vascular sources.[35] The cell bodies of these afferent fibers, or axons, are located in the spinal ganglia of the dorsal root.[35] The dorsal root ganglia is oval and is usually located between the perforation in the dura mater, by the dorsal root, and the intervertebral foramina (see Fig. 5-9).[35] The first and second cervical ganglia, however, are on the vertebral arches of the atlas and axis, respectively.[35] The cervical facet joints are in close proximity to the dorsal nerve roots.

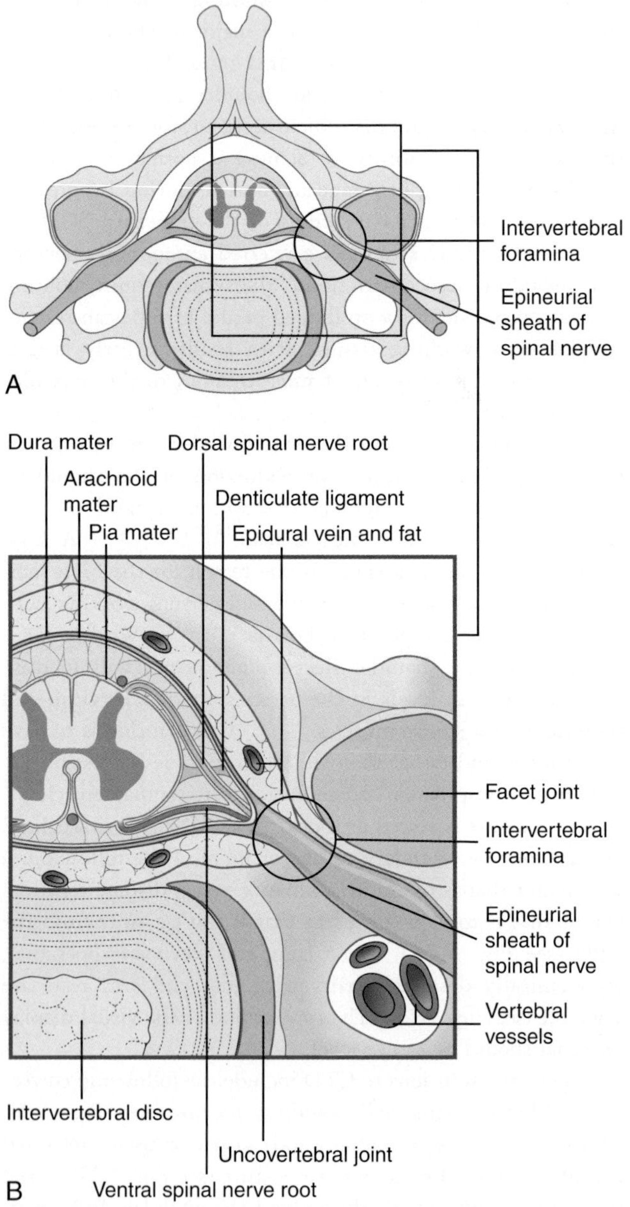

Figure 5-8 Anatomy of the spine. **A,** The cervical spinal nerve exits through the intervertebral foramina. The cervical spinal nerve forms through the convergence of the dorsal and ventral spinal nerves. **B,** A detailed view of anatomy. (Modified from Fitzgerald MJT: *Clinical neuroanatomy and neuroscience,* ed 5, Philadelphia, 2007, Saunders Elsevier.)

As the mixed spinal nerve emerges from the intervertebral foramina, it immediately diverges into several nerve branches. The recurrent meningeal (sinuvertebral) nerve branches off from the mixed spinal nerve just as it exits the intervertebral foramina.[22,35-37] The recurrent meningeal nerve then receives input from the gray rami communicantes.[22,35,37] This nerve, now a mixture of sensory and sympathetic nerves, returns back through the intervertebral foramina to innervate the dura mater, walls of blood vessels, periosteum, ligaments, uncovertebral joints, and intervertebral disks in the ventrolateral region of the spinal canal.[22,23,35-37] Occasionally, branches of the recurrent meningeal nerve innervate the dorsal dura, periosteum, and ligaments.[22,35,37]

After leaving the intervertebral foramina, the mixed spinal nerve divides into dorsal (posterior) and ventral (anterior) rami (see Fig. 5-9).[22,35] Near its origin, each ventral ramus receives a gray ramus communicans from the corresponding sympathetic ganglion.[22,35] The dorsal ramus of the cervical spinal nerve/divides, except the first cervical, into medial and lateral branches to supply the muscles and skin of the posterior regions of the neck.[22,35,36] The medial branch is also distributed to the capsules of the cervical facet joints, where it relays afferent input from fibers of type I, II, and III encapsulated mechanoreceptors and the type IV unencapsulated nociceptors back to the dorsal horn of the spinal cord.[22,36,37]

The type I receptors are most abundant in the joint capsules of the cervical facet joints, shoulder, and hip.[39] The actual number of active type I receptors may decline more rapidly in older patients or those who have suffered repeated traumas because of the superficial location of these mechanoreceptors within the joint capsule. One study did show a higher density of type II than type I mechanoreceptors in the cervical spine.[38] The subjects ($n = 3$) were few, however, and they were either deceased or had suffered traumatic

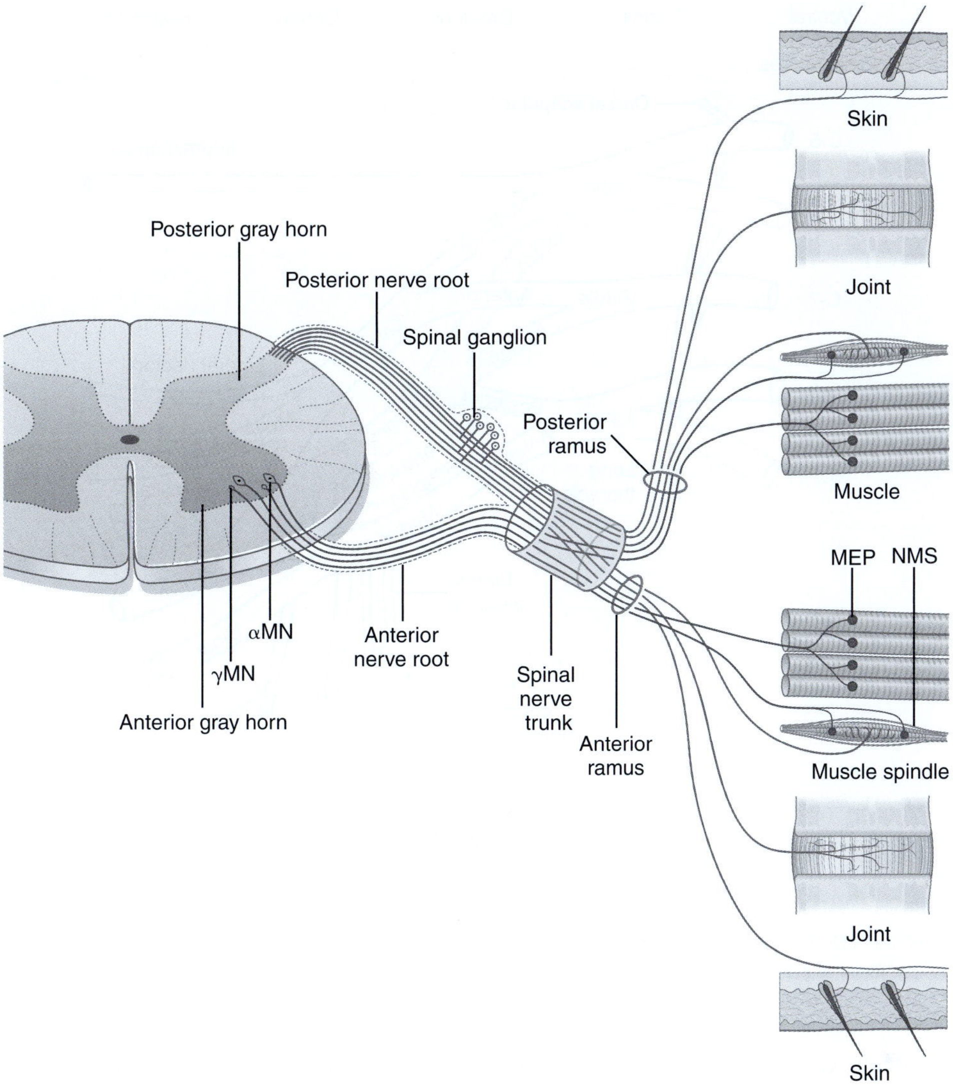

Figure 5-9 Composition and distribution of a cervical spinal nerve. The sympathetic component is not shown. MEP, motor end plate; MN, multipolar neurons; NMS, neuromuscular spindle. (From Fitzgerald MJT: *Clinical neuroanatomy and neuroscience,* ed 5, St. Louis, 2007, Saunders Elsevier.)

cervical spine injuries before the time of the study.[38] Type I receptors fire impulses for up to 1 minute (slowly adapting) after stimulation and are activated by deformation in the beginning or end range of tension for the capsule.[23] The type I receptors produce tonic reflexogenic effects on the neck and limb muscles, postural (low threshold) and kinesthetic sensation, and pain inhibition.[23,38-40]

The type II receptors, which are located deep in the joint capsule, fire an impulse for one-half second (rapidly adapting) after stimulation and are activated by deformation in the beginning or midrange of tension for the joint capsule.[23] These receptors are most abundant in the ankle and foot, wrist and hand, and temporomandibular joints.[39] Type II receptors are responsible for dynamic (phasic) reflexogenic effects on the muscles of the trunk and limbs.[23,38-40] They also provide information on joint acceleration and deceleration (low threshold).[39] Type II mechanoreceptors may also be activated to inhibit pain.

Type III receptors are also dynamic mechanoreceptors. Within the facet joint capsules of the cervical spine, these receptors are found at the junction between the dense fibrous capsule and the loose areolar subsynovial tissue.[38] These mechanoreceptors may also be found in ligaments and tendons.[38,39] They have a high threshold for activation and are very slow to adapt.[38,39] The type III mechanoreceptors have the lowest density in the facet joint capsules of the cervical spine when compared with types I and II.[38]

The type IV receptors are responsible for transmitting impulses that eventually reach the higher centers of the brain for perception as painful stimuli.[39] These nociceptors may be activated by trauma or chemical stimulation (mediators of inflammation).[23] In addition, the three encapsulated mechanoreceptors (types I to III) can produce a noxious stimulus in response to excessive joint motion.[39]

The cervical ventral rami supply the anterior and lateral portions of the neck.[22,35] The third cervical ventral ramus

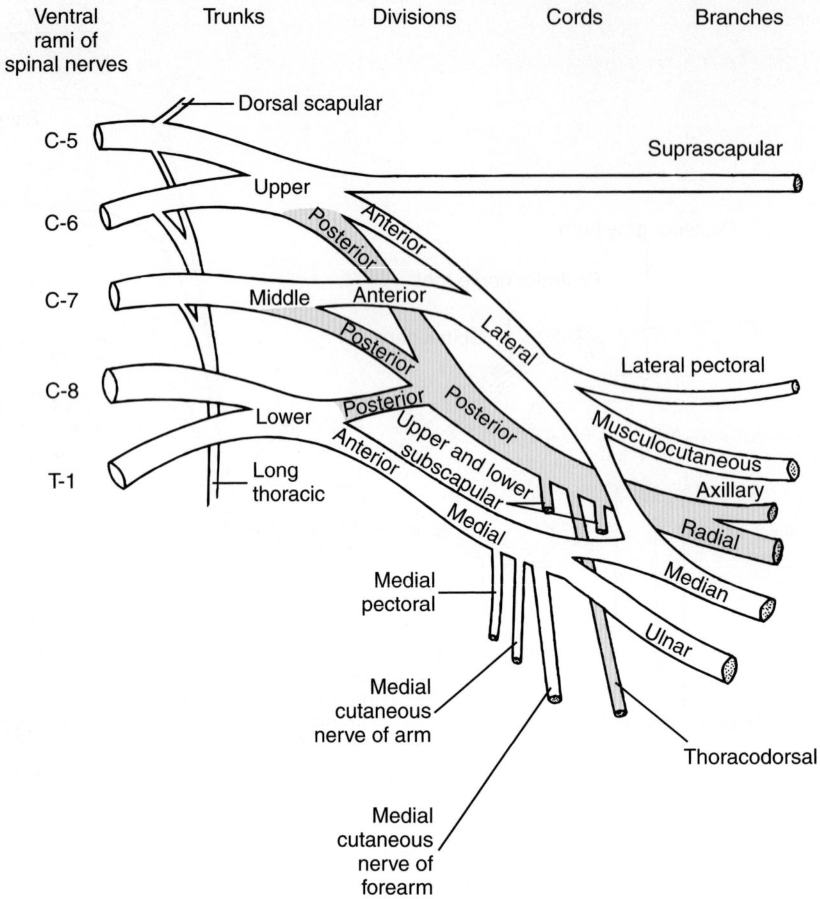

Figure 5-10 Diagram of the brachial plexus. The small nerve to the subclavius muscle, from the upper trunk, is omitted. (From Jenkins DB: *Hollinshead's functional anatomy of the limbs and back,* ed 9, St. Louis, 2009, Saunders Elsevier.)

appears between the longus capitis and the scalenus medius muscles.[22,35] The ventral rami of the fourth through eighth cervical spinal nerves emerge between the scalenus anterior and scalenus medius.[22,35]

The upper four cervical ventral rami form the cervical plexus. The lower four, including the first thoracic ventral ramus, form the brachial plexus (Fig. 5-10).[22,41] The cervical plexus supplies some nuchal muscles, the diaphragm, and areas of skin in the head, neck, and chest.[22,41] The formation of the brachial plexus allows for rearrangements of the efferent and afferent somatic and autonomic fibers so that they are redirected through the various trunks, divisions, and cords into the most appropriate channels (terminal branches) for distribution to the muscles, skin, vessels, and glands in the upper limbs.[22,41]

The dorsal scapular nerve (C5) arises from the uppermost root of the brachial plexus (see Fig. 5-10).[22,41] It pierces the scalenus medius muscle as it travels to supply the levator scapulae and the rhomboid major and minor muscles.[22,41] The suprascapular nerve (C5 and C6) arises from the superior trunk of the brachial plexus.[22,41] It supplies the supraspinatus and infraspinatus muscles, the glenohumeral and acromioclavicular joints, and the suprascapular vessels.[22,41] The axillary nerve (C5 and C6) originates from the posterior cord of the brachial plexus.[22,41] It supplies the glenohumeral joint and the deltoid and teres minor muscles.[22,41] The upper subscapular nerve (C5 and C6) arises from the posterior cord and innervates the subscapularis muscle.[2,22] The middle subscapular nerve, or thoracodorsal nerve (C7 and C8), arises from the posterior cord and innervates the latissimus dorsi muscle.[2,22] The lower subscapular nerve (C5 and C6) also arises from the posterior cord in proximity to the upper subscapular and the thoracodorsal nerves. The lower subscapular nerve innervates the subscapularis and teres major muscles.[2,22]

CENTRAL SENSITIZATION AND THE FACILITATED SEGMENT

Central sensitization (*central* referring to the central nervous system [CNS]; *sensitization* referring to its hypersensitivity and overreaction to incoming stimuli) refers to the changes in the nervous system (forebrain, brain, sympathetic nervous system [SNS], peripheral afferents, and dorsal horn of the spinal cord) that result in chronic pain, hyperalgesia, and allodynia long after tissue healing has occurred at the original site of injury. Repeated stimulation (e.g., reaching overhead, for a patient with shoulder impingement) of peripheral primary afferents including the unmyelinated C-fibers from group IV and the thinly myelinated Aδ-fibers from group III, leads to an increase in the hypersensitivity of neurons in the dorsal horn of the spinal cord.[42] Receptors on postsynaptic neurons in the dorsal horn of the spinal cord undergo changes secondary to this barrage of nociceptive afferent input. Presynaptic nociceptive afferent neurons have their terminals in the dorsal horn and release—on noxious stimulation—excitatory amino acids (glutamate) and excitatory neuropeptides (substance P and neurokinin A).[43-45] Glutamate receptors on the postsynaptic neurons, such as the α-amino-3-hydroxy-5-methyl-4-isoxazolepropionic acid (AMPA), kainite ligand–gated ion channels, and NMDA *N*-methyl-d-aspartate (NMDA), react to repeated glutamate stimulation by making the neuron more sensitive to incoming glutamate and therefore more sensitive to incoming impulses from peripheral afferent nociceptors.[43-45] Morphologic changes, such as an increase in the number of glutamate receptors on the postsynaptic neuron, may lead to an irreversible change in hypersensitivity.[46] This central sensitization is observed clinically as hyperalgesia (excessive pain from a noxious stimulus) and as mechanical allodynia (pain from a non-noxious stimulus). The change in sensitivity of the postsynaptic neuron in the dorsal horn is facilitated by a loss of supraspinal inhibition, part of which originates in the forebrain.[44,46]

Forebrain activity, such as fear, anxiety, and depression, can amplify and prolong the pain experience beyond the stages of tissue healing. Facilitory impulses descending down to the dorsal horn increase central sensitization by lowering the threshold for activation of the interneurons in the dorsal horn. Following a barrage of nociceptive afferent input from the periphery (e.g., a shoulder injury), negative thoughts and emotions from the forebrain decrease the normal pain inhibitory impulses that would otherwise descend down to the dorsal horn. This decrease in inhibitory impulses increases the chances of forming a facilitated segment. A *facilitated segment,* also referred to as central sensitization, may be defined as any segment of the spinal cord that has a lower than normal threshold for activation of the interneurons within the dorsal horn (Fig. 5-11).[47] This segment of the spinal cord (e.g., C5) facilitates, through a lowered threshold of activation for interneurons within the interneuron pool, the ability of incoming afferent stimuli to reach the critical threshold to elicit an efferent (motor) response, resulting in muscle guarding, or to ascend to the higher centers of the brain to be perceived as pain.

Depending on the stimulus they receive from the forebrain, descending neural pain pathways from the brainstem, specifically from the periaqueductal gray (PAG) and the rostral ventromedial medulla (RVM), can facilitate or inhibit the activity of the interneurons within the spinal cord.[48] These descending pathways are intimately connected with the forebrain and are influenced significantly by the activity and output coming from the forebrain.[42] Descending pathways from the brain to the dorsal horn include both the ventrolateral column and the lateral column of the PAG.[48] Nerves arising from the lateral column use norepinephrine (noradrenaline) as a neurotransmitter and are described as noradrenergic. This system of descending nerves controls the release of morphine (analgesic) in response to a mechanical

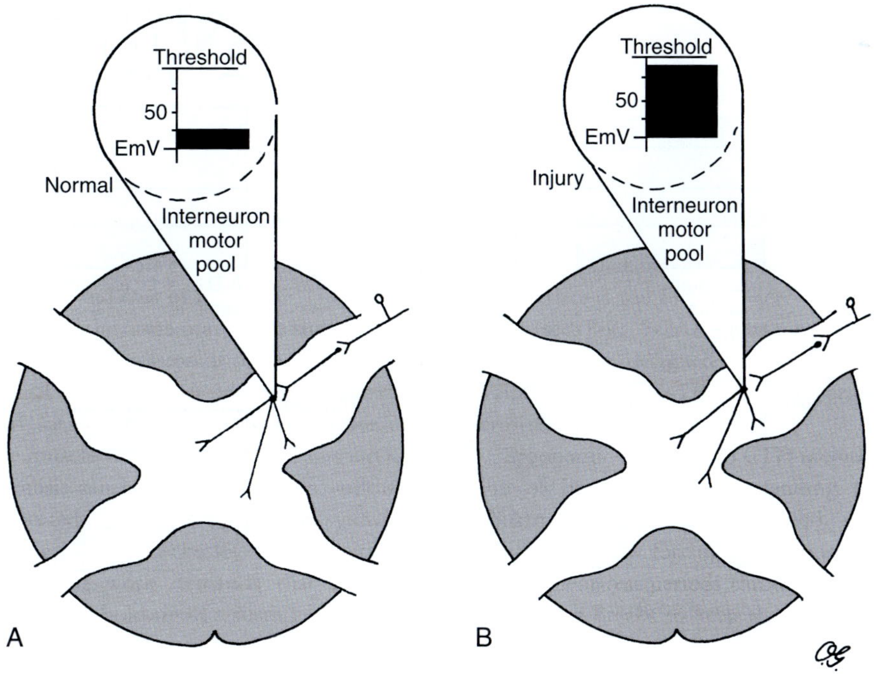

Figure 5-11 A normal and a facilitated segment of the cervical spinal cord. **A,** A normal segment with a low level of electrical activity and a high threshold for activation of the interneurons. **B,** A facilitated segment with a high level of electrical activity and a low threshold for activation of the interneurons.

nociceptive event. Nerves descending down through the ventrolateral column use serotonin as a neurotransmitter and are therefore described as serotonergic. These nerves control the release of morphine as a result of noxious thermal stimulation.[48] The release of substance P by presynaptic neurons in the dorsal horn, because of noxious mechanical stimulation, can be inhibited at the spinal cord level by descending inhibitory impulses from the PAG and the RVM.[48]

The modulation of pain by the forebrain depends on a person's state of attention, cognition, and emotion. Chronic symptoms in the extremities may not derive from ongoing microtrauma and inflammation (e.g., the diagnosis of supraspinatus tendinitis), but rather may originate from forebrain- and dorsal horn–mediated central sensitization that results in the perception of shoulder pain long after the tendon has healed. The actual site of pain production shifts as the patient leaves the acute stage of healing and inflammation, and most of the primary healing is completed, from the periphery (e.g., the supraspinatus tendon) to the dorsal horn (e.g., the C5 segment of the spinal cord). Pain continues to be perceived from the shoulder, but the real source of the pain is now in the dorsal horn because of changes in the glutamate receptors on the postsynaptic neurons that effectively lower the threshold of activation of the nerve impulses within the interneuron pool. At this point, allodynia is pervasive. The primary tissue in lesion is no longer the supraspinatus tendon; now it consists of the hyperreactive, sensitized, spinal cord interneurons in the dorsal horn with an extremely low threshold for activation. The primary role of the physical therapist becomes that of a desensitizer.[42] The goal is to try to desensitize the interneurons in the dorsal horn both directly, by using manual therapy and exercise, and indirectly, by minimizing inappropriate input from the periphery (e.g., excessive shoulder impingement motions and postures) and the forebrain (fear, anger, anxiety, and depression).

Another way that a facilitated segment, or central sensitization, can develop is through a loss of the almost constant barrage of inhibitory impulses from type I and type II mechanoreceptors.[23] Because of their superficial location, type I receptors within the facet joint capsules are at a greater risk of being damaged. As a result of spondylosis or trauma (e.g., after a motor vehicle accident), the number of type I mechanoreceptors available to produce inhibitory impulses in the dorsal horn declines.[23] This change may subsequently lead to a lowered threshold for activation of the interneurons within that segment of the spinal cord, thus producing a facilitated segment or central sensitization. Corpuscular mechanoreceptors in the skin and subcutaneous tissues also send inhibitory impulses to the spinal cord.[23] The loss of these receptors, because of scarring, burns, superficial wounds, or diseases, may also lead to lowering of the threshold and subsequent formation of a facilitated segment.[23] In this way, normally subliminal afferent stimuli, ADLs, for example (Fig. 5-12), may actually produce a motor or sympathetic efferent impulse, or they may reach the higher centers of the brain and be perceived as pain (shoulder), because the interneurons in that segment of the spinal cord (C5) have been facilitated (e.g., chronic spondylosis and acute injury to the C4-5 facet joint) by the loss of type I and possibly type II mechanoreceptors within the C4-5 facet joint capsule.[49]

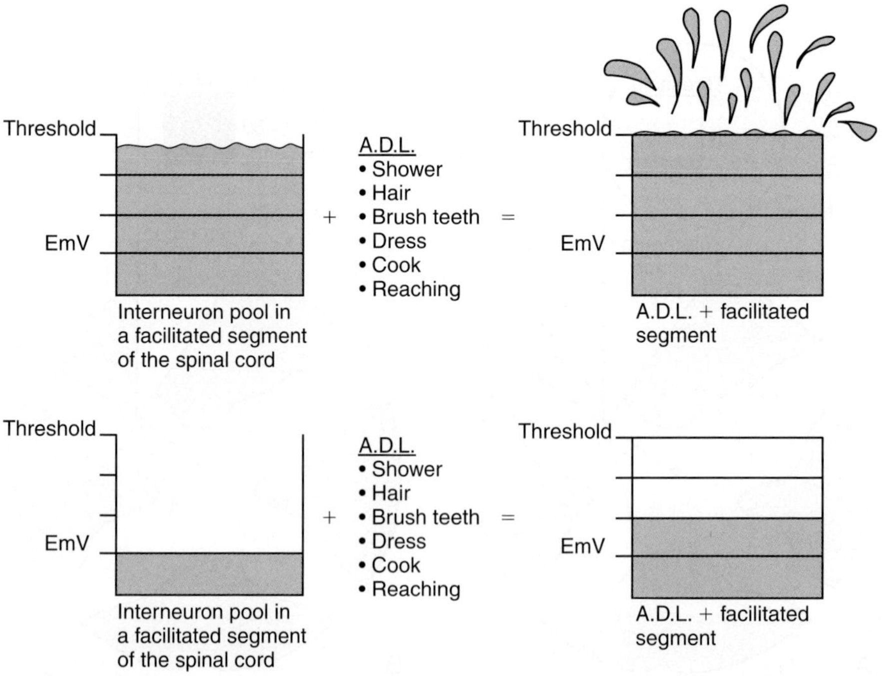

Figure 5-12 Electrical activity within the interneuron pool and the effect of activities of daily living (ADLs). On the *bottom* is a normal segment with a low level of electrical activity that increases with ADLs, but does not reach the threshold. On the *top* is a facilitated segment with a high level of electrical activity that easily reaches the threshold for activation following normal ADLs.

The segment of the spinal cord that is facilitated acts as a neurologic magnifying glass. The facilitated segment focuses and exaggerates the effects of all incoming afferent impulses on the tissues innervated from that segment.[50] Even ordinary innocuous events and ADLs may become relatively demanding and stressful to the neuromusculoskeletal system (see Fig. 5-12).[50]

Role of the Sympathetic Nervous System

The SNS can adjust circulatory, metabolic, and visceral activity depending on the postural and musculoskeletal demands.[51] For the SNS to perform this role, it must receive direct (by segmental somatic afferents) and indirect (by higher centers of the CNS) sensory input from the musculoskeletal system.[51] SNS hyperactivity has been associated with, and segmentally related to, musculoskeletal trauma and dysfunction.[51] Long-term hyperactivity of a particular sympathetic pathway can be deleterious to the associated tissue.[51] Some of the consequences of prolonged hyperactivity of the SNS are (1) ischemia because of vasoconstriction, (2) the shortening of tendons, (3) muscle atrophy, and (4) joint contractures.[51]

The cervical spine is capable of inducing real pathologic conditions (e.g., adhesive capsulitis, tendinitis, or bursitis) within the shoulder joint.[18,36,40,49,52-56] Wiffen,[57] in his review of adhesive capsulitis, suggested that this chronic painful condition of the shoulder may develop or be maintained by central sensitization in the dorsal horn of the spinal cord and by an overactive SNS. These pathologic conditions of the shoulder may be precipitated by vasoconstriction to the shoulder joint through cervical sympathetic activity as a result of cervical nerve root irritation.[40,49,54] Sympathetic cell bodies are found in spinal cord segments C4 to C8. The transmission of the preganglionic fibers, in the ventral roots of C5 to C8, has also been demonstrated.[53,58] The lowest somatic segmental supply to the upper extremities is T3, whereas the lowest sympathetic supply to the upper extremities is as low as T8.[58]

Synapses within the interneuron pool in the dorsal horn, between somatic and sympathetic neurons, can result in a sympathetically mediated vasoconstriction message that targets the shoulder.[49] These impulses may produce inflammation, exudation, fibrosis, adhesions, capsular thickening, degeneration, and calcification within the rotator cuff and joint capsule.[40,49] Cervical nerve root irritation may also give rise to complex regional pain syndrome type I (CRPS-I), with the changes mentioned previously to the capsule and tendons associated with the shoulder.[40] A previous asymptomatic event, such as active motion of the shoulder, may become symptomatic because of cervical spine–initiated vasoconstriction of the tissues in and around the shoulder. Another way that allodynia can develop in the shoulder is by the formation of a facilitated segment (C3, C4, C5, or C6) within the spinal cord. This may result from a chronic barrage of afferent nociceptive impulses, a loss of inhibitory impulses from type I or type II mechanoreceptors, or a loss of supraspinal inhibition from the forebrain.[23,30,49] The outcome is a lower threshold of activation of the interneurons responsible for relaying nociceptive impulses to the higher brain centers for the perception of pain.

MUSCULOSKELETAL SYNDROMES INVOLVING THE SPINE, RIBS, AND SHOULDER

Omohyoid Syndrome

Neck, shoulder, or arm pain may be the primary complaint of a patient with an omohyoid syndrome.[59-63] This syndrome is characterized by the sudden onset of a severe muscle spasm on one side of the neck.[59-63] The omohyoid muscle belly may contain myofascial trigger points.[63] The origin is often a contraction combined with a stretching of the omohyoid muscle.[60] An example is a yawn combined with an attempt to swallow as the head is bent to one side.[59] Forceful motions, such as vomiting, may also cause the omohyoid muscle to go into spasm.[63]

Symptoms

Patients report the sudden onset of pain and muscle spasms, often during yawning, swallowing, or vomiting.[59-61] The symptoms are typically aggravated by swallowing.[59-62] Pain is present on one side of the neck and may include the shoulder and arm.[59-63]

Signs

Patients often have their head flexed and bent ipsilaterally.[59,60] They have audible breathing and an alteration in the quality of the voice, such as slurred speech.[60] Swallowing is painful.[59-62] Neck flexion decreases the symptoms.[60] Pain is reproduced with stretching (extension, contralateral side bending, or contralateral rotation) or palpation of the omohyoid muscle.[59-61]

Levator Scapulae Syndrome

Another source of neck and shoulder pain is the levator scapulae syndrome.[64,65] This syndrome is proposed to consist of bursitis involving a bursa associated with the levator scapulae at its attachment to the scapula.[64] It is thought to occur because of friction among the levator scapulae, the serratus anterior, and the scapula as the muscles pull in opposite directions during repeated upper extremity tasks with the arm elevated.[64] A sustained head posture in rotation during prolonged typing or telephone calls may also precipitate a problem in the levator scapulae.[65] Additional risk factors include vigorous tennis or swimming.[65]

Symptoms

Patients complain of pain in the superior-medial angle of the scapula. They may report a "heaviness" or "burning" sensation, which radiates to the neck or shoulder.[64]

Signs

These patients have full AROM and passive ROM (PROM) at the neck and shoulder. Symptoms are reproduced through palpation or stretching of the levator scapulae muscle. Results of thoracic outlet, impingement, and neurologic testing are normal, as are plain radiographs of the shoulder.[64]

Droopy Shoulder Syndrome

The droopy shoulder syndrome, another source of neck and shoulder pain, may be considered a brachial plexus stretch injury. Drooping shoulders, a chronic postural strain, produce tension on the brachial plexus. This syndrome is normally exclusive to women.[66,67]

Symptoms

The patient may complain of head, neck, chest, and bilateral shoulder and arm pain. Patients often report paresthesias in the upper extremities, without objective numbness, weakness, or muscle atrophy. The patients may describe their symptoms as "tightness," "electrical," "jabbing," or "pulling."[66,67]

Signs

Postural examination shows a swan neck with low-set shoulders and horizontal clavicles. Symptoms are reproduced by palpation at the supraclavicular fossa or stretching of the brachial plexus (upper limb neurodynamic testing). Passive scapular depression increases the symptoms, whereas passive elevation decreases the symptoms. No vascular insufficiency, claudication, or Raynaud's phenomenon is present. Lateral radiographs of the cervical spine allow visualization of the second thoracic vertebra. Normally, a lateral radiograph of the neck allows visual inspection only down to the sixth cervical vertebra because of interference by the shoulder. Results of EMG studies are within normal limits (WNL).[66,67]

Snapping Scapula Syndrome

The snapping scapula syndrome is a source of scapulothoracic pain and dysfunction. Ten different muscles have attachment sites on the scapula that control its movement across eight ribs. Under normal circumstances, the scapula glides smoothly across the thorax, without interruption or interference, with the help of these 10 well-coordinated muscles. The scapula is curved to match the contour of the thoracic wall.

Symptoms

The patient complains of scapulothoracic pain and reports a grating or snapping sensation under the scapula during active movements of the upper extremity.[68,69] The complaints of pain are often diffuse and nonspecific in a region surrounding the scapula. The pain is thought to be the result of tendinosis of one or more of the scapula muscles or scapulothoracic bursitis.[68-70] The snapping or grating noise is thought to originate from a combination of poorly controlled scapula muscles, bony incongruity of the scapulothoracic "joint," and possibly the riding of the scapula over a fibrotic scapulothoracic bursa.[68-70]

Signs

The patient is able voluntarily to produce an audible and palpable grating, crepitus, or clunking noise with active movement of the scapula. The onset is thought to be secondary to various proposed factors such as the following: trauma; poor posture; poor scapulothoracic rhythm; a loss of muscle tone; atrophy of the serratus anterior muscle or subscapularis muscle; an adherent and fibrotic scapulothoracic bursa; or skeletal abnormalities that may include an abnormal angulation of the scapula or ribs, scapula exostoses and osteochondromas, and a bony or fibrocartilaginous protrusion or incongruity at the superior angle of the scapula.[68-71] A careful examination of the ribs (to rule out subluxation), spine (to exclude scoliosis), and scapula (to rule out hypomobility versus hypermobility) is indicated. This syndrome is more common in women. Although research into the use of conventional computed tomography (CT) scans in the diagnosis of snapping scapula has been contradictory, evidence indicates that three-dimensional CT scans are a valid tool in recognizing bony incongruity of the scapula in persons with this syndrome.[71,72]

CERVICAL SPINE TISSUES CAPABLE OF REFERRING PAIN AND DYSFUNCTION TO THE SHOULDER

Disk

Cervical disk disease (internal disruption, degeneration, herniation, or prolapse), without nerve root involvement, can be a source of shoulder pain.[52,53,73-79] The recurrent meningeal nerve receives afferent impulses from the posterior and posterior-lateral regions of the intervertebral disk and posterior longitudinal ligament (see Fig. 5-9). This nerve then joins the mixed spinal nerve and sends sensory information into the dorsal horn of the spinal cord.[22,35,37] In this way, referred pain at the shoulder may be experienced with disk abnormalities at the same segmental levels that innervate the shoulder. Degenerative disk disease can result in instability at that segment, which may lead to injury of ligaments or facet joint capsules.[80] In the late stages of this disease, osteophytes or a prolapsed disk can induce nerve root irritation.[80]

Symptoms

Pain, usually a dull ache, can vary in distribution from the occiput, mastoid, and temporomandibular joint (TMJ) to the anterior chest, upper back and scapula, and down to the elbow (Fig. 5-13).[78,79] Pain may be unilateral or bilateral. Grubb and Kelly[78] reported that bilateral symptoms occur 33% to 50% of the time, depending on the disk level. Pain normally does not travel below the elbow. Without nerve root involvement, patients have no complaints of numbness, pins and needles sensation, or specific muscle weakness. Pain is normally not referred to the biceps brachii muscle or anterior portions of the upper arm.

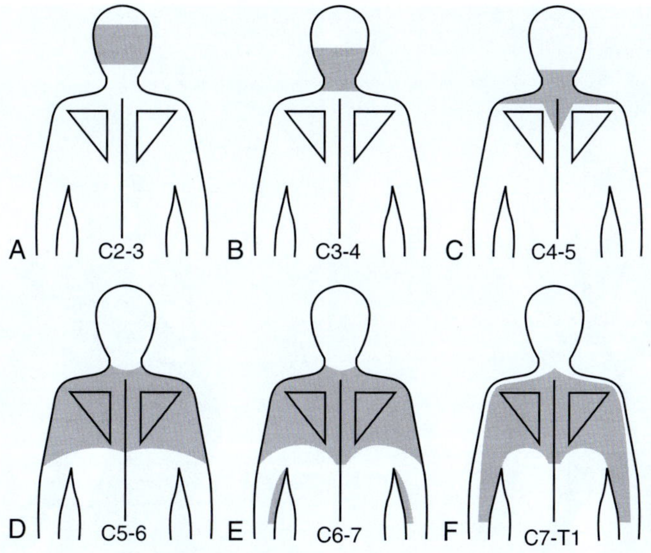

Figure 5-13 Referred pain patterns of specific cervical intervertebral disks following diskography. (Modified from Grubb S, Kelly CK: Cervical discography: clinical implications from 12 years of experience, *Spine* 25(11):1382, 2000.)

Signs

Reproduction of symptoms is expected during the following special tests (Fig. 5-14): compression of the cervical spine in neutral, flexed, and extended postures (Fig. 5-15); the segmental shear test (Fig. 5-16); coughing or sneezing; and Valsalva's test.[81] The shear test may also demonstrate increased shearing and hypermobility at the involved segment if the patient has degenerative disk disease or minimal muscle guarding, and the segment is not ankylosed. Often, no nerve root compression or irritation is present, in which case the results of the nerve root examination (sensation, strength, and deep tendon reflexes [DTRs]) and the nerve root special tests (Spurling's or cervical quadrant test, doorbell sign, upper limb neurodynamic testing) are normal. In general, the examiner may find that the symptoms are reproduced with provocation of the cervical spine and not the shoulder, although this may not always be the case.

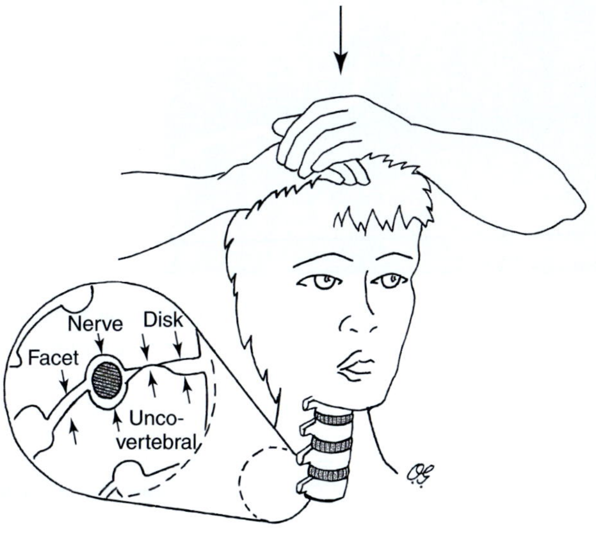

Figure 5-14 Axial compression of the cervical spine in neutral may produce pain from the intervertebral disk, vertebral body, uncovertebral joint, inflamed nerve root, or facet joint.

Imaging Studies

Plain radiographs, although helpful in examining the general morphologic features of the cervical spine, are not diagnostic. They may demonstrate decreased disk height or osteophytosis. Even in the presence of positive findings, the clinician must realize that many asymptomatic people have similar findings on plain film radiography. Myelography can demonstrate spinal cord or nerve root compression, but it cannot tell if whether a disk, an osteophyte, or a tumor is creating the compression. A CT scan following a myelogram allows the differential diagnosis of the tissue responsible for compression of neurologic tissues, but it cannot indicate whether a specific disk itself is symptomatic.[82,83] Magnetic resonance imaging (MRI) can identify a degenerated, desiccated, or herniated or prolapsed disk, but it cannot detect whether the disk is symptomatic.[78,79,82-84] CT diskography can clearly identify a symptomatic disk and determine the presence of internal disk disruption.[52,73,76,78,79,84,85] This diagnostic procedure, sometimes used to alleviate the patient's symptoms, is usually used to provoke and reproduce pain.[52,73,76,78,79,85]

Nerve

Irritation or partial compression of an inflamed cervical nerve root (dorsal root, ventral root, or the mixed spinal nerve) by an intervertebral disk, osteophytes from a facet or uncovertebral

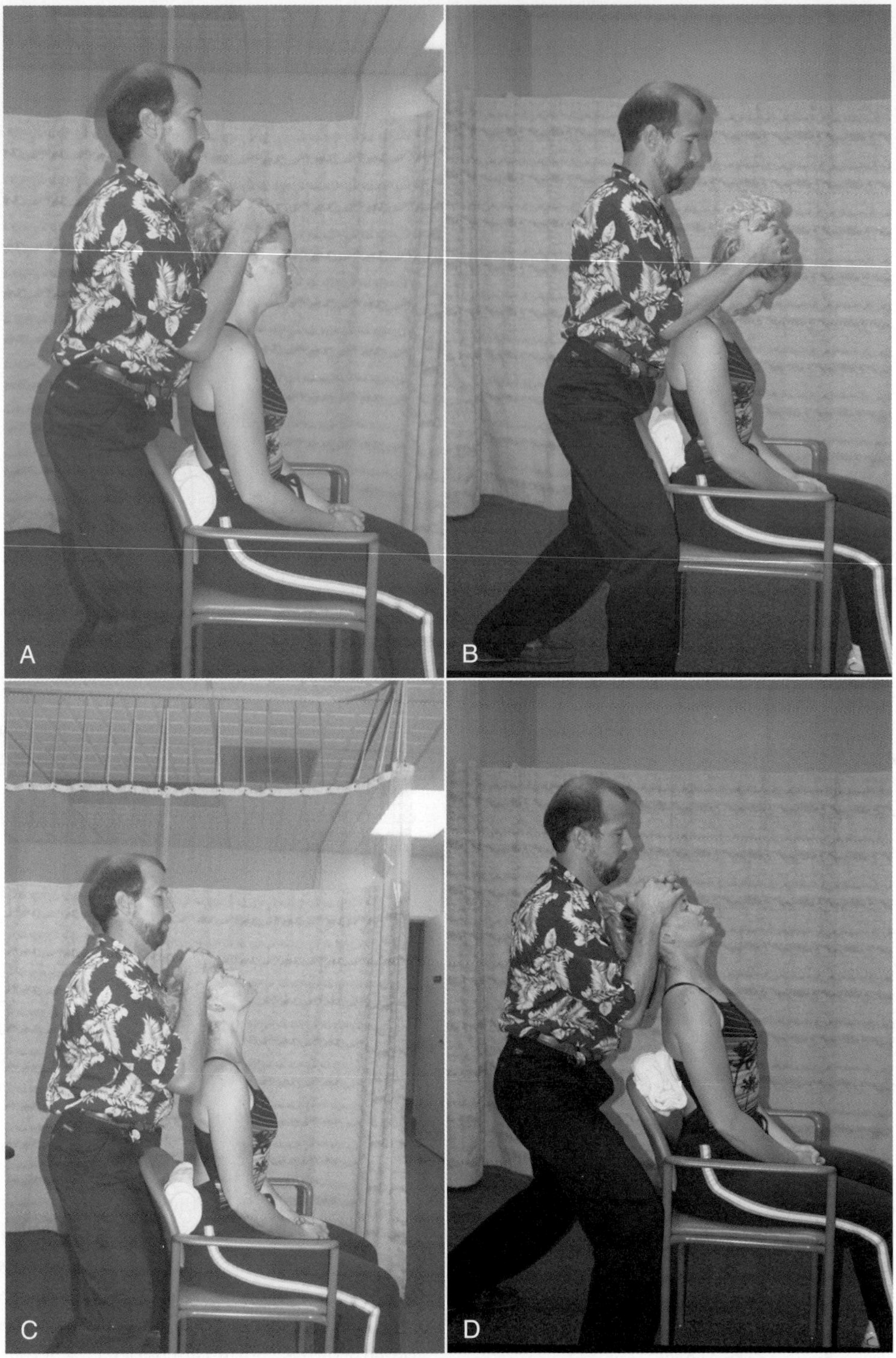

Figure 5-15 Differential diagnosis using axial compression testing of the cervical spine. **A,** Cervical spine in neutral. **B,** Flexion. **C,** Extension. **D,** Extension with retraction to target the lower cervical and upper thoracic segments. With the cervical spine in neutral, pain may be produced from the intervertebral disk, uncovertebral joint, nerve root, facet joint, or vertebral body. For disk-generated pain, symptoms are reproduced in all three positions (neutral, flexion, and extension). For uncovertebral–joint generated pain, symptoms are preferentially reproduced in a position of slight flexion combined with ipsilateral bending. For nerve root–generated pain, symptoms are reproduced in a position of extension. In severe cases, neutral may also be symptomatic. If an uninjured nerve root is being compressed, then one can expect to produce paresthesia into the upper extremity. If an inflamed nerve root is being compressed, then one can expect reproduction of pain often radiating down below the elbow. Other neurologic signs and special test results are also positive. For facet joint–generated pain, sharp pain is reproduced in a position of extension only. In severe cases, the patient may report discomfort in the neutral position as well. Facet-generated symptoms do not include paresthesia or pain radiating down below the elbow. For vertebral body–generated pain, symptoms are reproduced in all three positions, similar to discogenic pain. Vertebral body–generated pain may be preferentially stimulated by lightly tapping the spinous process (where accessible) with a reflex hammer or a tuning fork. A review of imaging studies also helps to rule out bone as a source of the patient's symptoms.

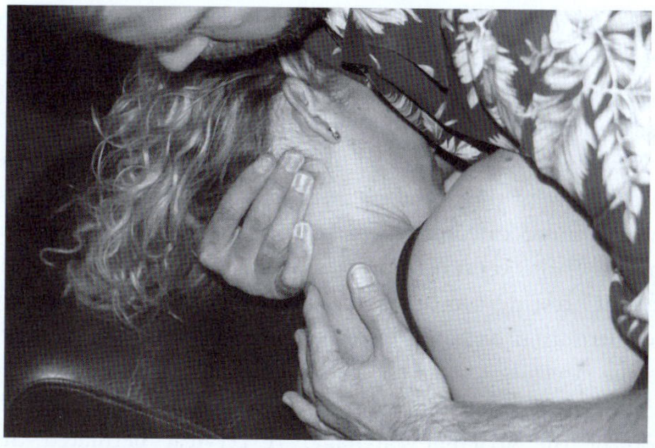

Figure 5-16 Shear test of the cervical intervertebral disk. Test of the C5-6 segment, for example: The patient is positioned in the side-lying position. The patient's head rests on the clinician's forearm with her forehead in contact with the clinician's biceps. The clinician's right hand supports the upper cervical spine and occiput. The cervical spine is flexed down through C4-5, but not C5-6. Keeping C4-5 and higher in flexion, the clinician oscillates his right forearm and humerus back and forth in an anterior-posterior (AP) shear motion as he palpates the amount of AP shear at C5-6 with his left index finger.

joint, or a tumor or other space-occupying lesion can be a source of neck, shoulder, and arm pain (Fig. 5-17).[36,40,73,74,86-88] Compression of an uninjured (without signs of inflammation) spinal nerve root normally does not give rise to pain. Paresthesias and complaints of itching, crawling, or varying degrees of numbness occur, depending on the degree of compression.[87]

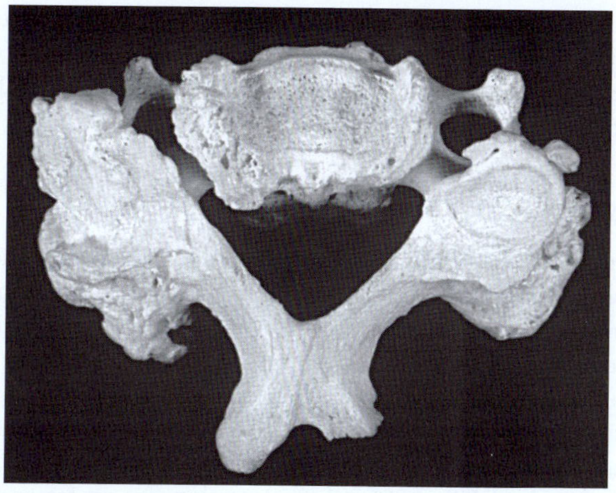

Figure 5-17 Degenerative joint disease and osteophytosis of the left cervical facet and uncovertebral joint. Note the narrowing of the intervertebral foramen and the bony encroachment toward the transverse foramen (vertebral artery). (From Tillmann B: *Slides in human arthrology,* Munich, 1985, Bergman Verlag.)

Symptoms

Patients often describe the pain as sharp, electrical, or "like a nerve is being pinched." Pain may start in the neck or shoulder and radiate as far as the fingertips (Fig. 5-18). Pain may also be felt in the posterior shoulder, scapula, or interscapular regions. The patient may complain of numbness, pins and needles, or weakness down the arm. Symptoms may be bilateral to the

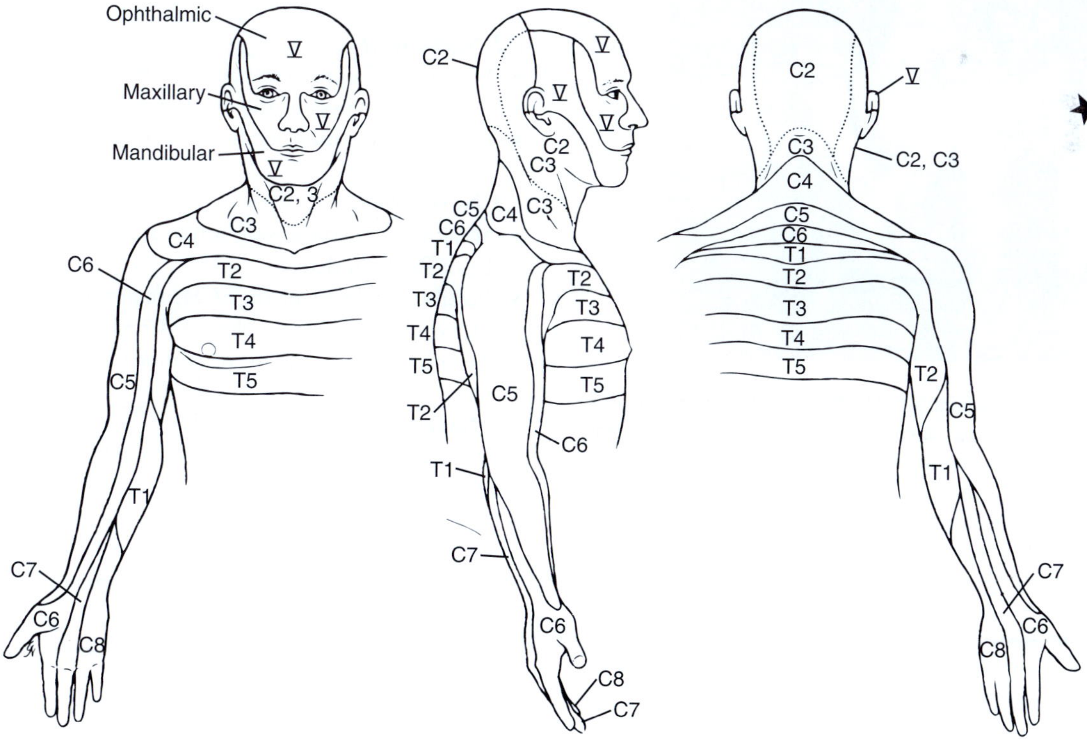

Figure 5-18 Dermatomes C2 through T5. (From Bland JH: Rheumatologic neurology. In *Disorders of the cervical spine: diagnosis and medical management,* ed 2, Philadelphia, 1994, Saunders.)

shoulder, but they are usually unilateral with respect to the upper extremities. Nerve root irritations and compressions are often associated with disk injury; some of these patients also experience discogenic pain.

Signs

Patients often obtain relief of symptoms by resting their involved hand on their heads.[79,89,90] Reproduction of symptoms is common during the following special tests: passive extension, ipsilateral side bending, or ipsilateral rotation of the cervical spine; the cervical quadrant test in extension, also known as Spurling's (Fig. 5-19)[53,79,89,90]; at least one abnormal finding with neurologic testing of motor or sensory reflexes or DTRs; cervical compression in an extended posture; and the doorbell sign[36] (palpation of the vertebral gutter outside the intervertebral foramina). Axial compression in the neutral posture of the cervical spine may be abnormal or normal, whereas compression in a flexed posture is normal. Cervical axial distraction, or traction in a flexed posture, often brings temporary relief of symptoms. However, symptoms can be aggravated if an inflamed and tethered nerve root is stretched over a bulging disk, osteophyte, or other space-occupying lesion.[79,86,89] If discogenic symptoms are present, then the results of tests for discogenic pain noted earlier will also be abnormal.

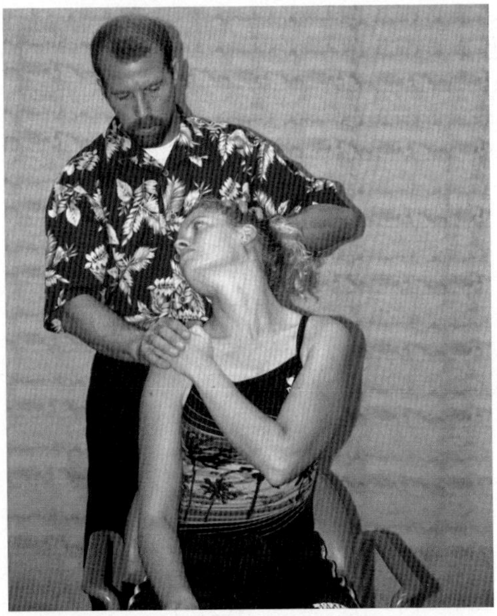

Figure 5-19 Cervical quadrant test in extension. The cervical spine is passively rotated, bent backward (ipsilateral side bending), and extended. This position maximally compresses the intervertebral foramen, facet, intervertebral disk, and vertebral body. The contralateral side experiences notable stretching strain to the soft tissues. Pain from the compressed side may be produced from the intervertebral disk (posterior-lateral compression), an inflamed spinal nerve root, the facet joint, or the vertebral body. Holding the position for at least 10 seconds helps the examiner to assess whether the initial pain subsides or whether neurologic signs and symptoms begin to appear. Slight overpressure may be applied if no symptoms occur initially. This position may also stress the vertebral artery. To test the lower cervical and upper thoracic segments sufficiently, especially for patients with a forward head posture, the examiner should ask patients to perform cervical retraction before starting the test.

Osteophytes from a cervical facet joint may hit the mixed spinal nerve or the dorsal (sensory) root only. In the latter case, the examiner can anticipate sensory, but no motor, disturbances. If the ventral (motor) root is spared, then the results of EMG testing can be expected to be normal.[91] If the nerve root irritation or compression is secondary to an osteophyte on the facet joint, then the patient may also demonstrate positive signs of facet joint pain or crepitus because of degeneration of the articular cartilage. A cervical herniated disk (contained bulging disk or complete prolapse), or osteophytes from the uncovertebral joint (see Fig. 5-17), may hit the mixed spinal nerve or the ventral root alone.[91] In this case, motor, but usually not sensory, signs and symptoms can be expected. (However, the motor nerve root is composed of up to 20% sensory nerve fibers.) If nerve root irritation or compression is secondary to a disk problem, the patient may demonstrate signs of discogenic pain. If the nerve root pathologic condition is caused by an osteophyte on the uncovertebral joint, then the patient may also display signs of this joint lesion. Signs of specific nerve root compression are noted in the following lists. Refer to Figure 5-18 (dermatomes) and Figure 5-20 (myotomes) as needed.[55,77,79,88,90,92-94]

C1 Nerve Root
- Weakness of upper cervical extension
- Possible weakness of the SCM
- Decreased sensation in the C1 dermatome

C2 Nerve Root
- Weakness of upper cervical flexion
- Possible weakness of the SCM and trapezius
- Decreased sensation in the C2 dermatome

C3 Nerve Root
- Weakness of cervical side bending, although weakness may be difficult to detect
- Possible weakness of the SCM, trapezius, and neck flexors
- Decreased sensation in the C3 dermatome; however, patients rarely complain of numbness

C4 Nerve Root
- Weakness of shoulder shrug, although weakness may be difficult to detect
- Possible weakness of the trapezius, neck flexors, rhomboids, and rotator cuff
- Decreased sensation in the C4 dermatome; however, patients rarely complain of numbness

C5 Nerve Root
- Weakness of shoulder abduction and external rotation
- Weakness of elbow flexion
- Decreased biceps or brachioradialis DTRs (inconsistent)
- Decreased sensation in the C5 dermatome

	C1	C2	C3	C4	C5	C6	C7	C8	T1
Sternocleidomastoid-trapezius	■	■	■	■	■				
Rectus capitis posterior major	■								
Rectus capitis posterior minor	■								
Obliquus capitis superior	■								
Obliquus capitis inferior	■								
Geniohyoid	■								
Thyrohyoid	■								
Rectus capitis lateralis	■	■							
Rectus capitis anterior	■	■							
Sternohyoid	■	■	■						
Sternothyroid	■	■	■						
Omohyoid	■	■	■						
Longus capitis	■	■	■	■					
Semispinalis capitis	■	■	■	■	■	■	■	■	■
Levator scapulae		■	■	■					
Longus colli		■	■	■	■	■	■	■	
Anterior intertransversarii		■	■	■	■	■	■	■	■
Posterior intertransversarii		■	■	■	■	■	■	■	■
Diaphragm			■	■	■				
Splenius capitis			■	■	■	■			
Scalenus medius			■	■	■	■	■		
Interspinales			■	■	■	■	■	■	■
Multifidus			■	■	■	■	■	■	■
Scalenus anterior				■	■	■	■		
Semispinalis cervicis				■	■	■	■	■	■
Rhomboids–major and minor				■	■				
Supraspinatus				■	■				
Infraspinatus				■	■	■			
Teres major					■	■			
Deltoid					■	■			
Teres minor					■	■			
Subscapularis					■	■			
Brachioradialis					■	■			

Figure 5-20 Muscles of the cervical spine, shoulder, and upper extremity, with their corresponding motor nerve innervation. (From Bland JH: Embryology: practical clinical implications and interpretation. In *Disorders of the cervical spine: diagnosis and medical management,* ed 2, Philadelphia, 1994, Saunders.)

C6 Nerve Root

- Weakness of elbow and finger flexors
- Weakness of shoulder internal rotation
- Weakness of pronation and wrist extension
- Occasionally, weakness in shoulder abduction
- Decreased biceps or brachioradialis DTRs
- Decreased sensation in the C6 dermatome

C7 Nerve Root

- Weakness of elbow extension and forearm supination
- Weakness in wrist and finger flexion or extension
- Decreased triceps DTRs
- Decreased sensation in the C7 dermatome

C8 Nerve Root

- Weakness in elbow and wrist extension
- Weakness in wrist flexion and intrinsic muscles of the hand; loss of grip strength
- Decreased triceps DTRs
- Decreased abductor digiti minimi DTRs
- Decreased sensation in the C8 dermatome
- Resemblance to brachial plexus injury, ulnar neuropathy, and neurogenic thoracic outlet syndrome

Note: Sensory changes and referred pain patterns are variable among patients and may not correspond to generally accepted dermatome maps.

Imaging Studies

Plain radiographs are not diagnostic, but they may show foraminal stenosis (oblique view) or osteophytes on the uncovertebral or facet joints. MRI (74% to 88% accuracy), CT scan (72% to 91% accuracy), myelography (67% to 92% accuracy), and CT-myelography (75% to 96% accuracy) are diagnostic tests used to determine the cause of nerve root irritation and compression.[83] EMG and nerve conduction velocity (NCV) tests can provide information on the extent of the nerve damage.[85,89]

Facet Joint

Irritation of a cervical facet (zygapophyseal) joint (C4-5, C5-6, C6-7, C7-T1) can refer pain to regions in and around the shoulder (Fig. 5-21).[75,95-100] Structures of the facet joint capable of provoking pain include the joint capsule and the meniscoids within the joint itself.[39,101] Investigators have suggested that the articular cartilage within the joint, normally considered to be avascular and without nervous innervation, may acquire nociceptive fibers if the tissue is undergoing "remodeling" because of injury or disease of the cartilage. Research has documented that it is much more likely for a patient to have a symptomatic cervical disk along with a symptomatic facet joint than it is for a patient to have either pathologic condition independently.[102]

Symptoms

Pain is unilateral and may be felt in the neck, top or posterior portions of the shoulder, scapula, or interscapular region. Patients often report a sharp pain or pinch if they quickly turn their head toward the painful side or look upward. Pain is generally not referred to the anterior shoulder, biceps brachii muscle, or below the elbow. No complaints of numbness, pins and needles, or specific weakness in the upper extremity are reported.

Signs

Reproduction of symptoms is expected during the following special tests: the cervical quadrant test in extension (Spurling's), passive cervical spine extension and often with ipsilateral passive side bending or rotation, the cervical spine compression test in extension and occasionally in neutral, and facet joint tenderness to palpation. Segmental mobility examination is usually abnormal at the suspected level. Quite often, the examiner finds that the symptomatic facet joint is part of a hypermobile segment. This segment, however, may initially test as hypomobile because of acute entrapment of a meniscoid or acute muscle guarding. The results of neurologic examination are normal, including nerve root compression and nerve tension tests. Discogenic examination results are normal with respect to Valsalva's test and cervical compression in flexion.

Imaging Studies

Plain radiographs, although helpful in examining the general morphology of the cervical spine, are not diagnostic. They may demonstrate decreased disk height or osteophytosis of the facets. Even in the presence of abnormal results, the clinician must realize that many asymptomatic people have similar findings on plain film radiography. MRI and CT scans are not diagnostic for the source of pain, but they may be helpful in terms of the general status of the spine, by revealing degenerative changes within the disk or facet joints. Myelography is not useful in this case. Facet joint injection blocks or anesthesia of the medial branch of the dorsal ramus are the most accurate, specific, and sensitive diagnostic examination techniques in the facet joints.[95,96,102]

Injury to the cervical facet joints, without consideration of referred pain patterns, can lead to intrinsic shoulder pain and dysfunction. Erl Pettman, a physical therapist and master clinician, often used the following case example to illustrate this point[103]:

A post-traumatic hypomobility of C3-C4 on the left leads to a compensatory hypermobility of C3-C4 on the right (a hypomobile C2-3 or C4-5 on the right may also lead to a hypermobile C3-C4 on the right). This facilitated C-4 segment creates a hypertonus of the right levator scapulae muscle because of the increased motor output from the ventral horn. This increased activity in the levator scapulae places the scapula in a position of relative adduction. In this new position, the rotator cuff muscles are forced to work more as stabilizers instead of the superior-glenohumeral joint capsule. The interscapular portion of the biceps tendon slackens and buckles, predisposing it to impingement. During elevation the levator scapulae muscle, hypertonic because of the C-4

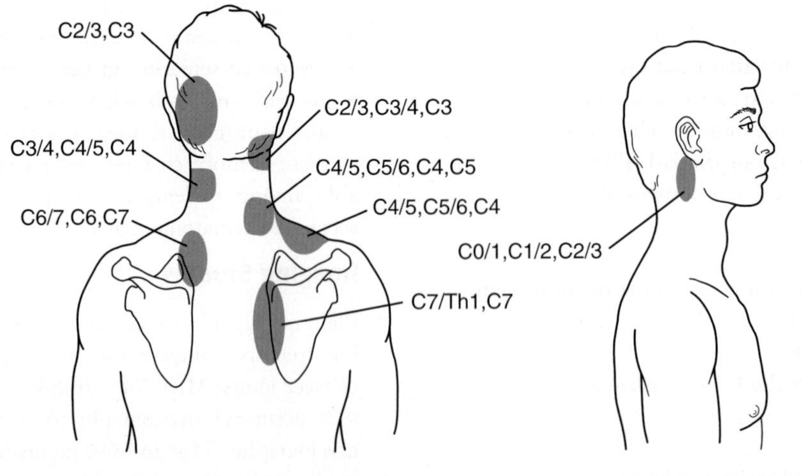

Figure 5-21 Referral distribution of cervical facet pain. Referred pain distribution is shown on one side only for each example. The pattern may be the same on the opposite side if the same structures are involved. (Redrawn from Fukui S, Ohseto K, Shiotani M, et al: Referred pain distribution of the cervical zygapophyseal joints and cervical dorsal rami, *Pain* 68:79–83, 1996 in Magee DJ: *Pathology and intervention in musculoskeletal rehabilitation*, St. Louis, 2009, Mosby Elsevier.)

facilitated segment, will limit the excursion of the scapula during the first 150° of ROM; this will require excessive motion from the glenohumeral joint, which can lead to glenohumeral joint laxity, instability, and possible labrum damage.

Other disorders within the cervical spine can also lead to an intrinsic shoulder problem, such as adhesive capsulitis, tendinitis, or bursitis.[18,36,40,49,52-56] Muscle guarding of the rotator cuff muscles, because of a lesion at the C5 or C6 segment of the spine, can lead to tendinosis.[40] Adhesive capsulitis of the shoulder may be caused by cervical disk disease or C5 or C6 radiculopathy.[40,54-56] One study reported that cervical spondylosis was found in 40% of patients with adhesive capsulitis.[74] When examined by thermography, 80% of these patients had hot spots on their cervical spine, and only 20% of them demonstrated hot spots on their shoulder.[74] Even though a patient may have reproduction of symptoms during a mechanical examination of the shoulder, a cervical disorder can lead to real shoulder dysfunction, and the patient is then likely to have dual pathologic conditions.[18,36,49,52]

Any tissue, from the skin and subcutaneous fat down to the center of the bones, with sensory afferent nerves feeding into the dorsal horn of the spinal cord between the C3 and T3 segments, is capable of referring pain and dysfunction to the shoulder.

THORACIC SPINE TISSUES CAPABLE OF REFERRING PAIN AND DYSFUNCTION TO THE SHOULDER

Disk

The thoracic spine often receives the least respect, in contrast to the cervical and lumbar spine. Primary sources of pain and injury are less common in the thoracic spine. This region typically receives less attention from clinicians in terms of evaluation and treatment, except in the case of postural analysis. Upper thoracic discogenic pain can be referred to regions of the posterior thorax, which can include the scapula, especially along the medial border.[104] Discogenic pain from as far down as T6-7 can refer pain to the inferior angle of the scapula. Disk injuries in the thoracic spine are much less common than in the cervical or lumbar spine. Upper thoracic disk injuries are often not diagnosed for many months or years after the onset of symptoms because most clinicians suspect that referred pain to the shoulder originates in the cervical spine. Subsequently, cervical spine imaging studies are ordered, and results may be normal, in which case the pain is thought to be myofascial. Conversely, subtle cervical degenerative joint disease (DJD) or subtle disk bulges are blamed for the pain. Thoracic disk injuries, bulges, and prolapses can be devastating because of the small diameter of the central spinal canal in the thoracic region and the close proximity of the spinal cord.

Lower thoracic disk ruptures have been associated with shoulder pain and dysfunction.[105] Wilke et al[105] discussed a case in which a woman was treated for chronic shoulder pain (diagnosed as supraspinatus calcific tendinitis). No success was reported after she had received 16 cortisone injections, 30 visits to a physical therapist, and finally subacromial decompression and debridement of the calcific deposit. The patient's shoulder and neurologic status grew progressively worse after surgery. A chronic, but recently exacerbated, T10-11 disk prolapse was then discovered. The patient improved rapidly after surgical decompression of the T10 disk prolapse. The authors of the study were convinced that the shoulder symptoms, if not a primary referral source of the T10-11 disk condition, were a direct result of changes in the dorsal horn of the thoracic spinal cord. This situation led to a central sensitization that hindered the rehabilitation of the shoulder symptoms.[105] In other words, the pathologic condition of the T10-11 disk was putting a strain on the shoulder, and this strain exacerbated the symptoms from the shoulder and interfered biomechanically, and probably neurophysiologically, with the rehabilitation of the shoulder.

Symptoms

Pain, usually a dull ache, is referred a short distance from the source to surrounding regions of the thoracic spine and scapular region (T1-6). Pain may be referred to the chest. Nausea or sweating with pain may be reported because of the connection between the sinuvertebral nerves (innervating the annulus fibrosus) and the sympathetic ganglion. Generally, the patient has no complaints of numbness, pins and needles sensation, or specific muscle weakness. Pain is usually not referred to the extremities or to the anterior or apical portions of the shoulder.

Signs

Reproduction of symptoms is expected during the following special tests: compression of the cervical and thoracic spine in neutral, flexed, and extended postures; segmentally specific posterior-anterior (PA) glides in a prone position (Fig. 5-22); coughing or sneezing; and Valsalva's test.[81] Neurologic indications are normal, including nerve root compression and nerve tension tests. In general, the examiner may find that the symptoms are reproduced with provocation of the thoracic spine and not the shoulder. Central sensitization, however, can produce the perception of pain during the examination of a relatively normal shoulder. In addition, chronic thoracic disk disease can induce true intrinsic disorders of the shoulder. In this example, the shoulder may respond with pain immediately during provocational testing, whereas the thoracic spine may become symptomatic only after prolonged activity.[80]

Imaging Studies

Plain radiographs, although helpful in examining the general morphologic features of the thoracic spine, are not diagnostic. They may demonstrate decreased disk height or osteophytosis. Even in the presence of abnormal findings, the clinician must realize that many asymptomatic people have similar findings on plain film radiography. Myelography can demonstrate spinal cord or nerve root compression, but it cannot indicate whether a disk, an osteophyte, or a tumor is creating the compression. A CT scan following a myelogram will allow for the differential diagnosis of the tissue responsible for compression of neurologic tissues, but it cannot show whether a specific disk is

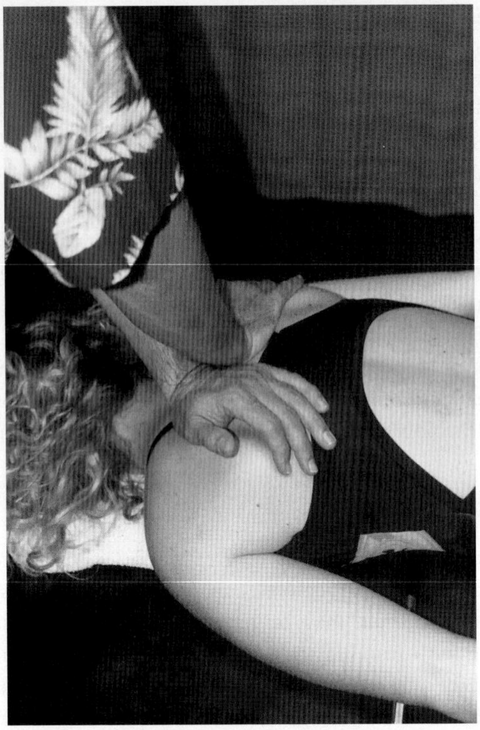

Figure 5-22 Prone thoracic posterior-anterior (PA) glides. This technique, in which the pisiform of each hand is placed on the transverse processes of the target vertebra, can be used in several ways: as a provocation to help rule out a symptomatic thoracic spine; to assess general thoracic (PA) mobility; as a mobilization technique (by using various speed and force techniques and oscillations or stretch) to inhibit pain and increase segmental mobility; and to deliver a high-velocity, low-amplitude thrust when appropriate.

symptomatic. MRI can identify a degenerated or herniated or prolapsed disk, but it cannot detect whether the disk is symptomatic. Diskography within a specific segment of the thoracic spine, however, can clearly identify a symptomatic disk.[106]

Nerve

First thoracic nerve root irritations and compressions (e.g., from a T1-2 disk injury) can produce neck, shoulder, and arm pain.[94,107,108] The differential diagnosis of these symptoms must include cervical radiculopathy (C8), thoracic outlet syndrome, ulnar neuropathy, and brachial plexus injuries, to name the most obvious neuromusculoskeletal choices. Visceral pain to consider includes the lung (Pancoast's tumor) and the heart (myocardial infarction).[107] Radiculopathy of T1 can therefore go undiagnosed for many months because the symptoms mimic those of other disorders, and most imaging studies will tend to focus on the cervical spine and miss the T1-2 segment. Nerve root injuries from T2 through T5 can also refer pain to the posterior shoulder and scapula (see Fig. 5-16).[109]

Symptoms

Patients often describe the pain as sharp, electrical, or "like a nerve is being pinched." Pain may start as a dull ache in the scapular region and progress to sharp radicular pain and paresthesia down the medial aspect of the arm, forearm, and hand.[107,108] The patient may also complain of a loss of grip strength. Because nerve root irritations and compressions are often associated with disk injuries, the patient may also complain of discogenic symptoms.

Signs

Reproduction of symptoms is expected during the following special tests: the cervical quadrant test in extension (Spurling's) with retraction[53,81,89,90]; passive extension, ipsilateral side bending, or ipsilateral rotation of the cervical-thoracic spine; compression in an extended posture; the T1 nerve root special test (Fig. 5-23); and at least one abnormal finding with neurologic testing of motor or sensory reflexes or DTRs. Findings from axial compression in the neutral posture of the cervical-thoracic spine may be abnormal or normal, whereas results from compression in a flexed posture are normal. Cervical-thoracic axial distraction or traction in a flexed posture often brings temporary relief of symptoms, but symptoms can be aggravated if an inflamed and tethered nerve root is stretched over a bulging disk or osteophyte.[81,86,89] The patient may have loss of sensation in the T1 dermatome, loss of strength in the T1 myotome (grip), and atrophy of the intrinsic muscles of the hand.[94,107,108] Because of the connection between the T1 nerve root and the SNS, Horner's syndrome may be present.[108] The signs of Horner's syndrome are miosis (pupil contraction), ptosis (partial drooping of the eyelid), enophthalmos (recession of the eyeball into the orbit), and loss of sweating on the side of the face. The standard upper extremity DTR examination is not affected. If discogenic symptoms are present, then the test results for discogenic pain noted earlier will also be abnormal.

Imaging Studies

Plain radiographs are not diagnostic, and results may be WNL, but they can show the morphologic features of the spine in terms of degenerative changes of the facets and vertebral end plates. MRI, CT scan, myelography, and CT-myelography can be diagnostic for nerve root irritation and compression. Examination using CT-myelography probably gives the most accurate and relevant information to help determine a rehabilitation strategy, prognosis, and the need for a surgical consultation. Information on the extent of the nerve root damage is best assessed by EMG and NCV studies.

Facet

Injuries to the upper thoracic facet joints (C7 to T1 to T5-6) can refer pain to the posterior regions of the shoulder and scapula (Fig. 5-24).[98,104,110,111] Menck et al[112] described a patient with CRPS-I who rapidly improved after receiving manipulation (high-velocity, short-amplitude thrust) to the facet and costotransverse joints from T3 to T5. In addition to the sympathetic symptoms, the patient had shoulder and upper extremity pain and dysfunction. Rapid improvement in shoulder ROM and pain was noted following the manipulations to the mid-thoracic and upper thoracic segments.[112] These investigators theorized that the increased ROM of the shoulder was the result of a decrease in the thoracic kyphosis.[112]

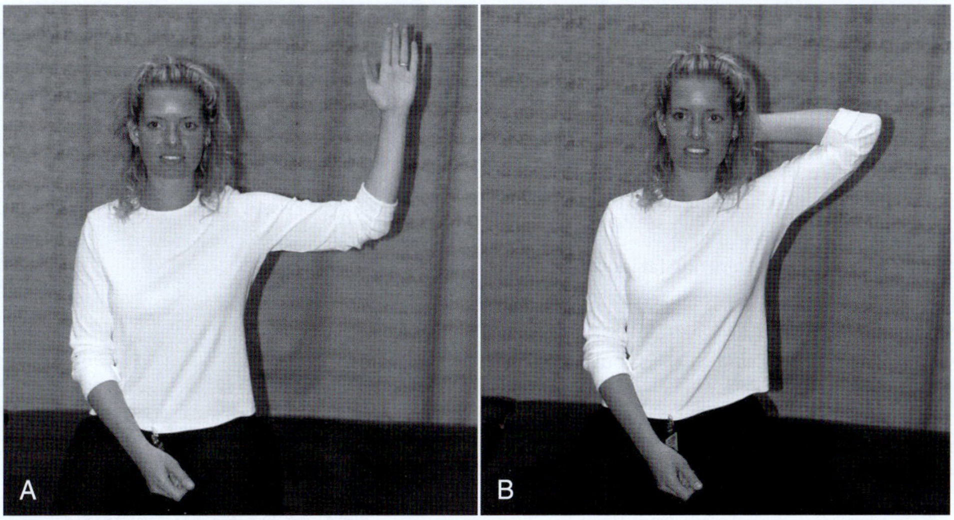

Figure 5-23 T1 nerve stretch test. **A,** The patient, seated, is instructed to rotate externally and abduct the involved extremity to 90° and to flex the elbow to 90° as well. This position should be relatively pain free, without a reproduction of the patient's primary complaints. **B,** The patient is then instructed to flex the elbow maximally by placing the hand behind the neck. The test result is positive if the patient's complaints of pain in the scapula and medially down the arm are reproduced. Paresthesia may also be exacerbated. This result of this test is also abnormal in persons with ulnar neuropathy.

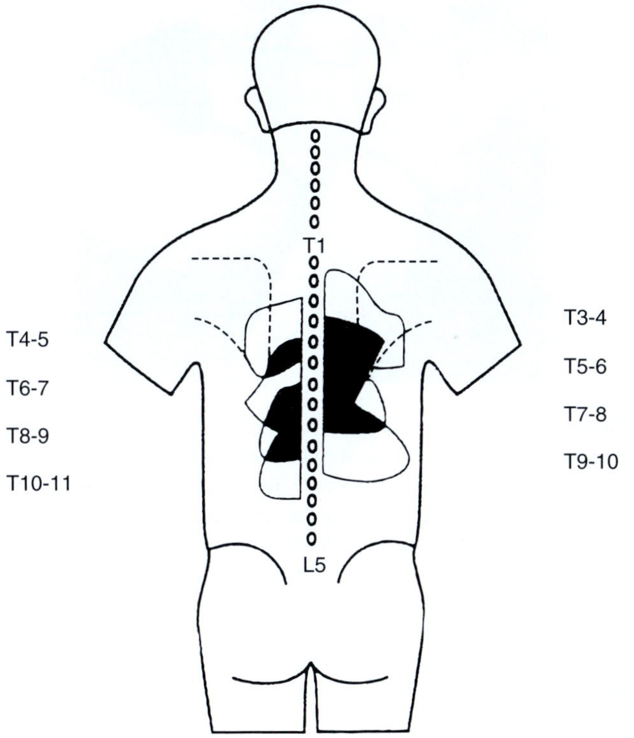

Figure 5-24 Referred pain patterns from specific thoracic facet joints. (From Dreyfuss P, Tibiletti C, Dreyer SJ, et al: Thoracic zygapophyseal pain: a review and description of an intraarticular block technique, *Pain Dig* 4:44, 1994.)

In addition to referral of pain directly to the shoulder from the thoracic spine, injury and dysfunction in the thoracic spine can lead to pain, injury, and dysfunction in the shoulder. Full elevation of the arm depends on elevation of the upper ribs, thoracic extension, thoracic side bending, and thoracic rotation. Restrictions in any of these motions put additional stress on the shoulder that may lead to repetitive strain injuries and a limitation in shoulder ROM and function.

Symptoms

Pain is unilateral and may be felt in the upper thoracic area and the posterior portions of the shoulder, scapula, or interscapular region. Patients may report a sharp pain or pinch if they quickly extend or turn toward the painful side. Pain is generally not referred to the anterior shoulder, biceps brachii muscle, or down the arm. No complaints of numbness, pins and needles, or specific weakness in the upper extremity are reported.

Signs

Reproduction of symptoms is expected during the following special tests: the thoracic quadrant test in extension; passive thoracic spine extension, and often with ipsilateral passive side bending or rotation; and the seated thoracic spine compression test, in extension and occasionally in neutral. Segment-specific PA glides in a prone position may also elicit pain. Segmental mobility examination is usually abnormal at the suspected level. Quite often, the examiner finds that the symptomatic facet joint is part of a hypermobile segment. This segment, however, may initially test hypomobile because of acute entrapment of a meniscoid or acute muscle guarding. Neurologic examination results are normal, including nerve root compression and nerve tension tests. Discogenic examination results are normal with respect to Valsalva's test and seated thoracic compression in flexion.

Imaging Studies

Plain radiographs, although helpful in examining the general morphologic features of the thoracic spine, are not diagnostic. They may demonstrate decreased disk height or osteophytosis of the facets. Even in the presence of abnormal findings, the clinician must realize that many asymptomatic people have similar results on plain film radiography. MRI and CT scans are not diagnostic for the source of pain, but they may be helpful in terms of the general status of the spine, by revealing degenerative changes within the disk or facet joints. Myelography is not useful in this instance. Facet joint injection blocks or anesthesia of the medial branch of the dorsal ramus are the most accurate, specific, and sensitive diagnostic examinations of the facet joints.[95,96,102]

Any tissue, from the skin and subcutaneous fat down to the center of the bones, with sensory afferent nerves feeding into the dorsal horn of the spinal cord between the C3 and T3 segments, is capable of referring pain and dysfunction to the shoulder.

RIB INJURIES THAT REFER PAIN AND DYSFUNCTION TO THE SHOULDER

The ribs and rib cage in general are often overlooked as a source of pain and dysfunction related to the shoulder. First rib injuries and diseases (e.g., costotransverse and costovertebral joint sprains, fractures, and bony tumors) refer pain to the shoulder almost exclusively.[113-115] First rib disorders often go undiagnosed for many months because the painful shoulder in the presence of a first rib injury can mimic shoulder impingement or rotator cuff tendinosis during evaluation. Imaging studies are often directed to the cervical spine and shoulder and therefore may not adequately visualize first rib injuries. Besides of the obvious problem of delaying an accurate diagnosis and appropriate treatment, fracture of the first rib can lead to devastating consequences because of the proximity of the subclavian artery, brachial plexus, and lung.

Injuries to the second or third rib at the costotransverse joint may also refer pain to the shoulder.[116] In these cases, patients are often incorrectly diagnosed with a rotator cuff tear, tendinosis, or impingement syndrome. The impingement test is thought to give a false-positive result secondary to the elevation and stress placed on the upper ribs during the Neer or Hawkins procedure.[116] The empty-can test (for supraspinatus tendinosis) may also give a false-positive result because of referred pain from the stress of the procedure on the upper ribs and motor weakness as a result of reflex inhibition.[116]

Symptoms

Pain is the primary complaint and may be perceived in the neck, chest, posterior shoulder, scapula, or arm.[113-115] The patient may report an episode of sharp pain during a particular motion, usually a fast motion such as during sports. If the rib injury is on the left, the pain may mimic the symptoms of angina or a myocardial infarction.[113]

Signs

The patient usually has full AROM of the shoulder with pain at the end range.[113-115] Full cervical AROM is common. Tenderness may be noted in the thoracic inlet on the first rib or deep in the axilla.[1,113] Results of provocational testing to the ribs (Figs. 5-25 and 5-26) are abnormal. Various rotator

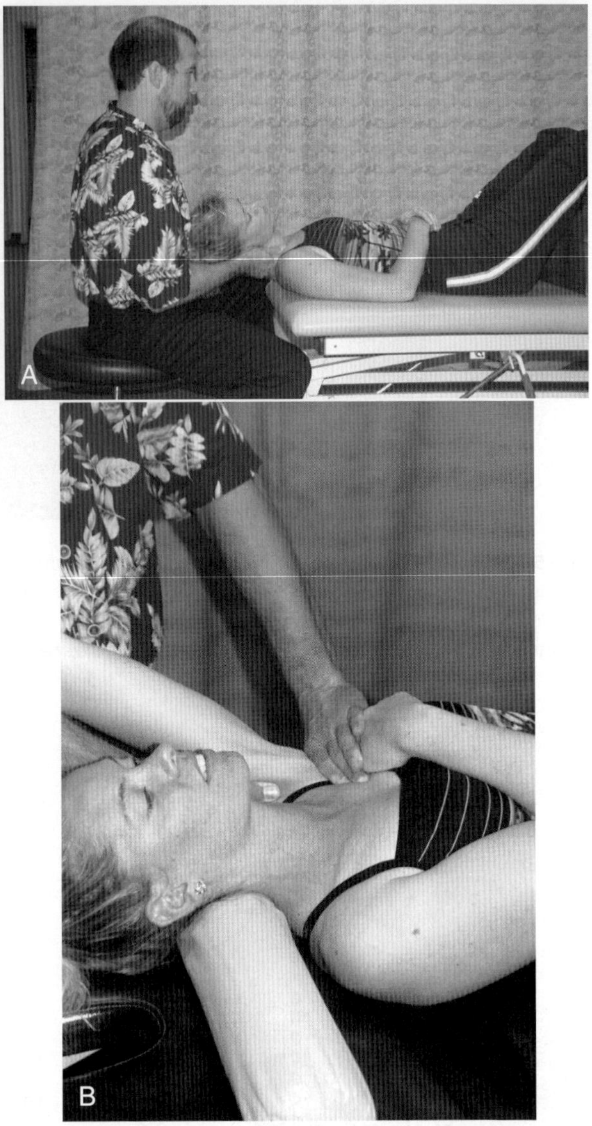

Figure 5-25 Mobility testing of the ribs. **A,** Mobility testing of the first rib. The patient, in a supine hook-lying position, is relaxed, with her head and neck passively rotated and side bent to the affected side to reduce the strain on the first rib from the scalenus muscle group and surrounding fascia. The clinician, using the lateral edge of the proximal phalanx of his index finger, gently mobilizes the first rib in an inferior and medial direction. This technique may be used in several ways: as a provocation test for first rib injuries, to test mobility, and to treat an elevated or restricted first rib. **B,** Mobility testing of ribs R2 to R6. The patient, in a supine hook-lying position, is using her right hand to cover her breast. The clinician, using the web space and the lateral portion of his index finger of his left hand, gently stabilizes the inferior rib (e.g., R3). His right hand has a firm hold of the proximal humerus that is passively guided into flexion as his left hand assesses the mobility between R2 and R3. This technique may be used in several ways: as a provocation test for rib injuries, to test mobility, and to treat restricted mobility between the ribs. Alternate techniques for ribs R4 to R12 include mobility testing the lateral portion of the rib cage in a side-lying position or the posterior portion of the rib cage with the patient prone.

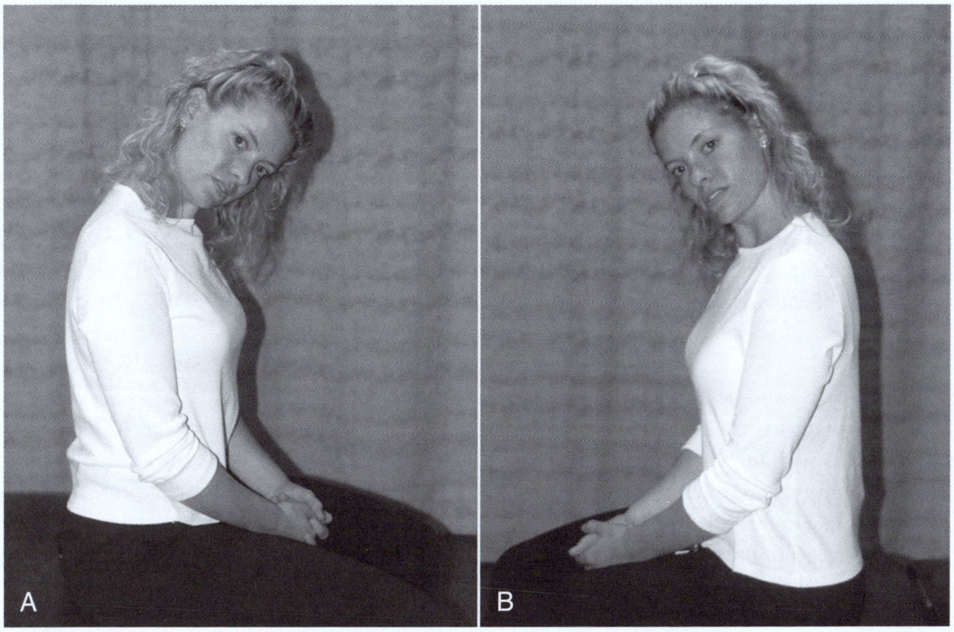

Figure 5-26 First rib special test. Cervical rotation lateral flexion (CRLF) is a special test to assess quickly whether a patient may have an elevated first rib or other possible first rib injuries and dysfunctions. The patient, seated, is asked to rotate his or her neck actively as far as possible. Then, holding that rotation, the patient actively laterally flexes the neck as far as possible. The test result is abnormal if the amount of lateral flexion is significantly different from one side to the other. **A,** Testing R1 on the left: right rotation with left lateral flexion. **B,** Testing R1 on the right: left rotation with right lateral flexion.

cuff special tests (e.g., Hawkins, Neer, and empty-can) may produce false-positive results because of the stress put on the upper ribs, especially the first rib, during these maneuvers.

Imaging Studies

Plain radiographs in an AP view of the cervical spine, chest, or shoulder are usually sufficient to visualize the first three ribs. Unfortunately, some clinicians fail to examine the upper ribs closely on a cervical spine radiograph.[113-115] On occasion, it may be necessary to obtain an oblique view of the shoulder or a supine chest radiograph. In cases of ambiguous or subtle stress fractures, a bone scan may be necessary.

Any tissue, from the skin and subcutaneous fat down to the center of the bones, with sensory afferent nerves feeding into the dorsal horn of the spinal cord between the C3 and T3 segments, is capable of referring pain and dysfunction to the shoulder.

LUMBAR SPINE AND PELVIC TISSUES CAPABLE OF REFERRING DYSFUNCTION TO THE SHOULDER

The most direct link to the shoulder from the low back is through the latissimus dorsi muscle. Injuries to the low back may cause muscle guarding or adaptive shortening in this muscle and may subsequently make it more difficult for the shoulder to achieve full elevation and full external rotation, thus causing stress to the tissues attempting to elevate the shoulder. Low back injuries that substantially alter spinal posture can also adversely affect shoulder function. Christie et al[117] found that persons with acute low back pain have a significant increase in thoracic kyphosis, both in sitting and standing positions, and demonstrate a forward head posture. The association between posture and shoulder dysfunction was made previously.

In erect standing, external loads applied to the spine through the upper extremity and shoulder (e.g., resisted horizontal adduction of the shoulder) must be counteracted by increased activity in muscles of the lumbar spine (e.g., multifidus and iliocostalis) for the body to remain erect and in its usual posture.[118] Movement of the shoulder in persons without low back pain is preceded by contraction of the transversus abdominis muscle.[119] In persons with chronic low back pain, the transversus abdominis contracts after the prime movers of the shoulder contract.[119] This finding indicates a decrease in motor control for spinal stability in persons with chronic low back pain. It also demonstrates the close relationship of the lumbar spine with the shoulder. Altered motor control and stability of the lumbar spine because of low back pain can adversely influence the dynamic control and coordination of the shoulder because the shoulder depends on proximal stability for its distal mobility. Therefore, any tissue injury in the low back that alters the posture, function, or stability of the lumbar spine or pelvis can have an adverse effect on shoulder function and can eventually lead to an intrinsic shoulder problem or injury.

CASE STUDY 5.1

Overview

The purpose of the initial examination is to evaluate the pain, the strain, and the brain. The rehabilitation program then focuses on treating the specific tissue producing the pain, the various tissues producing a strain, and the influence of the brain, by using the acronym WOMEN (*w*isdom, *o*ptimism, *m*anual therapy, *e*xercise, and *n*utrition).

Pain

Patients come for treatment because they are in pain. One of responsibilities of the therapist is to determine the source of the pain. This becomes a search for the primary "tissue in lesion." First, the therapist must determine the region (e.g., cervical spine versus shoulder) of the painful tissue, then the specific tissue (e.g., facet joint versus intervertebral disk) in that region that is the primary generator of the patient's pain. Specific provocational testing of all the tissues in a specific region allows for a reasonable differentiation of the tissue, or tissues, responsible for the pain. For example, a painful cervical facet joint injury is provoked by different stimuli (direct palpation and cervical axial compression in extension only) than a painful cervical disk injury (segmental disk shear test; cervical axial compression in a flexed, neutral, and extended posture; coughing or sneezing; and Valsalva's test). Once the therapist has found the tissue in lesion (e.g., left C5-6 facet joint impingement), he or she can provide specific treatment to the pain generator (the left C5-6 facet joint) to inhibit pain and to provide the optimal stimulus for regeneration of this tissue.

Strain

The next objective of the evaluation is to examine the patient for biomechanical and physiologic strains that may have caused the painful injury in the first place (pain of gradual or insidious onset) or that may be perpetuating the pain after direct trauma or surgery. The following are examples of biomechanical strains that can produce or perpetuate pain: postural dysfunction, poor spinal or extremity stability and motor control, significant leg length differences, lower kinetic chain dysfunction (hip, knee, foot, or ankle), adaptive shortening of musculotendinous tissue and fascia, and joint hypomobilities or hypermobilities above and below the pain generator.

Physiologic strains and comorbid diseases must be noted before treatment is initiated. Systemic problems such as rheumatoid arthritis, osteoporosis, diabetes, cardiovascular disease, medication abuse, and poor diet or nutritional habits can adversely affect the progress, prognosis, and eventual outcome of rehabilitation, especially if these strains are not identified and addressed while patients are under the therapist's care. Patient abuse of nonsteroidal anti-inflammatory drugs (NSAIDs) over a prolonged period can also be a strain. The prolonged use of NSAIDs, usually as a "pain killer," in patients who do not have an inflammatory disease, such as rheumatoid arthritis, can have the following consequences: (1) direct interference with the regeneration of bone and articular cartilage; (2) allowing of patients who would normally be limited by pain to overuse and overstress tissues that have not yet fully regenerated; and (3) death.[120-125] As many as 16,500 people die each year in the United States directly as a result of complications of NSAID use.[120]

Once the strains have been identified (e.g., thoracic kyphosis with forward head associated with adaptive shortening of the pectoralis minor, SCM, hip and knee flexion contractures; hypomobilities at C4-5 and C7-T4; hypermobility at L4-5; chronic right ankle instability; osteoporosis; and a pack-a-day smoker for the past 20 years), the therapist can provide specific treatment to these dysfunctions and decrease the adverse load on the primary tissue in lesion (left C5-6 facet joint impingement). Some patients have so many strains that it is not possible to give specific individualized attention to every little detail. In these cases, patient education and a comprehensive home instruction program can be extremely helpful.

Brain

The final objective in the initial examination process is to recognize how the patient's brain (frontal lobe: fear, anxiety, and depression versus motivation, determination, and optimism) and spinal cord (central sensitization) is reacting to the injury or disease. The treatment plan for one patient with a left C5-6 facet joint impingement may be different from the plan for another patient with the same diagnosis, depending on the status of their "brain." Issues such as fear and anxiety, chronic pain, prolonged medical leave from work, litigation, workers' compensation, signs of depression, low functional status, poor support network, poor self-motivation, and high dependence on others can dramatically alter both the progress and the prognosis of a patient if these issues are not recognized and addressed.

One of the greatest things therapists can do for their patients with chronic pain is to remove their fear and anxiety. Many of these patients experience high levels of pain, stress, and anxiety because they do not understand the source of their pain, why they have hurt for so long, and what they can do without risking reinjury. Therapists can help remove an enormous amount of fear and anxiety simply by educating these patients about their problem, their prognosis, and the realistic likelihood of reinjury during work and ADLs. Explaining the differences between pain and injury (i.e., "pain does not equal injury") goes a long way in terms of removing the activity and exercise avoidance issues that many patients with chronic pain exhibit because of their fears and anxieties. This approach is much

CASE STUDY 5.1—cont'd

better suited for the patient with chronic pain than for the patient with an acute injury or acute surgical repair. Patients who have an acute injury, have had recent surgery, or have persistent pain from tissues that are weak and not fully healed should respect pain for safety reasons. However, patients with chronic pain who complain long after their tissues have healed (those with central sensitization) are the ones who truly need to understand that reasonable activities that cause pain do not cause injury. The treatment approach involves providing wisdom and optimism for the patient, in hopes of altering this adverse or negative forebrain output. The goal is to help the patient increase the pain inhibitory impulses descending down from the forebrain, PAG, and RVM to the spinal cord and into the dorsal horn, to raise the threshold for activation of the interneurons responsible for nociceptive transmission.

Treatment may involve providing the patient with options for counseling, support groups and relaxation, or visualization techniques. Giving the patient relaxation and breathing techniques or visual imaging exercises can be very helpful. Patients can be taught to visualize themselves moving their injured arm as freely as the uninjured arm or to visualize themselves participating in full duty work or their favorite sport. In cases of severe, debilitating pain, the therapist can have the patient visualize the pain as a red balloon that slowly shrinks as it changes to blue. Staying upbeat and optimistic around the patient and being a cheerleader can do wonders. The therapist can give patients a realistic prognosis for increasing their function. The focus should move away from the pain and be placed on patients' functional abilities. "How are you functioning today?" versus "How much pain do you have today?" Any small doubts, hesitation, or negativity about recovery that the clinician has can be multiplied and exaggerated by the patient and used as a confirmation of the patient's own negative thoughts and fears about chronic pain and disability. The clinician should act and talk like an expert, without being phony, to take advantage of the placebo effect. If the patient perceives the therapist as an expert, then almost any treatment will help to some degree. If the clinician acts unsure, not confident, and without the appearance of expertise, then the patient may lose faith in the treatment approach, and even the best manual therapy program may be only marginally successful.

The other aspect of treatment to the "brain" involves the spinal cord and the plastic changes that happen within the dorsal horn in patients suffering from chronic pain. Changes in the glutamate receptors on the postsynaptic neurons can lead to a facilitated segment that now acts as the pain generator after the original primary tissue in lesion (e.g., supraspinatus tendinosis) has healed. Recognition of this source of chronic pain is the first step. Treatment involves the wisdom and optimism noted earlier along with manual therapy to segmentally related tissues (e.g., skin, fascia, muscle, and joints) to provide inhibitory impulses (through type I, II, and III mechanoreceptors) into the dorsal horn to raise the threshold for activation of the interneurons responsible for nociceptive transmission. These soft tissue and joint mobilizations of varying speeds and amplitudes, below the threshold for activation of pain or muscle guarding, have the potential to stimulate inhibitory interneurons within the dorsal horn that will subsequently alter the patient's perception of the pain experience. The laying-on of expert and caring hands to the patient can also help calm the forebrain's thoughts and perceptions and help to increase the amount of inhibitory impulses descending from the forebrain to the level of the facilitated segment in the spinal cord. In addition, positive imagery and a positive attitude by the patient can increase the amount of inhibitory impulses descending from the forebrain and into the facilitated segment to raise the threshold for activation of the interneurons responsible for nociceptive transmission.

Patient Presentation

This case study has been modified to enhance the learning experience and to fit the format of the *Guide to Physical Therapist Practice.*

Demographics

Bewell is a 49-year-old right-handed white woman and college graduate whose primary language is English. Her health maintenance organization (HMO) covers her medical and physical therapy care. Today, November 13, 2000, is her first visit with us.

Social History

Bewell lives with her husband and two teen-age daughters. She denies any cultural or religious beliefs that she feels may affect her care with us. Bewell is a legal secretary with a light physical demand level. Her job duties include the following: prolonged sitting; frequent speaking on the phone (no head set); prolonged keyboard and mouse use while sitting at a computer; occasional reaching, lifting, and carrying up to 20 lb; and infrequent lifting of up to 10 lb overhead. She has been out of work since May 1, 2000.

Living Environment

Bewell lives in a two-story home with one step and no railing leading to her front door. She denies the existence of any substantial obstacles in and around her home. She ascends and descends stairs with a railing in her home and ambulates freely without the use of assistive devices.

General Health Status

Bewell states that she is in good health and has had no major life changes in the past year.

Continued

CASE STUDY 5.1—cont'd

Social/Health Habits

Bewell drinks 3 to 4 cups of coffee a day, has smoked half a pack of cigarettes a day for the past 25 years, and has a couple of beers on the weekend. She does not supplement her diet with vitamins, minerals, herbs, or other health care products. Before surgery and the onset of her symptoms, Bewell's exercise routine included running, the Stairmaster, step aerobics, and lifting free weights.

Family History

Bewell's father died of prostate cancer, her grandmother died of a stroke, and she states that all the women in her family seem to suffer from osteoarthritis.

Medical/Surgical History

Bewell reports a history of allergies (to cats), a fractured fibula (1980), borderline hypoglycemia, and a neck injury at work in 1991 because of a tray table that hit her on the head. She complained of neck and shoulder pain for 1 year. She had an open-reduction and internal-fixation surgical procedure to her right fibula in 1980, a meniscectomy of her right knee in 1981, and a cesarian section in 1986. Concerning her left shoulder, Bewell reports that she had arthroscopic subacromial decompression surgery in 1998 because of a work-related injury. She received a total of at least 6 months of physical therapy (elsewhere) before and after her surgery. On May 5, 2000, she had another surgical procedure to her left shoulder in which the surgeon performed a bursectomy, acromioplasty, and excision of the distal clavicle. In the past year, she has complained of occasional headaches, weight gain because of a lack of exercise, difficulty sleeping, and pain at night from her shoulder. Bewell denies any current gynecologic difficulties but notes that she had endometriosis in 1992. She also denied a history involving motor vehicle accidents.

Current Condition(s)/Chief Complaint(s)

Bewell came to physical therapy (November 13, 2000) with a prescription for work hardening and the following diagnosis: status post left shoulder arthroscopy with decompression. She reports that surgery (May 5, 2000) was performed because of chronic pain in her shoulder. She denies experiencing any trauma to the shoulder between her first and second surgical procedure. Bewell states that her left shoulder pain gradually returned approximately 6 months before her last surgery. She received 2 months of physical therapy (at another facility) following surgery, but her symptoms progressively worsened. She then went for approximately 2 months without therapy, and her symptoms subsided. Three weeks ago, she started working out on her own by lifting weights up and over her head. Subsequently, she experienced a severe exacerbation of neck and left shoulder pain.

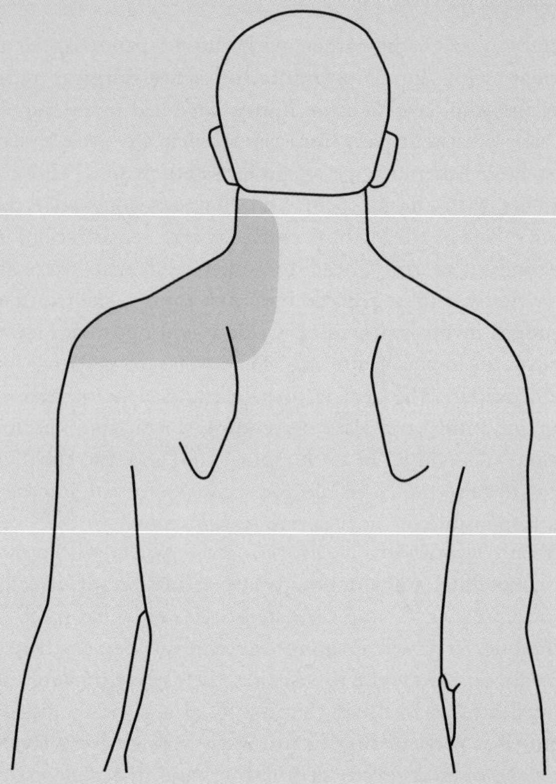

Figure 5-27 Pain diagram of a 49-year-old right-handed woman following surgery for subacromial decompression of her left shoulder.

Specifically, Bewell is complaining of periodic severe (0/10 to 8/10) neck and left shoulder pain (Fig. 5-27). She notes a periodic "slipping out" of her left shoulder. Bewell states that in certain positions her shoulder will pop or click. She also reports a grinding sound in her neck if she looks up and over her left shoulder. She denies headaches, dizziness, tinnitus, nausea, vision changes, swelling, radiation of pain down the upper extremities, weakness, or paresthesia in her upper extremities. Bewell reports that driving, talking on the telephone, and sitting increase her symptoms. Her symptoms decrease with rest. Her goal is to "get rid of the pain." She is under the care of her primary care physician for this problem.

Functional Status/Activity Level

Before surgery and the onset of her symptoms, Bewell's exercise routine included running, the Stairmaster, step aerobics, and lifting free weights. She scored 39 out of a possible maximum score of 100 on the Sharp Functional Activity Survey (Sharp FAS) for the Neck & Shoulder region (© Sharp HealthCare 1998). Because of her use of medications to control her pain, Bewell's Sharp FAS score of 39 overstates her true functional abilities. She reports moderate difficulty with most ADLs, with the exception of lifting and carrying, which give her severe difficulties,

CASE STUDY 5.1—cont'd

and sports (surfing and basketball with her daughter) or athletic activities (running, aerobics, weight lifting) that she cannot perform. She was placed on medical leave from work 6 months ago.

Medications

Bewell denies taking any prescription drugs other than birth control pills. She admits that she has been taking Tylenol (acetaminophen, an analgesic) and Advil (ibuprofen, an NSAID) almost daily since May.

Other Clinical Tests

The only tests reported by Bewell in the past year were a mammogram (results were normal), a blood test (normal), and radiographs: chest (normal) and shoulder (see "Imaging Studies," later in this case study).

Cardiovascular/Pulmonary System

Bewell has no symptoms related to her cardiopulmonary system. She does have risk factors associated with this system (decreased activity level, 13 pack-year smoking history, age, fear and frustration, and a family history of stroke). However, results from recent blood tests and a chest radiograph were normal. Therefore, evaluation of this system was deferred. Her cardiopulmonary system would have been evaluated if the results of examination of her musculoskeletal system had been normal. Bewell's cardiopulmonary system will be evaluated in the future if her symptoms change.

Integumentary System

Bewell's skin appears healthy, with good continuity of color and no substantial changes in temperature. Old surgical scars are noted at her right ankle and her right knee. Three small scars, well healed and almost white, are also noted on the left shoulder, the result of two previous arthroscopic surgical procedures.

Communication, Affect, Cognition, and Learning Style

No known learning barriers are identified for Bewell. She reports that she learns best when given a picture followed by a demonstration. Bewell does not show any deficits with regard to her cognition, orientation, or ability to communicate effectively. She is frustrated with her poor recovery from surgery 6 months ago and her inability to return to work. She is fearful of reinjuring her shoulder by doing too much. Bewell does not understand why she is still having shoulder pain, and she is upset because she cannot play basketball with her daughter, who just made the local high school team. The education needs identified for Bewell are as follows: an explanation of the source of her pain and what strains are feeding into it; an understanding that at this stage pain may not equal injury for her shoulder; nutritional and diet advice; ergonomic instructions for sitting at her computer at work; home care instructions; and home exercises.

Musculoskeletal System

Posture

In standing, Bewell has a forward head posture with rounded shoulders, protracted scapula, and a moderate increase in her thoracic kyphosis. Notable items are a slight increase in lumbar lordosis, mild right genu valgum, right calcaneal valgus with excessive pronation, and a moderate hallux valgus on the right.

Range of Motion

Cervical Spine Active Range of Motion

Bewell has moderate restrictions to cardinal movements of extension, left side bending, and left rotation. Pain is reproduced during each of these motions. Her head deviates to the left during flexion and to the right during extension. Repeated flexion, right side bending, or right rotation fails to reproduce her primary complaints of pain. Results from combined motions of flexion, left side bending, left rotation; flexion, right side bending, right rotation; and extension, right side bending, right rotation are all normal. Pain is reproduced with combined extension, left side bending, and left rotation.

Cervical Spine Passive Range of Motion

The same restrictions to movement are found as with AROM. The same movement patterns that reproduced Bewell's pain, as described earlier, are also noted during PROM testing.

Shoulder Active Range of Motion

Discomfort is reported with flexion and horizontal adduction only. No limitations to motion are present.

Shoulder Passive Range of Motion

Discomfort is reported in all directions except internal rotation. No limitations to motion are present.

Scapula and Elbow Range of Motion

Results from testing are normal and noncontributory.

Thoracic Spine Range of Motion

AROM and PROM testing fail to reproduce Bewell's primary complaint of pain. Moderate restrictions are noted with active and passive extension.

Rib Range of Motion

AROM and PROM testing fail to reproduce Bewell's primary complaint of pain. Full expansion of the rib cage during inhalation is inhibited by her thoracic kyphosis.

Lumbar Range of Motion

AROM is WNL with a slight deviation, variable from left to right on repeated examination, noted during active extension. Bewell reports pain, localized to the upper lumbar spine, at the end ROM of active extension.

Continued

CASE STUDY 5.1—cont'd

Muscle Performance

Cervical Spine Resisted Testing

Each resisted direction (six) is isometrically tested in three different muscle lengths: shortened, mid, and lengthened. The purpose of the test is to differentiate pain arising from contractile tissue (painful in all three muscle lengths tested) from noncontractile tissue (pain may occur only in a position that allows the contracting muscle to compress or stretch the truly injured tissue, such as the cervical facet joint or, when testing the shoulder, the supraspinatus tendon because of a position of impingement). For example, if resisted left side bending is abnormal in the shortened (cervical spine is side bent left into a pain-free range), middle (cervical spine is in neutral), and lengthened (cervical spine is side bent right into a pain-free range) positions, then it is reasonable to assume the pain is arising from the contractile tissues of the left scalenus, left SCM, or left upper trapezius muscle groups. If, however, resisted left side bending is painful (on the left side) only in the shortened muscle length, then the pain probably originates from compression of noncontractile tissue, such as the facet joint, uncovertebral joint, intervertebral disk, or a spinal nerve root.

For this case study, pain is reproduced in the shortened range of resisted extension, left side bending, and left rotation, tested separately. These same symptoms are reproduced in the lengthened range of resisted flexion, right side bending, and right rotation, tested separately. All these painful positions are compressive to noncontractile tissues, such as the facet joints on the left side of the cervical spine. Results of resisted testing to the cervical spine are normal when the facet joints on the left are not in a closed-pack position.

Shoulder Resisted Testing

Pain is reproduced during flexion and abduction testing only with the muscle in the shortened position (impingement posture). External rotation is painful only when the muscle is in the lengthened range. When pain is reported, it occurs only at the time resistance is released, a sign of instability.

Scapula and Elbow Resisted Testing

Results of testing are normal and noncontributory.

Thoracic Spine Resisted Testing

No reproduction of Bewell's primary complaint of pain occurs.

Rib Cage Resisted Testing

No reproduction of Bewell's primary complaint of pain occurs.

Note: No pain-free weakness is noted in the muscles of the spine and upper extremities.

Sensory Integrity

This part of the examination is deferred to save time during the evaluation and because Bewell denies having any neurologic symptoms.

Reflex Integrity

This part of the examination is deferred to save time during the evaluation and because Bewell denies having any neurologic symptoms.

Pain

Palpation

Pain and discomfort are reported with palpation of the C5-6 facet joint on the left. Tenderness is noted within the left supraspinatus and infraspinatus muscle bellies, left upper trapezius, bilateral scalenus (left more than right), and bilateral SCM.

Special Tests

Cervical Spine (Positive Tests)

Compression testing of the cervical spine in extension: pain
Posterior and superior traction force on the neck (facet distraction): relief
Left cervical quadrant test in extension (Spurling's): crepitus and left local pain only
Shear test at C5-6: mild increase in shearing, no pain

Cervical Spine (Negative Tests)

Compression tests with the cervical spine flexed and with the cervical spine in its normal neutral alignment
Coughing provocation test
Valsalva's test
Right cervical quadrant test in extension
Right and left cervical quadrant test in flexion
Doorbell sign (palpating spinal nerve at the foraminal gutter)

Shoulder (Positive Tests)

Sulcus sign: mild inferior capsular laxity; no pain
Anterior instability tests: all results indicate mild capsular laxity; no pain

- Anterior relocation test (90° abduction, 90° external rotation)
- Anterior fulcrum test (90° abduction, 90° external rotation)
- Anterior drawer (90° abduction)

Shoulder (Negative Tests)

Distraction and compression of the glenohumeral joint
Hawkins' impingement sign
Empty-can test
Speed's test
Acromioclavicular joint compression
Crank test (labrum)
O'Brien test (superior labrum anterior to posterior [SLAP])
Apprehension sign
Load and shift anteriorly (0°)
Load and shift posteriorly (0°)
Posterior instability tests

Thoracic Spine (Positive Tests)

Mobility and provocation testing using prone PA joint mobilization: limited mobility, no pain

CASE STUDY 5.1—cont'd

Thoracic Spine (Negative Tests)

Thoracic quadrant tests in flexion and extension; T1 nerve root tension test

Ribs (Positive Test)

Mobility and provocation testing of first rib: limited mobility on left, no pain

Cervical rotation lateral flexion (CRLF) test: limited mobility on left, no pain

Ribs (Negative Tests)

Deep inspiration and expiration (a measure of rib expansion and pain provocation)

Lateral compression of mid and lower ribs (supine)

Mobility and provocation testing of ribs R2 to R5 anteriorly

Mobility and provocation testing of ribs R6 to R12 (prone)

Joint Integrity and Mobility

Cervical Spine

Slight hypomobility at C5-6 in flexion, right side bending, and right rotation; severe hypomobility, with pain, at C5-6 in extension, left side bending, and left rotation.

Shoulder

Glenohumeral: Slight hypermobility (grade 4) in anterior and inferior glides and slight hypomobility in posterior glide

Sternoclavicular: Normal in all directions

Acromioclavicular: Not applicable (after excision of the distal clavicle)

Scapulothoracic: Normal in all directions

Thoracic Spine

Slight hypomobility in all directions except flexion from T1-4; slight hypomobility in extension from T4-9

Ribs

Slight hypomobility of the first rib on the left

Lumbar Spine

Slight hypermobility at L1-2 in extension

Neuromuscular System

Bewell has no gross gait, locomotion, or balance disorders. In general, she has good motor function. Specifically, however, she has only fair motor control and coordination of her scapula during elevation of her left arm.

Imaging Studies

Plain Radiographs

Cervical

1998 (June): Mild disk space narrowing at C5-6 with minimal anterior end-plate spurring and mild degenerative changes at the C5-6 facet joints bilaterally are noted. Ponticulus posticus is noted at C1. Other segments are relatively WNL.

1992 (February): Results are WNL, with an incidental note of a ponticulus posticus at C1.

Shoulder

2000 (March): Type II acromion with osteophyte formation at the inferior acromioclavicular joint and moderate acromioclavicular DJD are noted.

Chest

2000 (February): Results are WNL.

Diagnosis

Musculoskeletal pattern D: impaired joint mobility, motor function, muscle performance, and ROM associated with connective tissue dysfunction; and musculoskeletal pattern B: impaired posture

Bewell is a 49-year-old, right-handed legal secretary whose signs and symptoms suggest an irritable left C5-6 facet joint impingement with mild anterior and inferior instability of her left glenohumeral joint. In addition, she demonstrates the following: poor posture; mobility dysfunctions in her thoracic and lumbar spine and first rib; and biomechanical dysfunctions in her right knee, foot, and ankle. Bewell appears to be an independent self-motivator in chronic pain, with some fear and anxiety about her chronic pain and the fear of reinjury. She has a moderate intake of caffeine, tobacco, and ibuprofen (Advil).

Pain

The primary pain generator for Bewell is her left C5-6 facet joint.

Strain

The strains that are exacerbating the pain and dysfunction at C5-6 include poor posture, segmental hypomobilities in the thoracic spine, hypomobile first rib, hypermobile glenohumeral joint, hypermobility in the lumbar spine, mild genu valgum, and a notably pronated foot. The physiologic strains are excessive intake of caffeine, tobacco, and ibuprofen (Advil). No strains are identified as systemic diseases.

Brain

Bewell has experienced approximately 12 months of chronic shoulder pain, 6 of those months following surgery. Most of the primary tissue healing in her shoulder should have occurred after 3 months. She also has been suffering with persistent pain from an untreated and undiagnosed cervical facet joint impingement. She has been out of work for 6 months and is exhibiting signs of anger, frustration, fear of reinjury, and possibly symptoms suggestive of mild depression. The number of actively functioning type I mechanoreceptors in the collagen tissues surrounding her neck may have decreased because of her age and her history of neck trauma 9 years ago. The assumption that Bewell has developed some degree of central sensitization can be supported by the following: (1) a loss of supraspinal inhibitory impulses from her forebrain can be expected because of her visible anger, frustration, and fear; (2) nociceptive impulses have been hitting her dorsal horn at the same segment of the spinal cord for approximately 12 months, and (3) she

Continued

CASE STUDY 5.1—cont'd

may have a loss of inhibitory impulses from her type I mechanoreceptors in her midcervical spine.

Prognosis

Bewell has a very good prognosis for return to full duty work and a return to full function with ADLs, as well as a good long-term prognosis for returning to surfing and playing basketball with her daughter.

Plan of Care

Anticipated Goals

1. Bewell's goal: "Get rid of the pain." Reduce her pain experience to a minimal (3/10) level that is easily tolerated and allows her to focus on other aspects of her life.
2. Have minimal misalignment of her sitting and standing posture.
3. Minimize (3/10) her level of fear, frustration, and anger.
4. Perform full cervical AROM.
5. Have minimal loss of gross active thoracic spine extension.
6. Have minimal (3/10) difficulty carrying up to 20 lb, or lifting up to 10 lb overhead.
7. Return to meaningful employment.
8. Have a Sharp FAS score of (80/100) without the use of medications to control her pain.
9. Be independent with her home care instructions and her home exercises.

Expected Outcomes

At the time of discharge, Bewell is expected to have minimal difficulty with most functional ADLs and minimal difficulties returning to work and her previous athletic activities. In addition, she will be expected to take control and responsibility for her continued rehabilitation on her own, with a clear understanding of the realistic risks of reinjury and a realistic view of her prognosis.

Interventions

Wisdom

Bewell is educated on the anatomy and interrelationship of the spine and ribs to the shoulder. She is informed that most of her pain is actually coming from a joint in her neck and is referred toward her shoulder. Further explanation helps the patient realize that she can minimize discomfort to her neck and shoulder by correcting her posture and avoiding prolonged or repeated positions of cervical extension. Central sensitization is also explained to Bewell as a phenomenon that she may be experiencing in which she could be perceiving more frequent and more intense pain than is necessary, that is, her nervous system may be overreacting to some of her innocuous ADLs. The patient is also educated about all the strains feeding into her neck problem. She is told that although her primary pain generator is her neck, she does have some mild anterior and inferior instability in her glenohumeral joint that necessitates rehabilitation. With respect to her left shoulder, Bewell is advised to avoid the following: fast, ballistic movements; repetitive or sustained overhead reaching; and motions that combine abduction with external rotation.

Bewell is relieved to hear she will not need another surgical procedure, that the problem is not serious, and that her prognosis for returning to work is very good. She is given a home instruction packet (HIP) for her neck and shoulder that details activity modification, home and office ergonomics, sleeping and driving positions, pain management (hot and cold packs, light stretching, postures of comfort, self and partner massage, and visual imagery), nutritional advice, and a set of detailed home exercises. Because Bewell is not taking any physician-prescribed medications, the clinician takes the opportunity to discuss with her the rationale and side effects of taking an over-the-counter NSAID for her condition. She is encouraged to minimize her use of NSAIDs and to review the section in her HIP that offers several options for pain management. Because of the notable pronation of her right foot and the biomechanical consequences it may be causing up the kinetic chain, the patient is referred to a colleague for evaluation and, if necessary, casting for an orthotic.

Optimism

The clinician is upbeat during treatment sessions and realistically optimistic about Bewell's prognosis. Any level of improvement, related to functional improvements or musculoskeletal progress, is greeted with great enthusiasm by the clinician. The therapist had performed a very detailed evaluation that now allows every little detail of progress to be recognized. Bewell's focus is taken away from pain and put into function. Instead of "How are you feeling today?" or "Where is the pain today?" or "How bad is the pain today?" the clinician asks, "How are you functioning today, and what can you do now that you could not do a week or two ago?" The idea here is to refocus attention on function and away from the pain and injury.

Manual Therapy

Soft tissue mobilization (STM) is performed on the muscles and fascia of the spine, rib cage, and shoulder that are in guarding or demonstrating adaptive shortening. In this case, the targeted muscles are the SCM, pectoralis minor, scalenus, trapezius, and subscapularis. STM is performed with varying degrees of speed and force. In general, low velocity combined with high force gives the greatest gains in ROM. Conversely, high speed combined with low force can produce the greatest gains in pain reduction. This second approach involves rapid and repeated stimulation of mechanoreceptors in the various connective tissues (e.g., skin, muscle, tendon, fascia, ligament, and joint capsule) to provide a high-intensity afferent stimulus to the dorsal horn for inhibition. The ability to provide inhibitory impulses, versus facilitatory, to the dorsal horn depends

CASE STUDY 5.1—cont'd

on the clinician's ability to avoid overstimulating any hyperreactive or hyperirritable (e.g., acute injury or inflammation) tissues during the performance of STM. Techniques may include STM without joint motion (effleurage, petrissage, tapotement, vibration, transverse friction, skin rolling, and myofascial trigger point techniques), STM with joint motion (PROM, shorten-anchor-stretch, stripping, and tendon sheath gliding), passive pump massage (Fig. 5-28), active pump massage, and STM with a contract-relax or hold-relax component.

Joint mobilization is performed on the C5-6 segment to inhibit pain, decrease muscle guarding, and increase joint mobility. A stretch articulation, usually held for at least 10 seconds, is used in the direction of facet distraction (Fig. 5-29). This stretch of the facet joint collagen accomplishes several goals: (1) stretching for at least 10 seconds allows the collagen to creep, thereby increasing mobility; (2) the stretch stimulates fibroblasts, which, in turn, increase their production of collagen fiber and glycosaminoglycan (GAG); this increase in GAG production leads to an increase in elasticity and eventually mobility as well; and (3) stretching the joint capsule in distraction (versus a flexion or extension glide) stimulates the greatest number of mechanoreceptors (type I is preferentially activated by an end-range stretch versus type II) available to inhibit pain and muscle guarding.

An alternate technique is performed with the patient seated, using a method that unilaterally distracts only the involved facet joint (Fig. 5-30). This last technique can also be used for a short-amplitude, high-velocity thrust. A short-amplitude, high-velocity thrust is particularly helpful in patients with an acute meniscoid entrapment. Oscillatory articulations, gliding the facet joint back and forth at various speeds and amplitudes, are also part of Bewell's treatment plan. Oscillations accomplish several goals: (1) to help maintain newly gained ROM following a stretch articulation, (2) to inhibit pain by preferential activation of type II mechanoreceptors (most active in the beginning and midrange of capsular tension and an important emphasis in patients who may have lost some of their superficial Type I mechanoreceptors), and (3) to provide nutrition to the hyaline cartilage of the facet joint through repeated intermittent compression-decompression and gliding motions. This last goal is achieved by decreasing the viscosity of the synovial fluid, to allow greater absorption of the synovial fluid (nutrients) into the articular cartilage.

Joint mobilizations are also performed on the strains identified for Bewell. In particular, joint mobilizations are directed at the left first rib, the posterior glenohumeral joint (Fig. 5-31), and the thoracic spine (Fig. 5-32).

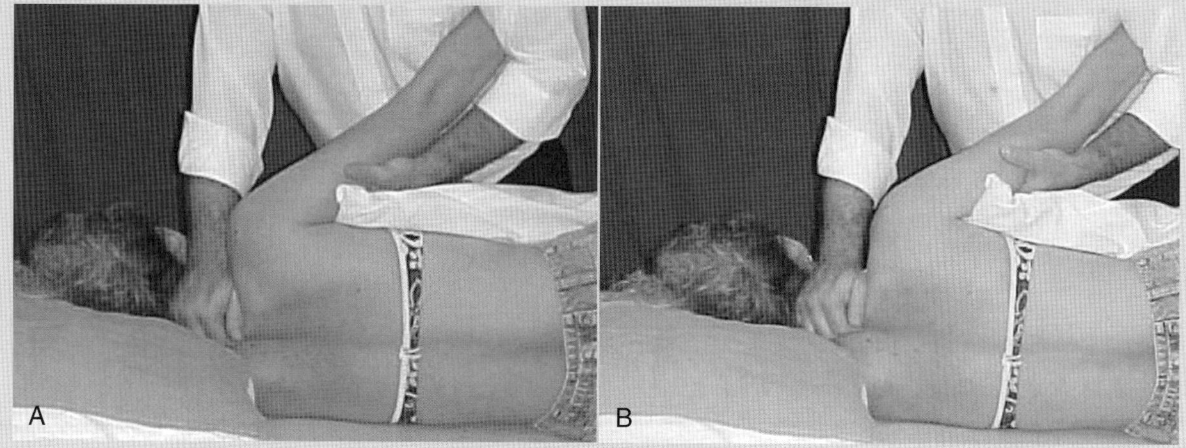

Figure 5-28 Passive and active pump massage of the upper trapezius muscle. Passive pump massage: **A,** The clinician uses his left hand, which has a firm grip just proximal to the patient's elbow, to shorten the upper trapezius. His right hand anchors a portion of the upper trapezius muscle belly. **B,** The clinician passively stretches the patient's upper trapezius muscle using his left hand to pull down on the humerus. The clinician progressively releases his right hand from the muscle belly, as the muscle tenses under his hand because of the stretch into a lengthened range of motion (ROM). This maneuver is repeated rhythmically. Active pump massage: **B,** The clinician uses his left hand, which has a firm grip just proximal to the patient's elbow, to lengthen the upper trapezius. His right hand anchors a portion of the upper trapezius muscle belly. **A,** The patient actively contracts her upper trapezius muscle, thus actively elevating the scapula, as the clinician supports, but offers no resistance to, her elbow. The clinician progressively releases his right hand from the muscle belly, as the muscle bulges under his hand because of the contraction into a shortened ROM. This maneuver is repeated rhythmically. (Courtesy of Yousef Ghandour.)

Continued

CASE STUDY 5.1—cont'd

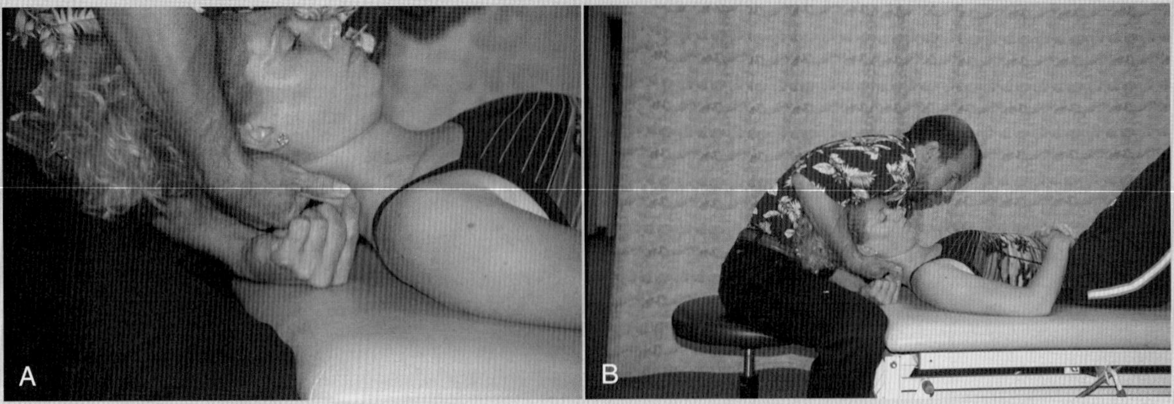

Figure 5-29 Bilateral distraction of the C5-6 facet joints. **A,** The clinician is stabilizing the laminae of C6 with the fleshy pads of his thumb and index finger of his left hand and is firmly grasping C5 with the thumb and index finger of his right hand. The spine is "locked" in flexion from the occiput down through C4-5. **B,** The patient relaxes in a supine hook-lying position with her head slightly off the edge of the table. Her head is held firmly between the clinician's forearm and the anterior portion of his shoulder. At this point, a distraction force is produced by the clinician's depressing his shoulder girdle down and back, which also allows the patient's occiput and C1 to C5 to move down and back, away from C6. With the occiput through C4-5 "locked" in flexion, movement occurs only at the C5-6 segment and perpendicular to the plane of the facet joints.

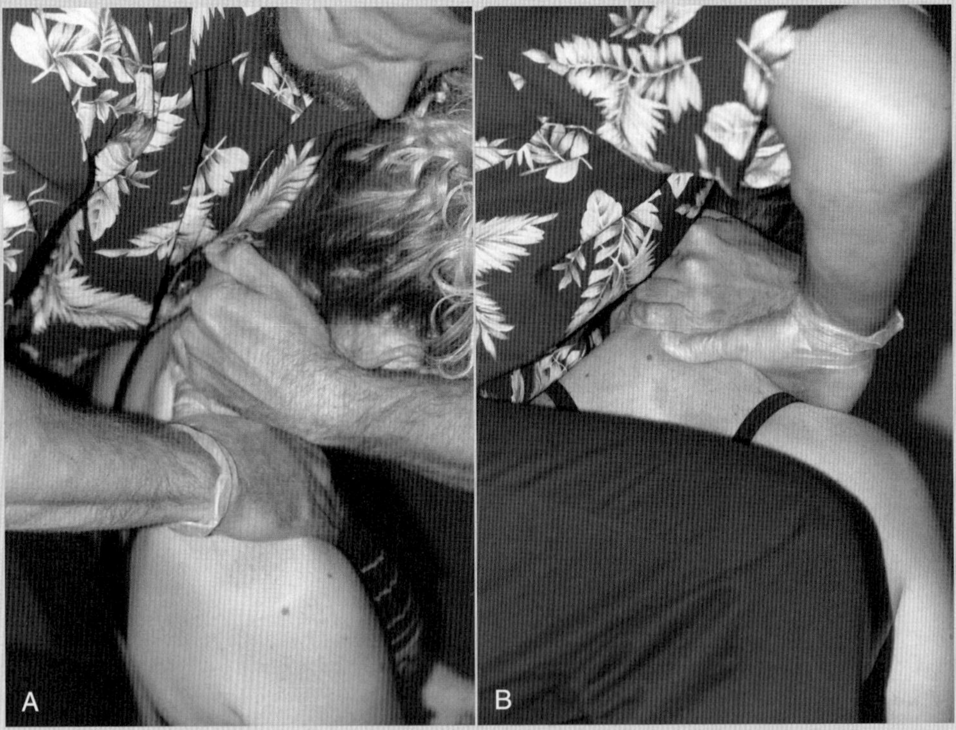

Figure 5-30 Unilateral distraction of the left C5-6 facet joint. **A,** The clinician "locks" the occiput down through C4-5 in flexion and right side bending (the midcervical spine naturally rotates to the right). The patient's forehead rests on the clinician's left biceps. **B,** The ulnar side of the clinician's left hand grasps the posterior arch of C5. The clinician's right thumb stabilizes the C6 segment by applying pressure to the right side of the C6 spinous process. A glove is used to improve traction and stabilization. Keeping the midcervical spine in flexion and the right side bending and in right rotation, the clinician uses the left arm to rotate occiput through C5 to the left as a single fixed unit. Because C2-3 through C4-5 is "locked" in flexion, right side bending, and right rotation, the mobilization force into left rotation is focused at the C5-6 segment.

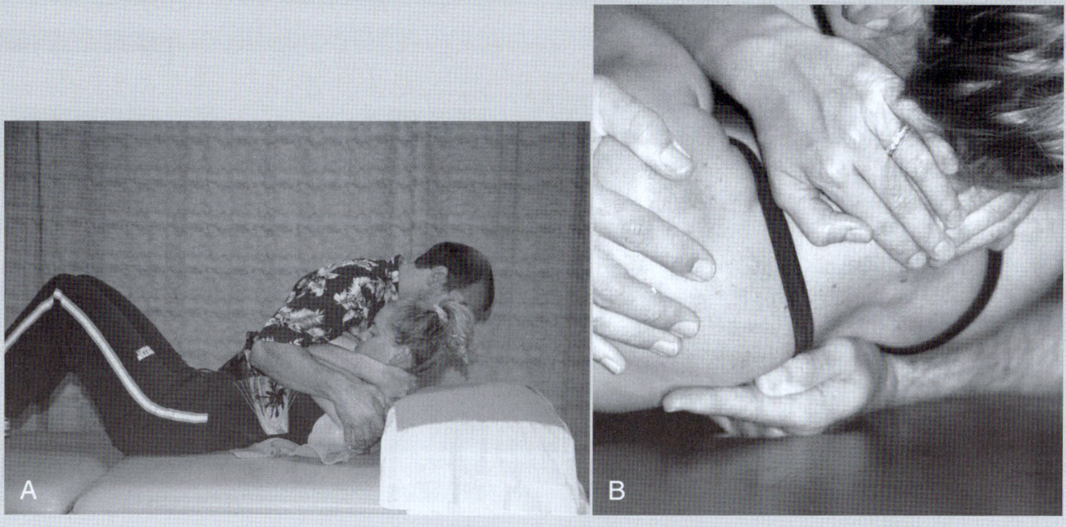

Figure 5-31 Bilateral distraction of the T3-4 facet joints. **A,** The patient is in a supine hook-lying position with her hands behind her neck and her elbows together. The clinician wraps his right arm around her elbows and grabs the posterior portion of her left shoulder with his right hand. The clinician "locks" C0-1 down through T2-3 in flexion by depressing or elevating his shoulder girdle as needed. When the clinician depresses his shoulder girdle against the patient's elbows, he induces thoracic flexion. Conversely, when the clinician elevates his shoulder girdle, he induces thoracic extension, **B,** The clinician makes a fist, or semifist, with his left hand and places it under the patient to stabilize the T4 segment. The spinous process of T4 falls between the clinician's thenar eminence and the middle phalanx of his middle finger. The right transverse process of T4 is stabilized by the thenar eminence of the clinician's left hand, and the left transverse process of T4 is stabilized by the middle phalanx of the same hand. **A,** Using his body weight and shoulder girdle, the clinician pushes through the patient's elbows, in the direction of her left humerus, posteriorly and superiorly. Because the occiput through T2-3 is "locked" in flexion, the distraction force is focused at the T3-4 segment. A wedge may be substituted for the hand for stabilization. This technique can also be performed as a high-velocity, short-amplitude thrust.

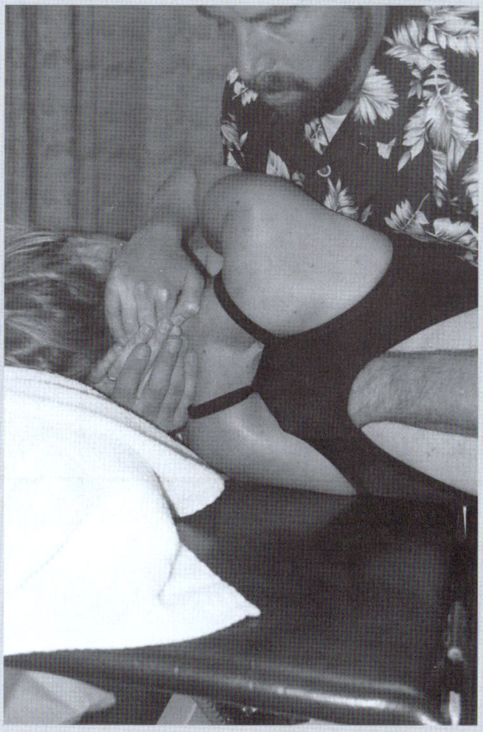

Figure 5-32 Extension mobilization of the T3-4 facet joints. The patient is in a side-lying position with her hands behind her neck and her elbows together. The clinician wraps his right arm around her elbows and grabs the posterior portion of her neck, on top of her hands, with his right hand. The distal portion of the patient's triceps is resting against the clinician's right biceps. His left hand is pinching, between his thumb and index finger, and stabilizing the T4 segment. The clinician gently shifts his weight to the right, thus pushing against the patient's arms and elevating them, to produce an extension mobilization specific to T3-4.

Continued

CASE STUDY 5.1—cont'd

Exercise

Following the manual therapy at each visit, Bewell completes a series of therapeutic exercises involving the principles of scientific therapeutic exercise progressions (STEP), which originated from medical exercise therapy (MET).[126-128] Initially, Bewell was instructed to exercise the joints for self-mobilization and coordination at 40% to 50% of her one repetition maximum (1RM), usually 40 to 50 repetitions per set. The purpose here is to build on the mobility gained during the manual therapy.[129] The light resistance allows for a greater number of repetitions without achieving muscle fatigue. Her self-mobilization exercises include supine cervical retraction, seated thoracic extension, and thoracic rotation exercises using a wedge and a mobilization bench (Fig. 5-33).[130, 131] In addition, exercise to vascularize the muscles and tissues that have been in guarding, ischemic, and full of lactic acid and other metabolic waste products is performed at 60% of 1RM, usually 25 to 30 repetitions per set (Fig. 5-34). Bewell should experience substantial muscle fatigue before reaching the thirtieth repetition. Rest for as long as a minute between sets may be necessary in some cases for the muscle to recover. The primary muscles in guarding for Bewell are the SCM, pectoralis minor, trapezius, scalenus, and subscapularis.

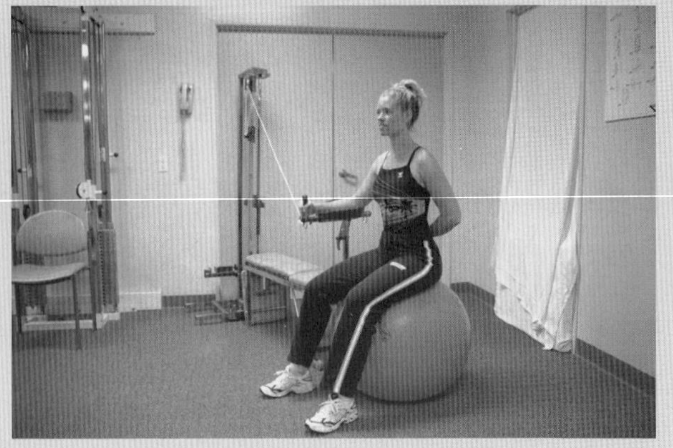

Figure 5-34 Exercising the internal rotators of the shoulder while placing a demand on the spine to maintain good postural alignment and stability.

Development of muscle coordination usually requires thousands and thousands of repetitions. To achieve this level of repetitions, six to eight different neck and shoulder exercises are often required with three to five sets per exercise. As weakness, muscle guarding, and joint limitations

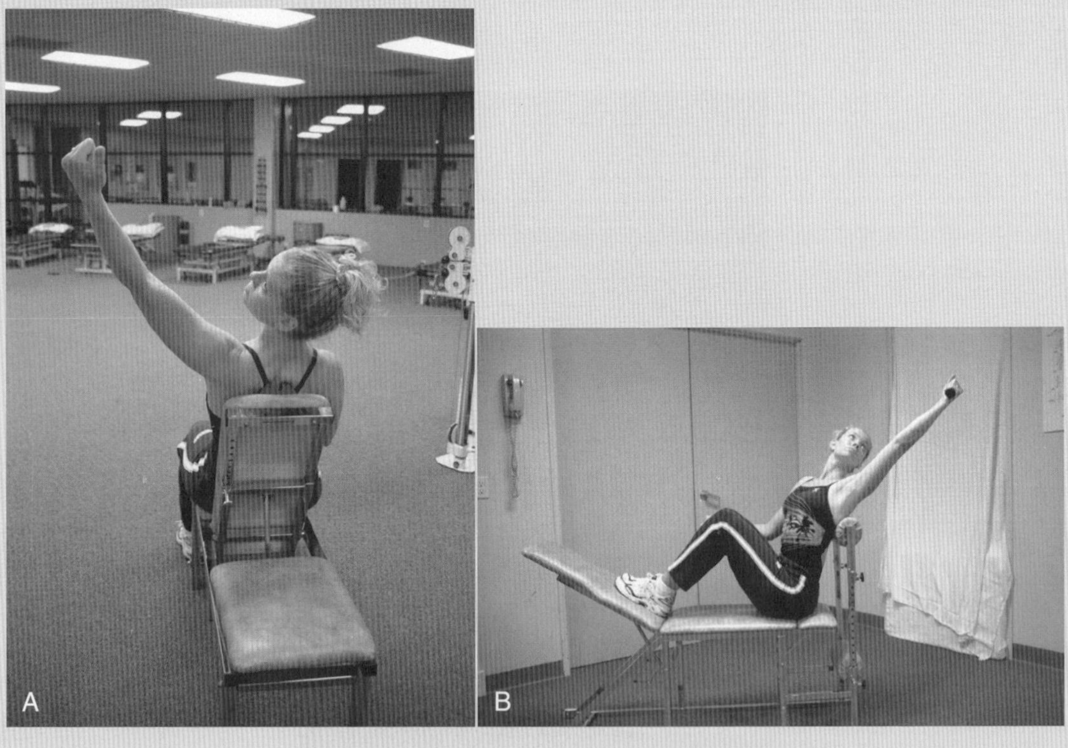

Figure 5-33 Self-mobilization exercises for the thoracic spine. Combining coordination exercise of the neck and shoulder with a mobilization technique to increase extension and left rotation of the upper thoracic spine. The initial progression for our patient, with mild anterior and inferior glenohumeral capsular laxity and the left C5-6 facet joint impingement, was to have her perform straight extension with her hands behind her neck and her elbows adducted. **A,** Progression of a self-mobilization technique for the upper thoracic spine that incorporates a greater demand on the patient's ability to control the movement of both her neck and her shoulder toward a range of motion associated with pain and instability. **B,** A less specific thoracic mobilization with a greater demand, the patient is holding a 2-lb weight, for coordinated motion of the neck and shoulder.

CASE STUDY 5.1—cont'd

subside, additional exercises may be added to the progression. Exercises in this stage of the rehabilitation process have a strong emphasis on the coordinated actions of the spine with the shoulder in functional movement patterns (Fig. 5-35). In general, exercises are progressed as follows: from supported to unsupported; non–weight bearing with gravity eliminated to weight bearing against gravity; from 40% to 50% 1RM to 80% 1RM; from high repetition (40 to 50) to low repetition (15 to 20); from endurance and coordination to power; from slow speed to fast; and from single-plane exercises to multiplane functional synergies.[129]

Nutrition

Bewell is provided with extensive nutritional advice and a few select high-quality research studies to support the advice given by her therapist. Specifically, Bewell is instructed to avoid the following: (1) tobacco—besides

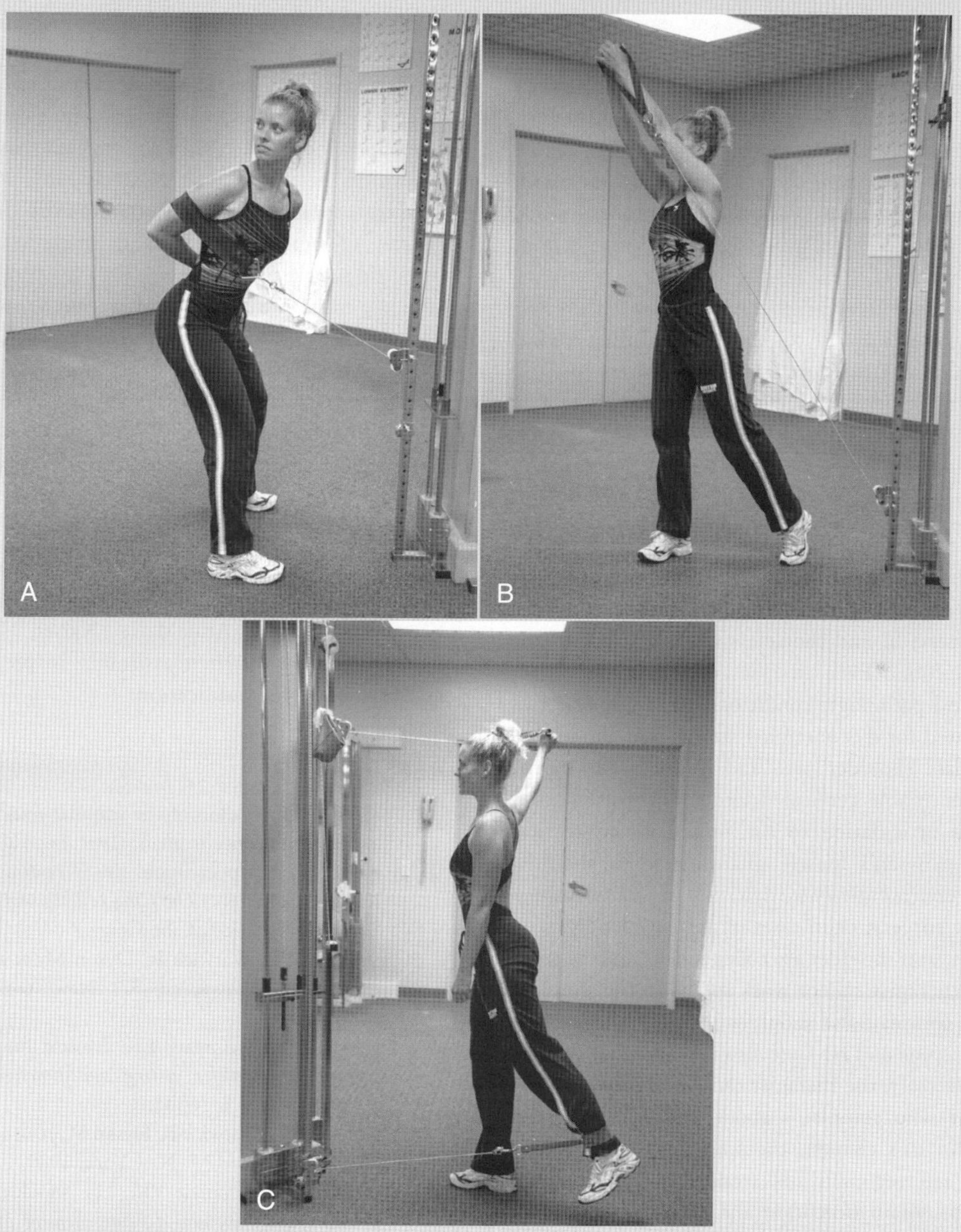

Figure 5-35 Examples of exercises integrating the coordinated efforts of the spine with the shoulder. **A,** Upper trunk rotation and scapula retraction with the pelvis and lower extremities stationary. **B,** The patient starts facing the pulley in a stooped posture with her spine in flexion and left rotation and then moves into spine extension and right rotation with accompanying shoulder flexion. **C,** The standing resisted "swimmers" exercise is one of the most challenging for coordinating movements of the spine and extremities.

Continued

CASE STUDY 5.1—cont'd

the well-known increased risk for cardiovascular disease, stroke, and lung cancer, smoking has also been associated with a loss of bone density, increased degenerative disk disease, and increased musculoskeletal pain[132-136]; (2) caffeinated drinks (e.g., coffee, tea, and soda) because caffeine increases the urinary loss of calcium and magnesium[137,138]; and (3) sources of arachidonic acid, the precursor to prostaglandin E_2, which stimulates the inflammatory response, nociceptors, and hyperalgesia.[139-142] Sources of arachidonic acid include red meats (beef, pork, lamb, and organ meats), shellfish (lobster, shrimp, and clams), and dairy fats (milk and cheese products). For this patient with chronic pain, no reason exists for her to be taking NSAIDs, especially considering all the potential side effects, the risk factors, and the interference with the regeneration process of her tissues. Safer methods of pain control are cold or hot packs, home STM and stretching, relaxation techniques, visual imagery, and a home transcutaneous electrical nerve stimulation (TENS) unit.

She is then advised to supplement her diet with the following: (1) glucosamine sulfate, chondroitin sulfate, vitamin E, and vitamin C to slow down the process of DJD at C5-6 and elsewhere; patients with diabetes or shellfish allergies should consult their physician before taking glucosamine sulfate, whereas those taking blood thinners should consult their physician before taking chondroitin sulfate[143-156]; (2) magnesium to support muscle performance, strength training, and bone density[157-160]; (3) microcrystalline hydroxyapatite (a source of calcium), zinc, copper, manganese, and vitamin D_3 to minimize the possible adverse effects on this 49-year-old woman's bone density, secondary to heavy tobacco and caffeine intake[156,161-165]; (4) bioflavonoids, which have been shown to inhibit the release of arachidonic acid, work as anti-inflammatory agents, and decrease tissue degeneration[166-168]; and (5) omega-3 fatty acids (eicosapentaenoic acid [EPA] and docosahexaenoic acid [DHA]), which have been shown to inhibit the metabolism of arachidonic acid and provide a mild long-term anti-inflammatory effect.[156,169,170] Sources of omega-3 fatty acids include cold-water fish (Atlantic mackerel, Atlantic herring, blue fin tuna, and salmon), nuts (butternuts and walnuts), and oils (flaxseed oil, soybean oil, canola oil, fish oil, cod liver oil, and walnut oil).

SUMMARY

Every patient who has a history of gradual onset shoulder pain, even occupational repetitive injuries, should receive a screening of the cervical and thoracic spine and ribs to rule out referred symptoms. Even in cases of irrefutable direct shoulder injury and pathologic conditions, the spine and ribs need to be evaluated for dysfunctional strains that can aggravate and perpetuate shoulder pain and dysfunction. In the absence of an identifiable cervical disorder, the patient may still benefit from articulation to the joints of the cervical spine to reduce pain and muscle guarding when shoulder mobilization is contraindicated, that is, in acute injury, immediately after surgery, or in cases of patient anxiety.

The spine, ribs, and shoulder are codependent and, as such, inseparable. The therapist cannot work solely on the shoulder of a patient who complains of shoulder pain. The joints and soft tissues of the spine and rib cage also need manual therapy and exercise. Conversely, the therapist cannot simply treat the neck of a patient who complains about his or her cervical spine. As noted in this chapter, the spine and ribs need to be evaluated for referred pain and strains. In addition, the contribution of the brain (forebrain and spinal cord) cannot be ignored. Treatment then is focused on rehabilitation for the pain, strains, and brain by using techniques incorporated in the acronym WOMEN (*w*isdom, *o*ptimism, *m*anual therapy, *e*xercise, and *n*utrition).

ACKNOWLEDGMENTS

Gray and Grimsby would like to thank Nancy Bresocnik, Yousef Ghandour, AnneMarie Kaiser, Jim Rivard, and Andrew Vertson for their assistance in preparing the figures in this chapter for publication.

REFERENCES

1. Kato K: Innervation of the scapular muscles and its morphological significance in man, *Anat Anz* 168:155, 1989.
2. Netter FH: Upper limb. In Woodburn RT, Crelin ES, Kaplan FS, editors: *The Ciba collection of medical illustrations*, Summit, NJ, 1987, Ciba-Geigy.
3. Williams PL, Warwick R, Dyson M, et al, editors: Myology. In *Gray's anatomy*, ed 37, New York, 1989, Churchill Livingstone.
4. Kendall FP, McCreary EK: Muscle function in relation to posture. In *Muscles: testing and function*, ed 3, Baltimore, 1983, Williams & Wilkins.
5. Williams PL, Warwick R, Dyson M, et al, editors: Arthrology. In *Gray's anatomy*, ed 37, New York, 1989, Churchill Livingstone.
6. Norkin CC, Levangie PK: The shoulder complex. In *Joint structure and function: a comprehensive analysis*, Philadelphia, 1985, Davis, p 164.
7. Norkin CC, Levangie PK: The shoulder complex. In *Joint structure and function: a comprehensive analysis*, Philadelphia, 1985, Davis, pp 178–186.

8. Kapandji IA: The shoulder. In *The physiology of the joints*, ed 5, New York, 1982, Churchill Livingstone.
9. Griegel-Morris P, Larson K, Mueller-Klaus K, et al: Incidence of common postural abnormalities in the cervical, shoulder, and thoracic regions and their association with pain in two age groups of healthy subjects, *Phys Ther* 72(6):425, 1992.
10. Pecina MM, Krmpotic-Nemanic J, Markiewitz AD: Scapulocostal syndrome. In *Tunnel syndromes*, Boca Raton, Fla, 1991, CRC Press.
11. Cailliet R: Mechanisms of pain in the neck and from the neck. In *Neck and arm pain*, ed 3, Philadelphia, 1991, Davis.
12. Cailliet R: Differential diagnosis of neck, arm, and hand pain. In *Neck and arm pain*, ed 3, Philadelphia, 1991, Davis.
13. Bateman JE: Lesions producing neck plus shoulder pain. In *The shoulder and neck*, Philadelphia, 1972, Saunders.
14. Norkin CC, Levangie PK: Posture. In *Joint structure and function: a comprehensive analysis*, Philadelphia, 1985, Davis.
15. Cailliet R: Posture in shoulder pain. In *Shoulder pain*, ed 3, Philadelphia, 1991, Davis.
16. Schultz K, Ekholm J, Harms-Ringdahl K, et al: Effects of changes in sitting work posture on static neck and shoulder muscle activity, *Ergonomics* 29:1525, 1986.
17. Kendall FP, McCreary EK: Muscle function in relation to posture. In *Muscles: testing and function*, ed 3, Baltimore, 1983, Williams & Wilkins.
18. Coventry MB: Problem of painful shoulder, *JAMA* 151:177, 1953.
19. Ayub E: Posture and the upper quarter. In Donatelli RA, editor: *Physical therapy of the shoulder*, ed 2, New York, 1991, Churchill Livingstone.
20. Bogduk N, Marsland A: On the concept of third occipital headache, *J Neurol Neurosurg Psychiatry* 49:775, 1986.
21. Lord SM, Barnsley L, Wallis BJ, et al: Third occipital nerve headache: a prevalence study, *J Neurol Neurosurg Psychiatry* 57:1187, 1994.
22. Williams PL, Warwick R, Dyson M, et al, editors: Neurology. In *Gray's anatomy*, ed 37, New York, 1989, Churchill Livingstone.
23. Wyke B: Neurology of the cervical spinal joints, *Physiotherapy* 65:72, 1979.
24. Wyke B: Cervical articular contributions to posture and gait: their relation to senile disequilibrium, *Age* 8:251, 1979.
25. Travell JG, Simons DG: Sternocleidomastoid muscle. In *Myofascial pain and dysfunction: the trigger point manual*, Baltimore, 1983, Williams & Wilkins.
26. Hebert LA: *The neck arm hand book: the master guide for eliminating cumulative trauma disorders from the work place*, Bangor, Me, 1989, Impacc.
27. Lannersten L, Harms-Ringdahl K: Neck and shoulder muscle activity during work with different cash register systems, *Ergonomics* 33:49, 1990.
28. Hagberg M: Occupational musculoskeletal stress and disorders of the neck and shoulder: a review of possible pathophysiology, *Int Arch Occup Environ Health* 53:269, 1984.
29. Palmer JB, Uematsu S, Jankel WR, et al: A cellist with arm pain: thermal asymmetry in scalenus anticus syndrome, *Arch Phys Med Rehabil* 72:237, 1991.
30. Larsson SE, Alund M, Cai H, et al: Chronic pain after soft-tissue injury of the cervical spine: trapezius muscle blood flow and electromyography at static loads and fatigue, *Pain* 57:173, 1994.
31. Travell JG, Simons DG: Subscapularis muscle. In *Myofascial pain and dysfunction: the trigger point manual*, Baltimore, 1983, Williams & Wilkins.
32. Chaffin DB, Andersson GBJ: Biomechanical considerations in machine control and workplace design. In *Occupational biomechanics*, New York, 1984, John Wiley & Sons.
33. Hagberg M, Wegman DH: Prevalence rates and odds ratios of shoulder-neck diseases in different occupational groups, *Br J Industrial Med* 44:602, 1987.
34. Travell JG, Simons DG: Trapezius muscle. In *Myofascial pain and dysfunction: the trigger point manual*, Baltimore, 1983, Williams & Wilkins.
35. Netter FH: Gross anatomy of brain and spinal cord. In Brass A, editor: *The Ciba collection of medical illustrations*, Summit, NJ, 1991, Ciba-Geigy.
36. Heller JG: The syndromes of degenerative cervical disease, *Orthop Clin North Am* 23:381, 1992.
37. Bogduk N, Windsor M, Inglis A: The innervation of the cervical intervertebral discs, *Spine* 13:2, 1988.
38. McLain RF: Mechanoreceptor endings in human cervical facet joints, *Spine* 19:495, 1994.
39. Wyke B: Articular neurology: a review, *Physiotherapy* 58:94, 1972.
40. Grieve GP: Clinical features. In *Common vertebral joint problems*, New York, 1981, Churchill Livingstone.
41. Netter FH: Nerve plexuses and peripheral nerves. In Brass A, editor: *The Ciba collection of medical illustrations*, Summit, NJ, 1991, Ciba-Geigy.
42. Zusman M: Forebrain-mediated sensitization of central pain pathways: "non-specific" pain and a new image for MT, *Man Ther* 7(2):80, 2002.
43. Strong J, Unruh AM, Wright A, et al, editors: *Pain: a textbook for therapists*, New York, 2002, Churchill Livingstone.
44. Woolfe CJ, Salter MW: Neuronal plasticity: increasing the gain in pain, *Science* 288:1765, 2000.
45. Basbaum AI: Spinal mechanisms of acute and persistent pain, *Reg Anesth Pain Med* 24:59, 1999.
46. Foley RA: *Neuroscience and pain: part of a neuro-orthopedic approach, Paper presented at the annual conference of the American Academy of Orthopaedic Manual Physical Therapists, St. Louis*, ; 1998.
47. Denslow JS, Korr IM, Krems AD: Quantitative studies of chronic facilitation in human motoneuron pools, *Am J Physiol* 150:229, 1947.
48. Wright A: Neurophysiology of pain and pain modulation. In Strong J, Unruh AM, Wright A, et al, editors: *Pain: a textbook for therapists*, New York, 2002, Churchill Livingstone.
49. Cinquegrana OD: Chronic cervical radiculitis and its relationship to "chronic bursitis"*Am J Phys Med* 47:23, 1968.
50. Korr IM: Clinical significance of the facilitated state, *J Am Osteopath Assoc* 54:277, 1955.
51. Korr IM: Sustained sympathicotonia as a factor in disease. In *The neurobiologic mechanisms in manipulative therapy*, New York, 1978, Plenum.
52. Hawkins RJ, Bilco T, Bonutti P: Cervical spine and shoulder pain, *Clin Orthop Relat Res* 258:142, 1990.
53. Wells P: Cervical dysfunction and shoulder problems, *Physiotherapy* 68:66, 1982.
54. Hargreaves C, Cooper C, Kidd BL, et al: Frozen shoulder and cervical spine disease, *Br J Rheumatol* 28:78, 1989.
55. Simeone FA: Cervical disc disease with radiculopathy. In Rothman RH, Simeone FA, editors: *The spine*, ed 3, Philadelphia, 1992, Saunders.
56. Macnab I, McCulloch J: Differential diagnosis of neck ache and shoulder pain. In *Neck ache and shoulder pain*, Philadelphia, 1994, Williams & Wilkins.

57. Wiffen F: What role does the sympathetic nervous system play in the development or ongoing pain of adhesive capsulitis? *J Man Manip Ther* 10(1):17, 2002.
58. Grieve GP: The autonomic nervous system in vertebral pain syndromes. In *Modern manual therapy of the vertebral column*, New York, 1986, Churchill Livingstone.
59. Caswell HT: The omohyoid syndrome, *Lancet* 1969:319, 1969.
60. Zachary RB, Young A, Hammond JDS: The omohyoid syndrome, *Lancet* 2:104, 1969.
61. Valtonen EJ: The omohyoid syndrome, *Lancet* 2:1073, 1969.
62. Wilmot TJ: The omohyoid syndrome, *Lancet* 2:1298, 1969.
63. Rask MR: The omohyoideus myofascial pain syndrome: report of four patients, *J Craniomandibular Pract* 2:256, 1984.
64. Menachem A, Kaplan O, Dekel S: Levator scapulae syndrome: an anatomic-clinical study, *Bull Hosp Jt Dis* 53:21, 1993.
65. Travell JG, Simons DG: Levator scapulae muscle. In *Myofascial pain and dysfunction: the trigger point manual*, Baltimore, 1983, Williams & Wilkins.
66. Swift TR, Nichols FT: The droopy shoulder syndrome, *Neurology* 34:212, 1984.
67. Clein LJ: The droopy shoulder syndrome, *CMAJ* 114:343, 1976.
68. Percy EC, Birbrager D, Pitt MJ: Snapping scapula: a review of the literature and presentation of 14 patients, *Can J Surg* 31 (4):248–250, 1988.
69. Carlson HL, Haig AJ, Stewart DC: Snapping scapula syndrome: three case reports and an analysis of the literature, *Arch Phys Med Rehabil* 78:506–511, 1997.
70. Nicholson GP, Duckworth MA: Scapulothoracic bursectomy for snapping scapula syndrome, *J Shoulder Elbow Surg* 11:80, 2002.
71. Mozes G, Bickels J, Ovadia D, et al: The use of three-dimensional computed tomography in evaluating snapping scapula syndrome, *Orthopedics* 22(11):1029, 1999.
72. de Haart M, van der Linden ES, de Vet HCW, et al: The value of computed tomography in the diagnosis of grating scapula, *Skeletal Radiol* 23:357, 1994.
73. Macnab I: Symptoms in cervical disc degeneration. In Sherk HH, Dunn EJ, Eismont FJ, et al, editors: *The cervical spine*, New York, 1989, Lippincott.
74. Middleditch A, Jarman P: An investigation of frozen shoulders using thermography, *Physiotherapy* 70:433, 1984.
75. Gunn CC, Milbrandt WE: Tenderness at motor points: an aid in the diagnosis of pain in the shoulder referred from the cervical spine, *J Am Osteopath Assoc* 77:196, 1977.
76. Roth DA: Cervical analgesic discography: a new test for the definitive diagnosis of the painful-disk syndrome, *JAMA* 235:1713, 1976.
77. Bogduk N: Neck pain, *Aust Fam Phys* 13(1):26, 1984.
78. Grubb S, Kelly CK: Cervical discography: clinical implications from 12 years of experience, *Spine* 25(11):1382, 2000.
79. Schellhas KP, Smith MD, Gundry CR, et al: Cervical discogenic pain: prospective correlation of magnetic resonance imaging and discography in asymptomatic subjects and pain sufferers, *Spine* 21(3):300, 1996.
80. Macnab I: Cervical spondylosis, *Clin Orthop Relat Res* 109:69, 1975.
81. Foreman SM, Croft AC: Physical examination. In *Whiplash injuries: the cervical acceleration/deceleration syndrome*, Baltimore, 1988, Williams & Wilkins.
82. Wesolowski D, Wang A: The radiology of cervical disc disease, *Semin Spine Surg* 1:209, 1989.
83. Bell GR, Ross JS: The accuracy of imaging studies of the degenerative cervical spine: myelography, myelo-computed tomography, and magnetic resonance imaging, *Semin Spine Surg* 7:9, 1995.
84. Schellhas KP, Smith MD, Gundry CR, et al: Cervical discogenic pain: prospective correlation of magnetic resonance imaging and discography in asymptomatic subjects and pain sufferers, *Spine* 21:300, 1996.
85. Bateman JE: Neurological and dystrophic disorders. In *The shoulder and neck*, Philadelphia, 1972, Saunders.
86. Campbell SM: Referred shoulder pain: an elusive diagnosis, *Postgrad Med* 73:193, 1983.
87. Chabot MC, Montgomery DM: The pathophysiology of axial and radicular neck pain, *Semin Spine Surg* 7:2, 1995.
88. Slipman CW, Plastaras CT, Palmitier RA, et al: Symptom provocation of fluoroscopically guided cervical nerve root stimulation: are dynatomal maps identical to dermatomal maps, *Spine* 23(20):2235, 1998.
89. Viikari-Juntura E, Porras M, Laasonen EM: Validity of clinical tests in the diagnosis of root compression in cervical disc disease, *Spine* 14:253, 1989.
90. Macnab I, McCulloch J: Cervical disc disease: clinical assessment. In *Neck ache and shoulder pain*, Philadelphia, 1994, Williams & Wilkins.
91. Cailliet R: Spondylosis: degenerative disk disease. In *Neck and arm pain*, ed 3, Philadelphia, 1991, Davis.
92. Cailliet R: Cervical disk disease in the production of pain and disability. In *Neck and arm pain*, ed 3, Philadelphia, 1991, Davis.
93. McQueen JD, Khan MI: Neurologic evaluation. In Sherk HH, Dunn EJ, Eismont FJ, et al, editors: *The cervical spine*, ed 2, New York, 1989, Lippincott.
94. Bland JH: Embryology: practical clinical implications and interpretation. In *Disorders of the cervical spine: diagnosis and medical management*, ed 2, Philadelphia, 1994, Saunders.
95. Barnsley L, Lord SM, Wallis BJ: The prevalence of chronic cervical zygapophysial joint pain after whiplash, *Spine* 20:20, 1995.
96. Bogduk N, Marsland A: The cervical zygapophyseal joints as a source of neck pain, *Spine* 13:610, 1988.
97. Dwyer A, Aprill C, Bogduk N: Cervical zygapophyseal joint pain patterns. Part 1. A study in normal volunteers, *Spine* 15:453, 1990.
98. Fukui S, Ohseto K, Shiotani M: Patterns of pain induced by distending the thoracic zygapophyseal joints, *Reg Anesth* 22 (4):332, 1997.
99. Fukui S, Ohseto K, Shiotani M, et al: Referred pain distribution of the cervical zygapophyseal joints and cervical dorsal rami, *Pain* 68:79, 1996.
100. Bogduk N: Innervation and pain patterns of the cervical spine. In Grant R, editor: *Physical therapy of the cervical and thoracic spine*, ed 3, New York, 2002, Churchill Livingstone.
101. Mercer S, Bogduk N: Intra-articular inclusions of the cervical synovial joints, *Br J Rheumatol* 32:705, 1993.
102. Bogduk N, Aprill C: On the nature of neck pain, discography and cervical zygapophyseal joint blocks, *Pain* 54:213, 1993.
103. Pettman E: *Spinal dysfunction and its effect on shoulder girdle function*. Paper presented at the annual conference of the American Academy of Orthopaedic Manual Physical Therapists, Orlando, 2002.
104. Bogduk N: Innervation and pain patterns of the thoracic spine. In Grant R, editor: *Physical therapy of the cervical and thoracic spine*, ed 3, New York, 2002, Churchill Livingstone.

105. Wilke A, Wolf U, Lageard P, et al: Thoracic disc herniation: a diagnostic challenge, *Man Ther* 5(3):181, 2000.
106. Wood KB, Schellhas KP, Garvey TA, et al: Thoracic discography in healthy individuals: a controlled prospective study of magnetic resonance imaging and discography in asymptomatic and symptomatic individuals, *Spine* 24(15):1548, 1999.
107. Alberico AM, Sahni KS, Hall JA, et al: High thoracic disc herniation, *Neurosurgery* 19(3):449, 1986.
108. Gelch MM: Herniated thoracic disc at T1-2 level associated with Horner's syndrome: case report, *J Neurosurg* 48:128–130, 1978.
109. Bland JH: Rheumatologic neurology. In *Disorders of the cervical spine: diagnosis and medical management*, ed 2, Philadelphia, 1994, Saunders.
110. Dreyfuss P, Tibiletti C, Dreyer SJ: Thoracic zygapophyseal joint pain patterns: a study in normal volunteers, *Spine* 19 (7):807, 1994.
111. Dreyfuss P, Tibiletti C, Dreyer SJ, et al: Thoracic zygapophyseal pain: a review and description of an intraarticular block technique, *Pain Dig* 4:44, 1994.
112. Menck JY, Requejo SM, Kulig K: Thoracic spine dysfunction in upper extremity complex regional pain syndrome type I, *J Orthop Sports Phys Ther* 30(7):401, 2000.
113. Woodring JH, Royer JM, Todd EP: Upper rib fractures following median sternotomy, *Ann Thorac Surg* 39(4):355–357, 1985.
114. Lankenner PA Jr, Micheli LJ: Stress fracture of the first rib: a case report, *J Bone Joint Surg Am* 67(1):159–160, 1985.
115. Hankin FM, Braunstein EM, Orringer MB: Timely evaluation of shoulder pain in a teenager, *Am Fam Physician* 33 (2):177–180, 1986.
116. Boyle JJW: Is the pain and dysfunction of shoulder impingement lesion really second rib syndrome in disguise? Two case reports, *Man Ther* 4(1):44, 1999.
117. Christie HJ, Kumar S, Warren SA: Postural aberrations in low back pain, *Arch Phys Med Rehabil* 76:218–224, 1995.
118. Ladin Z, Neff KM: Testing of a biomechanical model of the lumbar muscle force distribution using quasi-static loading exercises, *J Biomech Eng* 114:442–449, 1992.
119. Hodges PW, Richardson CA: Inefficient muscular stabilization of the lumbar spine associated with low back pain: a motor control evaluation of transversus abdominis, *Spine* 21 (22):2640–2650, 1996.
120. Wolfe MM, Lichtenstein DR, Singh G: Gastrointestinal toxicity of nonsteroidal anti-inflammatory drugs, *N Engl J Med* 340 (24):1888, 1999.
121. Giannoudis PV, MacDonald DA, Matthews SJ, et al: Nonunion of the femoral diaphysis: the influence of reaming and non-steroidal anti-inflammatory drugs, *J Bone Joint Surg Br* 82:655, 2000.
122. Solomon L: Drug-induced arthropathy and necrosis of the femoral head, *J Bone Joint Surg Br* 55:246, 1973.
123. Newman NM, Ling RSM: Acetabular bone destruction related to non-steroidal anti-inflammatory drugs, *Lancet* 6:11, 1985.
124. Palmoski MJ, Brandt KD: Effects of some nonsteroidal antiinflammatory drugs on proteoglycan metabolism and organization in canine articular cartilage, *Arthritis Rheum* 23(9):1010, 1980.
125. Dingle JT: The effects of NSAID on the matrix of human articular cartilage, *Z Rheumatol* 58:125, 1999.
126. Jacobsen F: Medical exercise therapy, *Sci Phys Ther* 3:1, 1992.
127. Torstensen TA, Meen HD, Stiris M: The effect of medical exercise therapy on a patient with chronic supraspinatus tendinitis: diagnostic ultrasound tissue regeneration: a case study, *J Orthop Sports Phys Ther* 20:319, 1994.
128. Grimsby O, Rivard J: Exercise theory. In *Science, theory and clinical application in orthopaedic manual physical therapy: applied science and theory*, vol 1, Taylorsville, 2008, The Academy of Graduate Physical Therapy, Inc.
129. Grimsby O, Rivard J: Exercise prescription. In *Science, theory and clinical application in orthopaedic manual physical therapy: applied science and theory*, vol 1, Taylorsville, 2008, The Academy of Graduate Physical Therapy, Inc.
130. Rivard J, Kring R, Gramont D, et al: Exercise rehabilitation of the cervical spine. In Grimsby O, Rivard J, editors: *Science, theory and clinical application in orthopaedic manual physical therapy: scientific therapeutic exercise progressions (STEP) - the neck and upper extremity*, vol 2, Taylorsville, 2008, The Academy of Graduate Physical Therapy, Inc.
131. Glatz C, Rivard J, Grimsby O: Exercise rehabilitation of the thoracic spine. In Grimsby O, Rivard J, editors: *Science, theory and clinical application in orthopaedic manual physical therapy: scientific therapeutic exercise progressions (STEP) - the neck and upper extremity*, vol 2, Taylorsville, 2008, The Academy of Graduate Physical Therapy, Inc.
132. Egger P, Duggleby S, Hobbs R, et al: Cigarette smoking and bone mineral density in the elderly, *J Epidemiol Community Health* 50:47, 1996.
133. Anderson H, Ejlertsson G, Leden I: Widespread musculoskeletal chronic pain associated with smoking: an epidemiological study in a general rural population, *Scand J Rehabil Med* 30 (3):185, 1998.
134. Fogelholm RR, Alho AV: Smoking and intervertebral disc degeneration, *Med Hypotheses* 56(4):537, 2001.
135. Battie M, Videman T, Gill K, et al: Smoking and lumbar intervertebral disc degeneration: an MRI study of identical twins, *Spine* 16(9):1015, 1991.
136. Eriksen WB, Brage S, Bruusgaard D: Does smoking aggravate musculoskeletal pain? *Scand J Rheumatol* 26:49, 1997.
137. Massey L, Wise K: Effects of dietary caffeine on mineral status, *Nutr Res* 4:43, 1984.
138. Bergman EA, Massey LK, Wise KJ, et al: Effects of dietary caffeine on renal handling of minerals in adult women, *Life Sci* 47:557, 1990.
139. Siekerka JR: Nutrition and biochemistry of the intervertebral disc: a clinical approach, *Chiropr Tech* 3:116, 1991.
140. Davies P, Bailey PJ, Goldenberg MM, et al: The role of arachidonic acid oxygenation products in pain and inflammation, *Annu Rev Immunol* 2:335, 1984.
141. Allen JW, Vicini S, Faden AI: Exacerbation of neuronal cell death by activation of group I metabotropic glutamate receptors: role of NMDA receptors and arachidonic acid release, *Exp Neurol* 169(2):449, 2001.
142. Yokotani K, Wang M, Murakami Y, et al: Brain phospholipase A_2–arachidonic acid cascade is involved in the activation of central sympatho-adrenomedullary outflow in rats, *Eur J Pharmacol* 398(3):341, 2000.
143. Vaz AL: Double-blind clinical evaluation of the relative efficacy of ibuprofen and glucosamine sulphate in the management of osteoarthrosis of the knee in out-patients, *Curr Med Res Opin* 8:145, 1982.
144. Pujalte JM, Llavore EP, Ylescupidez FR: Double-blind clinical evaluation of oral glucosamine sulphate in the basic treatment of osteoarthrosis, *Curr Med Res Opin* 7:110, 1980.

145. Drovanti A, Bignamini AA, Rovati AL: Therapeutic activity of oral glucosamine sulphate in osteoarthrosis: a placebo-controlled double-blind investigation, *Clin Ther* 3:260, 1980.
146. Tapadinhas MJ, Rivera IC, Bignamini AA: Oral glucosamine sulphate in the management of arthrosis: report on a multi-centre open investigation in Portugal, *Pharmatherapeutica* 3:157, 1982.
147. Bucci LR: Glycosaminoglycans. In *Nutrition applied to injury rehabilitation and sports medicine*, Boca Raton, Fla, 1994, CRC Press.
148. Pavelka K, Gatterova J, Olejarova M, et al: Glucosamine sulfate use and delay of progression of knee osteoarthritis: a 3-year, randomized, placebo-controlled, double-blind study, *Arch Intern Med* 162(18):2113, 2002.
149. Lippiello L, Woodward J, Karpman R, et al: In vivo chondroprotection and metabolic synergy of glucosamine and chondroitin sulfate, *Clin Orthop* 381:229, 2000.
150. Rovetta G, Monteforte P, Molfetta G, et al: Chondroitin sulfate in erosive osteoarthritis of the hands, *Int J Tissue React* 24 (1):29, 2002.
151. Machtey I, Ouaknine L: Tocopherol in osteoarthritis: a controlled pilot study, *J Am Geriatrics Society* 26:328, 1978.
152. Bucci LR: Fat-soluble vitamins. In *Nutrition applied to injury rehabilitation and sports medicine*, Boca Raton, Fla, 1994, CRC Press.
153. Hunt A: The role of vitamin C in wound healing, *Br J Surg* 28:436, 1941.
154. Krystal G, Morris GM, Sokoloff L: Stimulation of DNA synthesis by ascorbate in cultures of articular chondrocytes, *Arthritis Rheum* 25:318, 1982.
155. Bucci LR: Vitamin C (ascorbic acid). In *Nutrition applied to injury rehabilitation and sports medicine*, Boca Raton, Fla, 1994, CRC Press.
156. Sopler D: Nutritional implementation for better patient outcome. In Grimsby O, Rivard J, editors: *Science, theory and clinical application in orthopaedic manual physical therapy: applied science and theory*, vol 1, Taylorsville, 2008, The Academy of Graduate Physical Therapy, Inc.
157. Brilla LR, Haley TF: Effect of magnesium supplementation on strength training in humans, *J Am Coll Nutr* 11:326, 1992.
158. Wester PO, Dyckner T: The importance of the magnesium ion: magnesium deficiency, symptomatology and occurrence, *Acta Med Scand Suppl* 661:3, 1982.
159. Sojka JE, Weaver CM: Magnesium supplementation and osteoporosis, *Nutr Rev* 53:71, 1995.
160. Bucci LR: Calcium and magnesium. In *Nutrition applied to injury rehabilitation and sports medicine*, Boca Raton, Fla, 1994, CRC Press.
161. Epstein O, Kato Y, Dick R, et al: Vitamin D, hydroxy-apatite, and calcium gluconate in treatment of cortical bone thinning in postmenopausal women with primary biliary cirrhosis, *Am J Clin Nutr* 36:426, 1982.
162. Pines A, Raafat H, Lynn AH, et al: Clinical trial of microcrystalline hydroxyapatite compound ("Ossopan") in the prevention of osteoporosis due to corticosteroid therapy, *Curr Med Res Opin* 8:734, 1984.
163. Nilsen KH, Jayson MIV: Microcrystalline calcium hydroxyapatite compound in corticosteroid-treated rheumatoid patients: a controlled study, *BMJ* 2(6145):1124, 1978.
164. Finkelman RD, Butler WT: Vitamin D and skeletal tissues, *J Oral Pathol* 14:191, 1985.
165. Saltman PD, Strause LG: The role of trace minerals in osteoporosis, *J Am Coll Nutr* 12:384, 1993.
166. Bland J: *Bioflavonoids: the friends and helpers of vitamin C in many hard-to-treat ailments*, New Canaan, Conn, 1984, Keats Publishing.
167. Bucci LR: Nonessential dietary components: bioflavonoids and curcumin. In *Nutrition applied to injury rehabilitation and sports medicine*, Boca Raton, Fla, 1994, CRC Press.
168. Teixeira S: Bioflavonoids: proanthocyanidins and quercetin and their potential roles in treating musculoskeletal conditions, *J Orthop Sports Phys Ther* 32:357, 2002.
169. Lee TH, Hoover RL, Williams JD, et al: Effect of dietary enrichment with eicosapentaenoic and docosahexaenoic acids on in vitro neutrophil and monocyte leukotriene generation and neutrophil function, *N Engl J Med* 312:1217, 1985.
170. Simopoulos AP: Omega-3 fatty acids in health and disease and in growth and development, *Am J Clin Nutr* 54:438, 1991.

CHAPTER

6

Toby M. Hall and Robert L. Elvey

Neural Tissue Evaluation and Treatment

Since the previous edition of this chapter, considerable developments have occurred with respect to the understanding of the pathophysiology of pain disorders involving aberrant function of the nervous system. Indeed, dysfunction of the nervous system is now well recognized as an important contributing factor to many chronic musculoskeletal pain conditions. In addition, mobilization of the nervous system is a commonly used clinical treatment tool in current physical therapy practice. In clinical terms, however, it seems that not all neural pain disorders respond to hands-on physical therapy management. For example, one systematic review failed to find convincing evidence of therapeutic benefit for the use of neural mobilization in the most common peripheral nerve disorder, carpal tunnel syndrome.[1] To explain this disparity in treatment response requires an understanding of the basic mechanisms underlying neuropathic and nociceptive pain.

A mechanisms-based neural classification system has been described,[2] with an aim to identify patients suitable for neural mobilization. This classification system is based on pain mechanisms rather than on identification of the cause of nerve damage or disorder per se. This system requires careful consideration of information derived from the patient interview and physical examination to subclassify neuromuscular pain disorders of the upper quarter and is presented later in this chapter.

To understand better the basis for classification of neural pain disorders, a brief overview of pain mechanisms pertinent to the clinical evaluation and of the management approach taken is presented. Consequently, a comprehensive examination process incorporating evaluation of the neural system is presented that is fundamental to the clinical reasoning process necessary to evaluate upper quarter pain syndromes. Finally, classification-driven management techniques are described and are illustrated by a case study to outline the approach taken in this chapter.

Presentation of the topic in this way should not be construed as bias toward neural tissue as a major origin of pain or the tissue of involvement in most upper quarter pain neuromuscular syndromes. A detailed evaluation of each patient and interpretation of the findings are required before any clinical hypothesis or diagnosis regarding neural tissue as a pain source can be made. Even then, an open mind is essential, and continued critical assessment is necessary.

This chapter deals with shoulder and neck region pain disorders that are typically unaccompanied by significant neurologic deficit or evidence of neural compromise on radiologic imaging or other investigations. This type of disorder of the upper quarter is very common in physical therapy and manual therapy practice. The most apt descriptive term is nonspecific neck-shoulder-arm pain or *cervicobrachial pain syndrome*.

The diagnostic term *radiculopathy*, although technically incorrect for the cervical spine, is frequently and loosely used in referring to upper quarter pain disorders when pain radiates as far as the forearm or hand. Radiculopathy may therefore be considered an appropriate term for communication purposes within the context of neuromusculosketal pain, but it may also be considered incorrect in the absence of evidence of neurologic deficit of the peripheral nervous system.

INCIDENCE IN THE COMMUNITY

Cervicobrachial pain syndrome, a very common condition in the general population, causes suffering for individuals and has high societal costs. When measured in terms of lost productivity, medical treatment costs, and disability insurance claims, cervicobrachial pain syndrome represents a substantial burden.[3,4] To give some idea of the scale of the problem in the working population, neck and upper limb musculoskeletal disorders were estimated to cost up to 2.2% of the Nordic gross domestic product.[5]

The precise incidence of cervicobrachial pain is not known because of the lack of precision in the definition of cervicobrachial pain syndrome and the differences in the way in which population-based studies have been conducted. However, several investigators have tried to address this problem. Some reviews have reported the 12-month prevalence of neck pain to range from 14% up to 78%[6,7] and the 12-month prevalence of shoulder pain to range from 5% to 47%.[8] A large survey in the county of Stockholm, Sweden between 1990 and 2006 found the prevalence of self-reported neck-shoulder-arm pain higher in women than in men (25% and 15.4% prevalence rate ratio, respectively).[3] Furthermore, prevalence rates increased over the 16-year period of the investigation.[3] The authors of that study suggested that the increase in prevalence over time may result from increased exposure of physical stress during working life, random fluctuation, or general cultural awareness of reporting musculoskeletal symptoms. In addition to a higher prevalence in women, the prevalence increases with age in the general working-age population.[9]

The onset of cervicobrachial pain can either be traumatic or insidious. Frequently, in an older patient with preexisting cervical spondylosis, no single traumatic event is recalled, and the clinical picture develops insidiously. The most common trauma-induced cause is a motor vehicle accident involving "whiplash" injury of the cervical spine. Other much less common causes include radiation therapy–induced damage of the brachial plexus after mastectomy, open heart surgery, Pancoast's tumor of the lung, and vertebral artery loop formation, among many others.

UPPER QUARTER PAIN

In neuromuscular disorders, identification of the source of pain is essential before administration of physical treatment or prescription of patient-generated treatment programs. In this chapter, upper quarter pain includes cervicobrachial pain, as well as pain perceived in the upper back, upper chest, and suprascapular region.

In the evaluation of pain and the various types of pain patterns that may accompany disorders of the upper quarter, it is essential for the clinician to keep an open mind with respect to any judgment of the tissue of origin of pain. Although symptoms such as tingling, burning, pins and needles, and numbness are generally viewed as indicative of a pathologic condition affecting the nerve root or peripheral nerve trunk, when unaccompanied by paresthesia, pain may be very difficult to analyze in terms of tissue of origin. The pain may be of the following types:

1. Local pain, which may be an indication of pathologic conditions in musculoskeletal tissues immediately underlying the cutaneous area of perceived pain
2. Visceral referred pain, in which a visceral disorder may cause a perception of pain in cutaneous tissues distant to the viscera involved
3. Musculoskeletal referred pain, giving rise to perceived pain in cutaneous tissues distant to the musculoskeletal tissues
4. Neuropathic pain, which is perceived in cutaneous tissues that may be distant from pathologic neural tissues
5. Variable combinations of the preceding

Although detailed descriptions of nociception, the physiology of pain, and the mechanisms of musculoskeletal, visceral, and neuropathic pain are beyond the scope of this chapter, a brief outline is given to help gain an understanding of the topic.

Referred Pain

The phenomenon of referred pain is an added complexity when the clinician is trying to identify the source of symptoms.[10] This is particularly true during examination of a patient with a painful shoulder whose symptoms may arise from local structures including the glenohumeral joint and associated soft tissues or from cervical or thoracic vertebral segments. Determining the source of symptoms has important implications for correctly localizing treatment, particularly from a manual therapy perspective.

The topography and nature of referred pain in any one person are inadequate as factors in the differential diagnosis of both the tissue involved and the segmental level.[11] Two types of referred pain are recognized: musculoskeletal referred pain and radicular referred pain.

Musculoskeletal Referred Pain

Musculoskeletal referred pain is pain perceived in an area adjacent to (or at a distance from) its site of origin, but usually within the same spinal segment.[12] Several theoretical models have been put forward to explain musculoskeletal referred pain. One theory is that afferent impulses from different regions converge on the same viscerosomatotopic neurons in the central nervous system and cause mental projection of pain to the region corresponding to the spinal nerve.[10] This type of referred pain is not a homogeneous clinical entity because it may originate from a multitude of different structures including the cervical intervertebral disks, the facet joints, or other spinal structures. Figure 6-1 illustrates one of the physiologic mechanisms thought to be responsible for musculoskeletal referred pain. In this case, afferent input from an intervertebral disk is converging on the same neuron in the dorsal horn as neurons from the skin in a topographically separate area.

Landmark studies by Inman and Saunders[13] put forward the concept of myotomes and sclerotomes to explain segmentally referred pain from deep structures, a concept similar to that of the dermatomes for cutaneous sensation mapped by Foerster.[14] Dermatomic, sclerotomic, and myotomic charts published in standard texts should not be taken as patterns to which referred pain must invariably conform, nor do they necessarily provide insight into the source of symptoms. Wide variation exists among individuals in the patterns of referred pain, as well as much overlap from different anatomic structures. Examples include the patterns of referred pain from cervical intervertebral disks, muscles, and cervical facet joints.[15-22] In addition, the presence of significant central nervous system sensitization (frequently noted in patients seen in clinical practice) has a marked influence on the topography, nature, and intensity of referred pain; significant central sensitization makes it virtually impossible to identify the source of pain.[23,24]

Radicular Pain

Radicular or *projected pain* is pain perceived in a dermatomic or peripheral nerve distribution, depending on the site of the lesion. Radicular pain is evoked by stimulation of the peripheral nerve, the dorsal root ganglion, or the nerve root.[25] The perception that pain arises from the limb is caused by injury

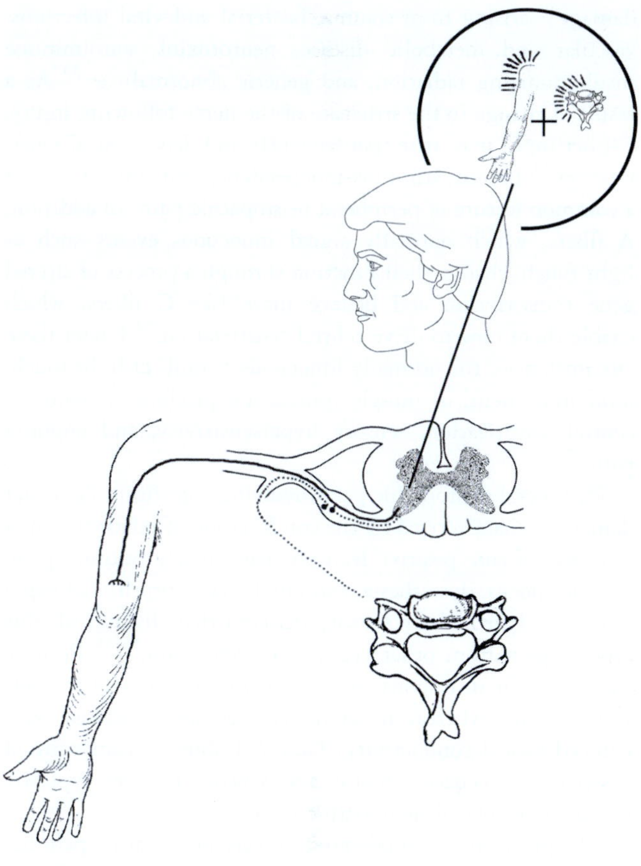

Figure 6-1 A schematic depicting the mechanism for musculoskeletal referred pain. Afferent fibers from the shoulder and arm and the cervical spine converge on the same neurons in the spinal cord. This convergence creates the mental illusion of shoulder pain as a result of noxious stimuli arising from disease in the cervical spine.

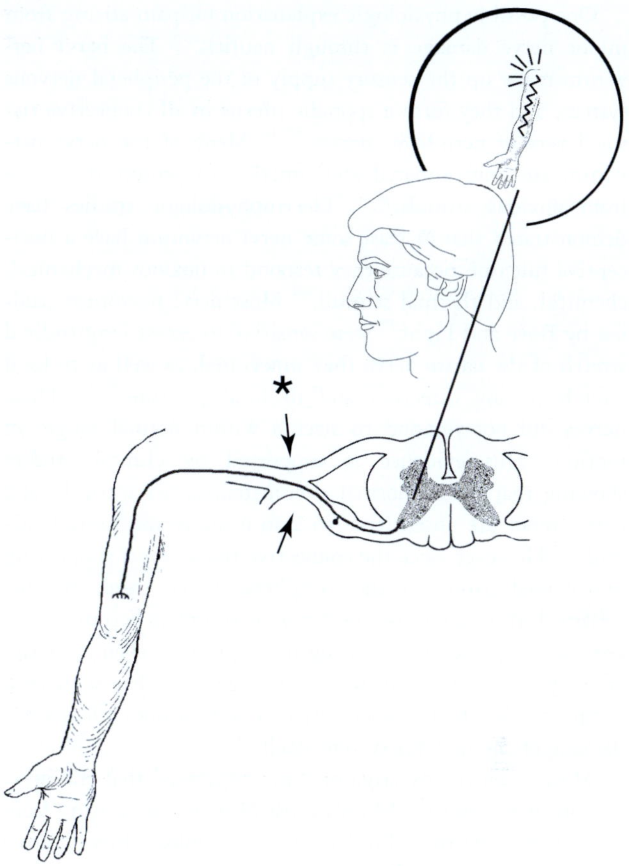

Figure 6-2 A schematic depicting the mechanism for radicular referred pain. Inflammation or damage of the nerve root, spinal nerve, or dorsal root ganglion *(asterisk, arrow)* results in radiating pain in the distribution of the damaged axons. This situation causes shoulder or arm pain in the absence of shoulder disease.

of the peripheral nerves proximal to their peripheral distribution.[26] An example of projected pain with segmental distribution is the pain of radiculopathy caused by herpes zoster or other diseases involving the nerve trunk before it divides into its major peripheral branches. Examples of projected pain with peripheral nerve distribution include trigeminal neuralgia, brachial plexus neuralgia, and meralgia paresthetica. Figure 6-2 illustrates one of the physiologic mechanisms thought to be responsible for *radicular referred pain*. Traditional orthopedic clinical practice attempted to distinguish between radicular referred pain and musculoskeletal referred pain by the distal extension of the pain in the limb.[27] More recently, however, investigators demonstrated that patients with typical symptoms consistent with radicular pain that extended down the whole limb had neurologic deficits similar to those patients with pseudoradicular pain, in which symptoms are only proximal.[28]

Neuropathic Pain

Pain is traditionally divided into two types: nociceptive and neuropathic.[29] Nociceptive pain arises from trauma or inflammation of musculoskeletal structures, whereas neuropathic pain arises from a lesion or disease affecting the nervous system itself. Of particular interest to this chapter is the distinction between nociceptive pain and peripheral neuropathic pain, although the difference between the two is becoming less clear both on a theoretical level[30] and in clinical practice.[31] This is particularly true for musculoskeletal conditions such as cervicobrachial pain or sciatica, in which both nociceptive pain and neuropathic pain may coexist. However, the clinical importance of differentiating between peripheral neuropathic pain and nociceptive pain must be emphasized because each condition requires a different treatment approach and each has a different prognosis.[32]

The fundamental cause of peripheral neuropathic pain is damage to the nervous system itself. It is both beguiling and confusing that nerve damage does not always cause pain.[33] Indeed, investigators have suggested that fewer than 10% of sudden-onset or gradual-onset peripheral nerve injuries cause significant pain.[34] Conversely, minor nerve damage, clinically difficult to detect on standard neurologic assessment, is capable of causing severe pain.[35-37] Complex regional pain syndrome is a good clinical example in which minor nerve trauma causes significant, even lifelong, pain.[38]

One possible physiologic explanation for pain arising from minor nerve damage is through neuritis.[33] The nervi nervorum make up the sensory supply of the peripheral nervous system, and they form a sporadic plexus in all connective tissue layers of peripheral nerves.[39,40] Many of the nervi nervorum are unmyelinated and function to protect the nerve from noxious stimuli.[40,41] Electrophysiologic studies have demonstrated that at least some nervi nervorum have a nociceptive function because they respond to noxious mechanical, chemical, and thermal stimuli.[39] Most nervi nervorum studied by Bove and Light[39] were sensitive to excess longitudinal stretch of the entire nerve they innervated, as well as to local stretch in any direction and to focal pressure.[40,41] These nerves did not respond to stretch within normal ranges of motion. This evidence is supported by clinical studies showing that, under normal circumstances, nerve trunks and nerve roots are insensitive to non-noxious mechanical stimuli.[42] However, once the connective tissue layers supporting undamaged axons in the peripheral nerve trunk become inflamed, this may cause the nervi nervorum to become sensitized and capable of generating nociception to even activities of daily living. Investigators have suggested that such pain should be classified as nociceptive because it does not involve damage of the nervous system itself.[33]

More recently, investigators have suggested that the nervi nervorum may not be the only cause of symptoms arising from mechanosensitization of inflamed nerve trunks.[43] Investigators have argued that if inflammatory mediators penetrate the connective tissue layers to the axons themselves, then physiologic changes will occur consistent with neuropathic pain.[30,33] Bove et al[35] demonstrated in a rat model that some intact nerve fibers become sensitive to pressure at the site of inflammation and that axons themselves develop properties of pressure mechanosensitivity.[35,36,43] Furthermore, Dilley et al[36] showed evidence of stretch sensitivity in a small proportion of structurally normal, but inflamed, A and C nerve fibers. Most responsive fibers fired to only 3% stretch, which is within the range of nerve stretch seen during normal limb movements. The mechanisms underlying mechanosensitivity of axons are complex, but they are believed to involve disruption to axoplasmic flow and axonal transport at the inflamed site.[44,45] Ongoing symptoms may arise from disruption to axoplasmic flow as a result of altered pressure around the nerve, rather than inflammatory mediators directly influencing the conducting elements.[46] In addition to these changes, ion channel expression is also altered, resulting in a change in type and density of ion channels produced by the cell body.[47,48] The consequence of these changes is that some axons generate impulses to mechanical stimuli when they would not normally do so. The studies by Bove et al[35,40,46] and Dilley et al[36,44,45] provide possible explanations for the frequent clinical finding of peripheral nerve trunk mechanosensitivity in a range of musculoskeletal disorders,[49] in which normal neurologic function is shown on electrodiagnostic tests and no apparent structural abnormality appears on any form of radiologic imaging.

In addition to pain caused by minor nerve trauma, peripheral neuropathic pain also occurs following significant nerve damage[50] arising from trauma, bacterial and viral infections, vascular and metabolic disease, neurotoxins, autoimmune insult, ionizing radiation, and genetic abnormalities.[33] As a result of change to the structure of the nerve following injury, C-fiber input may arise spontaneously and drive central sensitization.[51] Indeed, stimulus-independent, spontaneous pain is a common feature of peripheral neuropathic pain. In addition, A fibers, which normally signal innocuous events such as light touch, change their function through a process of altered gene transcription and behave more like C fibers, which enable them now to drive central sensitization.[52] Under these circumstances, the normally innocuous stimuli of light touch, joint movement, or muscle contraction produce or maintain central sensitization, sensory hypersensitivity, and ongoing pain.[47]

Peripheral neuropathic pain involving significant fascicular damage is characterized by the combination of relatively small numbers of core positive features (particularly burning pain, electric shocks, dysesthesia, and allodynia to brush) and negative signs (particularly sensory deficits) that distinguish this type of pain from other types of chronic pain.[53-55] Positive features occur in response to increased excitability of the nervous system, whereas negative features are associated with reduced axonal conductivity. Table 6-1 shows a composite of positive and negative motor and sensory features typically found in peripheral neuropathic pain.

The prevalence of moderate to severe neuropathic pain has been estimated by survey to be up to 5% in the general population.[56] Peripheral neuropathic pain is usually chronic and disabling and is the most challenging to treat, even from a medical perspective.[57] Hence the early identification of peripheral neuropathic pain is important for selecting appropriate management as well as for identifying patients who are unlikely to respond to particular types of intervention such as manual therapy.

Screening tools for the identification of peripheral neuropathic pain have been developed to help the clinician determine the predominance of neuropathic pain in a patient's presenting complaint. These tools include the Neuropathic

Table 6-1 Positive and Negative Features of Peripheral Neuropathic Pain

	Motor	Sensory

Positive	• Spasm
	• Dystonia
	• Cramp
		• Pain
		• Paresthesia
		• Hyperesthesia
		  • Allodynia (thermal and mechanical)
		  • Hyperalgesia
		  • Hyperpathia
		• Dysesthesia

Negative	• Weakness • Wasting • Hyporeflexia	• Anesthesia • Hypoesthesia

Pain Questionnaire,[58] the French Douleur Neuropathique 4 (DN4),[59] the Leeds Assessment of Neuropathic Symptoms and Signs (LANSS),[60] painDETECT,[61] and ID-pain.[62] Each tool attempts to identify the presence of neuropathic pain in a different way. For example, the ID-pain is purely subjective,[62] whereas the LANSS and DN4 consist of a questionnaire regarding pain description, together with items relating to the bedside clinical examination. The sensitivity and specificity of each questionnaire have been summarized elsewhere.[63]

Some preliminary evidence indicates that manual therapy is not effective for patients with low back–related leg pain who screen positive on the LANSS scale, a result indicating likely peripheral neuropathic pain.[64] Similarly, evidence indicates that physical therapy consisting of specific exercise is not effective for patients with whiplash-associated disorder with similar features of sensory hypersensitivity.[65] Hence the identification of these patients is important in clinical practice because it probably indicates a poor prognosis for exercise and manual therapy.

As stated previously, most nerve trauma does not cause symptoms. Hence not all nerve damage is associated with neuropathic pain. Clinically, however, some patients have significant signs of nerve trauma, correlated with significant pain but with an absence of positive features, and such patients test negative on neuropathic screening tools. The classic examples are spinal stenosis and some forms of cervical radiculopathy associated with osteoarthritic or degenerative change. Osteophytes progressively compress nerve roots and cause symptoms to develop gradually over time. Although pain is not always a feature of nerve root compression and spinal stenosis,[66-69] radicular pain in the absence of inflammation of the nerve root presumably results from chronic compression, which causes hypoxia and vascular compromise and subsequent damage of axons within the nerve root. Under these circumstances, the patient may have minimal evidence of axonal mechanosensitivity on clinical tests that lengthen the nerve[68,70] and few positive symptoms.[71]

Patients with nerve root or peripheral nerve compression typically present with pain associated with movement or postures that further compress the neural structures. In the example of spinal canal or foraminal stenosis, spine extension, ipsilateral rotation and lateral flexion, and combination movements are provocative because these movements further reduce the space available for the nerve root.[72] For these movements to compromise the neural structures, the volume of the canal or foramen must already have been reduced. This reduction usually occurs by some degenerative process or is caused by space-occupying lesion. Clinical evaluation of deep tendon reflexes, muscle power, skin sensation, and vibration perception reveal neurologic dysfunction. In addition, radiologic, and electrodiagnostic evidence of compressive neurologic compromise consistent with the clinical findings is also informative.

Peripheral nerve compression lesions in the shoulder region are relatively rare but include the brachial plexus, axillary nerve, long thoracic nerve, suprascapular nerve, and accessory nerve.[73] The identification of such conditions is based on a thorough clinical examination, with particular emphasis on the neurologic examination.

In summary, peripheral nerve damage at any point distal to and including the dorsal root ganglion may cause any combination of nociceptive and neuropathic pain, either local or referred. In addition, trauma sufficient to damage a peripheral nerve is also likely to traumatize adjacent musculoskeletal structures, so a complex mixture of pain mechanisms is likely to emerge.

EVALUATION

To evaluate a disorder for effective manual therapy management, the clinician must carry out a physical examination without presuming the source of symptoms and in a manner that results in a sufficient number of signs correlating with and supporting each other in the formulation of a clinical hypothesis or diagnosis.

In the evaluation of neural tissue for possible involvement in a disorder, clinical experience indicates that certain specific correlating signs must be present before any suggestion that neural tissue is involved can be made. This is necessary for an accurate treatment prescription when considering a manual therapy approach. Physical treatment, in the form of manual therapy, cannot be prescribed from imagery or nerve conduction studies, although it may well be strongly influenced and guided by such studies, even to the degree that the results of either investigative procedure may contraindicate manual therapy.

Physical Signs of Neural Tissue Involvement

1. Active movement dysfunction
2. Passive movement dysfunction, which must correlate specifically with 1
3. Adverse responses to neural tissue provocation tests (NTPTs), which must relate specifically and anatomically to 1 and 2
4. Hyperalgesic responses to palpation of specific nerve trunks, which must relate specifically and anatomically to 1 to 3
5. Hyperalgesic responses to palpation of cutaneous tissues, which relate specifically and anatomically to 4 and 6
6. Evidence in the physical examination of a local area of abnormality, which would involve the neural tissue showing the responses in 3 to 5

The physical therapist involved in treating disorders of the upper quarter must also consider visceral referred pain. Obviously, medical referral of patients should overcome this potential problem for the physical therapist. However, not all visceral conditions are readily diagnosed during a routine medical or clinical evaluation. Should a visceral condition be accompanied by strong shoulder pain and active shoulder movement restriction, the clinician may have some difficulty in making a clinical diagnosis involving viscera.

The liver, diaphragm, and heart are viscera requiring particular consideration when the physical therapist suspects the possibility of visceral referred shoulder pain. If any suspicion or doubt exists, medical opinion must be sought.

Hall and Elvey have seen many examples of this need in clinical practice. One example was a liver disorder in a middle-aged woman who saw her doctor because of increasing severity of pain in the right lower chest and upper right abdominal quadrant, pain that she said radiated from the middle of her back. She had pain on the right side of the neck, right shoulder, and upper arm and had difficulty elevating her arm above the shoulder level. She was very tender on palpation of the right upper abdominal quadrant and the midthoracic spine. Her doctor referred her for examination, including ultrasonography of the liver and plain radiographs of the thoracic spine. The ultrasonogram was reported as normal, and the plain radiographs indicated mild degenerative changes evident in the midthoracic levels. The patient was referred for physical therapy for treatment, with the thought that her chest pain was either musculoskeletal referred pain or radicular referred pain. Hall and Elvey were not happy with the situation and contacted the referring doctor, who investigated the patient further. The outcome was a diagnosis of liver disease. Of concern was the paucity of physical evaluation findings to suggest a neuromuscular disorder.

In the absence of other physical findings—in particular any spinal dysfunction—and in keeping with the severity of the pain, Hall and Elvey postulated that a liver disorder was likely because of the resultant diaphragm irritation, phrenic nerve sensitization, and subsequent facilitation of the related cervical dorsal horn neurons resulting in perceived shoulder and arm pain and sensitization of the upper trunk of the right brachial plexus. These findings excluded physical therapy as a treatment option, and a physician treated this patient.

Other cases of thoracic outlet area tumors have also been seen in practice and referred for treatment for "stiff painful shoulder" syndrome. These cases highlight the necessity of careful evaluation of accurate differential physical tests.

The clinician must consider the sensory innervation of the connective tissues by the peripheral nervous system and the relative dynamics of peripheral nerves to understand the structured scheme of evaluation for the presence of specific signs. As previously mentioned, peripheral nerves and their supporting structures can become mechanosensitized by pathologic events and can be a source of pain because of inherent sensory innervation. In addition, the target tissues of the affected neural tissues can become sensitized and tender.[74] Herpes zoster (shingles) and complex regional pain syndrome are good examples of the signs attributed to pathologic neural tissue, nerve as a pain source, and peripheral nerve trunks that can become hyperalgesic.

Peripheral nerve trunks are dynamic relative to the associated movement of anatomic surrounding tissue and structures. This means that nerve trunks have to adapt to positional changes of posture with movement of both the trunk and limbs. In other words, they have to be compliant with movement. Therefore, nerve trunks can be physically tested in a selective manner.

When nerve tissue becomes abnormal, and therefore tender and hyperalgesic, the outcome is pain associated with any trunk or limb movement in which the trunks of that nerve tissue have to adapt. The nerve trunks become noncompliant with movement because of the pain. This noncompliance is demonstrated by limitation of movement because of muscle tone and activity in groups of muscles antagonistic to the direction of movement. Muscles prevent pain by preventing movement. Muscle contraction, as measured by electromyography, in response to provocation of neural tissue has been demonstrated in both animal and in vivo human experiments.[42,75-81]

In more severe cases of pain of neural tissue origin, the increased tone of muscles becomes widespread and may involve muscles quite distant from the source of pain. In addition, a type of dystonia may be present, whereby an upper quarter pain syndrome of neural tissue origin may appear as a "painful stiff shoulder" or "frozen shoulder." This situation may explain the clinical finding of stiff painful shoulder or frozen shoulder in the presence of tumors in the thoracic outlet region (e.g., Pancoast's tumor).

The signs associated with the foregoing neural tissue abnormalities require very careful and precise evaluation, awareness of the significance of each sign, and an open mind with respect to the formulation of a clinical hypothesis.

Active Movement Dysfunction

Landmark studies[82] showed that a position of shoulder girdle depression, shoulder abduction and lateral rotation, elbow extension, and wrist or finger extension, with the cervical spine in contralateral lateral flexion, has the effect of placing the neural tissues of the brachial plexus and related cervical neural tissues and peripheral nerve trunks in the upper limb in a maximum anatomically lengthened state. Investigators also demonstrated that any movement of the upper quarter to attain this position influences the same neural tissues to variable degrees. Neural tissues as a structure slide within the anatomic surrounding tissues, or the surrounding anatomic tissues glide over the neural tissues, or both, as in functional movement. Hence when a nerve is mechanosensitized by whatever cause, the patient displays active movement dysfunction, and so does a patient with shingles when the herpes zoster virus affects a dorsal root ganglion of the brachial plexus. In the same manner, a patient with Pancoast's tumor affecting the lower trunk of the brachial plexus has a painful stiff shoulder.

With applied anatomy, it becomes clearly evident that different anatomic positions of the shoulder, elbow, and wrist influence the peripheral trunks of the brachial plexus in different ways. The median nerve is in its most lengthened state in the position described at the start of this section. The radial nerve is in its most lengthened position with abduction and medial rotation of the shoulder, elbow extension, wrist and finger flexion in the position of shoulder girdle depression, and cervical spine contralateral lateral flexion. The ulnar nerve is in its most lengthened position with abduction and lateral rotation of the shoulder, elbow flexion, wrist and finger extension, and again with the same common position of the shoulder girdle and cervical spine.

Although different anatomic positions of the upper limb influence the peripheral trunks of the brachial plexus in different ways, they do not do so without influencing other structures. For instance, movements that stress the median nerve also have some influence on other tissues and nerve trunks. Hence it is important to view a range of tests when examining a patient. Only by considering all aspects of the examination can a decision be made about the source of symptoms.

When any neural tissue tract of the upper quarter becomes involved in a painful disorder, various active movements are affected, depending on the involvement of the particular tract. Clearly, active shoulder abduction, with shoulder girdle depression and contralateral flexion of the cervical spine, affects all tracts of neural tissue from C5 to T1.

In testing a disorder to determine the possibility of neural tissue involvement, active shoulder abduction should be used in or behind the coronal plane. If pain is provoked, or if the range of movement is limited, the clinician can differentiate between shoulder joint and neural tissue abnormalities by gently resisting the concurrent shoulder girdle elevation occurring with active abduction and—at the same time—position the patient's head and neck in contralateral lateral flexion (Fig. 6-3). When neural tissue is involved, the response to active abduction is a more painful and further limited range of movement.

This is a basic approach to analysis of active movement in the physical evaluation of neural tissue. With some thought to applied anatomy, the clinician can evaluate active movements in different directions and in various ways to support a clinical hypothesis formed at this early stage of evaluation. For example, a disorder of the C4-5 motion segment may involve the C5 nerve roots or spinal nerve. This may cause an observable dysfunction of shoulder abduction and movement of the hand behind the back because of the increased tension that these movements place on the suprascapular and axillary nerve trunks. Contralateral lateral flexion of the head and neck would increase the dysfunction.

Passive Movement Dysfunction

Neural tissue tracts must comply with passive movement as they do with active movement. If a specific painful active movement dysfunction results from a disorder involving neural tissues, passive movement in the same directions will also be affected by pain and, as a consequence, limitation of range.

As with active movement, the clinician works through a differential evaluation process for a determination of possible neural tissue involvement associated with a painful limitation of range. When passive abduction is painfully limited in range, it correlates with painful active limitation of range. In addition, the pain increases and the range decreases when passive shoulder abduction is performed with the shoulder girdle fixed in depression or when the head and neck are positioned in contralateral lateral flexion.

This clinical approach applies to applicable passive movements in different directions that always correlate with active movement dysfunction. The quadrant position of shoulder joint examination described by Maitland[83] is of particular interest in passive movement evaluation. In the quadrant position, the humeral head has an upward fulcrum effect on the overlying neurovascular bundle in the region of the axilla.[82] Therefore, it is conceivable to use this method as a test not only of the shoulder articular structures, but also of the compliance of the neurovascular tissues and, in the context of this chapter, the neural tissues of the brachial plexus and its proximal and distal extensions. To do this, the quadrant test is performed as described by Maitland,[83] and with the shoulder girdle in elevation and depression, and the head and neck in ipsilateral and contralateral lateral flexion and the elbow in extension (Fig. 6-4).

These additional positions subtract or add distance over which the neural tissues travel and thereby afford the clinician the ability to determine whether the test responses represent neural tissue or shoulder joint signs.

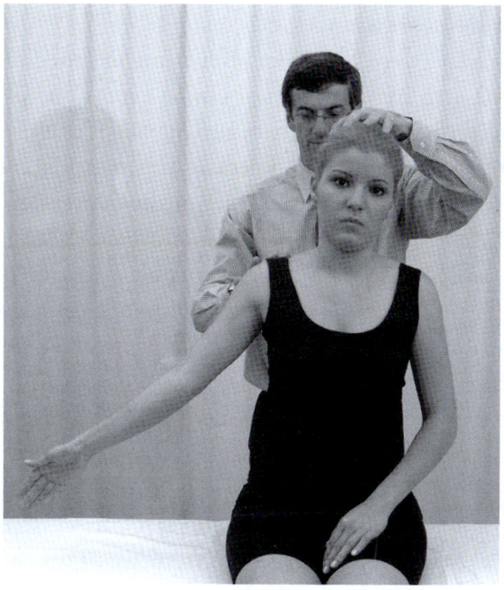

Figure 6-3 Active movement screening for peripheral nerve sensitization. Shoulder abduction without excessive scapula elevation is shown.

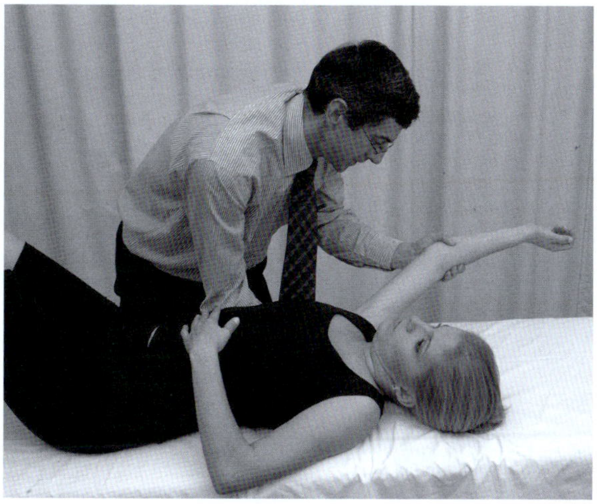

Figure 6-4 Passive movement testing for peripheral nerve sensitization. Shoulder quadrant position with cervical left lateral flexion and elbow extension is shown.

Adverse Responses to Neural Tissue Provocation Tests

Among a range of physical evaluation tests to assist in this task are NTPTs, also known as neurodynamic tests.[84] Tests used to diagnose upper quarter pain disorders, originally described by Elvey in 1979,[82,85] have been gaining popularity in the physical therapy literature.[86-88]

Provocation tests are passive tests that are applied in a manner of selectivity for the examination of compliance of different neural tissues with functional positions. This means that identifying a specific type of functional position noncompliance enables the clinician to form a hypothesis not only on the possible involvement of neural tissue in a disorder but also on the possible site of involvement.

In the past, NTPTs were criticized, and whether these tests could selectively stress nerve trunks was questioned.[89] Since that criticism, much research was undertaken to investigate the validity of NTPTs.[36,90-98] For example, an experimental pain model was used to determine the specificity of a median nerve NTPT in the differential diagnosis of hand symptoms.[93] Sensory responses to this test were unchanged by the presence of experimentally induced muscle pain in the hand, a finding illustrating high specificity for this test. Other studies similarly demonstrated high sensitivity for this test to identify patients with carpal tunnel syndrome[99] and cervical radiculopathy.

Provocation tests can be carried out only within the available range of passive movement, which is governed by the severity of pain associated with the disorder. An example for the radial nerve is shown in Figure 6-5. These passive movements are those that would lengthen the course over which the neural tissue extends to reach its maximum length. In more severe painful conditions involving neural tissue, it is obvious that passive movements and positions, well short of their maximum length, would result in a pain response sufficient to cause limitation of range or the inability to gain a functional position because of the pain and protective muscle.

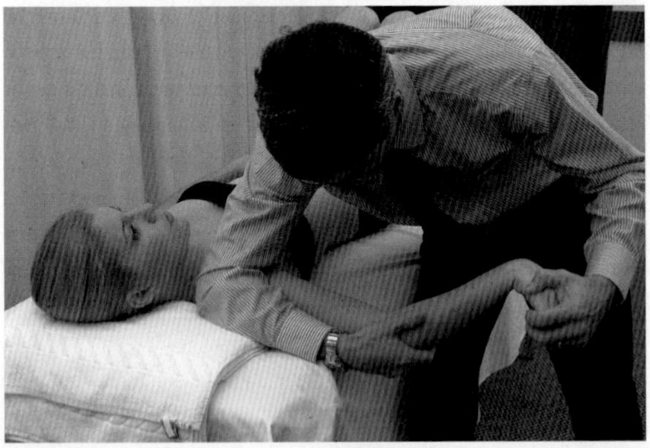

Figure 6-5 Neural tissue provocation test from distal to proximal for the radial nerve. The elbow is moved into extension with the forearm pronated, the finger and wrist flexed, the shoulder internally rotated, and the neck in left lateral flexion.

Therefore, it is unrealistic to develop a standard form of the provocation test technique. The clinician is required to formulate test techniques according to the each patient's unique symptoms and signs.

Test Technique from Distal to Proximal

The subject is supine, and the clinician's hands are positioned to control shoulder girdle elevation and elbow and wrist and finger flexion and extension, and also to alter shoulder rotation, head and neck lateral flexion, and forearm pronation and supination.

1. *By the median nerve.* Shoulder abduction and lateral rotation, forearm supinated, head and neck neutral, shoulder girdle neutral; extend elbow. Increase effects of the test with incremental wrist and finger extension, shoulder girdle depression, and head and neck contralateral lateral flexion.
2. *By the radial nerve.* Shoulder abduction and medial rotation, forearm pronation, head and neck neutral, shoulder girdle neutral; extend elbow. Increase effect with incremental wrist and finger (including thumb) flexion, shoulder girdle depression, and head and neck contralateral lateral flexion.
3. *By the ulnar nerve.* Shoulder abduction and lateral rotation, forearm pronation, head and neck neutral, shoulder girdle depression; flex elbow. Increase the effect with incremental wrist and finger flexion and head and neck contralateral lateral flexion.

Test Technique from Proximal to Distal

The subject is supine, and the clinician's hands are in a position to control head and neck lateral flexion, shoulder girdle elevation and depression, and shoulder abduction and rotation.

1. *By the median nerve.* Shoulder abduction and lateral rotation, with the arm comfortably in a position of elbow extension, slight wrist extension (positions naturally occurring as a result of the placement of the arm), head and neck contralateral lateral flexion. Increase the effect with shoulder girdle depression.
2. *By the radial nerve.* Shoulder abduction and medial rotation, with the arm in a position of elbow extension; slight wrist flexion (positions naturally occurring as a result of the placement of the arm); head and neck contralateral lateral flexion. Increase the effect with shoulder girdle depression.
3. *By the ulnar nerve.* Shoulder abduction and lateral rotation, elbow and wrist and finger extension, forearm pronation, shoulder girdle depression, head and neck contralateral lateral flexion. Increase the effect with increased shoulder girdle depression.

As the name implies, with passive NTPTs a response is the clinician's goal. Altered responses include resistance to movement, range, and pain.

- The clinician appreciates an increase in muscle tone in muscles to prevent further movement. This increase in tone should coincide with the first experience of the onset of pain in symptomatic patients[77] and later in range in asymptomatic patients.[76,81]

- The identification of the increased muscle tone amounts to a first limitation of range of the passive test movement. This is not a lack of range, as may be related to tethering or any other form of physical prevention of movement, but one directly related to an evoked pain response and resultant muscle activity to prevent further pain by the provoking movement.
- Having produced an initial adverse response, the test movement should be carefully taken further into range, to attempt to reproduce the reported pain. Reproduction of symptoms is always a requirement in manual therapy evaluation, to ensure that a condition is suited for a specific physical treatment.

Investigators have suggested that the sequence in which the various component movements are applied during NTPTs is important because it provides information on the site of neural tissue disease.[84,100] This conjecture is unsupported in the literature,[91,101] and it may be that responses to neurodynamic sequencing may simply result from the attention placed on the first of a combination of movements.[102] Again, the informed clinician combines information from the whole examination, rather than that from one test in isolation.

Hyperalgesic Responses to Nerve Trunk Palpation

If neural tissue responds with a painful reaction to a stimulus applied through its length in a longitudinal manner, such as with active movement or NTPTs, it must also follow that there would be a painful reaction to palpation.

Nerve trunks are selectively palpated. Although nerve palpation has not been investigated to a great degree, studies have shown that manual palpation is reliable in the upper limb[103] and lower limb.[104] The nerve trunks or neural tissues of the uninvolved or less severely affected side are palpated first, to allow the patient to make a comparison. Gently and precisely, gradually increasing pressure is applied until it is deemed sufficient to complete the examination. Palpation of neural tissue of the upper quarter is done in the following way:

Nerve Trunk Palpation in supine-Lying Position

Palpate:

1. The trunks of the brachial plexus in the posterior triangle of the neck. Selectively examine from the cranial to caudal and from the lateral margins of scalenus anterior and medius toward the middle third of the clavicle and hence the first rib.
2. The neurovascular bundle of the brachial plexus as it travels beneath the coracoid process.
3. The three major peripheral nerve trunks of the arm at their commencement in the axilla, where they may not be identifiable individually, but can certainly be identified as nerve trunks.
4. The median nerve, in the lower third of the medial upper arm, where it can be identified as a structure; and anterior at the level of the wrist, where it cannot be identified as a structure.
5. The radial nerve, in the posterolateral aspect of the upper arm, where in some individuals it can be identified as a structure. At the lower third of the lateral aspect of the upper arm, where it crosses into the anterior compartment. At the lateral aspect of the forearm below the elbow, and on the posterolateral region of the wrist.
6. The ulnar nerve, at the posteromedial aspect of the elbow, where it is readily identifiable, and at the anteromedial aspect of the wrist.

Nerve Trunk Palpation in Prone-Lying Position

Palpate:

1. The suprascapular nerve, through the trapezius on the superior border of the scapula.
2. The axillary nerve, through the posterior aspect of the deltoid and on the upper lateral border of the scapula as it enters teres minor.
3. The dorsal scapular nerve, through the rhomboids, midway between the medial border of the scapula and spine.

Hyperalgesic Responses to Palpation of Cutaneous Tissues

In disorders of pain involving neural tissue, it becomes readily apparent that palpation of tissue in regions anatomically related to the involved neural tissue detects marked tenderness to the point of being hyperalgesic. These tender points are predictably found in areas that appear to be target tissues of the involved nerve or its spinal anatomic segments of origin.

A suggestion exists that the tender points may represent ectopic pacemaker sites,[105] perhaps terminating cutaneous or subcutaneous branches of the nerve in question. The most common area found in disorders of the upper quarter, such as cervicobrachial syndrome, is medial to the medial border of the scapula.

Evaluation for Signs of a Local Area of Disease

In pathologic conditions of nerve tissue, all the features discussed may readily be found or determined during a physical evaluation. However, this does not mean that the condition is suited to manual therapy management. It is quite possible for *painful diabetic neuropathy*, painful neuropathy caused by a tumor infiltration, or carpal tunnel syndrome to cause all the features discussed thus far, including limitation of active and passive movement. Therefore, the clinician must determine a cause for the neural involvement.

As an example in the upper quarter, cervical intervertebral disk disease often results in radicular arm pain and specific cervical spine motion segment dysfunction. This disorder is manifested by abnormal responses to segmental movement tests. For example, C6 radiculopathy manifests with abnormal responses to segmental movement tests at C5-6.

Neurologic Examination

An important aspect of the evaluation of neural tissue disorders is assessment of neurologic function. In the clinical setting, the neurologic examination is the only means of determining the presence of axonal conduction loss. The neurologic examination incorporates both subjective inquiry and physical tests of nerve function.

The subjective examination must delineate the specific type and area of symptoms, including paresthesias and sensory loss. These areas can then be compared with typical dermatomal, sclerotomal, and myotomal maps. The clinician should not rely purely on dermatomal charts when determining the segmental origin of pain because these charts are not the ideal diagnostic reference,[106] given the significant overlap of innervation from adjacent nerve roots and the great variability among individuals.[107,108] In this respect, myotomal and sclerotomal charts[13] are more helpful.[106]

Physical neurologic examination procedures include tests for sensation, tendon reflexes, and muscle strength. Although some studies investigated the reliability and diagnostic validity of the neurologic examination, its value is still not well established.[109-112] Interobserver reliability and agreement are best achieved by incorporating the subjective history together with the physical examination findings.[110,113] Reliability was shown to be good for muscle strength[113-116] and sensory loss,[113] but controversial for reflex changes.[113,117,118] Wainner et al[111] investigated the diagnostic accuracy of a range of cervical physical tests (including range of motion, Spurling's maneuver, muscle strength, and reflexes, among others) to identify cervical radiculopathy and reported that a cluster of physical examination tests was more useful for identifying cervical radiculopathy than was any single test item.

The examination protocol presented in this chapter, together with neuropathic screening tools, enables the clinician to classify patients with upper quarter pain broadly into one of four categories.[71,119]

1. Sensory hypersensitivity comprising major features of nervous system sensitization (based on the LANSS scale[60])
2. Denervation arising from significant axonal compromise without evidence of significant sensory hypersensitivity changes (based on the neurologic assessment)
3. Peripheral nerve sensitization arising from nerve trunk inflammation without clinical evidence of significant denervation (based on active movement, NTPTs, and nerve palpation tests)
4. Musculoskeletal referred pain

Classification is based on dominant findings following an order of priority, with sensory hypersensitivity first, denervation second, peripheral nerve sensitization third, and musculoskeletal referred pain last. This classification system was shown to have good reliability,[119] as well as validity,[120] and is predictive of response to treatment.[64]

MANUAL THERAPY TREATMENT OF NEURAL TISSUE

In this chapter, a distinction is made among three types of disorders affecting peripheral neural tissue: sensory hypersensitivity, denervation, and peripheral nerve sensitization. This distinction is important for treatment options, which are different for each classification. Sensory hypersensitivity, as previously discussed, is a disorder categorized by abnormal processing of sensory information resulting from various central and peripheral nervous system pathologic mechanisms. Patients classified with this disorder are unlikely to respond to manual therapy techniques such as neural mobilization. Rather, cognitive-behavioral retraining programs, graded motor imagery, or mirror box therapy would be more appropriate management techniques,[121] and they are discussed in the literature.[122]

For patients fulfilling the denervation classification, neural tissue mobilization techniques, particularly those that attempt to lengthen or stretch the nerve such as "tensioners,"[88] are contraindicated. This is particularly important in the acute or subacute stage of the disorder in which the nerve trunk is physiologically vulnerable to hypoxia by lengthening.[123,124] For patients fulfilling this category, treatment techniques aimed at decompressing the affected nerve should be explored.[63]

Treatment in patients fulfilling the third category, peripheral nerve sensitization, should consist of gentle manual therapy involving passive movement techniques, in which the anatomic tissues or structures surrounding the affected neural tissue are gently mobilized. The cervical lateral glide is the technique of choice for patients with peripheral nerve sensitization involving the upper limb.

Cervical Lateral Glide

The patient lies supine, with the shoulder slightly abducted and elbow flexed to approximately 90° such that the hand rests on the chest or abdomen. The clinician gently supports the shoulder on the acromial region with one hand while comfortably holding and supporting the patient's head and neck (Fig. 6-6).

Technique

Gentle controlled lateral glide to the contralateral side occurs in a slow oscillating manner up to a point in range where the first resistance occurs in the form of antagonistic muscle activity.

The first resistance represents the treatment barrier. Should this barrier not be reached, the clinician must change the patient's arm position. This involves more abduction or possibly extending the elbow while maintaining the shoulder position.

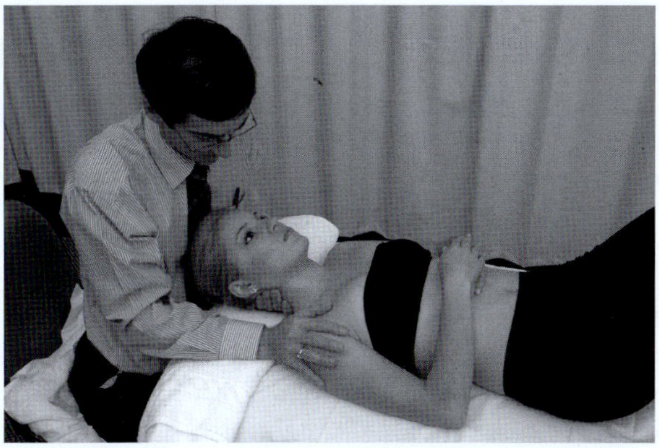

Figure 6-6 Cervical left lateral glide treatment technique for right arm symptoms. The therapist stabilizes the scapula over the acromion and glides the head and cervical spine to the contralateral side to the "treatment barrier."

The patient's arm must be fully supported on the treatment couch at all times. In more acute conditions, additional support should be given by using a pillow.

The technique progresses on subsequent treatment days, but only when indicated by a demonstrable improvement. If improvement can be detected, then the lateral glide is performed with the shoulder in gradually increased amounts of abduction. The most obvious indicator of successful treatment using this technique is an improvement in active shoulder abduction together with less pain.

The amount of time the technique is performed is variable, depending largely on the experience of the clinician and, as in any disorder, also depending on symptom severity and irritability. The composure of the patient is a prime consideration with regard to the amount of time devoted to a technique. Should the patient begin to show signs of lack of total relaxation, the technique should be temporarily ceased, and methods of soft tissue mobilization should be employed until composure is regained. Evidence of the efficacy of the cervical lateral glide was demonstrated in numerous studies in subjects with lateral elbow pain and cervicobrachial pain.[125-132]

As in so many disorders managed by manual therapy techniques, the clinician must consider treatment of tissues affected secondarily and as a consequence of the primary neural tissue abnormality. For example, cervical and shoulder girdle muscles may become maladaptive, and treatment to restore normality must be commenced. In addition, the cervical spine and the shoulder joint may require mobilizing treatment. The extent of the treatment to other tissues and structures depends on the chronicity of the disorder and its severity.

Self-treatment and management are most important. For neural tissue of the upper quarter, these techniques can be performed in various ways. A relatively simple treatment can be conducted by placing the hand of the involved side in a comfortable position against a wall, with a degree of elbow flexion. This is followed by very gentle and controlled contralateral flexion. This maneuver should not cause pain, but rather a pulling sensation in the shoulder and upper arm region. This movement is repeated three times daily. This technique may appear insubstantial, but it is essential to regard the movement as self-treatment and not exercise. Functional training in the form of graduated exercise to recondition the patient at a time deemed appropriate by the clinician also becomes essential to the self-management program to restore the patient to normal functional activity levels.

CASE STUDY

History

A 52-year-old female office secretary reported 18 months history of pain in the region of the right scapula radiating to the shoulder, with no other symptoms. She described the pain as a deep ache and rated the worst pain as 5 out of 10 on a verbal rating scale. The problem evolved insidiously, with no specific causal incident, but gradually worsened over the 18 months and was thought to relate to an increase in volume of computer work station use. She sought advice from a medical practitioner, who referred her for physical therapy and gave her nonsteroidal anti-inflammatory medication, which had no benefit. Typical aggravating activities included working for more than an hour on the computer, making beds in the morning, carrying heavy shopping bags in the right arm, and lying on the right side at night. Functional disability was rated as 5 out of 10 on the Patient-Specific Functional Scale.[133] Her sleep pattern was disturbed: she woke with pain at night, and she woke with pain in the morning. The LANSS scale result was negative, and she had no other signs of sensory hypersensitivity or other medical history of note.

Physical Evaluation

The patient had excessive scapular protraction and elevation at rest, together with poor dynamic scapular control on shoulder abduction and elevation. Active shoulder movement was restricted by pain at 120° of abduction and 160° of flexion. All other movements were full range and without pain. Shoulder abduction was more painful and more restricted in range when the head and neck were positioned in left lateral flexion and scapula elevation was controlled while the wrist and fingers were held in extension. The patient had no signs of articular dysfunction on testing the shoulder girdle articulations with accessory motion testing. Cervical active movement was neither restricted nor painful in any direction.

NTPTs were carried out from proximal to distal and vice versa for the median, radial, and ulnar nerve trunks.

Continued

CASE STUDY—cont'd

Significant evidence of sensitization of the median and radial nerve trunks was found. Mild pressure over the brachial plexus and the neurovascular bundle in the axilla, median, radial, and suprascapular nerve trunks of the right upper quarter produced painful responses that were not present on the left side. Manual diagnosis revealed dysfunction at C5-6, and the patient had no evidence of a neurologic deficit.

Assessment

In terms of classification, the negative LANSS, normal neurologic function, but significant signs of mechanosensitized median and radial nerve trunks provided convincing evidence to confirm peripheral nerve sensitization as the diagnostic classification for this patient.

Treatment

Treatment commenced with gentle cervical left lateral glide at the C5-6 segment. The right arm was positioned in 30° of abduction, with the elbow flexed to 90°, and the hand resting on the abdomen. Treatment was initially carried out twice weekly.

Subjective improvement occurred after the first treatment session, which coincided with improvements in shoulder abduction. Cervical lateral glide was continued with the arm in a progressively greater range of abduction but with the elbow maintained at 90° of flexion. A home exercise program was also introduced that involved sitting sideways at a table with the right arm supported on a pillow to achieve 30° of abduction. Active cervical left lateral flexion was performed without pain. Progression of this exercise was made by repeating the lateral flexion exercise but with the shoulder in a gradually greater range of abduction.

Treatment to restore normal scapula motor control was commenced after 3 weeks. After 6 weeks of treatment, the patient had regained 100% shoulder mobility and was able to undertake daily tasks without discomfort. She rated her pain as 0 out of 10, and disability had improved to 1 out of 10 on the Patient-Specific Functional Scale.

REFERENCES

1. Medina McKeon JM, Yancosek KE: Neural gliding techniques for the treatment of carpal tunnel syndrome: a systematic review, *J Sport Rehabil* 17(3):324–341, 2008.
2. Schäfer A, Hall TM, Rolke R, et al: Low back related leg pain – do sensory profiles differ between subgroups? *Manual Theraphy* (submitted for publication).
3. Leijon O, Wahlstrom J, Mulder M: Prevalence of self-reported neck-shoulder-arm pain and concurrent low back pain or psychological distress: time-trends in a general population, 1990–2006, *Spine* 34(17):1863–1868, 2009.
4. Picavet HS, Schouten JS: Musculoskeletal pain in the Netherlands: prevalences, consequences and risk groups, the DMC(3)-study, *Pain* 102(1–2):167–178, 2003.
5. Buckle P, Devereux J: for the European Agency for Safety and Health at Work: *Work related neck and upper limb musculoskeletal disorders*, Luxembourg, 1999, Office for Official Publications of the European Communities.
6. Fejer R, Kyvik KO, Hartvigsen J: The prevalence of neck pain in the world population: a systematic critical review of the literature, *Eur Spine J* 15(6):834–848, 2006.
7. Hogg-Johnson S, van der Velde G, Carroll LJ, et al: The burden and determinants of neck pain in the general population: results of the Bone and Joint Decade 2000–2010 Task Force on Neck Pain and Its Associated Disorders, *Spine* 33(4 Suppl): S39–S51, 2008.
8. Luime JJ, Koes BW, Hendriksen IJ, et al: Prevalence and incidence of shoulder pain in the general population: a systematic review, *Scand J Rheumatol* 33(2):73–81, 2004.
9. Walker-Bone K, Palmer KT, Reading I, et al: Prevalence and impact of musculoskeletal disorders of the upper limb in the general population, *Arthritis Rheum* 51(4):642–651, 2004.
10. Jinkins J: The anatomic and physiologic basis of local, referred and radiating lumbosacral pain syndromes related to disease of the spine, *J Neuroradiol* 31:163–180, 2004.
11. Grieve GP: Referred pain and other clinical features. In Boyling JD, Palastanga N, editors: *Grieves modern manual therapy*, ed 2, Edinburgh, 1994, Churchill Livingstone.
12. Bonica JJ, Procacci P: General considerations of acute pain. In Bonica JJ, editor: *The management of pain*, ed 2, Philadelphia, 1990, Lea & Febiger.
13. Inman VT, Saunders JB: Referred pain from skeletal structures, *J Nerv Ment Dis* 99:660–667, 1944.
14. Foerster O: The dermatomes in man, *Brain* 56:1–39, 1933.
15. April C, Axinn M, Bogduk N: Occipital headaches stemming from the lateral atlanto-axial (C1-2) joint, *Cephalalgia* 22:15–22, 2002.
16. Cooper G, Bailey B, Bogduk N: Cervical zygapophysial joint pain maps, *Pain Med* 8(4):344–353, 2007.
17. Dwyer A, Aprill C, Bogduk N: Cervical zygapophyseal joint pain patterns. Part I. A study of normal volunteers, *Spine* 15(6):453–457, 1990.
18. Dwyer A, Aprill C, Bogduk N: Cervical zygapophyseal joint pain patterns. Part II. A clinical evaluation, *Spine* 15(6):458–461, 1990.
19. Fukui S, Ohseto K, Shiotani M, et al: Referred pain distribution of the cervical zygapophyseal joints and cervical dorsal rami, *Pain* 68(1):79–83, 1996.
20. Grubb SA, Kelly CK: Cervical discography: clinical implications from 12 years of experience, *Spine* 25(11):1382–1389, 2000.
21. Schmidt-Hansen PT, Svensson P, Jensen TS, et al: Patterns of experimentally induced pain in pericranial muscles, *Cephalalgia* 26(5):568–577, 2006.
22. Windsor RE, Nagula D, Storm S, et al: Electrical stimulation induced cervical medial branch referral patterns, *Pain Physician* 6(4):411–418, 2003.

23. Koelbaek Johansen M, Graven-Nielsen T, Schou Olesen A, et al: Generalised muscular hyperalgesia in chronic whiplash syndrome, *Pain* 83(2):229–234, 1999.
24. Zusman M: Forebrain-mediated sensitization of central pain pathways: "non-specific" pain and a new image for MT, *Man Ther* 7(2):80–88, 2002.
25. Merskey H, Bogduk N: *Classification of chronic pain: descriptions of chronic pain syndromes and definitions of pain terms*, ed 2, Seattle, 1994, International Association for the Study of Pain.
26. Bogduk N, McGuirk B: Causes and sources of chronic low back pain. In *Medical management of acute and chronic low back pain: an evidence based approach*, Amsterdam, 2002, Elsevier, pp 115–125.
27. Bogduk N: *Clinical anatomy of the lumbar spine*, ed 4, Melbourne, Australia, 2004, Churchill Livingstone.
28. Freynhagen R, Rolke R, Baron R, et al: Pseudoradicular and radicular low-back pain: a disease continuum rather than different entities? Answers from quantitative sensory testing, *Pain* 135:65–74, 2008.
29. Backonja MM: Defining neuropathic pain, *Anesth Analg* 97(3):785–790, 2003.
30. Bennett GJ: Can we distinguish between inflammatory and neuropathic pain? *Pain Res Manage* 11(Suppl A):11A–15A, 2006.
31. Markman J, Dukes E, Siffert J, et al: Patient flow in neuropathic pain management: understanding existing patterns of care, *Eur J Neurol* 11:135–136, 2004.
32. Hans G, Masquelier E, De Cock P: The diagnosis and management of neuropathic pain in daily practice in Belgium: an observational study, *BMC Public Health* 7:170, 2007.
33. Zusman M: Mechanisms of peripheral neuropathic pain: implications for musculoskeletal physiotherapy, *Phys Ther Rev* 13(5):313–323, 2008.
34. Marchettini P, Lacerenza M, Mauri E, et al: Painful peripheral neuropathies, *Curr Neuropharmacol* 4(3):175–181, 2006.
35. Bove GM, Ransil BJ, Lin HC, et al: Inflammation induces ectopic mechanical sensitivity in axons of nociceptors innervating deep tissues, *J Neurophysiol* 90(3):1949–1955, 2003.
36. Dilley A, Lynn B, Pang SJ: Pressure and stretch mechanosensitivity of peripheral nerve fibres following local inflammation of the nerve trunk, *Pain* 117(3):462–472, 2005.
37. Greening J, Dilley A, Lynn B: In vivo study of nerve movement and mechanosensitivity of the median nerve in whiplash and non-specific arm pain patients, *Pain* 115(3): 248, 2005.
38. Rho RH, Brewer RP, Lamer TJ, et al: Complex regional pain syndrome, *Mayo Clin Proc* 77(2):174–180, 2002.
39. Bove G, Light A: Unmyelinated nociceptors of rat paraspinal tissues, *J Neurophysiol* 73:1752–1762, 1995.
40. Bove G, Light A: The nervi nervorum: missing link for neuropathic pain? *Pain Forum* 6(3):181–190, 1997.
41. Zochodne D: Epineural peptides: a role in neuropathic pain, *Can J Neurol Sci* 20:69–72, 1993.
42. Hall T, Quintner J: Responses to mechanical stimulation of the upper limb in painful cervical radiculopathy, *Aust J Physiother* 42(4):277–285, 1996.
43. Eliav E, Herzberg U, Ruda MA, et al: Neuropathic pain from an experimental neuritis of the rat sciatic nerve, *Pain* 83 (2):169–182, 1999.
44. Dilley A, Bove GM: Resolution of inflammation-induced axonal mechanical sensitivity and conduction slowing in C-fiber nociceptors, *J Pain* 9(2):185–192, 2008.
45. Dilley A, Bove GM: Disruption of axoplasmic transport induces mechanical sensitivity in intact rat C-fibre nociceptor axons, *J Physiol* 586(2):593–604, 2008.
46. Bove GM, Weissner W, Barbe MF: Long lasting recruitment of immune cells and altered epi-perineurial thickness in focal nerve inflammation induced by complete Freund's adjuvant, *J Neuroimmunol* 213(1–2):26–30, 2009.
47. Campbell JN, Meyer RA: Mechanisms of neuropathic pain, *Neuron* 52(1):77–92, 2006.
48. Costigan M, Woolf CJ: Pain: molecular mechanisms, *J Pain* 1(3 Suppl):35–44, 2000.
49. Nee R, Butler DS: Management of peripheral neuropathic pain: integrating neurobiology, neurodynamics, and clinical evidence, *Phys Ther Sport* 7:36–49, 2006.
50. Treede RD, Jensen TS, Campbell JN, et al: Neuropathic pain: redefinition and a grading system for clinical and research purposes, *Neurology* 70(18):1630–1635, 2008.
51. Woolf CJ: Dissecting out mechanisms responsible for peripheral neuropathic pain: implications for diagnosis and therapy, *Life Sci* 74(21):2605–2610, 2004.
52. Decosterd I, Allchorne A, Woolf CJ: Progressive tactile hypersensitivity after a peripheral nerve crush: non-noxious mechanical stimulus-induced neuropathic pain, *Pain* 100(1–2):155–162, 2002.
53. Attal N, Fermanian C, Fermanian J, et al: Neuropathic pain: are there distinct subtypes depending on the aetiology or anatomical lesion? *Pain* 138(2):343–353, 2008.
54. Baron R: Neuropathic pain: a clinical perspective, *Handb Exp Pharmacol* 194:3–30, 2009.
55. Baron R, Tolle TR, Gockel U, et al: A cross-sectional cohort survey in 2100 patients with painful diabetic neuropathy and postherpetic neuralgia: differences in demographic data and sensory symptoms, *Pain* 146(1–2):34–40, 2009.
56. Bouhassira D, Lanteri-Minet M, Attal N, et al: Prevalence of chronic pain with neuropathic characteristics in the general population, *Pain* 136(3):380–387, 2008.
57. Finnerup NB, Otto M, Jensen TS, et al: An evidence-based algorithm for the treatment of neuropathic pain, *Med Gen Med* 9(2):36, 2007.
58. Galer BS, Jensen MP: Development and preliminary validation of a pain measure specific to neuropathic pain: the Neuropathic Pain Scale, *Neurology* 48(2):332–338, 1997.
59. Bouhassira D, Attal N, Alchaar H, et al: Comparison of pain syndromes associated with nervous or somatic lesions and development of a new neuropathic pain diagnostic questionnaire (DN4), *Pain* 114(1–2):29–36, 2005.
60. Bennett M: The LANSS Pain Scale: the Leeds assessment of neuropathic symptoms and signs, *Pain* 92(1–2):147–157, 2001.
61. Freynhagen R, Baron R, Gockel U, et al: painDETECT: a new screening questionnaire to identify neuropathic components in patients with back pain, *Curr Med Res Opin* 22 (10):1911–1920, 2006.
62. Portenoy R: Development and testing of a neuropathic pain screening questionnaire: ID Pain, *Curr Med Res Opin* 22 (8):1555–1565, 2006.
63. Hall T, Elvey RL: Evaluation and treatment of neural tissue pain disorders. In Donatelli R, Wooden M editors: *Orthopaedic physical therapy*, ed 4, St. Louis, 2009, Churchill Livingstone Elsevier.
64. Schäfer A., Hall T.M., Muller G., Briffa K: Outcomes differ between subgroups of patients with low back abd leg pain

following neural manual therapy – a prospective cohort study, *Eur Spine J* (submitted for publication).

65. Jull G, Sterling M, Kenardy J, et al: Does the presence of sensory hypersensitivity influence outcomes of physical rehabilitation for chronic whiplash? A preliminary RCT, *Pain* 129 (1–2):28–34, 2007.
66. Kjaer P, Leboeuf-Yde C, Korsholm L, et al: Magnetic resonance imaging and low back pain in adults: a diagnostic imaging study of 40-year-old men and women, *Spine* 30(10): 1173–1180, 2005.
67. Macnab I: The mechanism of spondylogenic pain. In Hirsch C, Zotterman Y editors: *Cervical pain*, New York, 1972, Pergamon Press.
68. Olmarker K, Rydevik B, Holm S, et al: The effects of experimental graded compression on blood flow in spinal nerve roots: a vital microscopic study on porcine cauda equina, *J Orthop Res* 7:817–823, 1989.
69. Wiesel SW, Tsourmas N, Feffer HL, et al: A study of computer-assisted tomography. Part 1. The incidence of positive CAT scans in an asymptomatic group of patients, *Spine* 9:549–551, 1984.
70. Amundsen T, Weber H, Lilleas F, et al: Lumbar spinal stenosis: clinical and radiologic features, *Spine* 20(10):1178–1186, 1995.
71. Schäfer A, Hall T, Briffa K: Classification of low back-related leg pain: a proposed pathomechanism-based approach, *Man Ther* 14(2):222–230, 2009.
72. Takasaki H, Hall T, Jull G, et al: The influence of cervical traction, compression, and Spurling test on cervical intervertebral foramen size, *Spine* 34(16):1658–1662, 2009.
73. Neal S, Fields KB: Peripheral nerve entrapment and injury in the upper extremity, *Am Fam Physician* 81(2):147–155, 2010.
74. Elliot FA: Tender muscles in sciatica: EMG studies, *Lancet* 1:47–49, 1944.
75. Balster S, Jull G: Upper trapezius muscle activity during the brachial plexus tension test in asymptomatic subjects, *Man Ther* 2(3):144–149, 1997.
76. Boyd BS, Wanek L, Gray AT, et al: Mechanosensitivity of the lower extremity nervous system during straight-leg raise neurodynamic testing in healthy individuals, *J Orthop Sports Phys Ther* 39(11):780–790, 2009.
77. Hall T, Zusman M, Elvey R: Manually detected impediments during the straight leg raise test. In *Proceedings of the ninth biennial conference of the Manipulative Physiotherapists Association of Australia, Gold Coast, Queensland, 1995*, St. Kilda, Australia, 1996, Manipulative Physiotherapists Association of Australia, pp 48–53.
78. Hu JW, Vernon H, Tatourian I: Changes in neck electromyography associated with meningeal noxious stimulation, *J Manipulative Physiol Ther* 18(9):577–581, 1995.
79. Hu JW, Yu XM, Vernon H, et al: Excitatory effects on neck and jaw muscle activity of inflammatory irritant applied to cervical paraspinal tissues, *Pain* 55(2):243–250, 1993.
80. Jaberzadeh S, Scutter S, Nazeran H: Mechanosensitivity of the median nerve and mechanically produced motor responses during upper limb neurodynamic test 1, *Physiotherapy* 91:94–100, 2005.
81. van der Heide B, Allison GT, Zusman M: Pain and muscular responses to a neural tissue provocation test in the upper limb, *Man Ther* 6(3):154–162, 2001.
82. Elvey R: Brachial plexus tension tests and the pathoanatomical origin of arm pain. In Idczak R editor: *Aspects of manipulative therapy*, Melbourne, Australia, 1979, Lincoln Institute of Health Sciences, pp 105–110.
83. Maitland GD: *Peripheral manipulation*, ed 3, London, 1991, Butterworth-Heinemann.
84. Shacklock M: *Clinical neurodynamics*, Edinburgh, 2005, Butterworth-Heinemann.
85. Elvey R: Treatment of arm pain associated with abnormal brachial plexus tension, *Aust J Physiother* 32:225–230, 1986.
86. Butler D: *The sensitive nervous system*, Unley, 2000, NOI Group Publications.
87. Butler DS: *Mobilisation of the nervous system*, Melbourne, Australia, 1991, Churchill Livingstone.
88. Shacklock M: The normal response when the SLR is added to plantarflexion/inversion and the effect of passive neck flexion as support of a neural cause of symptoms. In *Proceedings of the seventh biennial conference of the Manipulative Physiotherapists' Association of Australia, Blue Mountains*, 1991, Manipulative Physiotherapists Association of Australia, pp 258–262.
89. Di Fabio R: Neural mobilisation: the impossible, *J Orthop Sports Phys Ther* 31(5):224–225, 2001.
90. Alshami AM, Babri AS, Souvlis T, et al: Biomechanical evaluation of two clinical tests for plantar heel pain: the dorsiflexion-eversion test for tarsal tunnel syndrome and the windlass test for plantar fasciitis, *Foot Ankle Int* 28(4):499–505, 2007.
91. Coppieters MW, Alshami AM: Longitudinal excursion and strain in the median nerve during novel nerve gliding exercises for carpal tunnel syndrome, *J Orthop Res* 25(7):972–980, 2007.
92. Coppieters MW, Alshami AM, Babri AS, et al: Strain and excursion of the sciatic, tibial, and plantar nerves during a modified straight leg raising test, *J Orthop Res* 24(9): 1883–1889, 2006.
93. Coppieters MW, Alshami AM, Hodges PW: An experimental pain model to investigate the specificity of the neurodynamic test for the median nerve in the differential diagnosis of hand symptoms, *Arch Phys Med Rehabil* 87(10):1412–1417, 2006.
94. Coppieters MW, Butler DS: Do "sliders" slide and "tensioners" tension? An analysis of neurodynamic techniques and considerations regarding their application, *Man Ther* 13(3):213–221, 2008.
95. Coppieters MW, Kurz K, Mortensen TE, et al: The impact of neurodynamic testing on the perception of experimentally induced muscle pain, *Man Ther* 10(1):52–60, 2005.
96. Coppieters MW, Stappaerts KH, Everaert DG, et al: Addition of test components during neurodynamic testing: effect on range of motion and sensory responses, *J Orthop Sports Phys Ther* 31(5):226–235, 2001.
97. Dilley A, Lynn B, Greening J, et al: Quantitative in vivo studies of median nerve sliding in response to wrist, elbow, shoulder and neck movements, *Clin Biomech (Bristol, Avon)* 18(10): 899–907, 2003.
98. Dilley A, Odeyinde S, Greening J, et al: Longitudinal sliding of the median nerve in patients with non-specific arm pain, *Man Ther* 13(6):536–543, 2008.
99. Wainner RS, Fritz JM, Irrgang JJ, et al: Development of a clinical prediction rule for the diagnosis of carpal tunnel syndrome, *Arch Phys Med Rehabil* 86(4):609–618, 2005.
100. Maitland G: The slump test: examination and treatment, *Aust J Physiother* 31(6):215–219, 1985.
101. Nee RJ, Yang CH, Liang CC, et al: Impact of order of movement on nerve strain and longitudinal excursion: a biomechanical study with implications for neurodynamic test sequencing, *Man Ther* 15(4):376–381, 2010.

102. Butler DS, Coppieters MW: Neurodynamics in a broader perspective, *Man Ther* 12(1):e7–e8, 2007.
103. Schmid AB, Brunner F, Luomajoki H, et al: Reliability of clinical tests to evaluate nerve function and mechanosensitivity of the upper limb peripheral nervous system, *BMC Musculoskelet Disord* 10:11, 2009.
104. Walsh J, Hall T: Reliability, validity and diagnostic accuracy of palpation of the sciatic, tibial and common peroneal nerves in the examination of low back related leg pain, *Man Ther* 14(6):623–629, 2009.
105. Devor M: Neuropathic pain and injured nerve: peripheral mechanisms, *Br Med Bull* 47(3):619–630, 1991.
106. Bove GM, Zaheen A, Bajwa ZH: Subjective nature of lower limb radicular pain, *J Manipulative Physiol Ther* 28(1):12–14, 2005.
107. Slipman CW, Plastaras CT, Palmitier RA, et al: Symptom provocation of fluoroscopically guided cervical nerve root stimulation: are dynatomal maps identical to dermatomal maps? *Spine* 23(20):2235–2242, 1998.
108. Wolff AP, Groen GJ, Crul BJ: Diagnostic lumbosacral segmental nerve blocks with local anesthetics: a prospective double-blind study on the variability and interpretation of segmental effects, *Reg Anesth Pain Med* 26(2):147–155, 2001.
109. Viikari-Juntura E: Interexaminer reliability of observations in physical examinations of the neck, *Phys Ther* 67(10):1526–1532, 1987.
110. Viikari-Juntura E, Porras M, Laasonen EM: Validity of clinical tests in the diagnosis of root compression in cervical disc disease, *Spine* 14(3):253–257, 1989.
111. Wainner RS, Fritz JM, Irrgang JJ, et al: Reliability and diagnostic accuracy of the clinical examination and patient self-report measures for cervical radiculopathy, *Spine* 28(1):52–62, 2003.
112. Wainner RS, Gill H: Diagnosis and nonoperative management of cervical radiculopathy, *J Orthop Sports Phys Ther* 30(12):728–744, 2000.
113. Vroomen PC, de Krom MC, Knottnerus JA: Consistency of history taking and physical examination in patients with suspected lumbar nerve root involvement, *Spine* 25(1):91–96, 2000.
114. Jepsen J, Laursen L, Hagert C, et al: Diagnostic accuracy of the neurological upper limb examination 1: interrater reproducibility of selected findings and patterns, *BMC Neurol* 6(8):1–11, 2006.
115. Jepsen J, Laursen L, Larsen A, et al: Manual strength testing in 14 upper limb muscles: a study of inter-rater reliability, *Acta Orthop Scand* 75(4):442–448, 2004.
116. Rainville J, Noto DJ, Jouve C, et al: Assessment of forearm pronation strength in C6 and C7 radiculopathies, *Spine* 32 (1):72–75, 2007.
117. Litvan I, Mangone CA, Werden W, et al: Reliability of the NINDS Myotatic Reflex Scale, *Neurology* 47(4):969–972, 1996.
118. Stam J, van Crevel H: Reliability of the clinical and electromyographic examination of tendon reflexes, *J Neurol* 237(7): 427–431, 1990.
119. Schäfer A, Hall TM, Ludtke K, et al: Interrater reliability of a new classification system for patients with neural low back-related leg pain, *J Man Manip Ther* 17(2):109–117, 2009.
120. Schäfer A, Hall TM, Briffa K, et al: *QST profiles of Subgroups of patients with low back related leg pain: do they differ?* Glasgow, 2008, International Association for the Study of Pain.
121. Daly AE, Bialocerkowski AE: Does evidence support physiotherapy management of adult complex regional pain syndrome type one? A systematic review, *Eur J Pain* 13(4):339–353, 2009.
122. Butler D, Moseley G: *Explain pain*, Adelaide, Australia, 2003, Noigroup Publications.
123. Kwan MK, Wall EJ, Massie J, et al: Strain, stress and stretch of peripheral nerve: rabbit experiments in vitro and in vivo, *Acta Orthop Scand* 63(3):267–272, 1992.
124. Topp KS, Boyd BS: Structure and biomechanics of peripheral nerves: nerve responses to physical stresses and implications for physical therapist practice, *Phys Ther* 86(1):92–109, 2006.
125. Allison GT, Nagy BM, Hall T: A randomized clinical trial of manual therapy for cervico-brachial pain syndrome: a pilot study, *Man Ther* 7(2):95–102, 2002.
126. Coppieters MW, Stappaerts KH, Wouters LL, et al: The immediate effects of a cervical lateral glide treatment technique in patients with neurogenic cervicobrachial pain, *J Orthop Sports Phys Ther* 33(7):369–378, 2003.
127. Coppieters MW, Stappaerts KH, Wouters LL, et al: Aberrant protective force generation during neural provocation testing and the effect of treatment in patients with neurogenic cervicobrachial pain, *J Manipulative Physiol Ther* 26(2):99–106, 2003.
128. Cowell IM, Phillips DR: Effectiveness of manipulative physiotherapy for the treatment of a neurogenic cervicobrachial pain syndrome: a single case study—experimental design, *Man Ther* 7(1):31–38, 2002.
129. Hall T, Elvey R, Davies N, et al: Efficacy of manipulative physiotherapy for the treatment of cervicobrachial pain. In *Proceedings of the tenth biennial conference of the Manipulative Physiotherapists Association of Australia, 1997, Melbourne*, 1997, Manipulative Physiotherapists Association of Australia.
130. Saranga J, Green A, Lewis J, et al: Effects of a cervical lateral glide on the upper limb neurodynamic test 1: a blinded placebo-controlled investigation, *Physiotherapy* 89(11):678–684, 2003.
131. Sterling M, Pedler A, Chan C, et al: Cervical lateral glide increases nociceptive flexion reflex threshold but not pressure or thermal pain thresholds in chronic whiplash associated disorders: a pilot randomised controlled trial, *Man Ther* 15(2): 149–153, 2010.
132. Vicenzino B, Collins D, Wright A: The initial effects of a cervical spine manipulative physiotherapy treatment on the pain and dysfunction of lateral epicondylalgia, *Pain* 68(1):69–74, 1996.
133. Westaway MD, Stratford PW, Binkley JM: The Patient-Specific Functional Scale: validation of its use in persons with neck dysfunction, *J Orthop Sports Phys Ther* 27(5):331–338, 1998.

CHAPTER

7

Kenji C. Carp

Sensory Integration and Neuromuscular Control of the Shoulder

Most rehabilitation professionals agree neuromuscular control (NMC) is how the nervous system produces coordinated movement appropriate to situational demands. Although many operational definitions exist, Williams et al[1] defined it thus in 2001:

> "NMC... involves the subconscious integration of sensory information that is processed by the central nervous system (CNS), resulting in controlled movement through coordinated muscle activity."

Computer modeling often serves as a useful analogy for the workings of the human nervous system. Therefore, a simple analogy using the terms "hardware" and "software" can assist in an overview of NMC. For example, a mouse and keyboard are types of hardware that mechanically input signals to the computer's central processor unit or CPU. The CPU processes the multiple streams of data into meaningful information about the desire of the user. For example, the CPU interprets the double clicking the mouse while the cursor is over a software icon as the user's desire to open the application. The CPU then recruits software (a series of stored code or commands) to drive the hardware into action. The hard drive spins, and the program opens.

The computer-based analogy for NMC of the shoulder works like this: peripheral sensory receptors or hardware such as the somatosensory mechanoreceptors, vestibular apparatus, and eyes transduce sensory input from the environment. Like the mouse, they translate sensory input into neural impulses that are carried to the central nervous system (CNS) by afferent peripheral nerves. Like a CPU, the CNS processes the vast amounts of data streaming to it. The term *sensory integration* refers to the accurate processing and weighting of the sensory data into meaningful information to form a perception of the environment.[2-11] Depending on situational demands, the CNS derives or selects specific programs or more generic software for the motor solution to the problem. The motor program software then recruits the specific motor units or hardware to execute a coordinated motor response.

FEEDBACK VERSUS FEEDFORWARD NEUROMUSCULAR CONTROL

Although feedback NMC and feedforward NMC are different mechanisms, they work concurrently and synergistically to produce coordinated shoulder movement.[1,2,4,6,9] For example, a painter producing a detailed brush stroke has very particular goals and thus requires specific patterning and grading of force. This task requires continuous real-time updating by the senses or what is referred to as a *feedback mechanism* of NMC. However, painting involves many sensory inputs, such as the image created, the texture of the canvas, and somatosensory input from the shoulder. Similarly, the movements of painting involve the combined interactions of all the joints of the shoulder girdle, elbow, wrist, and fingers, as well as the trunk if the painter is standing. The multiple sensory inputs, degrees of freedom, and grading of force all add up to a large number of data to be analyzed. This situation dictates extensive peripheral nervous system and CNS interneuron firing, all of which eats up time. Not surprisingly, the fastest possible speed at which feedback NMC can produce a specific volitional movement is approximately 120 milliseconds.[2] The painting example used here could require much more time.

The same meticulous painter would need a faster and more generalized shoulder response if he or she were to bobble the brush and attempt to catch it before it hit the floor. Feedforward NMC can produce relatively much faster movement by relying on selection of more generalized motor programs that predict the desired outcome. Feedforward NMC relies on afferent sensory input from multiple sources; however, because the neural impulses necessary for this lower-level processing cross fewer synapses, the movement is much faster.[1,2,4-7,9,11,12] The *monosynaptic stretch reflex* is the most direct form of feedforward NMC. As the name implies, this reflex crosses just one synapse and thus can occur in 30 milliseconds.[2,12] Long loop reflexes to the brainstem travel a little farther up the CNS and thus require 50 to 80 milliseconds.[2,11,12] Therefore, in this example, stimulation of the tactile receptors in the hand or peripheral visual stimulation results in afferent signals to brainstem that produce reflexive firing of the shoulder muscles and fast shoulder movement to bring the hand where the brush should fall.

Of great interest to shoulder rehabilitation specialists is the triggered response, or a blending of feedback and feedforward NMC. Research into eye-hand coordination has shown that, through practice, the CNS can sensitize the response to visual and somatosensory sensory cues and can allow more rapid selection of the correct motor program, sometimes within 80 to 120 milliseconds.[1,2,6,7,10,11,13] Sports performance research provides interesting insights that can also be used in rehabilitation. To be clear, training does not appear to rewire the interneuron connections of short or long loop reflexes because this would require a supernatural degree of neural plasticity. Rather, neuromuscular training (NMT) appears to result in more efficient processing of sensory input, as well as in faster selection of the correct motor program, with consequent relatively fast but appropriate movement.[3,4,6-9]

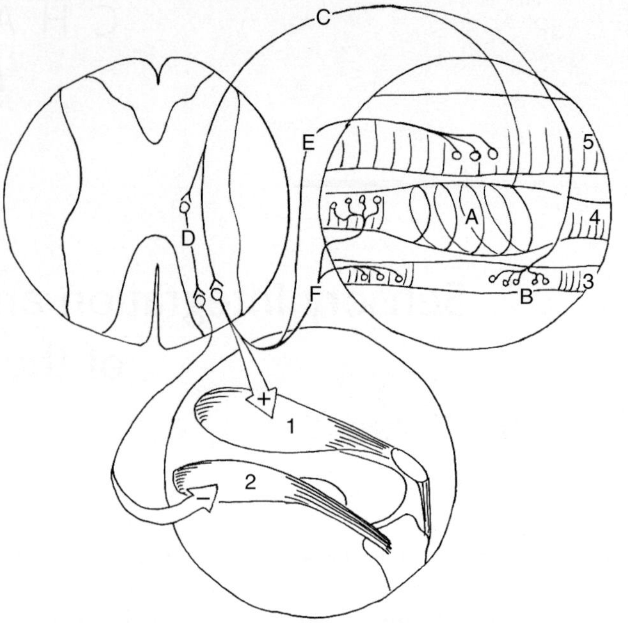

Figure 7-1 Muscle spindle diagram: A, annulospiral ending; B, flower spray ending; C, primary afferent fiber; D, inhibitory interneuron; E, alpha motor neuron; F, gamma motor neuron; 1, antagonist; 2, agonist; 3, nuclear chain fiber; 4, nuclear bag fiber; 5, extrafusal muscle fiber.

SENSORY INTEGRATION AND NEUROMUSCULAR CONTROL OF THE SHOULDER

Unfortunately but also commonly, orthopedic practitioners incorrectly refer to proprioception or "joint position sense" synonymously with NMC. However, as outlined earlier, NMC is actually the result of not only proprioception but also other sensory perceptions,[2-13] not to mention the motor end of the equation. Perhaps this misunderstanding is a product of the many and varied definitions of NMC. Ironically, the wealth of high-quality research describing the large role proprioception plays in NMC may have contributed to this misconception. Nevertheless, research clearly demonstrates that NMC of the shoulder is the product of sensory integration of somatosensory, visual, and even vestibular senses.[2-13] This section describes the neuroanatomy of somatosensory, visual, and vestibular sensation and research into their impact on NMC of the shoulder.

Somatosensory Sensation

The sensations of touch, pressure, vibration, and tension are all provided by specialized mechanoreceptors that lace the connective tissues. However, the muscle spindles and Golgi tendon organs contribute the most directly to the NMC of joint stability.[2-17]

Muscle Spindles

Muscle spindles, also known as intrafusal fibers, are embedded within the extrafusal fibers of the skeletal muscle (Fig. 7-1). In the center of the spindle lie clusters of nuclear bag fibers that mechanically deform in response to quick stretching of the spindle. Anulospiral sensory endings entwine the nuclear bag fibers, and when these fibers are stimulated by the quick stretching, the result is depolarization of the primary afferent fiber of the spindle.[2,3,5,6,12,14] The disklike nuclear chain fibers are arranged in series with the length of the spindle. The secondary afferent fibers innervate the proximal and distal aspects of the nuclear chain fibers by flower spray endings. Chain fibers are more responsive to slower prolonged stretch of the fiber. Each spindle afferent conducts its impulses upward through the mixed peripheral nerve, dorsal spinal nerve root, and then the spinal cord.[2,12]

While at the dorsal root ganglion, the ascending signal from the spindle sends an offshoot to excite the gamma motor neuron, and the result is concurrent contraction of the intrafusal fibers. This graceful design allows the intrafusal fiber to remain proportional to the extrafusal fiber so it can transduce stretch stimuli despite ongoing muscle activity. Once in the spinal cord, the ascending spindle signal triggers the monosynaptic reflex and results in recruitment of the agonist. In addition, however, the afferent signal stimulates an inhibitor interneuron that connects to the antagonist rotator cuff muscles, and the result is referred to as *reciprocal inhibition*.[2,12] For example, stretching of the posterior rotator cuff muscles causes reciprocal inhibition of the subscapularis muscle. The proportion of muscle spindles in smaller muscles such as the rotator cuff is much higher than larger prime movers such as the deltoid. This property suggests that these smaller muscles may serve a dual role as somatosensory receptors, by providing input used to modulate forces in the larger deltoid, pectoralis, and latissimus muscles, in addition to their mechanical role as restraints of the humeral head.[1-7]

Golgi Tendon Organs

The function of the Golgi tendon organs has long been thought to be the detection of dangerous levels of tension in the musculotendinous unit. The I beta afferent fibers perforate

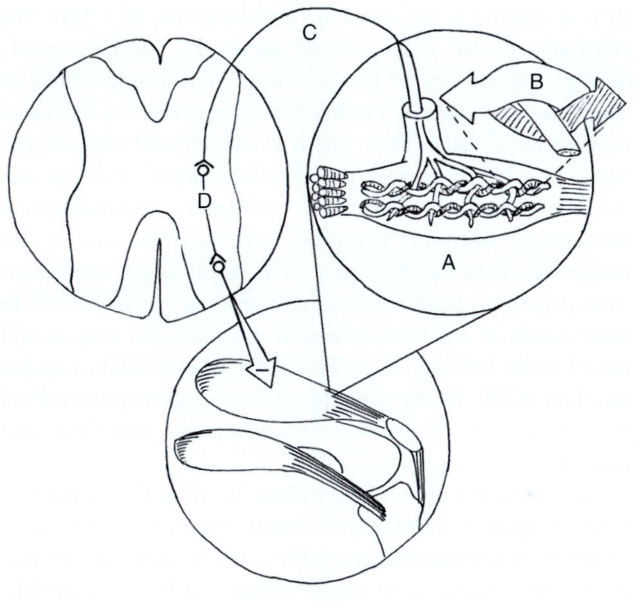

Figure 7-2 Golgi tendon organs. **A,** Sensory fibers interwoven with collagen fibers in a tendon. **B,** Tension deforms collagen and stimulates the sensory fibers. **C,** Afferent signal ascends to the spinal cord. **D,** Inhibitory interneuron reduces agonist recruitment, which reduces tendon tension.

capsules of fibrous collagen webs in the tendon and extend finger-like free afferent endings through the collagen fibers (Fig. 7-2). Tendon tension takes up creep in the collagen fibers, and this process pinches the free endings like a child's finger trap toy. The signal propagates up the I beta afferent to the CNS. Any perception of tension above the set point or perceived point of tendon failure results in stimulation of an inhibitory interneuron to the agonist alpha motor neuron as well as an excitatory interneuron to the antagonist alpha motor neuron. This process is referred to as the *inverse myotatic reflex* or *reflex inhibition,* and the net result is decreased tension on the tendon.[2,3,6,7,12]

Shoulder specialists often observe the effects of the inverse myotatic reflex with muscle tremors and even failure with eccentric training of deconditioned scapular thoracic or rotator cuff muscles. These tremors typically dissipate in a relatively short time, far before true muscular hypertrophy occurs. The reason is partly the neuromuscular adaptations to training; in other words, part of strength training is repeated exposure to tension on the tendons that results in habituation of the CNS. Consequently, the CNS no longer perceives the same tension as a threat and thus raises the threshold to trigger the inverse myotatic reflex. Advanced NMT activities such as shoulder plyometrics hold great potential for gains through CNS learning.

Unfortunately, many factors can adversely affect somatosensation about the shoulder. Studies show an age-related decrease in somatosensation in all joints that is attributed to atrophy of the mechanoreceptors.[5,7] Similarly, a wealth of research correlates abnormal somatosensation with common shoulder diagnoses such as acute dislocation, recurrent instability, impingement, and osteoarthritis.[12,14-18] For example, Myers et al[14] and other researchers documented abnormal kinesthesia in patients diagnosed with glenohumeral instability. This finding was initially hypothesized to be largely caused by the direct disruption of the somatosensory receptors with injury to the connective tissue of the shoulder capsule. More recent studies, however, suggested laxity of the capsule, rather than lyses of somatosensory receptors, as the cause. Although the studies of these disorders have not determined whether the pathologic process precedes the abnormal somatosensation, they do clearly correlate abnormal somatosensation with common orthopedic shoulder conditions. For example, numerous investigators linked scapular dyskinesis with abnormal somatosensation in the scapular girdle.[14-19] Studies by McClure et al[16] demonstrated abnormal scapular kinematics in subjects with impingement as compared with subjects without impingement. In addition, a plethora of studies attributed the abnormal NMC observed with most shoulder conditions to the confounding impact of pain or nociception on somatosensation. Hess et al[21] demonstrated delays in the firing of the subscapularis muscle during rapid shoulder external rotation in overhead throwers with increased nociception as compared with age-matched and activity level–matched subjects who were not in pain.

Vision

It almost goes without saying that vision is our preferred stream of sensory input for most upper extremity motor tasks. Patients understand what clinicians mean by the term hand-eye coordination. Similarly, research has demonstrated that visual sensation effects shoulder position, scapular postures, work-related ergonomics, throwing mechanics, and compensation for proprioceptive loss. Thus, a deeper understanding of visual perception allows the shoulder specialist to address the client's needs more effectively.

When patients use their shoulders, they are typically surrounded by light reflecting from objects in the environment. These waves of energy carry a high degree of bandwidth or data about the environment. To perceive visually, however, light must be captured by the eyes. The retina holds the rod and cones, which actually transduce photons of light into neural impulses. A healthy human retina has approximately 6 to 7 million cones, which are densely concentrated in the approximately 0.3-mm diameter fovea centralis or centermost aspect of the retina. Cones provide color vision and are responsible for high-acuity (detailed) vision. In contrast, a healthy retina has approximately 120 million rods, which are well adapted to provide night vision and peripheral vision and to detect motion. Rod density varies because rods are absent in the fovea, are most strongly concentrated in ring around the fovea, and then gradually dissipate toward the periphery of the retina.[21-28]

Retinal structure helps to explain visual perception in relation to shoulder movement. Arm movements that require visual perception of extrinsic motion in the peripheral visual field rely on the rods. For example, a mixed martial artist who attempts to block a blow to the side of the head does not need to know the color, fine texture, or exact location of the approaching hand. Instead, the martial artist needs to detect the hand quickly enough to drive feedforward NMC of the shoulder and to arrive at a generalized location to block the strike. The visual demands of an orthopedic surgeon differ greatly. Orthopedists use their shoulders routinely to preposition the hand for extremely fine motor tasks, as well as gross motor tasks such as moving the leg of a large patient. Orthopedists rely on foveal (also known as focal) vision because it provides the color perception to find stitches commonly placed as landmarks in tissues to be repaired, the acuity to judge objects that are millimeters in length, and the depth perception for tasks such as excising devitalized tissue.

One achieves foveal vision only if the light hits the extremely narrow fovea, however. Thus, complex NMC of the extraocular muscles is required for foveal visual perception (cones).[26,27] A useful analogy is that a photographer must first point and focus the camera to obtain a detailed color picture. Ocular NMC involves the interaction of smooth pursuits and saccades.[21,28] Smooth pursuits are quick to initiate tracking of a relatively slow moving target.[28] Saccades are used to catch the foveal vision up to faster moving targets or to move between targets. Although saccades are slower to initiate, they move the eye at much higher speeds than do smooth pursuits. Targets that outpace smooth pursuits result in "retinal slip" or drifting of the image to the periphery of the retina. This drift, in turn, stimulates peripheral vision (rods) and results in saccadic movements to reorient or "catch up" the foveal vision on target.[28]

Research demonstrates that smooth pursuits and saccades share common but modular CNS neuronal pathways. Visual neural impulses propagate through the optic nerves to the temporal, posterior parietal, and frontal cortices. From there, vast networks of interneurons connect the cortices to the pons, and cerebellum particularly the oculomotor vermis of the cerebellum, which communicates with the smooth pursuit and saccadic centers of the brainstem. These centers execute the motor programs through the oculomotor and abducens nuclei to time and grade extraocular muscle activity appropriate for the visual tracking task at hand.[28]

Humans enjoy binocular vision, meaning that they have two eyes slightly offset in the orbits in the front of the head. This position provides the CNS slightly different perspectives of the target that the CNS uses to calculate the distance to the target, or *depth perception*.[27] The ability to point each eye at the same target is referred to as *vergence,* which is also known as *teaming*. Again, foveal stimulation from the target image drives the oculomotor NMC to converge (point inward) or diverge (swivel outward), thus bringing both eyes to a position where the each eye captures a centered foveal image. CNS processing in the visual cortex allows for fusion of these slightly different perspectives into one image and the internal representation of the targets in a three-dimensional position in space.[27,28]

As mentioned earlier, the eyes sit in the orbits of the bony skull. So how do we maintain the aforementioned ocular NMC when the head moves with routine shoulder activities, such as driving a car, at oscillations in excess of 5 Hz? The vestibular ocular reflex (VOR) serves as "nature's steady cam" to stabilize visual gaze and thus minimize the effect of head motion on vision. The vestibular apparatus are described in more detail later. Their role is to detect head rotation and tilt. The CNS integrates the vestibular input and executes corrective eye movements by reflexive communication between the vestibular brainstem nuclei and the same oculomotor and abducens brainstem. The result is eye movement contralateral to head movement in the same plane.[4,27-30] In other words, if the head rotates to the right, the eyes should swivel to the left (Fig. 7-3). This knowledge is vital in understanding NMC of the shoulder during tasks requiring head movement such as driving, playing sports, shopping, and cooking.

A conundrum often plagues those learning the interaction between ocular NMC and visual perception. In most instances, when patients reach for a target, they do not perceive a microscopic focal target surrounded by vague peripheral objects. Put another way, if foveal vision is necessary for many volitional movements of the shoulder and complex ocular NMC is necessary to achieve this goal, then why do humans have such a rich visual perception of the environment? The answer is that, under normal circumstances, the CNS subconsciously, continually, and rapidly uses the ocular NMC mechanisms detailed earlier to update visual memory. These foveal images are stored in the internal representation of the environment until a given location is updated.[7,23,27-29] It helps to imagine the photographer described earlier placing pictures in a continually updating photo mosaic. In fact, the retina actually contains an anatomic blind spot in the fovea where the collection of fibers from the rods and cones exits to form the optic nerve. Humans do not perceive this blind spot, however, because of the continual updating of visual memory. The next section describes the way in which visual memory is vital in the NMC of the shoulder during reaching tasks.

Relevance of Visual Impairment to Physical Therapy of the Shoulder

Many patients with shoulder conditions have concurrent medical conditions, either diagnosed or undiagnosed, that affect their visual perception. For example, *strabismus* (commonly referred to as *crosseye)* is a condition in which one of the eyes deviates or turns off target, with a resulting lack of coordination of vergence. Studies suggest that the prevalence of strabismus is dramatically underreported or underdiagnosed. Studies also suggest that even subtle subclinical vergence abnormalities affect depth perception. Ptosis or drooping eyelid, often caused by paresis of the levator palpebrae muscle following viral neuronitis, causes monocular vision by direct occlusion of one eye.[23,24,27] *Amblyopia* (often called a *lazy eye*) is the inability to perceive visual sensation from the eye despite normal eye anatomy. Investigators believe that amblyopia can occur during early development following conditions such as strabismus or ptosis that eventually cause the CNS to

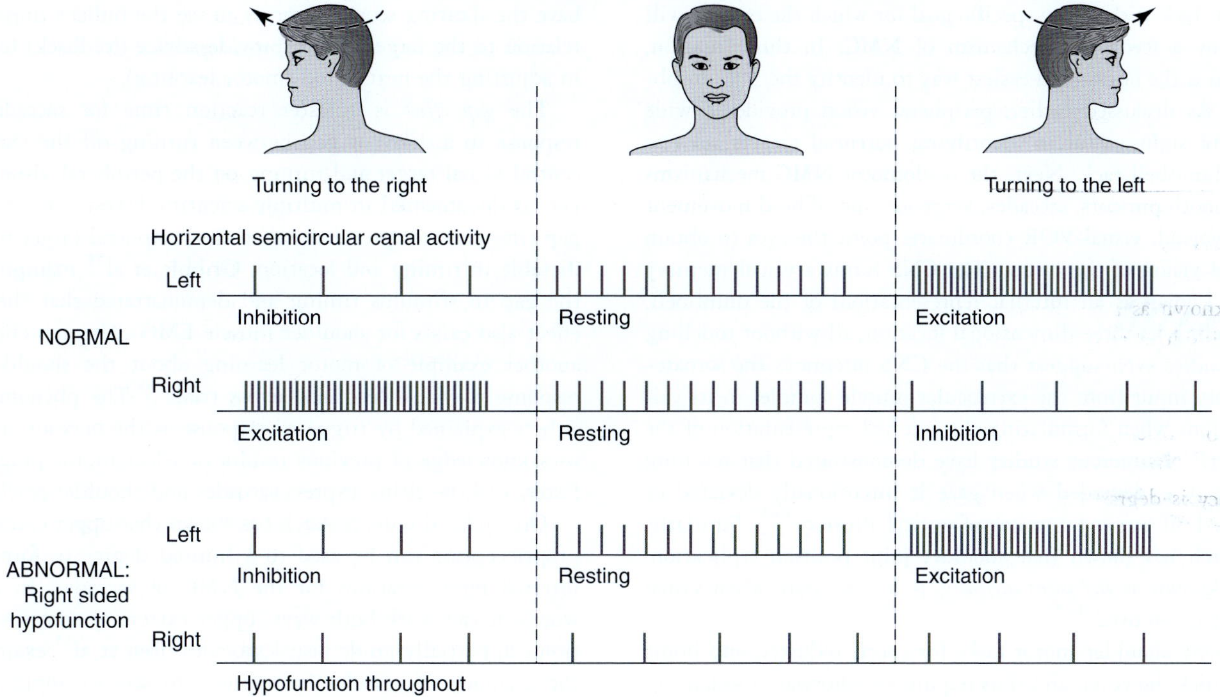

Figure 7-3 Responses of the horizontal semicircular canals to head turning to the right and left, with normal functioning *(top)* and with right-sided hypofunction *(bottom)*. (From Cameron MH, Monroe LG: *Physical rehabilitation: evidence-based examination, evaluation, and intervention,* St. Louis, 2008, Saunders Elsevier.)

perceive the world with monocular vision.[23,24] All these visual impairments adversely affect visual depth perception and thus shoulder reaching tasks.

Similarly, traumatic brain injury (TBI) is a condition linked to marked visual perceptual deficits. The modern profession of physical therapy began largely to meet the rehabilitation needs of soldiers injured in World War I. Sadly, at the time of this writing, military forces are again sustaining an alarming number of TBIs. The reason is the widespread use of improvised explosive devices, which can be inexpensively made and readily deployed. Available estimates of US military casualties place the incidence of TBI as high as 20% of all casualties sustained in the war in Iraq.[21-26] This incidence translates to high numbers of veterans who need treatment of often extensive upper extremity injuries that are compounded by marked visual impairment.

Mild TBI (MTBI), still commonly referred to as *concussion,* has come under increasing scrutiny as a medical problem in the national media because of the potential for catastrophic injury at all levels of sport. Research has shown that the incidence of MTBI remains dramatically underreported and that medial management of MTBI varies widely across regions.[31-42] Studies of MTBI showed that premotor regions of the brain involved in upper extremity tasks may be more susceptible than other brain regions to impairment with MTBI.[41,42] In addition, many patients with MTBI also have abnormal vestibular and visual sensation. As mentioned earlier, shoulder rehabilitation specialists often treat athletes and thus are often the first health care professionals to encounter individuals with MTBI. Therefore, the ability to assess and treat NMC of the upper extremity accurately will enhance the ability of these specialists to identify MTBI, to provide appropriate sensory cues specific to patients who are recovering from MTBI, and, when necessary, to advocate for patient access to appropriate care of MTBI.

Cerebrovascular accident or stroke is another concurrent diagnosis just about every shoulder specialist encounters. Roughly 780,000 people suffer new or recurrent strokes each year, and these strokes often result in marked hemiparesis or neurogenic weakness of one side.[43] This hemiparesis or weakness and other impairments make cerebrovascular accident the leading cause of long-term disability in the United States. Although many of these patients show favorable outcomes following rehabilitation, it is often by compensating for loss of the use of the hemiparetic upper extremity, as opposed to true recovery of limb function. Neuropsychological testing (which relies heavily on upper extremity motor response to sensory and cognitive processing) and sensorimotor measures were the best predictors of return of upper extremity function in a comprehensive review of literature.[43,44] Shoulder therapists can be assured they will encounter patients with painful and poorly functioning hemiparetic shoulders.

Visual Sensory Integration and Neuromuscular Control of Reaching

For example, a patient was recently cleared for strength training following partial-thickness rotator cuff repair. The cautious therapist asks the patient to grab the 3-lb dumbbell from the rack. The therapist has just assigned the patient a motor task with a very specific goal for which the patient will employ a feedback mechanism of NMC. In this situation, vision is the fastest and easiest way to identify the 3-lb dumbbell. As discussed earlier, peripheral vision provides a wide area of sight useful in identifying potential targets such as the dumbbell rack. Next, the oculomotor NMC mechanisms of smooth pursuits, saccades, vergence, and, if head movement is involved, visual-VOR coordinates point the eyes to obtain foveal vision of the target. The CNS forms a visual memory (also known as an internal representation) of the dumbbell, including its three-dimensional location, all without touching it. Studies even suggest that the CNS integrates the somatosensory input from the extraocular muscle spindles in its calculations when formulating the internal representation of the target.[45] Numerous studies have demonstrated that reaching accuracy is degraded when gaze is intentionally deviated or tricked off target by means of optical illusion.[46-50] Similarly, research has shown that shoulder joint position replication, also known as *end-point accuracy,* is less accurate when visual input is removed.[46,51]

Many shoulder motor tasks for sport, industry, and home are quick, however, and thus require a feedforward mechanism of NMC. Several researchers have examined the role of vision fast reaching by correlation of visual saccades (fast eye movements) with upper extremity movement and electromyography (EMG). In an elegant study by Gribble et al,[51] subjects began the test with their foveal vision on a central target, which was then turned off and replaced by a target in their peripheral vision. In response to the peripheral target, subjects were to point their arm as quickly as possible toward the target. The researchers positively correlated shoulder muscle EMG with the onset of saccades following the peripheral target stimulation.[50] A finding of shoulder EMG to following visual saccades would have suggested a "look then reach" motor program, as seen with feedback NMC of volitional reaching above. In fact, these investigators found that shoulder muscle activity slightly preceded the onset of saccades.[50] This finding confirms that, in the situational context of fast shoulder reaching, the nervous system can use peripheral visual input to form an internal representation of the target in space. The result is rapid activation of shoulder muscles to bring the hand to intercept. This finding is consistent with the results of other studies examining reach target preference that showed that subjects select a target and then move their gaze to the target, as opposed to looking and then reaching.[51]

These findings suggest a parallel shoulder and extraocular motor component of the feedforward NMC of fast reaching. Possible CNS centers involved in this parallel motor processing include reach neurons in the superior colliculus of the brainstem, aspects of the posterior parietal cortex, and neurons in the dorsal premotor cortex.[45-51] This parallel motor component appears necessary to provide visual feedback for learning across trials; namely, the saccades position the eyes to obtain visual feedback about the accuracy of the shoulder's reach. One could use the analogy of a sniper and spotter team working together. Once the sniper fires a round at the target, the bullet's path cannot be altered (feedforward). However, the spotter must have the spotting scope on target to see the bullet's impact in relation to the target and to provide advice (feedback) for use in adjusting the next round (motor learning).

The *gap effect* is a faster reaction time for saccades in response to a delay or gap between turning off the starting central visual target and turning on the peripheral visual target, as documented in multiple scientific investigations. The gap effect is most prevalent when the peripheral target is predictable in timing and location. Gribble et al[51] manipulated the gap in stimulus timing and demonstrated that the gap effect also exists for shoulder muscle EMG. The gap effect is another example of motor learning about the shoulder in response to visual feedback across trials.[50] The phenomenon is best explained by triggered response as the nervous system uses knowledge of previous results to select motor programs faster, with resulting express saccades and shoulder reach.

On a related note, research has shown that upper extremity proprioception can be used to a limited degree to form the internal representations for the NMC of saccades. In other words, it can work both ways: upper extremity somatosensation can partially guide visual saccades. Ren et al[31] examined the accuracy of saccades in response to sensory input from vision, visual memory, and upper extremity proprioception (by placing the visual target in the hand and moving the target in a darkened room). Their findings showed that upper extremity somatosensory input can update internal representation of saccade target locations. However, saccades based on somatosensory input were dramatically less accurate than were visual or visual memory–guided saccades.[51] Therefore, it appears that, under normal circumstances, the human nervous system heavily biases visual sensory input when controlling saccadic eye movement.

Vestibular Sensation

The vestibule of the inner chamber of the ear houses the delicate vestibular cochlear organs responsible for the transduction of sound waves and head position into sensory input.[2,4,8-11] For the purposes of this chapter, the discussion focuses only on the head position sense or purely vestibular sensation. Three semicircular canals arranged in plane with the X,Y, and Z dimensions shoot off from the inner ear. The horizontal canal is oriented with a 30° upward tilt to counteract the slight downward orientation of the head during most activities. Collectively, these canals are known as the labyrinth and are filled with a viscous endolymphatic fluid produced by the epithelial cells of the membranous portion of the labyrinth. The canals each have a larger-diameter ampulla just off the utricle that houses the hair cell receptors.[4,29,30] As the head rotates, inertia keeps the heavy endolymphatic fluid still while the hair cell deforms as it drags through the viscous fluid. The structure of the receptor cell membrane that dictates bending toward the larger kinocilium excites the vestibular nerve, whereas bending away from the kinocilium inhibits the vestibular nerve impulse.[4,29,30] See Figure 7-4 for a depiction of semicircular canal architecture. The utricle forms the central aspect of the vestibular apparatus and houses

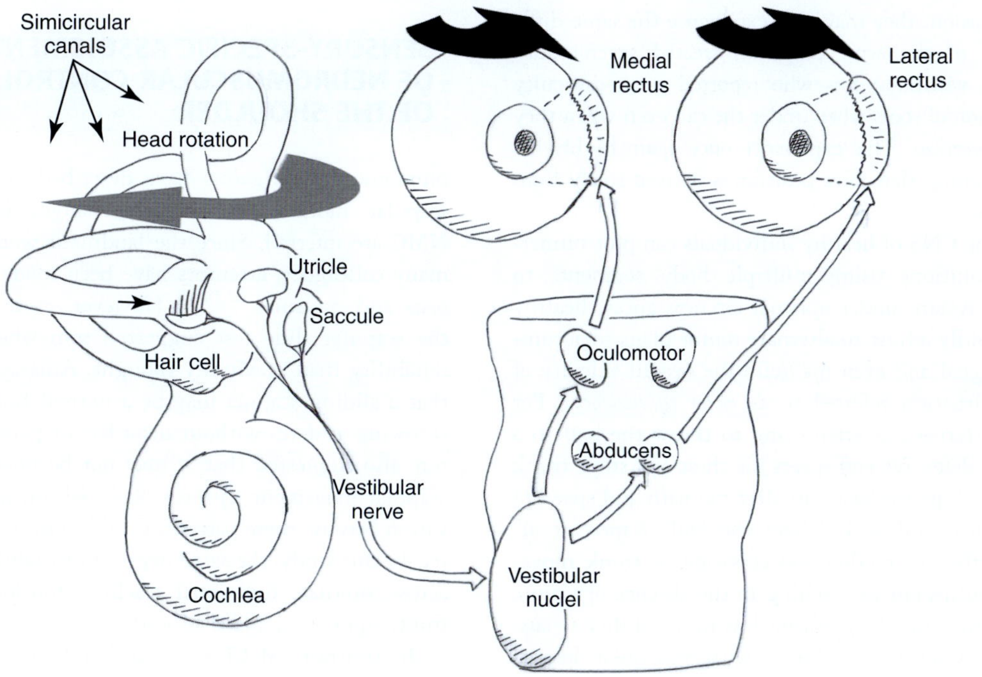

Figure 7-4 Vestibular apparatus.

the otoliths. The macula is a horizontally oriented gelatinous membrane with a similar hair cell receptor embedded in the gelatin. The saccule has the same design but is oriented vertically. The otoliths respond to linear acceleration, such as the pull of gravity when the head is tilted, or changes in speed, such as while riding in a car. The vestibular receptors are arranged in a "push-and-pull" relationship, meaning that rotation or tilt is excitatory to the vestibular nerve ipsilateral to the direction of movement while simultaneously inhibitory to the contralateral vestibular nerve.[4,29,30] The vestibular portion of cranial nerve XIII delivers the ascending signal to the vestibular nuclei, which comprise a "way station" in the brainstem. From there, a cascade of interneuronal connections links other brainstem nuclei, the cerebellum (particularly the vermis), and the cortex.[4,29,30]

Vestibular Sensory Integration and Shoulder Neuromuscular Control

Extensive research has documented the role of vestibular input in both feedback and feedforward NMC of balance and spinal stabilization. Similarly, investigators have shown that peripheral vestibular injury can degrade VOR from its normal gain (ratio of head to eye movement) of 0.75 to 0.35, resulting in the phenomenon of *oscillopsia,* often described as "jumpy" or even "double" vision by patients.[27,29,30] Thus, a patient with a shoulder disorder who has vestibular loss may experience the direct impact on upper extremity and trunk NMC described earlier, as well as an indirect effect because the decreased VOR gain results in concurrent alteration of visual sensation. Several more recent studies have further examined the links between vestibular sensory integration and NMC of the shoulder.

Borello-France et al[9] examined the effect of peripheral vestibular loss on the speed and kinematics of the shoulder girdle, head, neck, and trunk during volitional reaching tasks. These investigators found that subjects with vestibular loss demonstrated slower shoulder girdle motion than did uninjured controls. The subjects with vestibular loss also exhibited decreased head and neck movement. These observations were hypothesized to be expressions of overall motor strategy to minimize head movement and thus maintain gaze stability during the reaching tasks.[9]

Knox, Coppieters, and Hodges[10] researched the effect of galvanic vestibular stimulation to induce experimental peripheral vestibular imbalance on upper extremity position sense in the absence of vision. This clever study design allowed for examination of the impact of peripheral vestibular input on arm position sense while controlling for possible confounders from visual input and the input from cervical somatosensation that occurs during physical head movement, as seen in a previous study.[11] These investigators demonstrated that the vestibular-induced illusion of head movement significantly changed the subjects' ability to reposition the arm in space.[10] This study has numerous clinical implications, including further support of altered upper extremity NMC with vestibular loss and the need to include vestibular input in considerations of sensory integration when the arm is discussed.[10] Although therapists cannot directly project these findings to their patients with vestibular loss, it is a fairly safe assumption that patients with uncompensated vestibular loss are receiving abnormal vestibular input. If these patients are required to perform supine tasks with visual occlusion, they may well experience the same difficulty in NMC of the arm. Carp has treated several auto mechanics with vestibular loss who reported great difficulty with manipulation of tools when under the car, even when they did not report vertigo. This experience once again highlights the error in assuming that joint position is derived solely from somatosensation.

Normally, the CNS of healthy individuals can plot numerous possible solutions using multiple body segments to achieve a goal. Again, under optimal circumstances, healthy subjects can rapidly adjust to alternate motor plans to accomplish the same goal and even maintain the overall velocity of movement, a situation referred to as *motor equivalency*.[8] For example, a quarterback is attempting to throw the ball to a receiver when a defensive end spears his chest and stops trunk motion. A skilled quarterback can alter the path and speed of the throwing arm and still deliver the ball. Raptis et al[8] examined the effect of randomized cessation of trunk movement during multisegment reaching in the absence of vision. These investigators found significant loss in the ability to sustain motor equivalency in subjects with vestibular loss as compared with matched controls. This study also has clinical utility; as mentioned earlier, many athletic patients with shoulder disorders present with concurrent vestibular loss.[8] Thus, therapists should not be surprised if these patients demonstrate impaired NMC of full body motions such as throwing. Inversely, Raptis et al[8] demonstrated that even healthy subjects use vestibular input to guide multisegment arm motion when vision is unavailable.[8]

DYNAMIC JOINT STABILIZATION

Dynamic joint stabilization is the maintenance of optimal joint alignment by restraint of potentially destructive forces. Myers et al[14] provided the following excellent and specific definition of shoulder stability: "...glenohumeral stability is the state of the humeral head remaining or promptly returning to the proper alignment within the glenoid fossa through an equalization of forces."[14] The larger deltoid, pectoral, and latissimus muscles are capable of producing sufficient force to generate movement through the shoulder, but this comes at the expense of torque through the inherently unstable glenohumeral joint. Obviously, passive noncontractile tissues such as the ligamentous capsule and fibrocartilage glenoid labrum play a large role in stabilization of the shoulder.[12,14] However, research has demonstrated that restoration of NMC is a prerequisite for shoulder stability even when the anatomic integrity of the restraining tissues has been restored.[5-7,12,14] Dynamic stabilization of the shoulder is essential even when shoulders are not obviously clinically unstable because optimal muscle length–tension relationships must be maintained if efficient and functional shoulder motion is to continue. Such is the case with overhead-throwing athletes.[12,14-18] Thus, accurate clinical assessment of NMC of the shoulder becomes crucial in identifying the underlying impairments that prevent a return to function, as well as in documenting progress with therapy.

SENSORY-SPECIFIC ASSESSMENT OF NEUROMUSCULAR CONTROL OF THE SHOULDER

Numerous investigators have described clinical measures of scapular motion from which changes in scapulothoracic NMC are inferred. Since the landmark work of Kibler[18] and many colleagues, attempts have been made to quantify these tests and measures.[12,14-18] However, more recent studies of the scapular slide test suggested somewhat more equivocal reliability than previously thought. Amasay et al[20] suggested that a sliding scapula may be a normal finding in overhead-throwing athletes without disorders or pain. These investigators also suggested that it may not be possible to generalize scapular movement patterns observed during constrained elevation because these patterns exhibit a high degree of variability. In this study, the same degree of variability was consistent across alternate functional reaching motions (to belt, shelf, front, right, left, and overhead).[20]

In contrast, McClure et al[16] did demonstrate abnormal scapular movement in subjects with impingement as compared with controls. Later research by McClure et al[17] showed reliable assessment of visual classification of scapular dyskinesis defined as "the presence of either winging or dysrhythmia" when rated as "normal, subtle, or obvious dyskinesis."

Positioning Tests

Borstad[22] showed simple tape measurement of scapular surface anatomy to be a reliable clinical measure with the potential for great clinical utility. Tape measurement from the sternal notch to the coracoid process and the scapula index (the sternal notch to the coracoid process divided by the distance from the posterior lateral angle of the scapula to the thoracic spine) both correlated with internal scapular rotation by three-dimensional biomechanical analysis. Further study into normative ratios for the scapula index may provide clinicians with an economical assessment tool of real utility.[22]

Extensive research has described the use of joint angle replication as a reliable and valid measure of shoulder NMC under somatosensory-biased conditions. A cornerstone study by Davies and Dickoff-Hoffman[52] showed that uninjured male subjects can reproduce a joint angle within 3°, and uninjured female subjects can reproduce a joint angle within 4°. This study and one by Ellenbecker[53] were designed to examine the impact of proprioceptive input on NMC of the shoulder. The investigators typically occluded visual feedback by using a curtain or blindfold and then passively positioned the extremity to provide somatosensory input about the joint angle.[52,53]

These tests can be adapted to account for both visual and somatosensory input during specific functional shoulder repositioning and reaching. In the proposed "look and touch" test, the examiner places a novel target within reach of the extremity. The subject then rapidly moves the upper extremity to bring the index finger in contact with the target. With just

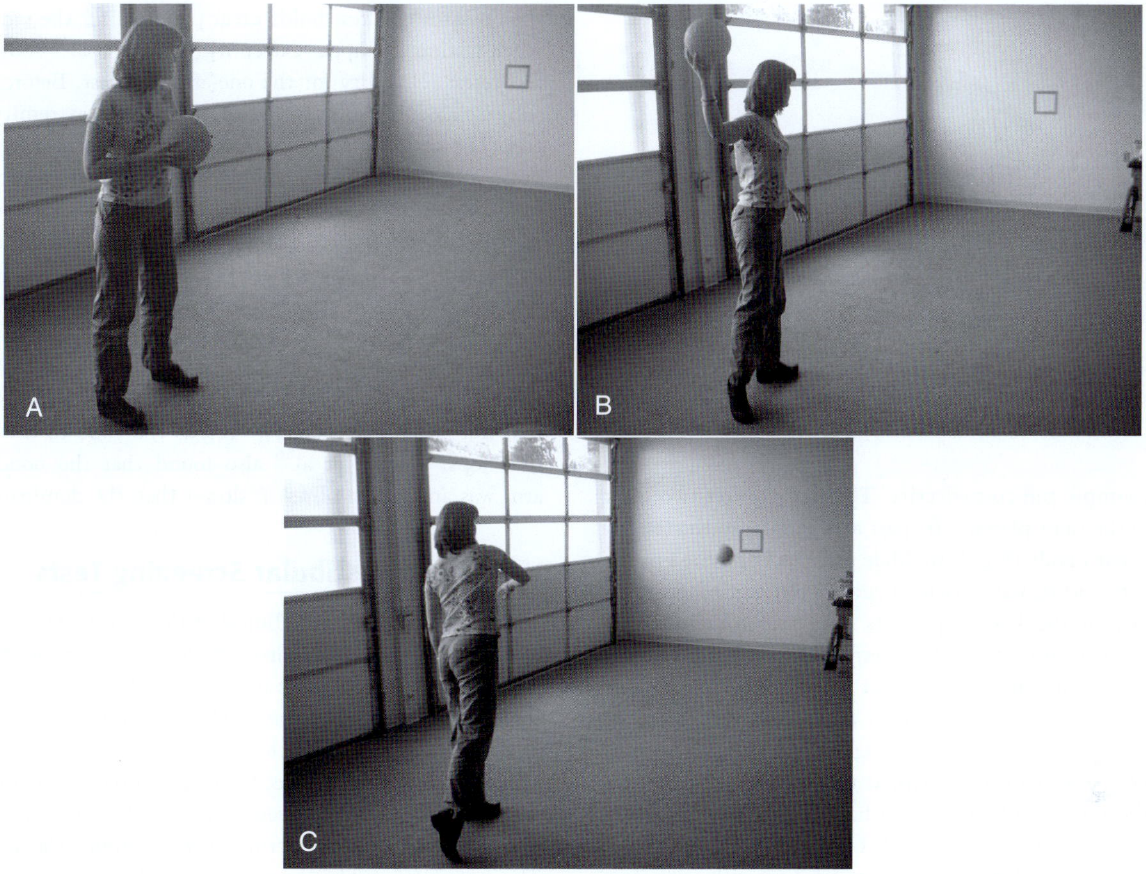

Figure 7-5 Functional throwing performance index (FTPI). **A,** Start. **B,** Crow hop to throw. **C,** Throw to target.

several repetitions, the subject will use the knowledge of visual feedback and learn the motor task, as evidenced by consistently hitting the target with the finger. The subject is then asked to close his or eyes and hit the target (visual sensory deprivation). Thus, in the second component of the test, the subject must rely on somatosensory input from the shoulder to match the internal representation of the target formed by previous visual and somatosensory input.

The functional throwing performance index (FTPI) is a clinical test that directly integrates the high degree of visual sensory input in NMC of the upper extremity (Fig. 7-5). Several investigators have cited good test-retest reliability with the FTPI, as well as normative data for athletes for clinically significant comparisons with patient performance. The FTPI requires a 1-ft^2 target placed on the wall at a height 4 ft from the floor and a 21-inch rubber playground-style ball. During the FTPI test, subjects should use their normal throwing mechanics, including a "crow hop" (short lateral jump before setting the feet for the throw). The subject is allowed to warm up with four submaximal throws, followed by five maximal warm-up throws while catching his or her own rebounds off the target wall. Once warm, the subject then performs three trials of as many controlled throws as possible in 30 seconds. The clinician counts both the number of total throws and the throws that hit in the target area. Results of the FTPI are expressed as the percentage of total throws on target over all three trials (Table 7-1).[52-54]

The closed kinetic chain upper extremity stability test (CKC UE stability test) provides an objective clinical measure of the NMC of shoulder stability. This test is similar to the Star excursion balance test for ankle stability because it is

Table 7-1 Functional Throwing Performance Index

	Trial 1	Trial 2	Trial 3	Totals	Average	Norms	
						Male	Female
Throws in target						15	13
Total throws						7	4
FTPI						47%	29%
Range						33%–60%	17%–41%

FTPI, Functional Throwing Performance Index.

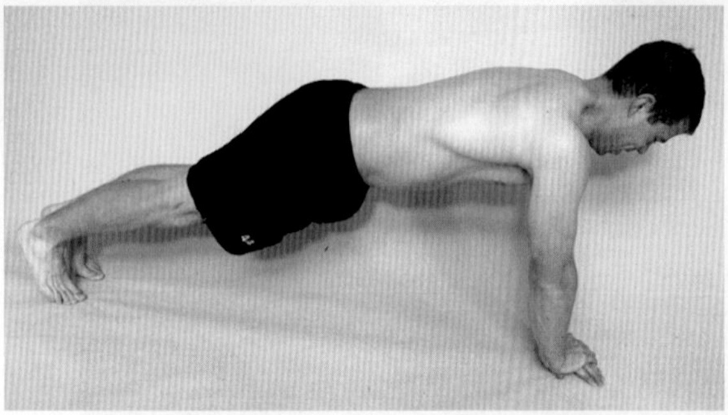

Figure 7-6 Closed kinetic chain upper extremity stability test touching the opposite hand. (From Magee DJ: *Orthopedic physical assessment,* ed 5, St. Louis, 2008, Saunders Elsevier.)

elegantly simple and cost effective. The test requires two lines of tape on the floor placed 3 ft apart and parallel to the length of the patient's body (Fig. 7-6). Male patients begin in a push-up position, and female patients begin in a modified push-up position (from the knees); patients have one hand on each taped line. The subject rapidly alternates placing both hands on one line by moving one hand at a time. This movement is similar to footsteps necessary to move the body between lines during a shuttle run. Following a submaximal warmup, the subject performs three maximal trials while the clinician records the number of times both hands are touching a line during a 15-second trial. The CKC UE stability test has been shown to have excellent test-retest reliability with interclass correlation coefficients of more than 0.92.[52-54]

Performance on the CKC UE stability test has been described in three ways: (1) simply the average number of touches completed in the three trials; (2) CKC UE stability scoring, calculated as the average number of lines touched over the three trials divided by the subject's height in inches and then multiplied by 100; this method normalizes the score for patients' height (because taller subjects have a wider wingspan); and (3) muscular power required to move the subject's body weight over the distance in the specified 15 seconds; power is calculated by multiplying the average number of touches over three trials by 68% of the subject's body weight (reported to represent the head, trunk, and arm segments) divided by 15.[52-54,55] A sample data collection table and normative values for the CKC UE stability test are displayed in Table 7-2.

Much as single-leg hop tests have been shown to have great clinical utility in assessing knee and lower extremity function, the one-arm hop test holds great potential for the same utility when testing the upper extremity. Falsone et al[56] showed good test-retest reliability for the one-arm hop test. Before the test, subjects are allowed to warm up on an upper extremity ergometer. The test begins with the subject in a one-arm push-up position with the feet a shoulder width apart, the back flat, and the weight bearing arm perpendicular to floor (Fig 7-7). A 10.2-cm step (typical height of most aerobics class and therapy gym plastic steps) is placed immediately lateral to the arm. The subject is then asked to hop with one arm only from the floor to the step and back five times as quickly as possible. Patients are given enough practice trials to perform five hops with the correct technique. The patient then performs a maximal test while the therapist records the time to complete all five hops. Falsone et al[56] also found that the nondominant arm was an average of 4.4% slower than the dominant arm.

Table 7-2 Closed Kinetic Chain Upper Extremity Stability Test

	Trial			Norms		
	1	2	3	Average	Score	Power
Touches						
Norms				18.5/20.5 (M/F)	Score: 26/ 31 (M/F)	Power: 150/ 135 (M/F)

M, male; F, female.

Visual and Vestibular Screening Tests

The Brock string test has clinical utility for qualitative screening of visual vergence. It requires a 6- to 10-ft string with three or more equally spaced beads on it. The subject holds one end of the string in front of the nose while the tester holds or ties the other end taut and just below eye level (Fig. 7-8). The subject is instructed to look at a specific bead. A subject with normal vergence should see one focused bead, as well as a blurry image of two crossed strings intersecting directly through the target bead. The cross is formed by the artifact of each eye's separate perspective of the string. Perception of the crossed strings through the target bead indicates that both eyes are correctly converging on the target. Perception of the cross in front of or behind the target bead suggests impaired vergence. Inability to perceive the visual artifact of the crossed strings may indicate lack of binocular vision. In either case, the altered depth perception could lead to abnormal NMC of the shoulder during reaching tasks and may warrant referral to an outside vision specialist.[26,27]

The head thrust test (HTT) is a simple, reliable, and valid clinical test of VOR function. It can give the shoulder specialist a good idea of vestibular function and the patient's related ability to use visual input during shoulder movements that also involve head rotation.[4,9,26,27,29,30] The subject's head is placed in 30° of downward tilt to align the horizontal semicircular canal. The subject maintains his or her gaze on a stationary target such as the clinician's nose. To relax the subject's neck, the clinician gently moves the subject's head in a 5° to 10° lateral rotation arc. The HTT involves an unpredictable rapid thrust to one side while the subject attempts to hold his or her gaze on the target (Fig. 7-9). A subject with a normally functioning VOR will maintain his or her gaze on the target regardless of the thrust, but subjects with vestibular loss will exhibit decreased VOR gain (ratio of eye to head movement). Thus, the eyes move with the head thrust off the target. The HTT result is considered positive if the clinician observes a corrective saccade to bring the subject's gaze back on target. The HTT was shown to be 71% sensitive for unilateral and 84% sensitive for bilateral peripheral vestibular hypofunctions. Its specificity of 82% is actually superior to the previous gold standard of

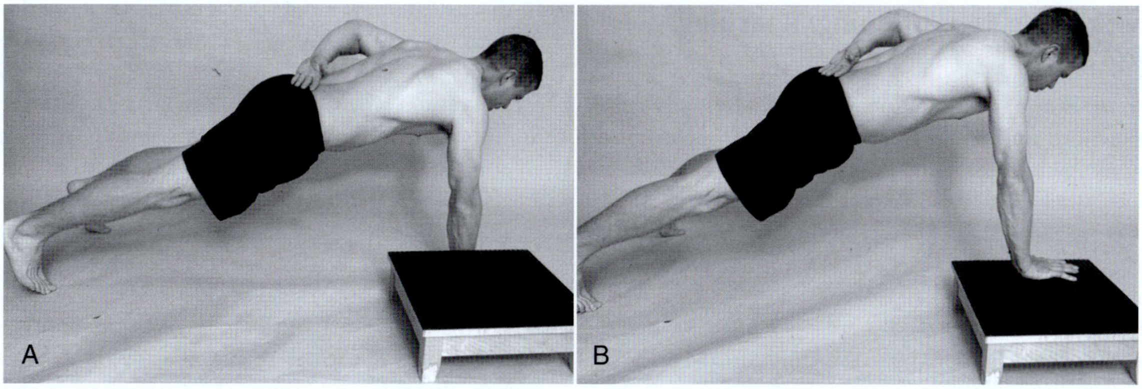

Figure 7-7 One-arm hop test. **A,** Start position. **B,** End position. (From Magee DJ: *Orthopedic physical assessment,* ed 5, St. Louis, 2008, Saunders Elsevier.)

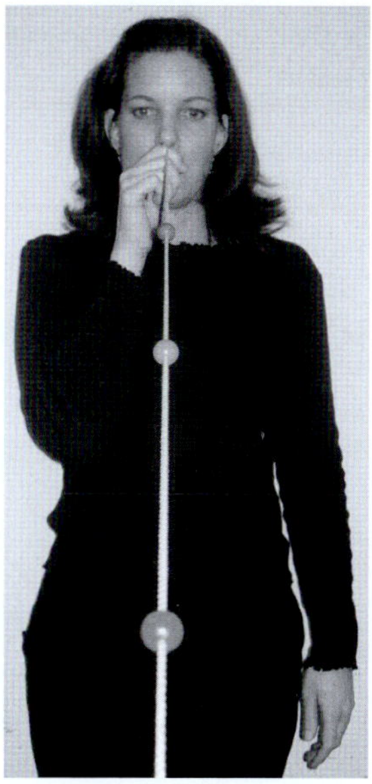

Figure 7-8 The Brock string test. (From Donatelli RA: *Orthopaedic physical therapy,* ed 4, St. Louis, 2010, Churchill Livingstone Elsevier.)

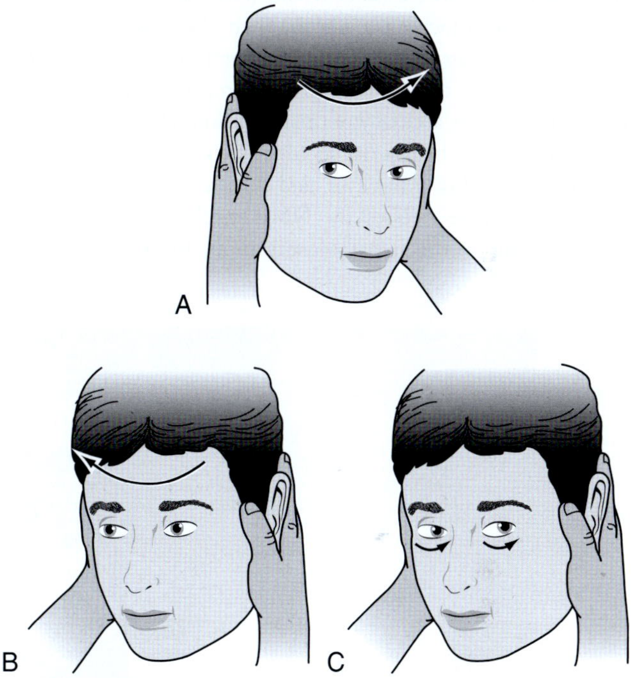

Figure 7-9 The head thrust test. The test is started with the eyes fixated on a target and the head in 30° of cervical flexion to improve test sensitivity. **A,** Normal response to rapid head thrust to the left: the eyes smoothly move to the right while maintaining fixation on the target. **B,** Abnormal response to rapid head thrust to the right: the eyes initially lose the target and move with the head and then (**C**) make small saccades to the left to regain fixation on the target. (From Cameron MC, Monroe LH: *Physical rehabilitation: evidence-based examination, evaluation, and intervention,* St. Louis, 2008, Saunders Elsevier.)

caloric electronystagmography.[30] Thus, the HTT may allow the shoulder specialist more accurately to identify the root cause of shoulder NMC control deficits that occur with concurrent head movements.

INTERVENTIONS TO ENHANCE NEUROMUSCULAR CONTROL OF THE SHOULDER

Generalized Exercise Programs

Evidence exists to support the use of generalized strength training programs to enhance shoulder NMC.[16,57,58] Lust et al[57] showed that a generalized 6-week training program focused on core stabilization drills and upper extremity strengthening can improve pitching accuracy. Similarly, McClure et al[16] showed that a 6-week program focused solely on rotator cuff strengthening and shoulder motion improved function. However, subjects in the strengthening-only protocol did not improved their elevation or scapular mechanics.[16] In a randomized clinical trial of 138 subjects with mechanical shoulder pain, Ginn et al[58] demonstrated improved function and pain with a 5-week exercise protocol focusing on strength, stretching, and stabilization; this regimen produced superior outcomes than those reported in control subjects.

Sensory-Specific Repositioning, Reaching, and Throwing

To adapt most clinical tests into training exercises is only natural. As described earlier, however, most shoulder repositioning tests are performed without visual feedback, at slow speeds, and using passive positioning of the joint to form the internal representation of the target necessary for NMC. Perhaps this is why many clinicians find limited gains with adaptations of these protocols to exercise.

An alternative NMT method is the use of a two-stage visual and then somatosensory-biased reaching drill. The drill begins by providing the patient a visual physical target. If the goal is to improve NMC of the shoulder during slower feedback types of tasks, such as painting, then the target should be in front of the patient, to use foveal vision. However, if the goal is to restore a faster feedforward type of NMC, such as for a boxer blocking a punch, then the target should be quickly flashed in the patient's peripheral vision. The patient reaches for the target at a goal-appropriate speed and is allowed to see the accuracy of the reach (knowledge of results). Next, the patient brings the shoulder back to a neutral resting position, closes his or her eyes, and then reaches for the target. The second stage stresses the NMC mechanism of reaching while relying on the somatosensory input from the shoulder. In this case, however, the CNS is still able to use the previous internal representation of the target formed with visual input.[45,47-51] This drill can be made more sport specific by incorporating task-specific implements, such as the fencing foil illustrated in Figure 7-10. Obviously, throwing drills are a natural extension of reaching. Subjects can safely throw a ball toward a wall in the second stage, but they should open their eyes after releasing the ball.

Visual training is fertile ground for enhancement of shoulder NMT programs. Several studies showed that visual targeting drills performed in conjunction with upper extremity tasks, such as shooting, produced gains in hand-eye tasks, such as shooting and tennis.[59,60] Clinical trials showed that the addition of visual training of saccades and vergence enhanced pistol target shooting in police cadets and improved the ability to hit curveballs in Little League baseball players as compared with normal sports practice alone.[61,62] However, it is not clear that visual training alone can improve performance of hand-eye tasks.[59,60]

Plyometrics

When paired with a medicine ball, throwing allows for plyometric training of the shoulder. In the short term, plyometrics allow for storing of mechanical energy in the parallel elastic

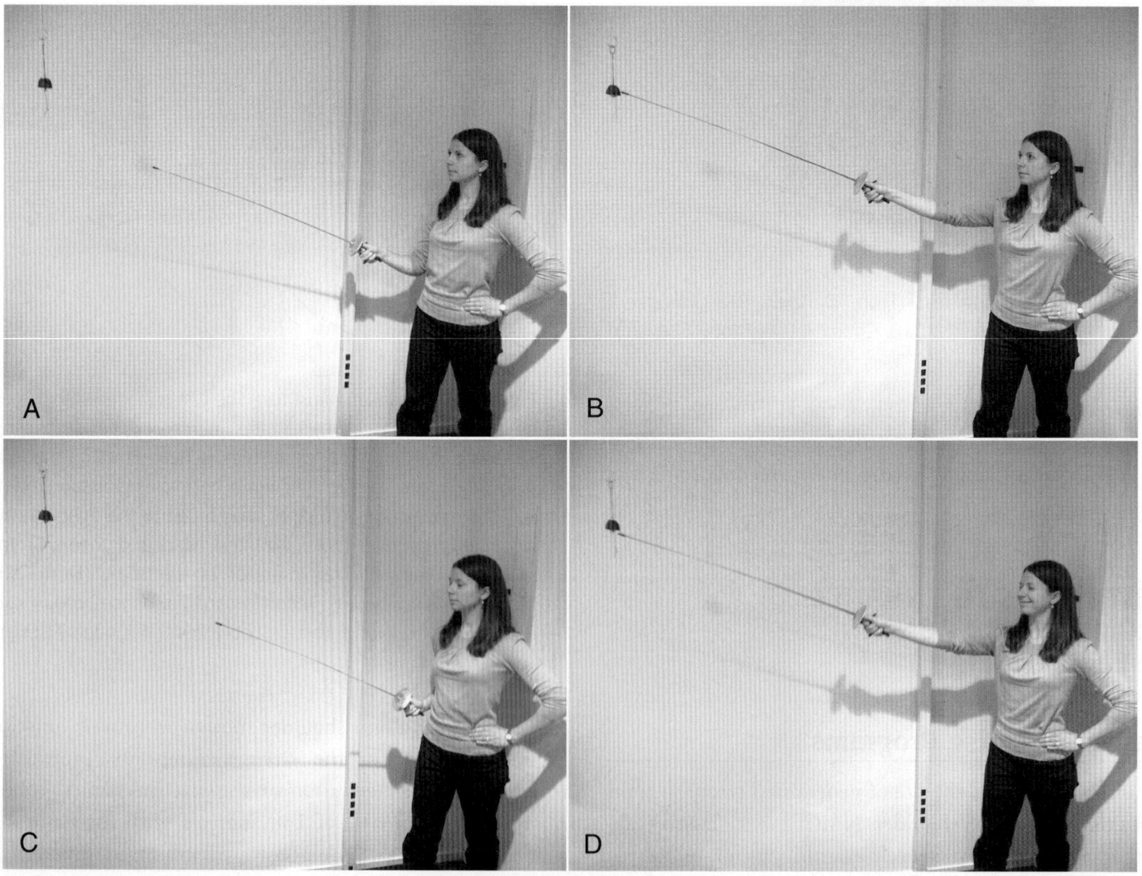

Figure 7-10 Look and reach drill. **A,** Forming the visual target. **B,** Reaching for the target using visual and somatosensory units. **C,** Return to the shoulder start position. **D,** Repeat drill without using visual feedback to emphasize somatosensory input.

component of shoulder girdle muscles that is soon rapidly released in the amortization phase. Over time, however, plyometrics provide a valuable neuromuscular response to training. For example, the pectoralis major muscle undergoes great amounts of tension during the eccentric phase or from the early to late cocking phase of throwing. With repeated plyometrics, the subject's CNS becomes habituated to the input from the pectoralis Golgi tendon organs. This habituation allows the patient's muscle to stretch more deeply into the eccentric phase of the throw without triggering the inverse myotatic reflex. This situation produces both greater storing of mechanical energy in the parallel elastic component of the muscles and a heightened effect of the stretch reflex. The net effect is heightened contractile force available to the thrower.[52-54,63-65]

Rhythmic Stabilization or Perturbation

Rhythmic stabilization drills are classic proprioceptive neuromuscular facilitation techniques historically described as having the therapist provide alternating manual pressures at various points on the arm while the patient meets these pressures with his or her own muscular force.[52-54,63] However, the term *rhythmic stabilization drills* is now commonly used to describe rapidly and randomly manually applied forces about the shoulder while the patient attempts to maintain a given shoulder position. Simply referring to the second technique as *perturbation* avoids the current unnecessary state of confusion.

Regardless of how it is delivered, perturbation is necessary to provide the error signal that drives CNS adaptation to feedforward NMT of dynamic stabilization of the shoulder. Sports activities such as scrum play in rugby and wrestling often require shoulder movement while the hand is fixed (closed kinetic chain), whereas throwing athletes operate almost exclusively in open kinetic chain mechanics (Fig. 7-11). Manual perturbations can be delivered in either condition. Just as in NMT of the lower extremity, devices such as tilt boards or the Shuttle Balance can provide ample perturbation for the shoulder joint.

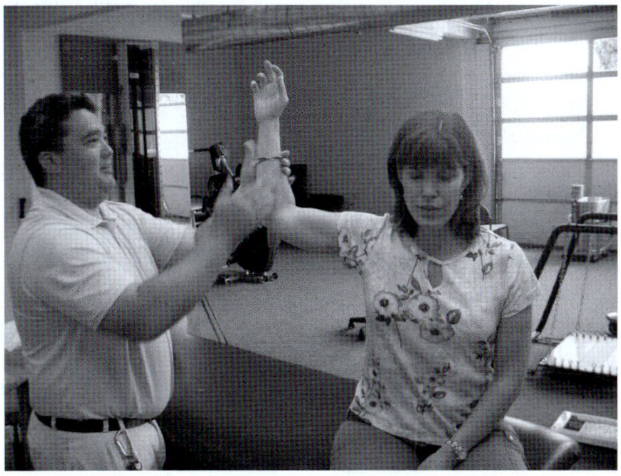

Figure 7-11 Open kinetic chain perturbation.

Again, applied sensory integration assists the shoulder specialist. For example, sports such as mixed martial arts place heavy stability demands on the shoulder, often when the subject cannot see the limb (many submission shoulder locks put the shoulder behind or to the side of the body). Thus, NMT of shoulder dynamic stabilization for these sports should include perturbation, in progressively more provocative positions, while the subject is deprived of vision. Maximization of somatosensory input dictates a firm surface to increase mechanoreceptor function. Similarly, research has suggested that shoulder specialists should consider exercising their patients in task-specific head positions because the resulting vestibular input partially forms the internal representation of shoulder position.[9-11] For example, both auto mechanics and soccer goalies spend an inordinate amount of time using their arms while their heads are in horizontal positions.

Tape as an Extrinsic Enhancer of Somatosensation

Selkowitz et al[66] examined the short-term effects of scapular taping on scapular girdle EMG. The tape technique used involved a strip of two-component strapping tape placed in the midbelly of the upper trapezius muscle perpendicular to the orientation of the muscle fiber (pulled medially and inferiorly). Patients with probable shoulder impingement exhibited decreased upper trapezius activity and increased lower trapezius activity while reaching overhead.[66] Miller and Osmotherly[67] performed a pilot randomized controlled trial examining the effect of a slightly different tape technique on patients with subacromial impingement. These investigators placed rigid strapping tape in two straps. One strap started at the anterior deltoid, moved posteriorly following the spine of the scapula, and ended at the spine. Another strap began at the coracoid process and then pulled posteriorly to simulate the action of the lower trapezius. The tape technique was applied to patients three times per week for the first 2 weeks. Assessment at 2 weeks showed a trend toward reduced pain and improved function as compared with controls. At the 6-week follow-up, however, the difference between the groups was insignificant.[67] In both studies, the researchers hypothesized that the outcome was largely the result of the increased somatosensory input provided by the tape on the skin that enhanced NMC of the scapular girdle.[66,67] Although these studies document only a short-term benefit in shoulder NMC, function, and pain, many clinicians will find the ability to provide tangible improvement in the earlier stages of shoulder rehabilitation invaluable in helping patients to understand and accept their overall treatment plan focusing on NMT exercises.

Virtual Reality and Video Games as Neuromuscular Training for the Shoulder

Previously, video games were controlled by pressing buttons on hand-held controllers. Typically, this could be done with finger motion alone and did not involve shoulder girdle movements. Devices such as the Nintendo Wii, however, now allow players

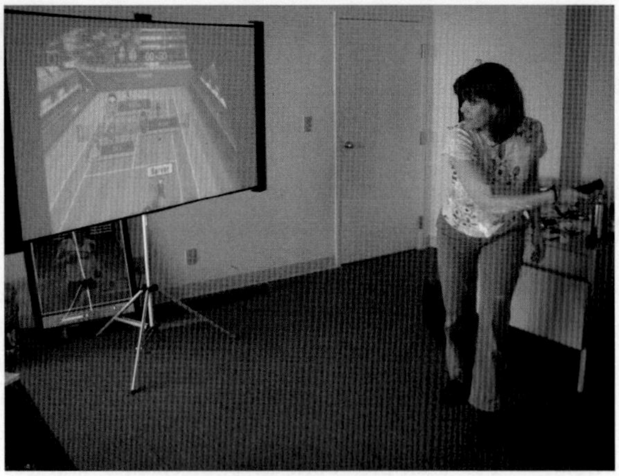

Figure 7-12 Shoulder Wiihab using a Nintendo Wii off-the-shelf video game device, which allows patients to input to the whole game by using upper extremity movements.

to send commands to the game system by using whole arm movements. This change has sparked widespread use of video games in physical therapy clinics and has even coined the term *Wiihab* (Fig. 7-12).[68-74] Numerous case studies have been published describing the potential uses of these largely shoulder movement–controlled video games. In general terms, these studies have described the benefits of improved compliance, enhanced motivation, and increased energy expenditure, particularly in adolescent or neurologically compromised subjects.[68-78]

While Carp has used these games in clinic and at home with his family, he urges caution. When subjects play a video game on the Wii, they are learning a specific motor task geared to the demands of the device. For example, many people learning to pitch on the Wii baseball game spontaneously discover that bringing the arm close to the body out of their normal throwing motion greatly improves their virtual pitching speed. This is because the shortened arm rotates faster (similar to an ice skater retracting the arms while spinning), the accelerometer in the Wii controller transduces the rapid change velocity, and the video game displays a very fast pitch. Therefore, although the lay video gamer considers this a hand-eye coordination activity, in essence he or she is learning an entirely different motor task from actual throwing. Carp hypothesizes minimal carryover of this type of training to functional shoulder motion. In other words, do people really think they will throw harder or more accurately just because they are good at the Wii?

It is even possible that the absence of normal somatosensory, visual, and vestibular sensory cues during virtual shoulder tasks could lead to abherent NMC. Some studies already examined movement patterns used during Wii boxing and other virtual gaming systems and found that these movement patterns are highly variable and do not necessarily simulate real-life motions.[76] Reports of tendinitis from excessive Wii play have been published, as has a report of a hemothorax injury in a patient who fell on her sofa while playing the Wii too frenetically.[77,78] Further research is required before a ringing endorsement of Wiihab for the shoulder can be made.

SUMMARY

In conclusion, shoulder specialists undoubtedly see patients with impaired somatosensory, visual, and vestibular sensation that directly affects these patients' ability to produce coordinated shoulder movement. Widening the definition of NMC to include the impact of sensory integration beyond somatosensation by incorporating visual and vestibular input can enhance the clinician's ability to identify reasons for abnormal NMC in all patients with shoulder disorders. Under most circumstances, visual input is weighted heavily in forming the internal CNS representation of the environment necessary to drive NMC of the shoulder for reaching and other coordinated upper extremity movements. Research also makes a strong case that vestibular input is vital in producing NMC of the shoulder when the head is in motion or positioned atypically. Sensory-specific and task speed–specific assessment and treatment approaches will allow physical therapists to assist their patients with shoulder conditions more effectively. Although video game–based technologies hold great promise in these areas, it is wise to exercise caution, and a need exists for strong evidence validating the use of these technologies in NMT of the shoulder.

REFERENCES

1. Williams GN, Chmielewski T, Rudolph KS, et al: Dynamic knee stability: current theory and implications for clinicians and scientists, *J Orthop Sports Phys Ther* 31(10):546–566, 2001.
2. Shumway-Cook A, Woolacoot M: *Motor control theory and practical applications*, Baltimore, 1995, Williams & Wilkins.
3. Shumway-Cook A, Horak FB: Assessing the influence of sensory integration on balance: suggestions from the field, *Phys Ther* 66:1548–1559, 1986.
4. Herdman SJ: *Vestibular rehabilitation*, ed 2, Philadelphia, 2000, Davis.
5. Forwell LA, Carnahan H: Proprioception during manual aiming in individuals with shoulder instability and controls, *J Orthop Sports Phys Ther* 23(2):111–120, 1996.
6. Suprak DN, Osternig LR, Donekarr PV, et al: Shoulder joint position sense improves with external load, *J Mot Behav* 39 (6):517–525, 2007.
7. Byle NN: Multisensory control of upper extremity function, *Neurol Rep* 26(1):32–43, 2002.
8. Raptis HA, Dannenbaum E, Paquet N, et al: Vestibular system may provide equivalent motor actions regardless of the number of body segments involved in the task, *J Neurophysiol* 97:4069–4078, 2007.
9. Borello-France DF, Gallagher JD, Furman JM, et al: Voluntary upper-extremity movements in patients with unilateral peripheral vestibular hypofunction, *Phys Ther* 82:216–227, 2002.
10. Knox JJ, Coppieters EMW, Hodges PW: Do you know where your arm is if you think your head has moved? *Exp Brain Res* 173:94–101, 2006.
11. Knox JJ, Hodges PW: Changes in head and neck position affect elbow joint position sense, *Exp Brain Res* 165:107–113, 2005.

12. Donatelli R: *Sports-specific rehabilitation*, ed 4, St. Louis, 2010, Churchill Livingstone Elsevier.
13. Shaffer SW, Harrison AL: Aging of the somatosensory system: a translational perspective, *Phys Ther* 87:193–207, 2007.
14. Myers JB, Wassinger CA, Lephart SM: Sensorimotor contribution to shoulder stability: effect of injury and rehabilitation, *Man Ther* 11:197–201, 2006.
15. Myers JB, Laudner KG, Pasquale MR, et al: Scapular position and orientation in throwing athletes, *Am J Sports Med* 33 (2):263–273, 2005.
16. McClure PW, Bialker J, Neff N: Shoulder function and 3-dimensional kinematics in people with shoulder impingement syndrome before and after a 6-week exercise program, *Phys Ther* 84:832–848, 2004.
17. McClure P, Tate AR, Kareha S, et al: A clinical method for identifying scapular dyskinesis. Part 1. Reliability, *J Athl Train* 44(2):160–164, 2009.
18. Kibler BW: The role of the scapula in athletic shoulder function, *Am J Sports Med* 26(2):325–338, 1998.
19. Laudner KG, Myers JB, Pasquale MR, et al: Scapular dysfunction in throwers with pathological internal impingement, *J Orthop Sports Phys Ther* 36(7):485–494, 2006.
20. Amasay T, Karduna AR: Scapular kinematics in constrained and functional upper extremity movements, *J Orthop Sports Phys Ther* 39(8):618–627, 2009.
21. Hess SA, Richardson C, Darnell R, et al: Timing of rotator cuff activation during shoulder external rotation in throwers with and without symptoms, *J Orthop Sports Phys Ther* 35:812–820, 2005.
22. Borstad JD: Resting position variable at the shoulder: evidence to support a posture-impairment association, *Phys Ther* 86:549–557, 2006.
23. Ciuffreda KJ, Kapoor N: Traumatic brain injury and the nation, *J Behav Optom* 18(3):58, 2007.
24. VanRoekel C: Military optometry in the care of traumatic brain injury patients, *J Behav Optom* 18(3):60–61, 2007.
25. Townsend JC: Traumatic brain injury: a new challenge for optometry neuro-optometric rehabilitation and our nation, *J Behav Optom* 18(3):63–66, 2007.
26. Ciuffreda KJ, Kapoor N, Rutner D, et al: Occurrence of oculomotor dysfunctions in acquired brain injury: a retrospective analysis, *Optometry* 78:155–161, 2007.
27. Schubert MC, Minor LB: Vestibulo-ocular physiology underlying vestibular hypofunction, *Phys Ther* 84:373–385, 2004.
28. Schubert MC, Tusa RJ, Grime LE, et al: Optimizing the sensitivity of head thrust for identifying vestibular hypofunction, *Phys Ther* 84:151–158, 2004.
29. Stelmack J: Measuring outcomes of neuro-optometric care in traumatic brain injury, *J Behav Optom* 18(3):67–71, 2007.
30. Ciuffreda KJ, Kapoor N: Oculomotor dysfunctions, their remediation, and reading-related problems in mild traumatic brain injury, *J Behav Optom* 18(3):72–77, 2007.
31. Ren L, Khan AZ, Blohm G, et al: Proprioceptive guidance of saccades in eye-hand coordination, *J Neurophysiol* 96:1464–1477, 2006.
32. Horstmann A, Hoffmann KP: Target selection in eye-hand coordination: do we reach to where we look or do we look to where we reach? *Exp Brain Res* 148:386–495, 2005.
33. Barnes BC, Cooper L, Kirkendall DT, et al: Concussion history in elite male and female soccer players, *Am J Sports Med* 26 (3):42–51, 1998.
34. Wojtys EM, Hovda D, Landry G, et al: Concussion in sports, *Am J Sports Med* 27(5):676–688, 1999.
35. Ferrara MS, McCrea M, Peterson CL, et al: A survey of practice patterns in concussion assessment and management, *J Athl Train* 36(2):145–149, 2001.
36. Guskiewicz KM, Bruce SL, Cantu RC, et al: National Athletic Trainers' Association position statement: management of sport-related concussion, *J Athl Train* 39(3):280–297, 2004.
37. Guskiewicz KM, Bruce SL, Cantu RC, et al: Research based recommendations of management of sport related concussion: summary of the National Athletic Trainers' position statement, *Br J Sports Med* 40:6–10, 2006.
38. Tommasone BA, Valovich McLeod TC: Contact sport concussion incidence, *J Athl Train* 41(4):470–472, 2006.
39. McCrea M, Guskiewicz KM, Marshall SW, et al: Acute effects and recovery time following concussion in collegiate football players: the NCAA Concussion Study, *JAMA* 290(19): 2556–2563, 2003.
40. McCrory P: When to retire after concussion, *Br J Sports Med* 35:380–382, 2001.
41. Mendez CV, Hurley RA, Lassonde M, et al: Mild traumatic brain injury: neuroimaging of sports-related concussion, *J Neuropsychiatry Clin Neurosci* 17(3):297–304, 2005.
42. Barr WB: Methodological issues in neuropsychological testing, *J Athl Train* 36(3):297–302, 2001.
43. Valovich McLeod TC, Barr WB, McCrea M, et al: Psychometric and measurement properties of concussion assessment tools in youth sports, *J Athl Train* 41(4):399–408, 2006.
44. Halterman CI, Langan J, Drew A, et al: Tracking the recovery of visuospatial attention deficits in mild traumatic brain injury, *Brain* 129:747–753, 2006.
45. Crawford JD, Medendorp WP, Marotta JJ: Spatial transformations for eye-hand coordination, *J Neurophysiol* 92:10–19, 2004.
46. Schubert MC, Herdman SJ, Tusa RJ: Vertical dynamic visual acuity in normal subjects and patients with vestibular hypofunction, *Otol Neurol* 23:372–377, 2002.
47. Tian J, Shubayev I, Demer JL: Dynamic visual acuity during passive and self-generated transient head rotation in normal and unilaterally vestibulopathic humans, *Exp Brain Res* 142: 486–495, 2002.
48. Brindle TJ, Nitz AJ, Uhl TL, et al: Measures of accuracy for active shoulder movement at 3 different speeds with kinesthetic and visual feedback, *J Orthop Sports Phys Ther* 34:468–478, 2004.
49. Mrotek LA, Soechting JF: Target interception: hand-eye coordination and strategies, *J Neurosci* 27(27):7297–7309, 2007.
50. Lee J, Donkelaar P: The human dorsal premotor cortex generates on-line error corrections during sensorimotor adaptations, *J Neurosci* 26(12):3330–3334, 2006.
51. Gribble PL, Everling S, Ford K, et al: Hand-eye coordination for rapid pointing movements: arm movement direction and distance are specified prior to saccade onset, *Brain Res* 145: 372–382, 2002.
52. Davies GJ, Dickoff-Hoffman S: Neuromuscular testing and rehabilitation of the shoulder complex, *J Orthop Sports Phys Ther* 18(2):449–458, 1993.
53. Ellenbecker TS: *Shoulder rehabilitation: non-operative treatment*, New York, 2006, Thieme.
54. Manske RJ, Davies GJ: Neuromuscular static and dynamic stability of the shoulder: the key to functional performance. In Manske R, editor: *Postsurgical orthopedic sports rehabilitation: knee and shoulder*, St Louis, 2006, Mosby Elsevier.
55. Goldbeck TG, Davies GJ: Test-retest reliability of the closed kinetic chain upper extremity stability test: a clinical field test, *J Sports Rehabil* 9(1):35–45, 2000.

56. Falsone SA, Gross MT, Guskiewicz KM, et al: One-arm hop test: reliability and effects of arm dominance, *J Orthop Sports Phys Ther* 32:98–103, 2002.
57. Lust KR, Sandrey MA, Bulger SM, et al: The effects of 6-week training programs on throwing accuracy, proprioception, and core endurance in baseball, *J Sport Rehabil* 18(3):407–426, 2009.
58. Ginn KA, Cohen ML: Exercise therapy for shoulder pain aimed at restoring neuromuscular control: a randomized comparative clinical trial, *J Rehabil Med* 37:115–122, 2005.
59. Rawstron JA, Burley CD, Elder MJ: A systematic review of the applicability and efficacy of eye exercises, *J Pediatr Ophthalmol Strabismus* 42:82–88, 2005.
60. Qevdedo L, Sole J, Palmi J, et al: Experimental study of visual training effects in shooting initiation, *Clin Exp Optom* 82 (1):23–28, 1999.
61. Bowen T, Horth L: Use of the EYEPORT vision training system to enhance the visual performance of Little League baseball players, *J Behav Optom* 16(6):143–148, 2005.
62. Liberman J, Horth L: Use of the EYEPORT vision training system to enhance the visual performance of police recruits: a pilot study, *J Behav Optom* 17(4):87–92, 2006.
63. Donatelli RA, Wooden MJ: *Orthopedic rehabilitation*, St. Louis, 2006, Mosby Elsevier.
64. Davies GJ, Matheson JW: Shoulder plyometrics, *Sports Med Arthrosc Rev* 9:1–18, 2001.
65. Pretz R: Plyometric exercises for overhead-throwing athletes, *Strength Cond J* 28(1):36–42, 2006.
66. Selkowitz DM, Chaney C, Stuckey SJ, et al: The effects of scapular taping on the surface electromyographic signal amplitude of shoulder girdle muscles during upper extremity elevation in individuals with suspected shoulder impingement syndrome, *J Orthop Sports Phys Ther* 37(11):694–702, 2007.
67. Miller P, Osmotherly P: Does scapula taping facilitate recovery for shoulder impingement symptoms? A pilot randomized controlled trial, *J Man Manip Ther* 17(1):E6–E14, 2009.
68. Deutsch JE, Borbely M, Filler J: Use of a low-cost, commercially available gaming console (Wii) for rehabilitation of an adolescent with cerebral palsy, *Phys Ther* 88:1196–1207, 2008.
69. Flynn S, Palma P, Bender A: Feasibility of using the Sony Play Station 2 gaming platform for an individual poststroke: a case report, *J Neurol Phys Ther* 31:180–189, 2007.
70. Widman LM, McDonald CM, Abresch T: Effectiveness of an upper extremity exercise device integrated with computer gaming for aerobic training in adolescents with spinal cord dysfunction, *J Spinal Cord Med* 29:363–370, 2006.
71. Yong JL, Soon YT, Xu D, et al: A feasibility study using interactive commercial off-the-shelf computer gaming in upper limb rehabilitation in patients after stroke, *J Rehabil Med Prev* 42:1–5, 2010.
72. Saposnik G, Mamdani M, Bayley M, et al: Effectiveness of Virtual Reality Exercises in Stroke Rehabilitation (EVREST): rationale, design, and protocol of a pilot randomized clinical trial assessing the Wii gaming system, *Int J Stroke* 5:47–51, 2010.
73. Lange B, Flynn S, Rizzo A: Initial usability assessment of off-the-shelf video game consoles for clinical game-based motor rehabilitation, *Phys Ther Rev* 14(5):355–364, 2009.
74. Graves LE, Ridgers ND, Stratton G: The contribution of upper limb and total body movement to adolescents' energy expenditure whilst playing Nintendo Wii, *Eur J Appl Physiol* 104 (4):617–623, 2008.
75. Hanneton S, Vaenne A: Coaching the Wii: evaluation of physical training experience assisted by a video game. In Altinsoy ME, Jekosch U, Bewster S, editors: *Haptic, audio, visual environments and games*, Berlin, 2009, Springer, pp 54–57.
76. Bianchi-Berthouze N, Kim WW, Darshak P: Does body movement engage you more in digital game play? and why? In Paiva A, Prada R, Picard RW, editors: *Affective computing and intelligent interaction*, LNCS 4738, Berlin, 2007, Springer, pp 102–113.
77. Bonis J: Acute Wiiitis, *N Engl J Med* 356(23):2431–2432, 2007.
78. Peek AC, Ibrahim T, Abunasra H, et al: White-out from a Wii: traumatic haemothorax sustained playing Nintendo Wii, *Ann R Coll Surg Engl* 90:W9–W10, 2008.

CHAPTER 8

Bruce H. Greenfield
and Kathleen Geist

Evaluation and Treatment of Brachial Plexus Lesions

The *Guide to Physical Therapist Practice* (the *Guide*) contains the preferred practice patterns of impaired joint mobility, motor function, muscle performance, range of motion, and reflex integrity associated with spinal disorders and impaired peripheral nerve integrity and muscle performance associated with peripheral nerve injury, including persons with injuries to their brachial plexuses.[1] Predicted impairments and functional losses related to these practice patterns include, but are not limited to, difficulty with manipulation skills, decreased muscle strength, impaired proprioception, impaired sensory integrity, abnormal neural tension signs, loss of motion, and postural changes. Consequently, physical and occupational therapists evaluate and identify the primary impairments and conditions contributing to injury to restore function.

The brachial plexus supplies both motor and sensory innervations to the upper extremities and the related shoulder girdle structures. Lesions to the brachial plexus compromise the neurologic integrity, and hence the function, of the shoulder and related upper extremities. Evaluation of shoulder dysfunction should include an assessment of the integrity and functional status of the brachial plexus. However, the complex structure of the brachial plexus requires a thorough understanding of the multiple innervation patterns to the various muscles. In addition, for proper and effective clinical management of the brachial plexus, the clinician should understand the mechanisms of injuries, the pathophysiologic changes of nerve fibers and nerve roots, and the potential for recovery.

Therefore, this chapter provides a review of the anatomy of the brachial plexus, classification of brachial plexus injuries, common musculoskeletal injuries that result in injuries to the brachial plexus, and descriptions of pathomechanical and pathologic changes to the specific nerve fibers and nerve roots. In addition, this chapter reviews an evaluation of the nature and extent of impairments and functional losses resulting from brachial plexus lesions. Clinical case studies offer combined physical and occupational therapy management of a person with a brachial plexus injury. The case studies incorporate the patient management schemes of the relevant preferred practice patterns in the *Guide.*

ANATOMY OF THE BRACHIAL PLEXUS

This review of the anatomy of the brachial plexus describes the gross anatomy of the plexus and its relationship with surrounding structures, as well as the microscopic anatomy of the nerve and nerve trunks.

Superficial Anatomy

The brachial plexus is composed of the anterior primary divisions of spinal segments C5, C6, C7, C8, and T1 (Fig. 8-1). The components of the brachial plexus include the following:

1. Undivided anterior primary rami
2. Trunks: upper, middle, and lower
3. Divisions of the trunks: anterior and posterior
4. Cords: lateral, posterior, and medial
5. Branches: peripheral nerves derived from the cords

Figure 8-2 shows the segmental motor innervation of the brachial plexus to the muscles of the shoulder. The fourth cervical nerve usually gives a branch to the fifth cervical nerve, and the first thoracic nerve frequently receives one from the second thoracic nerve. When the branch from C4 is large, the branch from T2 is often absent and the branch from T1 is reduced in size. This configuration constitutes the prefixed type of plexus. Conversely, when the branch from C4 is small or absent, the contribution of C5 is reduced in size and that of T1 is larger. The branch from T2 is always present. This arrangement constitutes the postfixed type of plexus.

The following is the typical arrangement of the brachial plexus (see Fig. 8-1). The fifth and sixth cervical nerves unite at the lateral border of the scalenus medius muscles to form the upper trunk of the plexus. The eighth cervical nerve and first thoracic nerve unite behind the scalenus anterior to form the lower trunk of the plexus, whereas the seventh cervical nerve constitutes the middle trunk. These three trunks travel downward and laterally and just above or behind the clavicle, and each trunk splits into an anterior and a posterior division. The anterior divisions of the upper and middle trunks combine to form a cord, which is situated on the lateral side

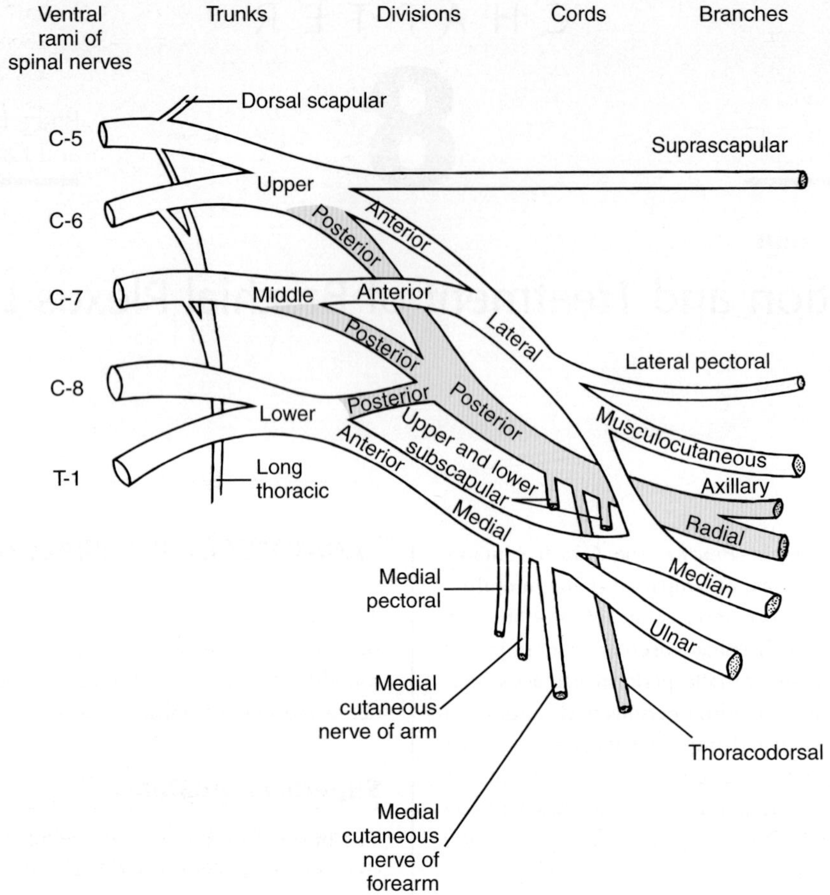

Figure 8-1 Segmental motor innervation of the muscles of the shoulder. (From Jenkins DB: *Hollinshead's functional anatomy of the limbs and back*, ed 9, Philadelphia, 2009, Saunders Elsevier.)

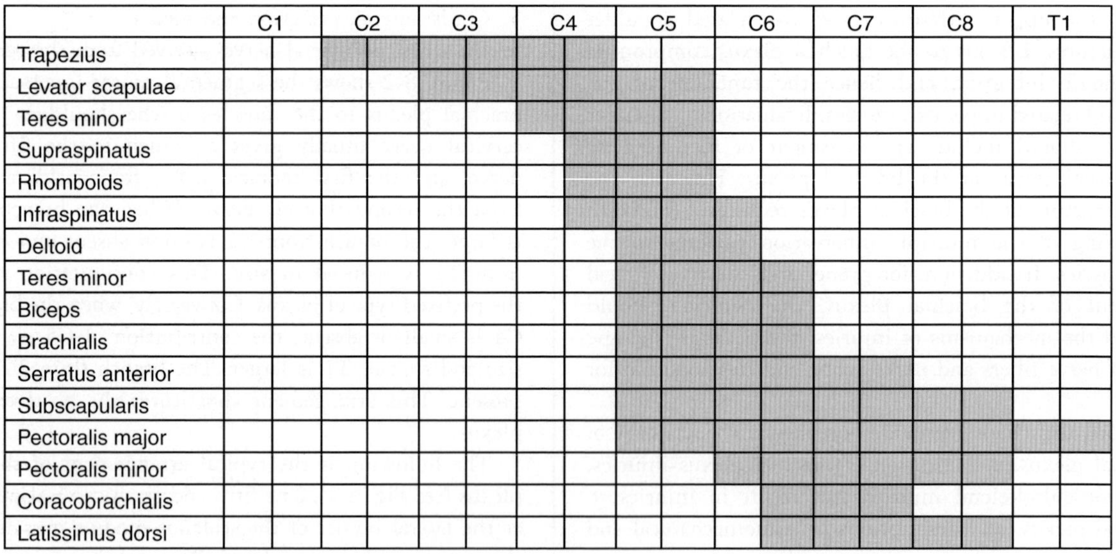

Figure 8-2 Additional segmental motor innervation of the muscles of the shoulder.

of the axillary artery and is called the *lateral cord.* The anterior division of the lower trunk passes downward, first behind and then on the medial side of the axillary artery, and forms the *medial cord.* This cord frequently receives fibers from the seventh cervical nerve. The posterior divisions of all three trunks join to form the *posterior cord,* which is situated at first above and then behind the axillary artery.[2]

The brachial plexus contains autonomic sympathetic nerve fibers consisting mostly of postganglionic fibers derived from the sympathetic ganglionated chain. The primary ramus T1 contains the only preganglionic fibers in the brachial plexus.[2] The sympathetic supply to the eye travels through the T1 nerve root. Horner's syndrome results from a traction injury with avulsion to that root. Constriction of the pupil and ptosis of the eyelid on the involved side characterize Horner's syndrome.[3]

Anatomic Relationships with the Brachial Plexus

To isolate a plexus lesion effectively, especially in the presence of open trauma, the clinician must identify the plexus and its relationship with the anatomic structures. For example, knowledge of the portion of the brachial plexus that lies between the clavicle and the first rib, in the presence of a clavicular fracture, can help the clinician to isolate the affected nerve and predict the affected muscles. Topographic relationships of the plexus are delineated in *Gray's Anatomy.*[2]

The *posterior triangle,* which is the angle between the clavicle and the lower posterior border of the sternocleidomastoid muscle, contains the brachial plexus. The plexus in this area is covered by skin, platysma, and deep fascia. The plexus emerges between the scalenus anterior and scalenus medius muscles, passes behind the anterior convexity of the medial two thirds of the clavicle, and lies on the first digitation of the serratus anterior and subscapularis muscles. In the axilla, the lateral and posterior cords of the plexus are on the lateral side of the axillary artery, and the medial cord is behind the axillary artery. The cords surround the middle part of the axillary artery on three sides: the medial cord lies on the medial side, the posterior cord behind, and the lateral cord on the lateral side of the axillary artery. In the lower part of the axilla, the cord splits into the nerves for the upper limb.

Anatomic variants identified within the axillary region may compress the nerves of the brachial plexus and create pain and paresthesias in the upper extremity. Anatomic anomalies of musculotendinous bands of the latissimus dorsi muscle have been found in cadaveric specimens and have been termed the *axillary arch* or the *axillary arch of Langer.* In a cadaveric dissection, Warwick and Williams described the presence of bilateral, musculotendinous bands, 8.0 cm in length from the superior-medial aspect of the latissimus dorsi, with a proximal insertion in the fascial aponeurosis to the anterior aspect of the coracobrachialis and with innervations from the thoracodorsal nerve. The axillary arch has been estimated to be present in 2% to 7% of the population The axillary arch includes a musculotendinous band that extends from the superior-medial aspect of the latissimus dorsi at the level of the third rib and can have various attachments to the pectoralis major, the coracoid process, or the fascial connection to the anterior surface of the coracobrachialis. The axillary arch passes anteriorly to the neurovascular bundle and can compress the median, musculocutaneous, and ulnar nerve and brachial vessels. Thus, when the shoulder is in a position of hyperabduction, the axillary arch can compress the underlying brachial plexus and cause impairment in circulation of the upper extremity, pain, and paresthesias into the arm, forearm, and hand.[4]

Serpel and Baum described the clinical presentation of an axillary arch as a visible fullness in the axillary region during full humeral abduction and external rotation, with a return of the axillary concavity when the shoulder is at the patient's side.[4] With the shoulder in a position of hyperabduction, the underlying neurovascular structures become compressed and cause upper extremity pain, edema, and paresthesias. Additional clinical manifestations of an axillary arch include upper extremity edema and median nerve entrapment in the infraclavicular region of the brachial plexus. Resisted manual muscle testing in shoulder adduction and internal rotation with the shoulder in a position of abduction is expected to reproduce upper extremity symptoms and to create a visible fullness in the axillary region. Symptoms may also be provoked by palpation of the neurovascular bundle of the distal attachment of the axillary arch when the shoulder is in full flexion and external rotation. The presence of an axillary arch should be another anatomic consideration in the differential diagnosis in those patients with symptoms mimicking thoracic outlet syndrome.[4]

Anatomy of the Nerve Trunks

The nerve trunks and branches contain parallel bundles (fasciculi) of nerve fibers comprising the efferent and afferent axons and their Schwann cells, which in some cases contain myelin sheaths (Fig. 8-3).[2] Fasciculi within each nerve trunk contain a few to many hundreds of nerve fibers. A dense, irregular connective tissue sheath, the epineurium, surrounds the whole trunk, and a similar but less fibrous perineurium surrounds the fasciculi within each nerve trunk. A loose, delicate connective tissue network—the endoneurium—penetrates the spaces between nerve fibers. These connective tissue sheaths serve as planes of access for the vasculature of peripheral nerves and as protective cushions for the nerve fibers.

Features of Nerve Trunks Providing Protection from Physical Deformation

Several factors protect the brachial plexus and nerve trunks from both traction and deformation injuries. First, with two notable exceptions—the ulnar nerve at the elbow and the sciatic nerve at the hip—the nerve trunks cross the flexor aspect of joints. Because extension is more limited in range than is flexion, the nerves are subjected to less tension during limb movements.

Second, the nerve trunks run an undulating course in its bed, the fasciculi run an undulating course in the epineurium, and the nerve fibers run an undulating course inside the fasciculi (Fig. 8-4). This means that the length of nerve fibers between any two fixed points on the limb is considerably greater than the distance between those points.

Third, the many elastic fibers within the perineurium impart a degree of elasticity in the nerve trunk in response to tensile forces. Fourth, the nerve trunk contains a large amount of epineurial connective tissue, which separates the fasciculi.

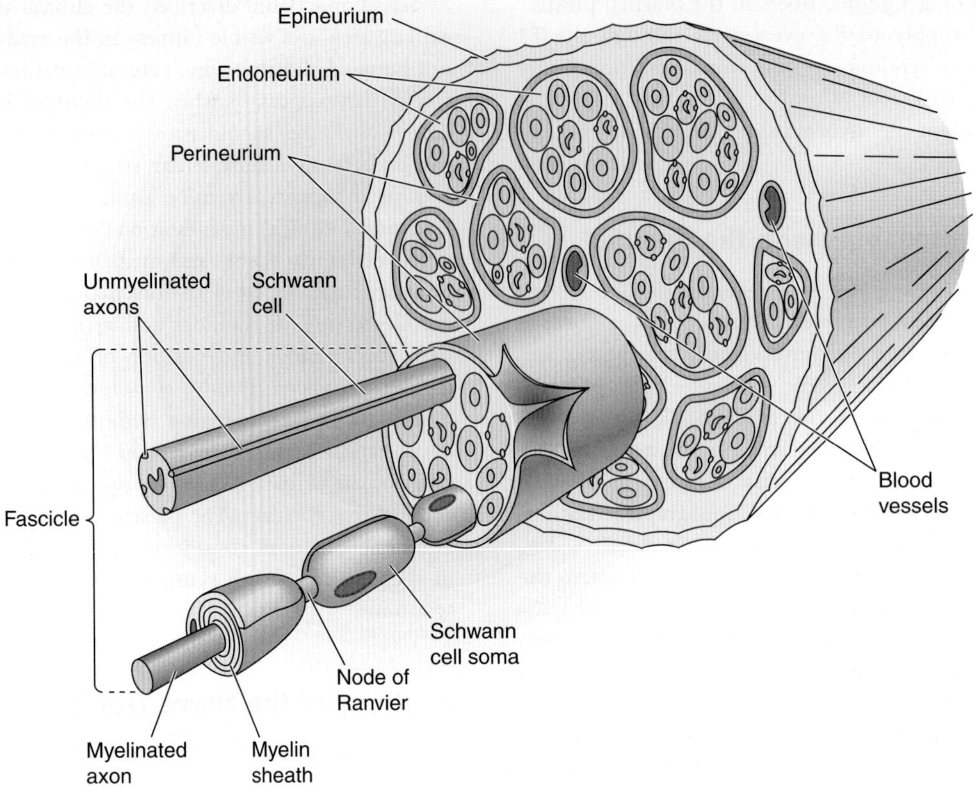

Figure 8-3 Structural features of peripheral nerve fibers and a nerve trunk (cut away) showing a large number of fasciculi, which individually contain many nerve fibers. (From Boron WF: *Medical physiology: a cellular and molecular approach,* ed 2, Philadelphia, 2009, Saunders Elsevier.)

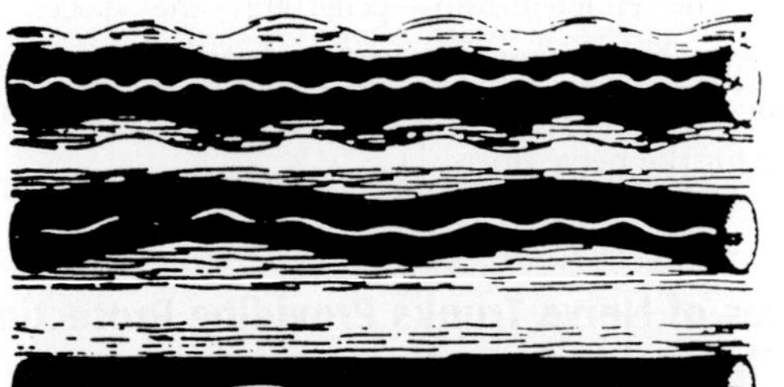

Figure 8-4 Example of the undulating structure of the funiculi, which contains nerve fibers of a nerve trunk to the point of failure. (From Sunderland S: Traumatized nerves, roots and ganglia: musculoskeletal factors and neuropathological consequences. In Korr IM, editor: *The neurobiologic mechanisms in manipulative therapy,* New York, 1978, Plenum.)

According to Sunderland,[5] values of epineurial connective tissue of various peripheral nerves range from 30% to 75% of the cross-sectional area of the total number of nerve fibers contained in each nerve trunk. Therefore, the epineurium provides a loose matrix for its fasciculi and cushions the nerve fibers against deforming forces.

Features of the Nerve Roots Providing Protection from Injury

The nerve roots at the intervertebral foramen are protected from traction injury by several mechanisms.[5] Normal cervical spine, shoulder girdle, and shoulder motions place repetitive strains on the nerve roots that form the brachial plexus. Overstretching of nerve roots by transmitted forces generated in this manner is normally prevented by the following factors.

First, the dura mater is adherent to, and part of, the nerve complex at the level of the intervertebral foramen. Therefore, when traction pulls the entire system outward, a dural funnel is drawn laterally into the foramen. The dura mater, being cone shaped at the junction of the intervertebral foramen, plugs the foramen in a way that guards against further displacement of the nerve (Fig. 8-5). Second, the fourth, fifth, sixth, and seventh cervical nerve roots are securely attached to the

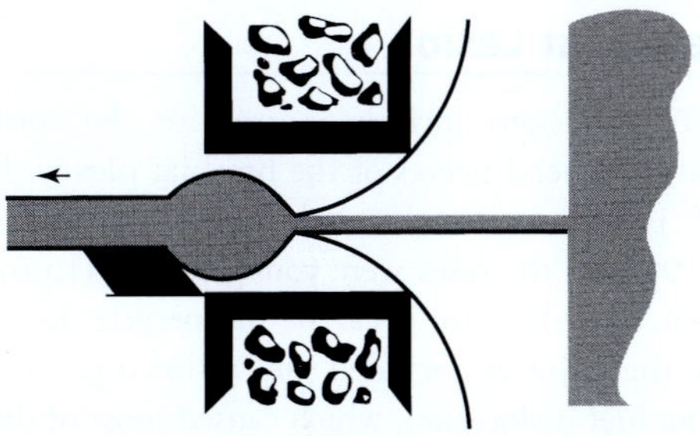

Figure 8-5 Displacement of the nerve complex laterally through the foramen is resisted by plugging the funnel-shaped dura mater and the dural attachment to the transverse process. (From Sunderland S: Traumatized nerves, roots and ganglia: musculoskeletal factors and neuropathological consequences. In Korr IM, editor: *The neurobiologic mechanisms in manipulative therapy,* New York, 1978, Plenum.)

vertebral column. Each nerve root, on leaving the foramen, is lodged into the gutter of the corresponding transverse process, bound securely by reflections of the prevertebral fascia and by slips from the dura mater attachment to the transverse processes (see Fig. 8-5). Sunderland[5] suggested that the significance of these attachments is to reduce the relative susceptibility to avulsion injury of the several nerve roots contributing to the brachial plexus. Traction injuries, which do not avulse nerve roots, more commonly involve the spinal nerves where these attachments exist. However, the incidence of avulsion injuries is much higher in the nerve roots, which do not have soft tissue attachments to the transverse processes.

CLASSIFICATION OF BRACHIAL PLEXUS INJURIES

Table 8-1 indicates numerous types of classifications of brachial plexus injuries. Most brachial plexus lesions result from either direct or indirect trauma, such as a strike from an instrument, or a traction lesion of the cervical spine or upper extremity.[6-13] Lesions are classified as either preganglionic or postganglionic. The term *preganglionic avulsion injury* indicates that the nerve root has been torn from the spinal cord, and it precludes the possibility of recovery. *Postganglionic lesions* may be either in continuity (root and sheath intact) or ruptured (root intact and nerve sheath ruptured).[6] Spontaneous recoveries may occur with the first injury. Without surgical repair of the rupture, however, no recovery will occur in the second lesion.

Postganglionic avulsions can be classified as supraclavicular or infraclavicular lesions. The roots and trunks of the brachial plexus comprise the supraclavicular plexus. The *retroclavicular plexus* is defined as the neural divisions of the brachial plexus that pass posterior to the clavicle. As the cords of the brachial plexus pass over the first rib, they are subclassified into the anterior, lateral, and posterior cords, based on the location of the nerves to the subclavian artery. Finally, the infraclavicular plexus comprises the cords and branches of the brachial plexus.[7] In a series of 420 brachial plexus lesions involving operations, Alnot[7] reported that 75% were supraclavicular lesions and 25% were infraclavicular lesions.

Table 8-1 Etiologic Classification of Brachial Plexus Injuries as Related to the Shoulder and Cervical Spine

Cause	Injury Type
Traumatic	Open injuries Fractures Closed injuries
Fractures	Obstetric injuries Postnatal exogenous injuries Sports injuries (e.g., burner syndrome, shoulder dislocations)
Compression	Exogenous (sometimes isolated branches) Anatomic predisposition (sometimes isolated branches) Genetically determined (sometimes isolated branches) Posture (muscle imbalances/spasms)
Tumors	Primary tumors of brachial plexus Secondary involvement of plexus by tumors of surrounding tissues
Vascular factors	Local vascular processes or lesions Participation in generalized vasculopathies (e.g., polyarteritis nodosa and systemic lupus erythematosus)
Physical factors	Radiation therapy Electric shock
Infectious, inflammatory, and toxic processes	Involvement of local sepsis Viral or infectious
Cryptogenic causes (neuralgic amyotrophy)	Parainfectious injury Related to serum therapy Genetic predisposition Cryptogenic injury

Modified from Mumenthaler M, Narakas A, Gilliat RW: Brachial plexus disorders. In Dyck PJ, Thomas PK, Lambert EH, et al, editors: *Peripheral neuropathy,* Philadelphia, 1984, Saunders.

Supraclavicular Lesion

Isolated supraclavicular lesions affect the upper, middle, or lower trunks of the brachial plexus. However, Alnot[7] reported that 15% of supraclavicular lesions are double level—affecting two trunks—or combined supraclavicular and infraclavicular lesions. The mechanism of injury in supraclavicular injuries involves forceful traction to the upper extremity that results in preganglionic avulsion of the involved nerve roots.[8] These lesions occur when the arm is forced violently into abduction and the middle part of the plexus is blocked temporarily in the coracoid region. Terminal branches tear and concomitant supraclavicular lesions occur when the head is jerked violently to the opposite side. Entrapment may occur lower down in the plexus in the musculocutaneous nerve, which is tightly attached near the origin of the coracobrachialis muscle. Entrapment also may occur in the axillary nerve in the quadrilateral space behind the shoulder or the suprascapular nerve in the suprascapular notch.[7,9] Patients with supraclavicular lesions usually have a poorer prognosis because of the location of the nerve injury, and they are not usually surgical candidates.[8]

Upper Trunk Lesion

Erb's palsy or Duchenne-Erb paralysis involves the C5 and C6 roots of the brachial plexus.[9] Palsy of C5 and C6 affects the strength of deltoid, biceps, brachialis, infraspinatus, supraspinatus, and serratus anterior muscles. Also involved are the rhomboids, levator scapulae, and supinator muscles. Therefore, this injury causes severe restriction of movement at the shoulder and elbow joints. The patient is unable to abduct or externally rotate the shoulder. The patient cannot supinate the forearm because of weakness of the supinator muscle. Sensory involvement is usually confined along the deltoid muscle and the distribution of the musculocutaneous nerve. According to Comtet et al,[10] partial or total spontaneous recovery of traumatic Duchenne-Erb paralysis is a frequent occurrence. The delay between injury and reinnervation of the corresponding muscle varies from 3 to 24 months. Therefore, the patient should undergo long-term rehabilitation with periodic reevaluation.

Middle Trunk Lesion

The middle trunk receives innervation from the C7 nerve root and extends distally to form a major portion of the posterior cord.[10] The middle trunk offers a major neural contribution to the radial nerve. Therefore, a lesion affecting the middle trunk of the brachial plexus weakens the extensor muscles of the arm and forearm, excluding the brachioradialis, which receives primary innervation from the C6 nerve root. Sensory deficit occurs along the radial distribution of the posterior arm and forearm and along the dorsal radial aspect of the hand. Brunelli and Brunelli[11] reported that 11% of a total series of brachial plexus injuries were isolated lesions to the middle trunk. Trauma to the shoulder in an anteroposterior location produces middle trunk lesions.

Lower Trunk Lesion

The lower trunk of the brachial plexus receives innervation from nerve roots C7 and T1. Therefore, Dejerine-Klumpke paralysis or injury to the lower trunk affects motor control in the fingers and wrist. Whether the plexus is prefixed or postfixed determines the extent of disability. The intrinsic muscles of the hand are only slightly affected in a lesion involving a prefixed plexus, whereas paralysis of the flexors of the hand and forearm occurs in a lesion in a postfixed plexus.[12] Sensory deficit occurs along the ulnar border of the arm, forearm, and hand. As indicated previously, Horner's syndrome occurs with injury to the sympathetic fibers contained within the anterior primary ramus.[3]

Infraclavicular Lesion

Infraclavicular lesions include injuries to the cords or the individual peripheral nerves of the brachial plexus. In Alnot's group of 105 patients with infraclavicular brachial plexus injuries,[7] 90% of the cases were young people (15 to 30 years of age) who had been in a car or motorcycle accident. The causes of the injuries included the following: (1) anterior-medial shoulder dislocation, which caused most of the isolated lesions of the axillary nerve and the posterior cord; (2) violent downward and backward movement of the shoulder, which caused stretching of the plexus; and (3) complex trauma with multiple fractures of the clavicle, scapula, or upper extremity of the humerus, which caused diffuse lesions affecting multiple cords and terminal branches. Patients with lesions to the infraclavicular portions of the brachial plexus tend to have a better prognosis and are candidates for nerve grafting surgical procedures if spontaneous recovery does not occur.[8]

Lateral Cord Lesion

Alnot[7] rarely found injury to the lateral cord. Injuries to the musculocutaneous nerve and the lateral head of the median nerve result in a motor deficit consisting of palsy in elbow flexion and a deficit of muscle pronators in the forearm, wrist, and finger flexors. A proximal lesion injures the lateral pectoral nerve and results in partial or total palsy of the upper portion of the pectoralis major muscle. Sensory deficit occurs in the forearm and at the thumb level.

Medial Cord Lesion

Isolated injuries to the medial cord are rare. Instead, upper medioulnar injury results in palsy, which is total in the distribution of the ulnar nerve and only partial in the distribution of the median nerve. Motor deficits occur in the flexor pollicis longus muscle and the flexor digitorum profundus muscle of the index finger. Partial palsy of the lower portion of the pectoralis muscle results in injury to the medial pectoral nerve.[7]

Posterior Cord Lesion

A posterior cord lesion involves the areas of distribution of the radial, axillary, subscapular, and thoracodorsal nerves. The lesion results in weakness of the extensors in the arm, with impairment of medial rotation and elevation of the arm at the shoulder.

Peripheral Nerve Lesion

Common peripheral nerve or branch injuries include, but are not limited to, lesions of the long thoracic nerve, axillary nerve, dorsal scapular nerve, and suprascapular nerve. Chapter 4 reviews injuries to the dorsal scapular and suprascapular nerves.

Long Thoracic Nerve Lesion

The long thoracic nerve originates from the anterior primary rami of C5, C6, and C7 nerve roots after these nerves emerge from their respective intervertebral foramina. The nerve reaches the serratus anterior muscle by traversing the neck behind the brachial plexus cords, entering the medial aspect of the axilla, and continuing downward along the lateral wall of the thorax.[2] Although isolated injuries to the long thoracic nerve are rare, traumatic wounds or traction injuries to the neck that result in isolated weakness of the serratus anterior muscle with winging of the medial border of the scapula are presumptive evidence of a long thoracic nerve lesion.[3] Normal shoulder abduction and flexion result from a synchronized pattern of movements between scapular rotation and humeral bone elevation. Variations in the scapulohumeral rhythm in the literature have been reported.[16-19] For every 15° of abduction of the arm, 10° occurs at the glenohumeral joint and 5° occurs from the rotation of the scapula along the posterior thoracic wall.[16] The rotation of the scapula results from a force couple mechanism combining the upward pull of the upper trapezius muscle, the downward pull of the lower trapezius muscle, and the outward pull of the serratus anterior muscle.[19] Therefore, palsy of the serratus anterior muscle in the presence of a long thoracic nerve injury, during abduction or flexion of the arm, results in partial loss of scapular rotation. The ability of the upper and lower trapezius muscles to compensate temporarily for the inability of the serratus anterior muscle to rotate the scapula externally allows for nearly full range (180°) flexion and abduction of the arm.[20] However, these muscles quickly fatigue after four or five repetitions, and the results are notable losses of full active shoulder flexion and abduction range of motion.

Axillary Nerve Lesion

The axillary nerve originates from spinal segments C5 and C6, travels to the distal aspect of the posterior cord of the brachial plexus, and advances laterally through the axilla.[2] The nerve bends around the posterior aspect of the surgical neck of the humerus to innervate the deltoid muscle and the overlying skin, as well as the teres minor muscle.

Anterior-medial shoulder dislocation is the most frequent cause of isolated axillary nerve lesions.[6,9] In 80% of cases, anterior-medial dislocation results in neurapraxia of the axillary nerve, with total recovery in 4 to 6 months.[7]

A complete lesion of the axillary nerve results in loss of active shoulder abduction. Sensory changes include an area of anesthesia along the deltoid muscle. However, some patients may have active shoulder abduction and external rotation in the presence of a total axillary nerve lesion. Residual shoulder abduction results from the actions of the supraspinatus and infraspinatus muscles, as well as the biceps muscle. The stabilization of the humeral head by the supraspinatus muscle combined with the action of the long head of the biceps muscle allows full overhead abduction in some cases. Specifically, by externally rotating the arm, the patient places the long head of the biceps muscle in the line of abduction pull. However, the strength of abduction under these conditions is poor, and loss of muscle power occurs quickly with repetitive movements.

PATHOMECHANICS OF TRAUMATIC INJURIES TO THE NERVES

According to Stevens,[21] traction or tensile strains produce most traumatic injuries to the brachial plexus. The brachial plexus stretches between two firm points of attachment: the transverse processes proximally and the clavipectoral fascia junction distally in the upper axilla. Stevens compared the cords of the plexus to a traction apparatus with a neutral axis at the C7 vertebra when the arm is at the horizontal position.

Specifically, Stevens compared the brachial plexus (Fig. 8-6) to a single cord with five separate points of attachment firmly snubbed at the transverse processes. According to Stevens, a traction apparatus must have a neutral axis and a line of resistance. When the force of traction falls through this neutral center of axis at the C7 vertebra, the traction is equally borne by all parts of the apparatus, as represented by nerve roots C5 through T1. A slight deviation from this neutral axis creates an unequal pull to one side or the other of the apparatus. In other words, if the line of traction falls outside the neutral axis of C7, the entire force is transmitted from the neutral axis, and all tension is released on the cords on the other side. Therefore, when tension is imparted to an arm elevated above the horizontal, stress is increased to the lower roots of the brachial plexus. Conversely, when tension is imparted to an arm depressed below the horizontal, stress is increased to the upper

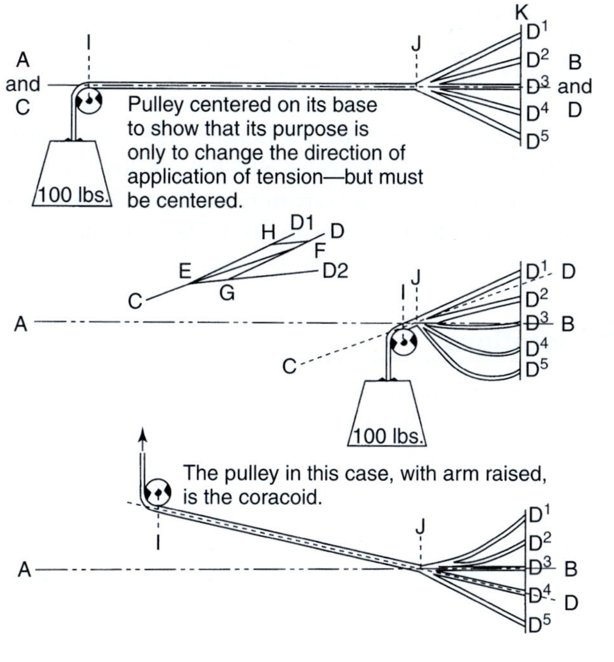

Figure 8-6 Traction apparatus representing the brachial plexus. (From Stevens JH: Brachial plexus paralysis. In Codman EA, editor: *The shoulder,* Melbourne, Australia, 1991, Krieger.)

roots of the brachial plexus (see Fig. 8-6).[21] In this way, the relative position of the shoulder and neck at the time of injury dictates the area and extent of the injury to the brachial plexus.

In addition to the position of the shoulder and neck, that magnitude of force affects the nature of a brachial plexus injury. Spinner et al[22] reported a substantial correlation between the experimental test weight imparted to restrained limbs in rats and the number of avulsed nerve roots. A lower force produced a higher percentage of avulsions at C6, whereas a higher force produced a higher number of avulsions at C7 and C8.

MUSCULOSKELETAL INJURIES

As previously mentioned, most brachial plexus injuries result from trauma, are complications of musculoskeletal injuries, or have viral or infectious causes. Examples of these injuries include the burner syndrome, shoulder dislocations, fractures, and obstetric injuries.

Burner Syndrome

The burner or stinger syndrome is one of the most common type of sports injuries that occur to the upper trunk of the brachial plexus.[9,13-15] This injury may occur secondary to traction in the brachial plexus when an athlete sustains a lateral flexion injury to the neck. Specifically, the syndrome results from an abrupt change in the neck and shoulder angle—as experienced by football players making a tackle—with depression of the shoulder and rotation of the neck to the contralateral shoulder.[9,13,14] Markey et al[13] reported a mechanism of injury in the area of Erb's point when a shoulder pad compressed the fixed brachial plexus and the superior medial scapula. Regardless of the mechanism of injury in burner syndrome, at the time of injury the athlete relates a stinging or burning pain, radiating from the shoulder into the arm.[13,14] Severe injury may result in cervical root avulsion.

Most burner injuries are self-limiting and resolve within minutes of the insult. Potential problems include persistent neck tenderness and upper extremity weakness. If these problems continue, electromyography should be performed at 3 to 4 weeks to test for serious nerve damage.[12-14]

Dislocations

Injuries to the brachial plexus can occur because of shoulder dislocation. The incidence of secondary brachial plexus injury after shoulder dislocation ranges from 2% to 35%, according to most literature. Guven et al[23] reported the unhappy triad at the shoulder of concomitant shoulder dislocation, rotator cuff tear, and brachial plexus injury. Axillary nerve injury sometimes occurs with acute anterior dislocation of the humeral head. Wang et al[24] described a case with concomitant mixed brachial plexus injury in the presence of inferior dislocation of the glenohumeral joint. Travlos et al[25] classified brachial plexus lesions caused by shoulder dislocation into diffuse infraclavicular, posterior cord, lateral cord, and medial cord injuries. The type of injury partly depends on the mechanism of injury and the direction of dislocation of the humeral head.

Fractures

Brachial plexus injuries occur with traumatic injuries associated with fractures of the shoulder girdle and humerus bones. Della Santa et al[26] reported 16 cases of costoclavicular syndrome related to compression of the subclavian artery and brachial plexus because of callus and scar formation as a result of fractures of the clavicle. Stromqvist et al[27] reported three cases of injury to the axillary artery and brachial plexus that complicated a displaced proximal fracture of the humerus. Blom and Dahlback[28] reported on 2 cases in a group of 31 cases of proximal humeral fractures with brachial plexus injuries. Silliman and Dean[9] reported suprascapular nerve injury as a complication of scapular fractures around the scapular spine.

Obstetric Lesions

van Ouwerkerk et al[29] reported that obstetric brachial plexus lesions occur in 0.5 to 3 of every 1000 live births. Most infants (75% to 90%) recover spontaneously within weeks or a few months, but 20% have incomplete recoveries. Risk factors include large or heavy babies, shoulder dystocia, instrument delivery, abnormal presentation, prematurity, and asphyxia. *Dystocia* refers to difficult births, and *shoulder dystocia* refers to abnormality of an infant's shoulder because of a difficult birth.

The most common mechanism is a stretch injury to the brachial plexus in cephalic presentations resulting in extreme lateral flexion and traction on the head. Lesions may produce either partial or full paralysis of the limb, depending on the level and extent of nerve root injury. Injuries may also include the following: hematomas to the sternocleidomastoid muscle; fracture of the clavicle, humerus, or ribs; lesions of the phrenic, facial, or hypoglossal nerves; and lesions of the spinal cord.

Physical therapy should begin within 3 weeks. The goal is to prevent contracture and joint deformities. The physical therapist instructs parents to perform gentle but frequent exercises to maintain full motion of the involved shoulder, elbow, wrist, and fingers. If spontaneous recovery does not occur within 2 months, referral to a specialized center is recommended. Failure to recover muscle function and evidence of severe Horner's syndrome after 3 months indicate likely avulsion of nerve roots. The diagnosis is confirmed by magnetic resonance imaging (MRI), myelographic computed tomography, and neurophysiologic studies. Surgical treatment is indicated for patients with nerve root avulsion.

Viral and Other Infectious Agents

The onset of acute brachial neuritis was first described by Spilane in 1943. Acute brachial neuritis is an uncommon disorder of unspecified origin. The clinical presentation can often be mistaken for cervical radiculopathy because shoulder and upper extremity pain, burning, and weakness are hallmarks of both disorders; however, the clinical manifestations vary in the sequential onset of symptoms.

Acute brachial neuritis has been referred to as "acute shoulder neuritis," "Parsonage-Turner syndrome," and "acute brachial plexitis." Plausible explanations of the onset of brachial neuritis include viral infection in 25% of cases and hepatitis B vaccinations. Most cases affect individuals between 20 and 60 years of age, with a strong male predominance from 2:1 to 11.5:1. The clinical manifestation of acute brachial neuritis includes a severe, insidious onset of burning pain of the affected shoulder and upper extremity. Over the course of several days, the severity of the pain decreases, and shoulder and upper extremity weakness, which begins abruptly, becomes the predominant clinical finding. The nerves of the upper brachial plexus are more often involved, with resulting weakness of the supraspinatus, infraspinatus, and deltoid muscles. However, cases involving mononeuritis have also been reported.

The diagnosis of acute brachial neuritis can be obtained by the clinical history and presentation with electromyographic and nerve conduction studies. The data from electromyographic studies for the diagnosis of brachial neuritis can be variable but more often include fibrillation potentials and positive waves suggestive of muscle denervation. MRI reveals an area of increased intensity within the involved muscles on T2-weighted images. Strength of the involved muscles typically returns 3 to 4 months after the initial onset of symptoms. Treatment during the recovery phase often includes analgesics or narcotics for pain management and physical therapy to improve range of motion, strength, and functional recovery.[30]

TUMORS OF THE BRACHIAL PLEXUS

Tumors arising from the nerves of the brachial plexus are rare. In a systematic review of primary neurogenic tumors over a 29-year period, 49% occurred within the nerve, 37% occurred within the neural sheath, and 14% were malignant peripheral nerve sheath tumors (MPNSTs).[31] Approximately 20% of tumors that affect peripheral nerves occur within the brachial plexus. Secondary tumors from anatomic sources external to the brachial plexus, such as apical tumors of the lung, osteosarcomas, and breast tumors, are more common.[32] An example of a secondary tumor that can affect the function of the brachial plexus is Pancoast's tumor. Pancoast's tumors are bronchogenic tumors that arise in the apex of the lung and can extend into the surrounding soft tissue to include the subclavian vessels, sympathetic chain, ribs, and spine. Bronchogenic tumors originate in the apex of the lung in the periphery; therefore, upper extremity symptoms are often early clinical manifestations that precede respiratory symptoms.[33]

Tumors of the brachial plexus can be classified by location, epidemiology, and pathogenesis of the lesion based on radiographic studies. The anatomic location of a lesion can assist in the differential assessment of a brachial plexus tumor. Tumors that arise from neural tissue follow the anatomic plane of the nerve. For instance, a tumor affecting the nerve trunk follows a superior-medial to inferior-lateral direction and lies between the anterior and middle scalene muscle. Tumors that are vertical on imaging studies are more likely to originate from surrounding anatomic structures. Neurogenic tumors tend to be oval, they follow the longitudinal axis of the nerve, and they can be differentiated based on the location within the nerve.[32]

Tumors of the brachial plexus can be benign or malignant. Primary neurogenic tumors that affect the peripheral nerve are benign in 85% to 90% of cases.[32] Neurofibromas and schwannomas are two types of benign, primary neurogenic tumors that affect the brachial plexus. Schwannomas develop from the Schwann cell of the nerve. Schwannomas are encapsulated tumors within the periphery that do not extend into the neural fascicles of the axon. Neurofibromas occur within the fascicles of the nerve and can interrupt neural conduction or damage the structure of the nerve. These types of primary neurogenic tumors have a high incidence in patients with neurofibromatosis type 1 (NF1).[32,33] MPNSTs are less common and comprise 14% of clinical cases over a 29-year period. MPNSTs are more prevalent in patients with neurofibromas associated with NF1 in the third of fourth decade of life. In the general population, MPNSTs are more prevalent in the seventh decade of life, with an incidence of 0.001%. The pathogenesis of MPNST remains inconclusive; however, these neural tumors have been thought to arise from Schwann cells. MPNSTs have been shown to arise 5 to 10 years following radiation treatments for disorders relating to Hodgkin's disease.[33]

Differential assessment of primary neurogenic tumors is performed using MRI. No standard MRI technique exists for identifying neural tumors, although a T1-weighted spin echo image, a short T1 inversion recovery (STIR) sequence, and a T2-weighted fat-suppressed sequence are adequate in the radiologic assessment of peripheral nerve tumors. The characteristics of benign, primary neurogenic tumors on MRI include a well-circumscribed, oval mass with the long axis of the tumor following the anatomic course of the nerve fibers. On T1-weighted imaging, a benign tumor has a homogeneous appearance with intermediate signal intensity. On T2-weighted imaging, a benign tumor has a heterogeneous appearance, with a peripheral margin of hyperintensity caused by the presence of myxoid tissue with a central hypointense area representative of fibrocollagenous tissue.[32]

The clinical presentation of peripheral nerve tumors includes pain in the involved upper extremity, paresthesias, numbness, tingling, palpable mass, muscle weakness, atrophy, or loss of neurologic function.[32,34] The clinical manifestations of malignant tumors can include the aforementioned signs and symptoms in addition to night pain that prevents the patient from sleeping and pain that is resistant to opiate medication.[34]

PATHOPHYSIOLOGY OF INJURY

The extent of injury to the nerve trunk, ranging from nondegenerative neurapraxia to severance of the nerve or plexus (neurotmesis), dictates the course of treatment, (surgical versus nonsurgical), the prognosis, and relative time frames for full recovery.

Sunderland[35] described five major degrees of injuries:

1. *First-degree nerve injury.* This injury is characterized by interruption of conduction at the site of the injury with preservation of the anatomic continuity of all components comprising the nerve trunk, including the axon. Clinical features include temporary loss of motor function in the affected muscles, but the presence of electric potential is retained because of axonal continuity. Cutaneous sensory loss may occur but recovers in advance of motor function. Most patients recover spontaneously within 6 weeks after injury.
2. *Second-degree nerve injury.* In this injury, the axon is severed and fails to survive below the level of injury, and, for a variable but short distance, the axon degenerates proximal to the point of the lesion. However, the endoneurium is preserved within the endoneurial tube. Histologic changes to the nerve include breakdown of the myelin sheath, Schwann cell degeneration, and phagocytic activity with eventual fibrosis. Clinical features include temporary complete loss of motor, sensory, and sympathetic functions in the autonomous distribution of the injured nerve. Several months pass before recovery begins, with proximal reinnervation occurring before distal reinnervation to the involved muscles.
3. *Third-degree nerve injury.* This condition is characterized by axonal disintegration, wallerian degeneration both distal and proximal to the site of the lesion, and disorganization of the internal structure of the endoneurial fasciculi. The general fascicular pattern of the nerve trunk is retained with minimal damage to both the perineurium and the epineurium. Because the endoneurial tube is destroyed, intrafascicular fibrosis may obviate axonal regeneration. Many axons fail to reach their original or functionally related endoneurial tubes and are instead misdirected into foreign endoneurial tubes. Motor, sensory, and sympathetic functions of the related nerves are lost. The recovery is long, up to 2 to 3 years, with a chance of notable residual dysfunction.
4. *Fourth-degree nerve injury.* This type of injury is similar to third-degree nerve injury, but the perineurium is disrupted. Therefore, the chance is high for residual dysfunction because of fibrosis and mixing of regenerating fibers at the site of injury, which may distort the normal pattern of innervation.
5. *Fifth-degree nerve injury.* In this injury, the entire nerve trunk is severed, and the result is the complete loss of function of the affected structures. Obviously, without surgical grafting, the recovery potential is negligible.

PATIENT MANAGEMENT

The five elements of patient management in the *Guide* are examination (history, systems review, and tests and measures), evaluation, diagnosis, prognosis (including patient care and expected number of visits), and interventions (including anticipated goals and expected outcomes).

The clinician evaluates the nature and extent of the brachial plexus lesion, to develop an appropriate and effective intervention using a thorough and systematic examination. Most brachial plexus lesions slowly improve over a long period of time, so the clinician must maintain and update accurate records concerning the progress of the patient. The clinician should use a chart like that shown in Figure 8-7 for recording results of the physical examination. Patient management is a joint effort by a physical and an occupational therapist that specializes in the treatment of hand and upper extremity injuries. Knowledge of hand management and rehabilitation is particularly important in patients with lower trunk injuries to the brachial plexus. Additionally, in the presence of fourth- and fifth-degree nerve injuries to the brachial plexus, occupational therapy offers strategies for splinting and equipment modification or assurance to assist permanently dysfunctional individuals.

History

Mechanisms of Injury

Because most brachial plexus injuries result from trauma, a thorough history should include questions concerning the nature and mechanisms of injury. According to Stevens,[21] the different varieties of stress and the relative position of the arm and head at the time of the stress make tremendous differences in the kinds of lesions suffered, in the location of the lesion, and in prognosis. The magnitude of forces, that is, high-speed versus slow-speed injuries, is important to ascertain. According to Framptom,[6] high-speed, large-impact accidents are commonly associated with preganglionic plexus injuries, whereas slow-speed, small-impact accidents are commonly associated with postganglionic injuries. An example of high-velocity injury is a fall from a speeding motorcycle, and an example of low-velocity injury is a fall down a stairway.

Pain

The clinician should document the area and nature of pain. Pain, described as a constant burning, crushing pain with sudden shooting paroxysms, is central. This pain results from deafferentation of the spinal cord at the damaged root level and leads to undampened excitation of the cells in the dorsal horn of the spinal cord. The confused barrage of abnormal firings is received and interpreted centrally as pain and is eventually felt in the dermatomes of the avulsed nerve root.[36] In a group of 188 patients with post-traumatic brachial plexus lesions, Bruxelle et al[36] reported that 91% experienced pain for at least 3 years after the injury. Pain may also result from secondary injuries to bones or related soft tissues. The clinician should note and document the report of any anesthesia or paresthesia, including the presence of Horner's syndrome. Questions concerning the course of events since injury or a change in the severity of the symptoms establish whether a lesion is improving or worsening. A condition that is resolving

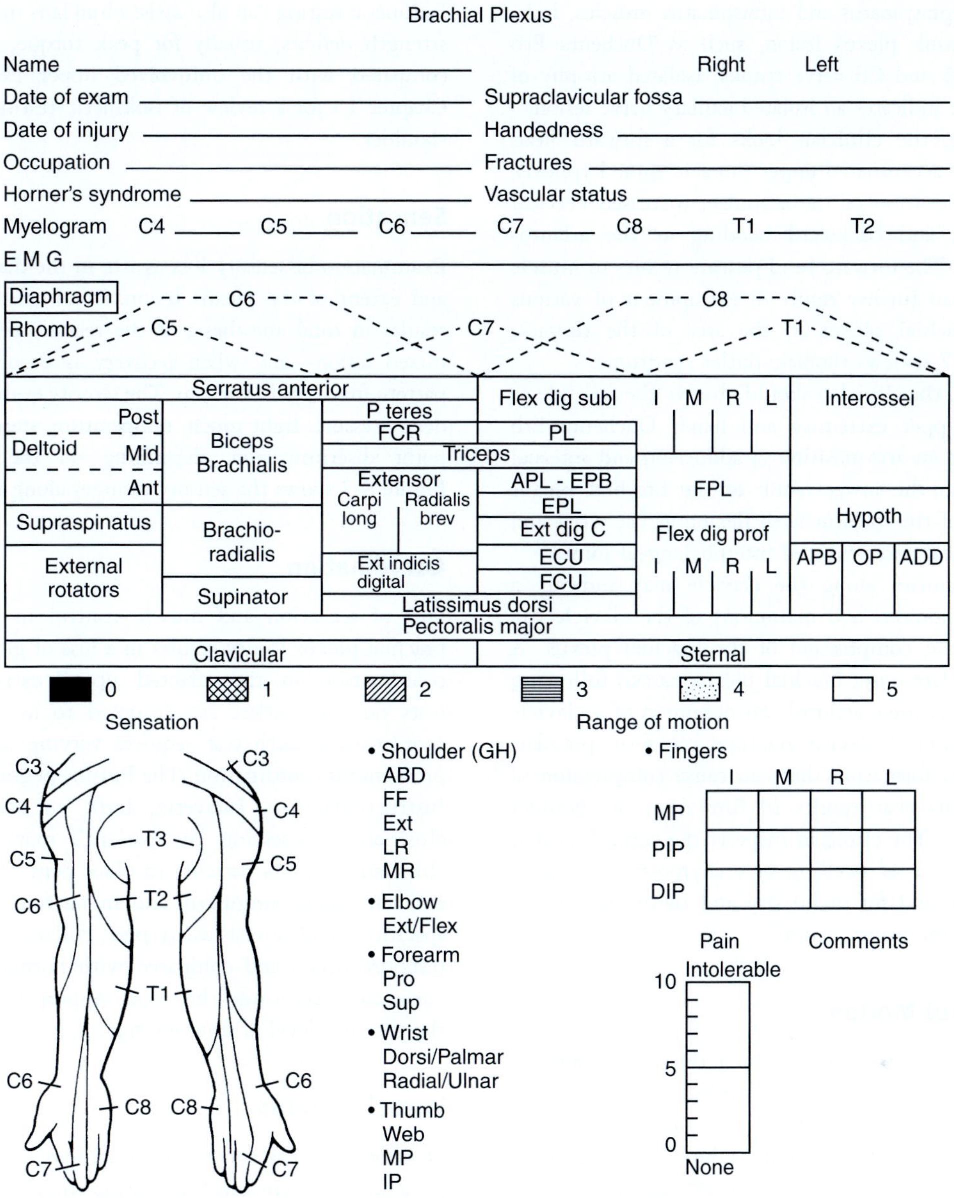

Figure 8-7 Chart for recording results of physical examination for brachial plexus injury. (From Leffert RD: Clinical diagnosis, testing, and electromyographic study in brachial plexus traction injuries, *Clin Orthop Relat Res* 237:24, 1988.)

spontaneously may indicate first- or second-degree nerve injuries, whereas a condition that has not changed for 6 weeks may indicate at least a third-degree nerve injury, according to Sunderland's classification. The clinician should record the patient's occupation, handedness, and previous state of health, to assist in establishing feasible goals for return to the patient's premorbid activity level.

Tests and Measures

The components of the physical examination include the following: (1) posture; (2) passive range of motion of the cervical spine, shoulder, and upper extremity; (3) motor strength; (4) sensation; (5) palpation; and (6) special tests. The occupational therapy evaluation includes assessment of (1) edema, (2) coordination, (3) activities of daily living, and (4) vocational and avocational pursuits. The physical evaluation should be repeated frequently during the process of rehabilitation, for careful assessment of subtle signs of nerve reinnervation.

Posture

The clinician observes the patient from the front, side, and behind. From behind, the clinician looks for muscle atrophy and "winging" of the scapula. Winging of the scapula signifies weakness of the serratus anterior muscle, which may indicate a lesion of the long thoracic nerve. Suprascapular nerve entrapment results in ipsilateral atrophy of the supraspinatus or infraspinatus muscles. Atrophy of the deltoid muscle, in addition to the supraspinatus and infraspinatus muscles, indicates an upper trunk plexus lesion, such as Duchenne-Erb paralysis of the C5 and C6 nerve trunks. Isolated atrophy of the deltoid muscle indicates an isolated axillary nerve lesion.

From the side, the clinician looks for a forward head posture, including accentuated upper thoracic spine kyphosis, protraction and elevation of the scapulae, increased cervical spine inclination, and backward bending at the atlanto-occipital junction. The forward head posture results in muscle imbalances that can further result in entrapment of various nerves of the brachial plexus in the area of the thoracic outlet.[37] Chapter 7 reviews thoracic outlet syndrome.

From the front, the clinician should observe the attitude or position of the upper extremity and hand. Duchenne-Erb paralysis results in an arm position of adduction and internal rotation. Injury to the lower trunk of the brachial plexus causes pronation of the forearm with flexion at the wrist and metacarpophalangeal and proximal interphalangeal joints.[9]

External deformities along the clavicle may indicate a fracture. Both nonunions and malunions of the clavicle can result in substantial compression of the brachial plexus. A common cause of late-onset brachial plexus paresis following a traumatic event is pseudarthrosis on nonunion of a clavicle fracture.[38] Nonunion of clavicle fractures can form pseudarthrosis with callus formation that can cause compression of the brachial plexus that results in limitation of shoulder motion and pain.[39] The clinician inspects the supraclavicular fossa for the presence of swelling or ecchymosis in patients with recent injury and for nodularity and induration in the brachial plexus if the injury is old.[6]

Passive Range of Motion

A standard goniometer is used to evaluate the passive range of motion of all joints of the shoulder girdle and upper limb. Deficits of joint motion from immobility result in contracture of the joint capsule, adhesions in the joints, and shortening of both muscle and tendons above the affected joints. The classic studies of Akeson et al[40] demonstrated the deleterious effects of 9 weeks of immobilization on periarticular structures, including the loss of water and glycosaminoglycan, randomization and abnormal cross-linking of newly synthesized collagen, and infiltration in the joint spaces of fatty fibrous materials.

Motor Strength

Several manuals are available that review proper isolation, stabilization, and grading procedures for manual muscle testing.[41,42] Most grading systems grade muscle from 0 to 5, with 0 being a flaccid muscle and 5 representing normal muscle strength.[42] The clinician should complete an upper extremity test to establish a database for measuring improvement. Therefore, the clinician performs repeated tests. A thorough manual muscle test assists the clinician in pinpointing the site and extent of the plexus lesion. Isolating and grading involved muscles help to establish an appropriate strengthening program. Isokinetic testing can also assist clinicians in measuring muscle strength deficits, usually for peak torque, power, and work, compared with the uninvolved upper extremity. Refer to Chapter 15 for a review of isokinetic testing protocols in the shoulder.

Sensation

Examination of sensory loss assists in the diagnosis of the level and extent of the plexus lesion. Total avulsion of the plexus results in total anesthesia of the related areas. However, in a mixed lesion—and when recovery is occurring—the sensory pattern may vary in the arm. The sensory evaluation may include deep pressure, light touch, temperature, stereognosis, and two-point discrimination, depending on the patient's status.[6] Figure 8-7 shows the sensory changes along dermatomes.

Coordination

Loss of sensation and muscle control in the presence of a brachial plexus injury results in a loss of gross and fine motor coordination in the affected upper extremity. Numerous tests on the market are designed to assess an individual's coordination. Each test requires varying amounts of fine or gross motor coordination. The Purdue pegboard test (Lafayette Instructional Co., Lafayette, Ind), for example, assists the clinician in assessing the patient's manual dexterity. The clinician instructs patients to place pegs with both the right and left hands, singularly and in tandem, and to perform a specific assembly task using pins, collars, and washers. These tests are timed and compared with normative values.[43] The clinician determines the most appropriate tests based on the patient's level of functioning.

Vascular Status

Disruption of the subclavian or axillary arteries occurs in the presence of severe brachial plexus injuries, particularly with associated fractures of the clavicle. The axillary artery can also become damaged with a posterior dislocation or fracture of the humerus. The degree of damage to the axillary artery with an anterior dislocation injury depends on the tautness of the artery as it exits laterally from the pectoralis minor. The mechanisms for most anterior shoulder dislocations occur with the glenohumeral joint in abduction and external rotation, a position that also places increased tension on the axillary artery. The portion of the axillary artery that is more predisposed to injury is the proximal division of the anterior circumflex artery. In an anterior shoulder dislocation, as the humerus is directed anteriorly, the axillary artery is also forced in an anterior direction, thus placing the artery as risk for disruption. Risk factors associated with axillary arterial injury include an older age of the patient (86% of patients are more than 50 years old) and recurring glenohumeral dislocation (27% of previous cases).[8]

Trauma to the axillary artery can also occur on relocation of an anterior glenohumeral dislocation. The incidence of arterial injury is also elevated in patients who are older and who have a history of a chronic glenohumeral dislocation. Axillary arterial damage can also occur in complex proximal humeral fractures with sequelae including a mass within the shoulder region. In the case of shoulder trauma with acute dislocation, the presence of distal upper extremity pulses does not eliminate the potential for poor arterial perfusion to the limb. Arterial damage can occur through intimal tearing, intra-arterial thrombus formation, or avulsion of a collateral branch of the arterial supply to the upper extremity. Venous damage can also cause signs of upper extremity edema and pain. In the case of suspected vascular injury, immediate referral to a specialist for a surgical consultation should be made, to prevent permanent nerve or ischemic damage to the upper limb.[8] Additionally, all patients who have had a substantial nerve injury have evidence of vasomotor changes.[3] The clinician inspects for dusky, cool skin indicating venous insufficiency and assesses the brachial and radial pulses.

The axillary artery can also become damaged by blunt trauma to the shoulder region with delayed onset of brachial plexus injury. Case studies have reported the development of a compressive hematoma formation following traumatic injury to the axillary artery. Murata et al[44] presented a case study in which a 16-year-old boy was evaluated for right shoulder pain following a motorbike accident. The clinical findings for this patient included generalized tenderness of the right shoulder and axillary regions, sensory deficit over the lateral aspect of the right arm, and active elevation of the right shoulder greater than 90°. Radiographic imaging revealed a nondisplaced fracture of the distal of the clavicle, without evidence of humeral fracture of glenohumeral dislocation. On physical examination, the patient had no focal motor weakness and no additional sensory deficits, and the radial and ulnar arteries were patent to palpation. The patient was diagnosed with axillary nerve palsy. Two days later, the patient developed swelling in his right arm with complete motor paralysis of his right upper extremity. An MRI scan of the right shoulder indicated the formation of a compressive hematoma measuring 4 by 5 cm that had developed between the subscapularis and the pectoralis minor. Angiography of the right axillary artery confirmed complete obliteration of the axillary artery and compression of the brachial plexus from the development of the compressive hematoma. An emergency surgical procedure was performed to evacuate the hematoma, with revascularization of the axillary artery. The patient had an excellent return to his previous functional activity without motor or sensory impairments.[44]

Edema

The clinician looks for edema, which can cause pain in the joints. Volumetrics are an established and accurate method to measure upper extremity edema. The clinician submerges the patient's hand in a Lucite container (Volumeter, Volumeters Unlimited, Idyllwild, Calif), and measures the amount of water displaced using a 500-mL graduated cylinder. Both extremities should be measured and the results recorded. Circumferential measurements of the hand and forearm are another method of measuring edema. This technique, however, is best suited for individual digit swelling or in open wounds, although open wounds may keep the patient from getting the extremity wet. Manual palpation is also used to measure edema. The severity of the edema is usually rated from 1 to 3, with 1 being minimal edema and 3 being severe or pitting edema.

Palpation

Manual palpation examines the patient for the presence of myofascial trigger points about the affected shoulder girdle and upper extremity musculature. Trigger points result from tight and contracted muscles or from partially denervated muscles that exhibit poor muscle control and altered movement patterns. Active trigger points refer pain into the affected upper extremity and the shoulder girdle, neck, and head.[45,46]

Special Tests

The presence of Tinel's sign, revealed by tapping over the brachial plexus above the clavicle, can be quite useful in distinguishing ruptures from a lesion in continuity.[3,6] Distal Tinel's sign indicates a lesion in continuity with intact axonal connections within the nerve trunk. This lesion may correspond to a first-degree nerve injury or a regenerating second- or third-degree nerve injury. Conversely, the presence of localized tenderness, revealed by tapping above the clavicle, indicates a possible neuroma resulting from disruption of part of the plexus. This type of injury corresponds to a fourth- or fifth-degree nerve injury. A significant change in blood pressure between the involved and uninvolved upper extremity could indicate damage to the proximal arteries of the shoulder girdle.[44]

Activities of Daily Living

The clinician questions the patient regarding all aspects of self-care to identify those specific tasks that the patient is not able to perform because of the extent of the brachial plexus injury. Such areas include feeding, bathing, grooming, and dressing. Based on the specific limitations of the patient, the occupational therapist determines whether to provide the patient with specific adaptive equipment or to instruct the patient in one-handed techniques.

Functional outcome measures are used at the initiation and throughout the rehabilitation process to determine a change in a patient's level of functioning. Four commonly used questionnaires that assess functional outcome measures are the DASH (Disabilities of the Arm, Shoulder, and Hand), the ASES (American Shoulder and Elbow Surgeons score), the SPADI (Shoulder Pain and Disability Index), and the SST (Simple Shoulder Test). A systematic review was conducted to assess the psychometric properties of each questionnaire.[47] All four functional outcome measures have been shown to have good test-rest reliability, and the construct convergent validity is high among the four instruments ($r \geq .70$). The responsiveness of each questionnaire depends on the patient population.

For example, the SPADI has better responsiveness in patients following rotator cuff surgery (SRM = 1.23) and in patients treated for shoulder impingement (SRM = 1.08; ES = 1.06). The value for the SRM is defined as the mean change in score divided by the standard deviation of the change in the score. The effect size (ES) is defined as the mean change in the score divided by the standard deviation of the pre-treatment score. The SPADI and the ASES have been shown to have superior responsiveness in patients following shoulder arthroplasty compared with the other shoulder questionnaires. The ASES and the SPADI are the more appropriate outcome measures for assessing pain and physical function, whereas the DASH is more beneficial to use if social and emotional constructs are to be evaluated.[47]

Assessment for Splinting

In the case of a complete brachial plexus injury, the occupational therapist fits the patient with a flail arm splint, which allows the patient to use the extremity at home and at work. The occupational therapist fits the splint early to prevent the patient from relying on one-handed methods as a means of performing specific activities.[6] In the case of a C5 to C7 injury, the patient may require a long-wrist and finger-extension assist splint (Fig. 8-8A). The occupational therapist may fit the patient with a resting-hand splint (see Fig. 8-8B) to wear at night to help maintain the wrist and fingers in a balanced position.

Vocational Issues

The occupational therapist obtains a detailed job description to assess the patient's potential to return to work. In addition, the patient may undergo a functional capacity examination later in the rehabilitation process to assess his or her physical demand level.

Avocational Issues

Because the brachial plexus–injured patient is unable to work, avocational pursuits are often an important source of much needed diversion. The occupational therapist questions the patient closely about premorbid hobbies or potential areas of interest. The occupational therapist develops activities of interest that encourage use of the affected extremity.

Laboratory Evaluations of Brachial Plexus Lesions

Laboratory evaluation involves electrodiagnostic testing, myelography, and radiographic assessment. These evaluations help the clinician diagnose the area and extent of the lesion and provide baseline measurements to help evaluate progress.

Radiographic Assessment

Every patient who has sustained a notable injury to the brachial plexus should have a complete radiographic series of the cervical spine and involved shoulder girdle, including the clavicle.[3] The physician rules out fractures of the clavicle with callus, which can impinge on the nerve trunks along the costoclavicular juncture, or fractures of the cervical transverse processes, which can indicate a root avulsion.[3,6]

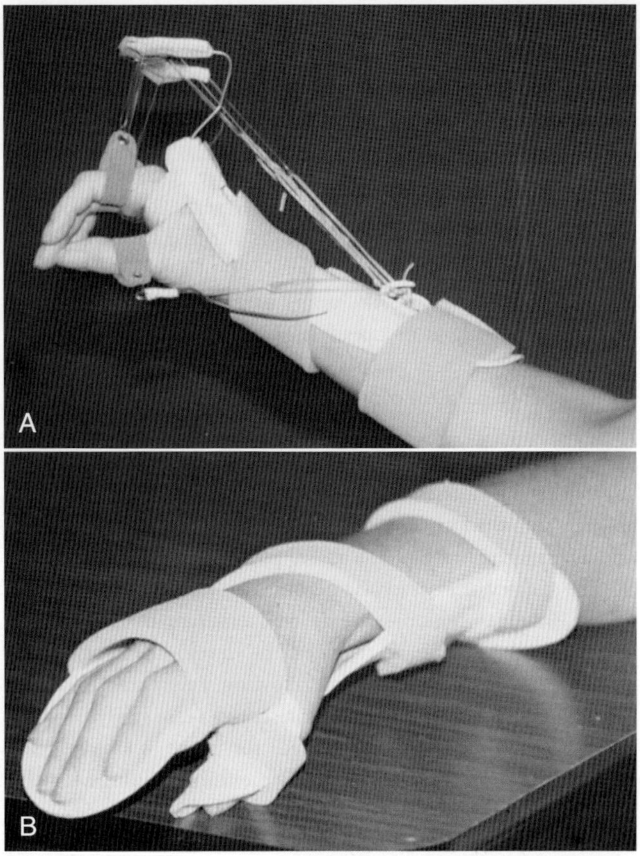

Figure 8-8 Splints. **A,** A long metacarpophalangeal extension splint used with a patient who has weak wrist extension and trace finger extension. **B,** A resting-hand splint used following a brachial plexus lesion to prevent overstretching of weak and finger extensor muscles by maintaining the wrist in approximately 20° of dorsiflexion.

MRI detects injuries to the brachial plexus. Bilbey et al[48] reported on 64 consecutive patients with suspected brachial plexus abnormalities of diverse causes that were diagnosed using MRI. MRI is 63% sensitive, 100% specific, and 73% accurate in demonstrating the abnormality in a diverse patient population with multiple causes of brachial plexus injuries. MRI is a useful diagnostic tool because of the multiplanar views and the ability to provide excellent delineation of the soft tissues that surround the brachial plexus. The anatomic structure of the brachial plexus is best viewed on a T1-weighted image with visualization in the axial and coronal views. The sagittal oblique view is the ideal view in which to visualize the trunks, divisions, cords, and terminal branches of the plexus. A normal anatomic finding of the nerve on a T1-weighted, transverse view is a rounded appearance of the nerve with the patterned architecture of the intraneural fascicles. The general appearance of the fascicles on T1-weighted imaging shows diffuse hypointense fascicles with hyperintense fibrofatty connective tissue surrounding the nerve.[39]

Myelography

Myelography identifies the condition of the nerve roots involved in traction injuries to the brachial plexus. According to Leffert,[3] root avulsion can be present in patients with a normal myelogram. However, Yeoman[49] indicated the efficacy of myelography as a valuable adjunct in the diagnosis of brachial plexus root lesions.

Electromyography

Because the loss of axonal continuity results in predictable, time-related electrical charges, knowledge and assessment of these electrical charges provide clinicians with information concerning muscle denervation and reinnervation.[3] For example, whereas normally innervated muscle exhibits no spontaneous electrical activity at rest with needle electrodes, denervated muscle produces readily recognizable small potentials (fibrillation) or large potentials (sharp waves), which are the hallmarks of denervation. These electrical discharges usually appear 3 weeks following injury to the plexus and signal the onset of wallerian degeneration of a specific nerve. The clinician localizes the lesion by sampling muscles innervated by different nerves and root levels.

The clinician should also perform an electromyographic evaluation of the posterior cervical musculature when root avulsion is suspected in a patient who has sustained a traction injury of the brachial plexus. The posterior cervical muscles are segmentally innervated by the posterior primary rami of the spinal nerves that provide the anterior primary rami to form the plexus. Denervation of the deep posterior cervical muscles is highly correlated with root avulsion. Conversely, if the electromyographic results are positive for the muscles innervated by the anterior primary rami, but not for the posterior cervical muscles, the clinician should suspect that whatever possible damage exists is infraganglionic.[50]

Nerve Conduction Studies

Nerve conduction velocity tests help to distinguish muscular weakness in the affected upper extremity from cervical intervertebral disk protrusion, anterior horn cell disease, or a brachial plexus lesion. Because anterior horn cell diseases and intervertebral disk protrusions do not influence nerve conduction latency, the clinician can be certain that a proximal nerve conduction delay is the result of a brachial plexus lesion.[51]

Another type of electrodiagnostic testing is the F response, an outgrowth of the measurement of velocity of conduction. This is a late reaction that potentially results from the backfiring of antidromically activated anterior horn cells. Electrical stimulation of motor points assesses the strength-duration curves of the affected muscles.[52] A denervated or partially denervated muscle requires more time and current than a normally innervated muscle. Serial strength-duration testing therefore allows the clinician to assess neuromuscular recovery.[52]

Rehabilitation Prognosis and Intervention

The clinician approaches rehabilitation for patients with brachial plexus lesions by maintaining or improving soft tissue mobility, muscle strength and function within the constraint of the nerve injury, and function. Because regeneration is excruciatingly slow, rehabilitation in severe cases is a long-term process, taking as long as 3 years. Therefore, patient and family education and home exercise programs are integral components of treatment.

The clinician should understand soft tissue healing after surgical grafting in the presence of fourth- and fifth-degree nerve injuries. The relatively high chance of residual upper extremity dysfunction in some cases necessitates vocational and avocational retraining, as well as occupational therapy intervention for assistance-providing devices and splints.

According to Framptom,[6] rehabilitation falls into three stages: (1) the early stage, consisting of diagnosis, neurovascular repair, and education regarding passive movement and self-care of the affected extremity; (2) the middle stage, when recovery is occurring, and intensive reeducation may be indicated; and (3) the late stage, when no future recovery is expected, and assessment for reconstructive surgery can take place.[6] The clinician bases the time frames and extent of each phase on the extent of the lesion and on the individual's own motivation and recuperative capabilities.

CASE STUDY 8-1

This case study presents a typical brachial plexus injury affecting the shoulder and upper extremity function. The evaluation presents the initial findings. The goals and phases of intervention combine a physical and occupational therapy approach with rationales.

Examination

History

A 22-year-old, right-handed man has sustained a traction injury to his right shoulder following a tackling injury while participating in a weekend football game. His primary complaints include an intermittent, diffuse ache over his right shoulder and arm. Electrodiagnostic testing indicates abnormalities in the right C5-6 myotomal distribution with an infraganglionic lesion to his right brachial plexus at Erb's joint, which is the portion of the brachial plexus where C5 and C6 unite to join the upper trunk. Radiologic studies indicate no fractures at the cervical spine or clavicle. The physician refers the patient to physical therapy 4 weeks after the initial injury.

Continued

CASE STUDY 8-1—cont'd

The patient reports numbness and tingling along the lateral aspect of his right shoulder, in the area of the deltoid muscle, and weakness in his right shoulder. He reports intermittent pain in his right shoulder and neck made worse with attempted elevation of his right arm. He reports less numbness and greater strength in his right arm since the initial injury.

Vocation

The patient works full time as a computer software programmer.

Tests and Measures

Postural/Visual Inspection

The clinician observes atrophy in the supraspinatus and infraspinatus muscles on the right compared with the left side, with sparing of the rhomboid, serratus anterior, and paraspinals on the right.

Passive Range of Motion

Elevation in the plane of the scapula measures 120°, external rotation in adduction measures 30°, external rotation in 45° abduction measures 60°, and external rotation in 90° abduction measures 70°. His elbow, forearm, wrist, and hand passive range of motion are within normal limits.

Active Range of Motion

Elevation in the plane of the scapula measures 60°, external rotation in adduction from full internal rotation measures 20°, and elbow, wrist, and hand active range of motion is normal.

Motor Strength

Motor strength is as follows:

- Grade 0 = no contraction
- Grade 1 = trace
- Grade 2 = poor
- Grade 3 = fair
- Grade 4 = good
- Grade 5 = normal

The clinician classifies the patient's muscle strength as follows: deltoid = 3, supraspinatus = 3, infraspinatus = 3, teres minor = 2, biceps brachii = 5, brachialis = 5, serratus anterior = 5, subscapularis = 3, extensor carpi radialis longus and brevis = 5, and supinator = 5. His grip strength is 100 lb bilaterally.

Sensation

The lateral aspect of the left shoulder, in the area of the deltoid muscle, and along the radial side of the forearm shows impaired sensation to light touch and to sharp or dull objects.

Reflexes

- Biceps, brachioradialis, and triceps: 2+ on the left
- Biceps and brachioradialis: 1+ on the right; triceps: 2+ on the right

Coordination

The clinician assesses coordination using the Purdue pegboard as follows: right hand, 14; left hand, 2; both hands, 4; assembly task, 6.

Edema

No edema is visible throughout the right upper extremity.

Vascular Status

The patient has 2+ pulses of the radial and brachial artery in the right upper extremity.

Palpation

The clinician palpates trigger points in muscle bellies of the left upper trapezius, left rhomboid, and left subscapularis muscles.

Functional Limitations

- The patient is unable to elevate his right arm overhead for dressing and grooming tasks.
- He is unable to use his right arm for driving tasks.
- He is unable to return to previous weekend sporting activities.

American Surgeon and Elbow Outcome Score

The patient has a score of 72.

Evaluation

This is a patient with a traction injury to the upper trunk of the brachial plexus involving nerve trunks C5 and C6. Because his affected muscles are spontaneously improving since the initial injury, the extent of the injury is between a first-degree and a second-degree injury.[35] In addition, the patient has impairments and functional losses associated with the preferred practice pattern: *impaired peripheral nerve integrity and muscle performance associated with peripheral nerve injury.* For example, he has decreased muscle strength and impaired nerve integrity. In this case, the patient has impaired passive range of motion. One can expect combined resolution of nerve function with full return of function of the right upper extremity.

Passive range of motion in the affected shoulder results from soft tissue changes described by Akeson et al,[40] Tabary et al,[53] and Cooper,[54] who reported on the effects of immobilization on the periarticular capsule, tendon, and muscle, respectively. The loss of motor control results in altered scapulohumeral rhythm. The rotator cuff muscles, particularly the supraspinatus, infraspinatus, and teres minor muscles, are unable to control gliding of the humeral head adequately during elevation of the shoulder. The resultant weakness, even in the presence of a weak deltoid muscle, leads to impingement of the suprahumeral soft tissues underneath the unyielding coracoacromial ligament. Chronic impingement results in inflammation and degeneration of the rotator cuff tendons.

CASE STUDY 8-1—cont'd

Prognosis

Based on this preferred practice pattern, the prognosis for recovery ranges from 4 to 8 months. The expected number of visits over that time period may range from 12 to 56. The *Guide* indicates that 80% of patients classified using this pattern achieve the anticipated goals.

Intervention: Early Stage

First Goal

The first goal is to reduce pain.

Intervention

The clinician applies heat, low-voltage surge stimulation, and spray and stretch techniques (see Chapter 10) to the active trigger points in the left upper trapezius and left rhomboid muscles. The clinician then applies transcutaneous neuromuscular stimulation, by using a high-rate, low-intensity conventional setting with dual channels and four electrodes around the left shoulder. The patient wears the transcutaneous neuromuscular stimulation device 8 hours per day.

Rationale

According to Travell and Simons,[45] myofascial trigger points in the shoulder girdle muscles refer pain into the left shoulder and arm in a consistent pattern. Therefore, the patient's pain reduces as trigger point tenderness subsides in the left upper trapezius and left rhomboid muscles. The conventional transcutaneous neuromuscular stimulation setting stimulates large A-beta sensory fibers that modulate impulses from the small A-delta fibers and C fibers in the dorsal horn of the spinal cord.[55,56] Irritation of nociceptor endings in the connective tissue sheaths surrounding the nerve fibers and trunks, because of the traction injury, produces pain impulses along the A-delta fibers and C fibers.[56]

Second Goal

The second goal is to restore full passive range of motion and soft tissue mobility.

Intervention

In this patient, the clinician applies low-voltage surge stimulation followed by spray and stretch techniques to the active trigger points in the muscle belly of the subscapularis. This treatment follows Maitland's grades III and IV mobilization of the various joints in the left upper extremity.[57]

The clinician instructs the patient in home range-of-motion exercises so the patient can preserve the range of motion for those joints that have no, or only limited, active range of motion. The exercises also preserve the range of motion for uninvolved joints so they do not become restricted as a result of disuse. The patient's family should be familiar with the exercise program so they can encourage the patient to follow through and become active participants in the patient's rehabilitation.

Rationale

A contracted subscapularis muscle results in the painful limitation of external rotation with the shoulder adducted along the lateral trunk. Therefore, spray and stretch, followed by distraction of the medial scapula border, elongate the subscapularis muscle and improve external rotation with the shoulder in the adducted position. Manual techniques at the shoulder mobilize the inferior and anterior capsules to promote abduction and external rotation movements, respectively. The scientific literature indicates no optimum time frames for applying grade IV manual stretching to the periarticular capsule. Clinically, three sets of 1-minute grade IV oscillations for the restricted tissue are recommended, preceded by heat and followed by ice.

Third Goal

The third goal is to prevent neural dissociation to the reinnervating muscles.

Intervention

The clinician applies high-frequency, low-voltage muscle stimulation with a pulse duration of 30 milliseconds, with a duty cycle of 10 seconds on and 20 seconds off, for a period of 30 minutes to the partially denervated muscle. The patient uses a home muscle stimulator three to four times daily.

Rationale

According to strength-duration studies, muscle stimulation to a partially denervated muscle requires a higher current and longer pulse duration than does stimulation to a normally innervated muscle.[49] In addition to maintaining reinnervating muscle tissue viability, electrically induced muscle contractions facilitate normal circulation, decrease edema, and present potential nutritional or tropic skin changes.[58,59]

Intervention: Middle Stage

First Goal

The first goal in the middle stage is to retrain reinnervating muscles.

Intervention

Three weeks after the initial evaluation, the clinician begins manual proprioceptive neuromuscular facilitation techniques emphasizing diagonal patterns, with the patient supine, followed by isotonic strengthening using adjustable cuff weights. Initial isotonic strengthening emphasizes external rotation movement patterns at the shoulder, flexion and extension movements at the elbow, and pronation and supination at the forearm. As strength improves, the patient progresses to isokinetic strengthening at slow speeds of approximately 60°, emphasizing rotational movement patterns in the shoulder. The patient progresses to isokinetic diagonal movement patterns in the supine position when

Continued

CASE STUDY 8-1—cont'd

isokinetic testing indicates a difference of left-to-right shoulder external rotation peak torque and power within 20%.

Vibration and tapping while the patient is exercising or performing functional activities facilitate purposeful movement.[60] Biofeedback and neuromuscular electrical stimulation help to retrain weak muscles.

Rationale

Manual proprioceptive neuromuscular facilitation diagonals allow the clinician to assess early subtle strength changes across treatments. Early isotonic strengthening builds up the shoulder rotator cuff muscles, specifically the supraspinatus, infraspinatus, and teres minor muscles. The restoration of rotator cuff muscle strength reestablishes the normal balance between these muscles and the upward pull of the deltoid muscle.[61] Isokinetic strengthening offers the advantage of accommodating resistance to load a contracting muscle maximally throughout the range of motion.[62] The patient exercises at slower speeds, so that he or she can consistently catch and maintain the speed of the dynamometer. External rotational strengthening restores the dynamic glide of the humeral head along the glenoid fossa by reestablishing strength in the supraspinatus, infraspinatus, and teres minor muscles. Isokinetic testing every 2 to 3 weeks assesses peak torque and power values of the involved, compared with the uninvolved, upper extremity. Isokinetic diagonal strengthening patterns eliminate the effect of the muscles working directly against gravity. Diagonal patterns are eventually performed with the patient sitting or standing after bilateral strength deficits between the left and right shoulder rotators are within 20%. Although this observation is not scientifically substantiated, when bilateral shoulder rotational strength deficits are greater than 20%, impingement and pain have occurred in the suprahumeral soft tissues during active shoulder elevation.

Intervention: Late Stage

First Goal

The first goal in the late stage is to optimize muscle strengthening within the constraints of reinnervation.

Intervention

Isokinetic strengthening continues to all major affected muscle groups in the left upper extremity, including rotational and diagonal strengthening at the shoulder. The clinician adds fast-speed training, at 180°, when bilateral slow-speed deficits, at 60°, are within 20%. The patient performs an aggressive home strengthening program using adjustable cuff weights and functional training, including lifting, carrying various size weights, hammering, and sawing activities.

Rationale

Strengthening continues to provide gains, with periodic isokinetic strength retests. Fast-speed training improves muscle endurance. The reason fast-speed training begins when slow-speed bilateral deficits are within 20% is that the patient cannot consistently catch and maintain the faster speeds of the dynamometer. Functional training for this particular patient simulates the working conditions and motor requirements of carpentry.

Second Goal

The second goal is optimizing joint and soft tissue mobility.

Third Goal

The third goal is to help the patient return to work.

Intervention

At 1-year after injury, a job analysis identifies those tasks that the patient needs to perform to be able to do his job safely and accurately. At that time, the patient starts on woodworking projects that require minimal fine motor tasks such as sanding or staining. At 15 months, he progresses to working on more intricate projects, and at 18 months, he returns to work.

CASE STUDY 8-2

The second case study demonstrates the differential diagnosis of a patient with shoulder pain and weakness. Considerations included in the physical therapy differential diagnosis include cervical radiculopathy, shoulder impingement, upper brachial plexopathy, and rotator cuff disease. Initial findings in the evaluation should be compared and contrasted with the findings in Case Study 1. The preferred practice pattern, with the prognosis, goals, interventions, and principles of treatment, is similar to that of Case Study 1.

Examination

History

A 24-year-old female patient reports that she woke up one morning 5 weeks ago with a constant, diffuse pain over the superior and posterior aspect of her left shoulder. She is a competitive swimmer, and her training routine consists of swimming 3 to 4 hours a day 6 days a week. She is right-arm dominant. She remembers waking up with her left arm abducted over her head during her sleep the previous night. Aggravating symptoms include pain with all swimming

CASE STUDY 8-2—cont'd

activity and while performing overhead activity. The patient presents to the physical therapist with a medical diagnosis of subacromial impingement of the left shoulder. The orthopedist prescribes nonsteroidal anti-inflammatory medication and refers the patient to physical therapy. No radiographic imaging studies have been performed on her left shoulder.

Vocation

The patient is a full-time student at a local university and is a competitive swimmer at the regional level.

Tests and Measures

Postural/Visual Inspection

The patient has marked atrophy over the left supraspinatus and infraspinatus.

Active and Passive Range of Motion

Cervical active range of motion is full and painless in flexion, extension, right and left rotation, and right and left sidebending. Left shoulder active range of motion is 170° in flexion and 140° in abduction with a painful arc from 80° to 120°. Passive range of motion is full in flexion and abduction on the left. Right shoulder active range of motion is 180° in flexion and abduction.

Special Tests

- Spurling's test: negative on the right and left
- Upper limb tension test: negative bilaterally
- Hawkins-Kennedy test: negative on the left
- Neer's test: positive on the left
- Relocation test: negative bilaterally
- External rotation lag sign: negative on the left

Reflexes

Reflexes for the C5, C6, and C7 are bilateral and symmetrical: 2+.

Motor Strength

Myotomal strength testing: manual muscle testing is 5/5 from C4 to T1, with the exception of 3+/5 in the supraspinatus and infraspinatus muscles in the left shoulder.

Sensation

Sensation is normal to light touch bilaterally throughout the upper extremities.

Palpation

The patient has tenderness to palpation of the long tendon of the biceps brachii and greater tubercle on the left.

Electrophysiologic Evaluation

Nerve conduction studies are performed with the electrical stimulation occurring at the supraclavicular fossa with the recording electrodes over the supraspinatus and infraspinatus on the left. The insertional activity of the infraspinatus and supraspinatus is increased. The patient has 3+ fibrillation potentials and positive sharp waves in both the supraspinatus and infraspinatus muscles.

Evaluation

Based on the examination findings, the more likely diagnosis includes suprascapular neuropathy. A diagnosis of cervical radiculopathy is ruled out because of the lack of positive test results with a negative upper limb tension test, negative distraction test, negative Spurling's test, and full cervical range of motion in rotation. The Hawkins-Kennedy test has a sensitivity of 0.92; thus, a negative test result would rule out subacromial impingement.[54] Neer's test has a specificity of 0.31, so the test is not a strong clinical test for subacromial impingement.[54] The clinical findings of a negative external rotation lag sign would not suggest a rotator cuff tear, with specificity of 1.0 and sensitivity of 0.70.[63]

Clinical findings include posterior shoulder or scapular pain, a mechanism of injury to include repetitive overhead activity or a traumatic traction force to the upper extremity, and weakness or atrophy of the supraspinatus and infraspinatus muscles. Fibrillation potentials with electromyographic examination, combined with clinical testing that produced a minimum strength grade of 3 in all affected muscle groups, indicate probable partial denervation of muscles affected by the C5 and C6 nerve roots. The diagnosis of suprascapular neuropathy is usually made based on exclusion within the differential diagnosis.[64] Spontaneous recovery occurs in case of axonotmesis, but axonal outgrowth takes a long time in these cases (at least 1 year) because of the limited growth rate and the long distance to their target muscles. Periodic electromyographic evaluations check for reinnervation characterized by polyphasic action potentials. After 1 year, a lack of recovery results in surgical exploration. Physical therapy interventions include patient education and a comprehensive rotator cuff strengthening program.

SUMMARY

The case studies illustrate the problem-solving approach to patient treatment. The clinician prioritizes signs and symptoms in order of their functional significance. The clinician establishes appropriate goals within the constraints of nerve reinnervation and uses the preferred practice patterns to predict the impairments and functional losses and to determine the prognosis. The preferred practice patterns provide only guidelines to intervention, so the clinician should use his or her clinical judgment with knowledge of evidence-based outcomes to individualize each program. The patient progresses through each phase based on the clinician's continued reevaluation of signs and symptoms, and discharge takes place when clinical tests and evaluation indicate no further improvement in the patient's motor capabilities. The clinician discharges the patient on a home program and periodically reevaluates the patient for improvement. Signs of motor reinnervation result in resumed intervention.

REFERENCES

1. American Physical Therapy Association: *Guide to physical therapist practice*, ed 2, Baltimore, 2001, American Physical Therapy Association.
2. Williams PL, Warwick R: *Gray's anatomy*, ed 36, Churchill Livingstone, 1980, Edinburgh.
3. Leffert RD: Clinical diagnosis, testing, and electromyographic study in brachial plexus traction injuries, *Clin Orthop Relat Res* 237:24, 1988.
4. Smith AR, Cummings JP: The axillary arch: anatomy and suggested clinical manifestations, *J Orthop Sports Phys Ther* 36 (6):425–429, 2006.
5. Sunderland S: Traumatized nerves, roots and ganglia: musculoskeletal factors and neuropathological consequences. In Korr IM, editor: *The neurobiologic mechanisms in manipulative therapy*, New York, 1978, Plenum.
6. Framptom VM: Management of brachial plexus lesions, *J Hand Ther* 115:120, 1988.
7. Alnot JY: Traumatic brachial plexus palsy in the adult: retro- and infraclavicular lesions, *Clin Orthop Relat Res* 237:9, 1988.
8. Zarkadas P, Throckmorton T, Steinmann S: Neurovascular injuries in shoulder trauma, *Orthop Clin North Am* 39: 483–490, 2008.
9. Silliman JT, Dean MT: Neurovascular injuries to the shoulder complex, *J Orthop Sports Phys Ther* 18:442, 1993.
10. Comtet JJ, Sedel L, Fredenucci JF: Duchenne-Erb palsy: experience with direct surgery, *Clin Orthop Relat Res* 237:17, 1988.
11. Brunelli GA, Brunelli GR: A fourth type of brachial plexus injury: middle lesions (C7), *Ital J Orthop Traumatol* 18:389, 1992.
12. Mumenthaler M, Narakas A, Gilliat RW: Brachial plexus disorders. In Dyck PJ, Thomas PK, Lambert EH, et al, editors: *Peripheral neuropathy*, Philadelphia, 1984, Saunders.
13. Markey KL, DiBendetto M, Curl WW: Upper trunk brachial plexopathy: the stinger syndrome, *Am J Sports Med* 21:650, 1993.
14. Hershman EB, Wilbourn AJ, Bergfeld JA: Acute brachial neuropathy in athletes, *Am J Sports Med* 17:655, 1989.
15. Speer KP, Bassett FH III: The prolonged burner syndrome, *Am J Sports Med* 18:591, 1990.
16. Inman VT, Saunders M, Abbot LC: Observations on the function of the shoulder joint, *J Bone Joint Surg Am* 26:1, 1944.
17. Freedman L, Munro RR: Abduction of the arm in the scapular plane: scapular and glenohumeral movements, a roentgenographic study, *J Bone Joint Surg Am* 48:1503, 1966.
18. Poppen NK, Walker PS: Normal and abnormal motion of the shoulder, *J Bone Joint Surg Am* 58:195, 1976.
19. Inman VT, Ralston HJ, Saunders JB, et al: Relation of human electromyograms to muscular tension, *Electroencephalogr Clin Neurophysiol* 4:187, 1952.
20. Kendall HO, Kendall FP, Wadsworth GE: *Muscles: testing and function*, ed 2, Baltimore, 1971, Williams & Wilkins.
21. Stevens JH: Brachial plexus paralysis. In Codman EA, editor: *The shoulder*, Melbourne, 1991, Krieger.
22. Spinner RJ, Khoobehi S, Kazmi, et al: Model of avulsion injury in the rat brachial plexus using passive acceleration, *Microsurgery* 20(2):94–97, 2000.
23. Guven O, Akbar Z, Yalcin S, et al: Concomitant rotator cuff tear and brachial plexus injury in association with anterior shoulder dislocation: unhappy triad of the shoulder, *J Orthop Trauma* 8:429, 1994.
24. Wang KC, Hsa KY, Shik CH: Brachial plexus injury with erect dislocation of the shoulder, *Orthop Rev* 21:1345, 1992.
25. Travlos J, Goldberg I, Boome RS: Brachial plexus lesions associated with dislocated shoulder, *J Bone Joint Surg Br* 72:68, 1990.
26. Della Santa D, Narakos A, Bonnard C: Late lesions of the brachial plexus after fracture of the clavicle, *Ann Chir Main Memb Super* 10:531, 1991.
27. Stromqvist B, Lidgren L, Norgren L, et al: Neurovascular injury complicating displaced proximal fractures of the humerus, *Injury* 18:423, 1989.
28. Blom S, Dahlback LO: Nerve injuries in dislocation of the shoulder joint and fractures of the neck of the humerus, *Acta Chir Scand* 136:461, 1970.
29. van Ouwerkerk WJ, van der Sluijs JA, Nollet F, et al: Management of obstetric brachial plexus lesions: state of the art and future development, *Childs Nerv Syst* 16:638–644, 2000.
30. Miller J, Pruitt S, McDonald T: Acute brachial plexus neuritis: an uncommon cause of shoulder pain, *Am Fam Physician* 62:2067–2072, 2000.
31. Saifuddin A: Imaging tumors of the brachial plexus, *Skeletal Radiol* 32:375–387, 2003.
32. Davis G, Knight S: Pancoast tumor resection with preservation of brachial plexus and hand function, *Neurosurg Focus* 22(6): E15, 2007.
33. Sughrue M, Levine J, Barbaro N: Pain as a symptom of peripheral nerve sheath tumors: clinical significance and future therapeutic direction, *J Brachial Plex Peripher Nerve Inj* 29 (3):6, 2008.
34. Gupta G, Maniker A: Malignant peripheral nerve sheath tumors, *Neurosurg Focus* 22(6):E12, 2007.
35. Sunderland S: *Nerves and nerve injuries*, ed 2, Churchill Livingstone, 1978, Edinburgh.
36. Bruxelle J, Travers V, Thiebaut JB: Occurrence and treatment of pain after brachial plexus injury, *Clin Orthop Relat Res* 237:87, 1988.
37. Janda V: Muscles, central nervous motor regulation and back problems. In Korr IM, editor: *The neurobiologic mechanisms in manipulative therapy*, New York, 1978, Plenum.
38. Krishnan K, Mucha D, Gupta R, et al: Brachial plexus compression caused by recurrent clavicular nonunion and space occupying pseudoarthrosis: definitive reconstruction using free vascularized bone flap—a series of eight cases, *Neurosurgery* 62 (5 Suppl 2):ONS461–ONS469, 2008.
39. Sureka J, Cherian R, Alexander M, et al: MRI of brachial plexopathies, *Clin Radiol* 64(2):208–218, 2009.
40. Akeson WH, Amiel D, Mechanis GI, et al: Collagen cross-linking alterations in joint contracture: changes in the reducible cross-links in periarticular connective tissue collagen after nine weeks of immobilization, *Connect Tissue Res* 5:15, 1977.
41. Highet WB: Grading of motor and sensory recovery in nerve injuries. In Seddon HJ, editor: *Peripheral nerve injuries*, Medical Research Council report series T2 282, London, 1954, Her Majesty's Stationery Office.
42. Daniels L, Worthingham C: *Muscle testing: techniques of manual examination*, ed 4, Philadelphia, 1980, Saunders.
43. Hamm NH, Curtis D: Normative data for the Purdue pegboard on a sample of adult candidates for vocational rehabilitation, *Percept Mot Skills* 50:309, 1980.
44. Murata K, Maeda M, Yoshida A, et al: Axillary artery injury combined with delayed brachial plexus palsy due to compressive hematoma in a young patient: a case report, *J Brachial Plex Peripher Nerve Inj* 28(3):9, 2008.

45. Travell JG, Simons DG: *Myofascial pain and dysfunction: the trigger point manual*, Baltimore, 1984, Williams & Wilkins.
46. Janda V: Some aspects of extracranial causes of facial pain, *J Prosthet Dent* 56:4, 1986.
47. Roy J, MacDermid J, Woodhouse L: Measuring shoulder function: a systematic review of four questionnaires, *Arthritis Rheum* 61(5):623–632, 2009.
48. Bilbey JH, Lamond RG, Mattrey RF: MR imaging of disorders of the brachial plexus, *J Magn Reson Imaging* 4:13, 1994.
49. Yeoman PM: Cervical myelography in traction injuries of the brachial plexus, *J Bone Joint Surg Br* 50:25, 1968.
50. Bufalini C, Pesatori G: Posterior cervical electromyography in the diagnosis and prognosis of brachial plexus injuries, *J Bone Joint Surg Br* 51:627, 1969.
51. Bonney G, Gilliat RW: Sensory nerve conduction after traction lesion of the brachial plexus, *Proc R Soc Med* 51:365, 1958.
52. Scott PM: *Clayton's electrotherapy and actinotherapy*, ed 7, London, 1975, Balliere Tindall.
53. Tabary JC, Tardieu C, Tardieu G, et al: Experimental rapid sarcomere loss with concomitant hypoextensibility, *Muscle Nerve* 4:198, 1981.
54. Cooper RR: Alterations during immobilization and regeneration of skeletal muscles in cats, *J Bone Joint Surg Am* 54:919, 1972.
55. Lampe GN, Mannheimer JS: *Stimulation characteristics of T.E.N.S.*, Philadelphia, 1984, Davis.
56. Guyton AC: *Organ physiology: structure and function of the nervous system*, ed 2, Philadelphia, 1976, Saunders.
57. Maitland GD: *Peripheral manipulation*, ed 2, London, 1977, Butterworth.
58. Gutman E, Guttman L: Effects of electrotherapy on denervated muscles in rabbits, *Lancet* 1:169, 1942.
59. Hatano E, Tsuge K, Ikuta Y, et al: Electrical stimulation on denervated skeletal muscles. In Goria A, Millesi H, Mingrino S, editors: *Posttraumatic peripheral nerve regeneration: experimental basis and clinical implications*, New York, 1981, Raven Press.
60. Trombly C, Scott A: *Occupational therapy for physical dysfunction*, Baltimore, 1977, Williams & Wilkins.
61. Saha AK: Dynamic stability of the glenohumeral joint, *Acta Orthop Scand* 42:491, 1971.
62. Hislop HJ, Perrine JJ: The isokinetic concept of exercise, *Phys Ther* 47:114, 1967.
63. Cleland J: *Orthopedic clinical examination: an evidence-based approach for physical therapists*, Philadelphia, 2007, Saunders Elsevier.

PART 3
SPECIAL CONSIDERATIONS

CHAPTER 9

Bruce H. Greenfield

Impingement Syndrome and Impingement-Related Instability

Impingement syndrome historically has been considered to be a continuum of a single pathologic condition involving the subacromial soft tissue.[1] As our understanding of this complex problem has developed, the simple continuum model has become less effective in guiding appropriate treatment. The purpose of this chapter is to provide the reader with more precise classifications of impingement syndrome and the impingement stability complex and their associated impairments, to provide more efficient and effective interventions that address the primary abnormality.

COMPRESSIVE CUFF DISEASE

Impingement syndrome, or compressive cuff disease, was originally described by Neer[1] as mechanical impingement of the supraspinatus and the long head of the biceps tendon underneath the acromial arch.[1,2] The primary pathologic condition involves a bursal surface lesion. Many investigators also classify mechanical impingement as an "outside-to-inside" lesion because the initial insult to the rotator cuff tendon occurs at its bursal surface, as opposed to its humeral surface ("inside-to-outside lesion"). The condition is often classified as primary impingement syndrome, in contrast to secondary impingement, which involves primary instability and is discussed later. Because primary impingement is recognized to involve a spectrum of lesions of tissues in the suprahumeral space, a working knowledge of its structural interrelationships will facilitate an understanding of the factors that result in abnormalities.

Suprahumeral Space

The *suprahumeral space,* also known as the subacromial space or supraspinatus outlet, is formed by the superior aspect of the humeral head below and the inferior surface of the acromion, the acromioclavicular joint, and the coracoacromial ligament above (Fig. 9-1). Within the subacromial space are the rotator cuff tendons (supraspinatus, infraspinatus, and teres minor), the long head of the biceps, and the subacromial-subdeltoid bursa. The subacromial distance is quite small, and it has been measured on radiographs and used as an indicator for proximal or superior humeral subluxation related to rotator cuff abnormality. The distance was found to be between 9 and 10 mm in 175 asymptomatic shoulders. A distance of less than 6 mm was considered indicative of rotator cuff disease.[3,4]

Coracohumeral Space

A second space for potential primary impingement was identified by Patte[5] as the coracohumeral compartment. The *coracohumeral space* is the space between the tuberosity and the lesser tubercle of the humerus. Within the confines of this space are situated the subscapularis bursa, subscapularis tendon, and subcoracoid bursa. In the resting position with the arm in medial rotation, the distance between the tip of the coracoid and the most prominent part of the lesser tuberosity has been measured at approximately 8.7 mm in healthy shoulders and 6.8 mm in the presence of subcoracoid impingement.[6] A decrease in the size of the subcoracoid space, caused by a fracture trauma to the tip of the coracoid process, has been implicated in primary subcoracoid impingement.[5] The clinician should be aware of this condition in the differential diagnosis of primary impingement, as well as in those patients who have not responded to conservative treatment, particularly after acromioplasty.

Because of the narrow confines of the subacromial space, a small margin of error exists to allow for normal excursion of the suprahumeral tissue to pass safely under the acromial process. Several factors have been implicated in abnormal narrowing of the subacromial space and in the resulting primary impingement syndrome.[7-14]

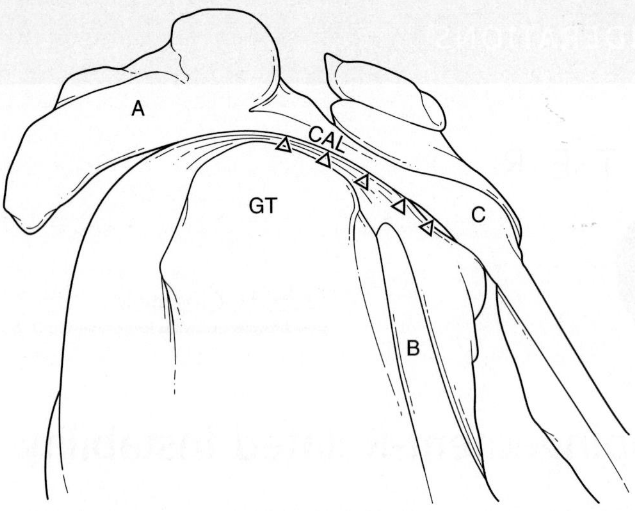

Figure 9-1 The subacromial space. A, acromion; B, biceps (long head); C, coracoid process; CAL, coracoacromial ligament; GT, greater tuberosity.

FACTORS RELATED TO PATHOLOGIC CONDITION

For purposes of description, factors related to this pathologic condition can be divided into intrinsic and extrinsic factors. *Intrinsic factors* directly involve the subacromial space and include changes in vascularity of the rotator cuff, degeneration, and anatomic or bony anomalies. *Extrinsic factors* include impairments associated with postural changes, muscle imbalances, and motor control problems of the rotator cuff (scapulohumeral) and thoracoscapular muscles, as well as precipitating factors, including training errors and occupational or environmental hazards.[14-23] Because several of these problems can coexist with primary impingement, isolating a specific factor as a cause is difficult. More likely, primary impingement has multiple causes, necessitating a thorough and circumspect evaluation of all possible intrinsic and extrinsic factors to injury.

Extrinsic Factors

According to Neer,[1] the anterior-inferior one third of the acromion is thought to be the causative factor in mechanical wear of the rotator cuff through a process called *impingement*. Neer believed that the supraspinatus and long head of the biceps are subjected to repeated compression when the arm is raised in forward flexion. Neer called this the *functional arc of elevation of the arm* (Fig. 9-2). Arthrokinematic movement dictates that forward flexion of the humerus causes concomitant internal rotation of the humeral head.[24] The result is that the suprahumeral tissue is effectively driven directly under the anterior-inferior one third of the acromion. The coracoacromial ligament and acromioclavicular joint can

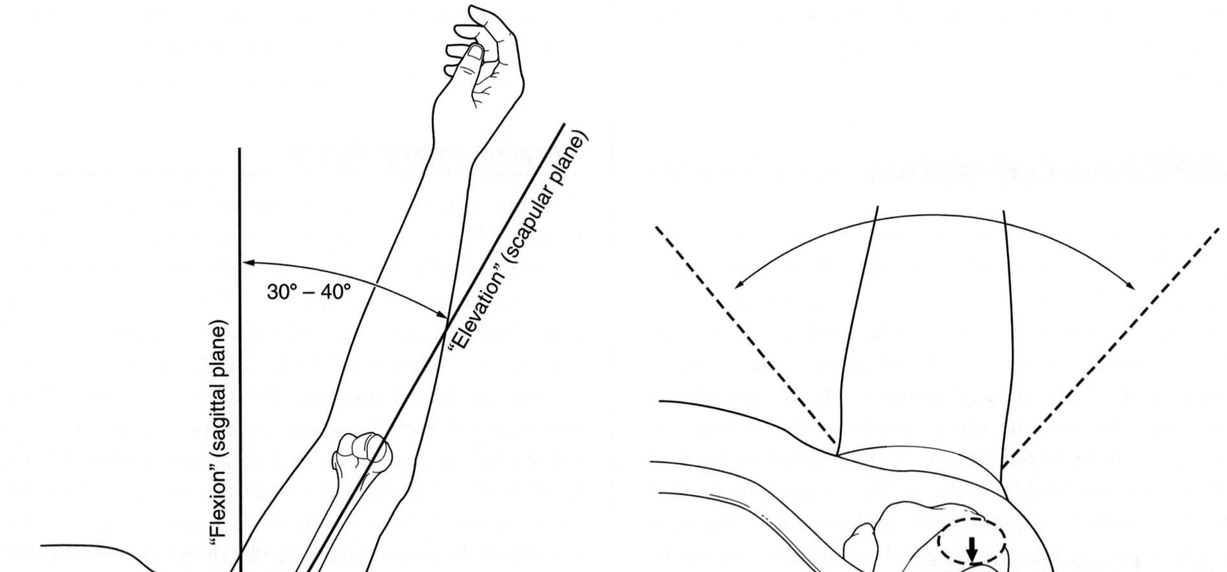

Figure 9-2 Functional arc. **A,** The functional arc of elevation occurs from the sagittal to the plane of the scapula. **B,** Superior view of anterior acromion. Elevation in the functional arc internally rotates the humerus under the anterior-inferior one third of the acromion.

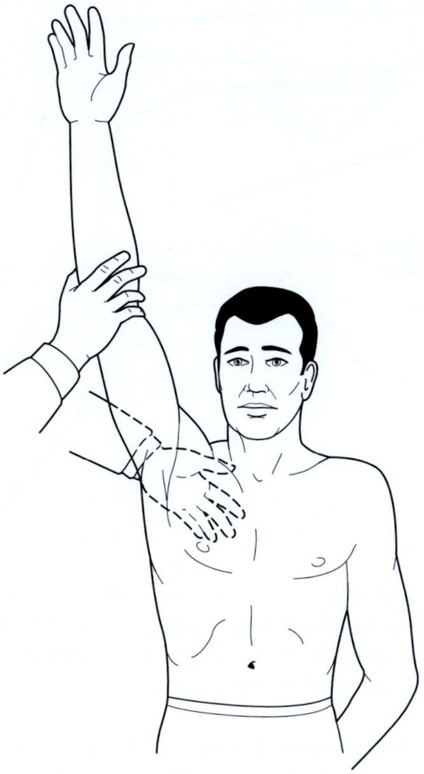

Figure 9-3 Neer's impingement test. Forceful elevation of the humerus with internal rotation results in impingement of the rotator cuff tendons and long head of the biceps underneath the anterior-inferior acromion. A positive result is provocation of subacromial pain.

also be involved in impingement during this functional movement. The Neer impingement test involves forced forward flexion with internal rotation of the humerus to simulate movement in the functional arc and to provoke pain in symptomatic individuals (Fig. 9-3). By focusing on the anterior acromion as the source of impingement rather than the entire acromion, Neer helped to target the technique and approach to acromial decompression to the area of the anterior-inferior acromion, thus avoiding excision of the lateral acromion and significant deltoid muscle morbidity. The overall result after acromial decompression or anterior acromioplasty is an accelerated and aggressive rehabilitation program.

Scapular Muscle Imbalances

Control of the scapula and humerus is primarily dictated by a series of muscle force couples.[25] A *force couple* is two forces of equal magnitude, but in opposite directions, that produce rotation on a body.[26] The scapula force couple is formed by the upper fibers of the trapezius muscle, the levator scapulae muscle, and the upper fibers of the serratus anterior muscle. The lower portion of the force couple is formed by the lower fibers of the trapezius muscle and the lower fibers of the serratus anterior muscle.[27] Simultaneous contraction of these muscles produces a smooth, rhythmic motion to rotate and protract (abduct) the scapula along the posterior thorax during elevation of the arm. The scapula functions to provide a stable base of support for the rotating humerus to allow the humeral head to maintain its normal pathway or rotation along the glenoid.[28] Weakness of the serratus anterior and the trapezius muscles can limit the upward (outward) rotation of the scapula, or it can result in an unstable base of support for the humerus. An unstable scapula, in turn, may produce inefficient action of the rotator cuff muscles to control the humeral head properly along the glenoid fossa during overhead elevation. In addition, the acromion may not elevate sufficiently to provide adequate clearance of the greater tuberosity of the humerus. Furthermore, weakness of the scapular retractors (adductors; the middle trapezius and rhomboid muscles) may increase protraction of the scapula that may narrow the space under the acromion and facilitate impingement of suprahumeral structures. The coordinated action of the scapula muscles is therefore believed by most clinicians to be indispensable to overall normal shoulder function, and current treatment programs are designed to restore normal parascapular muscle control.

Scapular Postural Changes and Altered Kinematics

Clinical researchers have examined the relationships among scapular muscle balance, position, movement, and shoulder pain, particularly as related to impingement. Kibler,[19] for example, observed consistent and abnormal scapular postural changes and altered scapular kinematics in overhead athletes with shoulder impingement and coined the term *scapular dyskinesis.* The best-known clinical test, developed by Kibler, is the *lateral scapula slide test,* which measures the ability of the scapular muscles to control the medial border of the scapula during three positions of the limb: adduction, hands on hips, and 90° of abduction.[19] In his clinical examination, Kibler found that an increase of 1 cm or more in two of the three positions correlated with shoulder impingement and instability in baseball players.

Similarly, Burkhart, Morgan, and Kibler[29] observed consistent asymmetrical malposition of the scapula in throwing athletes with shoulder impingement, and these investigators coined the term *SICK scapular syndrome.* The acronym SICK refers to their findings of *S*capular malposition, *I*nferior-medial border prominence, *C*oracoid pain and malposition, and dys-*K*inesis of scapular movement.

Sahrmann[30] classified scapular positional impairments in patients with selected shoulder conditions including impingement. Based on her years of clinical observations, she reported scapular postural changes of downward rotation and anterior tilting in patients with primary impingement. According to Sahrmann, downward scapular rotation syndrome occurs when the inferior-medial border of the scapula is closer to thoracic midline than the corresponding superior-medial border. Sahrmann observed that patients with a chronically downwardly rotated scapular position had insufficient scapular upward rotation during overhead elevation of the arm, with resulting subacromial pain and impingement.

Sahrmann theorized that long-term changes in muscle length correspond to long-term changes in scapular posture. In the case of a downwardly rotated scapula, for example, the lower trapezius and lower fibers of the serratus anterior muscle lengthen, whereas the levator scapulae and upper trapezius muscles shorten. Muscles that lengthen tend to gain sarcomeres in series and shift the abilities of those muscles to generate tension to the right of a standard length-tension curve. Conversely, muscles that shorten tend to lose sarcomeres in series and shift the abilities of those muscles to generate tension to the left of a standard length-tension curve.[31] The result is a change in muscle balance and force couple capabilities of the scapular muscles to produce outward scapular rotation.

Well-known orthopedic clinician researchers such as Kendall and McCreary,[18] and Janda,[16] have also observed consistent postural changes and muscle imbalances associated with shoulder conditions. Kendall and McCreary observed impaired shoulder elevation in patients with a pattern of muscle imbalances associated with chronic forward head and rounded shoulder posture that included shortness of the pectoralis major and minor and subscapularis muscles with lengthening of the middle trapezius and rhomboid muscles. Finally, Janda observed delays in recruitment of the lower trapezius and serratus anterior muscles in patients with postural impairment and shoulder conditions.

Sophisticated motion analysis studies of scapular kinematics in patients with shoulder impingement confirmed clinical findings related to scapular positional and movement changes.[32-34] Most of these studies indicated that identified deviations can be summarized by a loss of scapular outward rotation (excessive scapular downward rotation) and reduction of scapular posterior tilting (excessive scapular anterior tilting).

In summary, clinical and motion analysis studies confirm the role of scapular positional changes and movement changes as primary impairments related to shoulder pain in general, and impingement symptoms in particular. In view of these insights and research findings on the role the scapular in shoulder impingements, current approaches to interventions for shoulder impingement emphasize the importance of scapular muscle training as an essential component of shoulder rehabilitation.

Rotator Cuff Muscle Imbalance

Budoff et al[35] described the origin of impingement as a primary instability and with secondary impingement. The sequence of events that causes the instability is described as glenohumeral muscle imbalance. The supraspinatus is a small and relatively weak muscle in a key position and is susceptible to overuse injury. When repetitive eccentric overload occurs to the rotator cuff muscles, weakness of the musculotendinous unit results in damage to the tendon. Weak, fatigued, or injured rotator cuff muscles, infraspinatus, teres minor, and subscapularis are unable to oppose the superior pull of the deltoid muscle.

The inferiorly and horizontally directed rotator cuff muscle force vectors maintain the humeral head within the shallow glenoid and thereby resist the upward shear of the deltoid

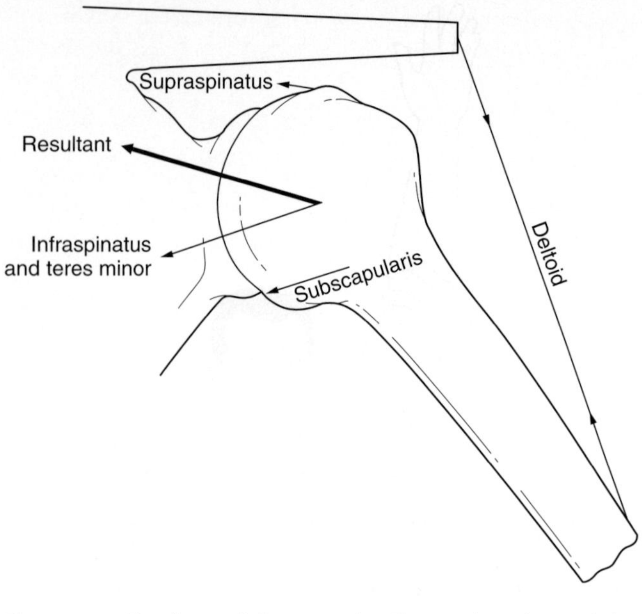

Figure 9-4 Glenohumeral force couple. The resultant force of the rotator cuff muscles results in compression and inferior glide of the humeral head during elevation of the arm.

generated during active elevation of the arm.[24] The result is that the rotator cuff muscles in effect "steer" the humeral head along the glenoid during movement of the humerus.[36] The combination of the resultant contractions of the rotator cuff muscles and the deltoid produces the glenohumeral joint force couple (Fig. 9-4). With an intact and normally functioning rotator cuff muscle group, the center of the humeral head is restrained in a very small arc of motion (within 3 mm) along the glenoid fossa. Poppen and Walker[24] and Weiner and MacNab[4] found that, in the presence of rotator cuff disease, the arc of motion of the humeral head increases to 6 mm or greater. The loss of the rotator cuff force couple results in superior migration of the humeral head, which causes the greater tuberosity and the rotator cuff to come in contact with the undersurface of the acromion and the coracoacromial ligament. The repetitive contact of the humeral head against the acromion causes reactive and degenerative osseous changes Osteophytic spurring occurs along the undersurface of the acromion. Additional traction spurs may form at the anterior medial corner of the acromion. The traction spur may easily be mistaken for an abnormal acromial hook, or type III acromion.[35] Therefore, superior migration of the humerus can produce repetitive impingement of the suprahumeral soft tissue. The result is an inflammatory cascade culminating in rotator cuff disease.

Anterior and Posterior Glenoid Impingement

Jobe[37] described the pathomechanics of posterior-superior labrum impingement. Overhead-throwing athletes are susceptible to forces that may result in impingement of the head of the humerus against the posterior-superior labrum. During throwing, the glenohumeral joint is between 60° and 90° of abduction, maximal external rotation, and horizontal extension. The head of the humerus is angulated in a posterior-superior direction relative to the glenoid. In addition, the greater tuberosity moves posteriorly, secondary to external rotation of the humeral head. Angulation of the humeral head on the glenoid is limited by the inferior glenohumeral ligament and the subscapularis. The cause of impingement is hyperangulation of the humeral head to the glenoid secondary to lack of resistance from a poorly conditioned and fatigued subscapularis muscle. The subscapularis is unable to control the excessive external rotation and extension angulation of the humeral head. Angulation, as opposed to translation, places an uneven stretch to the capsule. The failure of the capsule results from overstretching and instability of the anterior capsule causing subluxations. The deep surface of the supraspinatus is impinged between the humeral head and the posterior-superior labrum.[7]

Gerber and Sebesta[38] described impingement of the deep surface of the subscapularis tendon and the coracohumeral ligaments (reflection pulley) on the anterior-superior glenoid rim. With increasing internal rotation, the lesser tuberosity and biceps tendon are brought close to the anterior superior glenoid rim. Between 100° and 90° of shoulder flexion and full internal rotation, the subscapularis, the biceps tendon, and the superior and middle glenohumeral ligaments are impinging on the anterior glenoid labrum and rim. Patients who perform overhead movements, which are typical of racquet sports and overhead-throwing athletic activities, are more susceptible to anterior-superior glenoid rim impingement. Eccentric overload of the glenohumeral external rotator is common in overhead-throwing athletes. Poorly conditioned and fatigued infraspinatus and teres minor muscles result in excessive internal rotation of the humerus. In the final phase of pitching, the shoulder is in flexion and internal rotation. Excessive internal rotation of the humerus in the flexed position between 100° and 90° could result in impingement of the foregoing soft tissue structures on the anterior-superior glenoid rim.

Precipitating Factors

Precipitating factors to injury are any activities that involve repetitive use of the arm, usually overhead or above the shoulder level, that result in subacromial impingement.[21,22] The baseball pitcher who pitches a nine-inning game early in the season, the retiree who decides to spend the weekend painting her house, and the stock clerk who works two 12-hour shifts to stock inventory are examples of individuals with precipitating factors that result in overuse of the shoulder. A caveat to practicing clinicians is to identify these factors early during a comprehensive history and to modify activities appropriate to the stage of the pathologic condition of impingement and degree of clinical reactivity.

Intrinsic Factors

The primary intrinsic factors can be divided into vascular, degenerative, and anatomic. The original significance of rotator cuff tendon vascularity was described by Codman.[11] Codman referred to a critical zone in which a rupture occurred in the supraspinatus. This zone was located approximately 1 cm medial to the insertion of the tendon. Moseley and Goldie[39] noted that the anastomosis of the osseous and tendinous vessels in the supraspinatus occurred at this site. Rothman and Parke[9] believed that this location was relatively avascular, a condition intensified by aging. Microinjection studies of normal shoulders in cadavers showed an area of decreased vascularity within the tendinous portion of the supraspinatus tendon. Rathbun and Macnab[8] noted that the critical zone of the rotator cuff had an adequate blood supply when the vessels were injected with the arm in the abducted position, but this area was hypovascular when the injection was given with the arm in the adducted position. These investigators proposed a hypothesis of transient hypovascularity in the critical zone caused when vessels are "wrung out" when the arm is in the adducted position. These investigators also indicated that most degenerative rotator cuff tears occur within this zone, a finding suggesting that hypovascularity of the supraspinatus tendon may play a role in the pathogenesis of rotator cuff tears. Lohr and Uhthoff[40] found that the area of hypovascularity in the critical zone was more pronounced along the articular than the bursal surface of the supraspinatus tendon and within the site of early degeneration. Other investigators have disputed the hypovascularity findings.[41,42] A laser Doppler study of the rotator cuff vasculature showed substantial blood flow in the region of the critical zone and increased blood flow at the margins of rotator cuff tears.[42] Although definitive scientific evidence of a direct cause-and-effect relationship is not yet available, the finding seems to indicate a vascular predisposition to the pathogenesis of rotator cuff disease and impingement.

Degeneration

Evidence indicates natural age-related degeneration and tendinosis of the rotator cuff tendons. Codman[11] noted that rotator cuff tendon rupture in older patients normally occurred bilaterally and in the presence of preexisting tendon degeneration. Uhthoff et al[12] and Ozaki et al[13] found insertional tendinopathy or preexisting tendon degeneration in human specimens. These changes included histologic changes in the arrangement of tendon fibers, fiber disruption at their insertion site, and microcysts and osteopenia along the insertion site. These changes found along the articular side (humeral side) were not usually associated with changes in the acromial process.

Anatomic Anomalies

Morrison and Bigliani[7] studied the shape of the anterior-inferior acromion in anatomic specimens and in patients. They identified three types of acromions: type I (flat), type II (curved), and type III (hooked) (Fig. 9-5). The development of type II or II acromial processes remains controversial. The older theory is that these are congenital anomalies, although little evidence indicates that youngsters exhibit changes in

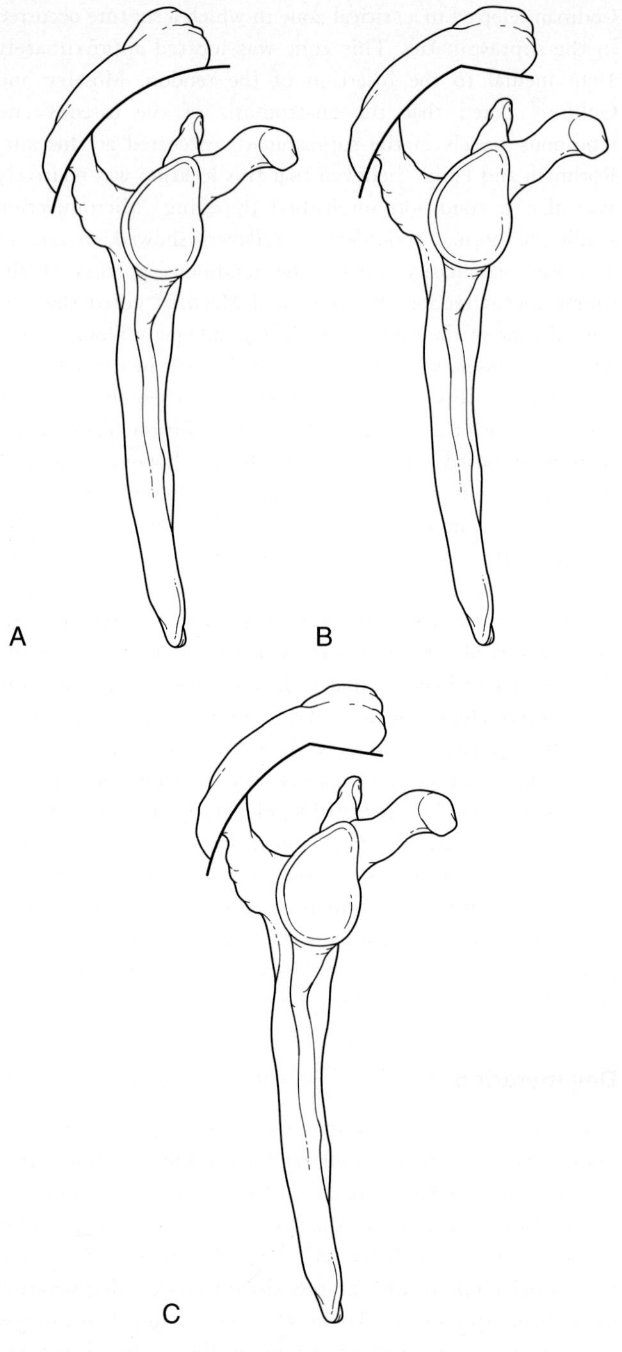

Figure 9-5 Three types of acromions. **A,** Type I, flat. **B,** Type II, curved. **C,** Type III, hooked.

acromial morphology. More logically, the development of type II or III acromial processes may result from excessive superior shear of the humeral head under the acromion, as a result of muscle imbalance in the parascapular or rotator cuff muscle. The repetitive impingement is thought to cause remodeling of the undersurface of the acromion.

Regardless of cause, in the anatomic specimen studies of Morrison and Bigliani,[7] 70% of rotator cuff tears were associated with type II or III acromions. None had type I acromions. Although no causal relationship between the shape of the acromion and rotator cuff tears or impingement can be concluded, the clinical findings support Neer's theory of impingement occurring primarily along the anterior-inferior acromion.

STAGES OF PATHOLOGY AND PRINCIPLES OF TREATMENT

Program design for conservative management of primary impingement syndrome is predicated on a problem-solving approach. This approach necessitates a thorough evaluation to clarify the nature and extent of the pathologic condition, the stage of reactivity, underlying impairments—including extrinsic problems to formulate a physical therapy diagnosis—and other factors that may affect treatment planning and outcome (e.g., age of the patient, motivation, and underlying disease). Classifying the pathologic condition based on the progression described by Neer can be correlated with clinical signs and symptoms and can provide a basic framework for preliminary treatment planning and progression. All program designs should be divided into treatment phases that include specific goals and criteria for progression and continual reevaluation of both subjective and objective findings. Table 9-1 presents a summary of the stages of pathologic conditions described by Neer. The stages are presented separately, but they represent a continuum of abnormality that in some cases overlap in a particular patient.

Stage I Impingement

Stage I of impingement is characterized by edema and hemorrhage (inflammation) of the rotator cuff and suprahumeral tissue. The patient is usually less than 25 years of age and normally has a precipitating factor of overuse of the shoulder. The clinical symptoms include pain along the anterior and lateral aspect of the shoulder, which when acute or reactive will extend below the elbow. The pain is usually described as a deep, dull ache, with sharp subacromial pain during elevation of the limb. The patient has full active range of motion (AROM) and passive ROM (PROM), a painful arc (pain between 60° to 90° and 120° of elevation of the limb), and an abnormal impingement sign. Muscle strength is usually normal for the abductors and external rotators of the glenohumeral joint, but muscles can be painful and weak in an acute state. Palpation elicits subacromial tenderness, usually along the greater tubercle and bicipital groove. Muscle spasms are often present along the ipsilateral upper trapezius, levator scapulae, and subscapularis muscles. Many of these patients exhibit scapular postural changes including excessive scapular downward rotation and anterior tilting.

Principles of Treatment

Principles of treatment for stage I are based on the stage of clinical reactivity and associated impairments. Because stage I primary impingement usually is acute, the goals of treatment

Table 9-1 Neer Stages of Impingement

Stages	Clinical Presentation	Treatment Principles
Stage I Age: less than 25 years Pathologic conditions: edema and hemorrhage	Subacromial pain and tenderness Painful arc Positive impingement and Neer's test Strong and painful for resisted abduction and external rotation	Reduction and elimination of inflammation Patient education Restoration of proximal control (parascapular muscular control)
Stage II Age: 25–40 years Pathologic condition: tendinitis, bursitis, and fibrosis	Add: capsular pattern of limitation at glenohumeral joint	Reestablishment of glenohumeral capsular mobility
Stage III Age: more than 40 years Pathologic conditions: bone spurs and tendon disruption	Add: weakness abduction and external rotation, "squaring" of acromion	Based on size of tear

are to reduce and eliminate inflammation, increase the patient's awareness of impingement syndrome, improve proximal (parascapular) muscle control, and prevent muscle atrophy or weakness caused by disuse at the glenohumeral joint. The patient should be instructed to rest from activity, but not function, and to perform all activities in front of the shoulder and below shoulder level. A thorough (but understandable) explanation of the impingement process is helpful for many patients to comprehend harmful positions. Forceful active elevation above the shoulder level can produce a painful arc and impingement and can perpetuate the inflammatory response. The patient would do well to take an oral nonsteroidal anti-inflammatory medication, in conjunction with anti-inflammatory modalities including ice, interferential stimulation, or pulsed or low-intensity ultrasound.[43] Soft tissue work and stretching should be used to alleviate muscle spasms. Exercise, including manual resistance, can be used early to facilitate scapular parascapular muscle control without further aggravation of the suprahumeral tissue (Fig. 9-6).

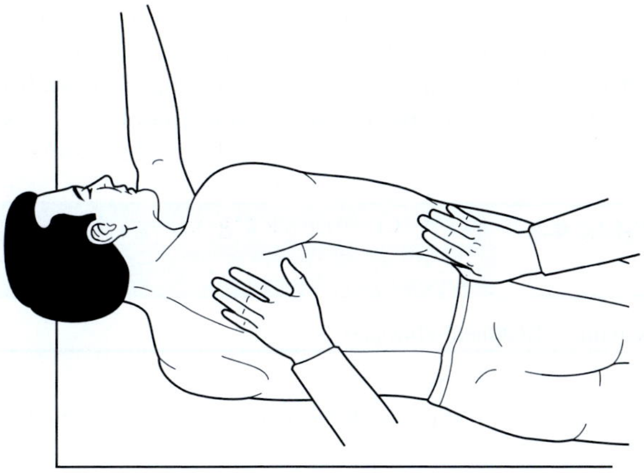

Figure 9-6 Manual technique illustrating resisted posterior scapular depression to facilitate early recruitment of the parascapular muscles.

As reactivity diminishes with elimination of rest pain and pain below the elbow, and with elimination of painful arc and subacromial tenderness, the patient progresses into a dynamic strengthening program that emphasizes reestablishment of the force couple mechanisms at both the scapulothoracic junction and the glenohumeral joint. Table 9-2 lists exercises that are normally effective at this stage. The emphasis should be on high repetitions (3 to 5 sets of 15 repetitions for each exercise), multiple sessions of 3 to 4 daily, working initially in a pain-free range, and using both concentric and eccentric muscle contraction. Exercises are slowly increased to 7 to 10 different movement patterns to isolate different muscle groups. The proper use of these exercises with a low-weight (never greater than 5 lb) and high-repetition format is recommended to enhance local muscle endurance of the rotator cuff muscle and parascapular muscles. Moncrief et al[44] studied the effects of a 5 times per week training program of rotator cuff exercises with 2 sets of 15 repetitions for 1 month in healthy,

Table 9-2 Shoulder-Strengthening Exercises

Muscle	Exercise
Supraspinatus	Prone horizontal abduction Scaption in internal rotation
Infraspinatus	Prone horizontal abduction in external rotation
Teres minor	Prone horizontal abduction in external rotation
Subscapularis	Scaption in internal rotation Military press with dumbbell
Anterior deltoid	Scaption in internal and external rotation
Posterior deltoid	Prone extension
Upper trapezius	Rowing (prone with dumbbell) Shrug
Middle trapezius	Prone horizontal abduction in neutral position
Lower trapezius	Prone horizontal abduction in external rotation
Rhomboids	Rowing (prone with dumbbell) Prone horizontal abduction in neutral position
Serratus anterior	Push-up with a plus

uninjured subjects. Subjects were pretested and post-tested on an isokinetic dynamometer to quantify internal and external rotation strength objectively. Results of the 1-month rotator cuff training program showed an 8% to 10% gain in isokinetically measured internal and external rotation strength in the training arms of the study and no significant improvement in strength in a control group.

Neer suggested that a patient should continue this conservative approach for several months before considering surgical treatment. If the patient is an athlete, as signs and symptoms permit, an additional program of sport-specific exercises and functional training should be incorporated into the program. More recent studies showed the effectiveness of a structured and supervised exercise program for patients with shoulder impingement that was comparable to surgical acromioplasties.

Stage II Impingement

Stage II impingement is characterized by fibrosis of the glenohumeral capsule and subacromial bursa and tendinitis of the involved tendons. The condition is normally seen in patients between 20 and 40 years old. The clinical presentation can be similar to that of stage I, except the patient has loss of AROM and PROM because of the capsular fibrosis. The loss of ROM normally appears in the *capsular pattern,* described by Cyriax[44,45] as a significant loss of external rotation and abduction, with less loss of internal rotation.

Principles of Treatment

The principles of treatment are similar to those for stage I impingement, except that a major goal is to restore full AROM and PROM to prevent further impingement and tissue damage. Cofield and Simonet[46] described how patients with adhesive capsulitis of the glenohumeral joint developed subacromial impingement. Specifically, posterior capsule tightness caused the humeral head to roll forward and superiorly into the subacromial arch and anterior-inferior acromion. Subsequent treatment should be directed at restoring capsular extensibility, to allow the humeral head to attain its normal center of rotation. Several manual techniques described in Chapter 14 are effective for mobilizing the glenohumeral joint capsule. The force and direction of the mobilizing force should be based on the stage of reactivity and clinical mobility testing. Treatment time in patients with a stage II pathologic condition is longer than in stage I, and the prognosis and functional outcome may be more limited.

Stage III Impingement

Stage III impingement is the most difficult to treat conservatively and is characterized by disruption of the rotator cuff tendons. The patient is normally more than 40 years old. Clinically, muscle testing yields weakness, usually for external rotation and abduction. Visual observation indicates a "squaring" of the acromion, a finding that indicates atrophy

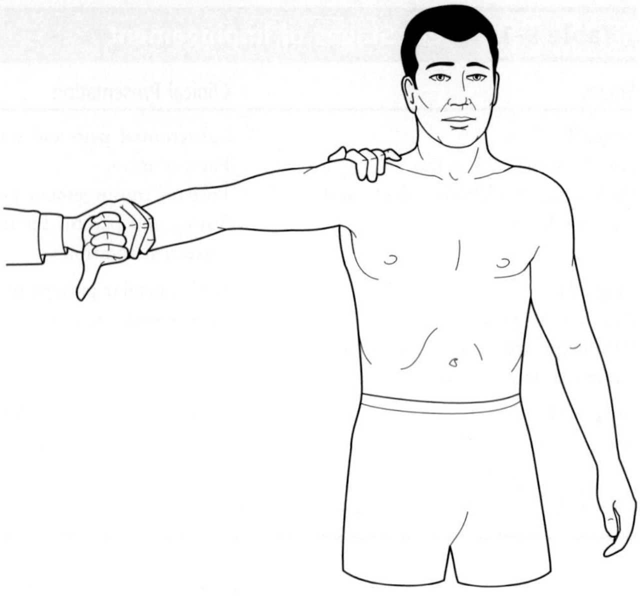

Figure 9-7 Supraspinatus test. The arm is abducted with internal rotation (thumb down) in the plane of the scapula. The patient is asked to resist downward pressure on the abducted arm. A test result is considered positive if the patient is unable to hold the arm against resistance.

of both the rotator cuff and deltoid muscles. Patients with significant tendon disruption have a positive "drop-arm" or supraspinatus test result (Fig. 9-7).

Principles of Treatment

Treatment principles are based partly on the size and location of the tear (Table 9-3). Tears are classified by size, diameter, location, or topography.[47] The small and moderate-size tears can do relatively well with limited functional goals. The patient progresses similarly to the previous treatment principles. If treatment is ineffective and the patient continues to have pain and inability to raise the arm overhead, surgical options include rotator cuff débridement and anterior acromioplasty, or a mini-open repair. For those with large and massive tears, surgery is usually the most effective option, followed by an extensive rehabilitation program incorporating the basic treatment principles for the impingement syndrome and adherence to soft tissue healing guidelines.

Table 9-3 Classification of Rotator Cuff Tear Based on Diameter

Size (cm)	Treatment Principles
1	Conservative
1–3	Conservative, acromioplasty, débridement, or mini-open repair
3–5	Mini-open repair
5	Open repair

CASE STUDY 9-1

This case represents a typical progression for a patient who has symptoms of primary impingement syndrome. Goals and treatment are based on some of the principles of treatment discussed in the previous sections.

General Demographics

Mr. Smith is a 40-year-old male construction worker with a 1-week history of right shoulder pain. He is right-hand dominant.

Social History

Mr. Smith is married with two teenage daughters. He smokes and drinks sparingly. He enjoys tennis.

Employment

He is a construction worker.

Living Environment

Mr. Smith lives with his wife and children in a ranch type of house.

Growth and Development

He is muscular with no external deformities.

Past Medical History

He has a history of arthritis in his cervical spine that occasionally results in tingling and pain into his right shoulder and arm. He reports that, at the age of 14 years, he had a "separated right shoulder" while playing football.

History of Chief Complaint

Mr. Smith spent the weekend painting his house. Since then, he reports pain in the anterior and lateral aspect of his right shoulder. He reports some tingling in his right hand. He describes the pain in his shoulder as a dull ache but sharp during active elevation of his arm. He had difficulty sleeping on his right shoulder at night.

Prior Treatment for this Condition

His family physician prescribed ibuprofen (Motrin) and referred him for a trial of physical therapy with a diagnosis of right shoulder muscle strain.

Structural Examination

During relaxed standing from behind, the scapulae are positioned between T2 and T8. The left scapular inferior-medial and superior-medial borders are in line and approximately 2 inches from the midthoracic spine. The right scapular inferior-medial border is closer to the mid-thoracic spine than is the corresponding superior-medial border. In addition, the inferior angles of the right and left scapulae are rotated posteriorly away from the thoracic chest wall.

Screening Tests

- Positive Spurling's test result: Testing of the right cervical spine reproduces tingling in the right hand.
- The result of Adson's test is negative.
- AROM: Scapulohumeral elevation in the scapular plane produces pain from 60° to full overhead elevation.
- PROM: The patient has full and pain-free PROM in all planes of motion.
- Accessory motion testing of the glenohumeral joint: Results show normal mobility and symmetry with the uninvolved side.
- Resisted testing: The response is painful and strong (empty can test [refer text for more details] and Speed's test).

Muscle Testing	Left	Right
Lower trapezius	4/5	3/5
Serratus anterior	4/5	3+/5
Rhomboids	5/5	4/5
Infraspinatus	5/5	4/5
Teres minor	5/5	4/5
Supraspinatus	4/5	3+/5

Flexibility and Soft Tissue

With the patient supine, both scapulae are elevated from the treatment table. Passive pressure applied to the anterior scapulae reveals tissue resistance associated with pectoralis minor muscle shortening and tightness.

Special Tests

The result of Neer's impingement test is positive.

Tenderness

Palpation elicits tenderness of the greater tubercle and along the bicipital groove.

Physical Therapy Evaluation

Based on presenting signs and symptoms, onset, and patient's age, the physical therapist classifies a stage I primary impingement. The stage of clinical reactivity is acute. The patient has pain to the elbow, is unable to sleep on the involved side, has a painful arc, pain with manual resistance, and a positive impingement sign. Resisted testing and palpation seem to indicate primary involvement of the supraspinatus muscle tendon and the long head of the biceps tendon (empty can and Speed's tests). A secondary problem of tingling in the right hand is likely related to cervical radiculopathy from long-term cervical arthritis (degenerative disk disease). This condition was also most likely exacerbated by painting.

Primary impairments (extrinsic) factors related to pathology include the following:

- Scapular downward rotation and anterior tilting syndromes

Continued

CASE STUDY 9-1—cont'd

- Weakness of the lower trapezius and serratus anterior resulting in inadequate scapular outward rotation
- Short and tight pectoralis minor muscles
- Weakness of the rotator cuff muscles of the right shoulder

Intervention

Initial treatment goals are to reduce and eliminate inflammation of the supraspinatus and long head of the biceps tendon, to educate the patient concerning his condition and helpful and harmful positions of the arm, and to improve parascapular muscle control (associated with chronic scapular downward rotation and anterior tilting) and increase rotator cuff muscle strength. The patient is instructed to monitor for an increase in his secondary symptoms of tingling in the hand because of suspected cervical radiculopathy.

One of the most useful educational techniques in primary impingement is to show this patient an illustration or photograph of the subacromial space and to demonstrate the narrow confines of the space and the mechanism of injury. After the therapist confirms the patient's understanding of the vulnerability of tissues in the subacromial space, the patient is instructed in positions that maximize the space by maintaining his arm below shoulder level and in front of the shoulder, to prevent impingement and stretching of the tendon. He is also instructed not to lift weights. He is instructed to try to maintain his arm in partial abduction and in the scapular plane to promote perfusion to the supraspinatus tendon. Early scapular exercises include manual resistance, simple shoulder shrugs, and scapular retraction exercises (see Fig. 9-6) and are used to promote parascapular muscle control and coordination.

Ice is applied along the greater tubercle to reduce inflammation and facilitate healing. The use of ice provides the strongest evidence base for reducing soft tissue inflammation and related acute pain, particularly over relatively superficial tissues at the shoulder.[43] Ice cups are used for 5 minutes three to four times daily to massage the greater tubercle and bicipital groove. In addition, stretching of the pectoralis minor muscle is accomplished through manual techniques, including the use of contraction and relaxation of the pectoralis minor as the scapula is pushed into a posterior tilting position.

Reexamination

The patient is seen for five sessions and improves considerably. Reevaluation indicates subjective reduction in both the intensity and area of pain, the ability to sleep on the right shoulder at night, elimination of painful arc, and pain with resisted abduction and external rotation.

Treatment goals are updated to facilitate dynamic humeral head control and muscle endurance and to optimize parascapular muscle control. The patient is instructed in a program of exercises (see Table 9-2) to be performed with 2-lb weights for 3 sets of 8 repetitions. He is instructed to exercise twice daily initially and in a pain-free range. Every two sessions, he is to increase 1 repetition per set to 20 repetitions for 3 sets. Ice is to be used after exercises. He is instructed not to perform other resistance exercises until he is completely pain free.

Summary

The patient continues this program for 1 month on a home program and is checked periodically by the physical therapist. He does quite well, and after 1 month returns to full activity with the warning not to overdo his weight lifting. The approach to this case is based partially on correct classification of the pathologic condition. Often in young, active individuals, an underlying glenohumeral joint instability is present that necessitates a slightly different approach and is reviewed in this chapter.

ROTATOR CUFF DISORDERS IN THE ATHLETE

Rotator cuff disease or impingement that results from glenohumeral joint instability is generally known as *secondary impingement.* Differentiating primary impingement from secondary impingement is crucial in the proper management of the two conditions. When secondary impingement is treated as primary impingement, the underlying impairment of instability fails to resolve. Instability in this case is defined as symptomatic hypermobility of the humeral head that occurs during function.[48] Instability is often contrasted with asymptomatic clinical laxity. The following sections review the classification of secondary impingement—which occurs primarily in the overhead-throwing athlete—the related clinical signs and symptoms, and approaches to treatment.

Classification

Rotator cuff abnormality in the athlete represents a continuum of problems that may coexist, thus making the primary diagnosis difficult. General classification of rotator cuff abnormality in athletes includes tensile overload, compressive impingement (Neer's classification), instability, and acute traumatic tears. Meister and Andrews[49] classified rotator cuff disease as (1) primary compressive cuff disease, (2) instability with secondary compressive disease, (3) primary tensile overload, (4) secondary tensile overload, and (5) macrotraumatic failure. Primary tensile overload is the result of deceleration forces in the absence of instability, whereas secondary tensile overload is precipitated by underlying instability. Neer's classification of compressive impingement is also observed in the athletic population and is described earlier in this chapter. Compressive rotator cuff disease can occur primarily, or it may be secondarily associated with other shoulder dysfunction. Jobe and associates[50,51] described a four-level classification of the impingement-instability complex that focuses on instability as the central process. This classification includes (1) pure impingement without instability, (2) impingement with instability, (3) impingemant with multidirectional instability, and (4) pure anterior instability without impingement. Finally, athletes sustain acute traumatic tears, a topic addressed in Chapter 12.

These problems occur principally in athletes involved in overhead sports, such as swimmers, tennis players, baseball and softball players, and volleyball players. Although rotator cuff dysfunction is seen most frequently in overhead sport athletes, individuals may have the same pathologic condition as a result of work-related activity. The same deceleration forces observed while serving in tennis can be found in various work environments. Repetitive overhead hammering or other construction activities produce problems similar to those encountered in swimming or throwing. The underlying mechanics, which result in overuse, must be analyzed relative to the respective signs and symptoms.

Primary Tensile Overload

Primary tensile overload can be defined as rotator cuff failure under tensile loads. These tensile loads are primarily the result of eccentric muscle contractions and are associated with activities such as throwing. In this case, the rotator cuff functions to decelerate the horizontal adduction, internal rotation, anterior translation, and distraction forces seen during deceleration.[52] During the early cocking phase of throwing, supraspinatus activity seen on electromyography (EMG) has been shown to be 40% of the maximum manual muscle test (MMT), with increases to 45% of the MMT during late cocking.[53] Peak infraspinatus and teres minor muscle activity has been found in the late cocking and follow-through phases of pitching.[53,54] DiGiovine et al[54] found that supraspinatus activity peaked in the early cocking phase at 60% of the MMT and diminished to 49% and 51% of the MMT during the late cocking and acceleration phases, respectively. Infraspinatus activity peaked at 74% of the MMT during late cocking, whereas teres minor activity was found to be 71% of the MMT during late cocking and 84% of the MMT during deceleration. Thus, repetitive throwing puts the rotator cuff at risk for failure. Andrews and Angelo[55] described rotator cuff tears in throwers located from the midsupraspinatus posterior to the midinfraspinatus, consistent with the deceleration function of these muscles. The mechanism of primary tensile overload is repetitive microtrauma during decelerative functions that results in fatigue and failure of the dynamic stabilizers.

In addition to the rotator cuff's function in deceleration and abduction, the supraspinatus, infraspinatus, and teres minor muscles also function to stabilize the humeral head on the glenoid. This is the dynamic component of shoulder stability, and static stabilization is provided by the labrum and capsuloligamentous structures. When the rotator cuff fatigues as a result of repetitive overload, not only is the decelerative function affected, but also the stabilization function is impaired. The result may be secondary overload on the capsulolabral structures (relative instability) or secondary compressive impingement. As pain persists, subtle changes in movement patterns can exacerbate the problem. Gowan et al[52] studied the patterns on EMG in amateur baseball pitchers and compared the patterns with those of professional pitchers. The professional pitchers used the shoulder muscles more efficiently than the amateurs, who used the rotator cuff and biceps brachii muscles during the acceleration phase.

Evaluation of the shoulder with primary tensile rotator cuff dysfunction reveals a stable shoulder without true compressive impingement. Resistive testing of the rotator cuff is painful, and the rotator cuff may be weak with single or multiple repetition testing. Andrews and Giduman[56] described the hallmark of primary tensile cuff disease to be a partial "undersurface" rotator cuff tear. As noted previously, this type of tear is described as an inside-outside tear. Frequently, no signs of compressive impingement are found at surgery.

The treatment principles are embedded in the knowledge of the underlying pathologic condition, the healing process of soft tissue, and functional demands of the shoulder. Given the premise that primary tensile overload is the result of excessive eccentric muscle contractions and resultant rotator cuff fatigue, the focus of rehabilitation should address these issues. Numerous training techniques challenge the rotator cuff eccentrically. The therapist should be familiar with these techniques and the muscle physiology of eccentric contractions. The problem can be exacerbated if eccentric work is initiated too vigorously in the early stages. Failure of conservative measures may result in surgical intervention to débride the rotator cuff tear. Subacromial decompression is rarely necessary because associated compressive cuff disease is uncommon.

Secondary Tensile Overload

Secondary tensile overload, like primary tensile overload, is defined as rotator cuff failure under tensile loads. In this case, excessive rotator cuff loading is caused by underlying instability. The concept of dynamic stability is important to appreciate in these patients. The subscapularis, supraspinatus, infraspinatus, and teres minor function to compress the humeral head into the glenoid and provide dynamic stability.[57-59] The rotator cuff muscles therefore must provide eccentric control of the humerus during throwing while steering the humeral head along the glenoid fossa. This double function leads to early fatigue failure, tendinitis, and possible secondary mechanical impingement.[60]

As a result of the demands placed on the rotator cuff muscles during throwing, secondary tensile load results from the simultaneous requirements of deceleration and stabilization. Although both demands are present and are generally tolerated in the normal shoulder, the unstable shoulder places an additional burden on the rotator cuff. Because the static stabilizers are compromised, the rotator cuff is overloaded, resulting in dysfunction and injury.

Evaluation of the shoulder with secondary tensile overload is similar to that of primary tensile overload, with the addition of underlying instability. Instability can be unidirectional or multidirectional and is evaluated by traditional instability testing. However, the symptoms may be those of pain rather than instability, and careful evaluation is necessary to delineate the underlying abnormality. Impingement signs may be positive if secondary compressive impingement coexists. Arthroscopic findings demonstrate instability and an associated undersurface rotator cuff tear.

As with primary tensile overload, the treatment principles should address the underlying pathologic condition. In this case, the emphasis is on dynamic stabilization. Again, supraspinatus, infraspinatus, and teres minor strengthening are important because of their role in both eccentric deceleration and stabilization. Additionally, the subscapularis muscle should be trained because of its role in opposing superior humeral head translation and in contributing to rotator cuff moment.[58,61]

Failure of conservative treatment may necessitate surgical intervention. Stabilization procedures and débridement of a partial rotator cuff tear are the appropriate surgical measures to address the underlying pathologic condition.

Instability-Impingement Complex

The scheme of instability and associated impingement noted by Jobe and associates[50-52,62] uses a four-group classification system, with instability as the central theme. In the young athlete, participation in overhead sports such as throwing, swimming, tennis, and volleyball requires large ranges, forces, and repetitions. These demands result in microtrauma to the static and dynamic structures, laxity in the anterior capsule, anterior humeral head subluxation, and posterior capsule tightness. This combination has been described as the *instability-impingement complex* and is discussed in the following scheme.[50]

Instability-Subluxation-Impingement-Rotator Cuff Tear

Individuals with pure compressive rotator cuff impingement whose examination findings include positive impingement signs and negative apprehension signs constitute group 1. Older recreational athletes are generally found in this group, whereas younger athletes are rarely in group 1. Arthroscopic examination reveals a stable shoulder with an undersurface rotator cuff tear and associated subacromial bursitis. The labrum and glenohumeral ligaments are normal. Treatment principles are based on clinical examination findings and follow the general guidelines presented in Neer's model of compressive cuff disease.

Group 2 consists of individuals with impingement-associated instability with labral or capsular injury, instability, and secondary impingement. Findings include positive impingement, apprehension and relocation signs and arthroscopic findings of instability, labral damage, and an undersurface rotator cuff tear. However, the instability findings are often so subtle, even when the patient is examined under anesthesia, that the underlying abnormality may be overlooked. As with group 1 impingement, most individuals respond to a conservative program that addresses the specific mobility, strength, and endurance deficits. Recognition of the underlying instability is the key to successful rehabilitation. In the event of failed conservative treatment, surgical intervention to stabilize the shoulder and débride any rotator cuff damage provides the best results. Isolated acromioplasty can exacerbate underlying instability.

Those individuals classified into group 3 have hyperelastic soft tissue resulting in anterior or multidirectional instability and associated impingement. Hyperelasticity, as evidenced by joint hyperextension, is the distinguishing characteristic between groups 2 and 3. In this case, results of impingement, apprehension, and relocation signs are positive. Arthroscopic examination reveals an unstable shoulder, an attenuated but intact labrum, and an undersurface rotator cuff tear. Jobe and Glousman[62] emphasized the difficulty in clarifying the diagnosis in groups 2 and 3. Once the diagnosis is made and the underlying pathologic condition is identified, appropriate rehabilitation measures are generally effective in returning the athlete to his or her sport. Group 4 consists of those individuals with pure anterior instability without associated impingement. Injury is caused by a traumatic event, resulting in an acute partial or complete dislocation. Clinical and arthroscopic examinations are consistent with an unstable shoulder, without impingement.

Posterior Impingement

As previously described, posterior-superior glenoid impingement (internal impingement) is an additional source of rotator cuff abnormality and is suggested to be the primary cause of rotator cuff disease in athletes.[63-67] In this case, the rotator cuff is impinged between the greater tuberosity and the posterior-superior glenoid labrum. This disorder often occurs in throwers and others involved in overhead activity. It is often associated with mild anterior instability, whereas patients with significant instability do not have posterior impingement. Some investigators have challenged the assumption that this problem is seen primarily in athletes and in those with mild instability and have found no statistically significant relationships among the position of contact and the mechanism of injury, ROM, throwers versus nonthrowers, or impingement signs.[67]

Several theories have been posited to explain the underlying mechanism of posterior-superior impingement.[68-70] Because many of these patients have a loss of internal rotation ROM greater than 20° (compared with their contralateral side), the thought is that internal rotation loss with a shortened posterior capsule creates a posterior-superior translation of the humeral head, particularly during the cocking phase of throwing.[70] As a result, the posterior cuff tendons are susceptible to entrapment between the posterior-superior humeral head and the corresponding glenoid fossa.

Patients with posterior impingement often complain of posterior pain, which is worse when in a position of abduction and external rotation. Results of anterior apprehension testing are positive for pain but may be negative for instability. Relocation testing relieves the symptoms. An arthroscopic study of patients with posterior impingement found 100% of these patients to have contact between the rotator cuff and the posterior-superior glenoid rim during apprehension testing.[65] The differential diagnosis includes posterior instability, anterior instability, and secondary tensile overload.

Rehabilitative Issues

Overview

Jobe and Pink[50] reported that approximately 95% of patients with the instability-impingement complex respond to conservative treatment. The remaining 5% will require a surgical procedure that addresses the primary pathologic condition. Anywhere from 2 to 3 to 6 to 12 months of *appropriate* conservative rehabilitation have been recommended before one should consider surgical intervention, depending on the specific impingement problem.[50,57,71,72] The rehabilitation program should be based on the underlying pathologic condition, the clinical examination results, and the patient's goals. The concept that everyone with impingement should be treated with a stretching and strengthening program neglects the spectrum of impingement problems. Jobe et al[51] emphasized this fact in suggesting that stretching should be performed judiciously and only on demonstration of specific musculotendinous tightness. In the presence of internal impingement, for example, Morgan et al[63] suggested a program of stretching the posterior capsule of the glenohumeral joint to increase internal rotation. In contrast, excessive stretching of already lax anterior shoulder structures may exacerbate the problem.

Rehabilitative exercises have been recommended for treating the unstable shoulder.[72,73] Burkhead and Rockwood[72] treated 115 patients with 140 unstable shoulders with an exercise program. Subjects had traumatic or atraumatic recurrent anterior, posterior, or multidirectional shoulder subluxation. In those individuals with atraumatic subluxation, 83% had a good or excellent result, compared with 15% of those with traumatic instability. These investigators emphasized the importance of continuing a maintenance strengthening program because several patients had recurrent symptoms when they stopped the exercises.

Mallon and Speer[73] recommended strengthening of the rotator cuff, specifically the supraspinatus, because of its role in preventing inferior subluxation. Short-arc strengthening is advocated, and stretching is generally avoided. Kronberg et al[74,75] evaluated the muscle activity and coordination in normal shoulders and concluded that muscle activity plays a significant role in stabilization through coordinated activation of prime movers and antagonists. A subsequent study analyzed shoulder muscle activity in patients with generalized joint laxity and shoulder instability compared with the control groups in the previous study.[76] Results in patients demonstrated increased anterior and middle deltoid activity during flexion and abduction and decreased subscapularis activity during internal rotation as compared with the control groups. A nonsignificant increase in supraspinatus activity was recorded during all movements except flexion, a finding suggesting compensatory muscle function. These findings support the role of the supraspinatus in stabilization and underscore the importance of training this muscle in rehabilitation.

Examination

The varying muscle function throughout any upper extremity activity underscores the importance of the evaluation process. The first and most fundamental rehabilitation issue is clarification of the problem through a thorough evaluation. Subjective information should include the painful position or motion, with estimation of the force, direction, and magnitude of muscle activity. In addition to the primary movers, muscles functioning as stabilizers and antagonists must be identified. The therapist must be aware that underlying instability may be subtle and unrecognized by the athlete. Moreover, instability testing may reproduce pain, but not a feeling of apprehension. The rehabilitation program varies, depending on the absence or presence of underlying hyperelasticity, frank instability, or secondary compressive impingement. In all cases, the primary underlying abnormality is the focus of rehabilitation, and secondary problems are addressed simultaneously. This situation is clearly more difficult than in the individual who has a single problem. Many athletes have returned to the clinic with a recurrence of impingement with a previously unrecognized underlying dysfunction. This underlying dysfunction may not be evident in the shoulder girdle, but it may manifest as weakness in another link in the kinetic chain, resulting in excessive load on the shoulder. A lower extremity or back injury may alter movement patterns, which are amplified at the shoulder.

Itoi et al[59] emphasized the importance of shoulder position in kinetic and kinematic analysis because muscle function changes depending on position. Moreover, an understanding of the differences in muscle activity between sports and among phases or positions of the same sport is the key to designing a rehabilitation program. Activity on EMG has been documented in swimming, throwing, golf, and tennis, as well as in painful and normal shoulders.[75,77-82] When evaluating data from EMG, the type of muscle contraction should be considered. The MMT on which data from EMG are based is generally performed isometrically, whereas acquired data from EMG may be from isometric, concentric, or eccentric muscle contractions, depending on the muscle's role at any point in time. Because of the efficiency of eccentric muscle activity, the same force can be generated with fewer motor units, and the result is a lower percentage of MMT. Incorrect interpretation of these data could affect the rehabilitation program design. The type of muscle contraction required at the painful position and the number of repetitions guide the rehabilitation program design.

An important aspect of the evaluation process is the determination of the specific return to activity goals. If strength and endurance are the primary issues, these should be the primary focus of rehabilitation. Dynamic stabilization and coordination drills should be at the program's core in athletes with underlying instability. Not all athletes require a plyometric program to return to their sport, and the program should differ from one individual to the next most dramatically in the late stages. As the rehabilitation program proceeds, the exercise program should begin to resemble the athlete's sport. This includes body posture, exercise range, type of muscle contraction, speed, load, and repetitions. Transition to the functional progression is facilitated by appropriate program design.

Role of the Scapula

As previously detailed, the scapular muscles place the scapula in a position for optimal glenohumeral function and provide a stable base for the glenohumeral rotator cuff muscles as well as the deltoid muscle. The scapular muscles include the rhomboid, trapezius, levator scapulae, serratus anterior, and pectoralis minor. Based on biomechanical and clinical studies, clinicians carefully evaluate and address scapular impairments as part of their overall treatment for impingement.[83-85]

Several of the scapular muscles have been studied in normal and in painful shoulders during functional activities to determine changes in firing patterns with pain. When investigators compared data from EMG during free-style swimming between individuals with normal and painful shoulders, significant differences were found.[79,80] Patients with painful shoulders demonstrated the following differences when compared with persons with normal shoulders: (1) less anterior and middle deltoid activity at hand entry and exit, (2) more infraspinatus activity at the end of pull-through, (3) less subscapularis activity at midrecovery, (4) less rhomboid and upper trapezius activity at hand entry, and (5) more rhomboid and less serratus anterior activity during pulling. Decreased serratus anterior activity during the pulling phase sets the stage for impingement symptoms because it positions the shoulder in protraction and upward rotation to prevent impingement. Increased rhomboid activity may partially substitute for the serratus anterior by attempting to create more subacromial space while preparing the shoulder for early hand exit. Similar findings were noted when comparing butterfly swimmers who had pain-free and painful shoulders.[77,78] Again, the serratus anterior, along with the teres minor, demonstrated decreased activity, a finding suggesting an unstable base of support and an inability to assist with propulsion. In persons with normal shoulders, the subscapularis, serratus anterior, teres minor, and upper trapezius maintained high levels of activity throughout the stroke, thus predisposing these muscles to fatigue. As such, training programs should focus on increasing the endurance of these muscles.

Glousman et al,[86] in a study of EMG in pitchers with normal shoulders and in those with anterior instability, noted decreased pectoralis major, latissimus dorsi, subscapularis, and serratus anterior muscle activity during throwing and especially during late cocking. During this phase, the serratus anterior functions to oppose the retractors while stabilizing and protracting the scapula. Additionally, the serratus anterior may assist in tipping the scapula to allow for maximal glenohumeral congruency during excessive external rotation.[54] Decreased serratus anterior activity in late cocking places an additional load on the anterior static stabilizers and may contribute to anterior instability. Strength and endurance of these muscles are the keystones for shoulder rehabilitation in this population.

Moseley et al[28] analyzed the activity on EMG in 8 scapular muscles during 16 rehabilitation exercises. Optimal exercises for each muscle were identified by the criteria of greater than 50% MMT over three consecutive arcs of motion. A group of four core exercises trained each of the eight muscles at the preset criteria and included scaption (elevation in the scapular plane), rowing, push-up with a plus (additional scapular protraction), and press-up. Closer evaluation of the data will allow the therapist to make appropriate choices regarding scapular-strengthening activities. For example, the criteria for the core exercise group necessitated that each muscle be used at the predetermined minimum level. The only qualifying exercise for the pectoralis minor was the press-up, so it was included in the core group. The press-up did not meet minimal criteria for any other muscle group. Additionally, the highest activity on EMG in the middle serratus anterior was produced during flexion and abduction, from 120° to 150°. Moreover, the standard deviations of some exercises are greater than 50% of the original value. As such, the therapist should choose exercises judiciously based on the examination and activity kinetics and should monitor the exercise quality carefully to ensure proper performance (Fig. 9-8).

Open and Closed Chain Exercise

Closed chain exercises have been advocated for lower extremity rehabilitation and have been suggested for the treatment of upper extremity problems.[87-90] Traditional physical therapy application of the closed kinetic chain concept assumes the distal segment to be fixed to an object that provides considerable external resistance, whereas in an open chain, the distal segment is free to move in space. The definition of "considerable external resistance" could potentially be met in a traditional open chain activity.[89] Dillman et al[89] suggested a new classification of this model because of inadequate standardized definitions, lack of quantitatively based definitions, classification of some exercises into opposing categories, and comparison of exercises with different mechanics. These investigators suggested the following three-level classification: (1) moveable boundary, no external load (MNL); (2) moveable boundary, external load (MEL); and (3) fixed boundary, external load (FEL). The MNL classification is like a traditional open chain exercise, the FEL is like a traditional closed chain exercise, and the MEL is like the "gray" area. Activities representative of the MEL classification are a resisted bench press, hack squat, and leg press. Matched MEL and FEL exercises in a single subject demonstrated that exercises with similar biomechanics result in comparable muscular activity.

Principles of closed chain exercise in the lower extremity have been applied to the upper extremity. Further study is necessary to determine whether this application is appropriate. The supposition that closed chain shoulder exercise enhances static stability during dynamic activity through mechanoreceptor education needs further testing.

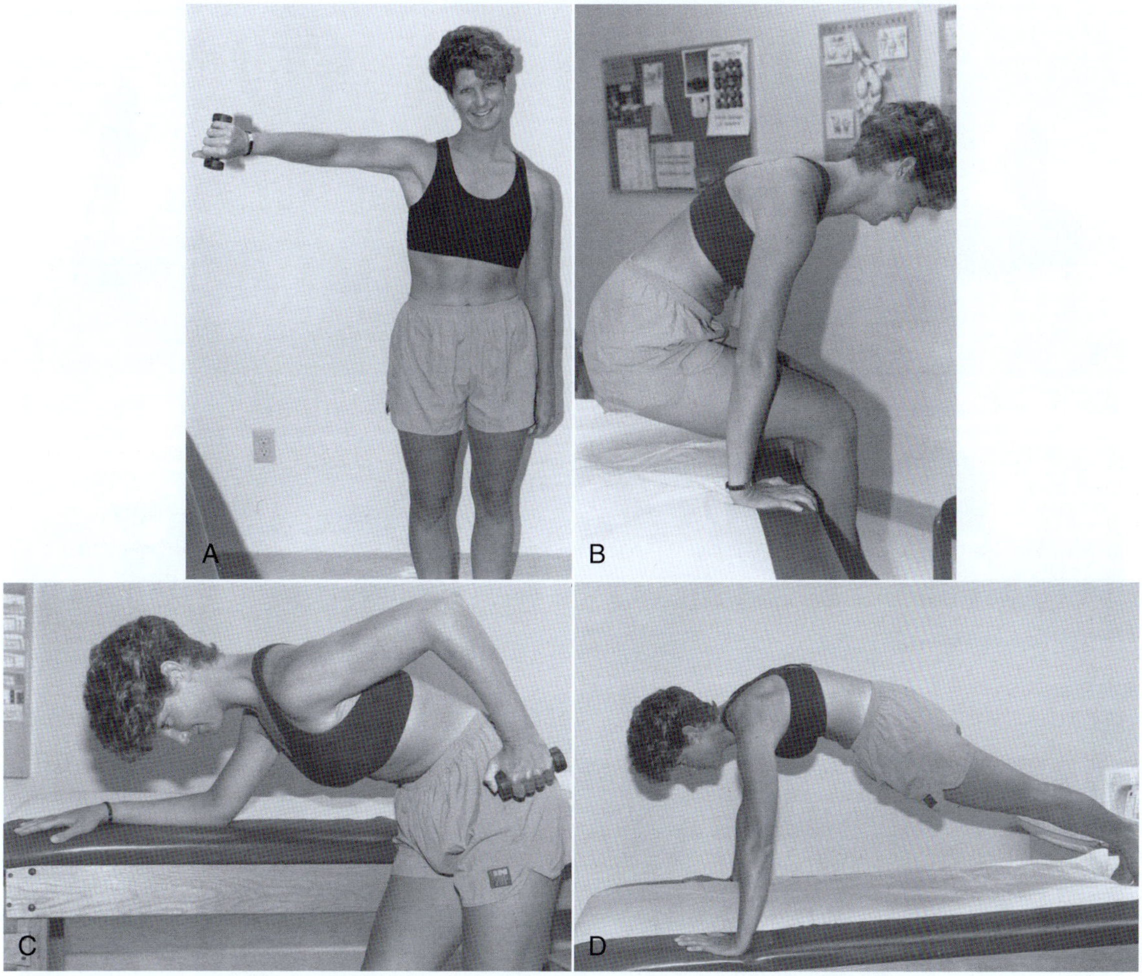

Figure 9-8 A, Scaption in internal rotation. **B,** Press-up. **C,** Rowing. **D,** Push-ups with a plus (additional scapular protraction).

Specificity of exercise guidelines would suggest little carryover from closed chain exercise to open chain activity. The value of closed chain exercise in the athlete participating in a closed chain sport is evident. Closed chain exercise training in an open chain sport may be of value for reasons yet to be clarified. Muscular cocontraction in closed chain activity can provide dynamic stabilization for the individual with an unstable shoulder. Carryover of this cocontraction into an open chain is essential for the open chain sport athlete and is discussed in further detail in the next section.

Closed chain exercise for the upper extremity includes activities such as wall push-ups, modified and full push-ups with a plus, weight shifts in weight-bearing positions, and press-ups (Fig. 9-9; see also Fig. 9-8). The progression should be from partial weight bearing against a wall, to increasing weight bearing on a table, to the quadrupedal position, to the modified and full push-up positions. Exercises may be progressed from two-arm to single-arm support, and eventually to plyometrics. Use of gymnastic balls, stair steppers, slide boards, treadmills, rocker boards, and other traditional lower extremity equipment challenges the shoulder dynamically. It is critical that the quality of the exercise be maintained throughout. As the scapular stabilizers fatigue, the scapulae may begin to wing, resulting in improper motor programming and possible injury. The therapist and athlete alike must be aware of and be able to recognize this situation.

The activity on EMG has been well documented during open and closed chain shoulder rehabilitation exercises.[90,91] Townsend et al[91] studied 9 muscles during 17 shoulder exercises. Exercises were considered a challenge if they produced more than 50% of the MMT over three consecutive arcs, and four exercises were found to load each of the nine muscles at least once at the given criteria. These exercises included (1) scaption in internal rotation, (2) flexion, (3) horizontal abduction in external rotation, and (4) press-up (Fig. 9-10; see also Fig. 9-8A and C). As with the data from Moseley and Goldie,[39] closer scrutiny can provide the therapist with a wealth of information to guide rehabilitation. Again, the press-up was included because of the preset criteria, whereas activity on EMG was noted only in the pectoralis major and latissimus dorsi. For the therapist wanting to train the rotator cuff selectively, other exercises tested would be more appropriate. Although the assumption is made that the exercise with the greatest activity on EMG should be chosen to strengthen a specific muscle, in rehabilitation that is not always the case. Occasionally, such an activity is too strenuous for the individual recovering from an injury or

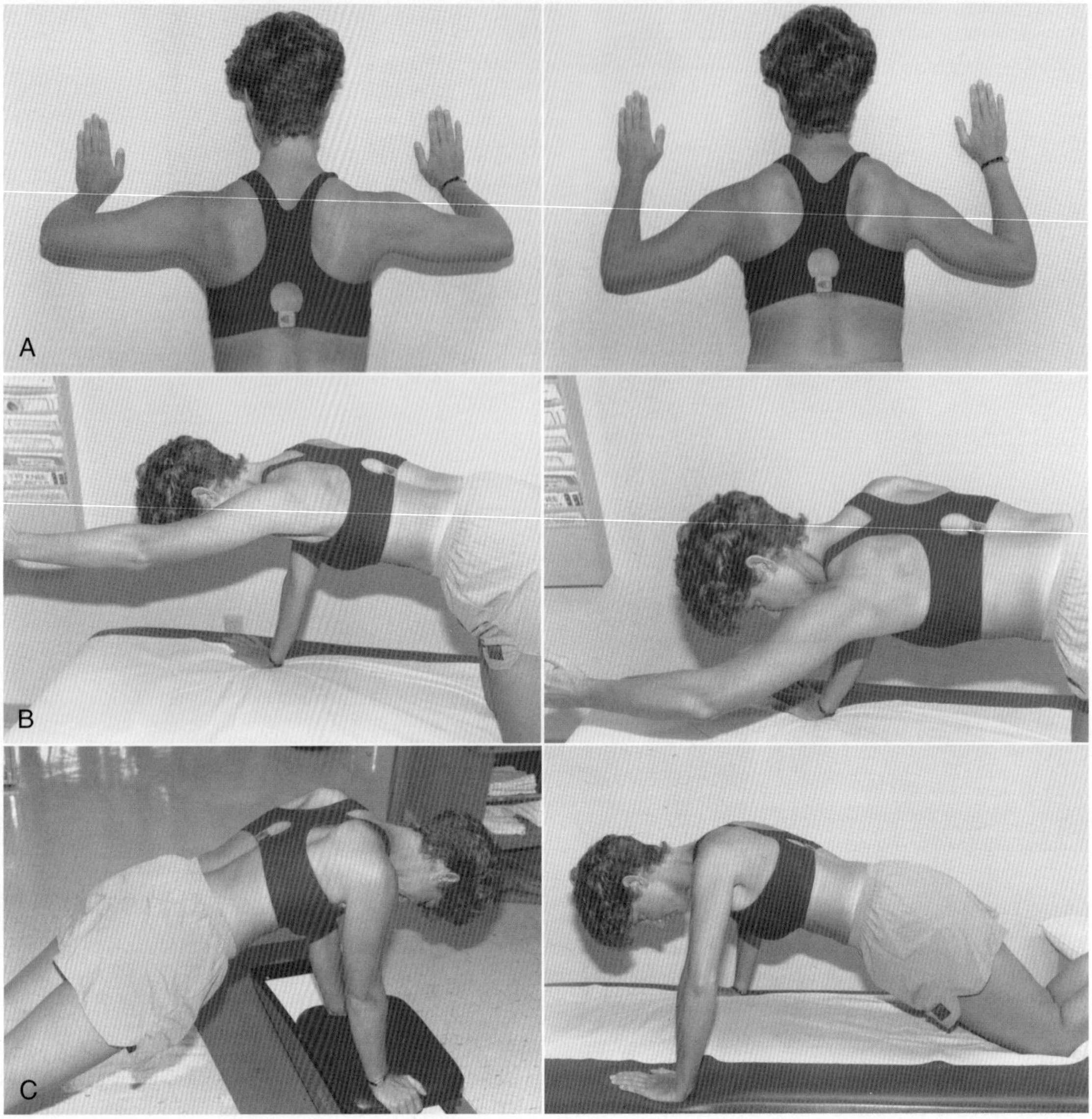

Figure 9-9 Proper and improper performance of exercises. **A1** and **A2,** Improper performance of a wall push-up with excessive scapular winging. The patient should be verbally cued for proper performance. **B1,** Proper performance of weight-bearing reaching activity with the lumbar spine neutral and proper scapular stabilization. **B2,** Improper performance of weight-bearing reaching activity with trunk rotation and poor scapular stabilization on the right. **C1,** Improper performance in modified push-up position during dynamic activity with excessive scapular winging during activity. **C2,** Return to lower-level static activity to reinforce proper performance of exercise.

surgery. In this case, the data from Townsend et al[91] provide the therapist with different choices that may be more appropriate. For example, if scaption in internal rotation is too weak or painful, scaption in external rotation will require less, but still significant, supraspinatus activity.

Neuromuscular Retraining

Neuromuscular retraining has been advocated by many investigators in the treatment of shoulder dysfunctions, especially the instability complex.[92-98] Lephart et al[94] found decreased passive repositioning sense and threshold to detection of passive motion in individuals with anterior shoulder instability. Following reconstruction, values for these same variables were the same as the normal control group. The relationship between static and dynamic structures was explored by Cain et al,[99] who found that contraction of the infraspinatus and teres minor muscles reduced strain on the anterior-inferior glenohumeral ligament at 90° of abduction. Guanche et al[100] noted a reflex arc from mechanoreceptors within the glenohumeral capsule to muscles crossing the joint. These findings reinforce the synergistic activity of the static and dynamic structures about the shoulder. However, Borsa et al[93] suggested that damage to the mechanoreceptors disables the reflexive dynamic stability and thus increases the instability problem.

Exercises purporting to facilitate development of proprioception should consider the multilevel aspect of nervous system training. Reflexive patterning at the spinal cord level

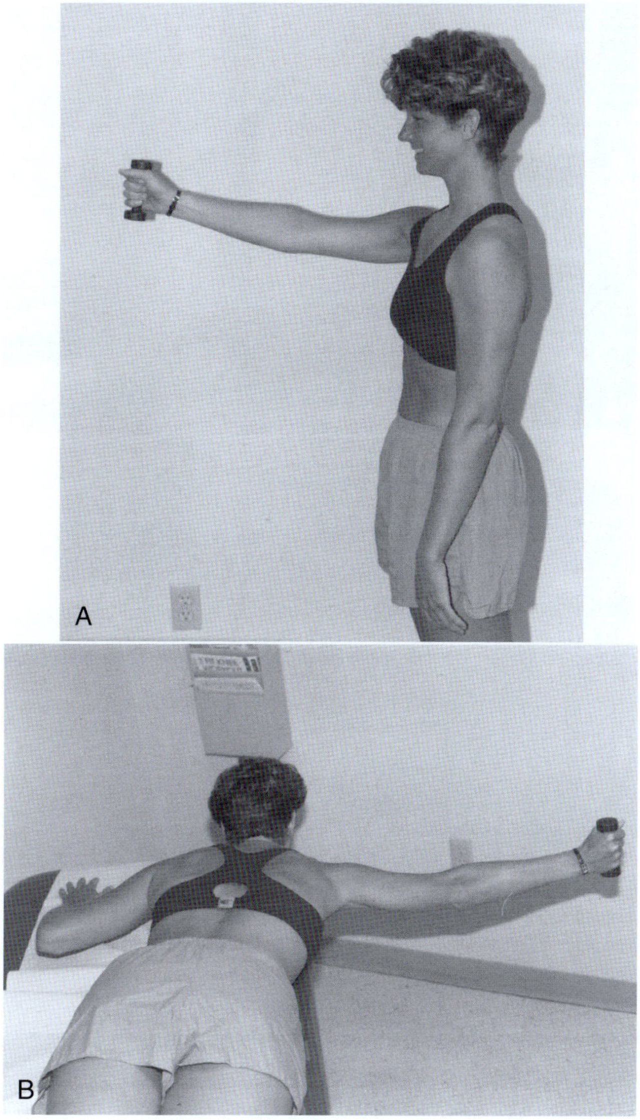

Figure 9-10 Shoulder exercises. **A,** Flexion. **B,** Horizontal abduction in external rotation.

occurs on a subconscious level and is only one aspect of neuromuscular retraining. Higher levels are involved with the planning and execution of motor tasks. The basal ganglia are involved in the more complex aspects of motor planning and ultimately influence the spinal motor neuron pool by forming a control loop with motor areas of the cortex involved with the planning and execution of voluntary motor tasks. The cerebellum regulates some of the specific parameters of motor control, including synergistic coordination and background muscle tone. The question of the cognitive role in proprioceptive training deserves attention. One purpose of a proprioceptive rehabilitation program is to enhance cognitive appreciation of the joint relative to position and motion, and most rehabilitation programs necessitate cognitive attention to the task.[94] However, when throwing a ball, serving volleyball, or swimming, the athlete is unlikely to be thinking about his or her shoulder. As such, removal of the cognitive aspect of activity must be incorporated at some time in the rehabilitation process. Mentally attending to something besides the task at hand will challenge the nervous system in a more realistic situation. Counting back by serial sevens, or engaging in unrelated conversation while performing challenging activities, will facilitate this skill. Conversion of a conscious task to unconscious motor programming, stored as central commands, is the goal.

Proprioceptive neuromuscular facilitation (PNF) exercises have been advocated for the development of kinesthetic awareness.[83,93] Additionally, Wilk and Arrigo[83] recommended several movement awareness drills to enhance neuromuscular control of the shoulder. These drills are performed in the advanced phase, and they place the athlete in a position that challenges the stabilizing mechanisms. When performing any kinesthetic or movement awareness exercises, the therapist must closely attend to additional information derived from other sensory systems that may assist in proprioception. These factors may include tactile cueing from the supporting surface, tactile cueing from the therapist, visual cueing, and predictability of movement pattern and speed based on previous experience. Additionally, the position during exercise becomes critical when considering the role of the cerebellum and basal ganglia in postural set and motor programming. An activity performed with the patient in the supine position on a table does not require the same neuromuscular coordination as when the same activity is performed when the patient is standing.

The Impulse Inertial Exercise System (IES; Newnan, Ga) was originally developed with neuromuscular training as the chief consideration. High-speed ballistic activities in numerous movement patterns can be repetitively performed on the IES. Rapid ballistic movements have patterns of agonist muscle and antagonist muscle contractions different from patterns seen with slower-speed activities. Synchronous activation of agonists and antagonists occurs with ballistic movements as a result of triphasic muscle activation.[101-105] The initial burst of agonist muscle contraction triggers the activity, and this activity ceases before the limb reaches its final position. Subsequently, the antagonist fires as a braking mechanism, and the final phase finds the agonist firing again to "clamp" the movement toward the target.[104] The same movement pattern at a slow speed demonstrates only agonist muscle contraction, with braking provided by the passive viscoelastic properties of the tissue. The timing and amplitude of antagonist activity are affected by the distance and speed of the movement. Small-amplitude movements at higher speeds result in substantial overlap of burst activity in agonist and antagonist during acceleration, whereas coactivation occurs in bursts during deceleration.[101] Finally, knowledge of the necessity for antagonist firing affects muscle activity. When a mechanical stop was placed in the testing apparatus, the antagonist burst disappeared within two to three trials, a finding suggesting some cognitive control over the braking mechanism. This work supports the use of high-speed ballistic activities to train open chain cocontraction in an unstable shoulder. Such activities can be achieved by use of the IES or resistive tubing (Figs. 9-11 and 9-12). Many different movement patterns can be trained, including shoulder rotation in abduction and PNF patterns.

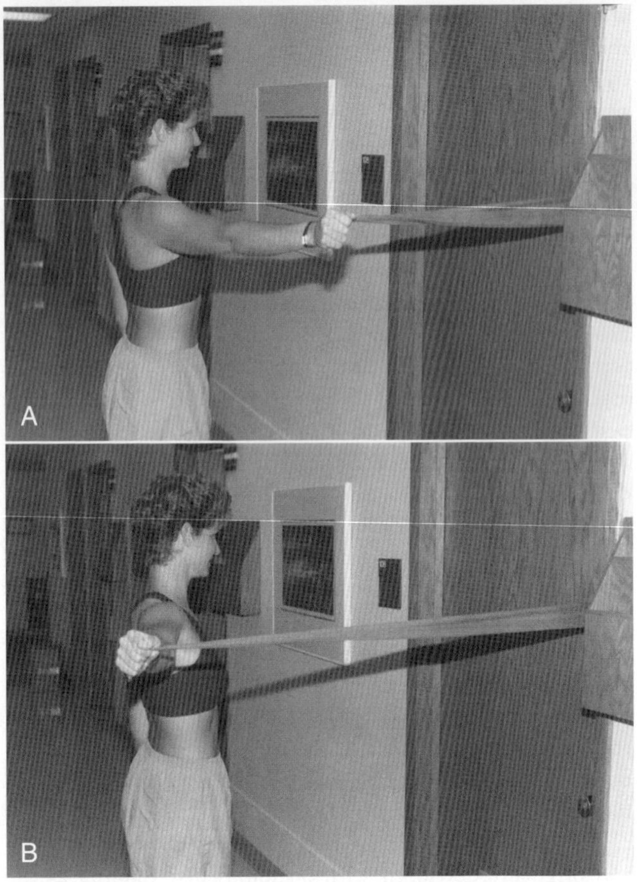

Figure 9-11 **A** and **B,** Starting and ending positions for dynamic ballistic horizontal abduction exercise using resistive tubing.

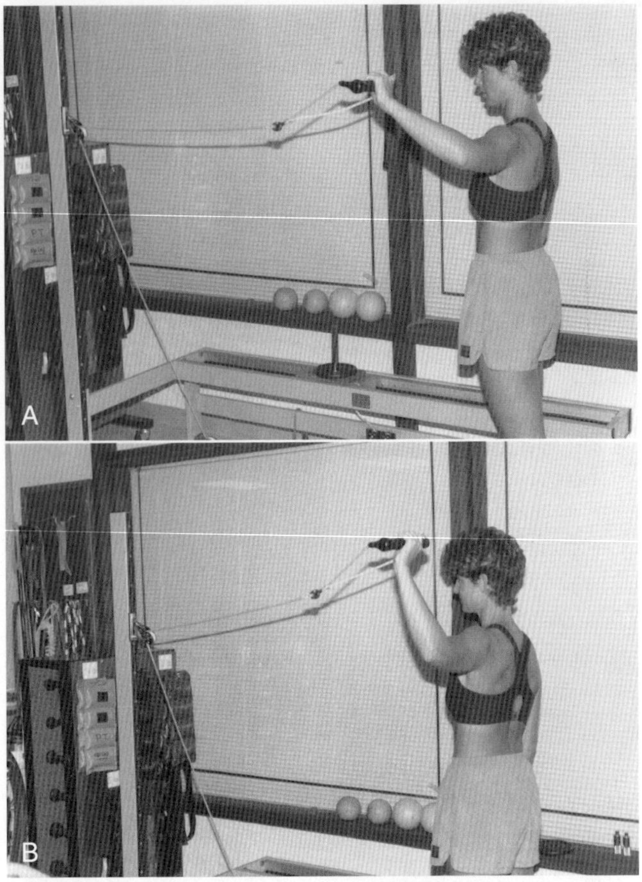

Figure 9-12 **A** and **B,** Starting and ending position for dynamic ballistic shoulder external rotation at 90° of abduction using the Impulse Inertial Exercise System.

CASE STUDY 9-2

General Demographics

Joan is a 16-year-old high school swimmer who comes to the clinic with a 4-month history of right shoulder pain. She is right-hand dominant.

Social History

Joan is single with no children. She does not smoke or drink.

Employment and Environment

She is a high-school student who swims competitively and also plays volleyball and softball.

Living Environment

She lives in a two-story house with her parents and younger brother.

Past Medical History

Joan has no history of shoulder or neck problems and no history of medical problems.

History of Chief Complaint

Joan is a butterfly swimmer who has been practicing, in her off-season, swimming and weight lifting to ready herself for her junior year in high school swimming. When she returned to swim practice, she noticed increasing pain in her right shoulder. Over the last month or so, the pain has becomes severe enough to interfere with her normal swimming regimen.

She is concerned because of the increasing pain and discomfort that may interfere with her upcoming swimming season, which begins in 3 weeks.

Prior Treatment for this Condition

She is currently taking a nonsteroidal anti-inflammatory drug prescribed by her primary physician. Other than that, she has received no additional treatment to her right shoulder.

Structural Examination

Physical Therapy Examination

On visual inspection, postural observation indicates that both scapulae are abducted approximately 4 inches from

CASE STUDY 9-2—cont'd

her thoracic midline. In addition, both her medial scapulae borders and inferior scapulae angles are prominent posteriorly.

Range of Motion

- AROM: Painful arc between 90° and 120° of elevation in the frontal plane; full ROM
- PROM: Full and pain free in all ranges

Accessory motion testing indicates that Joan's glenohumeral joint is hypermobile in all directions, particularly in an inferior direction, thus producing a sulcus sign bilaterally.

Tenderness

On palpation, Joan reports tenderness over the biceps tendon and rotator cuff tendon.

Muscle Performance

Resisted testing results show 4/5 strength in resisted abduction without pain. Results of all other testing are strong and pain free. However, Joan has only 3/5 strength in both lower trapezius muscles and 4/5 strength in both serratus anterior muscles.

Special Tests

Neer's and Hawkins' impingement signs are positive. Results of horizontal crossover testing are negative. Results of biceps tension testing and apprehension and relocation testing are positive.

Clinical Impression

Given the history and physical examination of the young athlete's shoulder, the physical therapist determines that she has impingement syndrome caused by underlying instability (impingement-instability complex). This problem is treated in a practice pattern focusing on impairments associated with connective tissue dysfunction. The stage of clinical reactivity is subacute. She has established good rotator cuff strength because of her cuff-strengthening program. However, she exhibits scapular postural changes and muscle weakness consistent with chronic scapular winging, anterior tiling, and abduction. As a result, underlying instability and scapular control have not been addressed, and they are the focus of the rehabilitation program.

Treatment Plan

The initial goal is to build on Joan's strength base without aggravating her secondary impingement syndrome. She is started on a high-speed, short ROM program with yellow resistive bands for shoulder external rotation and shoulder abduction and red bands for shoulder flexion and extension. All exercises are performed in neutral abduction. After a warm-up, she performs 1 set for 30 seconds and attempts to perform 30 to 50 repetitions in 30 seconds. She is instructed to add an extra set of 15 seconds or more as tolerated during the next week.

Immediate scapular manual PNF patterns are instituted for posterior depression to emphasize isolated activation of her lower trapezius muscle, anterior elevation, and isolated abduction (serratus anterior muscle). Resistance is modulated based on the patient's tolerance and her ability to complete smooth and synchronous scapular patterns. The resistance emphasizes both concentric and eccentric contractions. Furthermore, she is instructed to perform home exercises emphasizing scapular retraction with depression and scapular abduction (protraction), to fatigue.

On her return visit, she reports soreness for a day, with no fatigue in flexion and extension exercises after 2 days. Resisted external rotation is slightly sore but strong. Her flexion and extension exercises are progressed to 45° of abduction. One week later, she is improving steadily. She is up to 3 sets for 30 seconds of all exercises. Resisted external rotation is maintained in neutral, but with progression to red resistive bands. Flexion, extension, and abduction are discontinued, and horizontal abduction and adduction exercises are initiated at 90° of abduction with green bands. She is encouraged to try to perform up to 90 repetitions in 30 seconds.

By her fourth visit, she is feeling notably better. Internal and external rotation is initiated at 90° of abduction, and progress is made in the resistance of the bands. On her fifth visit, she has progressed to PNF D2 flexion exercises and reproduction of the throwing motion. She performs 3 sets each of more than 90 repetitions of each exercise in 30 seconds. On her sixth and final visit, the patient is placed on a functional progression for volleyball, as well as a maintenance strength and coordination program.

Summary

A 16-year-old high-school athlete is seen for a total of six visits to treat her impingement-instability complex. The key to successful rehabilitation is the recognition of the underlying instability, with exercise protocols addressing this problem. Rotator cuff strengthening alone is ineffective in this athlete, and the incorporation of dynamic stabilization exercises provides the needed dynamic control of her unstable shoulder.

SUMMARY

Impingement syndrome of the shoulder can result in a cascade of pathologic conditions that primarily affect the rotator cuff and result in subacromial pain and shoulder dysfunction. The causes of impingement presented in this chapter have multiple factors, but they can be divided into primary impingement and secondary impingement, depending on the presence of instability or impingement. These categories are further subdivided based on the pathomechanics of injury, the age of the patient, dysfunctions, and associated abnormalities. In the younger, athletic population, the basic problem is instability, which leads to subluxation, impingement, and rotator cuff disease. Treatment is based on accurate classification of the ailment and is logically focused on the signs, symptoms, and nature of the dysfunction. For example, treatment of impingement in younger athletes is designed to restore shoulder stability and control and to correct underlying mechanical problems associated with their sport. A systematic evaluation of the nature and extent of the injury is imperative for the clinician to classify the problem properly and to design an effective rehabilitation program.

ACKNOWLEDGMENTS

Greenfield is grateful to Anne Schwartz for providing the drawings on which the figures are based. He is also grateful to Lori Thein Brody for her contributions to the second part of this chapter concerning instability with impingement.

REFERENCES

1. Neer CS: Anterior acromioplasty for the chronic impingement syndrome of the shoulder, *J Bone Joint Surg Am* 54:41, 1972.
2. Neer CS: Impingement lesions, *Clin Orthop Relat Res* 173:70, 1983.
3. Peterson CJ, Redlund-Johnell I: The subacromial space in normal shoulder radiographs, *Acta Orthop Scand* 55:57, 1984.
4. Weiner DS, MacNab I: Superior migration of the humeral head: a radiological aid in the diagnosis of tears of the rotator cuff, *J Bone Joint Surg Br* 52:524, 1970.
5. Patte D: The subcoracoid impingement, *Clin Orthop Relat Res* 254:55, 1990.
6. Gerber C, Terrier F, Ganz R: The role of the coracoid process in the chronic impingement syndrome, *J Bone Joint Surg Br* 67:703, 1985.
7. Morrison DS, Bigliani LU: The clinical significance of variations in acromial morphology, *Orthop Trans* 11:234, 1987.
8. Rathbun JB, Macnab I: The microvascular pattern of the rotator cuff, *J Bone Joint Surg Br* 52:540, 1970.
9. Rothman RH, Parke WW: The vascular anatomy of the rotator cuff, *Clin Orthop Relat Res* 41:176, 1965.
10. Neviaser RJ, Neviaser TJ: Observations on impingement, *Clin Orthop Relat Res* 254:60, 1990.
11. Codman EA: *The shoulder*, ed 2, Boston, 1934, Thomas Todd.
12. Uhthoff HK, Hammond I, Sarkar K, et al: Enthesopathy of the rotator cuff. In *Proceedings of the fifth open meeting of American Shoulder and Elbow Surgeons*, Las Vegas, 1989, American Shoulder and Elbow Surgeons.
13. Ozaki J, Fujimoto S, Yoahiyuki N, et al: Tears of the rotator cuff of the shoulder associated with pathological changes in the acromion, *J Bone Joint Surg Am* 70:1224, 1998.
14. Griegel-Morris P, Larson K, Mueller-Klaus K, et al: Incidence of common postural abnormalities in the cervical, shoulder, and thoracic regions and their associations with pain in two age groups of healthy subjects, *Phys Ther* 72:6, 1992.
15. Greenfield B, Catlin P, Coats P, et al: Posture in patients with shoulder overuse injuries and healthy individuals, *J Orthop Sports Phys Ther* 21:287, 1995.
16. Janda V: Muscles, central nervous motor regulation and back problems. In Korr I, editor: *The neurobiologic mechanisms in spinal manipulative therapy*, New York, 1978, Plenum.
17. Kendall HD, Kendall FP, Boynton DA: *Posture and function*, Baltimore, 1958, Williams & Wilkins.
18. Kendall FP, McCreary EK: *Muscles, testing and function*, ed 3, Baltimore, 1988, Williams & Wilkins.
19. Kibler WB: Role of the scapula in the overhead throwing motion, *Contemp Orthop* 22:5, 1991.
20. Diveta J, Walker ML, Skibinski B: Relationship between performance of selected scapular muscles and scapular abduction in standing subjects, *Phys Ther* 70:470, 1990.
21. Hawkins RJ, Kennedy JC: Impingement syndrome in athletes, *Am J Sports Med* 8:151, 1990.
22. Herring SA, Nilson KL: Introduction to overuse injuries, *Clin Sports Med* 6:225, 1987.
23. Ludewig PM, Reynolds J: The association of scapular kinematics and glenohumeral joint pathologies, *J Orthop Sport Phys Ther* 39:90, 2009.
24. Poppen NK, Walker PS: Normal and abnormal motion of the shoulder, *J Bone Joint Surg Am* 58:195, 1978.
25. Inman VT, Saunders J, Abbott L: Observations on the function of the shoulder joint, *J Bone Joint Surg* 26:1, 1934.
26. Frankel VH, Nordin M: *Basic biomechanics of the skeletal system*, Philadelphia, 1980, Lea & Febiger.
27. Peat M, Culham E: Functional anatomy of the shoulder complex. In Andrews JR, Wilk KE, editors: *The athlete's shoulder*, New York, 1990, Churchill Livingstone.
28. Moseley BJ, Jobe FW, Pink M, et al: EMG analysis of the scapular muscles during a baseball rehabilitation program, *Am J Sports Med* 20:128, 1992.
29. Burkhart SS, Morgan CD, Kibler WB: The disabled throwing shoulder: spectrum of pathology. Part III. The SICK scapular, scapular dyskinesis, the kinetic chain, and rehabilitation, *J Arthrosc* 19:641, 2003.
30. Sahrmann SA: *Diagnosis and treatment of movement impairment syndromes*, St. Louis, 2002, Mosby.
31. Gossman MR, Sahrmann SA, Rose SI: Review of length associated changes in muscle: experimental evidence and clinical implications, *Phys Ther* 62:1799, 1982.
32. Ludewig PM, Cook TM: Alterations in shoulder kinematics and associated muscle activity in people with symptoms of shoulder impingement, *Phys Ther* 80:276, 2000.
33. McClure PW, Biakler J, Neff N, et al: Shoulder function and 3-dimensional kinematics in people with shoulder impingement syndrome before and after a 6-week exercise program, *Phys Ther* 84:832, 2004.
34. Endo K, Yukata K, Yasui N: Influence of age on scapular thoracic orientation, *Clin Biomech (Bristol, Avon)* 19:1009, 2004.
35. Budoff JE, Nirschl RP, Guidi EJ: Débridement of partial-thickness tears of the rotator cuff without acromioplasty, *J Bone Joint Surg Am* 80:733, 1998.
36. Saha AK: Dynamic stability of the glenohumeral joint, *Acta Orthop Scand* 42:491, 1971.
37. Jobe CM: Superior glenoid impingement, *Clin Orthop Relat Res* 330:98, 1996.
38. Gerber C, Sebesta A: Impingement of deep surface of the subscapularis tendon and the reflection pulley on the anterosuperior glenoid rim: a preliminary report, *J Shoulder Elbow Surg* 9:483, 2000.
39. Moseley HF, Goldie I: The arterial pattern of the rotator cuff of the shoulder, *J Bone Joint Surg Br* 45:780, 1963.
40. Lohr JF, Uhthoff HK: The microvascular pattern of the supraspinatus tendon, *Clin Orthop Relat Res* 254:35, 1990.
41. Chansky HA, Iannotti JP: The vascularity of the rotator cuff, *Clin Sports Med* 10:807, 1991.

42. Swiontkowski M, Iannotti JP, Boulas JH, et al: *Intraoperative assessment of rotator cuff vascularity using laser Doppler flowmetry*, St. Louis, 1990, Mosby-Year Book.
43. Miklovitz SL, Nolan TP Jr,: *Modalities for therapeutic intervention*, ed 4, Philadelphia, 2005, Davis.
44. Moncrief SA, Lau JD, Gale JR, et al: Effect of rotator cuff exercise on humeral rotation torque in healthy individuals, *J Strength Cond Res* 16:262, 2002.
45. Cyriax J: *Textbook of orthopaedic medicine: diagnosis of soft tissue lesions*, ed 8, Philadelphia, 1982, Bailliere Tindall.
46. Cofield RH, Simonet WT: Symposium in sports medicine. Part 2. The shoulder in sports, *Mayo Clin Proc* 59:157, 1984.
47. Patte D: Classification of rotator cuff lesions, *Clin Orthop Relat Res* 254:81, 1990.
48. Hayes K, Callanan M, Walton J, et al: Shoulder instability: management and rehabilitation, *J Orthop Sports Phys Ther* 32:1, 2002.
49. Meister K, Andrews JR: Classification and treatment of rotator cuff injuries in the overhand athlete, *J Orthop Sports Phys Ther* 18:413, 1993.
50. Jobe FW, Pink M: Classification and treatment of shoulder dysfunction in the overhead athlete, *J Orthop Sports Phys Ther* 18:427, 1993.
51. Jobe FW, Tibone JE, Jobe CM, et al: The shoulder in sports. In Rockwood CA, Matsen FA, editors: *The shoulder*, Philadelphia, 1990, Saunders.
52. Gowan ID, Jobe FW, Tibone JE, et al: A comparative electromyographic analysis of the shoulder during pitching, *Am J Sports Med* 15:586, 1987.
53. Bradley JP, Tibone JE: Electromyographic analysis of muscle action about the shoulder, *Clin Sports Med* 10:789, 1991.
54. DiGiovine NM, Jobe FW, Pink M, et al: An electromyographic analysis of the upper extremity in pitching, *J Shoulder Elbow Surg* 1:15, 1992.
55. Andrews JR, Angelo RL: Shoulder arthroscopy for the throwing athlete. In Paulos LE, Tibone JE, editors: *Operative techniques in shoulder surgery*, Gaithersburg, Md, 1991, Aspen.
56. Andrews JR, Giduman RH: Shoulder arthroscopy in the throwing athlete: perspectives and prognosis, *Clin Sports Med* 6:565, 1987.
57. Jobe FW, Moynes DR: Delineation of diagnostic criteria and a rehabilitation program for rotator cuff injuries, *Am J Sports Med* 10:336, 1982.
58. Sharkey NA, Marder RA: The rotator cuff opposes superior translation of the humeral head, *Am J Sports Med* 23:270, 1995.
59. Itoi E, Newman SR, Kuechle DK, et al: Dynamic anterior stabilizers of the shoulder with the arm in abduction, *J Bone Joint Surg Br* 76:834, 1994.
60. Silliman JF, Hawkins RJ: Current concepts and recent advances in the athlete's shoulder, *Clin Sports Med* 10:693, 1991.
61. Keating JF, Waterworth P, Shaw-Dunn J, et al: The relative strength of rotator cuff muscles: a cadaver study, *J Bone Joint Surg Br* 75:137, 1993.
62. Jobe FW, Glousman RE: Rotator cuff dysfunction and associated glenohumeral instability in the throwing athlete. In Paulos LE, Tibone JE, editors: *Operative techniques in shoulder surgery*, Gaithersburg, Md, 1991, Aspen.
63. Morgan CD, Burkhart SS, Palmeri M, et al: Type II SLAP lesions: three subtypes and their relationships to superior instability and rotator cuff tears, *Arthroscopy* 14:553, 1998.
64. Giombini A, Rossi F, Pettrone FA, et al: Posterosuperior glenoid rim impingement as a cause of shoulder pain in top level waterpolo players, *J Sports Med Phys Fitness* 37:273, 1997.
65. Paley KJ, Jobe FW, Pink MM, et al: Arthroscopic findings in the overhand throwing athletes: evidence for posterior internal impingement of the rotator cuff, *Arthroscopy* 16:35, 2000.
66. McFarland EG, Hsu CY, Neira C, et al: Internal impingement of the shoulder: a clinical and arthroscopic analysis, *J Shoulder Elbow Surg* 8:458, 1999.
67. Nielsen KD, Wester JU, Lorentsen A: The shoulder impingement syndrome: the results of surgical decompression, *J Shoulder Elbow Surg* 3:12, 1994.
68. Wilk KE, Miester K, Andrews JR: Current concepts in the rehabilitation of the overhead throwing athlete, *Am J Sports Med* 30:136, 2002.
69. Rizio L, Garcia J, Renard R, et al: Anterior instability increases superior labral strain in the late cocking phase of throwing, *Orthopedics* 30:544, 2007.
70. Burkhart SS, Morgan CD, Kibler WB: The disabled throwing shoulder: spectrum of pathology. Part 1. Pathoanatomy and biomechanics, *Arthroscopy* 19:404, 2003.
71. Tibone JE, Elrod B, Jobe FW, et al: Surgical treatment of tears of the rotator cuff in athletes, *J Bone Joint Surg Am* 68:887, 1986.
72. Burkhead WZ, Rockwood CA: Treatment of instability of the shoulder with an exercise program, *J Bone Joint Surg Am* 74:890, 1992.
73. Mallon WJ, Speer KP: Multidirectional instability: current concepts, *J Shoulder Elbow Surg* 4:54, 1995.
74. Kronberg M, Nemeth G, Brostrom LA: Muscle activity and coordination in the normal shoulder: an electromyographic study, *Clin Orthop Relat Res* 257:76, 1990.
75. Pink M, Jobe FW, Perry J, et al: The normal shoulder during the backstroke: an EMG and cinematographic analysis of twelve muscles, *Clin J Sports Med* 2:6, 1992.
76. Kronberg M, Brostrom LA, Nemeth G: Differences in shoulder muscle activity between patients with generalized joint laxity and normal controls, *Clin Orthop Relat Res* 269:181, 1991.
77. Pink M, Jobe FW, Perry J, et al: The painful shoulder during the butterfly stroke: an EMG and cinematographic analysis of twelve muscles, *Clin Orthop Relat Res* 288:60, 1993.
78. Pink M, Jobe FW, Perry J, et al: The normal shoulder during the butterfly stroke: an EMG and cinematographic analysis of twelve muscles, *Clin Orthop Relat Res* 288:48, 1993.
79. Pink M, Perry J, Browne A, et al: The normal shoulder during freestyle swimming: an EMG and cinematographic analysis of twelve muscles, *Am J Sports Med* 19:569, 1991.
80. Jobe FW, Moynes DR, Antonelli DJ: Rotator cuff function during a golf swing, *Am J Sports Med* 14:388, 1986.
81. Scovazzo ML, Browne A, Pink M, et al: The painful shoulder during freestyle swimming: an EMG and cinematographic analysis of twelve muscles, *Am J Sports Med* 19:577, 1991.
82. Ryu R, McCormick J, Jobe FW, et al: An electromyographic analysis of shoulder function in tennis players, *Am J Sports Med* 16:481, 1988.
83. Wilk KE, Arrigo C: Current concepts in the rehabilitation of the athletic shoulder, *J Orthop Sports Phys Ther* 118:365, 1993.
84. Paine RM, Voight M: The role of the scapula, *J Orthop Sports Phys Ther* 18:386, 1993.
85. Kelley MJ: Anatomic and biomechanical rationale for rehabilitation of the athlete's shoulder, *J Sport Rehabil* 4:122, 1995.

86. Glousman R, Jobe F, Tibone J, et al: Dynamic electromyographic analysis of the throwing shoulder with glenohumeral instability, *J Bone Joint Surg Am* 70:220, 1988.
87. Lutz GE, Palmitier RA, An KN, et al: Comparison of tibiofemoral joint forces during open-kinetic-chain and closed-kinetic-chain exercises, *J Bone Joint Surg Am* 75:732, 1993.
88. Livingstone BP: Open and closed chain exercises for the shoulder. In Tovin B, Greenfield BH, editors: *Evaluation and treatment of the shoulder: an integration of the guide to physical therapist practice*, Philadelphia, 2001, Davis.
89. Dillman CJ, Murray TA, Hintermeister RA: Biomechanical differences of open and closed chain exercises with respect to the shoulder, *J Sport Rehabil* 3:228, 1994.
90. Palmitier R, An KN, Scott S, et al: Kinetic chain exercise in knee rehabilitation, *Sports Med* 11:402, 1991.
91. Townsend H, Jobe FW, Pink M, et al: Electromyographic analysis of the glenohumeral muscles during a baseball rehabilitation program, *Am J Sports Med* 19:264, 1991.
92. Greenfield B: Proprioceptive neuromuscular facilitation for the shoulder. In Wilk KE, Reinold MM, Andrews JF, editors: *The athlete's shoulder*, ed 2, Philadelphia, 2009, Churchill Livingstone Elsevier.
93. Borsa PA, Lephart SM, Kocher MS, et al: Functional assessment and rehabilitation of shoulder proprioception for glenohumeral instability, *J Sport Rehabil* 3:84, 1994.
94. Lephart SM, Warner JJ, Borsa PA, et al: Proprioception of the unstable shoulder joint in healthy, unstable and surgically repaired shoulders, *J Shoulder Elbow Surg* 3:371, 1994.
95. Irrgang JJ, Whitney SL, Harner CD: Nonoperative treatment of rotator cuff injuries in throwing athletes, *J Sport Rehabil* 1:197, 1992.
96. Smith FL, Brunolli J: Shoulder kinesthesia after anterior glenohumeral joint dislocation, *Phys Ther* 69:106, 1989.
97. Blasier RB, Carpenter JE, Huston LJ: Shoulder proprioception: effect of joint laxity, joint position, and direction of motion, *Orthop Rev* 23:45, 1994.
98. Allegrucci M, Whitney SL, Lephart SM, et al: Shoulder kinesthesia in healthy unilateral athletes participating in upper extremity sports, *J Orthop Sports Phys Ther* 21:220, 1995.
99. Cain RP, Mutschler TA, Fu FH, et al: Anterior stability of the glenohumeral joint, *Am J Sports Med* 15:144, 1987.
100. Guanche C, Knatt T, Solomonow M, et al: The synergistic action of the capsule and the shoulder muscles, *Am J Sports Med* 23:301, 1995.
101. Freund HJ, Budingen HJ: The relationship between speed and amplitude of the fastest voluntary contractions of human arm muscles, *Exp Brain Res* 31:1, 1978.
102. Lestienne F: Effects of inertial load and velocity on the braking process of voluntary limb movements, *Exp Brain Res* 35:4407, 1979.
103. Marsden CD, Obeso JA, Rothwell JC: The function of the antagonist muscle during fast limb movements in man, *J Physiol* 335:1, 1983.
104. Wierzbicka MM, Wiegner AW, Shahani BT: Role of agonist and antagonist muscles in fast arm movements in man, *Exp Brain Res* 63:331, 1986.
105. Desmedt JE, Godaux E: Voluntary motor commands in human ballistic movements, *Ann Neurol* 5:415, 1978.

CHAPTER

10

Michael S. Zazzali
and Vijay B. Vad

Shoulder Instability

The shoulder is a complex joint that comprises the integration of four articulations: the glenohumeral, scapulothoracic, sternoclavicular, and acromioclavicular joints. These articulations need to work in tandem for proper arm elevation and function to occur without pain or excessive humeral head translation. Of these articulations, the glenohumeral joint permits a high degree of mobility, lacks inherent static stability, and exhibits the greatest amount of motion found in the body. This lack of inherent static stability places a greater demand on the dynamic stabilizers to help direct humeral motion in the glenoid and to protect against aberrant translation of the humeral head, which can possibly lead to shoulder instability.

Shoulder instability is a vague, nonspecific term that actually represents a wide spectrum of clinical pathologic conditions, ranging from gross and occult instability to symptomatic laxity or subluxation.[1] Matsen et al[1] described shoulder instability as a pathologic condition in which the laxity or the mobility of the joint increases abnormally. In other words, instability is the inability to maintain the humeral head centered in the glenoid cavity.[1] In all patients with shoulder instability, some component of the stabilizing matrix has become dysfunctional.

According to Pagnani and Warren,[2] typically no single "essential lesion" is responsible for all cases of shoulder instability. The pathophysiologic features of the shoulder produced may vary with the direction and the extent of the instability. The glenohumeral joint's static restraints include a negative intra-articular pressure gradient, which induces cohesion and adhesion between the humeral head and the glenoid fossa. During cadaveric sectioning, muscle activity is not required to hold the shoulder together, as long as the capsule is not vented.[3] Speer[3] reported that the magnitude of this pressure is small and is capable of producing an approximate stabilizing force of only 20 to 30 lb. This anatomic negative intra-articular pressure is often disrupted during open capsular surgery, thus leaving a postoperative joint pressure of approximately 0 mm Hg.[3]

The glenoid labrum and capsuloligamentous complex also play integral parts in the static glenohumeral restraints. The glenoid labrum is a fibrous rim that functions to slightly deepen the glenoid fossa and allows for attachment of the glenohumeral ligaments (Fig. 10-1). The function of the glenoid labrum is similar to a "chock-block" or buttress in controlling humeral head translation.[4] Biomechanical studies indicated that resection of the labrum can reduce the effectiveness of the concavity compression by 20%. Injury to the labrum is thought to disturb the negative intra-articular pressure gradient and thereby contribute to shoulder instability.[5]

The glenohumeral capsule was reported by Gohlke et al[6] to be thickest and strongest at the anterior-inferior region because of its dense organization of collagen and by the invagination of the inferior glenohumeral ligament complex. The anterior glenohumeral joint capsule exhibits three distinct ligaments consisting of the superior, middle, and inferior glenohumeral ligament complex.[7,8] The inferior glenohumeral ligament complex is the primary restraint at elevated positions such as in 90° of abduction, whereas the superior glenohumeral ligament is taut at 0° of abduction. The middle glenohumeral ligament tightens more so at the midrange of elevation when the arm is abducted and externally rotated.[7,8] The inferior glenohumeral ligament consists of an anterior band, which restricts anterior translation of the humeral head, and a posterior band, which is the primary contributor to posterior stability of the shoulder when the arm is in 90° of abduction.[7]

Proper treatment and management of the shoulder require an understanding of the pathophysiology of shoulder instability to direct clinical decision making regarding conservative rehabilitation or surgery. The following section of this chapter briefly describes the proposed mechanisms of injury and management guidelines for Bankart lesions, superior labrum anterior to posterior (SLAP) lesions, and rotator cuff interval injuries, and posterior instability, with the latest interventions suggested for these injuries and for those patients with recurrent instability. The postoperative

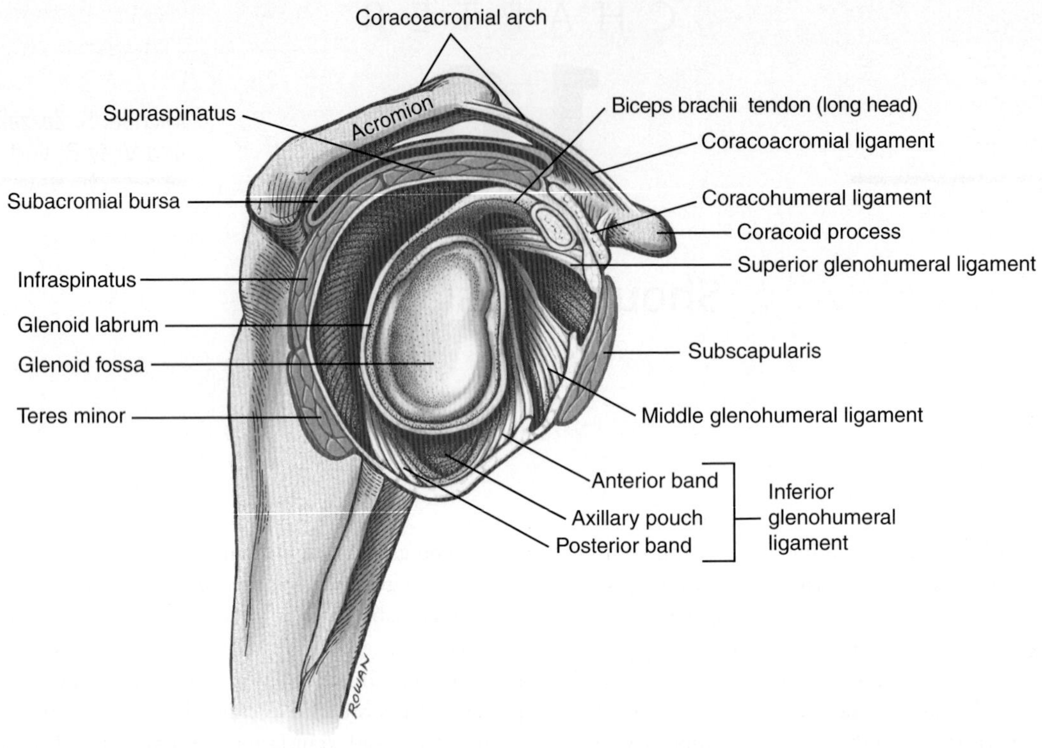

Figure 10-1 Lateral aspect of the internal surface of the right glenohumeral joint. The humerus has been removed to expose the capsular ligaments and the glenoid fossa. Note the prominent coracoacromial arch and underlying subacromial bursa *(blue).* The four rotator cuff muscles are shown in *red.* (From Neumann DA: *Kinesiology of the musculoskeletal system: foundations for rehabilitation,* ed 2, St. Louis, 2010, Mosby Elsevier.)

rehabilitation for each surgical procedure is demonstrated, including the most recent guidelines available and in a case study format.

On clinical examination, the patient with a Bankart lesion presents with a positive result on the apprehension test for anterior instability. The patient reports extreme feelings of vulnerability or pain as the shoulder is brought into end-range external rotation with the arm in 90° of abduction. A Bankart lesion results in anterior instability of the glenohumeral joint. The cadaveric model of Abboud and Soslowsky[9] suggested that a Bankart lesion alone reproduced only small amounts of anterior and inferior translations at all positions of abduction. These investigators believed that the amount of humeral head translation needed to produce clinical anterior glenohumeral dislocation required inferior glenohumeral ligament plastic deformation in addition to the Bankart lesion. Thus, they recommended surgical repair for recurrent instability and capsular laxity produced by the initial traumatic event and stated that the detachment of the glenoid insertion of the inferior glenohumeral ligament must be addressed to permit full stability.[9]

The operative indications for glenohumeral joint surgical stabilization are as follows: recurrent symptomatic instability, despite a minimum 3-month trial of a well-designed and supervised rehabilitation program; a requirement for stability for occupational reasons, such as in heavy manual laborers and military cadets; and connective tissue disorders in subgroups of patients, such as adolescents, who are at high risk for recurrence of instability. In the adolescent subgroup, it is important to rule out a psychological component through psychological testing before proceeding with the surgical intervention.

A Bankart lesion typically results from a traumatic anterior dislocation of the shoulder. The lesion itself is usually identified as a compromise or tear of the attachment site of the labrum to the glenohumeral ligaments. Thus, the definition of a *Bankart lesion* is an injury that occurs when the capsular-labral complex is torn from the glenoid rim (Fig. 10-2A).[10] Evidence suggests that patients between the ages of 21 and 30 years who sustained a primary shoulder dislocation and underwent physical therapy and immobilization did not reduce the risk of a recurrent dislocation of the shoulder.[11] The suggestion is that patients in this age group who participate in high-risk sports should undergo primary surgical stabilization because of the risk of a dislocation recurrence. Another objective sign of recurrent anterior instability is the presence of an osseous defect or lesion seen on a radiograph, commonly noted on the posterior-lateral portion of the humeral head, known as a *Hill-Sachs lesion* (see Fig. 10-2B).[12]

Occasionally, the dislocation may affect the axillary nerve, usually noticed as a change in sensation. At times, this lesion may have an effect on the motor branch of the deltoid, which has significant impact on functional lifting and reaching

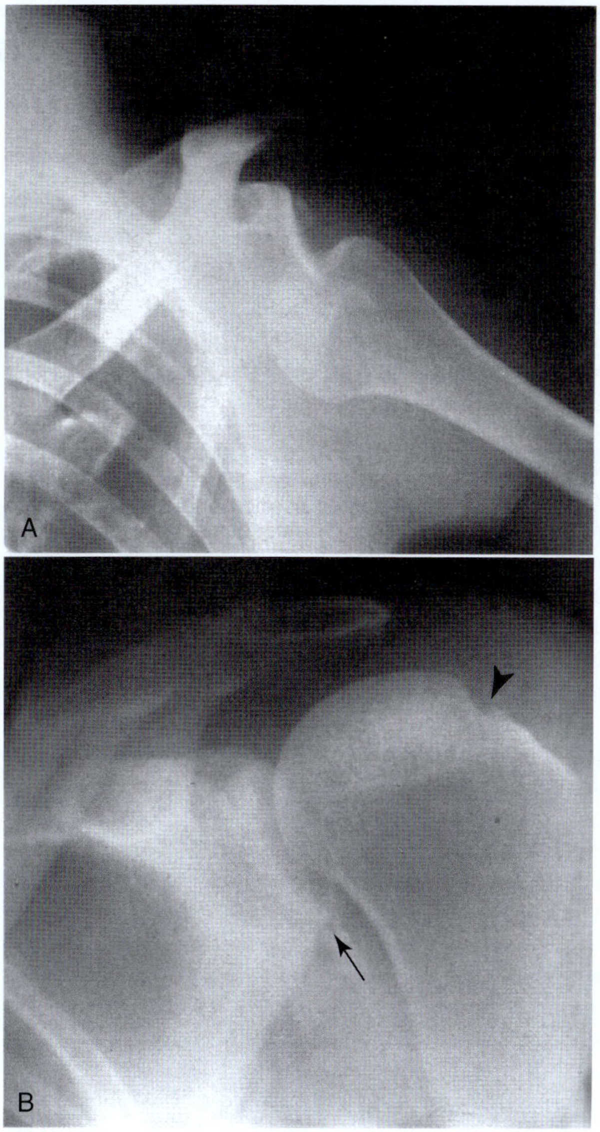

Figure 10-2 Plain radiographs demonstrate an anterior glenohumeral dislocation before (**A**) and after (**B**) reduction. Postreduction anterior-posterior view (**B**) demonstrates a Hill-Sachs lesion of the posterior-lateral humeral head *(arrowhead)* and a typical "bony Bankart" fracture of the anterior-inferior glenoid rim *(arrow)*. (From Stechschulte D, Warren R: Anterior shoulder instability. In Garrett W, Speer K, Kirkendall D, editors: *Principles and practice of orthopaedic sports medicine*, Philadelphia, 2000, Lippincott Williams & Wilkins.)

overhead. Indications for performing a Bankart surgical procedure also include decreasing the risk of future dislocations and avoiding the potential for more permanent injury to the axillary nerve.[13]

The open Bankart surgical stabilization technique for post-traumatic recurrent anterior stabilization has been referred to as the procedure of choice for patients who do not respond to nonoperative treatment.[14] This procedure is based on the premise that anterior instability is caused by detachment of the anterior-inferior labrum from the glenoid rim.[10]

Gill et al[15] reported on long-term results with patients after open stabilization for a Bankart repair for anterior instability of the shoulder. The study consisted of 60 shoulders in 56 patients, with a minimum follow-up of 8 years after a Bankart procedure. These patients had a mean follow-up period of 11.9 years and were examined for range of motion (ROM), stability, and strength according to the data form of the American Shoulder and Elbow Surgeons (ASES) for examination of the shoulder. The mean loss of external rotation was 12° (range, 0° to 30°). No significant differences were reported in elevation, abduction, or internal rotation between the involved shoulder and the contralateral, normal shoulder. Fifty-five of the 56 patients returned to their preoperative occupations without having to modify their activities. Fifty-two patients rated the result as good or excellent; 3 rated it as fair, and 1 rated it as poor.[15] Although this study demonstrated great patient satisfaction, the average loss of 12° of external rotation could be disabling for athletes. More recently, Randelli et al[16] also demonstrated an average loss of external rotation similar to the findings of Gill et al. Randelli et al quantified active ROM after arthroscopic Bankart repair with rotator interval closure and found a significant reduction in average active external rotation in the adducted position (12.14°) and a 7.21° reduction in 90° of abduction.[16]

Pagnani and Dome[17] reported their open stabilization procedure on 58 American football players over a 6-year period and noted the operation to be a predictable method to restore shoulder stability while maintaining an ROM approximating that found after arthroscopic repair. The average follow-up was 37 months after the surgical procedure; 55 patients reported good or excellent results, and 52 of the 58 returned to playing football for at least 1 year.[17] According to these investigators, the open stabilization procedure offers postoperative stability superior to that reported after arthroscopic techniques in this patient population.[17] The open Bankart repair, as described by Pagnani and Dome,[17] involves vertical tenotomy of the subscapularis tendon, which is performed with electrocautery approximately 1 cm medial to the tendon's insertion on the lesser tuberosity. The interval between the anterior aspect of the capsule and the subscapularis tendon is moved with blunt dissection to permit exposure to the anterior joint, and the capsular laxity and quality are assessed. Transverse capsulotomy is performed to permit exploration of the Bankart lesion. The glenoid neck is roughened with an osteotome to provide a bleeding surface. These investigators used two or three metallic suture anchors placed in the anterior-inferior aspect of the glenoid neck near, but not on, the glenoid articular margin. The capsule and labrum are reattached to the anterior aspect of the glenoid with slight medial and superior mobilization of the capsule. The goal of this surgical procedure is not to reduce external rotation, but to obliterate excess capsular volume to restore the competency of the inferior glenohumeral ligament at its glenoid insertion. These investigators also proposed performing anterior capsulorrhaphy to eliminate excess capsular laxity.[17]

CASE STUDY 1

This case presents a standardized postoperative rehabilitation protocol for the athlete after a Bankart repair, based on the latest literature and procedures.[17] The enhancement and the dynamic stabilization or concavity-compression mechanism are not addressed in surgery. Instead, neuromuscular exercises and training of the rotator cuff by means of a dedicated and essential rehabilitation program ultimately optimize functional recovery of the shoulder following capsulorrhaphy.[3]

General Demographics

Mr. C.M. is a 26-year-old professional football player, who is an offensive lineman. The patient injured his right (dominant side) shoulder during a blocking technique while his arm was in a position of abduction and external rotation. The resultant force stressed his shoulder quickly into horizontal abduction during the play, and he began feeling numbness and pain immediately thereafter in the arm. The team physician determined that Mr. C.M. had anteriorly dislocated his shoulder, which was manually relocated on the field and then placed in a sling. A magnetic resonance imaging (MRI) scan was taken in the locker room and displayed a Bankart lesion and tear of the anterior capsule. The patient underwent an open Bankart repair 1 week later.

Social History

Mr. C.M. is single, with no children. He does not smoke or drink alcohol.

Employment

He is a professional offensive lineman in the National Football League.

Living Environment

Mr. C.M. lives with his girlfriend in a bilevel home.

Growth and Development

He is an extremely muscular young man, with no external deformities noted.

Patient Medical History

He had right knee arthroscopy 2 years ago for a torn medial meniscus, with no complaints over the last year with respect to his knee.

History of Chief Complaint

Mr. C.M. is unable to resume football at the present time because of weakness, pain, and stiffness in his right shoulder. He comes to the physical therapy clinic 4 weeks after a right Bankart repair. He reports pain at the right upper trapezius and anterior-lateral shoulder that wakes him up at night, but he no longer feels numbness or "dead arm" symptoms. The patient has been immobilized for 4 weeks since surgery and has been taught only pendulum and elbow ROM exercises up to this time.

Prior Treatment for This Condition

The patient has not received prior treatment with respect to shoulder stability. Before his injury, the patient was active with a general weight training program with the team.

Structural Examination

The patient comes to physical therapy with his shoulder in a sling. Visual inspection reveals a well-healed anterior incision, and the patient is fully intact to light touch sensation surrounding the surgical incision. Mild ecchymosis and swelling are noted in the anterior shoulder region, as is tenderness along the lesser tuberosity at the insertion of the subscapularis. Mild atrophy is noted of the right deltoid, pectoralis major, and infraspinatus when compared with the contralateral side.

Range of Motion

Active Range of Motion

Active motion of the right shoulder is contraindicated at this time because of the tissue vulnerability from the surgery and the pull-out rate of suture anchors for stabilization. However, care must also be taken to protect the repair site with passive ROM (PROM), especially in the abducted and externally rotated position. Penna et al[18] examined the actual forces with PROM encountered at the glenoid-labrum interface after an isolated Bankart repair and a Bankart repair with a capsular shift. These investigators found that the greatest mean force experienced (17.7 N) was in shoulders undergoing the labral repair with capsular shift with the arm in abduction and external rotation. In this cadaveric study, the investigators concluded that the forces at the repair site were significantly less than those determined by previous authors to be necessary to result in failure of the Bankart repair. Thus, their data suggest that during the early postoperative period, rehabilitation must be modified to protect the repair site further than currently accepted guidelines indicate.[18]

Active motion testing is postponed at this time for the right shoulder. The left shoulder has full active ROM (AROM) with proper scapulohumeral rhythm with elevation. Right elbow flexion and extension, along with wrist flexion and extension, are full and pain free.

Passive Range of Motion

Initial PROM of the right shoulder is 80° of flexion, 50° of abduction, 0° of external rotation in the adducted position, and 45° of internal rotation. No hypermobility is noted at the contralateral upper extremity at the elbows or metacarpophalangeal joints. Again, care is taken to avoid stretching into external rotation in the abducted position until 6 weeks postoperatively, to protect the repair site.[18]

Accessory Motion Testing of the Glenohumeral Joint

Mr. C.M. has a moderately tight posterior capsule.

Muscle Testing

No further testing of the right shoulder is performed because of the acuteness of the patient's symptoms and the postoperative time frame.

Special Tests

The left shoulder does not demonstrate shoulder laxity in any direction with load and shift testing. No further special testing is performed at this time because of the acuteness of

CASE STUDY 1—cont'd

the patient's symptoms and nature of his postoperative time frame.

Palpation

Palpation elicits tenderness in the anterior shoulder along the subscapularis tendon insertion and along the anterior glenohumeral joint.

Physical Therapist's Clinical Impression

Based on the patient's signs and symptoms, and time frame from surgery (4 weeks), the main goal at this stage of rehabilitation is to begin restoration of PROM and active-assisted shoulder ROM while still protecting the surgical site. The main factor to consider at this stage is using a methodical yet progressive approach to restore shoulder external rotation while protecting against overstressing the anterior capsule, inferior glenohumeral ligament complex, and subscapularis musculotendinous junction. Therefore, anterior capsule joint mobilizations are contraindicated, along with aggressive pectoral stretching or stretching into external rotation in 90° of abduction.

Treatment Plan

Initial Treatment: 4 to 6 Weeks Postoperatively

Initial treatment goals are to reduce and eliminate inflammation of the anterior shoulder tissues with modalities as needed and graded manual scar tissue mobilization. The patient's external rotation should be limited to 30°, and forward flexion limited to 90° provided he has no signs or symptoms of impingement or rotator cuff symptoms. Proximal stabilization for the scapular rotators may begin at this time for retraction, posterior depression, and neuromuscular control exercises. Submaximal isometrics for the internal and external rotators are performed as tolerated. No strengthening isotonic exercises or repetitive exercises are started until after full ROM has been established.[19] By the sixth week, the patient demonstrates 160° of active forward flexion in the sitting position, with compensatory superior humeral migration and upper trapezius dominance. He demonstrates 55° of external rotation. At this time, a progression into graded resisted internal and external isometrics up in the plane of the scapula and prone shoulder extensions, serratus supine punches, rowing, and horizontal abduction with the weight of the arm may begin in modified arcs of motion while protecting the anterior restraints.

Treatment: 6 to 12 Weeks Postoperatively

At 8 weeks postoperatively, the patient demonstrates 175° of flexion, 160° of abduction, 65° of external rotation, and 65° of internal rotation. At this phase, he is tolerating rhythmic stabilization with the shoulder in varying degrees of flexion to enhance kinesthetic awareness and dynamic stability. He is now emphasizing his infraspinatus and teres minor strength, with side-lying external rotation, using progression to a 3-lb weight. His rotator cuff strengthening is advanced by week 10 to Thera-Band (Hygenic Corp., Akron, Ohio) exercises, and his abduction angles are slowly increased during rotator cuff and deltoid strengthening exercises. The scapular rotators are strengthened with the following: press-ups (seated dips), shrugs, horizontal abduction with modified arc to protect the anterior capsule, and open can exercises with continued prone rowing and shoulder extensions now at 5 lb.

Treatment: 12 to 18 Weeks Postoperatively

At this stage of the rehabilitation, the patient demonstrates 180° of flexion, 180° of abduction, 80° of external rotation, and 70° of internal rotation. On manual muscle testing, he demonstrates the following: abduction, 4+/5; flexion, 5/5; external rotation, 4/5 (fatigues with repetition); and internal rotation, 5/5. His scapulohumeral rhythm is comparable to his contralateral side. He has a positive Neer test result and mild posterior capsular tightness relative to the uninvolved side. During this phase of his rehabilitation, the focus is on restoration of terminal external rotation and further enhancement of neuromuscular control of the humeral head. The use of proprioceptive neuromuscular facilitation in dynamic patterns and in sport-specific patterns is initiated, along with plyometric exercises, such as medicine ball catches and chest passes. Use of Thera-Band exercises and isokinetics is elevated to the plane of the scapula and then to 90° of abduction. These exercises are performed at slow and fast speeds to prepare the anterior-posterior stabilizers properly for quick and prolonged stress and strain forces to the shoulder.

Assessment of anterior laxity and instability with load and shift testing is negative, as are apprehension test results. The end-range external rotation in the apprehension position is 95° by week 18 and pain free. An isokinetic evaluation to compare strength with the contralateral shoulder is performed at 17 weeks and demonstrates 5% and 15% deficits at the external and internal rotators, respectively.

Treatment: Past 18 Weeks Postoperatively

At this time, the patient has a negative Neer test result and 180° of flexion, 180° of abduction, 95° of external rotation, and 75° of internal rotation. The patient's program focuses on closed kinetic chain exercises, which are more sport specific for his profession as a lineman. He also progresses to a conventional weight-training program, with education placed on not overstressing the anterior capsule with end-range dips or chest presses. The patient is retested at 23 weeks postoperatively, with a second isokinetic evaluation demonstrating equal strength at his external rotators and 10% greater strength of his internal rotators relative to the contralateral side. At this time, the patient is cleared to progress from field to contact drills with the team. However, his surgeon suggests that he obtain an abduction harness initially as protection during blocking drills. The patient is cleared to return to full contact football by his

Continued

CASE STUDY 1—cont'd

physician and physical therapist by the 25th week postoperatively after he demonstrates good tolerance to contact drills with, and then without, the abduction brace and after he demonstrates symmetrical abduction and external rotation strength on isokinetic and manual muscle testing. Finally, the patient is instructed in posterior capsular (cross-body) stretching, as well as the "sleeper stretch," to maintain tissue extensibility and help reduce the likelihood of recurring impingement. The patient is checked periodically by the team physician for any recurring signs or symptoms of instability.

Summary of Case

The crucial phase of rehabilitation after the Bankart repair is the initial period of immobilization, followed by the beginning of ROM restoration. The biologic healing response of the repaired and imbricated tissue must be respected. The first goal is to maintain anterior-inferior stability. The second goal is to restore adequate motion, specifically external rotation, because it is well established that a significant lack of external rotation from capsular plication can hasten early degenerative arthritic changes at the glenohumeral joint.[9] The third goal is a successful return to sports or physical activity in a reasonable amount of time. Patients must be compliant and must understand the need to permit these anterior structures to heal, for adequate stabilization. This patient was not seen in physical therapy until the fourth week, so it was up to his physician to instill this point. The physical therapist must also respect the healing nature of the anterior stabilizers by not being too aggressive early on with restoring external rotation. This protocol is based on tendon-to-bone healing in a dog model and emphasizes avoidance of early resistance exercises, with aggressive early postoperative rehabilitation to help prevent compromise to the repair.[19,20] The approach to this case is typical for a patient after Bankart repair and emphasizes a safe progression through rehabilitation. The latter part of the rehabilitation is more sport specific and individualized, depending on the goals of the patient. However, as in this case when the patient demonstrated impingement signs, it is important to think critically and reassess, as the patient progresses, to be able to deter secondary complications. In this case, it appears the patient's impingement was related to residual posterior capsular tightness and limited external rotation in the abducted position, and possibly a concurrent increase in elevation with his graded strengthening exercises.

Originally, shoulder instability was corrected primarily through open procedures, whereas current technique allows correction of the entire spectrum of instability patterns by arthroscopic techniques. Speer et al[21] retrospectively investigated the outcomes of an arthroscopic technique for anterior stabilization of the shoulder that used a bioabsorbable tack in 52 patients with shoulder instability. The cause of the instability was a traumatic injury in 49 of the patients; 26 of these injuries were sustained during participation in a contact sport. Fifty of the shoulders had a Bankart lesion. The patients were evaluated at an average follow-up of 42 months postoperatively. Forty-one (79%) patients were asymptomatic and were able to return to their respective sport without restriction.[21] The repair had failed in 11 (21%) of the patients. In 4 of these patients, the failure resulted from a single traumatic reinjury during participation in contact sports, and 3 of the 4 patients were treated nonoperatively. The remaining 7 treatment failures occurred atraumatically.

The investigators reported that the rate of recurrent instability Speer et al[21] following this arthroscopic procedure (21%) greatly exceeded the rates of recurrence of open capsulorrhaphy (up to 5.5%).[10,22,23] The investigators believed that the wide discrepancy in results reflected this arthroscopic technique and did not address the coexistent capsular injury or plastic deformation reported to occur with Bankart lesions.[24] Therefore, they suggested that anterior stabilization with a bioabsorbable tack may be indicated for patients with anterior instability who do not need capsulorrhaphy to reduce joint volume.[21]

A prospective study by O'Neill[25] evaluated the results of an arthroscopic transglenoid suture stabilization procedure in athletically active patients who had recurrent unilateral, unidirectional anterior dislocations of the shoulder and an isolated Bankart lesion. The mean duration of follow-up was 52 months, within a range of 25 months to 7 years. The patients were evaluated annually with a physical examination, radiographs, isokinetic strength testing, the modified shoulder rating scale of Rowe and Zarins, and the scoring system of the ASES.[25]

The results of O'Neill's study determined that 40 (98%) of the 41 athletes returned to their preoperative sports after surgery. Thirty-nine patients (95%) had no additional dislocations or subluxations, and 2 (5%) had a single episode of subluxation. These last 2 patients were football players. These investigators concluded that arthroscopic transglenoid repair of an isolated anterior labral detachment or Bankart lesion restored stability of the shoulder and led to a favorable outcome in 39 (95%) of the 41 athletes. The only 2 patients who suffered a postoperative subluxation were the 2 football players, who also were the only patients to score less than 80 points on the ASES scale.[25]

The arthroscopic Bankart reconstruction, as described by Rook et al,[24] uses an anterior portal to ensure access to the inferior glenoid and to evaluate the lesion and anterior capsule. The anterior portal is also used for débriding and releasing the capsulolabral complex from the glenoid. The capsulolabral complex is released inferiorly to the 6 o'clock position of the glenoid. Rook et al then abrade the anterior and inferior glenoid to promote a bleeding surface on which

CASE STUDY 1—cont'd

the suture anchors will be placed at the 5 o'clock, 3 o'clock, and 1 o'clock positions (Fig. 10-3).

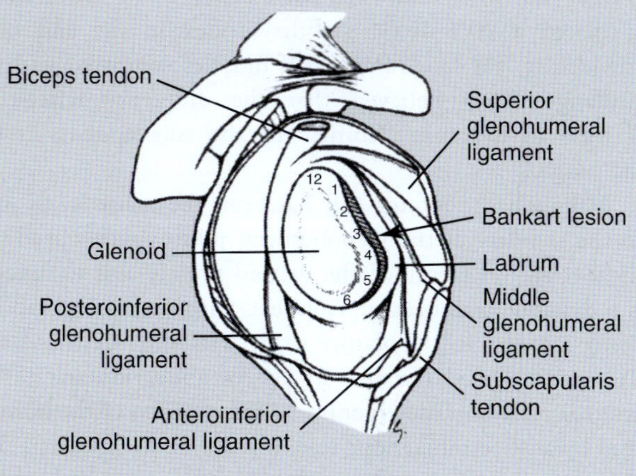

Figure 10-3 Drawing of the glenoid with numbers identifying anchor placement. (From Rook R, Savoie F, Field L, et al: Arthroscopic treatment of instability attributable to capsular injury or laxity, *Clin Orthop Relat Res* 390:52–58, 2001.)

Evidence indicates that arthroscopic treatment for shoulder instability may parallel the gold standard of open surgical techniques.[24] However, some studies may refute this claim and continue to suggest that arthroscopic treatment of shoulder instability has a greater failure rate than open procedures, especially in athletes who desire to return to contact sports postoperatively.[21,25-27] Ultimately, the need may exist for longer outcome studies of both approaches to determine which procedure (open versus arthroscopic) provides the highest success rate. Magnusson et al[14] suggested follow-up studies of up to 7 years and recommended that researchers consider incidences of subluxation and recurrent dislocations in their success rates. According to Magnusson et al,[14] a gold standard for reconstruction in patients with unidirectional, post-traumatic anterior instability does not appear to exist. Therefore, the choice of method for post-traumatic anterior instability must still be based on the experience of the surgeon and the patient's choice, rather than on scientific evidence from long-term prospective, randomized studies at the present time.[14]

MUSCLE MECHANICS: CONTRIBUTION TO SHOULDER DISLOCATION AND STABILITY

Increased understanding of the sequelae of and predispositions to shoulder dislocation may improve functional results during nonoperative treatment, surgical repair, and postoperative rehabilitation. McMahon and Lee[27] developed an in vitro, cadaveric model that investigated relevant shoulder musculature, its relationship with glenoid concavity compression for dynamic stability, and its role in contributing to dislocation. This research integrated work by Matsen et al,[28] who defined a muscle's function as a dynamic restraint related to a "stability ratio" between the displacing component (contributes to instability) of the joint force and the compressive component (contributes to stability). The Matsen model suggested that shoulder muscle dysfunction on one side of the joint not only may decrease the compression component, but also may increase the displacing component if forces on the other side are unbalanced.[28]

The term *concavity compression* refers to the stability afforded a convex object that is pressed into a concave surface.[29] This mechanism is particularly active in all glenohumeral positions, but most important in the functional midrange, in which the capsule and ligaments are slack.[30] The specialized anatomic features of the rotator cuff muscles and the intra-articular long head of the biceps are located ideally to compress the humeral head dynamically into the glenoid concavity.[31]

McMahon and Lee[27] assessed the alteration in glenohumeral joint forces with simulated shoulder muscle dysfunction. The joint was positioned in apprehension while the rotator cuff and deltoid were simulated and loaded. While the arm was in the apprehension position, the investigators altered the load in the infraspinatus and the pectoralis major tendons. The conditions were altered by first removing the load from the infraspinatus (infraspinatus muscle palsy) and then adding it to the pectoralis major; then these changes were repeated simultaneously, by removing the load from the infraspinatus as the load was added to the pectoralis major.

Compared with the intact condition, the magnitude of the compression force when the infraspinatus was unloaded decreased substantially by approximately 31%. The results also demonstrated a significant increase in the anteriorly directed force when the pectoralis major was loaded with and without infraspinatus muscle palsy of 143% and 142%, respectively. These simulated muscle dysfunctions resulted in a significant decrease in concavity compression of the humeral head into the glenoid cavity and a concomitant increase in the anteriorly directed force, a situation that could result in joint instability.[27] The investigators concluded that the large force developed in the pectoralis major muscle may be related to its ideal orientation to lever the humeral head effectively anteriorly and inferiorly out of the glenoid.[27]

An anatomic study by Ackland and Pandy[32] measured lines of action of 18 major muscles and "muscle subregions" crossing the glenohumeral joint of the shoulder and computed the potential contributions of these muscles to joint shear (instability) and compression (stability) during scapular plane abduction and sagittal plane flexion. The results demonstrated that, during flexion and abduction, the rotator cuff subregions were more favorably aligned to stabilize the glenohumeral joint in the transverse plane than in the scapular plane.

Overall, these investigators found that the anterior supraspinatus was most favorably oriented to apply glenohumeral joint compression. The pectoralis major and latissimus dorsi were the chief potential destabilizers of the scapular plane and demonstrated the most significant capacity to impart superior and inferior shear to the glenohumeral joint, respectively. These investigators also found the middle and anterior deltoid to be significant potential contributors to superior shear, and they believed that these muscles would act as a force couple to challenge the combined opposing "destabilizing" inferior shear potential of the latissimus dorsi and inferior subscapularis.[32] Ackland and Pandy[32] believed that the posterior deltoid and subscapularis had posteriorly directed muscle lines of action, whereas the teres minor and infraspinatus had anteriorly directed lines of action, and that both acted as potential stabilizers, depending on the directed instability. They suggested that knowledge of these lines of muscle actions and of the stabilizing potential of individual subregions of the shoulder musculature could assist clinicians in identifying muscle-related joint instabilities and aid in the development of rehabilitation designed to improve joint stability and the concavity-compression effect.[32]

Contrary to the study by Ackland and Pandy,[32] Gibb et al[33] demonstrated, with simulated supraspinatus muscle paralysis, that the glenohumeral kinematics were unaffected. This study suggested that joint compression was maintained through the remaining rotator cuff and was adequate to provide a stable fulcrum for concentric compression of the glenohumeral joint during abduction. This is typically what is seen clinically in that a patient with a massive supraspinatus tear with the remaining rotator cuff intact maintains abduction. However, a tear extending into the infraspinatus tendon disrupts the transverse force couple, and the stable platform for the glenohumeral abduction is lost.[33] It becomes even more important to strengthen the infraspinatus and teres minor in the patient with anterior-inferior instability because these muscles have been shown to reduce the strain on the anterior-inferior capsuloligamentous complex.[9,34] The subscapularis has been shown to be a primary dynamic restraint for stabilizing the glenohumeral joint anteriorly with the arm in abduction and neutral rotation, but it becomes less important in external rotation, in which the posterior cuff muscles reduce strain.[9]

Anterior dislocation of the glenohumeral joint occurs either by disruption of the glenohumeral ligaments and labrum or by rupture of the rotator cuff.[9] The rotator cuff acts as a force couple around the joint, by controlling or directing force through the joint. Abboud and Soslowsky[9] described two types of force couples that work around the glenohumeral joint. The first force couple is coactivation or simultaneous activation of the agonist and antagonist muscles around the joint. The second force couple is coordinated activation of the agonist with inhibition of the antagonist. According to Nichols,[35] this force couple increases joint torque and motion, increases forces through the joint, and allows transfer of forces through the joint. The coordinated muscle activation is necessary to produce torques and accelerations required for using the glenohumeral joint in a controlled and stable manner.[35]

Lee et al[29] hypothesized that dynamic factors can potentially stabilize the glenohumeral joint throughout the entire ROM. Investigators previously thought that the capsuloligamentous restraints were the only primary stabilizing factors at end range. Lee et al combined the force components with concavity-compression mechanics and a new entity, the *dynamic stability index,* was calculated. These investigators calculated a 20% lower stability index in the end range provided by the four rotator cuff muscles compared with the midrange. They believed that the difference reflected a decrease in dynamic stability for the subscapularis in the end range.[29]

Although the rotator cuff has been the mainstay of focus on the stability of the glenohumeral joint, another study, by Kido et al,[36] determined the deltoid muscle also to function as a dynamic stabilizer in shoulders with anterior instability. Using a controlled laboratory study with nine fresh cadavers, Kido et al placed the arm in 90° of abduction and 90° of external rotation. They monitored the position of the humeral head by an electromagnetic tracking device with 0 and 1.5 kg of anterior translation force. This device was applied with 0, 1, 3, and 5 kg of force to each of the anterior, middle, and posterior portions of the deltoid muscle with the capsule intact, vented, and with a simulated Bankart lesion. The results demonstrated that with the capsule intact, anterior displacement was significantly reduced by application of load to the middle deltoid muscle. After the capsule was vented, load application to the anterior, middle, or posterior deltoid muscle significantly reduced anterior displacement. With a simulated Bankart lesion, the effects of loading were most apparent in that anterior displacement was significantly reduced with loading of each muscle portion. These investigators concluded by stating that their model showed that the deltoid muscle is an anterior stabilizer of the glenohumeral joint with the arm in abduction and external rotation and that the deltoid takes on more importance and dynamic stabilizer as the shoulder becomes more unstable.[36]

Additional improvements in outcome after glenohumeral joint dislocation warrant improved understanding of the interplay of the static and dynamic restraints.[27] The therapist should attempt to focus the rehabilitation on those muscles found to contribute to concavity compression and enhance joint stability while appreciating those muscles that may contribute to dislocation and instability.

SLAP LESIONS

In 1990, Snyder et al[37] reported on a lesion that occurred at the anterior-superior labral-biceps complex, which they described as a tear located at the superior labrum that begins posteriorly and extends anteriorly (SLAP). This lesion involves the anchor of the biceps tendon to the labrum. Several investigators reported on the strong correlation between SLAP lesions and glenohumeral instabilities.[38-40] Pagnani et al[40] found that a complete lesion of the superior labrum was large enough to destabilize the insertion of the biceps tendon and was associated with significant increases in anterior-posterior and superior-inferior glenohumeral translation.

SLAP lesions are believed to be secondary to a traumatic event, and they can also be a sequela of repetitive stress, especially in the overhead athlete. One model that underwent two arthroscopic studies investigating clinical observations and biomechanical data questioned the role of microinstability as a cause of SLAP lesions in the throwing athlete.[38] Burkhart and Morgan[38] reported on 53 baseball players, 44 of whom were pitchers, who had type II SLAP lesions that were surgically repaired. Arthroscopic repair of these type II SLAP lesions returned 87% of these athletes to sport with a preinjury level of performance. This result was superior when compared with the 50% to 68% of athletes able to return to sport after open anterior capsulolabral repair. These investigators proposed that the mechanism of SLAP injuries is the Morgan-Burkhart *peel-back model,* which describes the pathologic lesion at the posterior-superior labrum.[38]

Unlike the Walch-Jobe-Sidles model[41] of internal impingement resulting from capsular laxity or microinstability, Burkhart and Morgan[38,42,43] believed that the underlying cause of SLAP lesions is not anterior instability or internal impingement, but rather contracture of the posterior-inferior capsule secondary to the follow-through in the throwing motion. Burkhart and Morgan demonstrated that a glenohumeral internal rotation deficit (GIRD) caused by a contracted posterior capsule would induce a posterior-superior shift of the glenohumeral contact point and thus permit a greater amount of external rotation to occur before internal impingement. Moreover, a GIRD reduces the cam effect of the anterior-inferior capsule and induces pseudolaxity. These investigators believed that this condition was misdiagnosed in the past in overhead-throwing athletes as anterior instability. The investigators defined GIRD as a loss in degrees of glenohumeral internal rotation of the throwing shoulder compared with the nonthrowing shoulder. Burkhart and Morgan emphasized the importance of evaluating GIRDS and believed that it is a priority to restore these deficits at least to symmetry with the nonthrowing shoulder, to prevent the pathophysiologic cascade that can lead to SLAP lesions.[38,42,43] (See Chapter 3 for more information on pathophysiology of the overhead-throwing athlete.)

Investigators have also postulated that SLAP lesions can result from a compressive force applied directly to the shoulder from a fall on an outstretched arm, with the humerus in a position of abduction and slight forward flexion.[44] This type of injury has the potential to drive the humeral head superiorly, thus avulsing the biceps or labral attachment from the glenoid.[45] This appears to be the most common mechanism of SLAP lesions and accounts for 23% to 31% of injuries.[46] Traction injuries have accounted for 16% to 25% of all SLAP lesions, and dislocation or subluxation has accounted for up to 19%.[45] Bey et al[47] made some generalizations about the possible causes of SLAP lesions and suggested that types I, III, and IV lesions may be the result of a shearing force between the humeral head and the glenoid.

The presence of a destabilizing SLAP lesion may have a profound impact on shoulder stability and function. Rodosky et al[48] demonstrated that the presence of superior labrum and biceps anchor injury diminished the force necessary to translate the humeral head anteriorly. According to Higgins and Warner,[45] the rotator cuff may be subject to internal impingement and may lead to tearing secondary to the instability sequelae of the SLAP lesion. Moreover, SLAP lesions have been found to occur more commonly in younger patients with acute rotator cuff tears.[49] Snyder et al[37] arthroscopically identified and classified SLAP lesions into four types (Fig. 10-4). In the type I lesion, the superior labrum is markedly frayed, but the attachments of the labrum and biceps tendon remain intact. The type I lesion is regarded by many orthopedic surgeons as benign, or not pathologic.[46,48] The type II lesion resembles the type I lesion, except that the attachment of the superior labrum is compromised, resulting in instability of the labral-biceps complex. Type III lesions consist of a bucket-handle tear of the labrum, which can be displaced into the joint space. However, the labral-biceps attachment remains intact. Type IV lesions are similar to type III lesions, except that the labral tear extends into the biceps tendon and permits it to subluxate into the joint.

Maffet et al[46] suggested expanding beyond the original four types of SLAP lesions, as suggested by Snyder et al,[37] after noting in a retrospective review of 712 arthroscopies that 38% were not classifiable as types I to IV. Maffet et al[46] suggested an expansion to seven categories and added descriptions for types V through VII. Type V SLAP lesions are characterized by the presence of a Bankart lesion of the anterior capsule that extends into the anterior superior

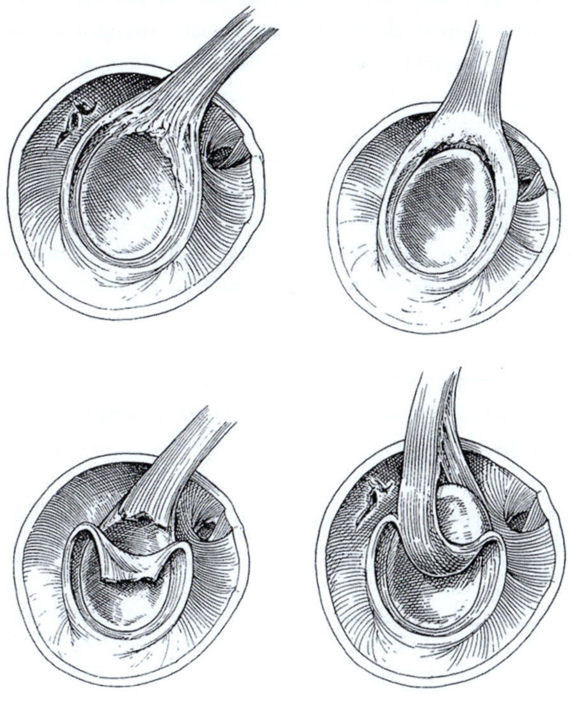

Figure 10-4 Superior labral tear classification. **A,** Type I. **B,** Type II. **C,** Type III. **D,** Type IV. (From Snyder SJ, Karzel RP, Del Pizzo W, et al: SLAP lesions of the shoulder, *Arthroscopy* 6:274–279, 1990.)

labrum. A type VI lesion indicates disruption of the biceps tendon anchor with an anterior or posterior superior labral flap tear. Type VII SLAP lesions are described as extensions of a SLAP lesion anteriorly to involve the inferior to the middle glenohumeral ligament.

Treatment of SLAP Lesions

Nonoperative Management

Conservative management of SLAP lesions is often unsuccessful, particularly when a component of glenohumeral instability is present. However, a few of patients with a type I SLAP lesion are amenable to conservative treatment.[50] The initial phase is to reduce the inflammation with short course of nonsteroidal anti-inflammatory drugs and cessation of throwing. Once the pain has subsided, physical therapy is initiated with a focus on restoring normal shoulder motion and strengthening the scapulohumeral rotators. Restoring glenohumeral internal rotation is critical, and thus emphasis should be placed on stretching the posterior capsule and external rotators to reduce the GIRD. Work by Izumi et al[51] suggested that the typical cross-body stretch and the sleeper stretch, as advocated by Burke and Morgan, may not be sufficient to stretch the entire posterior capsule. These investigators recommended that the arm be placed in 30° of elevation in the scapular plane with internal rotation for the middle and lower capsular tissues and stretching in 30° of extension with internal rotation for the upper and lower capsule.[51] (See Chapter 14 for further discussion of manual therapy techniques to stretch the posterior capsule.) The patient should be advanced as tolerated to a strengthening phase that includes the trunk, core, rotator cuff, and scapular musculature. Once the patient demonstrates adequate strength ratios of external to internal rotation of 70%, he or she is started on a throwing program for 3 months and continues with sport-specific strengthening.

Higgins and Warner[45] described an arthroscopic technique for repair of type II SLAP lesions. Historically, débridement alone did not provide adequate long-term results because the underlying instability was not addressed.[52] Currently, suture anchors are recommended, with an arthroscopic knot-tying technique instead of bioabsorbable tacks because of the risk of fragmentation of the tack and further complications.[45,49] Addressing any associated disorders at the time of arthroscopy, such as Bankart lesions or instability, is also important.

The technique advocated by Higgins and Warner[45] involves three portals: posterior, anterior (under the biceps tendon), and at the anterior-lateral acromion to allow for suture anchors and arthroscopic knots to be tied through this portal. The superior glenoid is removed of all fibrous material to prepare for repairing the labrum. The glenoid is decorticated, and the anchors are inserted through the working cannula. At least one anchor must be placed at, or posterior to, the biceps insertion to ensure solid fixation in this region. The sutures are tied off to the anchors with a sliding knot and are reinforced with several half stitches.

Type III SLAP lesions are treated similarly to type II lesions, except that the bucket-handle component of this lesion is excised, and no attempt is made to repair this lesion. While the patient is under anesthesia, the surgeon should attempt to discern whether any underlying instability predisposed the patient to the SLAP tear. Type IV SLAP lesions that compromise less than one third of the biceps tendon are débrided. If more than one third of the biceps tendon is involved, then the torn tendon is repaired back to the major fragment of the biceps.[45]

Postoperative Treatment for SLAP lesions

The rehabilitation following surgical intervention for a SLAP lesion should be specific to the type of lesion and the type of procedure performed (débridement versus repair), and it should also take into account other possible concomitant procedures, because of the underlying glenohumeral instability that is often present. The overall goal is to restore dynamic stability to the glenohumeral joint while simultaneously protecting the healing tissue from adverse stress, especially early postoperatively.

The surgical treatment and rehabilitation vary based on the concomitant disorders, but typically one should avoid the abducted and externally rotated position while the labrum is healing in those individuals with a SLAP lesion consistent with a peel-back lesion, as is often seen in the overhead athlete. In patients who sustained a compressive injury, such as a fall on an outstretched hand, weight-bearing exercises should be avoided, to minimize compression and shear on the superior labrum. Patients with traction injuries should avoid heavy resisted or excessive eccentric biceps contractions. These guidelines are crucial, especially in the early phase of recovery, because evidence has demonstrated failure rates as high as 32% in postoperative outcomes of SLAP repairs.[53]

CASE STUDY 2

This case represents the postoperative progression in a young patient who underwent repair for a type II SLAP lesion and supraglenoid cyst excision. Goals and treatment are based on soft tissue healing and on indications and contraindications postoperatively.

General Demographics

The patient, A.B., is a 10-year-old, English-speaking boy who comes to the clinic 4 weeks after right SLAP repair and supraglenoid cyst excision. He is right-hand dominant.

CASE STUDY 2—cont'd

Social History

A.B. lives with his mother and father. He does not smoke or drink.

Employment

He is a full time student in the fifth grade.

Living Environment

A.B. lives with his mother and father in a home in New Jersey.

Growth and Development

He is a lean boy, with hypermobile extremities.

Patient Medical History

He has a history of right shoulder pain, which occurred after too many innings and games as the starting pitcher for his traveling team that played all year round. He was treated for his SLAP tear and shoulder pain for 8 months of physical therapy before surgery and was doing reasonably well because his pain and dynamic stability improved. However, his glenoid cyst had grown in size and necessitates surgery.

History of Chief Complaint

A.B. reports that toward the last month of his summer baseball season, he began feeling right shoulder pain and paresthesias down into his right hand when he would try to pitch. He had been playing baseball all year because of his participation on a traveling team. He tried to stop pitching for a 2-week period, but still had pain trying to play second base to minimize the stress on his arm. He eventually sought a doctor's consultation and was diagnosed at the age of 9 years with supraspinatus tendinosis, a type II SLAP lesion, and a small paralabral ganglion cyst.

Prior Treatment for This Condition

His physician ordered an MRI scan that confirmed his diagnosis. Given his age, A.B. was first directed to begin a progressive course of physical therapy to see whether he could avoid surgery. His course of physical therapy initially tried to address his pain and gently begin rotator cuff and scapular strengthening and maintain his posterior capsular extensibility, which was not restricted at time of initial examination. Overall throughout his 8 months of physical therapy, he was able to progress with his strength and functional ROM and had minimal complaints of pain and paresthesias. However, he was asked to receive a repeat MRI scan before being cleared to resume a throwing program; the scan showed that his supraglenoid cyst had enlarged to a point that warranted arthroscopic surgery at this time.

Structural Examination

The patient is seen 2 weeks postoperatively, and visual inspection shows mild swelling along the anterior suture lines, but the sutures are intact and healing well. The right scapula is elevated relative to the left side.

Range of Motion

Shoulder Range of Motion

PROM is assessed at this time only for the shoulder: flexion, 75°; abduction, 60°; scaption, 80°; internal rotation, 45°; and external rotation, −10°. Elbow and wrist ROM are within normal limits.

Accessory Motion Testing of the Glenohumeral Joint

This motion is not assessed until 4 weeks postoperatively.

Muscle Testing

No resisted testing is permitted at this time, except for wrist motions and hand and finger motions, which are 5/5 grossly throughout.

Special Tests

No testing is done at this time.

Tenderness

The patient displays focal tenderness along the anterior-superior glenohumeral joint.

Palpation

Tenderness is found along the proximal biceps tendon and trigger points of the right upper trapezius.

Physical Therapist's Clinical Impression

The patient underwent a type II SLAP repair (two suture anchors) and supraglenoid cyst excision because of repetitive tensile loading to his capsuloligamentous restraints. His throwing mechanics were very poor on observation of video before his injury, which placed even greater shear forces at the glenohumeral joint and dynamic stability demand of his rotator cuff. A paralabral cyst invaginating into the glenoid and increasing in size is one of the possible sequelae of glenohumeral instability. His surgical procedure was necessary to help repair the detached labrum that was the underlying reason for his cyst formation. The main goals to consider in the early postoperative period are to permit proper soft tissue healing, to protect the biceps–superior labral complex from tensile stress, and to reduce pain, inflammation, and swelling. The early restrictions from 0 to 3 weeks are elevation to only 90° in the plane of the scapula, and external rotation to neutral to minimize strain on the labrum through the peel-back mechanism. This approach involves early avoidance of elbow flexion exercises, which are typically permitted after most shoulder procedures. Patients recovering from SLAP lesion repairs also require a longer period before they stress shoulder motion with external rotation in the abducted position. The reason is that as the biceps acts as a secondary anterior stabilizer in this position, it is also important to avoid the peel-back mechanism.[38,42]

Treatment Plan

The following is an overview of this patient's postoperative rehabilitation program. The patient is instructed on continued use of the sling for an additional 2 weeks at all

Continued

CASE STUDY 2—cont'd

times, except when he is doing his ROM exercises, to protect his biceps-labral complex. He is instructed to ice his shoulder three times a day for 10 to 15 minutes, to alleviate local inflammation and swelling, and to work on maintaining AROM of the elbow, wrist, and hand. He is instructed in middle and lower trapezius isometrics in the supine position to facilitate neuromuscular control at his scapular region. This protocol is reinforced during verbal and tactile cues instructing him to squeeze his shoulder blades down and inward, gently and slowly, while holding for 5 seconds. The patient's shoulder ROM is strictly passive at this time. He avoids pain and limits external rotation to 0° to 15° initially in the adducted position.

At 4 weeks postoperatively, the sling is removed, and PROM is progressed to 45° of external rotation and scaption (plane of the scapula) to 120°. The patient's initial PROM at this time is as follows: shoulder flexion, 105°; abduction, 100°; external rotation, 25°; and internal rotation, 50°. The initial phase of rehabilitation is to restore ROM, with particular attention paid to regaining proper length to the posterior capsule. When the posterior capsule is taut, the tendency is for the humeral head to shift anteriorly and superiorly, thus increasing the potential for augmenting compressive loading and shear at the biceps-labral complex. Modalities are used as needed to quell local postoperative inflammation and to prevent biceps or rotator cuff tendinitis. However, ultrasound is contraindicated, given the age of this patient and his open growth plates.

At 6 weeks postoperatively, strengthening of the rotator cuff and periscapular musculature is initiated, beginning first with isometrics and progressing to isotonic resisted training as tolerated in a pain-free arc of motion and in the adducted position. PROM is progressed as tolerated within the permissible range to protect the repair site. At this time, A.B.'s manual muscle testing demonstrates the following: shoulder flexion, 3+/5; abduction, 4−/5; external rotation, 3−/5; and internal rotation, 4/5; Biceps curls and resisted shoulder flexion are held for an additional 2 weeks.

At 8 to 12 weeks postoperatively, the patient progresses to light biceps curls. He is also instructed to begin shoulder scaption (0° to 90°) with 1-lb weights and to progress in 1-lb increments after he can perform 3 sets of 12 repetitions without altering the mechanics of the lift. Once he can perform external rotation with a 3-lb weight while side lying, he progresses to Thera-Band tubing beginning in the adducted position. Once he can tolerate Thera-Band scapular strengthening with rows and shoulder extensions, he progresses to prone scapular rotator exercises. The patient is instructed to avoid lifting his arm beyond his torso in the prone position, to avoid overstressing his anterior shoulder.

At 12 weeks after surgery, the patient demonstrates full restoration of AROM, with the exception of external rotation in abduction, which is 88°. This motion is not stressed actively or with resisted exercises until 6 months postoperatively, to avoid possibly overstressing the superior labral-biceps attachment. Manual muscle testing results are as follows: forward flexion, 5/5; abduction, 5/5; external rotation, 4+/5; internal rotation, 5/5; middle/lower trapezius, 5/5; and serratus anterior, 5/5. At this time, he is discharged and given a home exercise program. He is instructed to avoid overstressing his shoulder with throwing activities until he comes back in 4 weeks for a follow-up assessment. He is progressed with his home exercise program to include proprioceptive neuromuscular facilitation (D1, D2) diagonal patterns in standing with red and progressing to blue resistance. He is also progressed with Thera-Band strengthening for his external rotators in up in the plane of the scapula and demonstrates good form with sleeper stretch and ancillary stretches for posterior capsular extensibility.

Summary of Case

The patient continued his home program for a month and returns for a follow-up assessment that demonstrates 5/5 strength throughout his rotator cuff and scapular rotator musculature and full AROM. Although this patient does not demonstrate significant posterior capsule tightness before or after the procedure, it is still important to assess this region, based on work by Morgan et al.[42] Crockett et al[54] and Reagan et al[55] also suggested that as younger throwing athletes mature, their loss of internal rotation with concomitant increased external rotation is a function of skeletal changes at the humerus that induces greater humeral retroversion. Work by Liu et al[56] demonstrated the validity and accuracy of using a cluster of special tests, which have proven to be more accurate in predicting glenoid labral tears than MRI. The tests recommended by Liu et al include the apprehension, relocation, load and shift, inferior sulcus sign, and crank tests.[56] The use of the active compression test, as proposed by O'Brien et al[57] to diagnose the possibility of a SLAP lesion on examination more precisely, is also recommended. Several investigators believed that patients are predisposed to SLAP lesions when shoulder instability is present.[42,44,45] This condition is typically checked on physical examination and is confirmed when the patient is under anesthesia. This patient did not demonstrate any signs of instability; therefore, his surgical procedure did not warrant capsulorrhaphy, and he did not require further soft tissue healing time.

After SLAP repair surgery, the athlete typically is permitted to participate in sports 3 to 4 months postoperatively unless the sport involves throwing.[45] According to Higgins and Warner,[45] throwing short distances and at low

CASE STUDY 2—cont'd

velocity commences at approximately 4 months, with an emphasis on proper mechanics. Pitchers are permitted to practice low-velocity pitches from the mound at 6 months, and unrestricted throwing is held until at least 7 months postoperatively. Given the age of this patient, it seems prudent to wait closer to the 7- to 8-month postoperative period, to permit even more strength and soft tissue healing and thus prevent reinjury. He is also scheduled to work with a pitching coach to enhance his mechanics, to help avoid reinjury.

ROTATOR INTERVAL CAPSULE

Neer[58] was the first to use the term *rotator interval,* back in 1970. In 1981, Rowe and Zarins[23] documented the different sizes and variations in the rotator interval among patients with anterior instability. Fitzpatrick et al[59] suggested a wide patient spectrum involving potential laxity to instability of the rotator interval. Evidence suggests that the rotator interval region of the glenohumeral joint plays an integral role in the pathomechanics and intervention of patients with shoulder instability.[60-62] The term *rotator interval* has two distinct meanings when referring to the anterior-superior aspect of the shoulder. According to Gartsman and associates,[62] when the term is used in conjunction with repair of the rotator cuff, it is referring to the tendinous connection between the supraspinatus and subscapularis. When the term is used in reference to shoulder instability, it is defined as a triangular space bordered superiorly by the anterior margin of the supraspinatus tendon and inferiorly by the superior border of the subscapularis tendon (Fig. 10-5).[61,62] This triangular interval is bridged by capsular tissue and is reinforced superficially by the coracohumeral ligament and in its deepest segment by the superior glenohumeral ligament.[62-64]

Harryman et al[63] were among the first to investigate the role of the rotator interval in glenohumeral stability with a cadaveric model. These investigators determined that,

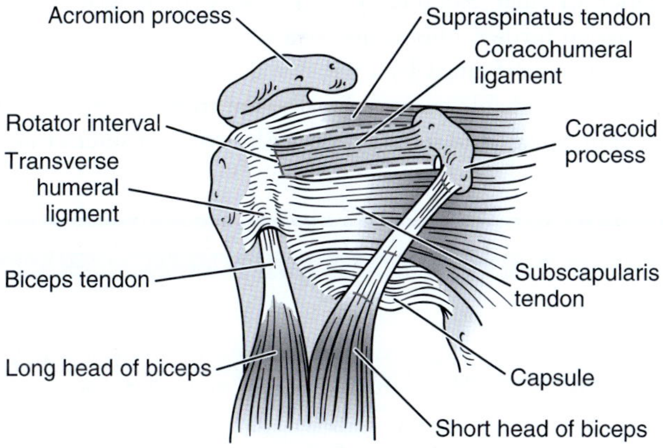

Figure 10-5 Rotator interval showing the relationship among the supraspinatus tendon, the subscapularis tendon, and the coracohumeral ligament. (From Magee DJ: *Orthopedic physical assessment,* ed 5, St. Louis, 2008, Saunders Elsevier.)

through operative sectioning of the rotator interval, a resultant increase in anterior, posterior, and inferior humeral head translation occurred. Conversely, imbricating the rotator interval decreased inferior and posterior translation compared with the intact state of the shoulder.[65] The studies by Harryman et al[63] and of Rowe and Zarins[23] suggested that the presence of defects in the rotator interval may be an important anatomic factor in shoulder instability.

Anatomy of the Rotator Interval

The triangular space also contains the biceps tendon. The quality of the capsular tissue varies in the rotator interval. Cole et al[60] did anatomic dissections of the rotator interval in 37 fetuses and found that 75% the capsular layer was not continuous, and a thin synovial membrane covered the rotator interval. The histologic examination of the covering of the rotator interval in both fetuses and adult populations revealed a loose and thin collagenous tissue that was poorly organized with a sparse population of fibroblasts. Because of Cole et al,[60] findings demonstrating that the tissue was relatively weak called into question the role of the rotator interval capsule in glenohumeral stability. Warner et al[66] confirmed the stabilizing and structural role of the rotator interval. These investigators showed that the inferior translation of the adducted arm was restricted by the superior glenohumeral ligament, the coracohumeral ligament, and the negative intra-articular pressure. A sealed glenohumeral capsule is necessary to maintain the negative intra-articular pressure, and the thin rotator interval capsule provides that seal.[66]

Field et al[61] retrospectively reported on an operative approach for patients with recurrent instability symptoms involving isolated closure of the rotator interval. These investigators determined a clinical relationship between a 2+ or more positive sulcus sign for inferior instability and rotator interval defects that influenced shoulder instability. These investigators also examined the shoulders for direction of instability while the patient was under anesthesia. They determined that, in all patients, the humeral head could be subluxated anteriorly to either grade 2+ (11 cases) or 1+ (4 cases), posterior translation had an average grade of 1+, and a positive sulcus sign was present in all patients. Zazzali and Vad observed that rotator interval defects are associated with a large sulcus sign combined with anterior instability. Both issues need to be addressed if they are found during surgical repair.

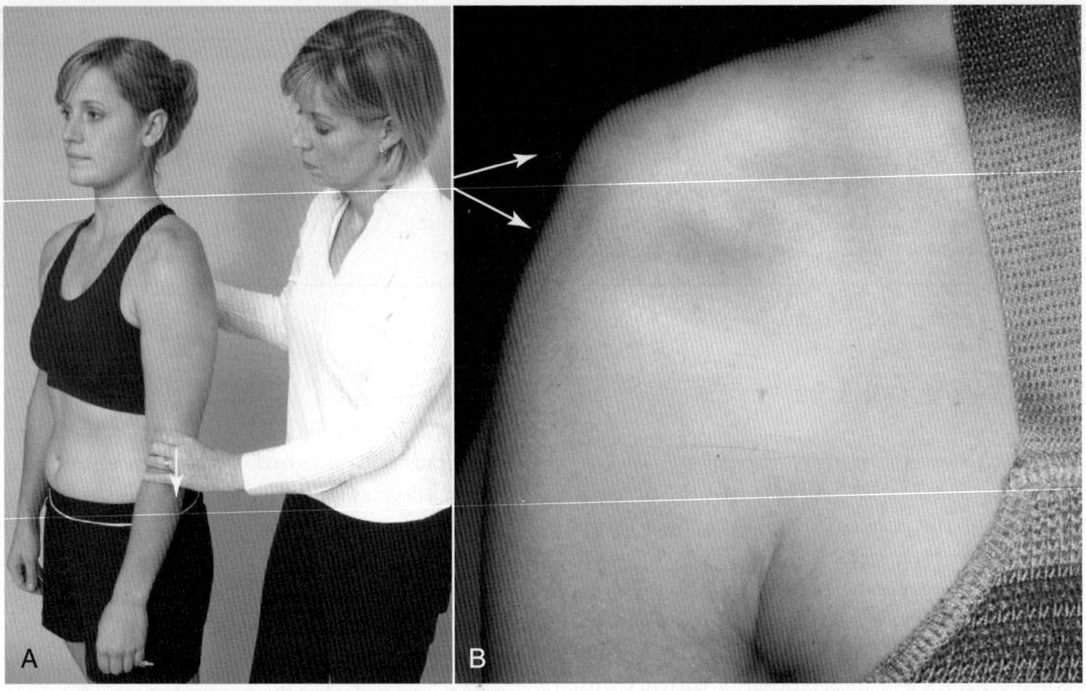

Figure 10-6 A, Test for inferior shoulder instability (sulcus test). **B,** Positive sulcus sign *(arrows).* (From Magee DJ: *Orthopedic physical assessment,* ed 5, St. Louis, 2008, Saunders Elsevier.)

Typically, before arthroscopic closure of the rotator interval, a supervised physical therapy regimen is implemented to attempt dynamic stabilization with a specific program to strengthen the rotator cuff and the scapular rotator. These exercises should be designed to enhance the concavity-compression effect of the rotator cuff at the glenohumeral joint without further compromising the static restraints of the shoulder. The physical therapy trial typically lasts 5 to 6 months before surgical intervention is considered.

According to Provencher and Saldua,[65] indications for surgical repair of the rotator interval remain poorly defined; however, evidence suggests that closure should be considered in the following: (1) patients with anterior instability and rotator interval lesion (incomplete sulcus), (2) patients with symptomatic shoulder instability and laxity in the inferior direction (positive sulcus) that does not obliterate with in external rotation with the arm at the side (Fig. 10-6), (3) patients who have significant laxity and a large sulcus finding with concomitant multidirectional instability, and (4) possibly some patients with posterior instability in whom prior surgical attempts at stabilization have failed.[65]

The surgical technique for isolated closure of the rotator interval defect, as described by Field et al,[61] involves an anterior arthroscopic technique, which necessitates release of the lateral 30% of the conjoined tendon insertion to permit access to the anterior capsule. The subscapularis tendon is released approximately 1 cm medial to its insertion on the lesser tuberosity; this approach also enhances visualization of the rotator interval. After delineation of the rotator interval, the defect edges are then approximated, typically with the patient's arm placed in 45° of abduction and external rotation. Imbrication is performed in a "pants-over-vest" fashion. The closure of the rotator interval defects reduces the anterior and inferior capsular redundancy. If necessary to reduce inferior translation further, imbrication of a lax superior glenohumeral ligament is performed by overlapping and suturing the ends with nonabsorbable sutures. Finally, the subscapularis tendon is reapproximated to its insertion with nonabsorbable sutures.

CASE STUDY 3

This case represents the progression postoperatively for a patient who underwent isolated closure of a rotator interval defect that induced shoulder instability. In general, the postoperative regimen follows the primary repair guidelines (i.e., for anterior, posterior or multidirectional instability). Patients are first placed in a sling for 4 weeks, and the primary procedure is allowed to dictate the postoperative regimen. Typically, patients are advised to limit forward flexion to 90° and external rotation to 0° for the first 4 weeks postoperatively.[67] After the sling is removed, AROM and active-assisted ROM exercises are begun, with a gradual progression to end-range stretches. By 8 weeks, most patients have regained full forward flexion and external rotation. The emphasis is then placed on restoring

CASE STUDY 3—cont'd

rotator cuff and scapular rotator strength, to enhance their dynamic stability and concavity-compression mechanism; full recovery and return to function are usually expected by 6 months.[65]

General Demographics

The patient, Mr. S.Y., is a 32-year-old, English-speaking, Asian man who comes to physical therapy 4 weeks after rotator interval closure. He is right-hand dominant.

Social History

Mr. S.Y. is single and lives alone. He does not smoke, and he drinks approximately twice per week.

Employment and Environment

He is a director of a nonprofit company, and he plays squash and tennis.

Living Environment

Mr. S.Y. lives alone on the fifth floor.

Patient Medical History

He has a history of right shoulder pain and "dead arm" symptoms, which occurred typically while playing recreational squash.

History of Chief Complaint

Mr. S.Y. reports that his chief complaint is a recurrent feeling of instability and clicking at the right shoulder, which occurs during tennis and squash, and pain that began approximately 4 months ago. He has ceased these sports activities secondary to exacerbation of his symptoms.

Prior Treatment for This Condition

The patient was seen by his orthopedic surgeon, who determined his symptoms to be associated with anterior instability based on his history and a positive apprehension test result, a positive sulcus test result that did not change with placing the shoulder in external rotation, and a 2+ load and shift test result for anterior instability grading. Standard radiographs of the affected shoulder showed no Bankart lesions or Hill-Sachs deformities. An MRI scan did not demonstrate the presence of capsular irregularities. The patient underwent arthroscopic exploratory surgery and was found to have a defect at the rotator interval capsule that was 2.75 cm in medial-to-lateral width and 2.1 cm in superior-to-inferior height. The patient underwent arthroscopy to close this defect and to reduce anterior and inferior capsular redundancy.

Structural Examination

The patient is seen 7 days postoperatively, and he is wearing a sling. Visual inspection reveals modest swelling along the anterior suture lines and ecchymosis, but the sutures are intact, clean, and dry. His right scapula is elevated relative to the right side and demonstrates some inferior angle winging at rest.

Range of Motion

Shoulder Active Range of Motion

AROM is not assessed because of the acuteness of his symptoms and contraindications relative to the postoperative time period. His PROM is assessed as follows: shoulder flexion, 80°; abduction, 60°; external rotation, −5°; and internal rotation, 50°. Elbow and wrist ROM are within normal limits.

Accessory Motion Testing of the Glenohumeral Joint

This motion is not assessed because of the acuteness of the patient's symptoms and the time frame from surgery.

Muscle Testing

No resisted testing is permitted at this time, except for elbow, wrist, and hand and finger motions, which are within normal limits.

Special Tests

No testing is done at this time.

Tenderness

The patient has focal tenderness along the anterior-superior glenohumeral joint and along the coracoid process.

Palpation

Tenderness is noted along the subscapularis tendon insertion and at the coracoid process.

Physical Therapist's Clinical Impression

The patient arrives for physical therapy for rehabilitation 1 week after right arthroscopy for isolated closure of the rotator interval. This surgical procedure was suggested to help reduce anterior-inferior instability.[61] The patient's ROM will need to be restored, with a priority to achieve a minimum of 35° of external rotation before advancing elevation beyond 90°, to prevent impingement.[68] However, external rotation will initially be limited to 0° for the first 4 weeks, to permit adequate fixation of the rotator interval region. Care will also need to be taken to avoid joint mobilization to the anterior or inferior capsules, to prevent overstressing the rotator interval repair site.

Treatment Plan

The following is an overview of this patient's postoperative rehabilitation program.

Pendulum exercises are started immediately postoperatively. The patient is instructed on continued use of the sling for an additional 3 weeks to protect the rotator interval when he is not in physical therapy or performing ROM exercises independently. Active-assisted external rotation exercises are initially limited to 0° for the first 4 weeks. He is instructed to ice his shoulder two to three times a day for 10 to 15 minutes to alleviate local inflammation and swelling and to work on maintaining AROM of the elbow, wrist, and hand.

Continued

CASE STUDY 3—cont'd

After the fourth postoperative week, the sling is removed, and forward flexion and external rotation exercises for ROM and motor control are progressing. The patient's initial AROM at this time is as follows: shoulder flexion, 90°; abduction, 75°; external rotation, 10°; and internal rotation, 50°. The initial phase of rehabilitation is to restore ROM, with graded physiologic stretching coupled with soft tissue mobilization to address periarticular fibrosis secondary to immobilization. Aggressive joint mobilizations are contraindicated at this time because of the possible risk of interfering with capsular length tension and shear to the repair site. Modalities are used as needed to quell local postoperative inflammation and to prevent manifestation of secondary rotator cuff tendinitis.

At 8 weeks postoperatively, he demonstrates the following: full forward flexion, 170°; abduction, 165°; internal rotation, 70°; and external rotation, 85°. At this time, a graduated strengthening program for the rotator cuff and periscapular musculature is initiated, beginning first with isometrics and progressing to isotonic resisted training as tolerated in a pain-free arc of motion and in the adducted position. At this time, Mr. S.Y.'s manual muscle testing results are as follows: shoulder flexion, 4/5; abduction, 4−/5; external rotation, 3+/5; and internal rotation, 4−/5.

At 12 weeks postoperatively, the patient progresses to Thera-Band rotator cuff exercises and prone scapular rotator exercises to address the middle and lower trapezius musculature. The patient is instructed to avoid lifting his arm beyond his torso in the prone position and to avoid overstressing the anterior shoulder. The rotator cuff exercises are gradually progressing to more provocative positions of elevated abduction for more sport-specific and functional patterns of motion.

By 16 to 20 weeks postoperatively, the patient demonstrates 5/5 strength throughout his right shoulder musculature on manual testing. He does not show any signs of laxity or symptoms of instability and is progressing to sport-specific exercises to prepare his arm for tennis and squash. Plyometric training is also instituted for proprioception and kinesthetic awareness, with the use of a medicine ball and quick Thera-Band repetitions in elevated positions of abduction for the internal rotators. The patient is permitted to return playing squash and tennis slowly by the sixth month postoperatively.

Summary of Case

The true incidence of rotator interval defects is unknown at the present time, but evidence suggests that these biologic insufficiencies may be congenital in origin.[60] The aforementioned patient was treated solely for surgical closure of a rotator interval defect. The surgeon determined by arthroscopic examination that the patient had no comorbidity to the labrum or anterior or posterior capsules. The therapist communicated with the referring surgeon to appreciate exactly which tissue was involved during the surgical procedure. Once the initial period of healing is permitted and a pragmatic approach is instituted, with the chief concern not to be aggressive with joint mobilization techniques (especially anteriorly and inferiorly before 6 weeks postoperatively), the patient progresses predictably with respect to strength and return to function.

POSTERIOR INSTABILITY

Posterior instability of the shoulder is uncommon and accounts for 2% to 5% of all cases of shoulder instability,[67,69] and for less than 2% of all shoulder dislocations. Posterior shoulder instability covers a continuum of disorders ranging from acute posterior dislocation at one end of the spectrum to chronic recurrent subtle posterior subluxations at the other end. Its origin has been classified as traumatic or atraumatic and its type as voluntary (individual can subluxate the shoulder posteriorly) or involuntary. The mechanism of injury for posterior instability has been described as the result of external force applications including posterior axial loads and forced hyperadduction.[69] Insufficient internal restraints that may play an etiologic part in posterior instability include glenoid retroversion,[70] glenoid hypoplasia,[71] and weakness in the external rotators.[72] Kim et al[73] found that the most common mechanism for posterior shoulder instability was a direct impact while the arm was in a horizontally adducted and flexed position during a fall to the ground. Steinmann[72] suggested that weakness in the external rotators is associated with posterior instability and theorized that progressively increasing forces on the static stabilizers with concomitant weak posterior cuff muscles can induce serial elongation of the posterior capsule that leads to instability.

Posterior dislocations can be associated with an acute traumatic event that can often create an impression defect on the anterior humeral head known as a *reverse Hill-Sachs lesion.* Symptomatic posterior shoulder instability is a condition in which symptoms are caused by an abnormal posterior translation of the humeral head relative to the glenoid cavity.[70] Posterior instability related to dislocations and recurrent subluxation may be associated with a posterior Bankart lesion, posterior capsular laxity or both.[69,70] The posterior Bankart lesion is described as a detachment of the posterior capsule and labrum below the glenoid equator.[70]

The mechanism of injury is typically a high-energy posteriorly directed force on an outstretched arm in the athlete.[74] Williams et al[70] theorized that a single traumatic episode, either alone or in conjunction with cumulative strain, may lead to excessive posterior head translation that can lead to detachment of the posterior capsulolabral complex.

Symptoms and Physical Examination

Individuals with posterior instability are typically men between the ages of 20 and 30 years and who are often involved in overhead-throwing or contact sports.[69,71] Patients typically have increased sensitivity and pain during weight-bearing activities and report pain, a feeling of weakness, and a sensation of abnormal mechanics including catching, clicking, and clunking.[70,74] On examination, pain is typically reproduced with the provocative position of 90° forward flexion combined with horizontal adduction and internal rotation. Patients usually describe posterior joint line tenderness, and they have excessive posterior translation of the humeral head with pain on posterior load-and-shift test, as well as a positive posterior apprehension sign. Patients may also have a positive result on a jerk test, which is performed by applying an axial load to the patient's arm while it is in 90° of abduction and internal rotation, after which the patient's arm is horizontally adducted while the axial load is maintained. The test result is positive if pain and a palpable or audible clunk are reproduced.[75] The jerk test has been reported to have a sensitivity of 73%, a specificity of 98%, a positive predictive value of 0.88%, and a negative predictive value of 0.95% for the detection of posterior-inferior labral lesions.[76]

Rehabilitation

Physical therapy is the primary recommended treatment intervention for individuals with symptomatic posterior instability.[70] A minimum of 6 weeks to 3 months is suggested for conservative physical therapy, consisting of a strong focus on rotator cuff strengthening (especially the infraspinatus) and scapular and rotator strengthening exercises.[77] To prevent increased symptoms, combined motions of shoulder internal rotation and flexion must be avoided, horizontal adduction motion must be limited, and posterior shear forces on the shoulder (applying weights in the hands with the shoulder flexed to 90°) must be minimized.[69,74] The postoperative rehabilitation following shoulder stabilization surgery allows the patient to regain proper balance of mobility and stability. ROM should be restricted to 90° of flexion for the first 4 weeks and then to 120° from weeks 4 to 6. Full shoulder ROM should be restored through progressive stretching by week 10. Stretching should be done with methodical care in the early postoperative period and tailored to the type of stabilization to prevent failure at the repair site. Posterior capsular stretching or mobilization is not begun until week 10 postoperatively. Neuromuscular and proprioception training are used to enhance strength and motor control, with an emphasis eventually on the end ROMs. Proper balance of the musculature is emphasized, with extra concern for the rotator cuff because of its effective role in providing dynamic stability.

OPEN INFERIOR CAPSULAR SHIFT

In 1980, Neer and Foster[78] were among the first to emphasize the importance of distinguishing between unidirectional and multidirectional instability because the standard repairs designed to correct unidirectional instability failed when they were performed on multidirectional unstable shoulders.[75,78] Neer and Foster described the inferior capsular shift procedure for treating patients with symptomatic multidirectional instability of the shoulder who had failed to respond to nonoperative management.[78] The inferior capsular shift is still considered the gold standard for multidirectional instability.[75,78,79]

Operative Technique

The operative approach is based on the predominant direction of instability in each case. This factor is determined by the preoperative symptoms and physical findings and is verified at the time of surgery while the patient is under anesthesia. The anterior approach is described here, as reported by Pollock et al.[75]

Once the superficial fascia is removed, the subscapularis tendon is incised 1 cm medial to its insertion on the lesser tuberosity. The incision proceeds from the superior rotator interval to the inferior border of the subscapularis tendon. The muscular portion of the subscapularis is also separated from the capsule. The capsule is then incised, starting superiorly in the region of the capsular cleft between the superior and middle glenohumeral ligaments and proceeding inferiorly around the anatomic neck of the humerus. The dissection of the capsule proceeds inferiorly until the redundant inferior pouch can be sufficiently reduced by pulling up on the traction sutures placed in the capsule and thus extruding the surgeon's index finger from the redundant inferior pouch. The surgeon must anchor the capsule medially to the glenoid with either nonabsorbable sutures or suture anchors. The capsule is then split in a T-shaped fashion just above the superior border of the inferior glenohumeral ligament (Fig. 10-7A). The patient's arm is now placed in 20° of abduction and external rotation. The inferior flap is pulled superiorly, thereby reducing the inferior capsular pouch, and is sutured to the lateral capsular remnant (see Fig. 10-7B). The capsular cleft between the superior and middle glenohumeral ligaments is closed, and this entire superior flap is then shifted inferiorly over the inferior flap in a cruciate fashion to reinforce the capsule anteriorly (see Fig. 10-7B. Finally, the subscapularis is repaired back to the lesser tuberosity, and the deltopectoral interval and skin are closed.

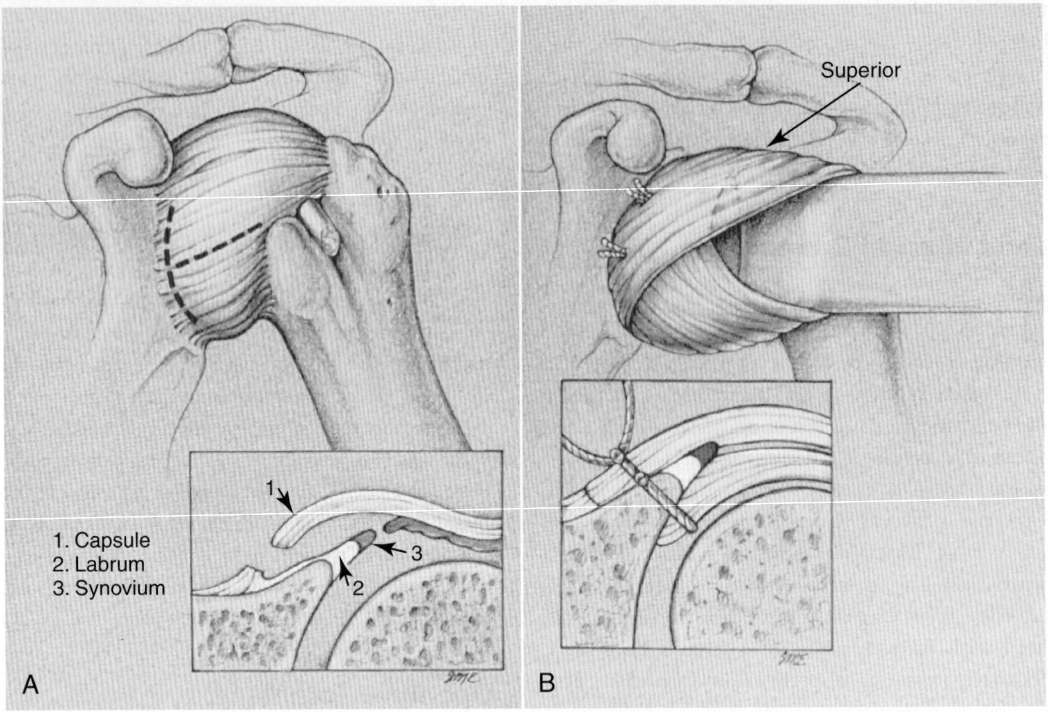

Figure 10-7 A, T-shaped incision in the glenohumeral joint capsule and synovial lining. **B,** Superior shift of the inferior flap and inferior shift of the superior capsular flap. (From Jobe F, Giangarra C, Kvitne R, et al: Anterior capsulolabral reconstruction of the shoulder in athletes in overhand sports, *Am J Sports Med* 19:428, 1991.)

CASE STUDY 4

This case represents the progression postoperatively for a patient who underwent an inferior capsular shift procedure to address anterior-inferior instability of the shoulder.

General Demographics

The patient, Mr. E.P., is a 29-year-old, English-speaking, Greek man who comes to physical therapy 4 weeks after inferior capsular shift of his right shoulder. He is right-hand dominant.

Social History

Mr. E.P. is single and lives alone. He does not smoke and drinks approximately twice per week.

Employment and Environment

He is a professor at a local university.

Living Environment

Mr. E.P. lives alone in a second-floor apartment.

Patient Medical History

He has a history of right shoulder pain and "dead arm" symptoms, which occurred after his first shoulder dislocation while playing recreational basketball. Over the course of a 3-year period, the patient dislocated his shoulder 8 to 10 times, with an increase in the ease of dislocation and subsequently greater difficulty with reduction of the shoulder. The patient reports intermittent paresthesia after each dislocation, which typically abates readily after relocation.

History of Chief Complaint

Mr. E.P. reports that his chief complaint is a recurrent feeling of instability and clicking at the right shoulder, which occurs during basketball and overhead weight training. The patient reports that the pain and instability symptoms are more frequent and recently have begun to occur during sleep. His goal is to function with activities of daily living (ADLs) without shoulder pain and instability and to return to recreational basketball after surgery.

Prior Treatment for This Condition

The patient was seen for physical therapy at another clinic to attempt dynamic stabilization of his shoulder, with a regimented and progressive exercise program addressing the rotator cuff and scapular rotators. He was seen for 4 months, which helped to decrease his pain considerably with ADLs. However, he still had frequent episodes of subluxation and dislocation with his right shoulder during sleep. He also was not able to resume basketball because of residual signs and symptoms of instability with overhead quick movements.

Structural Examination

The patient is seen 14 days postoperatively, and he is wearing a sling. Visual inspection reveals a well-healed anterior incision, which is intact to light touch. Moderate

CASE STUDY 4—cont'd

atrophy of the infraspinatus and supraspinatus is noted relative to the uninvolved side. His scapula is elevated on the right side when his arms rest at his side in the standing position.

Range of Motion

Shoulder AROM is not assessed at this time because of the acuteness of his symptoms related to the early postoperative time period. His PROM is assessed as follows: shoulder flexion, 90°; abduction, 60°; external rotation, −10°; and internal rotation, 50°. Elbow and wrist ROM were within normal limits.

Accessory Motion Testing of the Glenohumeral Joint

This motion was not assessed because of the acuteness of symptoms and the time frame from surgery.

Muscle Testing

No resisted testing is permitted at this time except for elbow, wrist, and hand and finger motions, which are of normal strength.

Special Tests

The load and shift test is performed for the left shoulder, and it demonstrates 1° of anterior and inferior translation. Hypermobility is also noted in the left and right elbows and the metacarpophalangeal joints.

Tenderness

The patient displays focal tenderness along the anterior glenohumeral joint and through the belly of the right upper trapezius muscle and subscapularis tendon insertion.

Physical Therapist's Clinical Impression

Given the patient's long history of instability, it is important to communicate with the referring surgeon regarding the patient's chief directions of instability at the time of the surgery. The surgeon reports using an anterior approach after determining, while the patient was under anesthesia, that the chief direction of instability was anteriorly and inferiorly. Furthermore, the surgeon states the patient's posterior capsule is tight, possibly augmenting the anterior capsular redundancy. Therefore, it is believed that posterior capsular mobilization techniques are indicated to reduce the stress at the anterior-inferior region of the shoulder and will not threaten posterior stability. The initial course of physical therapy is focused on addressing the impairments related to connective tissue dysfunction from immobilization and the surgical procedure.

Treatment Plan

Initial Treatment: Weeks 2 to 4

The patient is instructed on continued use of the sling for an additional 2 weeks to protect the anterior shoulder when he is not in physical therapy or performing ROM exercises independently. External rotation is limited to 30° for the first 6 weeks after repair. Submaximal isometrics for the rotator cuff are started at 3 weeks after surgery, along with manual resistance to the biceps, triceps, forearm, and wrist musculature. Manual resistance is also applied to the scapular retractors, with care to support and protect the glenohumeral joint.

Weeks 4 to 6

At the fourth postoperative week, the sling is removed, and forward flexion and external rotation exercises for ROM and motor control are begun, but external rotation is still progressing slowly, to prevent stretching the repair. Soft tissue mobilization and scapulothoracic mobilization are initiated along with glenohumeral posterior capsular mobilizations. The anterior and inferior joint glides are avoided to protect the healing anterior-inferior capsule. Rhythmic stabilization with the involved shoulder in varying planes of motion is initiated to promote proprioception, cocontraction, and kinesthetic awareness of the rotator cuff and scapular musculature.

Weeks 6 to 12

The patient's initial AROM at this time is as follows: shoulder flexion, 140°; abduction, 125°; external rotation, 40°; and internal rotation, 60°. At this time, isotonic strengthening exercises are initiated for the rotator cuff, scapular rotators, and deltoid. A format of low resistance and high repetitions is used to promote the circulatory phase of healing and to build endurance of the surrounding dynamic stabilizers. The goal at this phase is to continue progressing ROM, to attain end-range motion gradually. Continued passive stretching and posterior capsule joint mobilization techniques, and now caudal glides to restore flexion and internal rotation, are coupled with progressive strength training while the patient's signs and symptoms of tendinitis or instability are monitored.

Weeks 12 to 20

AROM by 12 weeks postoperatively is 170° of flexion, 165° of abduction, 75° of external rotation in 90° of abduction, and 70° of internal rotation. Results of manual muscle tests are as follows: forward flexion, 4+/5; abduction, 4+/5; external rotation, 4/5; internal rotation, 4+/5; and prone horizontal abduction with the thumb up (middle trapezius), = 4/5. At this time, the patient's strengthening program is advanced to plyometric exercises initially using therapeutic balls, including a basketball for chest passes and then progressing to a 5-lb medicine ball for chest and overhead passes. The patient is using Thera-Band tubing, with progressive resistance in the plane of the scapula to work his external rotators and in 90° of abduction to work his internal rotators. Proprioceptive neuromuscular facilitation patterns are initiated to promote functional and synergistic patterning of his scapulohumeral rotators with the deltoid. The initiation of isokinetic

Continued

CASE STUDY 4—cont'd

exercise for the internal and external rotator cuff in the "modified base position" is recommended at this time. The criterion for isokinetic progression is the tolerance of a 3-lb isotonic rotator cuff exercise in side-lying and standing external rotation, with at least blue Thera-Band resistance and full ROM within the training zones of motion. The isokinetic test on this patient is performed 16 weeks postoperatively and shows external rotation strength to be 10% weaker on the involved side and internal rotation strength to be 10% stronger on the involved side relative to the uninvolved, nondominant side.

Weeks 20 to 28

At week 20 postoperatively, the patient demonstrates full forward flexion of 175°, abduction of 170°, external rotation of 90°, and internal rotation of 70°. He does not show any signs of laxity or symptoms of instability and is progressing to sport-specific exercises to prepare for return to basketball. At 24 weeks postoperatively, a second isokinetic test shows equal external rotation strength at 60°, 180°, and 240° per second and 20% greater internal rotation strength on the involved, dominant side. At this time, he progresses with closed chain exercises for his home program, including modified arc push-ups with a plus to protect the anterior capsule, seated press-ups, and Swiss ball wall circles.

Summary of Case

The inferior capsular shift procedure that this patient underwent was specific for anterior and, to a lesser degree, inferior instability. The surgical approach is most often related to the primary direction of instability, to permit adequate visualization and stabilization. Adequate communication between the surgeon and the therapist is essential to avoid overstressing the repaired capsular component with directed joint mobilization techniques. This procedure is also used for multidirectional instability, which precludes the use of posterior capsular mobilizations early in the rehabilitation process. This patient has a long history of dislocations and needs adequate surgical fixation and postoperative rehabilitation to permit a safe return to sports without jeopardizing his glenohumeral stability and to perform ADLs pain free.

SCAPULAR KINEMATIC ALTERATIONS ASSOCIATED WITH GLENOHUMERAL JOINT INSTABILITY

Interest and study have increased with respect to the scapular kinematic abnormalities associated with glenohumeral joint instabilities.[80] A fairly consistent finding among investigations is that of significantly less scapular upward rotation or a significantly greater *scapulohumeral rhythm ratio* (defined as an indication of a lesser scapular upward rotation component) in subjects with instability.[81-84] *Scapular winging* is also reported to be significant in subjects with glenohumeral instability and is defined as a greater prominence of the scapular medial border that is also consistent with increased internal rotation of the scapula.[82,85] Paletta et al[86] examined patients with anterior instability with two-plane x-ray evaluation and determined that, early in ROM (0° to 90°), subjects with instability had lesser scapular upward rotation contribution to arm elevation, whereas later in the range of elevation, the scapular contribution was significantly greater. This finding is the reverse of what is typically expected in the normal scapulohumeral mechanics of the glenohumeral joint.

According to work by Bagg and Forrest,[87] who examined the electromyographic activity of the scapular rotators in the plane of the scapula during arm elevation, the scapula should set by the rhomboids in the first 30° of motion. During the ROM from 80° to 140° of elevation, the scapula should upwardly rotate and move in approximately a 1:1 ratio with the humerus. This is the critical phase of elevation, and the serratus anterior is very important throughout this phase, as are the middle and lower trapezius muscles, to provide proper glenohumeral contact to help facilitate inferior glenohumeral stability. Itoi et al[88] suggested that the reduction in scapular upward rotation in individuals with multidirectional instability does not represent a positive compensation but likely contributes to inferior glenohumeral joint instability. During the last 40° of elevation, (140° to 180°), the scapular body needs to sit back or tilt posteriorly and remain to provide proper acromiohumeral interval distance and stability. This positioning is possible with the help of the lower trapezius and middle trapezius and with concomitant extensibility of the pectoralis minor, latissimus dorsi, and subscapularis, to allow the scapula to dissociate from the humerus.

Based on the foregoing premise that the lower and middle trapezius muscles are important stabilizers of the scapula and that deficiencies in either of these muscles can compromise normal shoulder function and play a role in glenohumeral instability, the therapist should tailor exercises specific to these muscles. Work by Cools et al[89] investigated which exercises demonstrated high middle and lower trapezius activation with minimal upper trapezius output. These investigators established which exercises should be prescribed to restore scapular muscle balance and stability. The following four exercises met their criteria: (1) prone extension, (2) forward flexion in side lying, (3) external rotation in side lying, (4) and prone horizontal abduction with external rotation.[89]

De Mey et al[90] further evaluated this work by Cools et al to discern whether these exercises were activating the lower and middle trapezius before the upper trapezius as well as the posterior deltoid. De Mey et al[90] found that, of the four exercises, only the side-lying flexion exercise did not demonstrate significant timing differences in activation between portions of the trapezius.[90] These two studies demonstrated the importance of proper specificity of training with particular exercises to promote better scapular muscle balance, to augment scapular stability, and to enhance proper scapular kinematics in patients with shoulder disorders related to glenohumeral instability.

REFERENCES

1. Matsen F, Harryman D, Sidles J: Mechanics of glenohumeral instability, *Clin Sports Med* 10:783–788, 1991.
2. Pagnani M, Warren R: Stabilizers of the glenohumeral joint, *J Shoulder Elbow Surg* 3:173–190, 1994.
3. Speer K: Anatomy and pathomechanics of shoulder instability, *Clin Sports Med* 14:751–761, 1995.
4. Warner J: The "chock-block effect": the gross anatomy of the joint surfaces, ligaments, labrum, and capsule. In Matsen FA, Fu F, Hawkins R, editors: *The shoulder: a balance between mobility and stability*, Rosemont, Ill, 1993, American Academy of Orthopaedic Surgeons.
5. Vanderhooft E, Lippett S, Harris S, et al: Glenohumeral stability from concavity compression: a quantitative analysis, *Orthop Trans* 16:774, 1994.
6. Gohlke F, Essigkrug B, Schmitz F: The pattern of the collagen fiber bundles of the capsule of the glenohumeral joint, *J Shoulder Elbow Surg* 3:111–128, 1994.
7. O'Brien S, Schwartz R, Warren R, et al: The anatomy and histology of the inferior glenohumeral ligament complex of the shoulder, *Am J Sports Med* 18:449–456, 1990.
8. Turkel S, Panio M, Marshall J, et al: Stabilizing mechanisms preventing anterior dislocation of the glenohumeral joint, *J Bone Joint Surg Am* 63:1208–1217, 1981.
9. Abboud JA, Soslowsky LJ: Interplay of the static and dynamic restraints in glenohumeral instability, *Clin Orthop Relat Res* 400:48–57, 2002.
10. Bankart A: The pathology and treatment of recurrent dislocations of the shoulder-joint, *Br J Surg* 26:23–28, 1938.
11. Kralinger F, Golser K, Wischatta R, et al: Predicting recurrence after primary anterior shoulder dislocation, *Am J Sports Med* 30:116–120, 2002.
12. Hill H, Sachs M: The grooved defect of the humeral head: a frequently unrecognized complication of dislocations of the shoulder joint, *Radiology* 35:690–700, 1940.
13. Jackins S: Postoperative shoulder rehabilitation, *Phys Med Rehabil Clin N Am* 15:643–682, 2004.
14. Magnusson L, Kartus J, Ejerhed L, et al: Revisiting the open Bankart experience: a four-to nine-year follow-up, *Am J Sports Med* 30:778–782, 2002.
15. Gill T, Micheli J, Gebhard F, et al: Bankart repair for anterior instability of the shoulder, *J Bone Joint Surg Am* 79:850–857, 1997.
16. Randelli P, Arrigoni P, Polli L, et al: Quantification of active ROM after arthroscopic Bankart repair with rotator interval closure, *Orthopedics* 32(6):408, 2009.
17. Pagnani M, Dome D: Surgical treatment of traumatic anterior shoulder instability in American football players, *J Bone Joint Surg Am* 84:711–715, 2002.
18. Penna J, Deramo D, Nelson CO, et al: Determination of anterior labral repair stress during passive arm motion in a cadaveric model, *Arthroscopy* 24(8):930–935, 2008.
19. Wang R, Arciero R, Mazzocca A: The recognition and treatment of first-time shoulder dislocation in active individuals, *J Orthop Sports Phys Ther* 39(2):118–123, 2009.
20. Rodeo SA, Arnoczky SP, Torzilli PA, et al: Tendon-healing in a bone tunnel: a biomechanical and histological study in the dog, *J Bone Joint Surg Am* 75:1795–1803, 1993.
21. Speer K, Warren R, Pagnani M, et al: An arthroscopic technique for anterior stabilization of the shoulder with a bioabsorbable tack, *J Bone Joint Surg Am* 78:1801–1807, 1996.
22. Jobe F, Giangarra C, Kvitne R, et al: Anterior capsulolabral reconstruction of the shoulder in athletes in overhand sports, *Am J Sports Med* 19:428, 1991.
23. Rowe C, Zarins B: Recurrent transient subluxation of the shoulder, *J Bone Joint Surg Am* 63:863–872, 1981.
24. Rook R, Savoie F, Field L, et al: Arthroscopic treatment of instability attributable to capsular injury or laxity, *Clin Orthop Relat Res* 390:52–58, 2001.
25. O'Neill D: Arthroscopic Bankart repair of anterior detachments of the glenoid labrum: a prospective study, *J Bone Joint Surg Am* 81:1357–1366, 1999.
26. Cole B, L'Insalata J, Irrgang J, et al: Comparison of arthroscopic and open anterior shoulder stabilization: a two to six-year follow-up study, *J Bone Joint Surg Am* 82:1108–1114, 2000.
27. McMahon P, Lee T: Muscles may contribute to shoulder dislocation and stability, *Clin Orthop Relat Res* 403:18–25, 2002.
28. Matsen F, Thomas S, Rockwood C: Glenohumeral instability. In Harryman D, editor: *The shoulder*, Philadelphia, 1998, Saunders.
29. Lee SB, Kim KJ, O'Driscoll SW, et al: Dynamic glenohumeral stability provided by the rotator cuff muscles in the mid range and end range of motion: a study in cadavera, *J Bone Joint Surg Am* 82:849–857, 2000.
30. Lippitt SB, Matsen F: Mechanisms of glenohumeral joint instability, *Clin Orthop Relat Res* 291:20–28, 1993.
31. Lazarus MD, Sidles JA, Harryman DT II, , et al: Effect of a chondral-labral defect on glenoid concavity and glenohumeral stability: a cadaveric model, *J Bone Joint Surg Am* 78:94–102, 1996.
32. Ackland DC, Pandy MG: Lines of action and stabilizing potential of the shoulder musculature, *J Anat* 215 (2):184–197, 2009.
33. Gibb TD, Sideles JA, Harryman DT, et al: The effect of the capsular venting on glenohumeral laxity, *Clin Orthop Relat Res* 268:120–127, 1991.
34. Cain PR, Mutschler TA, Fu FH, et al: Anterior instability of the glenohumeral joint: a dynamic model, *Am J Sports Med* 271:249–257, 1987.
35. Nichols TR: A biomechanical perspective on spinal mechanisms of coordinated muscular action: an architecture principle, *Acta Anat* 151:1–13, 1994.
36. Kido T, Itoi E, Lee S, et al: Dynamic stabilizing function of the deltoid muscle in shoulders with anterior instability, *Am J Sports Med* 21(3):399–403, 2003.
37. Snyder S, Karzel R, Del Pizzo W, et al: SLAP lesions of the shoulder, *Arthroscopy* 6:274–279, 1990.
38. Burkhart SS, Morgan CD: The peel-back mechanism: its role in producing and extending posterior type II SLAP lesions and its effect on repair rehabilitation, *Arthroscopy* 14:637–640, 1998.

39. Kim SH, Ha KI, Ahn JH, et al: Biceps load test II: a clinical test for SLAP lesions of the shoulder, *Arthroscopy* 17:160–164, 2001.
40. Pagnani MJ, Deng XH, Warren RF: Effect of lesions of the superior portion of the glenoid labrum on glenohumeral translation, *J Bone Joint Surg Am* 77:1003–1010, 1995.
41. Walch G, Boileau J, Noel E, et al: Impingement of the deep surface of the supraspinatus tendon on the posterior superior glenoid rim: an arthroscopic study, *J Shoulder Elbow Surg* 1:238–243, 1992.
42. Morgan C, Burkhart S, Palmeri M, et al: Type II SLAP lesions: three subtypes and their relationships to superior instability and rotator cuff tears, *Arthroscopy* 14:553–565, 1998.
43. Burkhart S, Morgan C: The disabled throwing shoulder: spectrum of pathology. Part II. Evaluation and treatment of SLAP lesions in throwers, *Arthroscopy* 19:531–539, 2003.
44. Guidi E, Zuckerman J: Glenoid labral lesions. In Andrews J, Wilk K, editors: *The athlete's shoulder*, New York, 1994, Churchill Livingstone.
45. Higgins L, Warner J: Superior labral lesions: anatomy, pathology, and treatment, *Clin Orthop Relat Res* 390:73–82, 2001.
46. Maffett M, Gartsman G, Moseley B, et al: Superior labrum–biceps tendon complex lesions of the shoulder, *Am J Sports Med* 23:93–98, 1995.
47. Bey M, Elders G, Huston L, et al: The mechanism of creation of superior labrum, anterior, posterior lesions in a dynamic biomechanical model of the shoulder: the role of inferior subluxation, *J Shoulder Elbow Surg* 7:397–401, 1998.
48. Gartsman G, Hammerman S: Superior labrum, anterior and posterior lesions: when and how to treat them, *Clin Sports Med* 19:115–124, 2000.
49. Snyder S, Banas M, Karzel R: An analysis of 140 injuries to the superior glenoid labrum, *J Shoulder Elbow Surg* 4:243–248, 1995.
50. Dodson C, Altchek D: SLAP lesions: an update on recognition and treatment, *J Orthop Sports Phys Ther* 39(2):71–80, 2009.
51. Izumi T, Aoki M, Muraki T, et al: Stretching positions for the posterior capsule of the glenohumeral joint: strain measurement using cadaver specimens, *Am J Sports Med* 36(10):2014–2022, 2008.
52. Cordasco F, Steinmann S, Flatow E, et al: Arthroscopic treatment of glenoid labral tears, *Am J Sports Med* 21:425–430, 1993.
53. Katz LM, Miller H, Richmond JC: Poor outcomes after SLAP repair: descriptive analysis and prognosis, *Arthroscopy* 25 (8):849–855, 2009.
54. Crockett H, Gross L, Wilk K, et al: Osseus adaptation and range of motion at the glenohumeral joint in professional baseball pitchers, *Am J Sports Med* 30:20–26, 2002.
55. Reagan KM, Meister K, Horodyski M: Humeral retroversion and its relationship to glenohumeral rotation in the shoulder of college baseball players, *Am J Sports Med* 30:354–360, 2002.
56. Liu S, Henry M, Nuccion S, et al: Diagnosis of glenoid labral tears, *Am J Sports Med* 24:149–154, 1996.
57. O'Brien S, Pagnani M, Fealy S, et al: The active compression test: a new and effective test for diagnosing labral tears and acromioclavicular joint abnormality, *Am J Sports Med* 26:610–613, 1998.
58. Neer CS III, : Displaced proximal humeral fractures. I. Classification and evaluation, *J Bone Joint Surg Am* 52:1077–1089, 1970.
59. Fitzpatrick M, Powell S, Tibone J, et al: Instructional course 106. The anatomy, pathology, and definite treatment of rotator interval lesions: current concepts, *Arthroscopy* 19(Suppl 1):70–79, 2003.
60. Cole B, Rodeo S, O'Brien S, et al: The anatomy and histology of the rotator interval capsule of the shoulder, *Clin Orthop Relat Res* 390:129–137, 2001.
61. Field L, Warren R, O'Brien S, et al: Isolated closure of rotator interval defects for shoulder instability, *Am J Sports Med* 23:557–563, 1995.
62. Gartsman G, Taverna E, Hammerman S: Arthroscopic rotator interval repair in glenohumeral instability: description of an operative approach, *Arthroscopy* 15:330–332, 1999.
63. Harryman D, Sidles J, Harris S, et al: The role of the rotator interval capsule in passive motion and stability of the shoulder, *J Bone Joint Surg Am* 74:3–66, 1992.
64. O'Brien S, Arnoczky S, Warren R, et al: Developmental anatomy of the glenohumeral joint. In Rockwood C, Matsen F, editors: *The shoulder*, Philadelphia, 1990, Saunders.
65. Provencher M, Saldua NS: The rotator interval of the shoulder: anatomy, biomechanics, and repair techniques, *Oper Tech Orthop* 18:9–22, 2008.
66. Warner JJP, Higgins L, Parsons IM, et al: Diagnosis and treatment of anterosuperior rotator cuff tears, *J Should Elbow Surg* 10:37–46, 2001.
67. Wolf EM, CL Eakin CL: Arthroscopic capsular plication for posterior shoulder instability, *Arthroscopy* 14:153–163, 1998.
68. Browne A, Hoffmeyer P, Tananka S, et al: Glenohumeral elevation studied in three dimensions, *J Bone Joint Surg Br* 72:843–845, 1990.
69. Ekenrode B, Logerstedt D, Sennett B: Rehabilitation and functional outcomes in collegiate wrestlers following a posterior shoulder stabilization procedure, *J Orthop Sports Phys Ther* 39 (7):550–559, 2009.
70. Williams RJ 3rd, Strickland S, Cohen M, et al: Arthroscopic repair for traumatic posterior shoulder instability, *Am J Sports Med* 31:203–209, 2003.
71. Robinson CM, Aderinto J: Recurrent posterior shoulder instability, *J Bone Joint Surg Am* 87:883–892, 2005.
72. Steinmann SP: Posterior shoulder instability, *Arthroscopy* 19 (Suppl 1):102–105, 2003.
73. Kim SH, Ha KI, Park JH, et al: Arthroscopic posterior labral repair and capsular shift for traumatic unidirectional recurrent posterior subluxation of the shoulder, *J Bone Joint Surg Am* 85:1479–1487, 2003.
74. Mair SD, Zarzour RH, Speer KP: Posterior labral injury in contact athletes, *Am J Sports Med* 26:753–758, 1998.
75. Pollock R, Owens J, Flatow E, et al: Operative results of the inferior capsular shift procedure for multidirectional instability of the shoulder, *J Bone Joint Surg Am* 82:919–928, 2000.
76. Kim SH, Park JS, Jeong WK, et al: The Kim test: a novel test for posteroinferior labral lesion of the shoulder: a comparison to the jerk test, *Am J Sports Med* 33:1188–1192, 2005.
77. Pollock RG, Bigliani LU: Recurrent posterior shoulder instability: diagnosis and treatment, *Clin Orthop Relat Res* 291:85–96, 1993.
78. Neer C, Foster C: Inferior capsular shift for involuntary inferior and multidirectional instability of the shoulder: a preliminary report, *J Bone Joint Surg Am* 62:897–908, 1980.
79. Altchek D, Warren R, Skyhar M, et al: T-plasty modification of the Bankart procedure for multidirectional instability of the anterior and inferior types, *J Bone Joint Surg Am* 73:105–112, 1991.
80. Ludewig P, Reynolds J: The association of scapular kinematics and glenohumeral joint pathologies, *J Orthop Sports Phys Ther* 39:90–104, 2009.

81. IIlyes A, Kiss RM: Kinematic and muscle activity characteristics of multidirectional shoulder joint instability during arm elevation, *Knee Surg Sports Traumatol Arthrosc* 14(7):673–685, 2006.
82. Ogstoin JB, Ludewig PM: Differences in 3-dimensional shoulder kinematics between persons with multidirectional instability and asymptomatic controls, *Am J Sports Med* 35 (8):1361–1370, 2007.
83. Ozaki J: Glenohumeral movements of the involuntary inferior and multidirectional instability, *Clin Orthop Relat Res* 238:107–111, 1989.
84. von Eisenhart-Rothe R, Matson FA 3rd, Eckstein F, et al: Pathomechanics in atraumatic shoulder instability: scapular positioning correlates with humeral head centering, *Clin Orthop Relat Res* 433:82–89, 2005.
85. Warner JJ, Micheli LJ, Arslanian LE, et al: Scapulothoracic motion in normal shoulders and shoulders with glenohumeral instability and impingement syndrome: a study using Moire topographic analysis, *Clin Orthop Rel Res* 285:191–199, 1992.
86. Paletta GA Jr, Warner JJ, Warren RF, et al: Shoulder kinematics with two-plane x-ray evaluation in patients with anterior instability or rotator cuff tearing, *J Shoulder Elbow Surg* 6:516–527, 1997.
87. Bagg DS, Forrest WJ: Electromyographic study of the scapular rotators during arm abduction in the scapular plane, *Am J Phys Med* 65:111, 1986.
88. Itoi E, Motzkin NE, Morrey BF, et al: Scapular inclination and inferior instability of the shoulder, *J Shoulder Elbow Surg* 1:131–139, 1992.
89. Cools A, Dewitte V, Lanszweert F, et al: Rehabilitation of scapular muscle balance: which exercises to prescribe? *Am J Sports Med* 35:1744–1751, 2007.
90. De Mey K, Cagnie B, Van De Velde A, et al: Trapezius muscle timing during selected shoulder rehabilitation exercises, *J Orthop Sports Phys Ther* 39(10):743–752, 2009.

CHAPTER

11

Mollie Beyers
and Peter Bonutti

Frozen Shoulder

In this chapter, the term *frozen shoulder* describes the clinical entity in which a person has restricted passive mobility at the glenohumeral (GH) joint that often results in a loss of active range of motion (AROM) and pain. This loss of mobility can impose substantial disability for many patients. The cause of frozen shoulder is poorly understood. Much confusion exists in the medical population concerning terminology because the terms *adhesive capsulitis, capsulitis,* and *periarthritis* of the shoulder are often used synonymously. The purpose of this chapter is to provide a historical review of literature on the painful and stiff shoulder, characterize the clinical entity of frozen shoulder, supply a working definition of frozen shoulder, and provide a description of treatment approaches available for frozen shoulder.

HISTORICAL REVIEW

In 1896, Duplay was credited with the initial descriptions of the painful and restricted shoulder.[1] He termed the clinical entity of frozen shoulder *periarthritis scapulohumerale* and theorized that the pathologic condition occurred in the periarticular structures. The primary ailment was suspected to be located in the subacromial bursa. The recommended treatment approach was manipulation under anesthesia. In 1934, Codman[2] called the same disorder *frozen shoulder syndrome* and related the dysfunction to uncalcified tendinitis. He stated that the condition was "difficult to define, difficult to treat, and difficult to explain from the point of view of pathology."

Nevasier[3] introduced the concept of *adhesive capsulitis* in 1945, when he discovered a tight, thickened capsule that stuck to the humerus. He described an inflammatory reaction that led to adhesions, specifically in the axillary fold and in the attachment of the capsule at the anatomic neck of the humerus. Surgical exploration of 10 shoulders indicated an absence of GH joint synovial fluid and a redundant axillary fold of the capsule.

In 1949, Simmonds[4] speculated about a loss of motion at the GH joint related to degenerative changes and secondary inflammation of the supraspinatus tendon. He hypothesized that this situation resulted from repetitive wear against the acromion and coracohumeral ligament. Many of his patients experienced functional limitation, pain, and restriction in the shoulder for more than 5 years. Therefore, Simmonds concluded that the disease process was not self-limiting.

In 1954, Quigley[5] described a "pattern of pain-free passive motion sharply checked at about 45° of abduction (ABD) and half of the normal range of motion." He called the entity *checkrein shoulder* to describe this condition in a subgroup of individuals who had frozen shoulder but a good prognosis. This subgroup responded well to manipulation under anesthesia and was described "to present with an audible and palpable release" during the procedure.

In 1962, Nevasier[6] described four phases of frozen shoulder through the assistance of arthroscopic study. These stages are defined as follows: stage I, the preadhesive stage, found in patients with little to no restriction of GH motion; stage II, acute adhesive synovitis, characterized by with proliferative synovitis and early adhesiveness; stage III, the maturation stage, in which less synovitis is demonstrated with loss of the axillary fold; and stage IV, the chronic stage, manifesting with fully mature adhesions with notable restriction of ROM. Nevasier discussed a lack of explanation for the disease process and suggested that any condition requiring prolonged immobilization was a causative factor.

Reeves,[7] in a natural history study of frozen shoulder in 49 subjects that was conducted in 1975, reported a direct relationship between the duration of the stiff phase and the duration of the recovery phase. The observed population had an onset of disease at 42 to 63 years. The painful phase ranged from 10 to 36 weeks in length. The stiffness phase lasted from 4 to 12 months. Recovery of ROM ranged from 5 months to 26 months. The reported mean duration of symptom resolution without intervention was 30.1 months. Although Reeves[7] reported no intervention when following the natural history, the patients were instructed to use analgesics during the painful phase, to rest and wear a sling during the stiff phase, and "to exercise their shoulders to regain external rotation (ER) and abduction (ABD) during the recovery phase." This "advice" could have altered the true natural history.

In 1992, Itoi and Tabata,[8] in a study of 91 subjects, reported a positive correlation between ABD and the restriction of the axillary pouch through arthrographic measures. Chi-Yin et al,[9] in 1997, identified a statistically significant correlation between external rotation (ER) ROM and increased joint capacity in a study using arthrography following physical therapy. These investigators identified an increase in joint space in the acute frozen shoulder, but not in patients with chronic cases.

At present, frozen shoulder is a readily recognized clinical grouping of signs and symptoms. Specific descriptions of motion, pathologic condition, treatment, and recovery, however, are difficult to find and interpret.

DEFINITION

The suggested working definition of frozen shoulder is GH joint stiffness resulting from a noncontractile element unless it coexists with a noncontractile lesion. Both active motion and passive motion are painful and restricted. Passive mobility is limited in the capsular pattern, with ER the most limited, followed by ABD and internal rotation (IR). The GH capsular volume is less than 10 mL, and plain radiographic films are normal.

EPIDEMIOLOGY

In the United States, the prevalence of frozen shoulder is 2% to 5% of the population, and the condition is more common among women.[10,11] The affliction also occurs more frequently in the nondominant arm. The condition is most commonly reported between the ages of 40 and 64 years.[7,12-15] The cost of treatment for idiopathic adhesive capsulitis in the United States in the year 2000 was estimated to be $7 billion.[16]

CLINICAL PRESENTATION

Frozen shoulder is a grouping of multiple symptoms. Although not all patients follow the same course, awareness of the typical clinical course of frozen shoulder may be helpful.

Stages

Painful or Freezing Phase

The painful or freezing phase, as described by Reeves,[7] typically lasts 10 to 36 weeks. The patient has spontaneous onset of shoulder pain, which is often severe and disrupts sleep. The patient often rests the arm and notes an abatement of pain but increased stiffness with rest. At the end of the painful phase, the GH capsule volume is greatly reduced.[17]

Stiffening or Frozen Phase

The painful phase is often followed by a stiffening phase. This phase may last 4 to 12 months. The patient has restricted ROM in a characteristic pattern of loss of ER, IR, and ABD.[17]

Thawing Phase

The final phase is described as thawing and is characterized by the gradual recovery of ROM. The thawing phase lasts an average of 5 to 26 months and is reportedly directly related to the length of the painful phase.[17]

PRIMARY FROZEN SHOULDER

Primary frozen shoulder refers to the idiopathic form of a painful, stiff shoulder. The debate continues about the pathogenesis of idiopathic frozen shoulder. Possible causes include immunologic, inflammatory, biochemical, and endocrine alterations.[3,6,18]

Bunker and Anthony,[19] in 1995, reported that only 50 of 935 shoulders evaluated with restriction at the GH joint could be classified as primary frozen shoulder. In these 50 cases, loss of motion occurred from thickening and contracture of the coracohumeral ligament and rotator interval, thus acting as a tight "checkrein," which prevented ER. These investigators also confirmed a histologic similarity between Dupuytren's disease and frozen shoulder.

Also in 1995, Bunker and Esler[20] reported an association between hyperlipidemia, frozen shoulder, and Dupuytren's disease. The incidence of frozen shoulder in the diabetic population is reported to be 10.8%.[21] In 1993, Janda and Hawkins[22] reported a poor outcome in the diabetic population with frozen shoulder following treatment with manipulation under anesthesia.

SECONDARY FROZEN SHOULDER

Secondary frozen shoulder can follow a precipitating event or trauma, which can be identified to explain the loss of motion. Examples of such events leading to frozen shoulder include limitations following surgery, soft tissue trauma, and fracture. The three phases of frozen shoulder[17] may not always be recognizable in the patient with secondary frozen shoulder.

SCIENTIFIC RESEARCH

As with many poorly understood medical conditions, multiple approaches are used in the treatment of frozen shoulder. Historically, research on treatment has included the following: steroid injections, both intra-articular and extracapsular, with and without physical therapy; physical therapy, including certain modalities, AROM, stretching, exercise and mobilization, or a combination thereof; distention arthrography; closed manipulation, with and without steroid injections, and with and without physical therapy; and arthroscopy and open surgical release with physical therapy. The remainder of the chapter focuses on reviewing the scientific literature to date on the use and effectiveness of treatments for frozen shoulder.

Use of Steroid Injections with and without Physical Therapy

Many physicians use steroid injections in the treatment of frozen shoulder. Most often, this treatment approach is used in conjunction with physical therapy or home exercise. Scientific research supporting and refuting this approach is discussed in this section. Table 11-1 is a matrix summary of the research.

Quigley[5] conducted a prospective study on 29 subjects in 1954. Subjects who were classified into the inclusion for "checkrein" shoulder received manipulation, adrenocorticotropic hormone (ACTH), and steroid injections. The average age of the subjects was 50.5 years, with a mean duration of symptoms of 5.5 months before the intervention. Results reported were as follows: 10 subjects were pain free with normal ROM; 13 subjects reported little pain and loss of ROM, or both; and 6 showed no change. Quigley concluded that his definition of checkrein shoulder would delineate inclusion and exclusion criteria for those individuals who could be assigned a good prognosis.

In 1973 and 1974, Lee et al[12,23] performed the first study with a random clinical trial design. The preliminary study in 1973 included 4 groups, with 80 subjects randomly assigned to the groups. Individuals were included if they had periarthritis of the shoulder and pain in the shoulder with limitation of shoulder movement. In 1974, 45 subjects were randomly assigned to groups. Descriptions of treatments for each group are as follows:

- Group 1: active ROM and infrared heat
- Group 2: intra-articular hydrocortisone acetate and active ROM
- Group 3: hydrocortisone acetate to the bicipital groove
- Group 4: analgesics only

Chi-square for differences showed no differences among the groups for age, sex, or duration of symptoms. Physical therapy for groups 1, 2, and 3 was very specific and included a graduated exercise program. This included: (1) free-active exercise for 10 minutes three times a day of the following: assisted ROM,

Table 11-1 Research on Use of Steroid Injection and Physical Therapy for the Frozen Shoulder

Authors, Year, and Sample Size	Purpose	Use of Physical Therapy	Results
Quigley, 1954[5] N = 29	To determine the effectiveness of manipulation and ACTH, hydrocortisone acetate, or cortisone	Heat, exercise program	10 pain free with normal ROM 13 little pain and little loss of ROM or both 6 unimproved
Lee, Haq, and Wright, 1973[12] N = 80	To test the value of physical therapy and local injection of hydrocortisone acetate in periarthritis of the shoulder	Graduated active exercise for groups 1, 2, and 3	Active ROM and infrared Intra-articular hydrocortisone acetate and active ROM Hydrocortisone acetate to bicipital groove Analgesic only Improvement in ROM within first 3 wk; most change occurred with intra-articular hydrocortisone injections with ROM exercises No change in analgesic-only group
Lee, Lee, Haq, et al, Longton Wright 1974[23] N = 45	To test the effect of heat and exercise; intra-articular hydrocortisone and exercise; hydrocortisone to bicipital groove and exercise; analgesic control group on shoulder movement in periarthritis of the shoulder	Graduated active exercise for groups 1, 2, and 3	ROM of other groups improved over analgesics only; no significant change between the groups
Weiss and Ting,1978[24] N = 48	To report the authors' experience with intra-articular steroids and use of shoulder arthrography	None	16 pain free 11 painful No increase in glenohumeral ROM (no manipulation or ROM provided)
Binder, Hazelman, Parr, Roberts, 1986[25] N = 40	To ascertain whether a limited course of oral steroid therapy had any beneficial effects and to determine the treatment favored by local general practitioners	Home pendulum exercises for all	Decreased pain in steroid group; no difference in ROM between groups
Dacre, Beeney, Scott, 1989[26] N = 62	To determine effectiveness of physical therapy, steroid injections, or both	Physical therapy use varied for head for 4–6 wk	All groups showed decrease in pain and ROM increased 10% to 34% at 6 mo; no differences between groups

ACTH, adrenocorticotropic hormone; ROM, range of motion.

ROM-gravity counterbalance, and gravity-resisted ROM; and (2) proprioceptive neuromuscular facilitation (PNF): manual resistance and concentric contractions. The duration of follow-up was 6 weeks. Group 4 had inferior ROM results that led Lee et al to conclude that exercise was the beneficial component of treatment during the 6-week time period. These investigators also reported significant differences in ROM, the greatest change occurring in group 2. They noted the greatest improvement in ROM during the first 3 weeks. Overall, these investigators concluded that any treatment including exercise was superior to analgesics alone and that only 3 weeks of therapy should be prescribed, with physician follow-up to reassess the subject's status.

In a 1978 study performed by Weiss and Ting,[24] the investigators reported the effects of arthrographically assisted intra-articular injections on GH ROM in 48 subjects. These researchers reported success based on "total shoulder movement" rather than on pure GH joint motion. They did not describe the length of treatment, the numbers of injections received, or any statistical data. Outcomes were based on subjective reports of good, fair, or poor relief of pain. Motion was reported as improved or not improved, with no variance given if it was GH or total shoulder girdle movement. Four weeks following treatment, 16 patients reported pain-free shoulders, and 11 patients still had pain. No increase in GH motion was noted following only an injection. These researchers concluded that arthrographically assisted intra-articular injections should be attempted following failure of conservative therapy.

In 1986, Binder et al[25] studied the effects of oral prednisolone in treatment of frozen shoulder and reported a statistically significant decrease in pain, but no change in ROM when compared with nonintervention groups. Both groups performed a home pendulum exercise program.

In 1989 Dacre, Beeney, and Scott[26] found no significant advantage of physical therapy or steroid injection in the treatment of frozen shoulder. However, physical therapy treatment was not consistent among the 62 subjects.

Bal et al in 2008[27] evaluated the impact of intra-articular corticosteroids on home exercise program outcomes in patients with adhesive capsulitis. Eighty patients were randomly assigned; group 1 received intra-articular corticosteroid, group 2 received intra-articular serum physiologic, and both groups underwent a 12-week comprehensive home exercise program. Outcome measures were Shoulder Pain and Disability Index, University of California Los Angeles end-result scores, night pain, and passive ROM. Group 1 achieved better scores, at a statistically significant level, in all outcomes measured, at week 2. However, no significant differences between the groups were noted at week 12. The investigators concluded that intra-articular steroids provide rapid pain relief in the first weeks of an exercise program, and this effect could be useful for patients with predominant pain symptoms.

In 2009, Lorbach et al[28] compared the effectiveness of oral versus intra-articular injections of cortisone in the treatment of idiopathic adhesive capsulitis in a prospective randomized trial of 40 patients. Follow-up was performed at 4, 8, and 12 weeks and at 6 and 12 months. Data consisted of the Constant-Murley (CM) score, the Simple Shoulder Test (SST), and Visual Analog Scales (VAS) for pain, function, and satisfaction. Results showed that both oral and intra-articular steroids led to fast pain relief and improved ROM for treatment of adhesive capsulitis, but intra-articular injections of glucocorticoids showed superior results in objective shoulder scores, ROM, and patient satisfaction compared with a short course of oral corticosteroids.

Use of Physical Therapy

The debate on the effectiveness of physical therapy in treatment of the frozen shoulder continues. The length of physical therapy intervention and the stage at which it may be appropriate have not been identified thus far in the research literature. The research discussed here lacks well-controlled trials and useful outcome measurement tools. Because consistency among the studies does not exist, comparison is difficult. Table 11-2 is a matrix summary of the research.

In 1967, Parsons, Shepard, and Fosdic[29] performed a one-group pretest and post-test on seven subjects and reported the effects of dimethyl sulfoxide (DMSO), which has a vasodilation and anti-inflammatory action, with ultrasound in frozen shoulder. The researchers concluded that further studies on DMSO as an adjunct therapy for the treatment of frozen shoulder were needed. This study was terminated because of the adverse effects of the agent.

In 1976, Hamer and Kirk[30] performed a two-group pretest and post-test prospective study on 32 subjects to compare the effects of ultrasound and ice on outcome in patients with frozen shoulder. The mean age of subjects was 59, and the time between the onset of symptoms and discharge from physical therapy was 17.7 weeks. No demographic differences were reported between the groups at pretest. Both groups received active elevation and ER exercises twice daily for 10 minutes until discharge. Discharge was based on pain relief only, not ROM gains. No significant differences were reported between the groups. The researchers recommended including measurements of the contralateral shoulder for assessment of shoulder ROM gains.

Rizk et al,[14] in 1983, described a new method of therapy. Fifty subjects were assigned to groups. Group A received conventional physical therapy, including certain modalities, Codman's exercises, wall walks, shoulder wheel, pulley, rhythmic stabilization, and manipulation of the GH joint. Group B used transcutaneous electrical nerve stimulation (TENS), pulleys with up to 15 repetitions per exercise, and 2 hours of intermittent traction(15 minutes on and 5 minutes off). The mean age of the subjects was 56 years, and the duration of symptoms ranged from 3 to 8 months before the intervention. Treatment was administered for 8 weeks. The subjects' progress was assessed monthly for 6 months. Both groups performed a home exercise program consisting of Codman's exercises, wall walks, and wand ROM (five repetitions each, three times a day). Group B progressed faster

Table 11-2 Research on Use of Physical Therapy for the Frozen Shoulder

Authors, Year, and Sample Size	Use of Physical Purpose	Therapy	Results
Parsons, Shepard, and Fosdick, 1967[29] N = 7	Preliminary report on 5 mo; experimental study	DMSO with ultrasound	4 "better" 3 no change
Hamer and Kirk, 1976[30] N = 32	To compare the effectiveness of ultrasound and ice on frozen shoulder	Ice group, ultrasound group; all performed active external rotation and elevation exercises	No significant differences
Rizk, Christopher, Pinals, Higgins, and Frix, 1983[14] N = 56	To describe a new method of therapy that has been found to facilitate the recovery of patients with adhesive capsulitis	Group A: exercises and modalities Group B: pulley and traction	B group increased ROM faster first 2 wk
Bulgen, Binder, Hazleman, Dulton, and Roberts, 1984[31] N = 45	To study a carefully defined patient group and assess 3 treatment regimens: intra-articular steroids; mobilization; and ice PNF, and pendulum exercises.	See groups	Minimal differences between groups; injection may benefit pain and ROM in early stages; biggest improvement first 4 wk; after 6 mo decreased pain; no significant difference in ROM
Nicholson, 1985[32] N = 20	To determine the effects of passive mobilization and active exercises on pain and hypomobility in patients with painfully restricted shoulders Experimental group: mobilization and active exercises Control: active extension only	Mobilization, passive ROM, and strengthening; home exercise program	Mean improved over 4 wk, except internal rotation, with increased gains in experimental group
Shaffer, Tibone, and Kerlan, 1992[33] N = 62	To evaluate the long-term objective and subjective results in a carefully selected group of patients who had idiopathic frozen shoulder	Pendulum, modalities, and stretching following manipulation	See text
O'Kane, Jackins, Sidles, Smith, and Matsen, 1999[34] N = 41	To test the hypothesis that a simple home program can improve the self-assessed shoulder function and health status of a group of patients with frozen shoulder	Self-stretch flexion, abduction, external rotation, internal rotation	SF-36 showed almost all pretreatment deficits were reversed
Griggs, Ahn, and Green, 2000[35] N = 75	To evaluate the outcome of patients with idiopathic adhesive capsulitis who were treated with a stretching exercise program	Home exercise program: supine cane flexion, external rotation, internal rotation, pendulum; formal physical therapy	64 satisfactory: SF-36 7 not satisfied: SF-36 5 required manipulation or surgery ROM increased Pain decreased
Vermeulen, Obermann, Burger, Kok, Rozing, and Van der Ende, 2000[36] N = 7	To describe the use of end-range mobilization techniques in the management of patients with adhesive capsulitis	Mobilization	Increased ROM and decreased pain reported
Dogru, Basaran, and Sarpel, 2008[37] N = 49	To assess the effectiveness of therapeutic ultrasound in treatment of adhesive capsulitis	Home exercise program	Improved shoulder ROM: both groups Pain with ROM decreased: both groups SPADI significantly improved: both groups SF-36 improved at 3 mo: both groups

DMSO, dimethylsulfoxide; PNF, proprioceptive neuromuscular facilitation; ROM, range of motion; SF-36, Short Form (36) Health Survey, SPADI, Shoulder Pain and Disability Index.

and to a greater degree than did group A during the first 3 weeks of treatment. Both groups demonstrated the greatest gains in the initial 3 weeks, comparable to the findings of Lee et al.[12,23] Rizk et al[14] concluded that the treatment approach for group B was superior to conventional physical therapy. Random assignment was not used, and no statistical analysis was reported.

Bulgen et al[31] performed random controlled trials in 1984 that compared the following treatment groups: intra-articular steroids, once a week for 3 weeks; mobilization, three times a week for 6 weeks and PNF three times a week for 6 weeks; and pendulum exercises of only 2 to 3 minutes every hour. Forty-two subjects were recruited whose mean age was 55.8 years, with a symptom duration averaging 4.8 months before the intervention. Follow-up was performed weekly for 6 weeks and then monthly for 6 months. Statistical analysis showed no differences among the groups before treatment. Bulgen et al concluded that improvement in ROM was greatest during the initial 4 weeks of treatment and that no difference between groups was found when comparing the stage at which the patient joined the study and the severity of the subject's outcome. A correlation was reported between increasing age and decreasing ROM, except for ER. Final recommendations emphasized the need for well-designed, controlled prospective studies to test the efficacy of commonly used interventions.

In 1985 Nicholson[32] compared the effectiveness of active exercise with joint mobilization in 20 subjects. The mobilization group gained more IR and ABD than did the exercise-only group. The follow-up measurements were taken 4 weeks after initiation of the intervention.

Shaffer, Tibone, and Kerlan[33] evaluated the long-term subjective and objective results in 62 subjects who had shoulder pain and restriction for at least 1 month, ABD less than 100°, and less than 50% ER. The mean age was 52 years, with a mean duration of symptoms of 6 months before the intervention. All the subjects had previously received supervised physical therapy or a home stretching program. Ten patients had received manipulation under anesthesia, and 2 had undergone arthroscopic release. Conclusions from this study are as follows:

- The average total time from onset to resolution was 12 months.
- The average time to return to nearly normal motion (within 10° to 15°) was 6 months.
- Pain was resolved within an average of 6 months.
- Thirty-one percent of subjects had either mild pain or stiffness of the shoulder.
- Thirty-seven percent of subjects demonstrated restricted motion when compared with the control group (unaffected shoulder averages).
- Seven percent interference with function was reported.
- No association was reported between functional limitation and measurable restriction of motion.
- No association was reported between the objective ROM and duration of symptoms with the subjective outcome.

O'Kane et al[34] studied the effects of a home stretching program on self-assessed function. The researchers measured function with the Simple Shoulder Test and the Short Form (36) Health Survey (SF-36). All deficits identified with the SF-36 were reversed after treatment. The duration of follow-up was not reported.

Griggs et al[35] performed a prospective study on 41 subjects using home wand active assistive ROM (AAROM) exercises and pendulum exercises. The mean age of subjects was 56 years. The researchers concluded the SF-36 was not sensitive to the shoulder. No correlation was found between ROM gains and improvement in function.

Vermeulen et al,[36] in a case report of four subjects, observed increased ROM and decreased pain following physical therapy intervention. Physical therapy was provided for a maximum of 3 months. Treatment consisted of end-ROM mobilization techniques, with neither the use of modalities nor instruction in a home exercise program. All patients reported decreased pain and increased ROM. No statistical analysis was reported.

In 2008, Dogru, Basaran, and Sarpel[37] studied the effectiveness of therapeutic ultrasound in the treatment of adhesive capsulitis in a prospective, randomized trial of 49 patients. Each group received superficial heat and exercise, the study group received ultrasound, and the sham group received imitative ultrasound for 2 weeks. Shoulder ROM, pain, and Shoulder Pain and Disability Index were assessed at baseline, at 2 weeks, and at 3 months. Results of this study suggest that ultrasound compared with sham ultrasound gave no relevant benefit in the treatment of adhesive capsulitis.

Use of Physical Therapy with Interscalene Block or Local Anesthesia

The effectiveness of physical therapy mobilization during interscalene brachial plexus block or local anesthesia has been well supported in the literature. Table 11-3 is a matrix summary of the research.

In 1977, Weiser[15] reported on the treatment of frozen shoulder with gliding mobilization using local anesthesia in 100 subjects. Most subjects were 40 to 64 years old. Forty-five subjects had experienced symptoms for less than 3 months, and 55 subjects had experienced symptoms for more than 4 months before the intervention. The inclusion criteria were GH restriction only, ER less than 55°, and flexion less than 110°. Grade IV mobilization in all direction was performed for 5 to 10 minutes. The patients performed wand exercises and were instructed to perform these exercises 6 to 8 times per day for at least 20 minutes. Follow-up was at 2, 4, and 8 weeks. Seventy-eight of 100 subjects were reported to have no pain at their 2-, 4-, and 8-week follow-up visits. Sixty-one of the 78 patients had normal ROM. Seventeen of the 100 patients demonstrated a slight decrease in ROM. No statistical analysis was reported.

In 1995, Melzer et al[38] also studied the effects of manipulation while patients were under general anesthesia to "moderate mobilization." Eighty-nine subjects, 34 to 78 years old, participated. The duration of symptoms was not reported. The average postintervention follow-up for the groups was 1.4 and 1.7 years, respectively. The mobilization group showed an increase in pre-treatment to post-treatment ROM values as follows: ABD 78%, IR 81%, and adduction (ADD) 54%. The manipulation group showed an increase in pretreatment to post-treatment ROM values as follows: ABD 66%, IR 73%, and ADD 62%. No statistical analysis was reported. The researchers concluded that physical therapy with mobilization should be used before manipulation intervention.

Roubal et al[39] performed a similar study of 23 subjects in 1996. These researchers used an interscalene brachial plexus

Table 11-3 Research on Use of Interscalene Block or Local Anesthesia with Physical Therapy Techniques

Authors, Year, and Sample Size	Purpose	Use of Physical Therapy	Results
Weiser, 1997[15] N = 100	To report treatment of frozen shoulder using mobilization under local anesthesia	Cane flexion, abduction, internal rotation with extension and rotation	78 no pain 61 of 78 normal ROM 17 slight decreased ROM
Melzer, Wallny, and Hoffmann, 1995[38] N = 110	To compare moderate mobilization to manipulation in patients with frozen shoulder	Modalities, ROM, mobilization, stretching, isometric strengthening	Physical therapy: increased abduction 78%, internal rotation 81%, adduction 54% Mobilization under narcosis: increased abduction 66%, internal rotation 73%, adduction 62%
Roubal, Dobritt, and Placzek, 1996[39] N = 23	To develop and describe an alternative method that uses glide manipulation under interscalene brachial plexus block	Supine flexion, daily therapy, home exercise program flexibility	After manipulation: flexion increased 68°, abduction increased 77°, external rotation increased 49°, internal rotation increased 45°, flexion increased 67°, abduction increased 73°, external rotation increased 44°
Placzek, Roubal, Freeman, Kulig, Nasser, and Pagett, 1998[40] N = 31	To evaluate the long-term effects of glenohumeral joint transitional gliding, manipulation, ROM, pain, and function in patients with adhesive capsulitis	Not described	ROM increased significantly Pain decreased significantly

ROM, range of motion.

block and linear transitional gliding manipulation. Eight subjects demonstrated increased ROM when pretest and post-test measures of ROM were compared. No statistical analysis was performed.

In 1998, Placzek et al[40] performed a study similar to that of Roubal et al[39] that used linear transitional gliding manipulation on 31 subjects. The researchers reported a statistically significant improvement in ROM, pain reduction, and improved functional status at 5.3 to 14.4 weeks after the intervention. Placzek et al concluded that translational manipulation was more effective than traditional angular techniques used in manipulation. This conclusion was drawn because of increased accessory humeral head movement associated with translational techniques.

Use of Distention Arthrography

The use of distention arthrography, with or without the use of physical therapy, is addressed in scientific research. This slightly invasive technique has been attempted with local and general anesthesia. Table 11-4 is a matrix summary of scientific research.

Older et al[41] reported their experiences using distention arthrography on six subjects. Radiopaque contrast fluid was manually injected until the capsule ruptured by visualization on an arthrogram. The researchers reported full ROM at a 2.5-year follow-up and contributed this success to their treatment. ROM was reported as "full." However, all patients performed "exercises," and no attempt was made to control physical therapy between the intervention and the follow-up. The researchers did not perform a statistical analysis.

Arthrographic treatment progressed further when, in 1983, Loyd and Loyd[42] studied the effect of local anesthesia, arthrographic distention, and gentle manipulation in 31 subjects. The mean age of these subjects was 54 years, with a mean duration of 6 months for symptoms before arthrography. Subjects were included in the study if their capsular volume was less than 10 mL. Twenty-five subjects reported unrestricted function, whereas 9 subjects reported continued restrictions described as "slight weakness." No statistical analysis was reported. Loyd and Loyd reported the following advantages for use of their technique: increased diagnostic accuracy, arthrographically guided intra-articular injection, no morbidity, and better pain relief than with physical therapy and analgesics only. The researchers stated that 31 of the 33 subjects reported that the intervention had been beneficial and had provided excellent relief. No reliability or validity studies were discussed in regard to the outcome measurement tool.

Fareed and Gallivan,[43] in 1989, documented their results of hydraulic distention using under local anesthesia and AROM. No manipulation was performed. The mean age of the 20 subjects was 56 years. Subjects included in the study demonstrated exquisite pain on passive ER, IR, ABD, and night pain. An immediate increase in ROM to normal function was reported in 90% of the subjects. A 10° to 15° loss was reported at 2 weeks, which then increased to normal when receiving more than one intervention before the 4-week follow-up. Long-term follow up at 6 months and 10 years showed the same results. Statistical analysis was not reported.

Similar treatment intervention and results were reported by Ekeland and Rydell,[44] in a study in 1992. Follow-up in

Table 11-4 Research on Use of Distention Arthrography

Authors, Year, and Sample Size	Purpose	Use of Physical Therapy	Results
Older MWJ, McIntyre JL, Lloyd GJ 1976 N = 6	To report the researchers' experience with distention arthrography as a treatment of frozen shoulder	None	Reported full ROM 2.5 years after intervention; greatest change reported with abduction
Lloyd JA, Lloyd HM 1983 N = 31	To describe the efficacy of arthrographic diagnosis and treatment of the frozen shoulder	None	25 subjects reported unrestricted function, 9 subjects reported continued restrictions and weakness
Fareed DO, Gallivan WR 1989 N = 20	To document the effectiveness of hydraulic distention as a modality of treatment for frozen shoulder syndrome; no manipulation	Active external rotation, pendulum, resistive flexion and extension internal rotation and external rotation	90% return of function and ROM after first treatment 95%–100% function and ROM at 4 wk
Ekelund AL, Rydell N 1992 N = 22	To determine the effectiveness of distention arthrography and local anesthesia and steroids and manipulation	Flexion and abduction External rotation and internal rotation	All improved slightly or no pain
Van Royen and Pavlov, 1996[45] N = 40	To report the effectiveness of distention and manipulation under local anesthesia in treatment of the frozen shoulder	None	ROM increased 72%–95% Pain absent in 15
Buchbinder, Youd, Green, Stein, Forbes, Harris, Bennell, Bell, and Wright, 2007[47] N = 144	To evaluate value of active physical therapy program following arthrographic joint distention in adhesive capsulitis	Passive and active stretching, cervical and thoracic spine mob, GH joint mobilization, rotator cuff and scapular muscle strengthening	Physical therapy group sustained greater active shoulder ROM and perceived satisfaction at 6 mo

GH, glenohumeral; ROM, range of motion.

this study was 4 years. No attempt was made to control activity between the intervention and the follow-up. No statistical analysis was reported.

In a similar study in 1996, Van Royen and Pavlov[45] reported similar effects with a 72% to 95% increase in ROM with a reduction in pain. No statistical analysis was performed.

Buchbinder et al,[46] in a randomized placebo-controlled trial in 2004, studied the value of arthrographic distention with normal saline and corticosteroid in patients in the stiffening phase.. At 3 and 6 weeks, a significantly greater improvement in pain, function, and active ROM was reported in the group that received distention, but this result was not sustained at 12 weeks.

In 2007, these same investigators[47] performed a randomized placebo-controlled, blinded trial to determine whether an active physical therapy program following arthrographic joint distention augments the procedure's benefits. Study subjects received manual therapy and directed exercise twice per week for 2 weeks then once weekly for 4 weeks. The 144 of 156 subjects who completed the study were measured for pain, function, ROM, participant-perceived success, and quality of life at baseline and at 6, 12, and 26 weeks. Physical therapy following joint distention provided no additional benefits in terms of pain, function, or quality of life, but it resulted in sustained greater shoulder AROM and participant-perceived improvement for up to 6 months.

Quraishi et al,[48] in 2007, evaluated the outcome of therapeutic hydrodilatation compared with manipulation under anesthesia in a randomized prospective trial of 36 patients with stage II adhesive capsulitis. Visual Analog Scale and Constant scores in the hydrodilatation group were significantly better than in the manipulation group over the 6-month period of follow-up. ROM improved in all patients over the 6-month follow-up period, but the difference between the groups was not significant. At final follow-up, 94% of patients were satisfied or very satisfied with hydrodilatation treatment compared with 81% of those receiving manipulation.

Use of Closed Manipulation, Arthroscopic Release, or Open Release

Closed manipulation, arthroscopic release, or open capsular release may be attempted on failure of conservative treatment. Physical therapy is prescribed most often following the intervention. Scientific research concerning these more aggressive procedures is summarized in Table 11-5, which is a matrix summary of scientific research.

In 1988, Hill and Bogumill[49] compared manipulation under general anesthesia with the natural history of frozen shoulder. Fifteen subjects were retrospectively analyzed from August 1981 to November 1984. The mean age of the subjects was 51 years, and the mean duration of symptoms was 5.4 months.

Table 11-5 Research on Closed Manipulation and Arthroscopic or Open Release in Treatment of the Frozen Shoulder

Authors, Year, and Sample Size	Purpose	Use of Physical Therapy	Results
Hill and Bogumill, 1988[49] N = 15	To report the effects of manipulation and whether patients with this treatment regain full ROM sooner than by natural recovery	Active ROM	Significant difference in pretreatment to post-treatment ROM, but not post-treatment to discontinued treatment ROM, biggest change initially
Kivimaki and Pohjolainen, 2001[11] N = 24	To study the effects of manipulation with and without steroid injection	None	No enhancement with injection
Pollock, Duralde, Flatow, and Bigliani, 1994[50] N = 30	To determine the effectiveness of arthroscopy and manipulation under anesthesia	Immediate ROM while block active	50% unlimited function 33% satisfactory function 17% limited function
Segmüller, Taylor, Hogan, Saies, and Hayes, 1995[51] N = 24	To determine the effectiveness of inferior capsular release on frozen shoulder	In recovery	88% satisfied 76% return to normal or nearly normal function
Ogilvie-Harris, Bigop, Fitsiabolis, and Mackay, 1995[52] N = 40	To compare the effectiveness of manipulation versus anterior structure division in frozen shoulder pain, ROM, and function; 20 each group, not random groups: (1) manipulation with scope before and after and (2) divided contracted structures	Home exercise program and active assistive ROM; physical therapy within first wk	Manipulation group: pain: 8 none, 8 mild, 2 moderate ROM: abduction 11 normal, external rotation 10 normal Division group: pain: 16 none, 4 mild ROM: abduction 17 normal, external rotation 16 normal
Warner, Allen, Marks, and Wong, 1996[53] N = 23	To describe the results of arthroscopic release	Physical therapy first day and passive ROM; active assistive ROM; home exercise program	Flexion increase mean 49° External rotation at 0° increase mean 42° External rotation at 90° mean increase 53° Internal rotation increase 8 spinous process levels ROM increases not significant when compared with contralateral normal shoulder
Warner, Allen, Marks, and Wong, 1997[54] N = 18	To describe the authors' experience with arthroscopic release of the anterior shoulder capsule in treatment of postoperative stiffness	Physical therapy daily for ROM and strengthening	ROM mean significant increase Flexion increase 51° External rotation increase 31/40° Internal rotation increase 6 spinous process levels
Watson, Dulziel, and Story, 2000[55] N = 73	To determine the effectiveness of arthroscopic capsulotomy in treatment of frozen shoulder	Graduated	Significant decrease in pain Significant increase in ROM 5.5 wk
Gerber, Espinosa, and Perren, 2001[56] N = 45	To study the outcome of arthroscopic capsulotomy for treatment of shoulder stiffness after failure of conservative treatment and to determine whether different causes have a different prognosis	Passive ROM with block 2–4 days	Best results idiopathic, poorest result post-traumatic Functional 26% increase (68% of normal shoulder) statistically significant
Omari and Bunker, 2001[57] N = 75	To describe the effectiveness of surgical release of frozen shoulder in shoulders with severe disease that fail to release with manipulation under anesthesia	Formal physical therapy home exercise program for ROM	Flexion increased 97° External rotation increased 8° Internal rotation with extension increased from sacrum to T7
Wang, Huang, Hung, Ma, Wu, and Chen, 2007[58] N = 47	To compare short-term and long-term results of manipulation under anesthesia among primary, postinjury, and postsurgical frozen shoulders	Postoperative active and passive exercises with PT	Constant score 69.4 at 12 mo Less improvement overall in postoperative group compared with other two groups

PT, physical therapist; ROM, range of motion.

Physical therapy intervention averaged 2.2 months, and the mean follow-up was 22 months after manipulation. The study included patients who had not responded to "adequate" physical therapy. Significant pretreatment to post-treatment differences were found in ROM immediately following the manipulation. No change, however, was found after manipulation to the time of discharge. Flexion was found to increase significantly from before treatment to after treatment, but a decrease in ROM occurred from after treatment to discharge. No significant pretreatment to post-treatment differences were found in IR or ER. The researchers reported that 10% of the subjects returned to work between 2 and 6 months following manipulation, a shorter period than the reported natural history of the condition. The researchers did not report what "natural history" values they used to make their comparisons.

Kivimaki and Pohjolainen[11] performed a random clinical trial in 2001. Twenty-four subjects were randomly exposed to manipulation under anesthesia with or without steroid injection. No enhancement was found with steroid injection. Twenty-two of the 23 subjects demonstrated improved mobility. Pain was decreased in all but 3 subjects. The mean follow-up period was 4 months.

Pollock et al,[50] in 1994, used arthroscopy and manipulation under anesthesia for the resistant frozen shoulder. The mean age of the 30 subjects was 49 years, with an average symptom duration of 14 months before the intervention. The subjects received arthroscopic guided manipulation, débridement, and decompression. The subjects received physical therapy for ROM immediately following the procedure. The surgical procedures were individualized for each subject. At follow-up, the results were as follows: 50% of subjects reported unlimited function (flexion 170, ER 50, IR T10), 33% reported satisfactory function (flexion 160, ER 40, IR L1, slight pain), and 17% of subjects reported limited function (flexion less than 140°, moderate to severe pain). No statistical analysis was reported.

Segmüller et al[51] studied the effect of inferior capsular release without manipulation on 24 subjects with frozen shoulder. The mean age of the subjects was 50 years, and the mean follow-up was 13.5 months following intervention. Subjects were included in this study if no progress had been reported or if ROM had been lost during a 6-week period of physical therapy. Patients who had already undergone surgical procedures on the same shoulder were excluded from the study. Excellent results on the Constant-Murley shoulder tests were obtained following the procedure, with an average score of 87%. Eighty-eight percent of the subjects were satisfied, and 76% had a return to normal or nearly normal function.

Ogilvie-Harris et al[52] looked at the effectiveness of manipulation versus arthroscopic anterior structure division in frozen shoulder. Subjects were included if they had previously received physical therapy and cortisone injection or distention arthrography and continued to have difficulty for more than 1 year following intervention. Forty subjects, divided into two equivalent groups, were studied. One group received manipulation with arthroscopy before and after the procedure, whereas the other group underwent arthroscopic release of contracted anterior structures. All subjects performed hourly AAROM physical therapy and had 6 weeks of outpatient physical therapy. No differences were reported between the groups for ROM. Significant differences were reported for improved function in the group undergoing anterior structure division. Follow-up was reported in a range of 2 to 5 years. The researchers theorized that a significant difference in ROM between the groups would be found using a larger sample size, thus increasing the impact of the study.

In 1996, Warner et al[53] described similar increases in ROM in 23 subjects. The mean age of the subjects was 48 years, and the mean duration of symptoms was 48 months. Subjects included in the study had undergone conservative treatment and closed manipulation that had failed. Following arthroscopic release of chronic refractory frozen shoulder, increases were reported in both function and ROM. In a similar study in 1997, Warner et al[54] reported similar results using arthroscopic release in secondary frozen shoulder following rotator cuff tear repair.

Watson et al[55] performed arthroscopic capsulotomy on 73 subjects with a mean age of 52 years. The average duration of symptoms was 19.7 months before the intervention. Physical therapy intervention consisted of pendulum exercises, stretching, and AROM on days 1 through 4. Modalities and massage were initiated on day 10. Mobilization and isometrics were initiated at 2 weeks, and isotonic strengthening was begun at 4 weeks. Follow-up was reported on average 8.9 weeks following the intervention. Increased ROM and decreased pain were reported at 5.5 weeks. No statistical analysis was reported.

Gerber et al[56] compared arthroscopic outcomes for three groups of patients with frozen shoulder: idiopathic, postsurgical, and post-traumatic. The mean age of the 45 subjects was 50.8 years. The average follow-up occurred 26 months after the intervention. The researchers concluded that those patients with idiopathic frozen shoulder responded the best to arthroscopic treatment, with a 26% increase in function. The post-traumatic group demonstrated the worst outcome.

Omari and Bunker[57] reported improvements in pain and ROM following open release in patients in whom closed manipulation had failed to provide release. Seventy-five subjects, with a mean age of 52.6 years, were followed for an average of 19.52 months. These subjects demonstrated a mean increase in flexion of 97°, in ER of 8°, and in IR by 10 spinous process levels. Formal physical therapy was prescribed but not controlled. A significant increase in function was also reported. No statistical analysis was provided.

In 2007, Wang et al[58] compared the short-term and long-term results of manipulation under anesthesia among idiopathic, postinjury, and postsurgical frozen shoulders. Forty-seven cases with 51 frozen shoulders were evaluated retrospectively, by applying an adjusted Constant score. Data were collected at 3-week to 82-month follow-up times. The average adjusted Constant score at 12 months was 69.4. Researchers concluded that manipulation was an effective, simple, and noninvasive procedure for reducing the course of adhesive capsulitis; however, they found less improvement in the postoperative patient population compared with the idiopathic and postinjury groups.

In 2009, Jacobs et al[59] completed a prospective randomized study with a 2-year follow-up that compared the outcome of patients treated either by manipulation under anesthesia or by intra-articular steroid injections with distention. Fifty-three patients with primary adhesive capsulitis were randomized into each group. Outcome measures consisted of the Constant score, a Visual Analog Scale score, and the SF-36 questionnaire. No statistical differences were found between the two groups with regard to all outcome measures. The investigators recommended treatment using steroid injections with distention rather than manipulation under anesthesia because the attendant risks are fewer and the outcomes are equivalent.

Through this review of scientific research, it appears that in the very early stages of frozen shoulder, physical therapy—consisting of AROM exercises and end-ROM linear translation and mobilization techniques, especially using local or interscalene brachial plexus block—is beneficial.[4,42,52-57] Traction using TENS was noted in one case report, with improvements in ROM and pain.[14] Weiss and Ting[24] conducted arthrographically assisted intra-articular injections and reported no benefit on ROM. However, use of intra-articular steroid injections in the first 3 weeks of therapy may be beneficial for pain control.[12,14,23,32,49] Following failure of conservative treatment, distention arthrography—especially with gentle manipulation or mobilization and AROM exercises—led to successful increases in ROM.[21,41-43] Other measures may be needed for pain control.[41]

Closed manipulation of the GH joint has been studied extensively. Much controversy exists over the possible maladies associated with this intervention, such as fracture and nerve injury.[15,29,32,35,36,38,39] Two studies evaluated the effects of steroid injection during manipulation and the usefulness of oral steroids. No enhancement of ROM was reported with either treatment.[5,54] Surgical treatment, both arthroscopic release and open capsular release,[50-57] offered favorable results. However, the sample sizes were small. Researchers who are proponents of surgical release[44,50-57] argue against closed manipulation because of inconsistent results and unpredictable release of capsular structures. Arthroscopic release and open controlled release are favored by many surgeons to prevent the morbidities reported with closed manipulation.

The lack of a working definition of frozen shoulder has led to inconsistencies among inclusion and exclusion criteria used in scientific research. Because most studies reviewed reported no or minimal statistical analysis, comparison is difficult, and the credibility of results is questionable. The sample size in most studies was small, thus decreasing power. All studies reviewed were missing discussions about sources of secondary variance. The outcome measurement tools that were used were not consistent among the studies. Furthermore, the outcome measures used had no reliability or validity studies to support their use. Carefully controlled clinical trials need to be performed to evaluate treatment efficacy of the frozen shoulder further.

TREATMENT OBJECTIVES

The studies demonstrate that various forms of treatment are effective in increasing ROM and in reducing pain in patients with frozen shoulder. Physical therapy should play a major role in the initial treatment of frozen shoulder. After careful assessment and objective evaluation to confirm the diagnosis of frozen shoulder, to determine the current stage of the condition, and to identify any causal factors, physical therapists should be prepared to design an individual treatment program based on their assessment. The physician, in conjunction with the physical therapist, should direct each case if physical therapy is to be used alone or with other medical or surgical treatment.

The treatment objectives during the painful phases are pain control and reduction of inflammation. A combination of medical pharmaceutical management and exercise with certain modalities may help accomplish these objectives. The physical therapist should encourage the patient to use his or her arm as aggressively as the condition allows. A home exercise program should be recommended that promotes ROM in the pain-free range, especially in IR and ER. Promotion of elevation with compensatory scapular motion can increase impingement and inflammation, often causing a loss of GH mobility. The patient should be educated about GH elevation within a range to prevent impingement and compensatory motion. The physical therapist may provide gentle mobilization to promote accessory joint motion.

Heat application may be used to promote soft tissue pliability and pain reduction. Other investigators recommend heating the joint capsule before stretching, in the belief that increased circulation acts as an analgesic.[17] Cryotherapy may also be used before stretching to provide an analgesic effect or following stretching to prevent increased inflammation. This approach may be especially beneficial in the painful phase of frozen shoulder.

During the stiff or frozen and thawing phases, treatment objectives should focus on pain reduction and regaining ROM within a pain-free range. The exercise prescription should include active-assistive, active, and isometric activities. The physical therapist should provide mobilization to attempt to restore joint mobility. End-range linear translation or gliding techniques have been supported in research for treatment efficacy over traditional manipulative techniques.[15,35,39,40] Target-specific mobilization should be performed with prepositioning of the GH joint to address specific structures such as the posterior-inferior capsule or the coracohumeral ligament. The patient's capsular restrictions must be carefully assessed to determine the most effective techniques.

When designing any treatment program, the physical therapist should consider patient alignment and movement impairments so that optimal biomechanics can be achieved around the joint. Sahrmann[60] categorized key tests and signs that may assist the physical therapist in evaluation and treatment of frozen shoulder.

Movement impairments, which are especially helpful to identify to optimize the proper biomechanics of the shoulder, are categorized as follows:

1. Loss of both passive and active ROM in all directions, most commonly in the capsular pattern
2. Pain increases toward the limitations of motion
3. Excessive humeral superior glide during shoulder ABD and flexion
4. Decreased GH crease just distal to the acromion with the arm overhead
5. Compensatory movement: excessive scapular motion
6. Impairments of muscle recruitment: dominance of the deltoid over the rotator cuff; dominance of the upper trapezius over the lower trapezius
7. Impairments in muscle strength: weakened rotator cuff

OTHER TREATMENT

The patient is often required to perform a home stretching program to increase GH joint motion. Joint Active Systems (JAS, Effingham, Ill) provides an orthosis that is patient applied and directed for stretching of the shoulder; it is used as an adjunct to traditional physical therapy.[61] The system of stretching is based on the principles of stress-relaxation (Fig. 11-1) and static progressive stretching (Fig. 11-2), and it provides an ER or IR stretch from a range of neutral to 120° of ABD in the scapular plane. Impingement often associated with stretching into elevation can be avoided by using this orthosis. The recommended treatment protocol, based on published research showing permanent motion gains with use, consists of 30-minute sessions up to three times per day as tolerated.[61]

Donatelli et al,[62] following a pretreatment, post-treatment randomized prospective trial of 30 subjects, reported an increase of 1° of elevation for every degree gained in ER. Both groups received physical therapy, whereas group I performed a home exercise program in three planes of motion, and group II used the JAS shoulder orthosis twice a day for 30 minutes in ER only. Group II demonstrated twice the gain of ROM in ER and elevation compared with group I. The researchers also reported greater patient compliance (100%) and attributed this to the short wearing time requirement. The researchers concluded that the JAS shoulder orthosis is a useful adjunct at home for treatment of frozen shoulder (Fig. 11-3). Several studies using JAS static progressive stretch (SPS) orthoses have been published since the report by Donatelli et al; these studies demonstrated significant gains in ROM and functional outcomes with the use of SPS orthoses for patients with persistent joint stiffness for elbow, knee, wrist, and forearm joints.[17,63-67] All studies used the recommended 30-minute treatment protocol, which led to excellent compliance and statistically significant ROM gains compared with standard home exercise or use of alternative ROM orthoses such as dynamic splints.

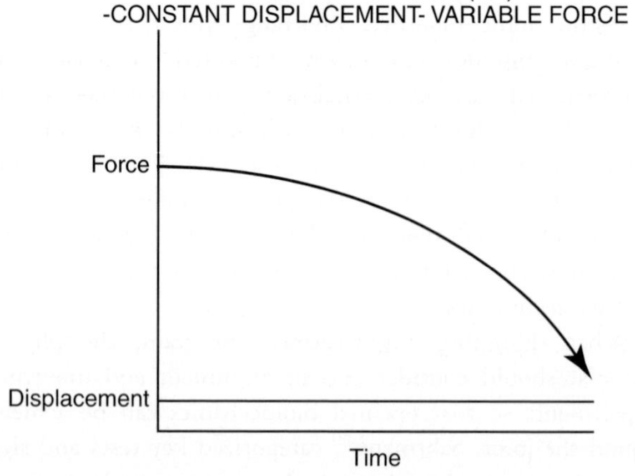

Figure 11-1 Loading conditions.

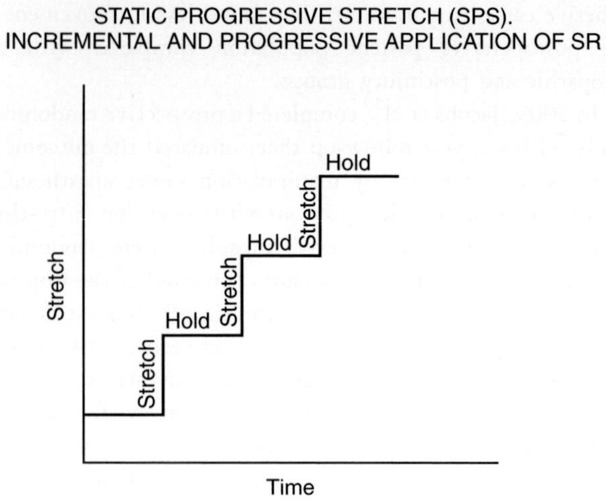

Figure 11-2 Static progressive stretch. Incremental and progressive application of stress relaxation (SR).

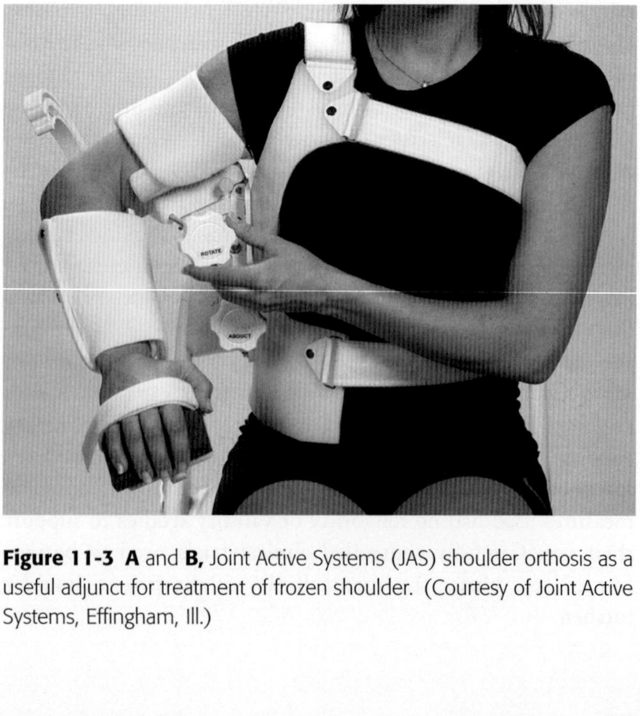

Figure 11-3 **A** and **B,** Joint Active Systems (JAS) shoulder orthosis as a useful adjunct for treatment of frozen shoulder. (Courtesy of Joint Active Systems, Effingham, Ill.)

SUMMARY

This chapter describes the distinct clinical entity of frozen shoulder and the confusion that exists about this condition. Clearly, in the clinical setting, the condition of frozen shoulder can be painful and debilitating to many patients. By understanding a typical presentation of primary frozen shoulder, and the literature supporting various treatment approaches, one can apply this knowledge to make treatment decisions based on evidence. The evidence at present supports varied treatment approaches, which largely depend on the stage at presentation for treatment and the failure of previous treatments. More clinical trials, with a clarified working definition for inclusion and exclusion criteria, will assist in promoting evidence-based practice and treatment of frozen shoulder.

REFERENCES

1. Rizk TE, Pinals RS: Frozen shoulder, *Semin Arthritis Rheum* 2:440, 1982.
2. Codman EA: *The shoulder*, Boston, 1934, Thomas Todd.
3. Nevasier JS: Adhesive capsulitis of the shoulder, *J Bone Joint Surg Br* 27:211–222, 1945.
4. Simmonds FA: Shoulder pain with particular reference to the "frozen" shoulder, *J Bone Joint Surg Br* 31(3):426–432, 1949.
5. Quigley TB: Checkrein shoulder: type of "frozen" shoulder: diagnosis and treatment by manipulation and ACTH or cortisone, *N Engl J Med* 164:4–9, 1954.
6. Nevasier JS: Arthrography of the shoulder joint, *J Bone Joint Surg Br* 44:1321–1330, 1962.
7. Reeves B: The natural history of frozen shoulder syndrome, *Scand J Rheumatol* 4:193–196, 1975.
8. Itoi E, Tabata S: ROM and arthrography in the frozen shoulder, *J Shoulder Elbow Surg* 1:106–112, 1992.
9. Chi-Yin M, Woan-Chwen J, Hui-Cheng C: Frozen shoulder: correlation between the response to physical therapy and follow-up shoulder arthrography, *Arch Phys Med Rehabil* 78:857–859, 1997.
10. Baums MH, Spahn G, Nozaki M, et al: Functional outcome and general health status in patients after arthroscopic release in adhesive capsulitis, *Knee Surg Sports Traumatol Arthrosc* 15(5):638–644, 2007.
11. Kivimaki J, Pohjolainen T: Manipulation under anesthesia for frozen shoulder with and without steroid injection, *Arch Phys Med Rehabil* 82:1188–1190, 2001.
12. Lee M, Haq AM, Wright V: Periarthritis of the shoulder: a controlled trial of physiotherapy, *Physiotherapy* 59(10):312–315, 1973.
13. Murnaghan JP: Frozen shoulder. In Rockwood C, Matsen FA, editors: *The shoulder*, Philadelphia, 1987, Saunders.
14. Rizk TE, Christopher RP, Pinals RS, et al: Adhesive capsulitis: a new approach to its management, *Arch Phys Med Rehabil* 4:29–33, 1983.
15. Weiser H: Painful primary frozen shoulder, mobilization under anesthesia, *Arch Phys Med Rehabil* 58:406–408, 1977.
16. Earley D, Shannon M: The use of occupation-based treatment with a person who has shoulder adhesive capsulitis: a case report, *Am J Occup Ther* 60(4):397–403, 2006.
17. Cyriax J: The shoulder, *Br J Hosp Med* 13:185–192, 1975.
18. Hazleman BL: The painful stiff shoulder, *Rheumatol Rehabil* 11:413–421, 1972.
19. Bunker TD, Anthony AA: The pathology of frozen shoulder syndrome, *J Bone Joint Surg Br* 77:677–683, 1995.
20. Bunker TD, Esler CN: Frozen shoulder and lipids, *J Bone Joint Surg Br* 77:684–686, 1995.
21. Bridgeman JF: Periarthritis of the shoulder and diabetes mellitus, *Am Rheum Dis* 31:69–71, 1972.
22. Janda DH, Hawkins R: Shoulder manipulation in patients with adhesive capsulitis and diabetes mellitus: a clinical note, *J Shoulder Elbow Surg* 2:36–38, 1993.
23. Lee PN, Lee AM, Haq AM, et al: Periarthritis of the shoulder: trial of treatments investigated by multivariate analysis, *Ann Rheum Dis* 33:116–119, 1974.
24. Weiss JJ, Ting M: Arthrography assisted intra-articular injection of steroids in treatment of adhesive capsulitis, *Arch Phys Med Rehabil* 59(6):285–287, 1978.
25. Binder A, Hazelman BL, Parr G, et al: A controlled study of oral prednisolone in frozen shoulder, *Br J Rheumatol* 25:288–292, 1986.
26. Dacre JE, Beeney N, Scott DL: Injections and physiotherapy for the painful stiff shoulder, *Ann Rheum Dis* 48:322–325, 1989.
27. Bal A, Eksioglu E, Gulec B, et al: Effectiveness of corticosteroid injection in adhesive capsulitis, *Clin Rehabil* 22(6):503–512, 2008.
28. Lorbach O, Anagnostakos K, Scherf C, et al: Nonoperative management of adhesive capsulitis of the shoulder: oral cortisone application versus intra-articular cortisone injections, *J Shoulder Elbow Surg* 19(2):172–179, 2010.
29. Parsons JL, Shepard WL, Fosdic WH: DMSO as an adjunct to physical therapy in the chronic frozen shoulder, *Ann N Y Acad Sci* 141(1):569–571, 1967.
30. Hamer J, Kirk JA: Physiotherapy and the frozen shoulder: a comparative trial of ice and US therapy, *N Z Med J* 83:191–192, 1976.
31. Bulgen DY, Binder AI, Hazleman DL, et al: Frozen shoulder: prospective study with an evaluation of three treatment regimens, *Ann Rheum Dis* 43:353–360, 1984.
32. Nicholson GG: The effects of passive joint mobilization on pain and hypomobility associated with adhesive capsulitis of the shoulder, *J Orthop Sports Phys Ther* 6:238–246, 1985.
33. Shaffer B, Tibone JE, Kerlan RK: Frozen shoulder: a long-term follow-up, *J Bone Joint Surg Am* 74(5):738–746, 1992.
34. O'Kane JW, Jackins S, Sidles JA, et al: Simple home program for frozen shoulder to improve patient's assessment of shoulder function and health status, *J Am Board Fam Pract* 22 (4):270–277, 1999.
35. Griggs SM, Ahn A, Green A: Idiopathic adhesive capsulitis: a prospective functional outcome study of non-operative treatment, *J Bone Joint Surg Am* 82(10):1398–1407, 2000.
36. Vermeulen HM, Obermann WR, Burger BJ, et al: End range mobilization techniques in adhesive capsulitis of the shoulder joint: a multiple subject case report, *Phys Ther* 80(12):1204–1213, 2000.
37. Dogru H, Basaran S, Sarpel T: Effectiveness of therapeutic ultrasound in adhesive capsulitis, *Joint Bone Spine* 75(4):445–450, 2008.
38. Melzer C, Wallny T, Writh CJ, et al: Frozen shoulder: treatment and results, *Arch Orthop Trauma Surg* 114:87–91, 1995.
39. Roubal PJ, Dobritt D, Placzek JD: Glenohumeral gliding manipulation following interscalene brachial plexus block in patients with adhesive capsulitis, *J Orthop Sports Phys Ther* 24(2):66–77, 1996.
40. Placzek JD, Roubal PJ, Freeman I, et al: Long-term effectiveness of transitional manipulation for adhesive capsulitis, *Clin Orthop Relat Res* 356:181–191, 1998.

41. Older MWJ, McIntyre JL, Lloyd GJ: Distension arthrography of the shoulder joint, *Can J Surg* 19:203–207, 1976.
42. Loyd JA, Loyd HM: Adhesive capsulitis of the shoulder: arthrographic diagnosis and treatment, *South Med J* 77(7):879–883, 1983.
43. Fareed DO, Gallivan WR: Office management of frozen shoulder syndrome: treatment with hydraulic distension under local anesthesia, *Clin Orthop Relat Res* 242:177–183, 1989.
44. Ekelund AL, Rydell N: Combination treatment for adhesive capsulitis of the shoulder, *Clin Orthop Relat Res* 282:105–109, 1992.
45. Van Royen BJ, Pavlov PW: Treatment of frozen shoulder by distension and manipulation under local anesthesia, *Int Orthop* 20:207–210, 1996.
46. Buchbinder R, Green S, Forbes A, et al: Arthrographic joint distension with saline and steroid improves function and reduces pain in patients with painful stiff shoulder: results of a randomized, double-blind, placebo controlled trial, *Ann Rheum Dis* 63:302–309, 2004.
47. Buchbinder R, Youd J, Green S, et al: Efficacy and cost-effectiveness of physiotherapy following glenohumeral joint distension for adhesive capsulitis: a randomized trial, *Arthritis Rheum* 57:1027–1037, 2007.
48. Quraishi NA, Johnston P, Bayer J, et al: Thawing the frozen shoulder: a randomized trial comparing manipulation under anesthesia with hydrodilatation, *J Bone Joint Surg Br* 89:1197–1200, 2007.
49. Hill JJ, Bogumill H: Manipulation in the treatment of frozen shoulder, *Orthopaedics* 11(9):1255–1260, 1988.
50. Pollock RG, Duralde XA, Flatow EL, et al: The use of arthroscopy in the treatment of resistant frozen shoulder, *Clin Orthop Relat Res* 304:30–36, 1994.
51. Segmüller HE, Taylor DE, Hogan CS, et al: Arthroscopic treatment of adhesive capsulitis, *J Shoulder Elbow Surg* 4:403–408, 1995.
52. Ogilvie-Harris DJ, Bigop DJ, Fitsiabolis DP, et al: The resistant frozen shoulder: manipulation versus arthroscopic release, *Clin Orthop Relat Res* 319:238–248, 1995.
53. Warner JJP, Allen A, Marks PH, et al: Arthroscopic release for chronic refractory adhesive capsulitis of the shoulder, *J Bone Joint Surg Am* 78(12):1808–1816, 1996.
54. Warner JJP, Allen A, Marks PH, et al: Arthroscopic release of postoperative contracture of the shoulder, *J Bone Joint Surg Am* 79(8):1151–1158, 1997.
55. Watson L, Dulziel R, Story I: Frozen shoulder: a 12-month clinical outcome trial, *J Shoulder Elbow Surg* 9:16–22, 2000.
56. Gerber C, Espinosa N, Perren TG: Arthroscopic treatment of shoulder stiffness, *Clin Orthop Relat Res* 390:119–128, 2001.
57. Omari A, Bunker TD: Open surgical release for frozen shoulder: surgical findings and results of the release, *J Shoulder Elbow Surg* 10:353–357, 2001.
58. Wang J, Huang T, Hung S, et al: Comparison of idiopathic, post-trauma and post-surgery frozen shoulder after manipulation under anaesthesia, *Int Orthop* 31:333–337, 2007.
59. Jacobs LG, Smith MG, Khan SA, et al: Manipulation or intra-articular steroids in the management of adhesive capsulitis of the shoulder? A prospective randomized trial, *J Shoulder Elbow Surg* 18(3):348–353, 2009.
60. Sahrmann S: *Diagnosis and treatment of movement impairment syndromes*, St. Louis, 2002, Mosby.
61. Bonutti PM, Windau JE, Ables BA, et al: Static progressive stretch to reestablish elbow range of motion, *Clin Orthop Relat Res* 303:128–134, 1994.
62. Donatelli R, Wilkes J, Hall W, et al: Frozen shoulder encapsulates therapy challenges, *Biomechanics* 2006.
63. Bonutti P, Marulanda G, McGrath M, et al: Static progressive stretch improves range of motion in arthrofibrosis following total knee arthroplasty, *Knee Surg Sports Traumatol Arthrosc* 18(2):194–199, 2010.
64. Doornberg J, Ring D Jupiter J: Static progressive splinting for post-traumatic elbow stiffness, *J Orthop Trauma* 20 (6):400–404, 2006.
65. Lucado A, Li Z: Static progressive splinting to improve wrist stiffness after distal radius fracture: a prospective, case series study, *Physiother Theory Pract* 25(4):297–309, 2009.
66. McGrath M, Ulrich S, Bonutti P, et al: Static progressive splinting for restoration of rotational motion of the forearm, *J Hand Ther* 22(1):3–9, 2009.
67. Ulrich S, Bonutti P, Seyler T, et al: Restoring range of motion via stress relaxation and static progressive stretch in posttraumatic elbow contractures, *J Shoulder Elbow Surg* 19 (2):196–201, 2010.

CHAPTER 12

Todd S. Ellenbecker

Etiology and Evaluation of Rotator Cuff Pathologic Conditions and Rehabilitation

The integral functions of the rotator cuff musculature, combined with the large multiplanar movement patterns inherent in both activities of daily living and sport activity in the glenohumeral joint, make the rotator cuff vulnerable to injury that commonly requires treatment in both orthopedic and sports physical therapy. The rotator cuff musculature functions to stabilize the glenohumeral joint in four primary ways: (1) by its passive bulk; (2) by developing muscle tension, which compresses the joint surfaces together; (3) by moving the humerus with respect to the glenoid and thus tightening the static stabilizers (capsular-ligamentous restraints); and (4) by limiting the arc of motion of the glenohumeral joint by muscle tension.[1] The rotator cuff muscles are among the primary dynamic stabilizing structures of the glenohumeral joint, and high-intensity concentric and eccentric rotator cuff muscular activity has been reported during simple elevation in the scapular plane,[2] and during the tennis serve[3-5] and throwing motion.[6,7] To understand the rehabilitation process required to restore normal shoulder joint arthrokinematics and pain-free glenohumeral joint function better, the etiology and classification must first be developed for rotator cuff injury.

ETIOLOGY AND CLASSIFICATION OF ROTATOR CUFF INJURY

The etiology of rotator cuff pathologic conditions can be described along a continuum, ranging at one end from overuse microtraumatic tendinosis to macrotraumatic full-thickness rotator cuff tears (Box 12-1). A second continuum of rotator cuff etiology consists of glenohumeral joint instability and primary impingement or compressive disease.[8] The clinical challenge of treating the patient with a rotator cuff injury begins with a specific evaluation and clear understanding of the underlying stability and integrity of not only the components of the glenohumeral joint, but also the entire upper extremity kinetic chain.

Rotator cuff injury can be classified in several ways. One classification method is based on the suspected or proposed pathophysiologic features.[9] For the purpose of this chapter, four classifications of rotator cuff pathologic conditions are discussed: primary compressive disease, secondary compressive disease, tensile disease or injury, and macrotraumatic failure. Additionally, this discussion includes the relatively new concept of undersurface or posterior impingement.

Primary Compressive Disease

Primary compressive disease or impingement is a direct result of compression of the rotator cuff tendons between the humeral head and the overlying anterior third of the acromion, coracoacromial ligament, coracoid, or acromioclavicular joint.[10,11] The physiologic space between the inferior acromion and superior surface of the rotator cuff tendons is termed the *subacromial space.* It has been measured using anterior-posterior radiographs and found to be 7 to 13 mm in size in patients with shoulder pain[12] and 6 to 14 mm in normal shoulders.[13]

Biomechanical analysis of the shoulder has produced theoretical estimates of the compressive forces against the acromion with elevation of the shoulder.[14-16] Poppen and Walker[14] calculated this force at 0.42 times body weight, and Lucas[15] estimated this force at 10.2 times the weight of the arm. Peak forces against the acromion were measured between 85° and 136° of elevation,[16] a position inherent in sport-specific movement patterns[7,17] and commonly used in ergonomic and daily activities. The positions of the shoulder in forward flexion, horizontal adduction, and internal rotation during the acceleration and follow-through phases of the throwing motion are likely to produce subacromial impingement caused by abrasion of the supraspinatus, infraspinatus, or biceps tendon.[7] These data provide scientific rationale for the concept of impingement or compressive disease as a cause of rotator cuff injury.

Neer[10,11] outlined three stages of primary impingement as it relates to rotator cuff injury. Stage I, *edema and hemorrhage,* results from the mechanical irritation of the tendon because of impingement that occurs with overhead activity. This stage is characteristically observed in younger patients who are more athletic and is described as a reversible condition with

BOX 12-1 Etiologic Factors Associated with Rotator Cuff Pathologic Conditions

- Microtrauma
- Tendinosis
- Instability
- Macrotrauma
- Rotator cuff tear
- Compressive disease

conservative physical therapy. The primary symptoms and physical signs of this stage of impingement or compressive disease are similar to those of the other two stages and consist of a positive impingement sign, painful arc of movement, and varying degrees of muscular weakness.[11]

The second stage of compressive disease outlined by Neer is termed *fibrosis and tendinitis*. This stage results from repeated episodes of mechanical inflammation and can include thickening or fibrosis of the subacromial bursae. The typical age range for this stage of injury is 25 to 40 years. Neer's stage III impingement lesion is termed *bone spurs and tendon rupture* and is the result of continued mechanical compression of the rotator cuff tendons. Full-thickness tears of the rotator cuff, partial-thickness tears of the rotator cuff, biceps tendon lesions, and bony alteration of the acromion and acromioclavicular joint may be associated with this stage.[10,11] In addition to bony alterations, which are acquired with repetitive stress to the shoulder, the native shape of the acromion is relevant.

The specific shape of the overlying acromion process, termed *acromial architecture,* has been studied in relation to full-thickness tears of the rotator cuff.[18,19] Bigliani et al[18] described three types of acromions: type I (flat), type II (curved), and type III (hooked). A type III or hooked acromion was found in 70% of cadaveric shoulders with a full-thickness rotator cuff tear, whereas type I acromions were associated with only 3% of cadaveric shoulders.[18] In a series of 200 clinically examined patients, 80% with an abnormal arthrogram had a type III acromion.[19]

Surgical treatment of primary compressive disease generally consists of decompression of 8 mm of the anterior acromion, with preservation of the insertion of the deltoid and beveling of approximately 2 cm posteriorly to provide additional space for the inflamed tendons.[9] Open repairs of associated full-thickness tears of the rotator cuff are routinely performed along with the decompression acromioplasty to address the offending overlying acromion and to repair the full-thickness defect in the rotator cuff. The method of open repair has specific ramifications on postoperative rehabilitation. Specifically, the type of open surgical approach can detach the deltoid origin from the lateral aspect of the clavicle and acromion, a procedure that can be referred to as the *traditional anterior approach,* or the deltoid can be split vertically along the direction of its fibers, a procedure commonly referred to as the *deltoid splitting approach* or *mini-open approach*. The preservation of the deltoid origin used during the deltoid splitting approach is of benefit because rehabilitation can commence sooner with active assistive range of motion (AAROM) and active ROM (AROM) as compared with the traditional deltoid detachment approach. The arthroscopic rotator cuff repair technique further minimizes tissue morbidity and allows access for rotator cuff repair in patients with trauma to the deltoid. This technique is fast becoming the method of choice for nearly all types of rotator cuff repairs as advances in instrumentation and suture anchors continue to develop. The traditional open approach often necessitates 6 to 8 weeks without active or resistive exercise to protect not only the healing rotator cuff, but also the healing deltoid origin, which is reattached following rotator cuff repair. Knowledge of the specific surgical technique used on a patient referred to physical therapy following an open repair of a full-thickness rotator cuff tear is imperative for optimal progression in postoperative rehabilitation.

Secondary Compressive Disease

Impingement or compressive symptoms may be secondary to underlying instability of the glenohumeral joint.[8,9] Attenuation of the static stabilizers of the glenohumeral joint, such as the capsular ligaments and labrum from the excessive demands incurred in throwing or overhead activities, can lead to anterior instability of the glenohumeral joint. Because of the increased humeral head translation, the biceps tendon and rotator cuff can become impinged secondary to the ensuing instability.[8,9] A progressive loss of glenohumeral joint stability is created when the dynamic stabilizing functions of the rotator cuff are diminished from fatigue and tendon injury.[9] The effects of secondary impingement can lead to rotator cuff tears as the instability and impingement continue.[8,9]

Tensile Overload

Another etiologic factor in rotator cuff injury is repetitive intrinsic tension overload. The heavy, repetitive eccentric forces incurred by the posterior rotator cuff musculature during the deceleration and follow-through phases of overhead sport activities can lead to overload failure of the tendon.[9,20] The pathologic changes referred to as "angiofibroblastic hyperplasia" by Nirschl[20] occur in the early stages of tendon injury and can progress to rotator cuff tears from the continued tensile overload.[9]

Research by Kraushaar and Nirschl,[21] in a histologic study of the extensor carpi radialis brevis, the primary tendon involved in lateral humeral epicondylitis, identified specific characteristics inherent in an injured tendon. Based on their histopathologic study, these investigators recommended that the term *tendinosis* be used, rather than tendinitis, to describe tendon injury more accurately. Histopathologic studies of tendons taken from areas of chronic overuse in the human body do not show large numbers of macrophages, lymphocytes, or neutrophils. "Rather, tendonosis [sic] appears to be a degenerative process, which is characterized by the presence of dense populations of fibroblasts, vascular hyperplasia, and disorganized collagen.[21] Kraushaar and Nirshl pointed out that investigators do not know why tendinosis is painful, given the absence of acute inflammatory cells, nor do they know why the collagen fails to mature.

In the biomechanical study of highly skilled pitchers,[7] the tensile stresses incurred by the rotator cuff during the arm deceleration phase of the throwing motion—to resist joint distraction, horizontal adduction, and internal rotation—were reported to be as high as 1090 N. The presence of acquired or congenital capsular laxity and labral insufficiency can greatly increase the tensile stresses to the rotator cuff muscle tendon units.[8,9]

Macrotraumatic Tendon Failure

Unlike the previously mentioned rotator cuff classifications, cases involving macrotraumatic tendon failure usually entail a previous or single traumatic event in the patient's clinical history.[9] Forces encountered during the traumatic event are greater than the normal tendon can tolerate. Full-thickness tears of the rotator cuff, with bony avulsions of the greater tuberosity, can occur from single traumatic episodes. According to Cofield,[22] injuries to normal tendons do not occur easily because 30% or more of the tendon must be damaged to produce a substantial reduction in strength. Although a single traumatic event, which resulted in tendon failure, is often reported by the patient in the subjective examination, repeated microtraumatic insults and degeneration over time may have created a substantially weakened tendon. The tendon ultimately failed under the heavy load described by the patient. Full-thickness rotator cuff tears require surgical treatment and aggressive rehabilitation to achieve a positive functional outcome.[9,11] Further specifics of rotator cuff surgical treatment are discussed later in this chapter.

Posterior or "Undersurface" Impingement

One additional cause for undersurface tear of the rotator cuff in the young athletic shoulder is termed *posterior, inside, or undersurface impingement*.[23,24] This phenomenon was originally observed by Walch et al[24] during shoulder arthroscopy with the shoulder placed in the 90/90 position. Placement of the shoulder in a position of 90° of abduction and 90° of external rotation causes the supraspinatus and infraspinatus tendons to rotate posteriorly. This more posterior orientation of the tendons aligns them such that the undersurfaces of the tendons rub on the posterior-superior glenoid lip and become pinched or compressed between the humeral head and the posterior-superior glenoid rim (Fig. 12-1).[23] Individuals having posterior shoulder pain brought on by positioning of the arm in 90° of abduction and 90° or more of external rotation, typically from overhead positions in sport or industrial situations, may be considered as potential candidates for undersurface impingement.

The presence of anterior translation of the humeral head with maximal external rotation and 90° of abduction, which has been confirmed arthroscopically during the subluxation relocation test, can produce mechanical rubbing and fraying on the undersurface of the rotator cuff tendons. Additional harm can be caused by the posterior deltoid if the rotator cuff is not functioning properly. The posterior deltoid's angle of pull pushes the humeral head against the glenoid and accentuates the skeletal, tendinous, and labral lesions.[23] Walch et al[24] arthroscopically evaluated 17 throwing athletes with shoulder pain during throwing and found undersurface impingement that resulted in 8 partial-thickness rotator cuff tears and 12 lesions in the posterior-superior labrum. Impingement of the undersurface of the rotator cuff on the posterior-superior glenoid labrum may be a cause of painful structural disease in the overhead athlete.

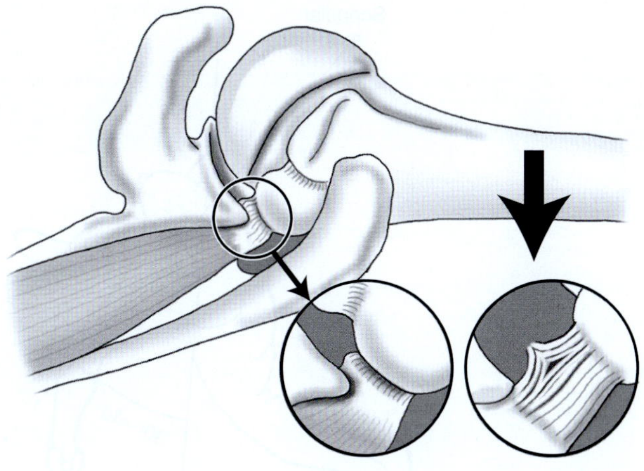

Figure 12-1 Schematic representation of posterior-superior glenoid impingement between the posterior edge of the glenoid and the deep surface of the supraspinatus and infraspinatus tendons. (From Loehr JF, Helmig P, Sojbjerg JO, et al: Shoulder instability caused by rotator cuff lesions: an in vitro study, *Clin Orthop Relat Res* 303:84, 1994.)

Additional research confirming the concept of posterior or undersurface impingement in the overhead athlete has been published.[25,26] By using magnetic resonance imaging (MRI) performed in the position of 90° of abduction and 90° of external rotation, Halbrecht et al[25] confirmed contact of the undersurface of the supraspinatus tendon against the posterior-superior glenoid in baseball pitchers with the arm placed in 90° of external rotation and 90° of abduction. Ten collegiate baseball pitchers were examined, and in all 10 pitchers, physical contact was encountered in this position. Paley et al[26] also published a series on arthroscopic evaluation of the dominant shoulder of 41 professional throwing athletes. With the arthroscope inserted in the glenohumeral joint, these investigators found that 41 of 41 dominant shoulders evaluated had posterior undersurface impingement between the rotator cuff and the posterior-superior glenoid. In these professional throwing athletes, 93% had undersurface fraying of the rotator cuff tendons, and 88% showed fraying of the posterior-superior glenoid.

Mihata et al[27] studied the effect of glenohumeral horizontal abduction during the cocking phase of throwing and its effect on posterior impingement in the abducted shoulder. Their findings confirmed that the articular portion of the supraspinatus

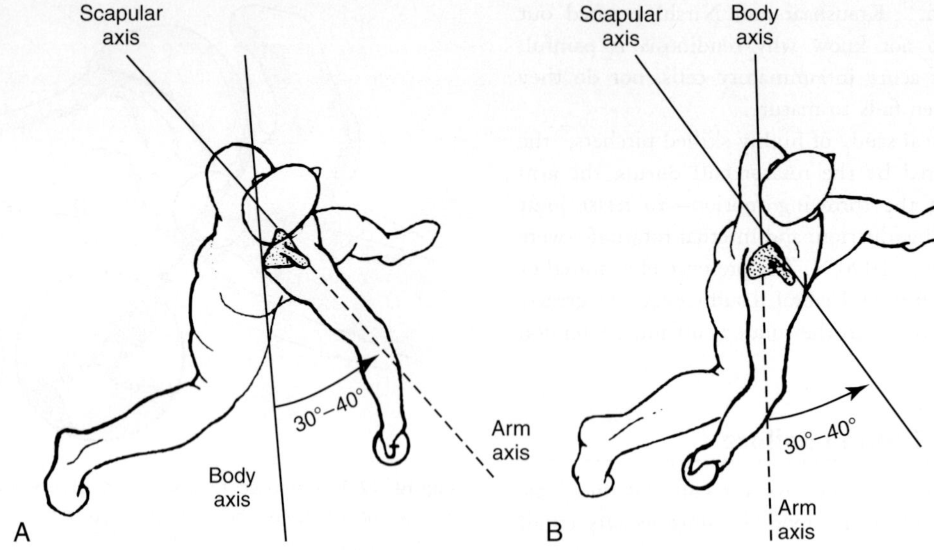

Figure 12-2 Hyperangulation.

and infraspinatus tendons underwent greater contact pressure against the posterior-superior glenoid with 30° and 45° of horizontal abduction as compared with the scapular plane and only 15° of horizontal abduction. This finding has significant clinical ramifications because throwing athletes with shoulder injury may have mechanics that place the shoulder in greater amounts of horizontal abduction (arm-lag or hyperangulation positions) (Fig. 12-2). Close evaluation of the amount of horizontal abduction in the 90° abducted shoulder is a critical aspect of the complete evaluation and rehabilitation of the injured throwing athlete with posterior or undersurface impingement, to minimize the contact pressures occurring at the articular surface of the rotator cuff.

Additional Etiologic Factors in Rotator Cuff Pathologic Conditions

In addition to the etiologic factors already mentioned for rotator cuff pathologic conditions, other factors inherent in the rotator cuff have relevance with respect to injury. The vascularity of the rotator cuff, specifically the supraspinatus, has been extensively studied beginning in 1934 by Codman.[28] In his classic monograph on ruptures of the supraspinatus tendon, Codman described a critical zone of hypovascularity located 0.5 inch proximal to the insertion on the greater tuberosity.[28] This region appeared anemic and infarcted. The biceps long head tendon was found to have a similar region of hypovascularity in its deep surface 2 cm from its insertion.[29] Rathburn and MacNab[30] reported the effects of position on the microvascularity of the rotator cuff. With the glenohumeral joint in a position of adduction, a constant area of hypovascularity was found near the insertion of the supraspinatus tendon. This consistent pattern was not observed with the arm in a position of abduction. These investigators termed this observation the "wringing out phenomenon" and also noticed a similar response in the long head tendon of the biceps. This positional relationship has clinical ramifications for both exercise positioning and immobilization. Brooks et al[31] found no significant difference between the tendinous insertions of the supraspinatus and infraspinatus tendons; both were hypovascular when they were studied by quantitative histologic analysis.

Contradictory research published by Swiontowski et al[32] does not support this region of hypovascularity or critical zone. Blood flow was greatest in the critical zone in living patients with rotator cuff tendinitis from subacromial impingement, as measured by Doppler flowmetry.

ANATOMIC DESCRIPTION OF ROTATOR CUFF TEARS

Several primary types of rotator cuff tears are commonly described in the literature. Full-thickness tears in the rotator cuff consist of tears that comprise the entire thickness (from top to bottom) of the rotator cuff tendon or tendons. Full-thickness tears are often initiated in the critical zone of the supraspinatus tendon and can extend to include the infraspinatus, teres minor, and subscapularis tendons.[33] Often associated with a tear in the subscapularis tendon is subluxation of the biceps long head tendon from the intertubercular groove, or either partial or complete tears of the biceps tendon. Histologically, full-thickness rotator cuff tears show various findings ranging from almost entirely acellular and avascular margins to neovascularization with cellular infiltrate.[33]

The effects of a full-thickness rotator cuff tear on glenohumeral joint stability were studied by Loehr et al.[34] Changes in stability of the glenohumeral joint were assessed by selective division of the supraspinatus or infraspinatus tendons. Findings indicated that a one-tendon lesion of either the supraspinatus or infraspinatus did not influence the movement patterns of the glenohumeral joint, whereas a two-tendon lesion induced notable changes compatible with instability of the glenohumeral joint.[34] Therefore, patients with full-thickness rotator cuff tears may have additional stress and dependence placed on the dynamic stabilizing function of the remaining rotator cuff tendons because of increased humeral head translation and the ensuing instability.

Additional research on full-thickness rotator cuff tears has had notable clinical ramifications. Miller and Savoie[35] examined 100 consecutive patients with full-thickness tears of the rotator cuff to determine the incidence of associated intra-articular injuries. Seventy-four of these 100 patients had one or more coexisting intra-articular abnormalities; anterior labral tears occurred in 62 patients, and biceps tendon tears were noted in 16. The results of this study clearly indicate the importance of a thorough clinical examination of the patient with a rotator cuff injury.

A second type of rotator cuff tear is an incomplete or partial-thickness tear. Partial-thickness tears can occur on the superior surface (bursal side) or undersurface (articular side) of the rotator cuff. Although both bursal and articular side tears are partial-thickness tears of the rotator cuff, notable differences in causes are proposed for each type.[9]

Neer[10,11] and Fukuda et al[36] emphasized that superior surface (bursal side) tears in the rotator cuff are the result of subacromial impingement. In the classification scheme listed earlier in this chapter, tears on the superior or bursal side of the rotator cuff are generally associated with both primary and secondary compressive disease and macrotraumatic tendon failure. The progression of the mechanical irritation on the superior surface can produce a partial-thickness tear, which can ultimately progress to a full-thickness tear.[9-11]

Partial-thickness tears on the undersurface or articular side of the rotator cuff are generally associated with tensile loads and glenohumeral joint instability.[9,37] Tears on the undersurface of the rotator cuff are commonly found in overhead-throwing athletes, in whom anterior instability, capsular and labral insufficiency, and dynamic muscular imbalances are often reported. To understand the differing causes of rotator cuff tears further, Nakajima et al[37] performed a histologic and biomechanical study of the rotator cuff tendons. Biomechanically, their results showed greater deformation and tensile strength of the bursal side of the supraspinatus tendon. The bursal side of the supraspinatus tendon was composed of a group of longitudinal tendon bundles, which could disperse a tensile load and generate greater resistance to elongation than the articular or undersurface of the tendon. These investigators found the articular surface to be composed of a tendon, ligament, and joint capsule complex that elongated poorly and tore more easily.[37] The results of this study further reinforce tensile stresses as the proposed causes of undersurface rotator cuff tears.

One final type or classification of rotator cuff tear is the intratendinous or interstitial rotator cuff tear. This tear develops between the bursal and articular side layers of the degenerated tendon.[38] Shear within the tendon appears to be responsible in the pathogenesis of this rotator cuff tear.

Rotator cuff injury has several underlying etiologic factors, as evidenced by the classification schemes and scientific research in literature. Although it is imperative to understand the common causes and classifications of rotator cuff injury and types of rotator cuff tears, it is of paramount importance that a structured, scientifically based evaluation procedure is used not only to diagnose rotator cuff injury, but also ultimately to identify the cause.

CLINICAL EVALUATION OF THE SHOULDER FOR ROTATOR CUFF INJURY

It is beyond the scope of this chapter to cover a comprehensive evaluation of the shoulder completely. This is provided in Chapter 4. A brief discussion is warranted, however, on the specific aspects of the evaluation process that are of critical importance in identification and delineation of rotator cuff injury. The multiple causes and specific types of rotator cuff ailments are reflected in the types of clinical tests routinely employed.

During the subjective examination, specific questioning—particularly for the overhead athlete—can greatly assist in understanding the probable cause and type of rotator cuff injury. Merely establishing that the patient has pain with overhead throwing or during the tennis serve does not provide the optimal level of information elicited by more specific questioning aimed at identifying the stage or phase of the overhead activity. Specific muscular activity patterns and joint kinetics inherent in each stage of these sports activities can assist in the identification of compressive disease or tensile-type injuries. The presence of instability, however subtle, during the cocking phase of overhead activities can produce impingement or compressive symptoms.[9,23,24] In contrast, a feeling of instability or loss of control during the follow-through phase and during the predominantly eccentric loading, can indicate a tensile rotator cuff injury.[9] Additional questions regarding a change in sport equipment, ergonomic environment, and training history provide information that is imperative in understanding the stresses leading to injury.

Scapular Examination

Objective examination of the patient with rotator cuff injury must include postural testing and observation.[39] Tests are indicated to diagnose scapular posterior displacement in multiple positions (at waist level and at 90° of flexion or greater) with an axial load through the arms. Testing for scapular dyskinesia can be performed using the Kibler scapular slide test in both neutral and 90° elevated positions.[40] A tape measure is used to measure the distance from a thoracic spinous process to the inferior angle of the scapula. A difference of more than 1 to 1.5 cm is considered abnormal and may indicate scapular muscular weakness and poor overall stabilization of the scapulothoracic joint.[40]

Greater understanding of the importance the scapulothoracic joint plays in rotator cuff injury led to the development of a more advanced and detailed classification system of scapular dysfunction. Several movements and translations occur in the scapulothoracic joint during arm elevation. These include scapular upward and downward rotation, internal and external rotation, and anterior and posterior sagittal plane tilting. In addition to those three rotational movements, two translations occur, superior and inferior translation, as well as protraction and retraction.[40] During normal, healthy arm elevation, scapular upward rotation, posterior tilting, and external rotation occur.[40] Although scapular movement and biomechanics are very technical and complex, clinical evaluation of the scapulothoracic joint is an integral part of the complete evaluation of the patient with shoulder dysfunction. Kibler et al[41] outlined three primary scapular dysfunctions. This classification system proposed by Kibler can assist the clinician in evaluating the patient with more subtle forms of scapular malady. Zeier[42] described the massive dissociation of the scapula from the thoracic wall that result from injury to the long thoracic nerve. This severe dissociation has been termed *scapular winging*.[42] However, few patients with a rotator cuff condition clinically display true scapular winging.

To address and define the types of scapular pathologic conditions seen clinically in patients with rotator cuff injury more clearly, Kibler et al[41] developed a classification system for subtle scapular dysfunction. This classification system consists of three primary scapular conditions and is named for the portion of the scapula that is most pronounced or most prominently visible when viewed during the clinical examination. The scapular examination valuation recommended by Kibler et al includes visual inspection of the patient from as follows: the posterior view in resting stance; again in the hands on hips position (hands placed on the hips such that the thumbs are pointing backward on the iliac crests); and during active movement bilaterally in the sagittal, scapular, and frontal planes.[41] These scapular dysfunctions are termed *inferior angle, medial border,* and *superior*.[41]

In the *inferior angle scapular dysfunction,* the patient's inferior border of the scapula is extremely prominent (Fig. 12-3). This configuration results from anterior tipping of the scapula in the sagittal plane. It is most commonly seen in patients with rotator cuff impingement because the anterior tipping of the scapula causes the acromion to be positioned in a more offending position relative to an elevating humerus.[41] The *medial border dysfunction* causes the patient's entire medial border to be posteriorly displaced from the thoracic wall (Fig. 12-4). This condition results from internal rotation of the scapula in the transverse plane and is most often witnessed in patients with glenohumeral joint instability. The internal rotation of the scapula results in an altered position of the glenoid that is commonly referred to as *antetilting,* which allows for an opening up of the anterior half of the glenohumeral articulation.[40] The antetilting of the scapula was shown by Saha[43] to be a component of the subluxation-dislocation complex in patients with microtrauma-induced glenohumeral instability. Finally, *superior scapular dysfunction,* as described by Kibler et al,[41] involves early and excessive superior scapular elevation during arm elevation (Fig. 12-5). This dysfunction typically results from rotator cuff weakness and force couple imbalances.[40]

Kibler et al[41] tested the Kibler scapular classification system using videotaped evaluations of 26 individuals with

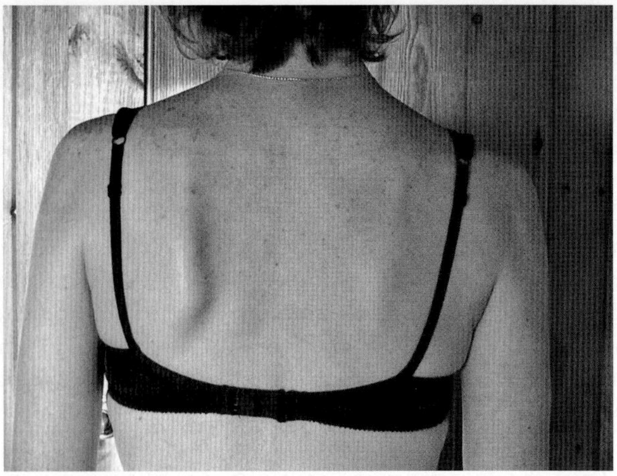

Figure 12-4 Medial border scapular dysfunction.

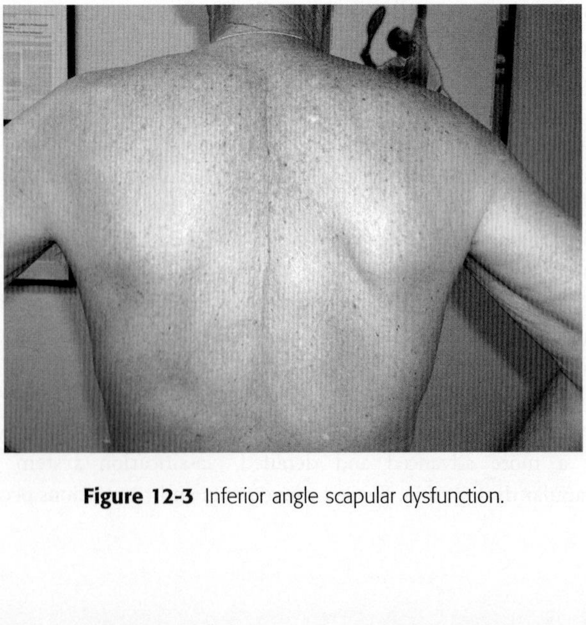

Figure 12-3 Inferior angle scapular dysfunction.

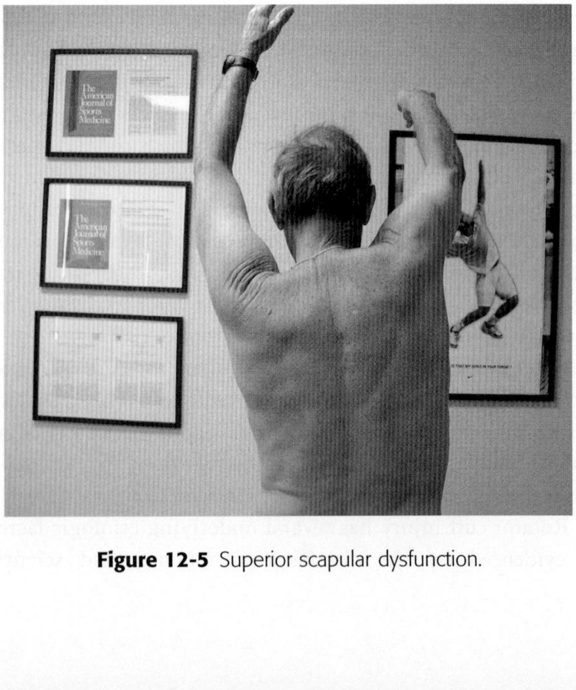

Figure 12-5 Superior scapular dysfunction.

and without scapular dysfunction. Four evaluators, each blinded to the other evaluators' findings, observed individuals and categorized them as having one of the three Kibler scapular dysfunctions or normal scapulohumeral function. Intertester reliability measured using a kappa coefficient was slightly lower (kappa = 0.4) than intrarater reliability (kappa = 0.5). The results of this study support the use of this classification system to categorize subtle scapular dysfunction by careful observation of the patient in static stance positions and during active goal-directed movement patterns.

Additional studies were performed to test the effectiveness of visual observation of scapular movement. McClure et al[44] measured athletes during forward flexion and abduction by using a 3- to 5-lb weight and visual observation of scapular mechanics. These investigators graded the scapular disorder as obvious, subtle, or normal. Multiple examiners viewed the subjects, and reported coefficients of agreement ranged from 75% to 80% among examiners with this method (kappa coefficients, 0.48 to 0.61). Their findings support the visual observation of scapular disease. Further support for this method of clinically applicable scapular evaluation comes from research by Uhl et al.[45] These investigators measured 56 subjects (35 with disorders) during arm elevation in the shoulders in the scapular and sagittal planes. They reported coefficients of agreement of 71% (kappa = 0.40) when grading the scapula as "yes pathology" (Kibler types I, II, or III), as opposed to "no pathology" (Kibler type IV); the coefficient of agreement was 61% (kappa = 0.44) when the four-part Kibler classification was used.[45] Additionally, Uhl et al[45] calculated specificity and sensitivity values by comparing scapular mechanics measured directly with three-dimensional tracking and visual observation. Specificities of 31% to 38% were calculated for the yes/no classification method with 62% to 85% values generated for the four-part Kibler classification method. Sensitivities for the yes/no method were 74% to 78%, whereas sensitivities of 10% to 47% were measured when observers attempted to classify the scapula into one of the four Kibler classes. This research supports the use of the visual observation method for determining scapular disease and highlights the need for further application of basic science research on scapular biomechanics to clinical practice.

Additional clinical tests can be used during the scapular evaluation of the patient with shoulder dysfunction. These include the scapular assistance test (SAT), scapular retraction test (SRT), and the flip sign. Each of these tests helps the clinician to establish the important role scapular stabilization and muscular control play in shoulder function and to highlight the role or involvement of the scapula in shoulder disease.

Kibler[46] described the SAT. This test (Fig. 12-6) involves the assistance of the scapula through the examiner's hands; one hand is applied to the inferior-medial aspect of the scapula, and the other hand is positioned at the superior base of the scapula, to provide an upward rotation assistance type motion while the patient actively elevates the arm in either the scapular plane or the sagittal plane. A negation of symptoms or increased ease in arm elevation during the application of this pressure as compared with the response when the patient performs the movement independently without the assistance of the examiner determines a positive or negative test result. A positive SAT result occurs when greater ROM or decreased pain (negation of impingement type symptoms) occurs during the examiner's assistance of the scapula. Rabin et al[47] tested the interrater reliability of the SAT and found coefficient of agreements ranging between 77% and 91% (kappa range, 0.53 to 0.62) for flexion and scapular plane movements. These investigators concluded that the SAT is

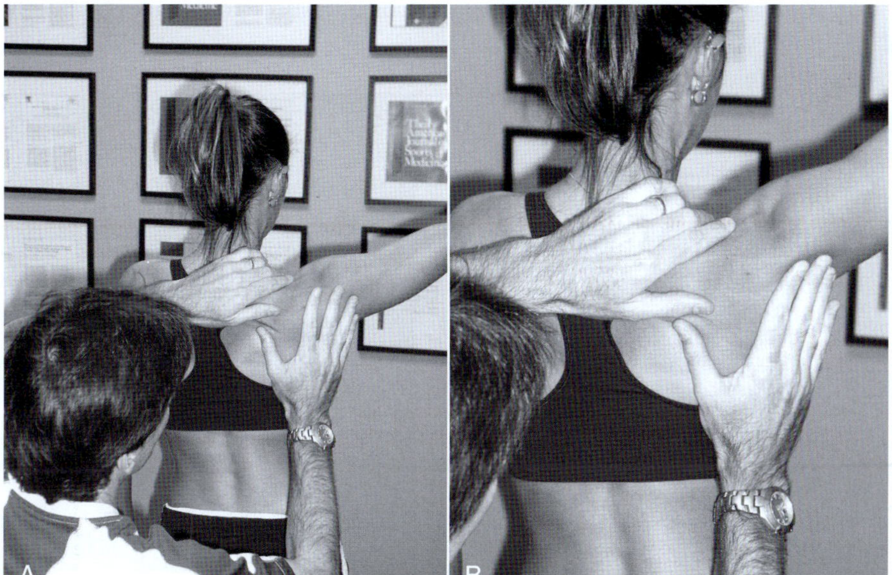

Figure 12-6 Scapular assistance test. **A,** Start position. **B,** Demonstration of movement.

acceptable for clinical use with moderate test-retest reliability. Additional research on the SAT by Kibler et al[48] showed an increase in the posterior tilt of the scapula by 7° during application of the clinician's stabilization and movement, with a decrease in pain ratings of 56% (8-mm Visual Analog Scale). This study demonstrated the favorable changes in scapular kinematics that can reduce symptoms in patients with shoulder pain.

Another test developed by Kibler et al[48] is the SRT. This test involves retraction of the scapula manually by the examiner during a movement that previously was unable to be performed secondary to weakness or loss of stability or a movement that was painful. Manual retraction of the scapula is performed using a cross-hand technique (Fig. 12-7). Figure 12-7 illustrates this test performed during internal and external rotation at 90° of abduction, a common motion provoking pain in overhead athletes with posterior impingement and rotator cuff disease.[27] Research by Kibler et al,[48] profiling the kinematic and neuromuscular actions during the SRT, showed an increase of 5° of scapular retraction during application of the clinician's pressure. Additionally, mean increases of 12° of posterior tilting and a reduction of internal rotation by 8° occurred during the performance of the SRT. Observed kinematic changes during the SRT place the glenohumeral joint in a biomechanically favorable position for function.

One final scapular test or sign that can be used during evaluation of the shoulder is the flip sign. Kelley et al[49] originally described this test, which consists of resisted external rotation at the side by the examiner with close visual monitoring to the medial border of the scapula during the external rotation resistance applied by the examiner (Fig. 12-8). A positive flip sign is present when the medial border of the scapular "flips" away from the thorax and becomes more prominent. This sign indicates a loss of

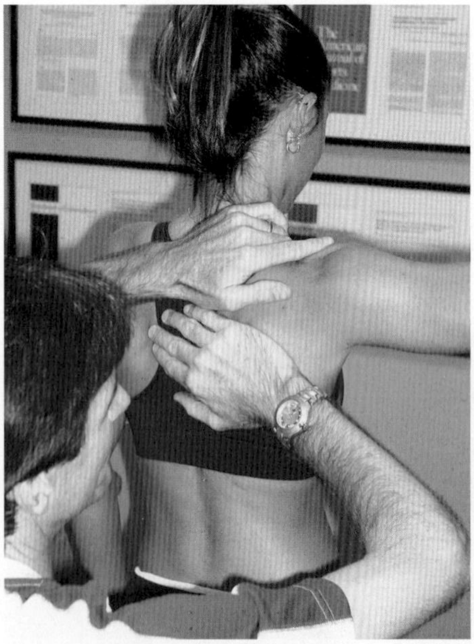

Figure 12-7 Scapular retraction test.

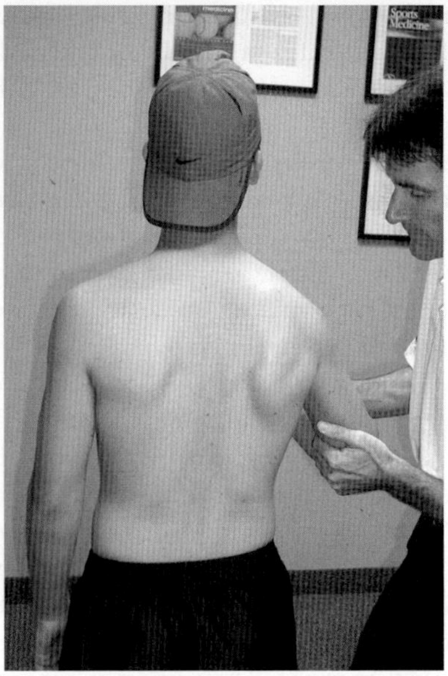

Figure 12-8 Flip sign.

scapular stability and should direct the clinician to evaluate the scapula further and to integrate exercise progressions aimed at the serratus anterior and trapezius force couple to stabilize the scapula.[49]

Glenohumeral Joint Range of Motion Measurement

A detailed, isolated assessment of glenohumeral joint ROM is a key ingredient of a thorough evaluation. Selective loss of internal rotation ROM on the dominant extremity is consistently reported in elite tennis players[50,51] and professional baseball pitchers. A goniometric method using an anterior containment force by the examiner (Fig. 12-9) to minimize the scapulothoracic contribution and or substitution is recommended by Ellenbecker et al.[52] The loss

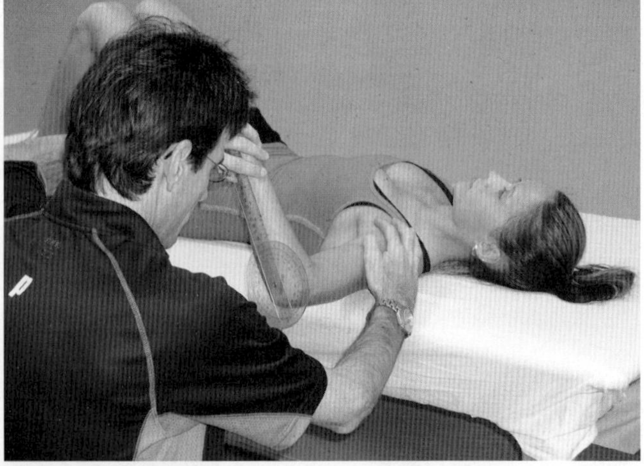

Figure 12-9 Goniometric measurement of internal rotation range of motion.

of internal rotation ROM is notable for two reasons. The relationship between internal rotation ROM loss (tightness in the posterior capsule of the shoulder) and increased anterior humeral head translation has been scientifically identified. The increase in anterior humeral shear, as reported by Harryman et al,[53] was manifested by a horizontal adduction cross-body maneuver similar to that incurred during the follow-through of the throwing motion or tennis serve. Tightness of the posterior capsule has also been linked to increased superior migration of the humeral head during shoulder elevation.[54]

Research by Koffler et al[55] studied the effects of posterior capsular tightness in a functional position of 90° of abduction and 90° or more of external rotation in cadaveric specimens. These investigators found that humeral head kinematics were changed or altered with imbrication of either the inferior aspect of the posterior capsule or imbrication of the entire posterior capsule. In the presence of posterior capsular tightness, the humeral head shifted in an anterior-superior direction as compared with a normal shoulder with normal capsular relationships. With more extensive amounts of posterior capsular tightness, the humeral head was found to shift posteriorly and superiorly.

Muraki et al[56] tested the effect of posterior-inferior capsular tightness on the contact area beneath the coracoacromial arch during the throwing motion. The findings were somewhat consistent with those of other studies showing that posterior-inferior capsular tightness not only increased the subacromial contact of the rotator cuff but also increased the contact area or size of the area of contact compared with normal capsular conditions. This study also showed that the peak subacromial contact forces occurred during the follow-through phase of the pitching motion.

Anterior translation of the humeral head and superior migration are two key factors in rotator cuff injury.[8,9] Loss of internal rotation ROM has also been consistently identified in a population of patients with glenohumeral joint impingement.[57] Tyler et al[58] reported that correction of posterior shoulder tightness in patients who had the diagnosis of posterior impingement and an average glenohumeral internal rotation deficit of 35° on initial evaluation was accomplished through the application of stretching and mobilization of the posterior shoulder. The application of stretches to the posterior shoulder and glenohumeral joint mobilization resulted in improvements in internal rotation deficiency of 9° in cross-arm adduction range motion of 8°. This study showed that these interventions of posterior shoulder stretching and glenohumeral joint mobilization can lead to symptom reduction in patients with posterior impingement.

Careful assessment of glenohumeral joint ROM is an important part of the clinical evaluation. Wilk et al[59] compared the difference in glenohumeral internal rotation measures by using three distinct levels of scapular stabilization and a condition with no scapular stabilization. Their study showed significant differences in internal rotation values in subjects when three methods of evaluating ROM were used. Careful and consistent use of a method to measure glenohumeral joint internal rotation is recommended and should include scapular stabilization.

Measurement of active and passive internal and external rotation at 90° of abduction—along with scapular plane elevation, forward flexion, and abduction—is performed during the examination of the patient with rotator cuff injury. Documentation of combined functional movement patterns (Apley's scratch test),[60] such as internal rotation with extension, and abduction and external rotation, is important. However, specific, isolated testing of glenohumeral joint motion is necessary to identify important glenohumeral joint motion restrictions.[50]

Research performed on elite junior tennis players and professional baseball pitchers that used a new concept called the *total rotation range-of-motion concept* has clinical ramifications for clinicians treating overhead athletes with glenohumeral joint injury.[52] Ellenbecker et al[52] measured internal rotation, external rotation, and total rotation ROM with 90° of glenohumeral joint abduction in 163 asymptomatic overhead athletes (117 elite junior tennis players and 46 professional baseball pitchers). The total rotation ROM is obtained simply by summing the internal and external rotation measures together. Results indicated significantly greater dominant-arm external rotation ROM (103° dominant arm versus 94° nondominant arm) and significantly less internal rotation ROM (42° dominant arm versus 54° nondominant arm) in the professional baseball pitchers. However, despite these significant differences in internal and external rotation, the total rotation ROM was not significantly different between extremities (145° versus 146°).[52] In the elite junior tennis players, significantly less internal rotation ROM was found on the dominant arm (45° versus 56°), as well as significantly less total rotation ROM on the dominant arm (149° versus 158°).[52]

This total rotation ROM has specific clinical ramifications for treating athletes from this population. If during the initial examination of a high-level baseball pitcher, the clinician finds an ROM pattern of 120° of external rotation and only 30° of internal rotation, some uncertainty may exist about whether that represents an ROM deficit in internal rotation that requires rehabilitative intervention by stretching and specific mobilization. However, if measurement of that patient's nondominant extremity rotation reveals 90° of external rotation and 60° of internal rotation, the current recommendation based on the total rotation ROM concept would be to avoid extensive mobilization and passive stretching of the dominant extremity because the total rotation ROM in both extremities is 150° (120° of external rotation + 30° of internal rotation = 150° dominant arm/90° of external rotation and 60° of internal rotation = 150° total rotation of the nondominant arm). In elite tennis players, the total active rotation ROM can be expected to be up to 10° less on the dominant arm.[52]

This total rotation ROM concept can be used as illustrated to guide the clinician during rehabilitation, specifically in the area of application of stretching and mobilization. This approach allows the clinician to determine most accurately which glenohumeral joint requires additional mobility and which extremity should not have additional mobility because of the obvious harm induced by increases in capsular mobility and increases in humeral head translation during aggressive upper extremity exertion.

Muscular Strength Testing

Determination of isolated and gross muscular strength during the examination of the patient with rotator cuff injury not only has a major impact on the determination of the underlying cause, but also assists in the formulation of a specific, objectively based rehabilitation program. Isolated testing in the "empty can" position for the supraspinatus is performed in the scapular plane, 30° anterior to the coronal plane (Fig. 12-10).[43,61] Testing for the infraspinatus and teres minor muscles is done with resisting external rotation in both the neutral adducted position and the 90° abducted position.[61] Resisted internal rotation in the neutral adducted position is generally recommended for the subscapularis.[61] Care must be taken when interpreting normal grade static manual muscle tests of the internal and external rotators.[62]

Normal grade 5/5 muscular strength has varied when compared with isokinetic testing in patients with rotator cuff injury and in normal control groups.[62] Regardless of this reported variability, the consistent application of manual muscle testing is highly recommended for the rotator cuff, deltoid, scapular stabilizers, and distal upper extremity muscle groups. For the patient with subtle symptoms and apparently normal muscular strength, more specific, dynamic, isokinetic testing is indicated to diagnose muscular weakness or unilateral strength imbalances more accurately.[63] It is beyond the scope of this chapter to outline fully the specific isokinetic testing principles and interpretation of isokinetic tests for evaluation and rehabilitation of the patient with rotator cuff dysfunction. The reader is referred to reference 64 for a detailed isokinetic review for shoulder rehabilitation.

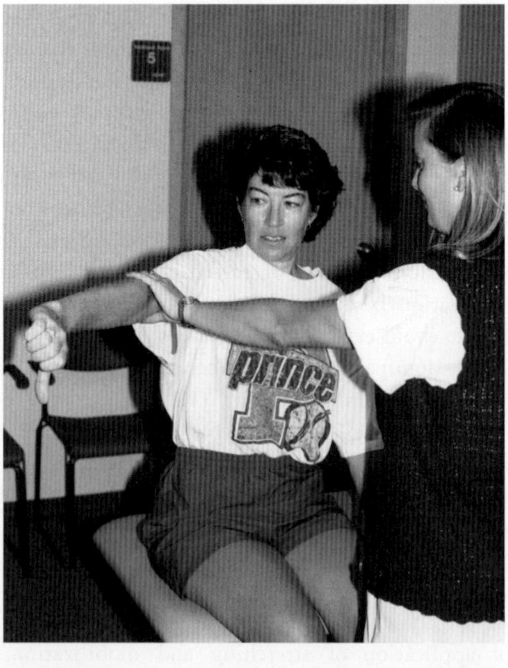

Figure 12-10 Supraspinatus manual muscle test position.

Special Tests

The classic tests for evaluation of a patient with rotator cuff injury are the impingement tests. The impingement test reported by Neer[10,11] places the shoulder in full forward flexion with overpressure. This position places the supraspinatus under the coracoacromial arch and can compress the tendon and reproduce the patient's symptoms. A second impingement test, reported by Hawkins and Kennedy,[65] involves 90° of forward flexion with full internal rotation. This test passes the rotator cuff under the coracoacromial arch; pain and a facial grimace indicate an abnormality. A final impingement test is the crossed-arm adduction test, which involves horizontally adducting the humerus starting in 90° of elevation. These impingement tests primarily indicate the presence of rotator cuff injury from compression or impingement.[10,65]

Tests to determine the integrity of the static stabilizers of the glenohumeral joint are a vital part of the comprehensive evaluation.[8,9] Rotator cuff injury caused by instability of the glenohumeral joint is a common occurrence in younger individuals and in overhead athletes.[8,9]

Clinical tests for instability must be routinely performed on the patient with rotator cuff injury to determine the underlying mobility status or the degree of instability in the glenohumeral joint. Clinical tests for instability of the glenohumeral joint include the apprehension and multidirectional instability (MDI) sulcus signs, and the fulcrum, load and shift, and subluxation relocation tests. (Further description of these clinical tests can be found in Chapter 4.) The subluxation relocation test popularized and originally described by Jobe and Kivitne[8] and by Jobe and Pink[23] is performed with the patient supine, with 90° of glenohumeral joint abduction and 90° of external rotation. The examiner pushes the humeral head forward, by using one hand on the posterior aspect of the patient's shoulder. This maneuver places tension on the anterior capsule and can produce a subtle anterior subluxation of the humeral head that often reproduces the patient's shoulder pain.[8] The relocation portion of the test consists of a posteriorly directed force produced by the examiner, who places the heel of his or her hand over the patient's humeral head anteriorly. This posterior force centralizes the humeral head in the glenoid fossa. A positive subluxation relocation sign consists of provocation of the patient's symptoms—with the anterior translation in the position of 90° of abduction and external rotation—with cessation of the symptoms during relocation (posterior centralization force).

Modification of the relocation test was recommended by Hamner et al,[66] who used the position of 90° of abduction and full end-range external rotation, rather than only 90° of external rotation, as Jobe originally described to provoke the rotator cuff further. Additionally, testing is performed with subluxation and relocation forces not only in 90° of abduction, but also at 110° and 120° of abduction. Arthroscopic confirmation of contact between the undersurface of the rotator cuff and the posterior-superior glenoid was confirmed using the modified subluxation relocation test in overhead athletes with shoulder dysfunction.[66] This test is the primary method used to diagnose individuals with posterior or undersurface impingement of the rotator cuff.

Capsular mobility testing—with the patient supine at 30°, 60°, and 90° of abduction—is also performed with both anterior and posterior stresses imparted. The anterior stress applied at 30°, 60°, and 90° of abduction tests the integrity of the superior, middle, and inferior glenohumeral ligaments, respectively.[67] The degree of translation of the humeral head relative to the glenoid, and the end feel, are bilaterally compared and recorded.[9,68] Ellenbecker et al[67] tested the intrarater and interrater reliability of the anterior humeral head translation test at 90° of abduction. Significantly greater intrarater and interrater reliability was achieved when examiners simply graded the movement of the humeral head relative to whether the head traversed the glenoid rim. Estimating end feel and further delineating humeral head translation grades complicated and jeopardized both intrarater and interrater reliability. Research recommendations call for the primary delineation during humeral head translation tests to be whether the humeral head stays within the glenoid when stress is applied (grade I) or whether the humeral head traverses up and over the glenoid rim with spontaneous reduction on removal of anterior load or stress (grade II). Capsular mobility testing with the shoulder in 90° of abduction is particularly important because of the hammock-like stabilizing function of the inferior glenohumeral ligament complex. The anterior band of the inferior glenohumeral ligament provides critical reinforcement against anterior translation of the humeral head (subluxation) with the arm in a position of 90° of abduction and 90° of external rotation.[67]

An additional test to determine the degree of anterior capsular laxity is the Lachman test of the shoulder.[9] With the patient supine and the shoulder abducted 90°—with 45° of external rotation—an anterior force is applied to the humeral head to assess anterior translation of the glenohumeral joint and to note the end point of the anterior capsule.[9]

The consistent use of these instability tests will provide the clinician with greater insight into the relationship, if any, between the patient's rotator cuff injury and glenohumeral joint instability. The identification of either anterior or multidirectional glenohumeral joint laxity should lead to a treatment plan addressing the instability.[9] The special tests listed previously are by no means comprehensive. Many other areas of emphasis are of paramount importance, such as tests to determine the integrity of the biceps and glenoid labrum. Interpretation of the results of a comprehensive evaluation allows the clinician to develop an objectively based rehabilitation program for rotator cuff injury.

BIOMECHANICAL CONCEPTS FOR REHABILITATION OF ROTATOR CUFF INJURY

Several biomechanical concepts have notable applications in the formulation and application of rehabilitative exercise for the patient with rotator cuff injury. One important concept is the force couple. A *force couple* consists of a pair of forces acting on an object that tends to produce rotation even though the forces may act in opposite directions.[69] An example of a force couple in the shoulder is the deltoid rotator cuff force couple outlined by Inman et al.[70] The force vector of the deltoid is superior, if contracting unopposed, which would create superior migration of the humeral head.[71] The supraspinatus muscle has a compressive function while contracting that creates an approximation of the humerus into the glenoid (Fig. 12-11). The infraspinatus, teres minor, and subscapularis produce a caudal force that resists the superior migration of the humeral head. One key factor when clinically interpreting the force couple concept is the muscle's force potential in relation to its physiologic cross-sectional area.[69] Research shows the subscapularis to have the greatest force potential, followed closely by the infraspinatus teres minor group.[69] The smallest physiologic cross-sectional area is exhibited by the supraspinatus. These small rotator cuff cross-sectional areas pale in comparison to the larger force-generating capacities of the deltoid muscle. The presence of a force couple imbalance is often identified on initial evaluation of the patient with rotator cuff injury.[39,57] Weakness of the rotator cuff, coupled with hypertrophy or training enhancement of the deltoid through uneducated exercise prescription in a patient who has used traditional "large shoulder muscle group dominant" resistive training exercises, further perpetuates this force couple imbalance.

Further application of this deltoid rotator cuff force couple was presented in research comparing normal subjects with patients with primary glenohumeral joint impingement.[72]

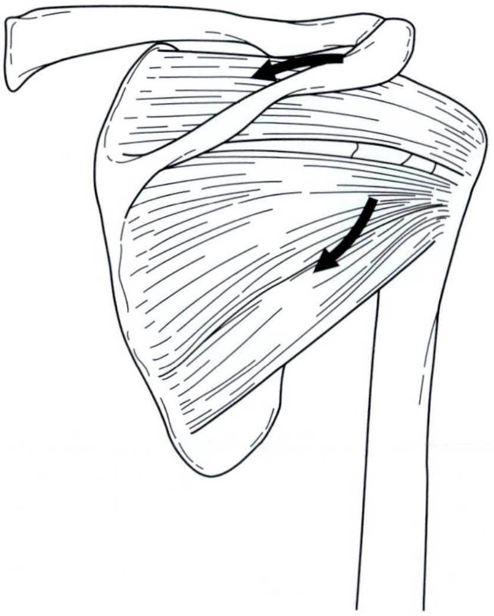

Figure 12-11 Deltoid rotator cuff force couple.

Electromyography (EMG) showed a substantial reduction in infraspinatus and subscapularis activity during the critical first stage of elevation of the shoulder in the scapular plane between 30° and 60°. Further decreases in infraspinatus activity on EMG were noted between 60° and 90° of elevation in the impingement group. The study by Reddy et al[72] showed decreases in the inferior force vector provided by the rotator cuff in patients with subacromial impingement.

The coordinated interplay between the rotator cuff and deltoid musculature was further demonstrated by EMG by Kronberg et al.[2] This study illustrated that all the rotator cuff muscles are involved, to some extent, in basic shoulder movements. These muscles act to assist movement and counterbalance the micromotions of the humeral head to keep it stable within the glenoid.

Additional force couples described in literature[8,69] are the serratus anterior trapezius and internal-external rotator couples. The serratus anterior trapezius force couple is also important in rotator cuff injury because it produces upward rotation of the scapula,[8] thus moving the overlying acromion superiorly out of the path of the elevating proximal humerus. The internal-external rotator force couple is another commonly imbalanced pair in the overhead athlete because of selective development of internal rotation strength, which overpowers the controlling and decelerating influence of the external rotators.[69,73,74]

Cain et al[75] and Blaiser et al[1] demonstrated further evidence of the rotator cuff's vital function in glenohumeral joint arthrokinematics in cadaveric studies. These studies showed the rotator cuff's ability to reduce the strain on the anterior capsule (inferior glenohumeral ligament) with the shoulder in 90° of abduction and external rotation. This important stabilizing function of resisting anterior translation demonstrates the rotator cuff's critical contribution to joint stability. Additional biomechanical research by Clark et al[76] identified the intimate, adherent association of the rotator cuff with the capsuloligamentous structures. It also identified the ability of rotator cuff muscular contraction to create tension and affect the orientation of the capsuloligamentous complex.

Muscular force vectors have been studied with the shoulder in the functional position of 90° of abduction and external rotation.[77] In this abducted position, the subscapularis functions as a flexor and internal rotator, the supraspinatus is an extensor, and the infraspinatus is an adductor. This study demonstrated the importance of working the dynamic stabilizers of the shoulder in both neutral and functional positions to simulate most closely the actual muscular length, tension, and contraction specificity incurred in activities of daily living and overhead sport movement patterns.

REHABILITATION OF ROTATOR CUFF INJURY

Both nonoperative rehabilitation and postoperative rehabilitation of the rotator cuff involve the following principles.

Reduction of Overload and Total Arm Rehabilitation

The initial goal of any treatment program includes the reduction of pain and inflammation by protection of the extremity from stress, but not from complete function.[20] Application of modalities, or modification or complete cessation, is often required in sport and ergonomic movement patterns. Care should be taken to identify the presence of any compensatory actions in the upper extremity kinetic chain, such as excessive scapular movement or elbow kinematics.[78] Early use is indicated for the distal strengthening of the elbow, forearm, and wrist, particularly in postoperative cases in which the degree and length of immobilization are greater. Mobilization of the scapulothoracic joint and submaximal strengthening of the scapular stabilizers are indicated, with great care taken not to impart inappropriate stresses or loads onto the injured tissues. One early technique used throughout rehabilitation phases is pictured in Figure 12-12. It involves a side-lying position and specific hand placements to resist scapular protraction and retraction without stress applied by the glenohumeral joint. This technique, performed with

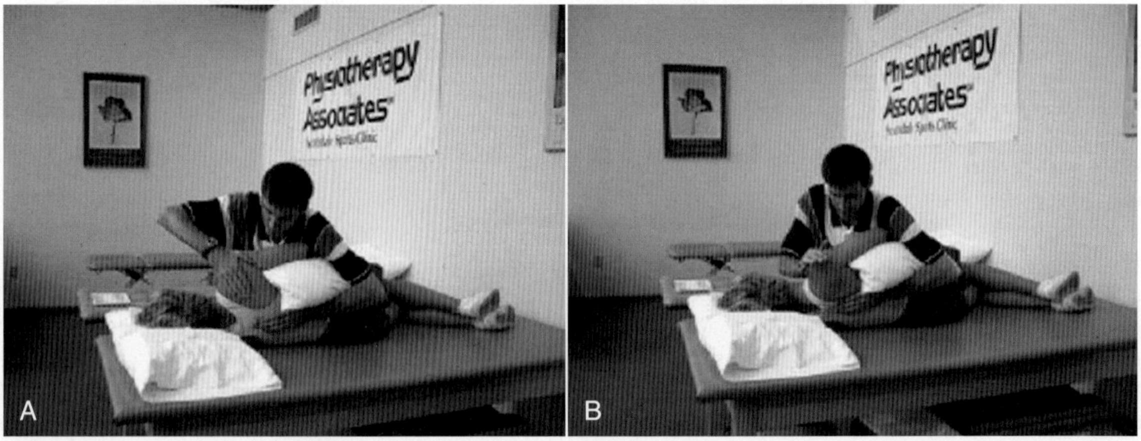

Figure 12-12 Side-lying manual scapular protraction (**A**) and retraction (**B**) resistance exercise to promote scapular stabilization.

manual resistance and a pillow, both to place a barrier between the patient and therapist and to position the glenohumeral joint in slight abduction and forward flexion during scapular motion, is performed using a relatively low initial resistance level. It emphasizes increased repetitions to build local muscular endurance of the serratus anterior during protraction, particularly of the lower trapezius and rhomboids during retraction.

Restoration of Normal Joint Arthrokinematics

Thorough evaluation to determine the degree of hypermobility or hypomobility of the glenohumeral joint, coupled with isolated joint ROM measurements, predicates the progression of and inclusion of stretching and joint mobilization in treatment. The presence of increased anterior capsular laxity and underlying instability of the glenohumeral joint, a finding consistently found in overhead athletes, contraindicates the application of joint accessory mobilization and stretching techniques that attenuate the anterior capsule. Posterior capsular mobilization and stretching techniques are often indicated and applied to improve internal rotation ROM. The consequences of posterior capsular tightness are outlined earlier in the chapter.

In postoperative rehabilitation of rotator cuff repairs, the use of joint mobilization techniques is recommended both to retard and to address the effects of immobilization. In addition to the posterior capsular mobilization described, specific emphasis on the caudal glide in varying positions of abduction is applied assertively to stress the inferior capsule and to prevent both adhesions and loss of functional elevation ROM.[39]

Promotion of Muscular Strength Balance and Local Muscular Endurance

The addition of resistive exercise is begun as inflammation and pain levels allow. Early submaximal resistance exercise in the rotator cuff and scapular muscles is initiated in the form of multiple-angle isometrics and progresses rapidly to submaximal isotonic exercises because of their inherent dynamic characteristics.[63] The presence or lack of pain over the joint or affected tendon or tendons determines the speed of progression and the intensity of exercise. Resistive exercises are used that emphasize concentric and eccentric muscular contributions from the key dynamic stabilizers of the shoulder. The movement patterns applied require high activation levels from the rotator cuff based on confirmation by EMG and biomechanical study.[79-81] The proper use of these patterns using a low-resistance (never greater than 5 lb and typically initiated with either no weight or as little as 1 lb), high-repetition format is recommended to enhance local muscular endurance[82] of the rotator cuff musculature. The movement patterns pictured in Figure 12-13 have been biomechanically studied and produce high levels of rotator cuff activation. These positions neither place the shoulder in a potential position of impingement nor place excessive stress on the often attenuated anterior capsuloligamentous complex. The movement patterns recommended for strengthening the rotator cuff do not place the shoulder in elevation beyond 90° or posterior to the coronal plane.

Research has confirmed the use of the rotator cuff exercise patterns outlined in Figure 12-13. Moncrief et al[83] studied the effects of a 5 times per week training program in which healthy, uninjured subjects performed the exercises for 2 sets of 15 repetitions for 1 month. Subjects were pretested and post-tested on an isokinetic dynamometer to quantify internal and external rotation strength objectively. Results of the 1-month rotator cuff training program showed 8% to 10% gains in isokinetically measured internal and external rotation strength in the training arms of the study and no significant improvement in strength in the control group arms. This fine study showed the effectiveness of using a low-resistance, high-repetition format with specific exercises that create high levels of activation in the rotator cuff muscles.

Bitter et al[84] reported the inherent advantages of using low-resistance exercise strategies to target the infraspinatus during external rotation exercise. These investigators reported specifically on external rotation exercise using a 40% maximal voluntary isometric contraction to be superior to higher loads in preferentially recruiting the infraspinatus muscle over conditions with higher maximal voluntary isometric contraction loading. Increased loading leads to a relative increase in the amount of middle deltoid muscle activation. This finding has significant clinical applications. Patients often attempt to use loads that are too high with their rotator cuff exercise, or patients are progressed too quickly to use loads that lead to greater amounts of substitution during external rotation exercise. Care must be taken to use exercise loading that allows for the highest relative activation of the rotator cuff without substitution during rehabilitation.

Similar positional limitations are applied in this stage of rehabilitation for strengthening the scapular stabilizers. Patterns resisting scapular protraction and retraction, elevation, and depression produce considerable muscular activity in the serratus anterior, trapezius, and rhomboids.[85] Kibler et al[86] published EMG research on low-level scapular exercises such as the robbery, low row, and lawn mower exercises and profiled the amount of lower trapezius and serratus anterior activation inherent in these exercises. This research provides an excellent reference for clinicians for prescribing exercises early in the rehabilitation following injury or surgery because these exercises all use low positions of abduction and minimally stress the rotator cuff and capsular stabilizers. Wilk et al[87] published EMG research measuring the timing of trapezius activation during rehabilitative exercises such as prone horizontal abduction, prone extension, side-lying external rotation, and forward flexion in side lying. The findings support the use of prone extension and prone horizontal abduction exercises in rehabilitation because of the generous and early contribution from the middle and lower portions of the trapezius. Use of closed chain exercise, which approximates the glenohumeral joint and produces cocontraction of the proximal stabilizing musculature of the scapulothoracic joint, is also recommended for both postoperative

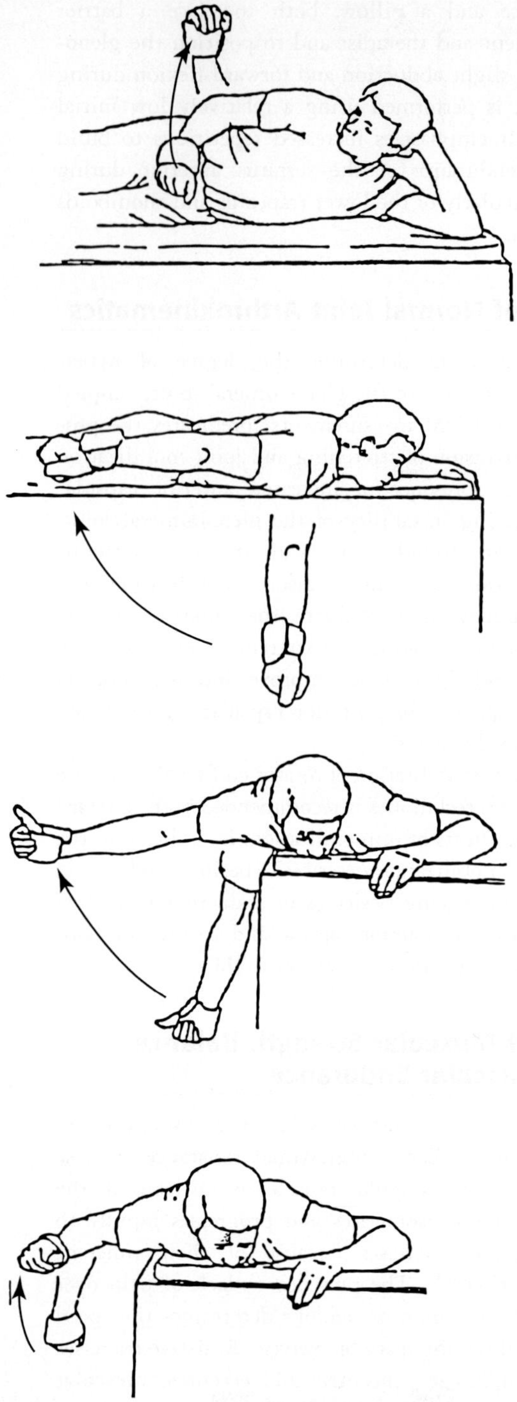

Figure 12-13 Rotator cuff exercise patterns.

rehabilitation of the rotator cuff and rehabilitation that is not postoperative. An example of a commonly used closed chain exercise is pictured in Figure 12-14, in which the therapist applies rhythmic stabilization or perturbation stresses with the patient's shoulder placed in the scapular plane and 90° of elevation. Progression to advanced-level plyometric exercises is also indicated for the upper extremity. Common applications are medicine balls and therapeutic Swiss balls in exercise patterns that use the stretch-shortening cycle of the scapulothoracic musculature, such as chest passes, and various throw and catch maneuvers that alter the position of the glenohumeral joint.[87]

Resistive exercises, with emphasis on the biceps muscle, are recommended in rotator cuff rehabilitation because of the glenohumeral joint stabilizing and humeral head depression actions.[88-90] Strengthening of the biceps in neutral and 90° of shoulder flexion is recommended, with concentric and eccentric contractions implemented.

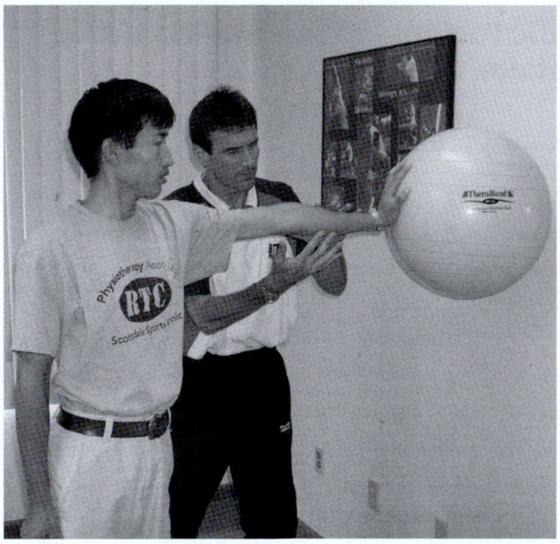

Figure 12-14 Closed chain scapular exercise: ball on wall.

The use of isokinetic exercise is warranted in later stages of both postoperative rehabilitation and rehabilitation that is not postoperative. As patients tolerate medium-resistance elastic tubing exercises, and can perform isolated rotator cuff exercises with a 2- to 3-lb weight, they are considered for this progression. The Davies modified base position is initially used for all patients for internal and external rotation.[39,47,64] Submaximal intensities at speeds ranging from 210° to 300°/second are used in active athletic patients, and a more intermediate contractile velocity range of 120° to 210°/second is used for less active and general orthopedic patients. Specific emphasis is placed on the external rotators because of their important role in functional activities[3,5,7] and in the maintenance of dynamic glenohumeral joint stability.[1,76]

Progression from the modified position in patients who will return to aggressive overhead activity is observed, by using tissue tolerance as the guide. Isokinetic internal and external rotation in the scapular plane, with 80° to 90° of abduction using fast contractile velocities, has been used successfully as an end-stage rotator cuff exercise to prepare the rotator cuff musculature for the demands of overhead activity (Fig. 12-15).

Interpretation of isokinetic test data typically focuses on bilateral comparisons and unilateral strength ratios.[63,64] Unilaterally dominant upper extremity athletes often demonstrate 15% to 30% greater internal rotation strength on the dominant arm, with bilaterally symmetrical external rotation strength.[39,63,64,73,74] Although bilateral comparison does provide important baseline comparison for the individual, the unilateral strength ratio may be of even greater importance.[39,63,64] The unilateral ratio of external rotation to internal rotation ratio in healthy shoulders has been reported at 66% throughout the velocity spectrum.[63,64] A goal in rehabilitation of patients with rotator cuff injury is to bias this ratio to range between 66% and 75%. This goal has been referred to as a *posterior dominant shoulder* and ensures that the strength of the external rotators is present to stabilize the humeral head in the glenoid and to provide stability.[65] Patients with rotator cuff impingement and glenohumeral joint instability have significant alterations of this normal 66% ratio.[57] The unilateral strength ratio is also altered (less than 66%) in the dominant arm in overhead throwing and racquet sport athletes because of the selective internal rotation strength development.[39,63,64,73,74] Isokinetic exercise and isolated joint testing are objectively quantifiable methods to address the force couple imbalances often inherent in the shoulder with rotator cuff injury.

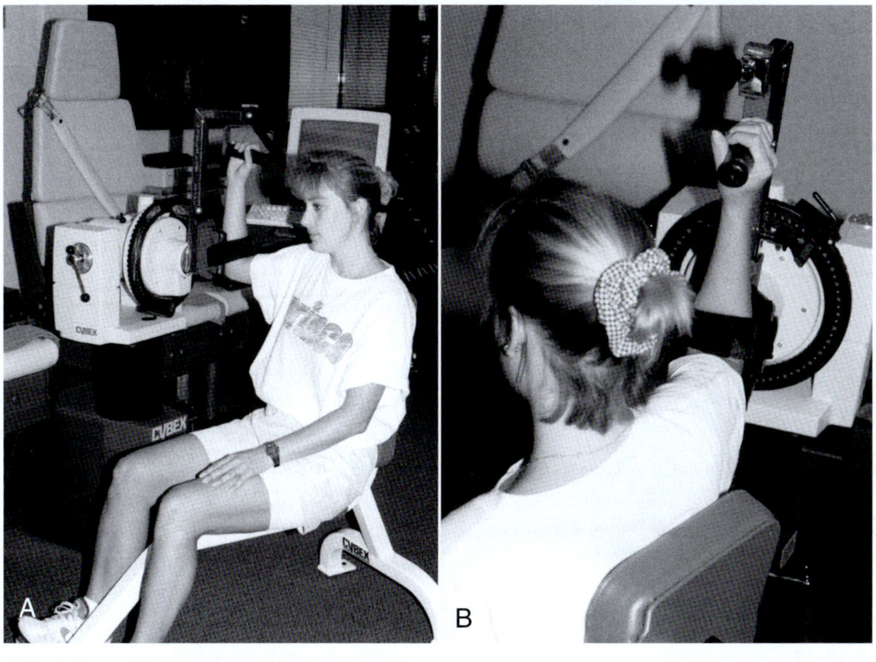

Figure 12-15 **A** and **B,** Isokinetic internal/external rotation with 90° of abduction in the scapular plane.

Finally, patients are placed on a home exercise program to maintain ROM gained during their rehabilitation program. This is particularly true for overhead athletes for whom a return to throwing or overhead sports can often mean a gradual reduction in internal rotation ROM.[91] McClure et al[92] studied the effects of two stretches used to improve glenohumeral joint internal rotation ROM in a prospective fashion. The stretches used and recommended in their study were the cross-arm stretch (Fig. 12-16A) and the sleeper stretch (Fig. 12-17). Subjects performed the stretches during a 4-week period, and both stretches produced favorable increases in glenohumeral joint internal rotation. In the short-term, the sleeper stretch produced 3.3° of internal rotation ROM increase immediately following the performance of the exercise.[93] These studies support the use of stretches such as the cross-arm and sleeper stretch to maintain glenohumeral joint internal rotation ROM, to prevent loss of internal rotation ROM in the human shoulder.

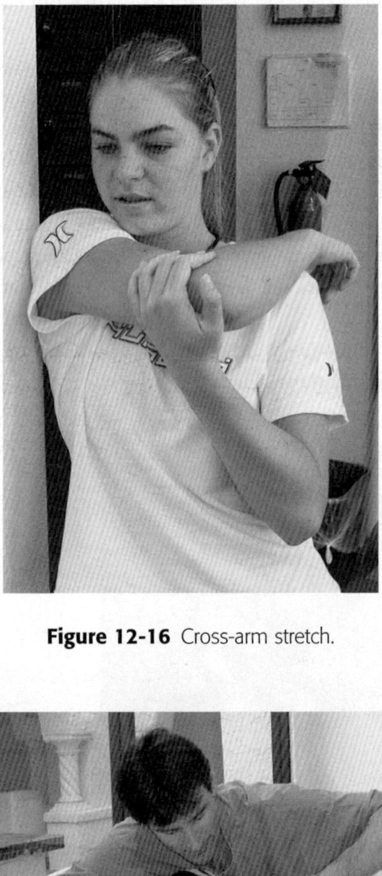

Figure 12-16 Cross-arm stretch.

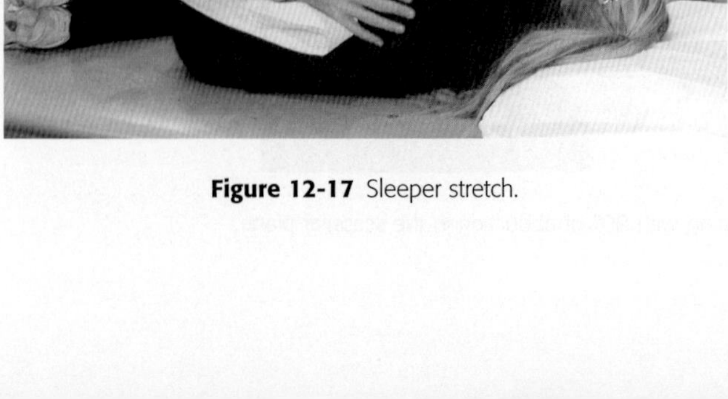

Figure 12-17 Sleeper stretch.

Specific Factors Influencing the Rehabilitation of Rotator Cuff Tears

Surgical Approach

Two of the most common surgical approaches commonly seen in rehabilitation are discussed briefly in this portion of the chapter. These include the mini-open approach and the all-arthroscopic approach. However, the traditional anterior approach, consisting of an anterior-lateral incision beginning just below the middle one third of the clavicle, crossing the coracoid tip, and continuing distally in an oblique lateral fashion to the anterior aspect of the humerus, is still used in some larger rotator cuff tears.[78] This traditional open approach has the greatest tissue morbidity and is used less often in today's surgical approaches when repair of a full-thickness rotator cuff tear is desired. In most cases, use of this anterior surgical exposure of the shoulder necessitates detachment of the deltoid origin from the anterior aspect of the acromion.[94] This is particularly common if an open subacromial decompression is performed. The subacromial decompression is used to remove a portion of the overlying offending structure and to provide both protection for the rotator cuff and prevention of further disease progression following its repair.[94]

The most commonly used open surgical exposure for rotator cuff repair is now the lateral deltoid splitting approach. This surgical approach begins with a transverse incision through the skin, 4 to 6 cm in length, beginning at the anterior-lateral corner of the acromion and continuing posteriorly to the posterior-lateral corner.[95] A straight longitudinal incision, based off the lateral aspect of the acromion and along the line of the deltoid fibers, is also frequently used. Regardless of the orientation of the skin incision, the deltoid is then split in line with its fibers near the anterior-lateral corner of the acromion. The deltoid's origin is protected and is not detached. The deltoid is not split farther distally than 5 cm, to avoid damage to the axillary nerve.[95]

The type of surgical approach used in an open rotator cuff repair dictates the progression of both ROM and resistance exercise following surgery. With the anterior deltopectoral approach (in which the deltoid can be detached from its origin), restrictions regarding the application of active or resistive exercise are normally recommended to allow the deltoid's origin to heal and become viable before the larger stresses of active or resistive movements are applied. Active assistive movement following surgery with the mini-arthrotomy or mini-open technique, using the lateral deltoid splitting approach, can normally commence on the first postoperative day.[95] Preservation of the deltoid's origin allows more aggressive ROM and earlier application of strengthening exercises during the rehabilitation process.

Most current rotator cuff repairs are now performed using an all-arthroscopic approach. This approach allows for complete protection of the deltoid and affords excellent exposure and visualization of the rotator cuff and labrum.

It also allows for performance of a subacromial decompression and distal clavicular excision, to minimize tissue morbidity. Ellenbecker's protocol for rehabilitation following the all-arthroscopic rotator cuff repair is presented in Case Study 2, later in this chapter.

Progression of both ROM and resistive exercise is much faster following arthroscopic rotator cuff débridement (see Case Study 1, later). AROM, AAROM, and passive ROM (PROM) all commence on the first postoperative day following arthroscopy unless associated surgical procedures were performed such as anterior plication, repair of a Bankart or SLAP (superior labrum anterior to posterior) lesion with suture tacks, laser capsulorrhaphy, or extensive subacromial decompression. Submaximal intensity resistive exercise is also initiated rapidly, following débridement of partial rotator cuff tears. Because arthroscopic approaches to the shoulder do not disturb the deltoid origin or the trapezius-deltoid fascia, resistive exercise using a low-resistance, high-repetition format is recommended early, to retard atrophy and to begin to normalize muscular strength imbalances.[95]

Length of Immobilization

The degree and length of immobilization of the shoulder following rotator cuff repair can greatly affect early rehabilitation emphasis. Traditional immobilization in a sling, or a sling and swathe, for up to 6 weeks following rotator cuff repairs results in a capsular pattern of ROM limitation that necessitates extensive joint mobilization and passive stretching. Extensive limitation in active and passive elevation, and external rotation of the shoulder, is commonly present following this degree and length of immobilization. Patients seen following arthroscopic débridement of partial rotator cuff tears often receive no immobilization other than a sling for 1 to 2 postoperative days. They often require minimal accessory mobilization to restore normal joint arthrokinematics. The common finding of associated instability and capsular laxity in the overhead athlete with partial undersurface rotator cuff tears, coupled with minimal immobilization time following arthroscopic débridement, often deemphasizes the importance of accessory joint mobilization, especially of the anterior capsule. As stated earlier, the loss of internal rotation ROM is an indication for the application of posterior capsular mobilization and passive stretching techniques in this population.[53,54]

Surgical Procedure

Debate exists in literature regarding the surgical management of rotator cuff tears. Open repair of the torn rotator cuff tendon and arthroscopic débridement with subacromial decompression are two frequently discussed options.[96-98] Rockwood and Burkhead[96] observed 93 patients who underwent open débridement and subacromial decompression for irreparable rotator cuff tears. Minimal deterioration in function and no degenerative changes were reported with an 8-year average follow-up evaluation. Burkhart[98] studied 25 patients who underwent arthroscopic débridement and subacromial decompression of massive rotator cuff tears with an average 30-month follow-up. Eighty-eight percent of the patients in this series were found to have good or excellent results, with no deterioration over time. Finally, Montgomery et al[97] compared the results of open surgical repair with arthroscopic débridement in 87 consecutive patients with full-thickness rotator cuff tears. A 2- to 5-year follow-up indicated that the open surgical repair group had superior results as compared with the arthroscopic group. The literature contains an extensive array, far beyond the scope of this chapter, of research demonstrating the efficacy of various surgical procedures for rotator cuff injury. One consistent finding is the important role of physical therapy in both the conservative treatment[99,100] and the postoperative management of rotator cuff disease.

Factors Influencing the Results of Nonoperative Rehabilitation of Rotator Cuff Tears

Several factors are consistently reported in the literature as having a notable relationship with the outcome of nonoperative treatment of rotator cuff disease. The following clinical findings and prognostic factors were associated with unfavorable clinical outcomes in a sample of 136 patients with impingement syndrome and rotator cuff disease: (1) a rotator cuff tear larger than 1 cm^2, (2) a history of pretreatment symptoms for more than 1 year, and (3) significant functional impairment at initial evaluation.[100] Itoi and Tabata[99] reported on the clinical outcome of conservative treatment of 124 shoulders with a full-thickness rotator cuff tear with a follow-up of 3 years. The primary factors relating to an unsatisfactory result were identified in their sample as limited abduction ROM and significant abduction muscular weakness on initial evaluation of the patient. Factors not associated with clinical outcome included the patient's age, gender, occupation, associated instability, dominance, and chronicity of onset.

Summary

Rehabilitation of rotator cuff pathologic conditions necessitates an extensive, objectively based evaluation and a thorough understanding of the complex biomechanical principles and etiologic factors associated with rotator cuff injury. A rehabilitation program aimed at restoring normal joint arthrokinematics and normal muscular strength, endurance, and balance is supported by the scientific principles currently present in the literature. Isolated treatment and evaluative focus on the rotator cuff and glenohumeral joint must be combined with a more global upper extremity kinetic chain approach to address rotator cuff injury comprehensively.

CASE STUDY 1

Subjective Information

The patient is a 27-year-old professional baseball pitcher who started having left anterior shoulder pain in early April following normal, uneventful spring training. Although the patient denies any particular incident of injury, he reported initially decreased recovery following pitching and pain in the anterior aspect of his shoulder during the acceleration phase and continued pain during follow-through of his pitching motion. In addition to localized anterior left shoulder pain, the patient complained of weakness, loss of velocity in his throwing, and eventually an inability to tolerate repeated repetitions of overhead activity. His pertinent history includes previous bouts of what he calls impingement dating back to his high school and collegiate baseball years. He denies any dislocations of his left shoulder. After 2 months of nonoperative treatment, including nonsteroidal anti-inflammatory medication and physical therapy for rotator cuff and general upper extremity strengthening, he was scheduled for further diagnostic testing.

Diagnostic testing revealed an undersurface (articular side) tear in the supraspinatus tendon. He underwent an arthroscopic procedure to débride the margins of the partial-thickness tear. He is referred to physical therapy 1 day following arthroscopic surgery.

Initial Findings

Examination of the patient postoperatively shows no obvious atrophy, with the exception of a hollowing in the infraspinous fossa on the left. Passive motion on the second day following surgery is 120° in forward flexion, 100° of abduction, 75° of external rotation, and 20° of internal rotation. Good distal strength is present along with confirmation of intact neurologic status. Passive accessory mobility of the patient's left shoulder indicates a 2+ anterior translation at 60° and 90° of abduction, as compared with a 1+ on the right uninjured shoulder. Posterior and caudal mobility are equal bilaterally. Additional special tests, such as labral and impingement, are deferred because of the patient's early postoperative status.

Treatment

Week 1

Modalities (electrical stimulation and ice) are applied to decrease pain and swelling, with a primary goal initially of restoring normal joint motion. PROM, AAROM, and AROM are used as tolerated to terminal ranges. Accessory mobilization is applied in the posterior and caudal directions to facilitate the return of flexion, abduction, and internal rotation ROM. Anterior glides are not indicated because of the hypermobility assessed on initial evaluation. Application of isometric and manually resisted rotator cuff strengthening is initiated along with scapular stabilization techniques (rhythmic stabilization, manual protraction and retraction). At the end of the first postoperative week, the patient has 175° of forward flexion and abduction, 90° of external rotation, and 35° of internal rotation measured with 90° of abduction.

Weeks 2 to 4

Continued use of ROM techniques is indicated at terminal ROMs, with posterior glides and emphasis on stretching of the posterior musculature to increase internal rotation. Progression of the patient's rotator cuff strengthening program includes concentric and eccentric isotonic exercise using the patterns with high levels of scientifically documented rotator cuff activation. Initially, a 1-lb weight is tolerated, with progression to 3 lb by the third week after surgery. Advancement of the patient's scapular strengthening program includes the use of closed chain Swiss ball exercise, seated rows, shrugs, and serratus anterior dominant activities, including a protraction punch movement pattern with tubing and manual resistance. Distal strengthening is of key importance, and biceps-triceps and forearm-wrist isotonics are performed both in the clinic and in the home program. Continued progress of this patient is noted with average ROM of the left shoulder at 175° of forward flexion and abduction, 95° of external rotation, and 40° of internal rotation.

Weeks 4 to 8

Addition of isokinetic exercise in the modified base position is warranted in this patient. Tolerance of a minimum of 3-lb isolated rotator cuff exercises, normal results of impingement tests, and functional ROM make him a candidate for isokinetic exercise between 4 and 6 weeks postoperatively. A submaximal introduction to the isokinetic form of resistance is recommended, with an isokinetic test to document internal and external rotation strength applied during this time frame. Results of the patient's initial isokinetic test show 10% to 15% greater internal rotation strength when compared with the uninjured extremity and 5% to 10% weaker external strength at 5 weeks postoperatively. External/internal rotation ratios range between 45% and 50%, a finding revealing a relative weakness or imbalance of external rotation strength on the dominant extremity. A pylometric program, with medicine balls to simulate functional muscular contractions and to facilitate scapulothoracic strength, is initiated during this stage.

Weeks 8 to 12

Continued mobilization and PROM are performed to normalize glenohumeral joint motion, with continued emphasis on the posterior capsule and posterior musculature. Isotonic rotator cuff exercise is progressed to not more than 5 lb, and advancement of the scapular programs in isotonic,

CASE STUDY 1—cont'd

closed chain, and plyometric venues continues. Isokinetic testing at 8 to 9 weeks postoperatively shows 25% greater internal rotation strength and equal external rotation strength measured in the modified position. At this time, the patient progresses to an interval-throwing program carried out at the clinic on alternate days beginning with tossing at a 30-foot distance and progressing during the next 3 to 4 weeks to 60-, 90-, and 120-foot distances. Once the patient tolerates 120 feet with as many as 75 to 100 repetitions, he is progressed to throwing off the mound at 50% intensities. The isokinetic strengthening progresses to a more functional 90° abducted position in the scapular plane. The continuation of a total arm strength program is followed both in the clinic and at home.

CASE STUDY 2

Subjective History

The patient is a 51-year-old male competitive tennis player with a 1-year history of shoulder tendinitis with impingement symptoms reported as intermittent based on his level of activity. One month ago, the patient was hitting a serve early in a match with minimal warm-up and felt a deep, sharp pain in the anterior-lateral aspect of his shoulder as his arm was accelerating forward just before hitting the ball. He was unable to continue playing and was unable to abduct or flex his arm more than 90°. Continuous pain was reported, even with rest and sleep, and he was examined by an orthopedic surgeon 2 days later. An MRI was scheduled, and results showed a full-thickness tear of the supraspinatus tendon. He subsequently underwent an arthroscopic surgical repair of the supraspinatus and was referred for rehabilitation 2 days following surgery.

Initial Findings

The patient appears with his right arm immobilized in a sling. Initial treatment called for immobilization and limited ROM at home using Codman's exercises for the first 2 weeks. He presents to the clinic for his first physical therapy visit 2 weeks postoperatively. Initial evaluation reveals no distal radiation of symptoms and full light touch sensation and strong distal grip. The initial examination consists primarily of a neurologic screening and PROM measurement of the involved extremity and measurement of baseline AROM of the contralateral extremity. The patient has a 1° load and shift, and a negative MDI sulcus sign in bilateral shoulders. The patient expressly denies any instability in either shoulder before this injury.

Initial Phase

Weeks 2 to 6

Modalities consisting of electrical stimulation and ice are applied as needed to control pain and to increase local blood flow. PROM and AAROM are performed to the patient's tolerance with no limitation on ROM. Evaluation of the patient's accessory movement shows a decreased caudal glide and posterior glide relative to the contralateral extremity. Accessory mobilizations are applied, using the caudal and posterior directions along with passive stretching. Scapulothoracic joint mobilization also is used. Passive stretching of the elbow, particularly into extension because of the continued use of a sling for immobilization, is indicated, as is the use of grip putty to prevent disuse atrophy of the forearm and wrist musculature during the immobilization period. The patient's initial PROM at 2 weeks after open rotator cuff repair is 140° of flexion and 120° of abduction, 50° of internal rotation, and 40° of external rotation measured at 45° of abduction. During the second to sixth postoperative week, PROM exercise progresses to AAROM and finally to AROM. The use of overhead pulleys and the upper body ergometer are added. Submaximal multiple-angle isometrics are performed for shoulder internal rotation and external rotation, as is manual resistance exercise for the biceps and triceps, the scapular protractors and retractors and elevators, and the distal forearm and wrist musculature.

Phase II: Total Arm Strength

Weeks 6 to 12

The patient's ROM is advanced to terminal ranges and approaches full ROM in all planes. Current ROM of the patient is 160° of flexion, 145° of abduction, 65° of external rotation, and 70° of internal rotation, again measured at 45° of abduction. Continued mobilization of the glenohumeral joint is combined with end-range passive stretching techniques to restore normal joint arthrokinematics. Resistive exercise in the form of isotonic internal and external rotation, prone extension, and horizontal abduction is begun, using a low-load, high-repetition format (i.e., 3 sets of 15 repetitions). The resistance level progresses as tolerated. Scapular stabilization exercise is applied at this time, with eventual advancement of the scapular strengthening program to include plyometrics, with a Swiss ball and eventually a medicine ball. Concentric work and eccentric muscular work are performed using

Continued

CASE STUDY 2—cont'd

elastic tubing and controlled execution of the resistive exercise patterns with isotonic resistance. At 10 weeks postoperatively, this patient has 175° of forward flexion, 165° of abduction, and 85° of external rotation with 90° of abduction. Sixty degrees of internal rotation is present with 90° of abduction. Tolerance is demonstrated using 3-lb isolated rotator cuff exercises (mentioned earlier). The patient progresses to isokinetic internal and external rotation in the modified base position for a trial of submaximal isokinetic exercise. Continued home exercise for the rotator cuff and scapular stabilizers using elastic tubing and light isotonic loads is performed. Additionally, elastic tubing and light weights are continued to prepare the distal upper extremity for the return to tennis play in the later stages of rehabilitation.

Return to Activity Phase

Weeks 12 to 16

Continued accessory mobilization to achieve full range of elevation is applied to this patient, as is passive stretching in physiologic ROM patterns. An isokinetic test is performed in the modified base position, indicating equal internal rotation strength bilaterally, with a 35% external rotation deficit identified. The patient's ratio of external rotation to internal rotation is 54%, much lower than the desired 66% balance. ROM for this patient has continued to improve to 175° of flexion and 170° of abduction, 95° of external rotation, and 60° of internal rotation. Advancement of the patient's strengthening program includes the 90° abducted position for both isokinetic internal rotation and external rotation and surgical tubing strengthening. Pylometric exercise with medicine balls intensifies, as does the entire scapular program, including the use of closed chain push-ups and step-ups, with emphasis on protraction for serratus strengthening. The patient continues with rehabilitative exercise and close adherence to a home program to reinforce the concept of total arm strength in preparation for the interval return to playing tennis. Achievement of greater external rotation muscular strength and endurance is recommended before this patient begins the interval tennis program. The guided return to tennis will include ground stroke activity initially, with progression to volleys and serving based on tolerance to the forehand and backhand ground strokes. Typically, the interval tennis program following a repair of a full-thickness rotator cuff tear takes up to 6 to 8 weeks before protected match play can resume. The emphasis is on continued use of the rotator cuff and scapular strength maintenance program following discharge of the patient from formal physical therapy.

REFERENCES

1. Blaiser RB, Guldberg RE, Rothman ED: Anterior stability: contributions of rotator cuff forces and the capsular ligaments in a cadaver model, *J Shoulder Elbow Surg* 1:140, 1992.
2. Kronberg M, Nemeth F, Brostrom LA: Muscle activity and coordination in the normal shoulder: an electromyographic study, *Clin Orthop Relat Res* 257:76, 1990.
3. Rhu KN, McCormick J, Jobe FW, et al: An electromyographic analysis of shoulder function in tennis players, *Am J Sports Med* 16:481, 1988.
4. Vangheluwe B, Hebbelinck M: Muscle actions and ground reaction forces in tennis, *Int J Sports Biomechan* 2:88, 1986.
5. Miyashita M, Tsunoda T, Sakurai S, et al: Muscular activities in the tennis serve and overhead throwing, *Scand J Sports Sci* 2:52, 1980.
6. Jobe FW, Moynes DR, Tibone JE, et al: An EMG analysis of the shoulder in pitching, *Am J Sports Med* 12:218, 1984.
7. Fleisig GS, Andrews JR, Dillman CJ, et al: Kinetics of baseball pitching with implications about injury mechanisms, *Am J Sports Med* 23:233, 1995.
8. Jobe FW, Kivitne RS: Shoulder pain in the overhand or throwing athlete: the relationship of anterior instability and rotator cuff impingement, *Orthop Rev* 28:963, 1989.
9. Andrews JR, Alexander EJ: Rotator cuff injury in throwing and racquet sports, *Sports Med Arthroscop Rev* 3:30, 1995.
10. Neer CS: Anterior acromioplasty for the chronic impingement syndrome in the shoulder: a preliminary report, *J Bone Joint Surg Am* 54:41, 1972.
11. Neer CS: Impingement lesions, *Clin Orthop Relat Res* 173:70, 1983.
12. Golding FC: The shoulder: the forgotten joint, *Br J Radiol* 35:149, 1962.
13. Cotton RE, Rideout DF: Tears of the humeral rotator cuff: a radiological and pathological necropsy survey, *J Bone Joint Surg Br* 46:314, 1964.
14. Poppen NK, Walker PS: Forces at the glenohumeral joint in abduction, *Clin Orthop Relat Res* 135:165, 1978.
15. Lucas DB: Biomechanics of the shoulder joint, *Arch Surg* 107:425, 1973.
16. Wuelker N, Plitz W, Roetman B: Biomechanical data concerning the shoulder impingement syndrome, *Clin Orthop Relat Res* 303:242, 1994.
17. Elliot B, Marsh T, Blanksby B: A three dimensional cinematographic analysis of the tennis serve, *Int J Sports Biomechan* 2:260, 1986.
18. Bigliani LU, Ticker JB, Flatow EL, et al: The relationship of acromial architecture to rotator cuff disease, *Clin Sports Med* 10:823, 1991.
19. Zuckerman JD, Kummer FJ: Cuomo, et al: The influence of coracoacromial arch anatomy on rotator cuff tears, *J Shoulder Elbow Surg* 1:4, 1992.
20. Nirschl RP: Shoulder tendonitis. In Pettrone FP, editor: *Upper extremity injuries in athletes, American Academy of Orthopaedic Surgeons Symposium, Washington, DC, 1988*, St. Louis, 1988, Mosby.

21. Kraushaar BS, Nirschl RP: Current concepts review: tendonosis of the elbow (tennis elbow): clinical features and findings of histological, immunohistochemical, and electron microscopy studies, *J Bone Joint Surg Am* 81(2):259, 1990.
22. Cofield R: Current concepts review of rotator cuff disease of the shoulder, *J Bone Joint Surg Am* 67:974, 1985.
23. Jobe FW, Pink M: The athlete's shoulder, *J Hand Ther* 7(2):107, 1994.
24. Walch G, Boileau P, Noel E, et al: Impingement of the deep surface of the supraspinatus tendon on the posterosuperior glenoid rim: an arthroscopic study, *J Shoulder Elbow Surg* 1:238, 1992.
25. Halbrecht JL, Tirman P, Atkin D: Internal impingement of the shoulder: comparison of findings between the throwing and nonthrowing shoulders of college baseball players, *Arthroscopy* 15(3):253–258, 1999.
26. Paley KJ, Jobe FW, Pink MM, et al: Arthroscopic findings in the overhand throwing athlete: evidence for posterior internal impingement of the rotator cuff, *Arthroscopy* 16(1):35–40, 2000.
27. Mihata T, McGarry MH, Kinoshita M, et al: Excessive glenohumeral horizontal abduction as occurs during the late cocking phase of the throwing motion can be critical for internal impingement, *Am J Sports Med* 38(2):369–374, 2010.
28. Codman EA: *The shoulder*, ed 2, Boston, 1934, Thomas Todd.
29. Chansky HA, Iannotti JP: The vascularity of the rotator cuff, *Clin Sports Med* 10:807, 1991.
30. Rathburn JB, MacNab I: The microvascular pattern of the rotator cuff, *J Bone Joint Surg Br* 52:540, 1970.
31. Brooks CH, Revell WJ, Heatley FW: A quantitative histological study of the vascularity of the rotator cuff tendon, *J Bone Joint Surg Br* 74:151, 1992.
32. Swiontowski MF, Iannotti JP, Boulas HJ, et al: Intraoperative assessment of rotator cuff vascularity using laser Doppler flowmetry. In Post M, Morrey BF, Hawkins RJ, editors: *Surgery of the shoulder*, St. Louis, 1990, Mosby–Year Book.
33. Iannotti JP: Lesions of the rotator cuff: pathology and pathogenesis. In Matsen FA, Fu FH, Hawkins RJ, editors: *The shoulder: a balance of mobility and stability*, Rosemont, Ill, 1993, American Academy of Orthopaedic Surgeons.
34. Loehr JF, Helmig P, Sojbjerg JO, et al: Shoulder instability caused by rotator cuff lesions: an in vitro study, *Clin Orthop Relat Res* 303:84, 1994.
35. Miller C, Savoie FH: Glenohumeral abnormalities associated with full-thickness tears of the rotator cuff, *Orthop Rev* 23:159, 1994.
36. Fukuda H, Hamada K, Yamanaka K: Pathology and pathogenesis of bursal side rotator cuff tears viewed from en bloc histologic sections, *Clin Orthop Relat Res* 254:75, 1990.
37. Nakajima T, Rokumma N, Kazutoshi H, et al: Histologic and biomechanical characteristics of the supraspinatus tendon: reference to rotator cuff tearing, *J Shoulder Elbow Surg* 3:79, 1994.
38. Fukuda H, Hamada K, Nakajima T, et al: Pathology and pathogenesis of the intratendinous tearing of the rotator cuff viewed from en bloc histologic sections, *Clin Orthop Relat Res* 304:60, 1994.
39. Ellenbecker TS: Rehabilitation of shoulder and elbow injuries in tennis players, *Clin Sports Med* 14:87, 1995.
40. Kibler WB: Role of the scapula in the overhead throwing motion, *Contemp Orthop* 22:525, 1991.
41. Kibler WB, Uhl TL, Maddux JWQ, et al: Qualitative clinical evaluation of scapular dysfunction: a reliability study, *J Shoulder Elbow Surg* 11:550–556, 2002.
42. Zeier FG: The treatment of winged scapula, *Clin Orthop Relat Res* 91:128–133, 1973.
43. Saha AK: Mechanism of shoulder movements and a plea for the recognition of "zero position" of glenohumeral joint, *Clin Orthop Relat Res* 173:3, 1983.
44. McClure PW, Tate AR, Kareha S, et al: A clinical method for identifying scapular dyskinesis, part 1: reliability, *J Athl Train* 44:160–164, 2009.
45. Uhl TL, Kibler WB, Grecewich B, et al: Evaluation of clinical assessment methods for scapular dyskinesis, *Arthroscopy* 11:1240–1248, 2009.
46. Kibler WB: The role of the scapula in athletic shoulder function, *Am J Sports Med* 26:325–337, 1998.
47. Rabin A, Irrgang JJ, Fitzgerald GK, et al: The intertester reliability of the scapular assistance test, *J Orthop Sports Phys Ther* 36(9):653–660, 2006.
48. Kibler WB, Uhl TL, Cunningham TJ: The effect of the scapular assistance test on scapular kinematics in the clinical exam, *J Orthop Sports Phys Ther* 39(11):A12, 2009.
49. Kelley MJ, Kane TE, Leggin BG: Spinal accessory nerve palsy: associated signs and symptoms, *J Orthop Sports Phys Ther* 38(2):78–86, 2008.
50. Ellenbecker TS, Roetert EP, Piorkowski P: Shoulder internal and external rotation range of motion of elite junior tennis players: a comparison of two protocols [abstract], *J Orthop Sports Phys Ther* 17:65, 1993.
51. Chandler TJ, Kibler WB, Uhl TL, et al: Flexibility comparisons of elite junior tennis players to other athletes, *Am J Sports Med* 18:134, 1990.
52. Ellenbecker TS, Roetert EP, Bailie DS, et al: Glenohumeral joint total rotation range of motion in elite tennis players and baseball pitchers, *Med Sci Sports Exerc* 34(12):2052–2056, 2002.
53. Harryman DT, Sidles JA, Clark JM, et al: Translation of the humeral head on the glenoid with passive glenohumeral joint motion, *J Bone Joint Surg Am* 72:1334, 1990.
54. Matsen FAIII, Artnz CT: Subacromial impingement. In Rockwood CA Jr, Matsen FA III, editors: *The shoulder*, Philadelphia, 1990, Saunders.
55. Koffler KM, Bader D, Eager M, et al: *The effect of posterior capsular tightness on glenohumeral translation in the late-cocking phase of pitching: a cadaveric study*, Paper presented at the Arthroscopy Association of North America annual meeting, Washington DC, 2001, abstract SS–15.
56. Muraki T, Yamamoto N, Zhao KD, et al: Effect of posterior-inferior capsule tightness on contact pressure and area beneath the coracoacromial arch during the pitching motion, *Am J Sports Med* 38(3):600–607, 2010.
57. Warner JJP, Micheli LJ, Arslanian LE, et al: Patterns of flexibility, laxity, and strength in normal shoulders and shoulders with instability and impingement, *Am J Sports Med* 18:366, 1990.
58. Tyler TF, Nicholas SJ, Lee SJ, et al: Correction of posterior shoulder tightness is associated with symptom resolution in patients with internal impingement, *Am J Sports Med* 38(1):114–119, 2010.
59. Wilk KE, Reinold MM, Macrina LC, et al: Glenohumeral internal rotation measurements differ depending on stabilization techniques, *Sports Health* 1(2):131–136, 2009.
60. Hoppenfeld S: *Physical examination of the spine and extremities*, Norwalk, Conn, 1976, Prentice-Hall.
61. Daniels L, Worthingham C: *Muscle testing: techniques of manual examination*, ed 5, Philadelphia, 1986, Saunders.

62. Ellenbecker TS: Muscular strength relationship between normal grade manual muscle testing and isokinetic measurement of the shoulder internal and external rotators [abstract], *J Orthop Sports Phys Ther* 19:72, 1994.
63. Davies GJ: *A compendium of isokinetics in clinical usage*, ed 4, LaCrosse, Wis, 1992, S & S Publishers.
64. Ellenbecker TS, Davies GJ: The application of isokinetics in testing and rehabilitation of the shoulder complex, *J Athl Train* 35(3):338–350, 2000.
65. Hawkins RJ, Kennedy JC: Impingement syndrome in athletes, *Am J Sports Med* 8:151, 1980.
66. Hamner DL, Pink MM, Jobe FW: A modification of the relocation test: arthroscopic findings associated with a positive test, *J Shoulder Elbow Surg* 9:263–267, 2000.
67. Ellenbecker TS, Bailie DS, Mattalino AJ, et al: Intrarater and inter-rater reliability of a manual technique to assess anterior humeral head translation of the glenohumeral joint, *J Shoulder Elbow Surg* 11:470–475, 2002.
68. Altchek DW, Skyhar MJ, Warren RF: Shoulder arthroscopy for shoulder instability. In *Instructional Course Lectures: the shoulder*, Rosemont, Ill, American Academy of Orthopaedic Surgeons.
69. Dillman CJ: Biomechanics of the rotator cuff, *Sports Med Arthroscop Rev* 3:2, 1995.
70. Inman VT, Saunders JB, de CM Abbot LC: Observations on the function of the shoulder joint, *J Bone Joint Surg Am* 26:1, 1994.
71. Weiner DS, MacNab I: Superior migration of the humeral head, *J Bone Joint Surg Br* 52:524, 1970.
72. Reddy AS, Mohr KJ, Pink MM, et al: Electromyographic analysis of the deltoid and rotator cuff muscles in persons with subacromial impingement, *J Shoulder Elbow Surg* 9:519–523, 2000.
73. Ellenbecker TS: Shoulder internal and external rotation strength and range of motion of highly skilled junior tennis players, *Isokinet Exerc Sci* 2:1, 1992.
74. Ellenbecker TS, Mattalino AJ: Concentric isokinetic shoulder internal and external rotation strength in professional baseball pitchers, *J Orthop Sports Phys Ther* 25(5):323–328, 1997.
75. Cain PR, Mutschler TA, Fu F, et al: Anterior stability of the glenohumeral joint: a dynamic model, *Isokinet Exerc Sci* 15:144, 1987.
76. Clark J, Sidles JA, Matsen FA: The relationship of the glenohumeral joint capsule to the rotator cuff, *Clin Orthop Relat Res* 254:29, 1990.
77. Bassett RW, Browne AO, Morrey BF, et al: Glenohumeral muscle force and moment mechanics in a position of shoulder instability, *J Biomech* 23:405, 1990.
78. Cooper JE, Shwedyk E, Quanbury AO, et al: Elbow joint restriction: effect on functional upper limb motion during performance of three feeding activities, *Arch Phys Med Rehabil* 74:805, 1993.
79. Ballantyne BT, O'Hare SJ, Paschall JL, et al: Electromyographic activity of selected shoulder muscles in commonly used therapeutic exercises, *Phys Ther* 73:668, 1993.
80. Blackburn TA, McLeod WD, White B, et al: EMG analysis of posterior rotator cuff exercises, *J Athl Train* 25:40, 1990.
81. Townsend H, Jobe FW, Pink M, et al: Electromyographic analysis of the glenohumeral muscles during a baseball rehabilitation program, *Am J Sports Med* 19:264, 1991.
82. Fleck S, Kraemer W: *Designing resistance training programs*, Champaign, Ill, 1987, Human Kinetics.
83. Moncrief SA, Lau JD, Gale JR, et al: Effect of rotator cuff exercise on humeral rotation torque in healthy individuals, *J Strength Cond Res* 16(2):262–270, 2002.
84. Bitter NL, Clisby EF, Jones MA, et al: Relative contributions of infraspinatus and deltoid during external rotation in healthy shoulders, *J Shoulder Elbow Surg* 16(5):563–568, 2007.
85. Moesley JB, Jobe FW, Pink M: EMG analysis of the scapular muscles during a shoulder rehabilitation program, *Am J Sports Med* 20:128, 1992.
86. Kibler WB, Sciascia AD, Uhl TL, et al: Electromyographic analysis of specific exercises for scapular control in early phases of shoulder rehabilitation, *Am J Sports Med* 36:1789–1798, 2008.
87. Wilk KE, Voight ML, Keirns MA, et al: Stretch shortening drills for the upper extremities: theory and clinical application, *J Orthop Sports Phys Ther* 17:225, 1993.
88. Glousman R, Jobe FW, Tibone JE, et al: Dynamic electromyographic analysis of the throwing shoulder with glenohumeral joint instability, *J Bone Joint Surg Am* 70:220, 1988.
89. Itoi E, Kuechle DK, Newman SR, et al: Stabilizing function of the biceps in stable and unstable shoulders, *J Bone Joint Surg Br* 75:546, 1993.
90. Rodosky MW, Harner CD, Fu FH: The role of the long head of the biceps muscle and superior glenoid labrum in anterior stability of the shoulder, *Am J Sports Med* 22:121, 1994.
91. Reinold MM, Wilk KE, Macrina LC, et al: Changes in elbow and shoulder passive range of motion after pitching in professional baseball players, *Am J Sports Med* 36:523–527, 2008.
92. McClure P, Balaicuis J, Heiland D, et al: A randomized controlled comparison of stretching procedures for posterior shoulder tightness, *J Orthop Sports Phys Ther* 37:108–114, 2007.
93. Laudner KG, Sipes RC, Wilson JT: The acute effects of sleeper stretches on shoulder range of motion, *J Athl Train* 43(4):359–363, 2008.
94. Kunkel SS, Hawkins RJ: Open repair of the rotator cuff. In Andrews JR, Wilk KE, editors: *The athlete's shoulder*, New York, 1994, Churchill Livingstone.
95. Timmerman LA, Andrews JR, Wilk KE: Mini open repair of the rotator cuff. In Andrews JR, Wilk KE, editors: *The athlete's shoulder*, New York, 1994, Churchill Livingstone.
96. Rockwood CA Jr, Burkhead WZ: Management of patients with massive rotator cuff defects by acromioplasty and rotator cuff debridement, *Orthop Trans* 12:190, 1988.
97. Montgomery TJ, Yerger B, Savoie FH: Management of rotator cuff tears: a comparison of arthroscopic debridement and surgical repair, *J Shoulder Elbow Surg* 3:70, 1994.
98. Burkhart SS: Arthroscopic debridement and decompression for selected rotator cuff tears: clinical results, pathomechanics, and patient selection based on biomechanical parameters, *Orthop Clin North Am* 24:111, 1993.
99. Itoi E, Tabata S: Conservative treatment of rotator cuff tears, *Clin Orthop Relat Res* 275:165, 1992.
100. Bartolozzi A, Andreychik D, Ahmad S: Determinants of outcome in the treatment of rotator cuff disease, *Clin Orthop Relat Res* 308:90, 1994.

CHAPTER

13

John C. Gray

Visceral Referred Pain to the Shoulder

An important component of the initial orthopedic evaluation is the differentiation of the causes of the patient's pain complaints between a musculoskeletal origin and a visceral pathologic condition or disease. Screening for visceral disease is important for several reasons, including the following: (1) many diseases mimic orthopedic pain and symptoms, and a subsequent delay in diagnosis and treatment may lead to severe morbidity or death; (2) a notable increase is reported in the number of people who are more than 60 years old who seek orthopedic medical care, and this patient population is at the greatest risk for visceral disease; (3) as of June 2010, 46 states in the United States had unlimited or provisional direct access to physical therapy services; (4) the physical therapy profession is committed to entry-level Doctor of Physical Therapy degree programs and complete autonomous practice by the year 2020[1]; (5) an aggressive managed care environment in some states encourages primary care physicians to limit the number of referrals to specialists, as well as to limit referrals for diagnostic testing; and, finally, (6) comorbid medical problems are important to identify because they have an impact on treatment planning with respect to safety issues, selection of the appropriate interventions (manual therapy, exercise, modalities, home management strategies, ergonomic advice, diet and nutritional advice), and prognosis. The physical therapist in an outpatient orthopedic setting is evaluating and treating patients who may have greater morbidity and may be more acutely ill than the patients who were referred for outpatient physical therapy 20 years ago. Boissonnault and Koopmeiners[2] found, in their study, that approximately 50% of all the patients referred for outpatient orthopedic physical therapy have at least one of the following diagnoses: high blood pressure, depression, asthma, chemical dependency, anemia, thyroid problems, cancer, diabetes, rheumatoid arthritis, kidney problems, hepatitis, or heart attack.

Pain may be defined as an unpleasant sensory and emotional experience associated with actual or potential tissue damage.[3] True visceral pain can be experienced within the involved viscus.[4,5] It is often described as deep, dull, achy, colicky, and poorly localized.[4-6] Visceral injury or disease can elicit a strong autonomic reflex phenomenon, including sudomotor changes (increased sweating), vasomotor responses (blood vessel), changes in arterial pressure and heart rate, and an intense psychic or emotional reaction.[3,5,7] Viscera are innervated by nociceptors (see Fig 13-2).[4,8] These free nerve endings are found in the loose connective tissue walls of the viscus, including the epithelial and serous linings, and in the walls of the local blood vessels in the viscus.[4] After activation of these nociceptors by sufficient chemical or mechanical stimulation, neural information is transmitted along small unmyelinated type C nerve fibers within sympathetic and parasympathetic nerves.[4,8-10] This information is subsequently relayed to the mixed spinal nerve, the dorsal root, and into the dorsal horn of the spinal cord. Second-order neurons in the dorsal horn project into the anterior-lateral system.[8] In the anterior-lateral system, nociceptive impulses ascend through the spinothalamic, spinoreticular, and spinomesencephalic tracts.[8] The targets in the brain for these tracts are the thalamus, reticular formation, and midbrain, respectively.[8]

Chemical stimulation of nociceptors may result from a buildup of metabolic end products, such as bradykinins or proteolytic enzymes, secondary to ischemia of the viscus.[4] Prolonged spasm or distention of the smooth muscle wall of viscera can cause ischemia secondary to a collapse of the microvascular network within the viscus.[4] Chemicals, such as acidic gastric fluid, can leak through a gastric or duodenal ulcer into the peritoneal cavity, with resulting local abdominal pain.[4,11] Mechanical stimulation of visceral nociceptors can occur secondary to torsion and traction of the mesentery, distention of a hollow viscus, or impaction.[3-7] Distention may result from a local obstruction, such as a kidney stone, or from local edema caused by infection or inflammation.[4] Spasm of visceral smooth muscle may also be a sufficient mechanical stimulus to activate the nociceptors of the involved viscus.[4,6,11]

Visceral pain is not uncommon in patients suffering from neoplastic disease. Pain complaints in patients with cancer have several origins. *Somatic pain* results from activation of nociceptors in cutaneous and deep tissues (e.g., tumor metastasis to bone) and is usually constant and localized.[3] Visceral pain results from stretching and distending, or from the production of an inflammatory response and the release of algesic chemicals in the vicinity of nociceptors.[3-5] This inflammation can provoke a central sensitization phenomenon (see Chapter 5) that results in a lowering of the threshold of activation of neurons in the dorsal horn, which can subsequently produce referred hyperalgesia (exaggerated response to a painful stimulus).[12] Metastatic tumor infiltration of bone and gastrointestinal and genitourinary tumors that invade abdominal and pelvic viscera are very common causes of pain in patients with cancer.[3] *Deafferentation pain* results from injury to the peripheral or central nervous system as a result of tumor compression or infiltration of peripheral nerves or the spinal cord. This type of pain also results from injury to peripheral nerves as a result of surgery, chemotherapy, or radiation therapy for cancer.[3] Examples are metastatic or radiation-induced brachial or lumbosacral plexopathies, epidural spinal cord or cauda equina compression, and postherpetic neuralgia.[3]

Investigators have observed that visceral disease produces not only orthopedic-like pain, but also true orthopedic dysfunction.[13,14] For example, pain referred to the T4 spinal segment from cardiac tissue (angina) may cause reflex muscle guarding of the tonic muscles surrounding T4 and may therefore interfere with normal mobility. This process may then produce movement around a nonphysiologic axis at that segment that predisposes the segment to injury. Even in the absence of acute injury, hypomobility at T4, induced by muscle guarding, can inhibit full flexion and abduction at the shoulder. Subsequently, this situation could initiate a cascade of events leading to shoulder impingement and rotator cuff tendinopathy (see Fig. 5-6). This patient, for example, with signs and symptoms consistent with supraspinatus tendinosis, may experience a prolonged rehabilitation effort if the T4 dysfunction and cardiac symptoms are not addressed.

A thorough physical examination of the cervical and thoracic spine, ribcage, and shoulder is important to identify impairments and to determine whether a musculoskeletal reason for the patient's shoulder pain exists. Two important aspects of the orthopedic evaluation that help the clinician to screen for visceral pathologic condition or disease are a careful history and palpation (Box 13-1).

A self-administered patient questionnaire (Fig. 13-1) is also useful as a quick screen for a possible visceral pathologic condition or disease. For example, if a patient has a few checks under the "yes" column for pulmonary, then the physical therapist should refer to the "Lung" section later in this chapter. This approach allows the physical therapist to analyze the patient's signs and symptoms to see whether they correlate with a possible medical disorder in the lung. The idea is not to diagnose visceral disease, which should be left to the physician, but rather to assess whether the patient's symptoms

BOX 13-1 Questions During a Patient Visit and Warning Signs That Can Be Garnered from Those Questions

Questions that Should Be Part of Your Standard Interview

- Describe the first and last time you experienced these same complaints.
- Are your symptoms the result of a trauma, or are they of a gradual or insidious onset?
- Was it a macrotrauma (motor vehicle accident, fall, or work or sports injury) or repeated microtrauma (overuse injury or cumulative trauma disorder)?
- What was the mechanism of injury?
- Do you have any other complaints of pain throughout the rest of your body: head, neck, temporomandibular joint (TMJ), chest, back, abdomen, arms, or legs?
- Do you have any other symptoms throughout the rest of your body: headaches, tinnitus, vision changes, nausea, vomiting, dizziness, shortness of breath, weakness, fatigue, fever, bowel or bladder changes, numbness, tingling, or pins or needles?
- Is your pain worse while sleeping?
- Do certain positions or activities change your pain, by either aggravating or relieving your symptoms?
- Does eating or digesting a meal affect your pain?
- Does bowel or bladder activity affect your pain?
- Does coughing, laughing, or deep breathing affect your pain?
- Does your shoulder pain get worse with exertional activities, such as climbing stairs, that do not directly involve your shoulder?

Warning Signs that May Indicate a Possible Visceral Pathologic Condition or Disease

- Pain is constant.
- The onset of pain is not related to trauma or chronic overuse.
- Pain is described as throbbing, pulsating, deep aching, knifelike, or colicky.
- Rest does not relieve pain or symptoms.
- Constitutional symptoms are present: fever, night sweats, nausea, vomiting, pale skin, dizziness, fatigue, or unexplained weight loss.
- Pain is worse during sleep.
- Pain does not change with changes in arm position or upper extremity activity.
- Pain changes in relation to organ function (eating, bowel or bladder activity, or coughing or deep breathing).
- Indigestion, diarrhea, constipation, or rectal bleeding is present.
- Shoulder pain increases with exertion that does not stress the shoulder, such as walking or climbing stairs.

Data from Boissonnault WG, Bass C: Pathological origins of trunk and neck pain: pelvic and abdominal visceral disorders, *J Orthop Sports Phys Ther* 12:192, 1990; and Goodman CC, Snyder TEK: Introduction to differential screening in physical therapy. In *Differential diagnosis in physical therapy,* ed 2, Philadelphia, 1995, Saunders.

are orthopedic in origin, to acknowledge comorbid disease, and to refer the patient for medical follow-up for an undiagnosed disorder that is not musculoskeletal.

The second important aspect of the evaluation is palpation. Palpation should include the lymph nodes (for infection or neoplasm)—which are normally 1 to 2 cm—in the cervical (medial border of sternocleidomastoid, anterior to upper trapezius muscle), supraclavicular, axillary, and femoral triangle regions.[4,15,16] Abnormal findings are swollen, tender, or immovable lymph nodes.[16] The physical therapist palpates the abdomen for muscle rigidity and significant local tenderness (possible visceral disease) or for a large, pulsatile mass (indicative of an aortic aneurysm).[4,16,17] The right upper abdominal quadrant is palpated to assess the liver, gallbladder, and portions of the small and large intestines, whereas the left upper abdominal quadrant is palpated to assess the stomach,

Patient Questionnaire

Name ________________ Date ________

	Yes		No
Age		______	
Height		______	
Weight		______	
Fever and/or chills	______		______
Unexplained weight change	______		______
Night pain/disturbed sleep	______		______
Episode of fainting	______		______
Dry mouth (difficulty swallowing)	______		______
Dry eyes (red, itchy, sandy)	______		______
History of illness prior to onset of pain	______		______
History of cancer	______		______
Family history of cancer	______		______
Recent surgery (dental also)	______		______
Do you self inject medicines/drugs	______		______
Diabetic	______		______
Pain of gradual onset (no trauma)	______		______
Constant pain	______		______
Pain worse at night	______		______
Pain relieved by rest	______		______
Pulmonary			
History of smoking	______		______
Shortness of breath	______		______
Fatigue	______		______
Wheezing or prolonged cough	______		______
History of asthma, emphysema or COPD	______		______
History of pneumonia or tuberculosis	______		______
Cardiovascular			
Heart murmur/heart valve problem	______		______
History of heart problems	______		______
Sweating with pain	______		______
Rapid throbbing or fluttering of heart	______		______
High blood pressure	______		______
Dizziness (sit to stand)	______		______
Swelling in extremities	______		______
History of rheumatic fever	______		______
Elevated cholesterol level	______		______
Family history of heart disease	______		______
Pain/symptoms increase with walking or stair climbing and relieved with rest	______		______
Pregnant women only			
Constant backache	______		______
Increased uterine contractions	______		______
Menstrual cramps	______		______
Constant pelvic pressure	______		______
Increased amount of vaginal discharge	______		______
Increased consistency of vaginal discharge	______		______
Color change of vaginal discharge	______		______
Increased frequency of urination	______		______

A

Figure 13-1 A and **B**, Self-administered patient questionnaire.

(Continued)

Patient Questionnaire

Female urogenital system (women only)

	Yes	No
Date of last menses		
Are you pregnant		
Painful urination		
Blood in urine		
Difficulty controlling urination		
Change in the frequency of urination		
Increase in urgency of urination		
History of urinary infection		
Post-menopausal vaginal bleeding		
Vaginal discharge		
Painful menses		
Painful intercourse		
History of infertility		
History of venereal disease		
History of endometriosis		
Pain changes in relation to menstrual cycle		

Gastrointestinal

	Yes	No
Difficulty in swallowing		
Nausea		
Heartburn		
Vomiting		
Food intolerances		
Constipation		
Diarrhea		
Change in color of stools		
Rectal bleeding		
History of liver or gallbladder problems		
History of stomach or GI problems		
Indigestion		
Loss of appetite		
Pain worse when lying on your back		
Pain change due to bowel/bladder activity		
Pain change during or after meals		

Male urogenital system (men only)

	Yes	No
Painful urination		
Blood in urine		
Difficulty controlling urination		
Change in frequency of urination		
Increase in urinary urgency		
Decreased force of urinary flow		
Urethral discharge		
History of urinary infection		
History of venereal disease		
Impotence		
Pain with ejaculation		
History of swollen testes		

B

Figure 13-1—cont'd

spleen, tail of the pancreas, and portions of the small and large intestines.[17] The kidneys lie deep posteriorly in the left and right upper abdominal quadrants. The appendix and large intestine are found in the right lower quadrant, whereas other portions of the large intestine may be found in the left lower quadrant.[17] A tender mass in the femoral triangle or groin area may indicate a hernia.[17] When evaluating abdominal tenderness, the physical therapist must differentiate the source as the superficial myofascial wall or the deep viscera. If palpable tenderness is elicited at rest and again with the abdominal wall contracted, then the symptoms are probably originating from the myofascial abdominal wall.[17] If, however, the palpable tenderness disappears when the abdominal muscles are contracted, then deep visceral disease should be suspected.[17] Again, the objective is not to diagnose medical disease, but to know when to refer the patient for medical follow-up. Even though the patient's shoulder pain may not be visceral in origin, the physical therapist may be the first to discover a comorbid medical problem.

The ability to palpate and interpret peripheral pulses is another important diagnostic tool for the physical therapist. Palpating the arterial pulses can help to identify cardiovascular and peripheral vascular disease. The arterial pulses may be palpated in the upper extremity (axillary artery in the axilla, brachial artery in the cubital fossa, and ulnar and radial arteries at the wrist) and lower extremity (femoral artery at the femoral triangle, popliteal artery at the popliteal fossa, posterior tibialis artery posterior to the medial malleolus, and dorsal pedis artery at the base of the first and second metatarsal bones).[4,16,18,19] When palpating a pulse, the therapist needs to compare the amplitude and force of pulsations in one artery with those in the corresponding vessel on the opposite side.[18] Palpation of the artery should be performed with a light pressure and a sensitive touch. If the pressure is firm, then the physical therapist risks not being able to perceive a weak pulse or misinterpreting his or her own pulse as that of the patient's.[18] Pulsations may be recorded as normal (4), slightly (3), moderately (2), or markedly reduced (1), or absent (0).[18]

The physical therapist must be alert and aware of older elderly patients who have osteoarthritis, degenerative joint disease (DJD), degenerative disk disease (DDD), or spondylosis. One should not assume that the DJD seen on the patient's imaging studies is the source of the pain. Many asymptomatic older persons have abnormal radiographs indicating the presence of these diseases. The older members of society are at a greater risk for visceral abnormalities and disease. In addition, previously healed orthopedic injuries may appear to be symptomatic, but the pain could be a "misinterpretation" by the brain as a result of facilitation from a segmentally related visceral organ in a diseased state.[20,21]

THEORIES ON VISCERAL REFERRED PAIN

1. Referred pain is pain experienced in tissues that are not the site of tissue damage and whose afferent or efferent neurons are not physically involved in any way.[22]
2. Pain happens within the central nervous system, not in the damaged tissue itself. Pain does not really happen in the hands, feet, or head. It happens in the images of the hands, feet, or head that are held in the brain.[22]
3. Referred pain from deep somatic structures is often indistinguishable from visceral referred pain.[23]
4. Visceral pain fibers constitute less than 10% of the total afferent input to the lower thoracic segments of the spinal cord and are activated rarely.[8] In this way, a visceral stimulus may be mistaken for the more familiar somatic pain.[8]
5. Visceral referred pain may be caused by misinterpretation by the sensory cortex.[24] Over the years, specific cortical cells are repeatedly stimulated by nociceptive activity from a specific area of the skin. When nociceptors of a viscus are eventually stimulated chemically or mechanically, these same sensory cortex cells may become stimulated, and the cortex may interpret the origin of this sensory input based on past experience. The pain therefore is perceived to arise from the area of skin that has repeatedly stimulated these cortical cells in the past. The referred pain may lie within the dermatome of those spinal segments that receive sensory information from the viscera.[24]

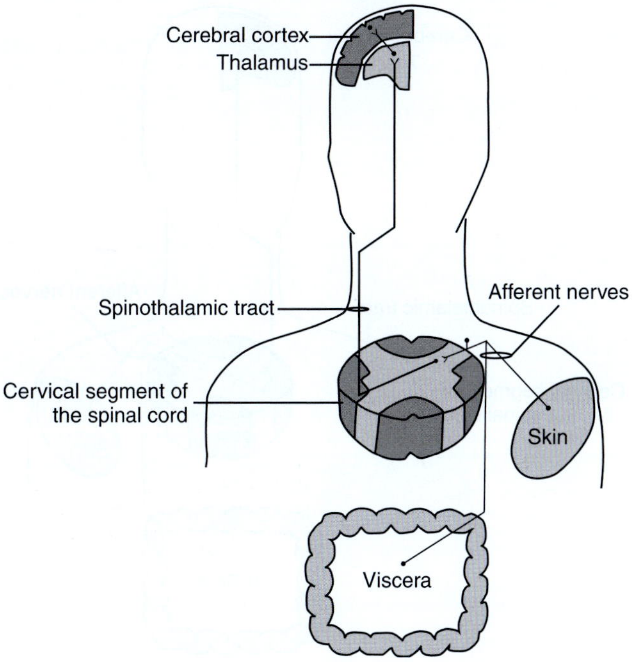

Figure 13-2 Schematic drawing of a single afferent nerve fiber receiving input from both skin and viscera.

6. Sensory fibers dichotomize as they "leave" the spinal cord, with one branch passing to a viscus as the other branch travels to a site of reference in muscle or skin (Fig. 13-2).[25,26]
7. Visceral nociceptor activity converges with input from somatic nociceptors into common pools of spinothalamic tract cells in the dorsal horn of the spinal cord. Visceral pain is then referred to remote cutaneous sites because the brain misinterprets the input as coming from a peripheral cutaneous source, which frequently bombards the central nervous system with sensory stimuli (Fig. 13-3).[3,5-8,17,23,27-29]

VISCERA CAPABLE OF REFERRING PAIN TO THE SHOULDER

Diaphragm

Although the diaphragm is a musculotendinous structure and not a viscus, it is interesting in terms of the distance it refers its pain to the shoulder. In addition, many viscera (lung, esophagus, stomach, liver, and pancreas) can refer pain to the shoulder through contact with the diaphragm (Fig. 13-4).[4] The central portion of the diaphragm, which is segmentally innervated by cervical nerves C3 to C5 through the phrenic nerve, can refer pain to the shoulder.[4,25,29-36] The peripheral portion of the diaphragm is innervated by the lower six or seven intercostal nerves and does not refer pain to the shoulder.[37] In the rat, cervical (C3, C4) dorsal root ganglion cells were seen that had collateral nerve fibers, which emanated

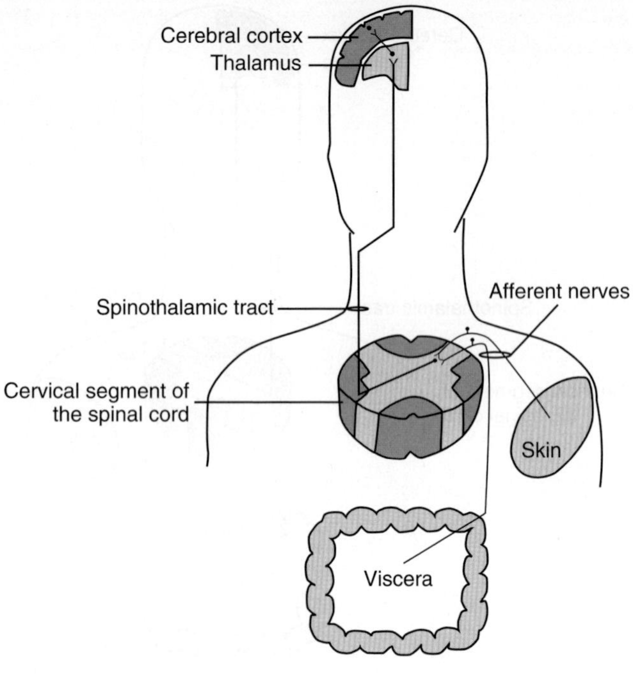

Figure 13-3 Schematic drawing of a visceral afferent nerve and a somatic afferent nerve converging onto the same spinothalamic tract cell in the dorsal horn of the spinal cord.

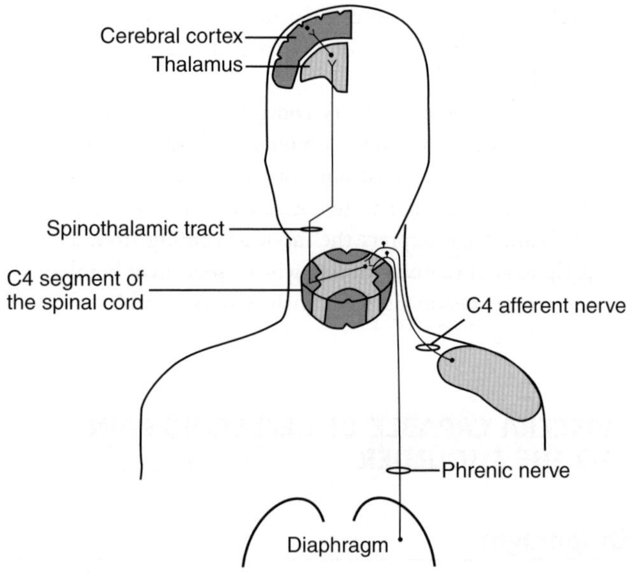

Figure 13-4 Schematic drawing of an afferent nerve from the diaphragm converging onto the same spinothalamic tract cell as a somatic afferent nerve from the skin of the shoulder.

from both the diaphragm and the skin of the shoulder (see Fig. 13-2).[25] Patients usually have a history of direct or indirect (e.g., severe twisting motions) trauma to the rib cage and diaphragm. Diaphragmatic strain may occur secondary to strong, sudden bursts of trunk rotation in a poorly conditioned athlete playing golf, tennis, or racquetball, for instance.

Symptoms

Pain in the shoulder is most often felt at the top or posterior portions of the shoulder, that is, at the superior angle of the scapula, in the suprascapular region, or along the upper trapezius muscle.[30,31] The upper arm and anterior portions of the shoulder are not common areas of referred pain for the diaphragm. Normally, the patient has no complaints of pain in the region of the diaphragm, unless the patient suffered trauma or a musculoskeletal strain to the surrounding tissues.

Signs

Shoulder pain is reproduced or exacerbated by deep breathing, coughing, or sneezing.[32,35,36] The patient may note local tenderness during palpation of the diaphragm, but generally no shoulder pain is elicited because it is difficult to reach the central portion of the diaphragm, and the peripheral portion does not refer pain to the shoulder. Full active and passive shoulder elevation in standing may cause pain because this motion changes the shape of the rib cage and subsequently puts tension on the diaphragm.[32] If the diaphragm is the primary source of the patient's referred shoulder pain, then active range of motion (AROM), passive ROM (PROM), and special tests of the shoulder with the patient seated and the thoracic spine in a slumped or flexed posture (to minimize stress on the diaphragm) should not increase the patient's pain.

Pneumoperitoneum

Pneumoperitoneum, or air in the peritoneal cavity, can refer pain to the shoulder because of pressure on the central portion of the diaphragm by trapped air (see Fig. 13-4).[30-32,38-43] Patients have a history of acute visceral pain (before perforation), recent abdominal or vaginal surgery, current pregnancy, or recent parturition. Air may be released into the peritoneal cavity in several different ways. Perforation of an abdominal viscus can release air into the peritoneum.[30,40,44] Examples include peptic ulcer, acute pancreatitis, perforated appendix, and splenic infarct or rupture.[32,40,44] Abdominal or vaginal surgical procedures that allow free air to enter and become trapped within the peritoneal cavity, or operations that necessitate insufflation of the peritoneum, are another source of referred pain to the shoulder.[45] Although rare, certain activities during pregnancy, within 6 weeks post partum, or following abdominal or vaginal surgery can lead to pneumoperitoneum. These include menstruation, effervescent vaginal douching, knee to chest stretching exercises, vigorous sexual intercourse, and orogenital insufflation.[38,39,41,42] The last two activities in rare cases can be fatal because of air embolism.[38,39,41-43] To create pneumoperitoneum under these circumstances, air must first enter the vagina before it passes through a patent os cervix to enter the body cavity of the cervix and must subsequently travel through the uterine tube before escaping into the peritoneal cavity (Fig. 13-5). To create air embolism, the air under positive pressure is introduced through the endometrium into dilated vessels of the uterine wall. The greatest risk is to

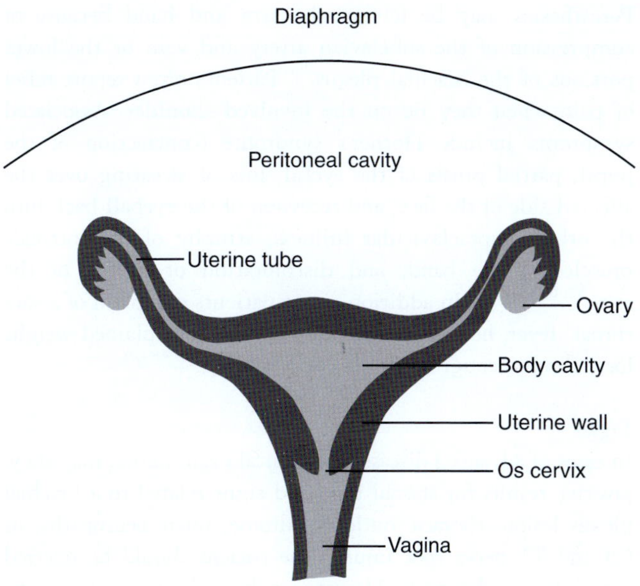

Figure 13-5 Schematic drawing of the pathway that air must travel to create pneumoperitoneum.

women who have had trauma to their uterine wall (e.g., recent surgery, biopsy or an intrauterine device) that would allow blood vessels to come in contact with air forced into the uterus. Once the air has entered the venous drainage of the uterus, it travels up the inferior vena cava. If large amounts of air reach the heart rapidly, the air bubbles will prevent the blood from flowing into the pulmonary artery; cardiac arrest is then possible.

Symptoms

The patient may complain of acute or spasmodic shoulder or abdominal pain, especially in the case of perforated abdominal viscus. In the case of splenic infarct or rupture, the pain is in the left shoulder.[44] Symptoms vary depending on which viscus is perforated.

Pain in the shoulder is most often felt at the top or posterior portions of the shoulder, that is, at the superior angle of the scapula, in the suprascapular region, or along the upper trapezius muscle.[30,31] The upper arm and anterior portions of the shoulder are not common areas of referred pain for the diaphragm. Normally, the patient has no complaints of pain directly attributable to the diaphragm.

Signs

Shoulder pain may be reproduced or exacerbated by deep breathing, coughing, or sneezing.[32,35,36] The patient often notes no local tenderness during palpation of the diaphragm because the peripheral portion has not been traumatized. Full active and passive shoulder elevation in standing may cause pain because this motion changes the shape of the rib cage and subsequently puts tension on the diaphragm.[32] If the diaphragm is the primary source of the patient's referred shoulder pain, then AROM, PROM, and special tests of the shoulder with the patient seated and the thoracic spine in a slumped or flexed posture (to minimize stress on the diaphragm) should not increase the patient's pain. In the case of perforated viscus, pain or rigidity are noted with abdominal palpation. An upright plain anterior-posterior radiograph demonstrates free intraperitoneal air under one or both hemidiaphragms.[38]

Lung

The lung, which is innervated by thoracic nerves T5-6, is capable of referring pain from two distinct diseases to the shoulder.[4,30,32,33,36,46-59] The first is pulmonary infarction, which is often secondary to pulmonary embolism. The second is Pancoast's tumor.[32,49]

Pulmonary Infarction

The most common cause of pulmonary embolism is deep venous thrombosis (DVT) originating in the proximal deep venous system of the lower legs.[49] Risk factors for DVT include recent surgery, blood stasis caused by bed rest, endothelial (blood vessel) injury from surgery or trauma, and a state of hypercoagulation.[49] Other risk factors include congestive heart failure, trauma, surgery (especially of the hip, knee, and prostate), age greater than 50 years, infection, diabetes, obesity, pregnancy, and oral contraceptive use.[49] Pain is normally referred to the shoulder because of contact with the central portion of the diaphragm (see Fig. 13-4).[30-32] This potentially fatal condition necessitates rapid referral for emergency medical attention.

Symptoms

When the inferior lobe of the lung is involved and is in contact with the diaphragm, the referred pain is most often felt at the top or posterior portions of the shoulder, that is, at the superior angle of the scapula, in the suprascapular region, or along the upper trapezius muscle.[30,31] The upper arm and anterior portions of the shoulder are not common areas of referred pain for the diaphragm. The region surrounding the diaphragm may be free of pain. When the diaphragm is not involved, pain may be referred to the scapula or interscapular region. Patients usually report the relief of pain when they are lying on the involved shoulder. Symptoms related directly to pulmonary embolism may include swollen and painful legs with walking, acute dyspnea or tachypnea, chest pain, tachycardia, low-grade fever, rales, diffuse wheezing, decreased breath sounds, persistent cough, restlessness, and acute anxiety.[49-51]

Signs

Shoulder pain may be reproduced or exacerbated in cases with diaphragmatic irritation by deep breathing, coughing, or sneezing.[32,35] The patient often notes no local tenderness during palpation of the diaphragm because the peripheral portion has not been traumatized. Full active and passive shoulder elevation in standing may cause pain because this motion changes the shape of the rib cage and subsequently puts tension on the diaphragm.[32] If the diaphragm is the primary source of the patient's referred shoulder pain, then AROM, PROM, and special tests of the shoulder with the patient seated and the thoracic spine in a slumped or flexed posture (to minimize stress on the diaphragm) should not increase the patient's pain. Chest radiographs, arterial blood gas studies, pulmonary angiography, and ventilation-perfusion scintigraphy are the most common diagnostic tools.[52] Plain radiographs can miss the pulmonary infarct if it is in the inferior lobe of the lung and is hidden by the dome of the diaphragm.[32]

Pancoast's Tumor

Pancoast's tumor occurs in the apical portion of the lung.[30,32,36,46,48,49,53,54] Lung cancer is the most common fatal cancer in both men and women.[53] It commonly refers pain to the supraclavicular fossa, usually on the right side.[32] Pain from Pancoast's tumor may be referred to the shoulder because of the involvement of the upper ribs.[54] Shoulder and arm pain may also occur secondary to contact between the cancerous lobes of the lung and the eighth cervical (C8) and first thoracic (T1) nerves. This contact results in shoulder and upper extremity symptoms similar to those of myocardial infarction, brachial plexus lesion, thoracic outlet syndrome, ulnar neuropathy, and C8 or T1 nerve root injury.[36,46,48,49,53,54] The chest wall and subpleural lymphatics are often invaded by the tumor.[54] Other structures that may be involved include the subclavian artery and vein, internal jugular vein, phrenic nerve, vagus nerve, common carotid artery, recurrent laryngeal nerve, sympathetic chain, and stellate ganglion.[46,48,54] Cancer can metastasize to the lungs from carcinomas in the kidney, breast, pancreas, colon, or uterus.[49] Smoking is a risk factor.[36,49] The peak incidence occurs in smokers who are approximately 60 years of age.[36] Suspicions should be raised in patients who are more 50 years of age, have a long history of smoking, and present with vague or equivocal musculoskeletal signs.

The lung itself is a common source of metastatic cancer to the bone, liver, adrenal glands, and brain.[49,53] Symptoms associated with cancer of the spine include a deep, dull ache that may be unrelieved by rest.[53] Pain often precedes a pathologic fracture.[53] If a fracture is present, then the pain may be sharp, localized, and associated with swelling.[53] Pain is often reproduced by mechanical stress, which simulates pure musculoskeletal dysfunction. Neurologic signs and symptoms, present in some patients, are caused by compression of the spinal cord, C8, or T1 nerves. Percussion of a spinous process with a reflex hammer exacerbates pain from the involved vertebrae.[53] A tuning fork may also be used to elicit symptoms from the involved vertebrae.

Symptoms

Shoulder pain is the symptom present in more than 90% of patients with Pancoast's tumor.[46,49] Arm pain is also common, often involving the medial aspect of the forearm and hand, including the fourth and fifth digits.[46,48,54] Paresthesias may be felt in the arm and hand because of compression of the subclavian artery and vein or the lower portions of the brachial plexus.[54] Patients often report relief of pain when they lie on the involved shoulder. Associated symptoms include Horner's syndrome (contraction of the pupil, partial ptosis of the eyelid, loss of sweating over the affected side of the face, and recession of the eyeball back into the orbit), supraclavicular fullness, atrophy of the intrinsic muscles of the hand, and discoloration or edema of the arm.[32,46,48,49,54] In addition, some patients complain of a sore throat, fever, hoarseness, bloody sputum, unexplained weight loss, chronic cough, dyspnea, or wheezing.[36,48-50]

Signs

In cases of advanced disease, the clinical examination may show positive results for special tests and signs related to a brachial plexus lesion, thoracic outlet syndrome, ulnar neuropathy, or C8 and T1 nerve root injury. The patient should be referred for a chest radiograph. However, a bone lesion of the spine may be detected before a lung lesion on a plain radiograph because lung cancer metastasizes to the bone early.[49-53]

Esophagus

The esophagus, which is segmentally innervated by thoracic nerves T4 to T6, can refer pain to the shoulder through contact with the central portion of the diaphragm (see Fig. 13-4).[4,17,55] Esophageal pain is transmitted by afferents in the splanchnic and thoracic sympathetic nerves.[8] The primary afferent fibers, both A-delta and C-fiber neurons, pass through the paravertebral sympathetic chain and the rami communicantes to join the spinal nerve and enter the dorsal root ganglia before they enter the dorsal horn of the spinal cord.[8] Referred pain is thought to occur through convergence of visceral (cardiac and esophageal) and somatic afferents onto the same dorsal horn neurons (see Fig. 13-3).[8,56]

Symptoms

When the diseased esophagus is in contact with the diaphragm, the referred pain is most often felt at the top or posterior portions of the shoulder, that is, at the superior angle of the scapula, in the suprascapular region, or along the upper trapezius muscle.[30,31] The upper arm and anterior portions of the shoulder are not common areas of referred pain for the diaphragm. The region surrounding the diaphragm may be free of pain. When the diaphragm is not involved, pain may be referred to the scapula or interscapular region. Patients often report that the pain in the shoulder is exacerbated during or following meals.[4] They may also complain of substernal chest, neck, or back pain.[50] Other symptoms include difficulty swallowing, weight loss, and (in the late stages) drooling.[50] Symptoms associated with esophageal cancer are bloody cough, hoarseness, sore throat, nausea, vomiting, fever, hiccups, and bad breath.[50] Symptoms associated with reflux esophagitis are regurgitation, frequent vomiting, and a dry nocturnal cough.[50]

The patient complains of heartburn that is aggravated by strenuous exercise or by bending over or lying down and is relieved by sitting up or taking antacids.[50]

Signs

Diagnostic tests include a positive result of 24-hour intraesophageal pH and pressure recordings, acid perfusion, edrophonium stimulation, balloon distention, and ergonovine stimulation.[4,57,58] Shoulder pain, in cases with diaphragmatic irritation, may be reproduced or exacerbated by deep breathing, coughing, or sneezing.[32,35,36] The patient often notes no local tenderness during palpation of the diaphragm because the peripheral portion has not been traumatized. Full active and passive shoulder elevation in standing may cause pain because this motion changes the shape of the rib cage and subsequently puts tension on the diaphragm.[32] If the diaphragm is the primary source of the patient's referred shoulder pain, then AROM, PROM, and special tests of the shoulder with the patient seated and the thoracic spine in a slumped or flexed posture (to minimize stress on the diaphragm) should not increase the patient's pain.

Heart

The heart, which is innervated by thoracic nerves T1 to T5, can refer pain to the shoulder.[4,30-33,55,59] Cardiac afferent fibers have shown evidence of convergence with esophageal afferents and somatic afferents in the upper thoracic spinal cord.[23] In fact, esophageal chest pain is known to mimic angina pectoris.[57] In addition, convergence has been demonstrated among cardiac afferents, abdominal visceral afferents (e.g., gallbladder), and somatic afferents in the lower thoracic spinal cord.[23,56] Convergence has also been noted with proximal somatic afferents (shoulder), phrenic (diaphragm), and cardiopulmonary spinal afferents onto the cervical spinothalamic tract neurons (Fig. 13-6).[29] This explains how diaphragmatic disease and cardiac disease are both able to refer pain to the shoulder and to other cervical-related dermatomes. Heart disease is most common in men more than 40 years old and is associated with smoking, obesity, high blood pressure, diabetes, and physical inactivity.[36,60] Timely recognition of a cardiac problem cannot be overstated. Coronary artery disease may manifest as angina, myocardial infarction, heart failure, or sudden death.[36]

Symptoms

The patient may complain of pain in the left shoulder that is often associated with reports of numbness and tingling in the left hand.[19,31,50,60] Pain may also be felt in the chest, neck, arm (usually the left, and along a C8 and T1 distribution), jaw, posterior thorax, or epigastrium.[19,36,50,60] The patient may describe tightness, pressure sensations, throbbing, cramping, or aching in the foregoing areas.[19,36] Other symptoms include exertion and nocturnal dyspnea, ankle edema, palpitations, easy fatigability, syncope, weakness, anxiety, profuse sweating, nausea, vomiting, tachycardia, and bradycardia.[19,36,50]

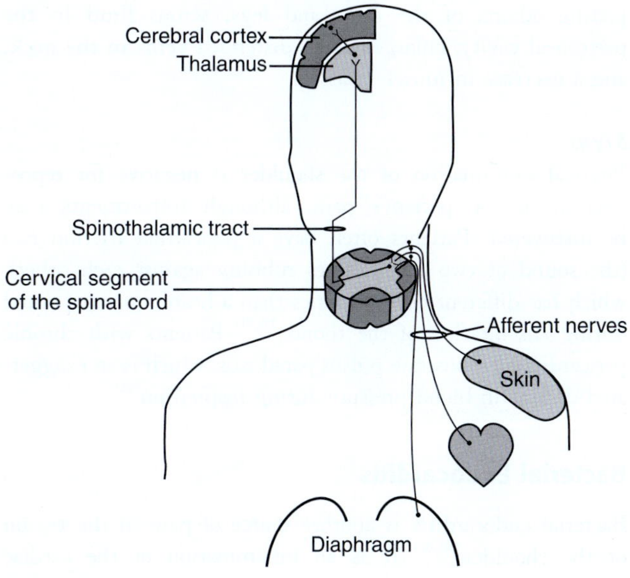

Figure 13-6 Schematic drawing of a somatic afferent nerve (shoulder), a phrenic nerve (diaphragm), and a cardiopulmonary afferent nerve all converging onto the same spinothalamic tract neuron.

Signs

The patient has a history of shoulder or chest pain (angina) on effort or exercise, such as a brisk walk or climbing stairs, not associated with movements of the shoulder.[19] Symptoms are relieved by rest.[19] The patient may have a resting pulse greater than 100 or less than 50 beats per minute.[36] Blood pressure consistently higher than 160/90 mm Hg is a positive sign.[36] Nitroglycerin provides immediate relief of symptoms. Physical examination of the shoulder is negative for reproduction of the patient's pain, although impairments may be discovered. The patient should be referred for electrocardiogram, blood test (increased creatine phosphokinase levels), treadmill with echocardiogram, or angiography.

Pericarditis

The heart, which is innervated by thoracic nerves T1 to T5, is capable of referring pain to the shoulder in cases of pericarditis.[4,36,60] *Pericarditis* is an inflammation of the sac surrounding the heart.[36,60] This disorder has numerous causes, including viral and bacterial infection, trauma, cancer, collagen vascular disease, uremia, cardiac surgery, myocardial infarction, radiation therapy, and aortic dissection.[19,36,60]

Symptoms

The patient usually has a sharp, burning pain in the chest or left shoulder.[36,50,60] Pain may be evoked by deep breathing, coughing, or lying flat and relieved by sitting up and leaning forward.[19,36,50,60] Other symptoms include fever, tachycardia, and dyspnea.[50] Symptoms of chronic pericarditis include pitting edema of the arms and legs, serous fluid in the peritoneal cavity, enlarged liver, distended veins in the neck, and a decrease in muscle mass.[50]

Signs

Physical examination of the shoulder is negative for reproduction of the patient's pain, although impairments may be discovered. Patients often have a pericardial friction rub (the sound of two dry surfaces rubbing against each other), which has different characteristics than a heart murmur, noted during auscultation of the thorax.[19,50] Patients with chronic pericarditis demonstrate pulsus paradoxus, which is an exaggerated decline in blood pressure during inspiration.[50]

Bacterial Endocarditis

Bacterial endocarditis is another source of pain in the region of the shoulder.[60-62] It is an inflammation of the cardiac endothelium overlying a heart valve that is caused by a bacterial infection.[19,60] If left undiagnosed and untreated, bacterial endocarditis can be fatal.[61,62] The patient's history often indicates no trauma or previous occurrence of these symptoms. Pain is most common in the glenohumeral, sternoclavicular, or acromioclavicular joints, and symptoms are usually confined to one joint.[60-62] Symptoms are not caused by referred pain; therefore, the patient has a positive musculoskeletal examination of the involved joint. Articular involvement is thought to be secondary to deposition of large particulate masses (emboli) that contain immune complexes.[60-62] Risk groups for this illness include the following: patients with abnormal cardiac valves, congenital heart disease, and degenerative heart disease (calcific aortic stenosis); parenteral drug abusers; and those with a history of bacteremia.[60-62] Treatment is with antibiotics.[60-62]

Symptoms

Pain is often localized to one of the three true joints of the shoulder. Low back pain, which may mimic a herniated disk and sacroiliac joint pain, is often reported.[60] In approximately 25% of patients, musculoskeletal complaints are the first symptoms of this disease.[60-62] The patient may have an abrupt onset of intermittent shaking chills with fever.[50,60] The patient may also complain of dyspnea and chest pain with cold and painful extremities.[60] Other symptoms include pale skin, weakness, fatigue, night sweats, tachycardia, and weight loss.[19,50,60]

Signs

Palpation of the involved joint reveals warmth, redness, and tenderness.[60-62] Acute synovitis in a single joint, especially the metacarpophalangeal, sternoclavicular, or acromioclavicular joint, which is not commonly involved in other diseases, should raise suspicions of bacterial endocarditis.[61,62] The patient has a heart murmur, positive results of a blood test for anemia, elevated erythrocyte sedimentation rate (ESR), decrease in serum albumin levels, increase in serum globulin concentration, and microhematuria (blood in the urine).[61,62] Symptoms are relieved by antibiotics. Fever is present at some time during the illness.[60-62] Associated signs are dyspnea, peripheral edema, fingernail clubbing, enlarged spleen, anorexia, Roth's spots (small white spots in the retina, usually surrounded by areas of hemorrhage), petechiae (small purplish hemorrhagic spots on the skin), and Janeway's lesions (small red-blue macular lesions) on the palm of the hands or the soles of the feet.[50] Diagnosis may be difficult in older patients, who have a higher frequency of nonpathologic heart murmurs and are less likely to have a fever develop in response to infection.[60-62] A plain radiograph may show destructive changes within the joint (glenohumeral, acromioclavicular, or sternoclavicular) indicative of an infection.[61,62]

Vascular System

Aneurysm

An aneurysm within a subclavian vessel can result in pain at the shoulder.[30-32,50,55] This is a potentially dangerous arterial condition.[36] An *aneurysm* is an abnormal widening of the arterial wall caused by the destruction of the elastic fibers of the middle layer of that wall or by a tear in the inner lining of the arterial wall that allows blood to flow directly into the wall and subsequently widen it.[36] Aortic aneurysms can enlarge and compress pain-sensitive structures in the upper mediastinum and can lead to shoulder pain.[30] These aneurysms generally occur in older patients and slowly enlarge over many years.[36] Rapid morbidity or mortality is expected if an aneurysm ruptures.[36]

Symptoms

Pain in the shoulder may include throbbing and cramping. The patient may also report paresthesia, neck pain, or chest pain.[50] Other symptoms include night sweats, pallor, nausea, weight loss, Raynaud's phenomenon, diplopia, dizziness, and syncope.[50] Symptoms may be aggravated by an increase in activity level (climbing stairs, fast walk, or upper extremity repetitive motions) and relieved by rest.[32]

Signs

Physical examination of the shoulder, especially elevation above 90°, may give a false-positive response to a musculoskeletal test because of stress on the subclavian vessels. Upper extremity repetitive motions that stress the vascular system, but not the shoulders (e.g., elbow flexion and extension with the arms at the side), may help to distinguish this disorder. The patient has a prolonged capillary refill time for the fingers, systemic hypotension, and a weak or absent distal pulse (radial and ulnar arteries at the wrist).[50] Bilateral dilation of the pupils occurs late.[50] A plain radiograph of the chest may or may not allow visualization of the aneurysm.

Arterial Occlusion

Arterial occlusion is usually caused by atherosclerosis or compression of an artery, such as the subclavian artery in thoracic outlet syndrome. Arterial occlusion can manifest as a deep, constant pain in the shoulder, or it can lead to ischemic pain with exercise.[30,63]

Symptoms
Patients complain of pain in the region of the shoulder that may mimic nerve root compression.[64] Other symptoms include paresthesia, coldness, weakness, and fatigue in the involved extremity.[50,64]

Signs
Physical examination of the shoulder, especially elevation above 90°, may give a false-positive response to a musculoskeletal test because of stress on the subclavian vessels. Upper extremity repetitive motions that stress the vascular system, but not the shoulders (e.g., elbow flexion and extension with the arms at the side), may help to distinguish this disorder. Systolic blood pressure is higher, whereas diastolic blood pressure remains unchanged in the involved extremity.[50] The patient has a weak or absent distal pulse (radial and ulnar arteries at the wrist).[50,64] The extremity is cool and cyanotic, and it demonstrates a prolonged capillary refill time.[50] Tachycardia and angina pectoris may also be present.[50] Contrast angiography demonstrates arterial occlusion, which is best seen with the extremity elevated.[64] In the case of thoracic outlet syndrome, results of one of the following tests is abnormal: Adson's test; costoclavicular, hyperabduction, and pectoralis minor stress tests; and the 3-minute flap-arm test (Roo's test).[63-65]

Thrombophlebitis

Thrombophlebitis of the axillary and subclavian veins can also cause shoulder pain (Fig. 13-7).[30,55,66-69] *Thrombophlebitis* is an inflammation of a vein in the presence of a blood clot. This is a serious situation, because emboli may break free and travel to the lung, a potentially fatal condition. The risk of pulmonary embolization for persons with subclavian thrombosis is approximately 12%.[66] DVT of the upper extremity is often caused by venous trauma from repetitive motions of the shoulder, referred to as *effort thrombosis,* in persons with an abnormal thoracic outlet.[66-68] The most common site of compression is near the clavicle, the costocoracoid ligament, and the first rib.[67,68] Repeated compression of the vein can lead to injury and inflammation, which then puts the vein at risk for the formation of a thrombus.[67,68] Other causes of venous thrombosis include the presence of indwelling venous catheters (central lines or pacemaker leads), local compression, radiation, and hypercoagulability.[66-68]

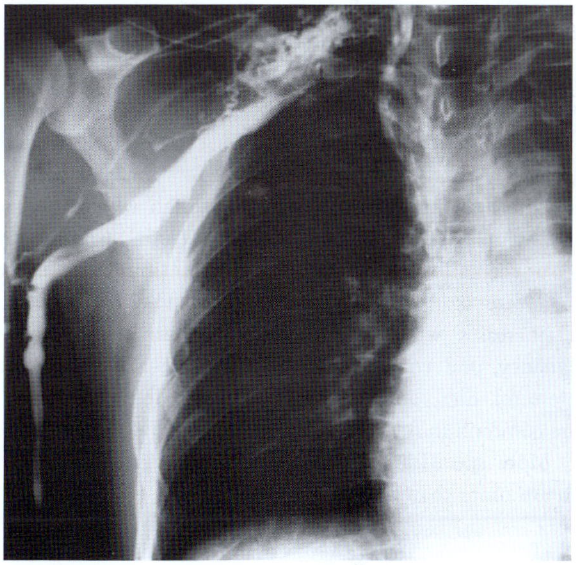

Figure 13-7 Thrombosis of the subclavian vein at the level of the thoracic outlet. (From Rohrer MJ: Vascular problems. In Pappas AM, editor: *Upper extremity injuries in the athlete,* New York, 1995, Churchill Livingstone.)

Symptoms
The patient usually complains of a dull pain in the shoulder and down the arm that may include paresthesia. Fever and chills may be present.[50] The patient may complain of cold and swollen fingers.[67] Patients with effort thrombosis complain of the sudden onset of swelling and cyanosis involving the entire arm.[66] These patients often report a history of upper extremity exertion such as weight lifting or prolonged repetitive motions.[66-68] Symptoms of shortness of breath (SOB), pleuritic chest pain, hemoptysis (expectoration of blood), or a new nonproductive cough suggest pulmonary embolus.[66]

Signs
Physical examination of the shoulder, especially elevation above 90°, may give a false-positive response to a musculoskeletal test because of stress on the axillary and subclavian vessels. Upper extremity repetitive motions that stress the vascular system, but not the shoulders (e.g., elbow flexion and extension with the arms at the side), may help to distinguish this disorder. Edema, coldness, and cyanosis may be noted in the fingers, hand, or upper arm.[50,66-69] Distention of the superficial veins is usually seen in the hand, upper arm, shoulder, or anterior chest wall.[66-69] Effort thrombosis is usually seen in young, healthy individuals with an athletic physique.[66,67] It is also seen frequently in hikers who carry backpacks.[66] Exertion of the involved extremity leads to a notable exacerbation of the pain and swelling.[66] The patient may have a loss of ROM at the shoulder. Conservative treatment usually consists of heat, elevation, and anticoagulation medication. The heat is used to dilate the veins so that the fluid may pass by the thrombus. Diagnostic tests include duplex ultrasound scanning and venography.[67] Thoracic outlet tests and arteriograms show no abnormalities.

Additional diagnostic tests, which may be indicated for certain vascular disorders, include Allen's test of the radial and ulnar arteries at the wrist, Doppler ultrasonic flow detector, systolic blood pressure, pulse volume recording, angiography, and auscultation of the major arteries.[18,65]

Liver

The liver, which is segmentally innervated by thoracic nerves T7 to T9, can refer pain to the right shoulder through its contact with the central portion of the diaphragm (see Fig. 13-4).[4,17,32,55,70] Cancer of the liver is more common in men and women who are more than 50 years old.[4] The liver is one of the most common sites of metastasis from primary cancers elsewhere in the body (colorectal, stomach, pancreas, esophagus, lung, and breast cancers).[70] *Hepatitis,* or inflammation of the liver, can range from the subclinical stage to the rapidly progressive and fatal stage.[17,70]

Symptoms

The referred pain is most often felt at the top or posterior portions of the right shoulder, that is, at the superior angle of the scapula, in the suprascapular region, or along the upper trapezius muscle.[30,31] The upper arm and anterior portions of the shoulder are not common areas of referred pain for the diaphragm. The region surrounding the diaphragm may be free of pain. Right shoulder pain may be acute or spasmodic.[4] The patient may also complain of headache, myalgia, and arthralgia.[17] Other symptoms include indigestion, nausea, vomiting, unexplained weight loss, and fatigue.[4,17,50,70] Pain from cancer of the liver may also be described as deep, gnawing, and poorly localized to the upper abdomen or back.[4]

Signs

The patient often notes no local tenderness during palpation of the diaphragm because the peripheral portion has not been traumatized. Full active and passive shoulder elevation in standing may cause pain because this motion changes the shape of the rib cage and subsequently puts tension on the diaphragm.[32] If the diaphragm is the primary source of the patient's referred shoulder pain, then AROM, PROM, and special tests of the shoulder with the patient seated and the thoracic spine in a slumped or flexed posture (to minimize stress on the diaphragm) should not increase the patient's pain. Shoulder pain may be reproduced or exacerbated, in cases with diaphragmatic irritation, by deep breathing, coughing, or sneezing.[32,36] However, the patient may have a mass in the upper right abdominal quadrant (liver) or an enlarged liver, or the liver may be tender to palpation.[4,17,50,70] Associated signs include jaundice, pale skin, purpura (red and purple hemorrhage into the skin), ecchymosis, spider angiomas (hemorrhagic pattern in the skin), palmar erythema, anorexia, and the accumulation of serous fluid in the peritoneal cavity.[17,50,70] The patient should be referred for a plain radiograph, diagnostic ultrasound, computed tomography (CT) scan, or magnetic resonance imaging (MRI) of the abdomen.[70]

Pancreas

The pancreas, which is segmentally innervated by thoracic nerves T6 to T10, can refer pain to the left shoulder through contact with the central portion of the diaphragm (see Fig. 13-4).[4,17,30,55] *Pancreatitis,* or inflammation of the pancreas, may be caused by heavy alcohol use, gallstones, viral infection, or blunt trauma.[17,44] Acute pancreatitis can be fatal.[44] Pancreatic cancer has been linked to diabetes, alcohol use, a history of pancreatitis, and a high-fat diet.[44] Cancer of the pancreas is more common in men and women older than 50 years of age.[4]

Symptoms

Shoulder pain is usually referred to the left scapula, supraspinous area, midepigastrium, or back.[17,44] Patients with a pancreatic abscess, cancer, or pancreatitis may complain of fever, weight loss, jaundice, tachycardia, nausea, or vomiting.[44,50] Patients with a pancreatic abscess may also report an abrupt rise in temperature, diarrhea, and hypotension.[50] Patients with pancreatic cancer may also complain of fatigue, weakness, and gastrointestinal bleeding.[50] A patient with pancreatitis often bends forward or bring the knees to the chest to relieve the pain.[44,50] These patients report an exacerbation of pain with walking or lying supine.[44] In addition, patients with pancreatitis complain of waxing and waning pain in the epigastric and left upper quadrant of the abdomen.[17] Pain is exacerbated by eating, alcohol intake, or vomiting.[17]

Signs

The patient often notes no local tenderness during palpation of the diaphragm because the peripheral portion has not been traumatized. Full active and passive shoulder elevation in standing may cause pain because this motion changes the shape of the rib cage and subsequently puts tension on the diaphragm.[32] If the diaphragm is the primary source of the patient's referred shoulder pain, then AROM, PROM, and special tests of the shoulder with the patient seated and the thoracic spine in a slumped or flexed posture (to minimize stress on the diaphragm) should not increase the patient's pain. Shoulder pain may be reproduced or exacerbated in cases with diaphragmatic irritation by deep breathing, coughing, or sneezing.[32,36] The patient may have an abdominal mass, enlarged liver or spleen, or tenderness in the epigastric area.[4,17,50] Diagnostic ultrasound, CT scan, or MRI may be necessary for an accurate diagnosis.

Gallbladder

The gallbladder, which is innervated by thoracic nerves T7 to T9, can refer pain to the right shoulder (see Figs. 13-2 and 13-3).[4,17,30-32,50,55,70] Afferent fibers (T6 to T11) from the gallbladder pass into hepatic and celiac plexuses and then enter the major splanchnic nerves, through which they pass to the sympathetic chain into the spinal cord.[27] Common diseases of the gallbladder include *cholecystitis* (inflammation) and *cholelithiasis* (stones).[4] Risk factors for cholelithiasis include age (increases with age), sex (more common in women), pregnancy, oral contraceptive use, obesity, diabetes, a high-cholesterol diet, and liver disease.[70] Gallbladder cancer is more common in men and women who are more than 50 years old. More specifically, it is most common in obese women who are more than 40 years of age.[4,17]

Symptoms

Cramping pain or a deep, gnawing, poorly localized pain in the back of the right shoulder may be the first symptoms of gallbladder involvement.[4,17,50,70] Pain is usually referred to the right scapula.[4,17,70] Other symptoms include chronic epigastric or right upper abdominal pain after meals, nausea, vomiting, and fever.[17,50,70] Patients suffering with cholelithiasis, the passage of a stone through the bile or cystic duct, complain of sudden and severe paroxysmal pain, in addition to chills and restlessness.[50]

Signs

Physical examination of the shoulder is negative for reproduction of the patient's pain, although impairments may be discovered. Gallbladder cancer is characterized by weight loss, anorexia, or jaundice.[50,70] Patients with cholecystitis have fever, jaundice, tenderness over the gallbladder, and abdominal rigidity.[50,70] Cholelithiasis produces a low-grade fever.[17,50] Fatty or greasy foods exacerbate the symptoms of gallbladder disease.[4,70] The patient has tenderness, and occasionally a palpable mass, in the right upper abdominal quadrant.[17] The patient should be referred for a plain radiograph, diagnostic ultrasound, or CT scan.[70]

Kidney

Although pain referred from the kidney is rare, the kidney, which is innervated by thoracic nerves T10 to L1, may refer pain to the shoulder region (see Figs. 13-2 and 13-3).[4,32,71] Several pathologic conditions must be considered with respect to the kidney, including cancer, perinephric abscess, and other disease processes such as kidney stones. Chronic kidney disease may be associated with poor calcium deposits in bone, which lead to a weak bone structure.[4] Associated disorders include pyelonephritis, nephritis, nephropathy, nephrotic syndrome, renal artery occlusion, renal failure, renal infarction, and renal tuberculosis.[50] Cancer of the kidney is most common between the ages of 55 and 60 years.[53] It can metastasize to the lung, brain, or liver.[53] Metastasis to bone occurs late in the disease process.[53]

Symptoms

Musculoskeletal pain is rarely the primary complaint. Some of the following symptoms may be noted: acute or spasmodic ipsilateral shoulder; lower abdominal, groin, low back, or flank pain; weakness, fatigue, or generalized myalgia; unexplained weight loss; nausea, vomiting, or chills; or painful, frequent, and urgent urination, with or without hematuria.[4,50,71,72] Kidney stones may produce severe cramping pain.[4]

Signs

Tenderness is noted at the costovertebral angle, and patients with inflammation have a fever.[50,71] Patients with a perinephric abscess have no tenderness over the renal areas of the back, and only mild distention is noted during abdominal palpation.[72] The ESR, white cell count, and temperature are all elevated.[72] A plain anterior-posterior KUB (view of the kidney, ureters, and bladder) radiograph demonstrates the following: (1) difficulty identifying the psoas stripe, (2) absence of the renal outline, and (3) curvature of the spine toward the side of the disease.[72] For all the diseases of the kidney discussed here, patients may benefit by referrals for intravenous pyelogram, diagnostic ultrasound, CT scan, or MRI.

Stomach

The stomach, which is segmentally innervated by thoracic nerves T6 to T10, can refer pain to the shoulder through contact with the central portion of the diaphragm (see Fig. 13-4).[4,30] Risk factors for ulcer or gastritis include heavy alcohol use, smoking, and the use of nonsteroidal anti-inflammatory drugs (NSAIDs).[17,44] Cancer of the stomach is more common in men and women who are more than 50 years of age.[4]

Symptoms

Pain is most often felt in the right shoulder at the superior angle of the scapula, in the suprascapular region, and in the upper trapezius muscle.[30,31,44] The patient may also complain of epigastric or right upper abdominal quadrant pain.[17,44] Patients with cancer, an ulcer, or gastritis may complain of weight loss, night pain, or chronic dyspepsia (painful digestion), a sense of fullness after eating, heartburn, nausea, vomiting, and a loss of appetite.[17,44,50] Patients with stomach cancer may complain of a deep, gnawing, and poorly localized pain in the upper abdomen or back.[4] Persons with an ulcer may also complain of gastrointestinal bleeding and epigastric pain 1 to 2 hours after a meal that may occur with vomiting, fullness, or abdominal distention.[44,50] Patients with gastritis may also report belching, fever, malaise, anorexia, or bloody vomit.[50]

Signs

The patient often has no local tenderness during palpation of the diaphragm because the peripheral portion has not been traumatized. Full active and passive shoulder elevation in standing may cause pain because this motion changes the shape of the rib cage and subsequently puts tension on the diaphragm.[32] If the diaphragm is the primary source of the patient's referred shoulder pain, then AROM, PROM, and special tests of the shoulder with the patient seated and the thoracic spine in a slumped or flexed posture (to minimize stress on the diaphragm) should not increase the patient's pain. Full active and passive right shoulder elevation in standing may cause pain because this motion changes the shape of the rib cage and subsequently puts tension on the diaphragm.[32] Right shoulder pain may be reproduced or exacerbated by deep breathing, coughing, or sneezing.[32,36] The patient may have an abdominal mass or tenderness noted on palpation.[4,50] Abdominal CT scan or MRI may be necessary for an accurate diagnosis.

Colon or Large Intestine

The colon or large intestine, which is innervated by thoracic and lumbar nerves T11 to L1, can refer pain to the right shoulder, although this is a rare event (see Figs 13-2 and 13-3).[4,73] The gastrointestinal tract has dual innervation. Certain afferent fibers join sympathetic nerves, and other afferent fibers that join parasympathetic nerves.[74] Pain from the gastrointestinal tract is predominantly mediated by afferent activity in sympathetic nerves, such as the splanchnic and hypogastric nerves.[74] These afferent nerve fibers have their cell bodies in thoracolumbar spinal ganglia, and their central projections enter the spinal cord at levels between T2 and L3.[74] Disorders relevant to this region include ulcerative colitis, irritable bowel syndrome, spastic colon, obstructive bowel disease, diverticulitis, and cancer. Colon cancer is the most frequently diagnosed cancer in the United States.[17] Cancer in this region is most common in men and women who are more than 50 years old.[4,53] Metastasis to the spine, liver, and lung is common.[17,53] Smoking, alcohol, NSAIDs, and caffeine may increase the risk of disease.[4] NSAIDs may also mask the symptoms.[4] Other risk factors include a prior history of inflammatory bowel disease, prior cancer of another organ, and benign polyps of the colon.[17]

Symptoms

Pain is referred to the right shoulder from the hepatic flexure of the colon.[73] Cramping pain is often described in the lower mid-abdominal region.[17,44,50] The patient may also note fluctuation of pain with eating habits, painful bowel movements, diarrhea, indigestion, nausea, vomiting, change in bowel habits, bloody stools, jaundice, and weight loss.[4,50] *Irritable bowel syndrome* is the most common gastrointestinal disorder in Western society.[44] Symptoms are aggravated or precipitated by emotional stress, fatigue, alcohol, eating a large meal with fruit, roughage, or high fat content.[44] In addition to the foregoing symptoms, the patient may have constipation, foul breath, and flatulence.[44] The predominant symptoms of *ulcerative colitis* are rectal bleeding and diarrhea.[44] In *obstructive bowel disease,* the patient complains of constipation, rapid heart rate, and short episodes of intense, cramping pain.[50] *Diverticulitis,* an inflammation in the wall of the colon, produces constant left lower abdominal pain with radiation commonly to the low back, pelvis, or left leg.[17] Patients with cancer may note a change in the frequency of bowel movements, a sense of incomplete evacuation, bloody stools, unexplained weight loss, weakness, fatigue, exertional dyspnea, and vertigo.[17,50,53]

Signs

Physical examination of the shoulder is negative for reproduction of the patient's pain, although impairments may be discovered. Patients may exhibit signs of abdominal distention, abdominal tenderness, rectal bleeding, anorexia, and abnormal bowel sounds.[50] The primary diagnostic test is colonoscopy.

CASE STUDIES

The case studies in this chapter have been modified slightly for instructional purposes and to fit the format of the *Guide to Physical Therapist Practice.* The patients' names are fictitious.

CASE STUDY 13-1

Demographics

Robert is a 24-year-old, right-handed, white male college graduate whose primary language is English. He came to physical therapy on September 9, 2009, without a physician's diagnosis or referral and complaining of periodic left shoulder pain. He denied previous treatment of any kind for his current complaints.

Social History

He shares an apartment with two of his friends. Robert denies any cultural or religious beliefs that he thinks may affect his care. He has been unemployed for 3 months.

Living Environment

Robert lives in a three-bedroom apartment on the second floor. He denies the existence of any major obstacles in and around his apartment. He ascends and descends one flight of stairs every day. He does not use assistive devices of any kind for his activities of daily living (ADLs).

General Health Status

He states that he is in excellent health and has had no major life changes in the past year. The medical screening questionnaire that he completed did not produce any notable "red flags" to indicate visceral involvement (Fig. 13-8).

Social/Health Habits

Robert reports that he eats a healthy diet that excludes red meat. He takes a multivitamin and protein shake daily and denies any substantial intake of caffeine or tobacco. He drinks a few beers on the weekends. He states that he is a competitive racquetball and volleyball player. He lifts weights occasionally, but surfs on a regular basis.

Family History

Both his parents and all his grandparents are still alive. Both his father and his grandfather suffered heart attacks. His grandmother had a cerebrovascular accident (CVA). He notes that his mother and grandmother both suffer from rheumatoid arthritis.

CASE STUDY 13-1—cont'd

Patient Questionnaire

Name Case Study #1 Date 02/15/92

	Yes		No
Age		24	
Height		5' 11"	
Weight (lbs)		165	
Fever and/or chills			X
Unexplained weight change			X
Night pain/disturbed sleep			X
Episode of fainting			X
Dry mouth (difficulty swallowing)			X
Dry eyes (red, itchy, sandy)			X
History of illness prior to onset of pain			X
History of cancer			X
Family history of cancer			X
Recent surgery (dental also)			X
Do you self inject medicines/drugs			X
Diabetic			X
Pain of gradual onset (no trauma)	X		
Constant pain	X		
Pain worse at night			X
Pain relieved by rest			X
Pulmonary			
History of smoking			X
Shortness of breath			X
Fatigue			X
Wheezing or prolonged cough			X
History of asthma, emphysema or COPD			X
History of pneumonia or tuberculosis			X
Cardiovascular			
Heart murmur/heart valve problem			X
History of heart problems			X
Sweating with pain			X
Rapid throbbing or fluttering of heart			X
High blood pressure			X
Dizziness (sit to stand)			X
Swelling in extremities			X
History of rheumatic fever			X
Elevated cholesterol level			X
Family history of heart disease	X		
Pain/symptoms increase with walking or stair climbing and relieved with rest			X
Pregnant women only			
Constant backache			
Increased uterine contractions			
Menstrual cramps			
Constant pelvic pressure			
Increased amount of vaginal discharge			
Increased consistency of vaginal discharge			
Color change of vaginal discharge			
Increased frequency of urination			

Figure 13-8 Patient questionnaire for Case Study 1.

Medical/Surgical History

- 2008: Muscle injury to the left side of his rib cage after a weekend volleyball tournament
- 2007: Muscle injury to the left side of his rib cage after a weekend volleyball tournament
- 2004: Low back muscle injury from racquetball

He denies a history of surgery. The only illness or other complaints he has had in the past year are related to the flu, which he had 6 to 9 months ago.

Current Condition(s)/Chief Complaint(s)

Robert comes to physical therapy complaining of periodic, severe (2/10 to 7/10), localized left shoulder pain at the acromioclavicular joint (Fig. 13-9). He reports a constant, low-intensity ache (2/10), which never goes away regardless of what he does. He is able, however, to produce a sudden and sharp pain with certain movements. The movements that consistently reproduce his pain are full flexion or full abduction of his shoulder overhead. He also reports sharp

Continued

CASE STUDY 13-1—cont'd

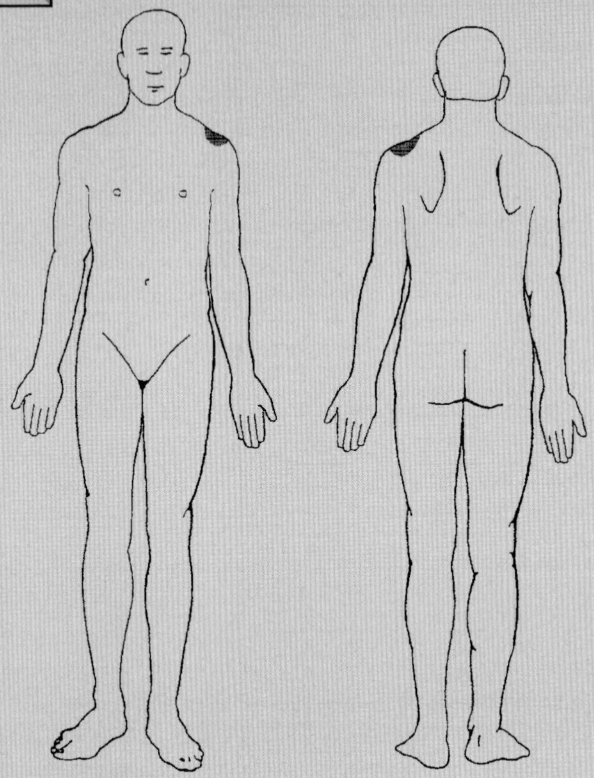

Figure 13-9 Pain diagram from a 24-year-old, right-handed man experiencing left shoulder pain.

pain with powerful or forceful movements, such as hitting a racquetball hard or spiking a volleyball. He is able to sleep on his left side without much difficulty. He denies neck pain, headaches, dizziness or vertigo, vision changes, tinnitus, nausea, upper extremity symptoms (radiating pain, weakness, or paresthesia), night pain, and SOB. He reports no change in his shoulder pain related to eating, associated with bowel or bladder activity, or during exertional activities (light jog) that do not directly involve his shoulder. He also denies having constitutional symptoms (fever, night sweats, nausea or vomiting, dizziness, fatigue, or unexplained weight loss). He states that the sharp pain is not constant and that he can get immediate relief if he rests his shoulder. He admits having shoulder pain if he laughs out loud or takes a deep breath. He is not sure whether coughing is a problem. He denies a history of a motor vehicle accident (MVA), fractures, or falls. His pain started 6 days ago. He denies any incidents of specific trauma. Nine days ago, he participated in a 2-day walleyball tournament (volleyball on a racquetball court); and 6 days ago, he was involved in two competitive racquetball league matches.

Functional Status/Activity Level

Before the onset of his shoulder pain, Robert was a competitive racquetball and volleyball player who played either sport three to four times a week. He also lifted weights occasionally and surfed on a regular basis. Robert scores 92 out of a possible maximum score of 100 on the Sharp Functional Activity Survey (Sharp FAS) for the neck and shoulder region (Sharp HealthCare, San Diego, 1998). He reports no difficulties performing all of his ADLs. He does state, however, that he has severe difficulty playing volleyball and racquetball at a competitive level because of the periodic sharp pains in his left shoulder.

Medications

Robert denies taking any medications, prescription or nonprescription, of any kind.

Other Clinical Tests

No clinical tests of any kind were performed on this patient in the past year. He has never had any imaging studies performed on his shoulder or neck. Robert did have radiographs taken of his low back in 1994, which he reported were read as normal.

Cardiovascular/Pulmonary System

Although it is well known that the heart and lungs can refer pain to the left shoulder, there is no indication that this patient's symptoms may be cardiopulmonary in origin. Robert is a very fit and very young (24-year-old) man with no risk factors and no specific symptoms of heart or lung disease. His medical screening questionnaire does not raise any red flags for the pulmonary and cardiovascular sections (see Fig. 13-8). Therefore, a physical examination of his cardiopulmonary system is deferred.

Integumentary System

Robert's skin appears healthy, with a good continuity of color and no significant changes in temperature. No joint effusion, soft tissue edema, or scars are noted.

Communication, Affect, Cognition, Learning Style

No known learning barriers are identified for this patient. Robert reports that he learns best when given a demonstration of the procedure or exercise. He does not show any deficits with regard to his cognition, orientation, or ability to communicate effectively.

Musculoskeletal System

Posture

In standing, he has good posture with only a slightly forward head and a slight increase in his lumbar lordosis.

CASE STUDY 13-1—cont'd

Range of Motion

Cervical Spine

AROM and PROM are within normal limits (WNL) and pain free.

Shoulder

Left shoulder AROM and PROM are WNL. Pain is reproduced at the end ROM in active flexion or abduction, with the patient standing. PROM, tested in the sitting position with the thoracic spine flexed, is pain free.

Scapula and Elbow

AROM and PROM are WNL and pain free.

Thoracic Spine

Thoracic AROM and PROM are minimally limited in flexion and extension. Sharp left shoulder pain, however, is noted with movement into the end range of active or passive flexion or extension.

Rib

Active deep inhalation reproduces the patient's left shoulder pain. Passive lower rib cage compression is normal.

Lumbar Spine

Moderate restriction of AROM is noted in the upper lumbar region during active flexion, and a mild, sharp angulation into extension is observed at approximately the L4-5 segment.

Muscle Performance

Symptoms are not reproduced during resisted testing in each of the shortened, middle, and lengthened ranges for muscles of the cervical and thoracic spine, shoulder, or rib cage. Specific myotome testing is deferred to save time and because the patient has no neurologic complaints.

Sensory Integrity

This part of the examination is deferred to save time. The patient denies having any neurologic symptoms.

Reflex Integrity

This part of the examination is deferred to save time. The patient denies having any neurologic symptoms.

Pain

The patient has no tenderness or reproduction of symptoms on palpation of musculoskeletal structures throughout the cervical and thoracic spine, chest, shoulder, and upper ribs. Palpation of the lymph nodes in the cervical, supraclavicular, and axillary regions is normal. Palpation of the abdomen indicates local pain and tenderness along the left anterior-lateral border of the diaphragm and costal margin, just under the rib cage. Palpation of this peripheral portion of the diaphragm does not reproduce the patient's shoulder pain. The central portion of the diaphragm is out of reach for palpation. Palpation of Robert's upper extremity pulses is deferred because he reports no symptoms during his history or on his medical screening questionnaire that suggest cardiovascular disease.

Special Tests

Musculoskeletal Structure	Test
Cervical spine (positive tests)	None
Cervical spine (negative tests)	Compression testing of the cervical spine in flexion, neutral, and extension (see Fig. 5-15) Cervical quadrant test in flexion and extension Valsalva's maneuver
Shoulder (positive tests)	None
Shoulder (negative tests)	Distraction and compression of the glenohumeral joint Hawkins' impingement sign Load and shift test (anterior and posterior instability) Distraction and compression of the acromioclavicular joint O'Brien's test (superior labrum anterior to posterior [SLAP]) Crank test (labrum) Empty can test (supraspinatus tendon) Speed's test (biceps tendon)
Thoracic spine (positive tests: shoulder pain)	Thoracic quadrant test in flexion to the left Thoracic quadrant test in extension to the left Thoracic quadrant test in extension to the right
Thoracic spine (negative tests)	Segmental joint mobility and provocation testing (prone posterior to anterior glides) (see Fig. 5-22) T1 nerve root tension test (see Fig. 5-23)
Ribs (positive test: shoulder pain)	Coughing and deep inhalation
Ribs (negative tests)	Lateral compression testing of the middle and lower ribs (supine) Mobility and provocation testing of the first rib (see Fig. 5-25) Cervical rotation lateral flexion (CRLF) test (see Fig. 5-26) Mobility and provocation testing of ribs R2 to R5 anteriorly (see Fig. 5-25)

Joint Integrity and Mobility

Cervical Spine

Examination is deferred to save time because the patient has full cervical AROM without pain (will examine during a future appointment as needed).

Continued

CASE STUDY 13-1—cont'd

Shoulder

- Glenohumeral: Normal in all directions, with no complaints of pain
- Sternoclavicular: Normal in all directions, with no complaints of pain
- Acromioclavicular: Normal in all directions, with no complaints of pain
- Scapulothoracic: Normal in all directions, with no complaints of pain

Thoracic Spine

Slight hypomobility is noted in the middle and lower thoracic spine in extension, with muscle guarding and no pain.

Ribs

Slight hypomobility of R7 to R10 is observed on the left, with muscle guarding and no pain.

Neuromuscular System

Robert has no gross gait, locomotion, or balance disorders.

Imaging Studies: Radiographs

- Lumbar (2004): The films and the radiologist's report are not available.

Diagnosis

Musculoskeletal Pattern D: Impaired joint mobility, motor function, muscle performance, and ROM associated with connective tissue dysfunction.

This is a 24-year-old, right-handed male patient with signs and symptoms consistent with an extrinsic source of shoulder pain. Shoulder AROM at the end of range for flexion or abduction, which deforms the rib cage and can put stress on the diaphragm, is the only test of the shoulder that gives rise to pain. Results of all other tests of the shoulder—palpation, PROM, resisted testing, special tests, and specific mobility tests—are negative. This extrinsic source appears to be from an irritation of his central left hemidiaphragm, with subsequent referred pain to the left shoulder. Although end ROM of the thoracic spine, thoracic quadrant tests, coughing, and deep inhalation produce shoulder pain, motions that also deform the rib cage and produce stress on the diaphragm, no collaborative findings of thoracic or rib injury from resisted testing, palpation, special tests, or specific mobility testing of the thoracic spine and ribs are present.

In cases involving the diaphragm, suspicion of visceral disease or tumor-induced inflammation of the diaphragm is high. Even though no signs, symptoms, patient history, or family history suggest a possible medical disease involving the diaphragm, it must be part of the differential diagnosis.

Pain

The primary pain generator for this patient appears to be his left hemidiaphragm.

Strain

The biomechanical strains that may be exacerbating the pain and dysfunction are mild hypomobilities in the thoracic spine and ribs with possible lumbar instability. No physiologic strains or comorbidities are noted.

Brain

The patient has experienced his current pain episode for only 1 week. He is in the early stage of healing and has not demonstrated any signs of fear, anger, or frustration. He has no indication of a primary central sensitization disorder or adverse forebrain activity at this time.

Prognosis

Robert has a very good prognosis for returning to competitive volleyball and racquetball.

Intervention

Anticipated goals are as follows:

1. Robert's goal: "Get back to a competitive level of volleyball and racquetball."
2. The patient will be independent with his home exercise program (HEP).
3. Thoracic spine and rib mobility will return to WNL.
4. The patient will return to competitive volleyball and racquetball with minimal discomfort (3/10).

Robert receives a comprehensive treatment program incorporating the WOMEN (*w*isdom, *o*ptimism, *m*anual therapy, *e*xercise, and *n*utrition) plan of care concept outlined in Chapter 5. He was expected to achieve at least a 50% reduction in pain after 7 to 10 days. If not, the clinician was prepared to refer the patient to an internal medicine specialist for further medical evaluation. Fortunately, this patient is 90% improved with respect to his symptoms after 1 week. He is able to play racquetball at a competitive level after 2 weeks, with only minimal discomfort. At a 1-year follow-up with the patient, he reports that his left shoulder pain has not returned and he has reported no illnesses or adverse symptoms over the past year. Although it is difficult to verify the source of the patient's pain, the only structure that seems a likely candidate is his diaphragm. Instances of diaphragmatic inflammation from physical strain that is not related to surgery, viscera, or tumor are rare. Therefore, it is strongly suggested that with a similar patient presentation, serious consideration should be given to a differential diagnosis of visceral disease or musculoskeletal tumor.

CASE STUDY 13-2

Demographics

Lucy is a 66-year-old, right-handed Hispanic female college professor whose primary language is Spanish, although she is fluent in English. She is referred to physical therapy on August 27, 2007, from her primary care physician with a diagnosis of "frozen shoulder." She denies previous treatment of any kind for her current complaints.

Social History

Lucy lives at home with her husband of 34 years. She denies any cultural or religious beliefs that she thinks may affect her care. She is employed as a professor of biology at a local university. Her job requires her to reach overhead and to perform repetitive motions with her arm elevated, including writing on the chalkboard, lifting and carrying less than 10 lb, prolonged sitting, and prolonged standing. She has not missed any time from work because of her current complaints.

Living Environment

Lucy lives in a two-story house in which she ascends and descends one flight of stairs every day. She denies the existence of any major obstacles in and around her house. She does not use assistive devices of any kind for her ADLs.

General Health Status

Lucy rates her general health as fair. In the past year, both her sister and her father died of cancer. The medical screening questionnaire that Lucy filled out on her first visit indicated a family history of cancer (Fig. 13-10). Her grandmother died of throat cancer, her father died of prostate cancer, and her sister died of pancreatic cancer. Questioning her on her smoking habits uncovers that she is a 50-pack-year smoker (1 pack per day for 50 years). The miscellaneous questions of the medical screening questionnaire document a significant number of items that may not be related to somatic injury and dysfunction, including unexplained weight change, history of cancer, extensive family history of cancer, insidious onset of pain, constant pain, and pain that is worse at night—therefore raising a red flag. In addition, half of the questions under the pulmonary section of the questionnaire are answered "yes," again raising a red flag. The cardiovascular section is of only mild concern because the items checked are not strong indicators of cardiovascular disease. At this point, one should have concerns about the patient's pulmonary system and how this may relate to her family's history of cancer and her history as a heavy smoker. If her symptoms correlate with a known visceral disease, and the physical therapist is unable to provoke her symptoms and come up with a meaningful musculoskeletal explanation, then she will have to be referred for further medical evaluation.

Social/Health Habits

Lucy reports that she has smoked approximately one pack of cigarettes a day for the past 50 years (50-pack-year smoker). She takes a multivitamin pill daily, drinks one to two cups of coffee a day, and has two to three glasses of wine each week. She is not a vegetarian and eats at least two meals a day, usually skipping breakfast. Her normal physical activity level involves walking 5 days a week for approximately 40 minutes. She does not participate in sports or any other forms of physical exercise.

Family History

She reports that three members of her family have died of various forms of cancer, and congestive heart failure has been diagnosed in one other family member. Her parents are both deceased.

Medical/Surgical History

- 2007: Surgery to right temporomandibular joint (TMJ) 2 months ago for malignant melanoma
- 2005: Diagnosis of osteoporosis
- 2004: Fall onto right shoulder, no fracture; symptoms resolved in 4 months
- 1990: Lumbar disk surgery

In the past year, she has had episodes of chest pain, cough, SOB, pain at night, loss of appetite, weight loss, and nausea.

Current Condition(s)/Chief Complaint(s)

Lucy comes to physical therapy on August 27, 2007, with a diagnosis of "frozen shoulder." Her main complaint is constant, severe (7/10 to 9/10) right shoulder pain that radiates down her arm and along the ulnar border of her forearm and hand and includes the third through fifth digits (Fig. 13-11). Approximately 6 weeks before her evaluation, she reported an episode in which her whole right arm felt numb. This symptom has not returned. She does report, however, a periodic mild tingling sensation along the ulnar border of her right hand. On further discussion, she admits that she forgot to tell her physician about the tingling. She denies neck pain, headaches, chest pain, dizziness or vertigo, vision changes, tinnitus, nausea, and upper extremity weakness. She reports no change in her shoulder pain related to eating or bowel or bladder activity or during exertional activities (light jog) that do not directly involve her shoulder. Laughing, coughing, or taking a deep breath does not seem to alter her constant, severe pain. She also denies having constitutional symptoms (fever, night sweats, nausea or vomiting, dizziness, or fatigue). She denies a history of neck pain, fracture, or MVA. Other than what she has stated earlier, Lucy denies any other complaints or symptoms throughout the rest of

Continued

CASE STUDY 13-2—cont'd

Patient Questionnaire

Name Case Study #2 Date 5/31/95

		Yes		No
Age			66	
Height			5' 4"	
Weight (lbs)			85	
Fever and/or chills				X
Unexplained weight change		X		
Night pain/disturbed sleep				X
Episode of fainting				X
Dry mouth (difficulty swallowing)				X
Dry eyes (red, itchy, sandy)				X
History of illness prior to onset of pain				X
History of cancer		X		
Family history of cancer		X	(3)	
Recent surgery (dental also)		X		
Do you self inject medicines/drugs				X
Diabetic				X
Pain of gradual onset (no trauma)		X		
Constant pain		X		
Pain worse at night		X		
Pain relieved by rest				X
Pulmonary				
History of smoking		X		
Shortness of breath		X		
Fatigue				X
Wheezing or prolonged cough		X		
History of asthma, emphysema or COPD				X
History of pneumonia or tuberculosis				X
Cardiovascular				
Heart murmur/heart valve problem				X
History of heart problems				X
Sweating with pain		X		
Rapid throbbing or fluttering of heart		X		
High blood pressure				X
Dizziness (sit to stand)				X
Swelling in extremities				X
History of rheumatic fever				X
Elevated cholesterol level				X
Family history of heart disease		X	(1)	
Pain/symptoms increase with walking or stair climbing and relieved with rest				X
Pregnant women only				
Constant backache				
Increased uterine contractions				
Menstrual cramps				
Constant pelvic pressure				
Increased amount of vaginal discharge				
Increased consistency of vaginal discharge				
Color change of vaginal discharge				
Increased frequency of urination				

Figure 13-10 Patient questionnaire for Case Study 2.

her body. She states that her shoulder pain started gradually, with no trauma or overuse noted, sometime in January of 2007. Her pain is evoked by reaching into the back seat of her car from the driver's seat. She gets relief when she lies down on her right side.

Functional Status/Activity Level

Her normal physical activity level involves walking 5 days a week on her lunch hour for approximately 40 minutes. She does not participate in sports or any other forms of physical exercise. Lucy scores 66 out of a possible maximum

CASE STUDY 13-2—cont'd

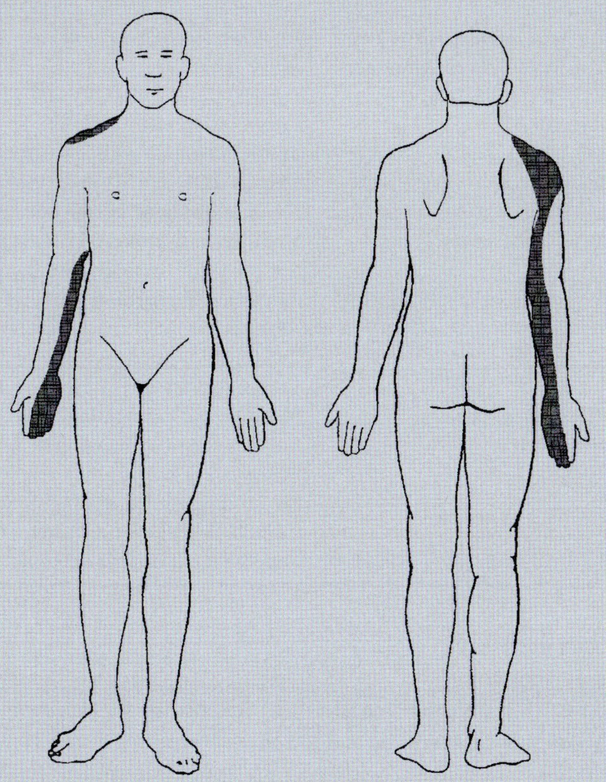

Figure 13-11 Pain diagram from a 66-year-old, right-handed woman with a diagnosis of "frozen shoulder."

score of 100 on the Sharp FAS for the neck and shoulder region. She reports moderate difficulties with her job, looking up or reaching overhead, dressing, and her domestic duties around the house.

Medications

- Prescription: alendronate (Fosamax) for osteoporosis
- Nonprescription: ibuprofen (Advil) and acetaminophen (Tylenol) daily for the past 6 months

Other Clinical Tests

- 2005: She underwent a CT bone density scan of the spine: T-score of −2.7 (osteoporosis).
- 2004: Cervical spine and right shoulder plain radiographs showed a "normal cervical spine" and a "normal right shoulder," according to the radiologist.

Cardiovascular/Pulmonary System

- Heart rate (resting): 75 beats per minute
- Respiratory rate (resting): 16 breaths per minute (shallow)
- Blood pressure: 130/80 mm Hg
- Edema: none

Integumentary System

Lucy's skin appears healthy, with good continuity of color and no significant changes in temperature. She has very mild swelling and a surgical scar around her right TMJ, and mild swelling is also noted in the right supraclavicular fossa. A well-healed, thin, white scar is noted in her lower lumbar spine.

Communication, Affect, Cognition, Learning Style

No known learning barriers are identified for this patient. She states that she learns best when given a diagram and a demonstration. Lucy does not display any deficits with regard to her cognition, orientation, or ability to communicate effectively.

Musculoskeletal System

Posture

In standing, she has a forward head, rounded and protracted shoulders, and moderately increased thoracic kyphosis. Her iliac crest is high on the right, with right genu recurvatum, collapsed arches bilaterally, and bilateral hallux valgus (right more than left).

Range of Motion

Cervical Spine

Active and passive extension and right rotation reproduce her shoulder pain. Both motions are limited by pain.

Shoulder

AROM and PROM are equally limited. Abduction and external rotation are moderately limited, with minimal limitations in internal rotation and flexion. Minimal shoulder pain, but no arm pain, is reproduced at end ROM in all directions.

Scapula and Elbow

AROM and PROM are WNL and pain free.

Thoracic Spine

Thoracic AROM and PROM are severely limited in extension and moderately limited in side bending and rotation. This patient's primary complaint is not reproduced.

Rib

Active deep inhalation is limited and accompanied by a cough and a dull ache in her shoulder. Gentle (because of Lucy's age and diagnosis of osteoporosis), passive middle and lower rib cage compression is performed, and she reports no pain (full PROM is not tested).

Lumbar Spine

Moderate restrictions in AROM are noted in all directions, without complaints of pain.

Muscle Performance

Shoulder pain and arm pain are reproduced with resisted testing of the cervical spine when the neck is held in extension (shortened position for the neck extensors and lengthened position for the neck flexors) or right side bending (shortened position for the scalenus and upper trapezius on the right and lengthened position for the

Continued

CASE STUDY 13-2—cont'd

scalenus and upper trapezius on the left). No reproduction of symptoms is elicited for all the cardinal directions tested in each of the shortened, middle, and lengthened ranges for muscles of the thoracic spine and shoulder. Manual muscle testing (isometric; 5/5 is WNL) of the upper extremities is as follows: right triceps (4/5), wrist flexion and extension (4/5), and the intrinsics of the hand (3/5).

Sensory Integrity

Her sensation to light touch and pinprick is decreased in the right C8 and T1 dermatomes.

Reflex Integrity

Her deep tendon reflexes (DTRs) are 2+ and equal at the biceps, brachioradialis, and triceps tendons. The right abductor digiti minimi tendon reflex is 1+. The scapulohumeral reflex (SHR) and Hoffmann's sign show normal results. Both these tests are upper motor neuron–mediated reflexes used to help rule out cervical central canal stenosis.

Pain

Palpation

Swelling and tenderness are noted in the right supraclavicular fossa and the right TMJ. No edema or skin discoloration is noted in the extremities. Palpation of the lymph nodes (sternocleidomastoid, supraclavicular, and axillary), arterial pulses (brachial and radial), and abdomen is normal.

Special Tests

Cervical spine (positive tests: reproduction of symptoms)	Cervical quadrant test in extension to the right or flexion to the left (see Fig. 5-19) Compression testing of the cervical spine positive only in extension (see Fig. 5-15) Upper limb neurodynamic testing (ULNT) brachial plexus and median nerve and ulnar nerve bias techniques
Cervical spine (negative tests)	Cervical quadrant test in flexion to the right or extension to the left ULNT radial nerve bias technique Thoracic outlet syndrome Valsalva's maneuver
Shoulder (positive tests: reproduction of symptoms)	Hawkins' impingement sign
Shoulder (negative tests)	Distraction and compression of the glenohumeral joint Load and shift test (anterior and posterior instability) Distraction and compression of the acromioclavicular joint O'Brien's test (SLAP) Crank test (labrum) Empty can test (supraspinatus tendon) Speed's test (biceps tendon)
Thoracic spine (positive tests: reproduction of symptoms)	T1 nerve root tension test (see Fig. 5-23)
Thoracic spine (negative tests)	Segmental joint mobility and provocation testing (prone posterior-anterior glides) (see Fig. 5-22) Thoracic quadrant tests
Ribs (positive test)	Mobility and provocation testing of the right first rib: local pain and muscle guarding (see Fig. 5-25) CRLF test: limited mobility on the right (see Fig. 5-26)
Ribs (negative tests)	Mobility and provocation testing of ribs R2 to R5 anteriorly (Fig. 5-25) Lateral compression testing of the middle and lower ribs (supine) Coughing and deep inhalation

Joint Integrity and Mobility

Cervical spine

Loss of segmental mobility is present in all directions throughout the middle and lower cervical spine. Severe limitations are evident, with pain and muscle guarding from C6 to T1 in extension, right side bending, and right rotation. The result of the disk shear test at C5-6 is positive (see Fig. 5-16).

Shoulder

- Glenohumeral: Normal in all directions except distraction, which causes muscle guarding and pain
- Sternoclavicular: Normal in all directions, with no complaints of pain
- Acromioclavicular: Normal in all directions, without a primary complaint of pain
- Scapulothoracic: Normal in all directions, without a primary complaint of pain

Thoracic Spine

The patient has severe hypomobility at all levels in extension, and the upper segments are associated with local pain and muscle guarding.

Ribs

The patient has slight hypomobility of R1 on the right, with pain.

Neuromuscular System

Lucy has no gross gait, locomotion, or balance disorders.

Imaging Studies

- Cervical (2004): A review of Lucy's cervical spine radiographs reveals the following: mild DDD at C5-6 and DJD at C5-6 and C6-7.
- Shoulder, right (2004): A review of her shoulder radiographs reveals the following: WNL with a type II acromion.

CASE STUDY 13-2—cont'd

Diagnosis

Suspicions are raised of a possible disorder that is not musculoskeletal because of the insidious onset of symptoms, age of the patient, constant pain, night pain, family history of cancer, patient history of cancer, pulmonary symptoms, and 50-pack-year smoking history.

Musculoskeletal Pattern F: Impaired joint mobility, motor function, muscle performance, ROM, and reflex integrity associated with spinal disorders; or Neuromuscular Pattern F: Impaired peripheral nerve integrity and muscle performance associated with peripheral nerve injury. Also, Musculoskeletal Pattern A: Primary prevention/risk reduction for skeletal demineralization; and Musculoskeletal Pattern B: Impaired posture.

Pain

The primary pain generator for this patient appears to be her right C8 or T1 nerve root or nerve.

Strain

The physiologic strains that may be exacerbating the pain and dysfunction are heavy smoking, osteoporosis, and signs of possible pulmonary disease or dysfunction. The biomechanical strains are poor posture and hypomobility in the cervical and thoracic spine and the ribs.

Brain

The patient has experienced her symptoms only for a few weeks, and she has no overt signs of anger, frustration, hopelessness, depression, or denial. No indication of a primary central sensitization disorder or adverse forebrain activity is present at this time.

Prognosis

Prognosis is uncertain and depends on the presence or absence of visceral disease.

Plan of Care

Anticipated goals are as follows:

1. Lucy's goal: "Get rid of the pain!"
2. The patient will have minimal restrictions, less than a 15° loss, with active and passive shoulder abduction and external rotation.
3. Active and passive thoracic extension will improve so that the restrictions are no longer severe.
4. The patient will have minimal difficulty (3/10) with her job and domestic duties.
5. The Sharp FAS score will be 85/100 without the dependence on pain medication.
6. The patient will be independent, with a comprehensive HEP.

Intervention

Lucy's primary physician is contacted and made aware of concerns regarding her pulmonary status. She receives five treatments (WOMEN) of physical therapy while waiting for her follow-up visit with her physician. Minimal progress is made during this initial course of physical therapy. Following a chest radiograph and further medical examination, Pancoast's tumor is diagnosed in her right lung. After radiation treatment and surgery to remove the cancerous tumor from her lung, Lucy reports a moderate decrease in her complaints of neck and right upper extremity symptoms. This patient does not have Horner's syndrome.

CASE STUDY 13-3

Demographics

Joe is a 48-year-old, obese, left-handed, white male. He is referred to physical therapy on May 12, 2006, by his primary care physician with a diagnosis of "shoulder pain—bursitis." He received approximately six treatments from a chiropractor without relief. The treatments consisted of massage and ultrasound to his shoulder, followed by a chiropractic adjustment to his cervical spine at each visit.

Social History

Joe is recently divorced and has 50% custody of his two children, whom he sees mainly on weekends. He denies any cultural or religious beliefs that he thinks may affect his care. He is employed as an architect, a job that requires him to sit for a prolonged time. He occasionally has periods of driving and prolonged standing at construction sites. He lifts and carries up to 20 lb, but rarely has to reach over his head and normally does not perform repetitive motions. He does, however, spend hours at a time on his computer. He has not missed any time from work because of his current complaints.

Living Environment

He lives in a two-bedroom condominium on the fourth floor and has the choice of stairs or an elevator when he comes and goes. He denies the existence of any major obstacles in and around his house. He does not use any assistive devices for his ADLs.

General Health Status

Joe rates his general health as good. In the past year, he went through a painful and costly divorce, a beloved family pet died, and he moved into a condominium in a different

Continued

CASE STUDY 13-3—cont'd

part of town. The medical screening questionnaire, which Joe fills out on his first visit, is notable in the pulmonary and cardiovascular sections (Fig. 13-12). At the time of his evaluation, he is a 33-pack-year smoker and has a history of heart problems (palpitations and tachycardia), and both his father and grandfather died prematurely of heart attacks.

Social/Health Habits

Joe reports that he has smoked an average of one pack of cigarettes a day since he was 15 years old (33-pack-year smoker). He drinks one to two cups of coffee in the morning, and has a couple of beers or other type of alcohol usually just once during the week. He is not a vegetarian, does not skip any meals, does not take any vitamins or

Patient Questionnaire

Name Case Study #3 Date 12/11/94

	Yes		No
Age		48	
Height		5' 10"	
Weight (lbs)		245	
Fever and/or chills			X
Unexplained weight change			X
Night pain/disturbed sleep			X
Episode of fainting			X
Dry mouth (difficulty swallowing)			X
Dry eyes (red, itchy, sandy)			X
History of illness prior to onset of pain			X
History of cancer			X
Family history of cancer			X
Recent surgery (dental also)			X
Do you self inject medicines/drugs			X
Diabetic			X
Pain of gradual onset (no trauma)	X		
Constant pain			X
Pain worse at night			X
Pain relieved by rest	X		
Pulmonary			
History of smoking	X		
Shortness of breath	X		
Fatigue	X		
Wheezing or prolonged cough			X
History of asthma, emphysema or COPD			X
History of pneumonia or tuberculosis			X
Cardiovascular			
Heart murmur/heart valve problem			X
History of heart problems	X		
Sweating with pain	X		
Rapid throbbing or fluttering of heart			X
High blood pressure	X		
Dizziness (sit to stand)			X
Swelling in extremities			X
History of rheumatic fever			X
Elevated cholesterol level	X		
Family history of heart disease	X		
Pain/symptoms increase with walking or stair climbing and relieved with rest	X		
Pregnant women only			
Constant backache			
Increased uterine contractions			
Menstrual cramps			
Constant pelvic pressure			
Increased amount of vaginal discharge			
Increased consistency of vaginal discharge			
Color change of vaginal discharge			
Increased frequency of urination			

Figure 13-12 Patient questionnaire for Case Study 3.

CASE STUDY 13-3—cont'd

supplements, and usually eats at a fast food restaurant several times a week. Joe does not participate in regular physical activity or sports other than playing "catch" with his sons on the weekends.

Family History

His mother is still alive and in reasonably good health. His grandmother died of a pulmonary embolus, at the 65 years of age, following hip surgery. Both his father (56 years old) and grandfather (46 years old) died prematurely of heart attacks. Diabetes and rheumatoid arthritis appear to "run" in his family.

Medical/Surgical History

- 2005: Arthroscopic surgery to the right knee: lateral meniscectomy, still stiff and painful, according to the patient
- 2005: Fall and sprain of left shoulder; resolved in 3 months
- 2004: Diagnosis of high cholesterol (345 mg/dL)
- 2000: Diagnosis of non–insulin-dependent (type 2) diabetes mellitus
- 1997: Lumbar disk surgery

In the past year, he has reported fatigue, SOB, sweating with pain, difficulty sleeping, chest pain, and dizziness without vertigo or blackouts.

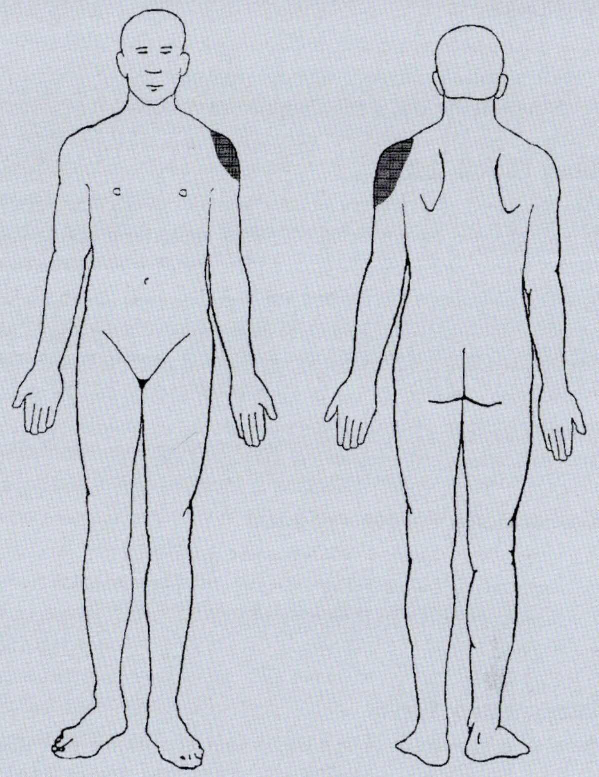

Figure 13-13 Pain diagram from a 48-year-old, left-handed man with a diagnosis of "shoulder pain—bursitis."

Current Condition(s)/Chief Complaint(s)

Joe is a 48-year-old, obese, left-handed man who comes to physical therapy on May 12, 2006, with a diagnosis of "shoulder pain—bursitis" and complaining of periodic moderate (0 to 6/10) pain in his left shoulder (Fig. 13-13). He states that the pain is not constant and does not radiate down his arm. He does admit that his left hand "tingles" every once in a while. He denies neck pain, headaches, nausea, tinnitus, dizziness or vertigo, vision changes, upper extremity numbness, and upper extremity weakness. He also denies chest pain, but admits to muscle soreness in his chest after playing "catch" with his sons. He denies a change in symptoms after eating a greasy meal, bowel movement, coughing, or laughing or during a deep inhalation. He also reports no change in his shoulder pain related to eating or bowel and bladder activity. He notes that exertional activity—climbing four flights of stairs to his condominium—gives him SOB, fatigue, and an ache in his left shoulder. He denies having the following constitutional symptoms: fever, night sweats, nausea or vomiting, dizziness, or unexplained weight loss. Other than what is reported here, he denies any other complaints or symptoms throughout the rest of his body. Joe reports that his symptoms started 2 days after an afternoon of throwing and catching a football with his sons approximately 2 months ago. He reports that his shoulder pain is made worse by activities such as waxing his car or carrying groceries. He states that his symptoms change with his activity level, but not with changes in his posture. He notes that, with repeated overhead use, he has shoulder pain and fatigue, which is quickly resolved if he stops that particular activity.

Functional Status/Activity Level

Joe does not participate in regular physical activity or sports other than playing "catch" with his sons on the weekends. He used to use the four flights of stairs up to his condominium as a source of exercise; however, he had to give that up a couple of months ago because of SOB and significant fatigue. Joe reports that he can throw 8 or 10 good passes with the football without pain. Then his shoulder rapidly fatigues and begins to ache. He states that he can lift 10 lb or more over his head without difficulty, but he has problems with repeated overhead activities such as painting his garage or washing and drying his camper. He has difficulty carrying groceries if his car is parked too far away from the grocery store, and he has noted fatigue and shoulder pain if he vacuums more than one room of his condominium. Joe scores 73 out of a possible maximum score of 100 on the Sharp FAS for the neck and shoulder region. He reports no difficulties with sleeping, looking up or reaching overhead, driving, dressing, personal care, or work.

Continued

CASE STUDY 13-3—cont'd

Medications

- Prescription: atorvastatin (Lipitor) for high cholesterol and insulin for type 2 diabetes mellitus
- Nonprescription: acetaminophen (Tylenol)

Other Clinical Tests

According to his last physician visit 2 weeks ago, Joe's blood glucose level was WNL. His cholesterol level was high, but much improved at 250 mg/dL. No imaging studies have been performed on Joe's cervical or thoracic spine or shoulder. In 1997, he had a plain radiograph of his lumbar spine followed by an MRI scan (films and the radiologist's report are not available). In 2005, he also had a plain radiograph and MRI scan of his right knee (films and the radiologist's report are not available).

Cardiovascular/Pulmonary System

- Heart rate (resting): 80 beats per minute
- Respiratory rate (resting): 18 breaths per minute
- Blood pressure: 135/88 mm Hg
- Edema: none

Integumentary System

Joe's skin appears healthy, with good continuity of color and no significant changes in temperature. White, well-healed scars are noted around the right knee and the lower lumbar spine. No swelling is noted.

Communication, Affect, Cognition, Learning Style

No known learning barriers are identified for this patient. He states that he can remember things best if they are clearly explained to him with a good rationale and if he is allowed to take notes. Joe does not reveal any deficits with regard to his cognition, orientation, or ability to communicate effectively.

Musculoskeletal System

Posture

In standing, he has a slightly forward head, a flat thoracic and lumbar spine, a protruding belly (obese), slight genu valgum bilaterally, and bilateral pes planus.

Range of Motion

Cervical Spine

AROM and PROM are WNL and pain free.

Shoulder

AROM and PROM are WNL and pain free.

Scapula and Elbow

AROM and PROM are WNL and pain free.

Thoracic Spine

AROM and PROM are pain free. Mild to moderate limitations are noted in flexion.

Rib

AROM and PROM are WNL and pain free.

Lumbar Spine

AROM is painful and limited in extension and left side bending. Pain is localized to the lower lumbar spine.

Muscle Performance

No reproduction of symptoms is elicited for all the cardinal directions tested in each of the shortened, middle, and lengthened ranges for muscles of the cervical and thoracic spine and left shoulder. Manual muscle testing (isometric; 5/5 is WNL) of the upper extremities is WNL (5/5).

Sensory Integrity

Upper extremity light touch and pinprick sensation is WNL.

Reflex Integrity

Upper extremity DTRs are equal and brisk (2+). The SHR and Hoffman's sign are normal.

Pain

Palpation

No reproduction of symptoms is elicited on palpation of musculoskeletal structures throughout the cervical and thoracic spine, chest, shoulder, and upper ribs. No edema or skin discoloration is noted in the extremities. Palpation of the lymph nodes (sternocleidomastoid, supraclavicular, and axillary), arterial pulses (brachial and radial), and the abdomen is normal.

Special Tests

Musculoskeletal System	Test
Cervical spine (positive tests: reproduction of symptoms)	Thoracic outlet syndrome: Roo's 3-minute flap arm test reproduces left shoulder pain
Cervical spine (negative tests)	Compression testing of the cervical spine in flexion, neutral, and extension (see Fig. 5-15)
	Thoracic outlet syndrome: Adson's test, costoclavicular test, and pectoralis minor stress test
	Cervical quadrant test in flexion and extension (see Fig. 5-19)
	ULNT = 3
	Valsalva's maneuver
Shoulder (positive tests)	None
Shoulder (negative tests)	Distraction and compression of the glenohumeral joint
	Hawkins' impingement sign
	Load and shift test (anterior and posterior instability)
	Distraction and compression of the acromioclavicular joint
	O'Brien's test (SLAP)
	Crank test (labrum)
	Empty can test (supraspinatus tendon)
	Speed's test (biceps tendon)

CASE STUDY 13-3—cont'd

Musculoskeletal System	Test
Thoracic spine (positive tests)	None
Thoracic spine (negative tests)	Segmental joint mobility and provocation testing (prone posterior-anterior glides) (see Fig. 5-22)
	T1 nerve root tension test (see Fig. 5-23)
	Thoracic quadrant tests
Ribs (positive test)	None
Ribs (negative tests)	Mobility and provocation testing of ribs R2 to R5 anteriorly (see Fig. 5-25)
	Mobility and provocation testing of the right first rib (see Fig. 5-25)
	CRLF test (see Fig. 5-26)
	Lateral compression testing of the middle and lower ribs (supine)
	Coughing and deep inhalation

Joint Integrity and Mobility

Cervical Spine

Examination is deferred (full gross AROM and PROM without pain; will examine segmental mobility at a future appointment as needed).

Shoulder

- Glenohumeral: Normal in all directions, with no complaints of pain
- Sternoclavicular: Normal in all directions, with no complaints of pain
- Acromioclavicular: Normal in all directions, with no complaints of pain
- Scapulothoracic: Normal in all directions, with no complaints of pain

Thoracic Spine

Examination is deferred to save time (will examine at a future appointment as needed).

Ribs

Results are normal for first ribs bilaterally, with no complaints of pain.

Neuromuscular System

Joe has no gross gait, locomotion, or balance disorders.

Imaging Studies

No imaging studies are taken of this patient's cervical or thoracic spine or shoulder.

Diagnosis

Cardiovascular/Pulmonary Pattern D: Impaired aerobic capacity/endurance associated with cardiovascular pump dysfunction or failure.

Joe's symptoms do not appear to be musculoskeletal in origin. Except for positive Roo's test for thoracic outlet syndrome with a vascular bias, the patient's symptoms are not reproduced during a thorough musculoskeletal examination. A return to the interview process reveals that the patient periodically feels a tightness or pressure on his chest at the same time he feels the shoulder pain. Both symptoms rapidly go away when he sits down and relaxes. Of concern was the number of "yes" answers on his medical screening questionnaire in the sections for pulmonary and cardiovascular disease. He also has risk factors related to cardiovascular disease, such as his age (48 years old), sex (male), diet (fast food), smoking (33-pack-year history), high cholesterol, diabetes, and family history (father and grandfather died of myocardial infarction). In addition, he notes that exertional activities give him SOB, fatigue, and a shoulder ache. Finally, he has reported cardiovascular type symptoms in the past year: SOB, fatigue, sweating with pain, chest pain, and dizziness.

Pain

The primary pain generator in this case appears not to be musculoskeletal in origin. A diagnosis of cardiovascular disease must be excluded.

Strain

The biomechanical strain that may be exacerbating Joe's pain and dysfunction is restricted mobility in the thoracic spine. The physiologic strains that may be exacerbating his pain are smoking, obesity, lack of regular exercise, and signs of possible cardiopulmonary disease.

Brain

Because his symptoms are not chronic, a primary central sensitization disorder was not suspected initially. However, because most of his musculoskeletal examination is negative, the possibility of a central sensitization disorder must be reexamined if he has no visceral disease or medical condition to explain his symptoms. Joe does not exhibit any overt signs of fear, anger, or frustration. He has, however, had several recent and significant life-changing events (divorce, move to a new residence, death of a pet). To facilitate the rehabilitation process, Joe may benefit from a referral for counseling.

Prognosis

Prognosis is uncertain and depends on the presence of visceral disease.

Intervention

The patient is referred back to his primary care physician for follow-up to rule out cardiopulmonary disease. Subsequently, myocardial ischemia, with associated angina pectoris, is diagnosed. His shoulder symptoms disappear immediately with the use of nitroglycerin.

CASE STUDY 13-4

Demographics

Vinaka is a 64-year-old, right-handed Fijian female interpreter who speaks fluent English, French, and several Fijian dialects. She is referred on March 16, 2007, by a physical therapist at another facility, for a consultation and second opinion on her right shoulder pain. She denies previous treatment of any kind for her current complaints.

Social History

She is married with five adult children and six grandchildren. Vinaka states that she comes from a very modest culture with strict religious beliefs. If she were to receive ongoing care, then she would feel more comfortable with a female therapist. Because of the nature of her job as an interpreter, she spends approximately 6 months in Fiji, 3 months in Europe, and 3 months in the United States each year.

Living Environment

In Fiji, she lives in a modest one-story, two-bedroom house. In Europe, she lives in a one-bedroom apartment on the second floor, and in the United States, she divides her time between a two-bedroom condominium on the first floor and a one-bedroom apartment on the third floor. She denies the existence of any major obstacles in and around any of her living quarters, except for the stairs leading up to her apartments. She does not use any assistive devices for her ADLs.

General Health Status

Vinaka states that she is in very good health for her age. In the past year, she learned that her sister was diagnosed with cancer. She has had no other major life changes, and she states that she enjoys the amount of traveling her job requires. The medical screening questionnaire, which Vinaka fills out on her first visit, is notable for the general and cardiovascular sections (Fig. 13-14). Specifically, the patient questionnaire reveals recent surgery, fever, SOB, and a prosthetic cardiac valve. On further questioning, this patient admits to an episode of chest pain 2 weeks ago, but she relates this to muscle soreness from washing her windows.

Social/Health Habits

Vinaka reports that she has never used tobacco products. She drinks a cup of decaffeinated coffee in the morning and has approximately three sodas with caffeine throughout the day. She does not drink alcohol. She takes a multivitamin supplement, extra calcium, fish oil tablets, and glucosamine sulfate. She is not a vegetarian, but she avoids red meat in favor of chicken or seafood and has a limited intake of dairy products. Vinaka does not participate in any sports or regular forms of physical activity other than her daily walks between 1 and 2 miles.

Family History

Vinaka's grandfather died, at the age 65, of a myocardial infarction and her grandmother died, at the age of 77, following her second CVA in 2 years. Her mother died of breast cancer at the age of 69 years; her father died of a massive myocardial infarction at age 73 years; non-Hodgkin's lymphoma was diagnosed in her 62-year-old sister; and her brother, 66 years old, received coronary artery bypass surgery, involving four arteries, 10 years ago.

Medical/Surgical History

- 2007: Surgery (August) root canal
- 2007: Surgery (March) implant of a prosthetic heart valve
- 2000: Diagnosis of high blood pressure/hypertension
- 2000: Diagnosis of high cholesterol (300 mg/dL)
- 1989: Hysterectomy

In the past year, she has reported fatigue, SOB, swelling in the extremities, heart palpitations, difficulty sleeping, nausea, and dizziness without vertigo or blackouts.

Current Condition(s)/Chief Complaint(s)

Vinaka, a 64-year-old, right-handed woman, comes to physical therapy on September 3, 2007, with a complaint of constant, severe (7/10 to 10/10) right shoulder pain. She reports that she has had a low-grade fever for the past 2 weeks. She denies neck pain, headaches, chest pain, dizziness or vertigo, vision changes, tinnitus, nausea, radiating arm pain, upper extremity paresthesia, and upper extremity weakness. She denies a history of right shoulder pain, neck pain, falls, fractures, or MVA. She reports no change in her shoulder pain related to eating, bowel or bladder activity, coughing, laughing, or deep inspiration or during exertional activities (e.g., long walks) that do not directly involve her shoulder. She also denies having the following constitutional symptoms: night sweats, nausea or vomiting, dizziness, fatigue, or unexplained weight loss. Other than what she reports here, she denies any other complaints or symptoms throughout the rest of her body. She reports the sudden onset, without trauma, of right shoulder and upper trapezius pain approximately 1 month before her initial evaluation (Fig. 13-15).

Functional Status/Activity Level

Vinaka does not normally participate in any sports or regular forms of physical activity other than her daily walks between 1 and 2 miles. She works full time as an interpreter, which involves a lot of traveling (planes, trains, and automobiles), prolonged standing, and a moderate degree of sitting. Her job does not require her to stress her shoulders or upper extremities to any significant degree. However, she is required to carry a briefcase and a suitcase when traveling, and this does put stress on her shoulder. She cannot sleep on her right side and has moderate

CASE STUDY 13-4—cont'd

Patient Questionnaire

Name Case Study #4 Date 9/16/93

	Yes		No
Age		64	
Height		5' 5"	
Weight (lbs)		125	
Fever and/or chills	X		
Unexplained weight change			X
Night pain/disturbed sleep			X
Episode of fainting			X
Dry mouth (difficulty swallowing)			X
Dry eyes (red, itchy, sandy)			X
History of illness prior to onset of pain	X		
History of cancer			X
Family history of cancer	X		
Recent surgery (dental also)	X		
Do you self inject medicines/drugs			X
Diabetic			X
Pain of gradual onset (no trauma).... sudden onset	X		
Constant pain			X
Pain worse at night			X
Pain relieved by rest	X		
Pulmonary			
History of smoking			X
Shortness of breath	X		
Fatigue			X
Wheezing or prolonged cough			X
History of asthma, emphysema or COPD			X
History of pneumonia or tuberculosis			X
Cardiovascular			
Heart murmur/heart valve problem	X		
History of heart problems	X		
Sweating with pain			X
Rapid throbbing or fluttering of heart			X
High blood pressure	X		
Dizziness (sit to stand)			X
Swelling in extremities	X		
History of rheumatic fever			X
Elevated cholesterol level	X		
Family history of heart disease	X		
Pain/symptoms increase with walking or stair climbing and relieved with rest			X
Pregnant women only			
Constant backache			
Increased uterine contractions			
Menstrual cramps			
Constant pelvic pressure			
Increased amount of vaginal discharge			
Increased consistency of vaginal discharge			
Color change of vaginal discharge			
Increased frequency of urination			

Figure 13-14 Patient questionnaire for Case Study 4.

difficulties with all ADLs (reaching overhead, driving, dressing, personal care, lifting or carrying, and domestic duties) because of pain in her right shoulder. Vinaka scores 63 out of a possible maximum score of 100 on the Sharp FAS for the neck and shoulder region.

Medications

- Prescription: hydrochlorothiazide (Lotensin) for hypertension, ibuprofen (NSAID), and fluvastatin (Lescol) for high cholesterol
- Nonprescription: acetaminophen (Tylenol)

Continued

CASE STUDY 13-4—cont'd

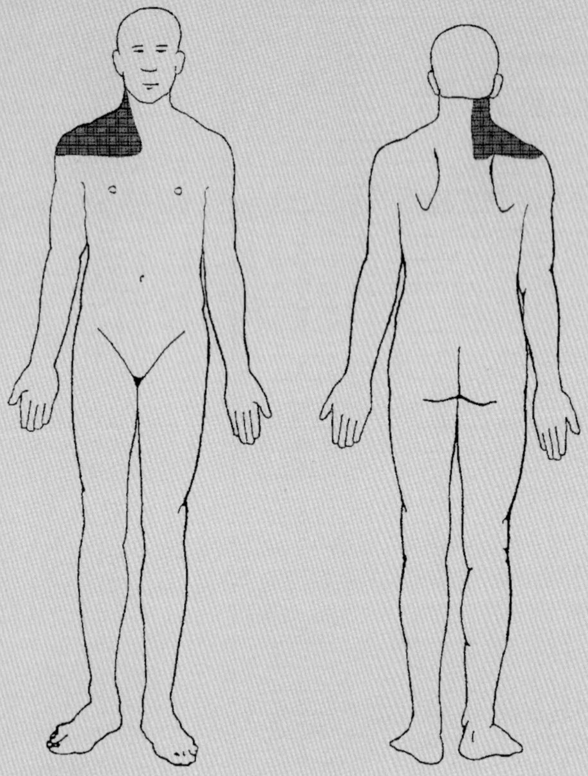

Figure 13-15 Pain diagram from a 64-year-old, right-handed woman with a diagnosis of "right shoulder pain."

Other Clinical Tests

At her last visit to her primary care physician 2 months ago, her blood pressure was 125/85 mm Hg, and her total cholesterol was 245 mg/dL. Vinaka has had no imaging studies, other than those at the dentist's office, in the past 10 years.

Cardiovascular/Pulmonary System

- Heart rate (resting): 75 beats per minute
- Respiratory rate (resting): 15 breaths per minute
- Blood pressure: 130/90 mm Hg
- Edema: mild bilateral ankle edema

Integumentary System

Vinaka's skin appears generally healthy. The area surrounding her right sternoclavicular joint is slightly swollen, warm, red, and tender. A well-healed surgical scar is noted across her sternum. Mild bilateral ankle edema is noted.

Communication, Affect, Cognition, Learning Style

No known learning barriers are identified for this patient. She states that she can remember things best if they are written down clearly and, in the case of home exercises, if she is also given a chance to perform them under supervision for the first time. Vinaka does not reveal any deficits with regard to her cognition, orientation, or ability to communicate effectively.

Musculoskeletal System

Posture

In standing, she has a slightly forward head, slight scoliosis (concave right through the midthoracic spine), and an elevated and slightly winging left scapula. She also has a high left iliac crest high, left posterior superior iliac spine, left gluteal, and left popliteal fossa, as well as a pronated left foot with moderate hallux valgus.

Range of Motion

Cervical Spine

AROM and PROM are limited slightly in flexion and left side bending with complaints of a "stretching ache" in the region of the right upper trapezius only during left side bending. The patient is able to perform pain-free cervical left side bending, through a full ROM, with the right scapula passively elevated and the upper trapezius placed on slack.

Shoulder

Active and passive flexion, extension, abduction, horizontal adduction, and horizontal abduction reproduce pain. AROM in these directions is minimally limited. PROM is WNL.

Scapula

Active and passive elevation, depression, protraction, and retraction also reproduce the patient's complaints of pain. AROM is mildly limited in all directions. PROM is WNL.

Elbow

AROM and PROM are WNL and pain free.

Thoracic Spine

AROM and PROM are pain free. In general, moderate limitations are noted in left side bending, right rotation, and extension.

Rib

AROM and PROM are WNL and pain free for general inhalation and exhalation and passive compression. First rib mobility on the right is slightly hypomobile, but pain free.

Lumbar Spine

AROM is pain free, but limited in all directions.

Muscle Performance

No reproduction of symptoms is elicited for all the cardinal directions tested in each of the shortened, middle, and lengthened ranges for muscles of the cervical and thoracic spine and right shoulder. Because this patient reports no history of upper extremity symptoms suggestive of neurogenic injury or irritation, specific manual muscle testing is deferred on the myotomes of the upper extremity.

Sensory Integrity

Tests are deferred because no neurogenic symptoms are reported and also to save time.

Reflex Integrity

Tests are deferred because no neurogenic symptoms are reported and also to save time.

CASE STUDY 13-4—cont'd

Pain

Palpation

The right sternoclavicular joint is slightly swollen, warm, red, and exquisitely tender. A palpable band of tender tissue is noted in the right upper trapezius muscle. Palpation of the lymph nodes (sternocleidomastoid, supraclavicular, and axillary), arterial pulses (brachial and radial), and abdomen is normal. No petechiae or Janeway's lesions are present on her skin. Ankle edema is noted bilaterally.

Special Tests

Musculoskeletal System	Test
Cervical spine (positive tests: reproduction of symptoms)	Cervical quadrant test in flexion left: "stretch" pain in the right upper trapezius) Cervical quadrant test in extension left: pain in right sternoclavicular joint (see Fig. 5-19)
Cervical spine (negative tests)	Compression testing of the cervical spine in flexion, neutral, and extension (see Fig. 5-15) Cervical quadrant test in flexion right and extension right (see Fig. 5-19) Valsalva's maneuver
Shoulder (positive tests: pain at the sternoclavicular joint)	Hawkins' impingement sign Acromioclavicular joint compression (horizontal adduction of humerus)
Shoulder (negative tests)	Distraction and compression of the glenohumeral joint Load and shift test (anterior and posterior instability) O'Brien's test (SLAP) Crank test (labrum) Empty can test (supraspinatus tendon) Speed's test (biceps tendon)
Thoracic spine (positive tests)	None
Thoracic spine (negative tests)	Segmental joint mobility and provocation testing (prone posterior-anterior glides) (see Fig. 5-22) Thoracic quadrant tests
Ribs (positive test)	Mobility and provocation testing of right first rib: hypomobile with local tenderness (see Fig. 5-25) CRLF test: hypomobile on the right (see Fig. 5-26).
Ribs (negative tests)	Mobility and provocation testing of ribs R2 to R5 anteriorly (see Fig. 5-25) Lateral compression testing of the middle and lower ribs (supine) Coughing and deep inhalation

Joint Integrity and Mobility

Cervical Spine

The cervical spine is severely hypomobile at C6 in extension, left side bending, and left rotation, but without pain. It is mildly hypermobile at C5 in extension and left rotation, also without pain. The result of the disk shear test is positive at C5 (see Fig. 5-16).

Shoulder

- Glenohumeral: Normal in all directions, without pain
- Sternoclavicular: Hypomobile, mild in all directions, with pain
- Acromioclavicular: Normal in all directions, without pain
- Scapulothoracic: Normal in all directions, without pain

Thoracic Spine

The thoracic spine is mildly hypomobile from T1 to T4 for left side bending and right rotation, without pain, and is severely hypomobile from T1 to T7 in extension, also without pain.

Ribs

The patient has rib hypomobility, mild for the right first rib, without complaints of shoulder pain.

Neuromuscular System

Vinaka has no gross gait, locomotion, or balance disorders.

Imaging Studies

No imaging studies are taken of this patient's cervical or thoracic spine or shoulder.

Diagnosis

Musculoskeletal Pattern E: Impaired joint mobility, motor function, muscle performance, and ROM associated with localized inflammation.

This patient's signs and symptoms are consistent with an irritable, and probably inflamed, right sternoclavicular joint. She demonstrates classic signs of inflammation: pain, tenderness, swelling, warmth, and redness. Because of the multiple "yes" answers in the cardiovascular section of her medical screening questionnaire, and because of her history of prosthetic valve surgery, recent surgery, recent illness, SOB, fever, chest pain, and the sudden onset of pain without trauma, the plan is to refer her back to her primary care physician to rule out cardiac symptoms and disease. If nothing else, this is thought to be a musculoskeletal problem with comorbid cardiac disease.

Pain

The primary pain generator for this patient appears to be her right sternoclavicular joint.

Strain

The biomechanical strains that may be exacerbating her pain and dysfunction at the sternoclavicular joint are poor posture, segmental instability of the cervical spine, and hypomobilities in the first rib and thoracic spine. The physiologic strain that may be exacerbating her pain and dysfunction is the possibility of heart disease.

Continued

CASE STUDY 13-4—cont'd

Brain

The patient has experienced her symptoms only for a few weeks, and she has no overt signs of anger, frustration, hopelessness, depression, or denial. No indication of a primary central sensitization disorder or adverse forebrain activity is present at this time.

Prognosis

Prognosis is uncertain and depends on the presence of visceral disease and whether the visceral disease is comorbid or the primary generator of her symptoms.

Intervention

Anticipated goals are as follows:

1. Vinaka's goal: "Learn an exercise program I can do on my own."
2. Cervical AROM will return to WNL.
3. The patient will have minimal restrictions for thoracic spine motion.
4. The patient will have minimal difficulty (3/10) with ADLs.
5. The Sharp FAS score will be 85/100 without dependence on pain medication.
6. The patient will be independent, with a comprehensive HEP.

Because Vinaka was referred for a consultation and second opinion, treatment is not initiated. She is referred back to her primary care physician with concerns regarding her cardiac status. A report is sent to her primary physical therapist with a recommendation to hold physical therapy until after Vinaka sees her physician. After a referral to a rheumatologist and then a cardiac specialist, bacterial endocarditis is eventually diagnosed. After a week on antibiotics, her right shoulder pain is minimal (3/10), and she is scheduled to begin physical therapy elsewhere.

CASE STUDY 13-5

Demographics

Alex is a 51-year-old, right-handed, obese, African American female patent attorney whose primary language is English. She is referred for physical therapy by her primary care physician on September 24, 2008, with a diagnosis of "right shoulder strain." She denies previous treatment of any kind for her current complaints.

Social History

Alex is single, never married, and lives with her partner. She denies any cultural or religious beliefs that she thinks may affect her care. She works as a patent attorney, which involves prolonged sitting and long periods on her computer. She has minimal physical stress, however, in terms of lifting, carrying, and overhead activities.

Living Environment

She lives in a two-story, three-bedroom house. She denies the existence of any major obstacles in and around her house. She denies the use of assistive devices during her ADLs.

General Health Status

Alex reports that she is in "pretty fair" health. She states she started her own law firm 6 months ago and has only recently been able to keep her work week to less than 60 hours. The medical screening questionnaire, which Alex fills out on her first visit, is notable for the general and gastrointestinal sections (Fig. 13-16). Further questioning reveals that she has had a low-grade fever for the 3 weeks before her evaluation in physical therapy. In addition, she also admits to having occasional upper abdominal and right shoulder blade pain after meals.

Social/Health Habits

Alex reports that she stopped smoking 10 years ago. Before then, she had smoked a half to a full pack of cigarettes a day for approximately 26 years. She drinks two to three cups of coffee and two to three cans of soda with caffeine a day. She drinks a beer or glass of wine 3 to 4 nights a week. She takes a multivitamin and extra calcium. She is not a vegetarian, eats red meat several times a week, dairy products daily, and shellfish occasionally. Lately, she has been avoiding greasy or fried foods. Her only form of exercise—she does not participate in athletic activities or sports—is walking on a treadmill for 20 minutes three times a week.

Family History

Her father died at the age of 71 years of progressive heart failure. Her mother is still alive, but diabetes, lupus, and rheumatoid arthritis have been diagnosed. Her sister, who is 54 years old, has fibromyalgia.

Medical/Surgical History

2007: Arthroscopic decompression of right shoulder (August)
2006: Diagnosis of hepatitis

CASE STUDY 13-5—cont'd

Patient Questionnaire

Name Case Study #5 Date 5/21/95

	Yes		No
Age		51	
Height		5' 3"	
Weight (lbs)		175	
Fever and/or chills	X		
Unexplained weight change	X		
Night pain/disturbed sleep	X		
Episode of fainting			X
Dry mouth (difficulty swallowing)			X
Dry eyes (red, itchy, sandy)			X
History of illness prior to onset of pain			X
History of cancer			X
Family history of cancer	X	(1)	
Recent surgery (dental also)	X		
Do you self inject medicines/drugs	X		
Diabetic	X		
Pain of gradual onset (no trauma)			X
Constant pain			X
Pain worse at night	X		
Pain relieved by rest			X

Gastrointestinal

	Yes	No
Difficulty in swallowing		X
Nausea	X	
Heartburn		X
Vomiting		X
Food intolerances	X	
Constipation		X
Diarrhea	X	
Change in color of stools		X
Rectal bleeding		X
History of liver or gallbladder problems	X	
History of stomach or GI problems	X	
Indigestion	X	
Loss of apetite		X
Pain worse when lying on your back		X
Pain change due to bowel/bladder activity		X
Pain change during or after meals	X	

Figure 13-16 Patient questionnaire for Case Study 5, modified to show notable portions of both pages.

2003: MVA with diagnosis of cervical sprain and strain and whiplash; resolved

1996: Diagnosis of non–insulin-dependent (type 2) diabetes mellitus

In the past year, Alex has complained of joint pain, difficulty sleeping, nausea, indigestion, diarrhea, unexplained weight change, headaches, and fever.

Current Condition(s)/Chief Complaint(s)

Alex, a 51-year-old, right-handed, obese woman, comes to the office on September 24, 2008, with a diagnosis of "right shoulder strain." She complains of a periodic, severe (0 to 8/10), deep, and generalized ache across the back of her right shoulder (Fig. 13-17). She reports that her right shoulder pain is worse at night. After asking her directly, she does admit that there seems to be an exacerbation of her right shoulder pain an hour or so after lunch. Alex reports that she often has lunch with clients at a local restaurant. Her lunchtime meals vary from hamburger with fries, fried chicken, and mashed potatoes to the occasional soup and salad. She denies neck pain, headaches, TMJ dysfunction, chest pain, dizziness or vertigo, vision changes, tinnitus, radiating right arm pain, paresthesia in the right upper extremity, and right upper extremity weakness. She reports no change in her right shoulder pain related to bowel and bladder activity or during prolonged walks or climbing stairs. She admits to having the following constitutional symptoms: fever, unexplained weight change, night pain, indigestion, diarrhea, and nausea. She denies night sweats, vomiting, dizziness, and fatigue. Alex reports the sudden onset of a severe ache in her right shoulder

Continued

CASE STUDY 13-5—cont'd

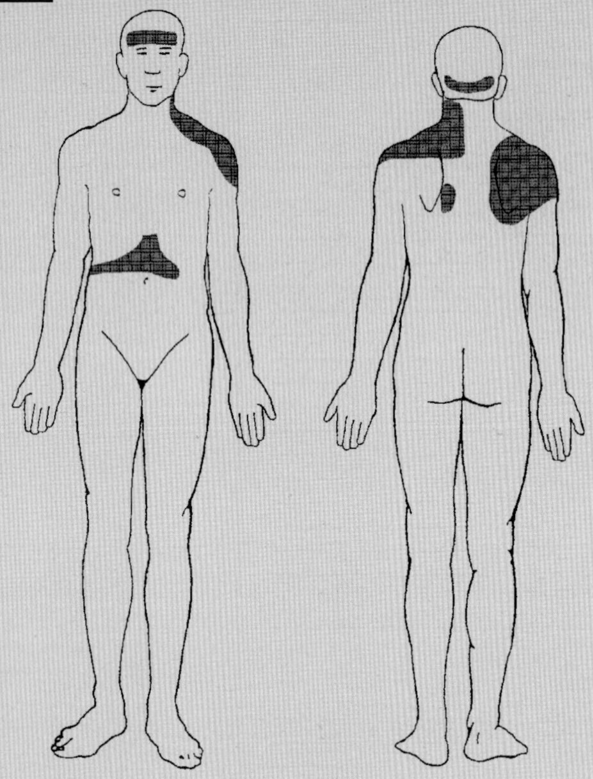

Figure 13-17 Pain diagram from a 51-year-old, right-handed woman with a diagnosis of "right shoulder strain."

after a day of housecleaning 2 weeks ago. She also admits to a long history (5 years) of headaches, neck pain, and left shoulder pain with tingling in her left hand. The symptoms in her neck and left shoulder do not change after cleaning her house, and they remain mild in intensity. The pain in her left shoulder is not the same as the pain in the right. The left shoulder pain is sharp, shooting, and localized. She does admit to an occasional ache in her right shoulder blade during the past 2 months before she came to physical therapy. She denies a history of falls or fractures. Other than what she reports here, she denies any other complaints or symptoms throughout the rest of her body.

Functional Status/Activity Level

Alex's only form of exercise—she does not participate in athletic activities or sports—is walking on a treadmill for 20 minutes three times a week. She scores 58 out of a possible maximum score of 100 on the Sharp FAS for the neck and shoulder region. She reports severe difficulty looking up or reaching overhead; moderate difficulty with sleeping, driving, dressing, personal care, lifting or carrying, and domestic duties; and minimal difficulty with leisure activities and work. She is working full time and has not had to miss any time from work because of her neck and shoulder complaints.

Medications

- Prescription: celecoxib (Celebrex, an NSAID), hydrocodone and acetaminophen combination (Vicodin) for pain, carisoprodol (Soma) for insomnia, and amitriptyline (Elavil) for depression
- Nonprescription: aluminum hydroxide and magnesium hydroxide combination (Maalox) as needed

Other Clinical Tests

She has regular tests for blood glucose levels. Her most recent test was 3 weeks ago and was reported as WNL. A mammogram last year was reported as normal according to the patient. A review of a plain radiograph of her cervical spine that was taken 4 years ago shows mild to moderate degenerative changes throughout her cervical spine. A review of a plain radiograph of her right shoulder taken last week reveals no significant abnormalities.

Cardiovascular/Pulmonary System

Although it is well known that the heart and lungs can refer pain to the left shoulder and can cause indigestion and nausea, the right shoulder is not a common area of the body for referred cardiac pain and symptoms. No clear indication existed that this patient's symptoms may be cardiopulmonary in origin. Her medical screening questionnaire does not raise any red flags in the pulmonary or cardiovascular sections (see Fig. 13-16). Therefore, a specific cardiopulmonary physical examination is deferred.

Integumentary System

Alex's skin appears healthy, with good continuity of color and no significant changes in temperature. No swelling is present. White, well-healed surgical scars are noted around her right shoulder.

Communication, Affect, Cognition, Learning Style

No known learning barriers are identified for this patient. She states that she can remember things best if they are explained clearly and she is given a good rationale to back up the advice or instruction. Alex does not reveal any deficits with regard to her cognition, orientation, or ability to communicate effectively.

Musculoskeletal System

Posture

In standing, she has a slightly forward head, exaggerated lumbar lordosis, and bilateral pes planus.

Range of Motion

Cervical Spine

Active and passive cervical extension, left side bending, and left rotation reproduce neck and left shoulder pain. No reproduction of right shoulder pain is elicited.

CASE STUDY 13-5—cont'd

Shoulder (Right)

AROM and PROM of the right shoulder do not reproduce pain, although mild restrictions are noted with flexion, abduction, and external rotation.

Scapula and Elbow (Right)

AROM and PROM are WNL and pain free.

Thoracic Spine

AROM and PROM are pain free. Moderate limitations are noted in upper thoracic left side bending and extension.

Rib

AROM and PROM are WNL and pain free for general inhalation and exhalation and passive compression. First rib mobility on the left is slightly hypomobile.

Lumbar Spine

AROM is pain free, with a moderate limitation in flexion and extension and a mild limitation in all other directions.

Muscle Performance

No reproduction of right shoulder pain is elicited for all the cardinal directions tested in each of the shortened, middle, and lengthened ranges for muscles of the cervical and thoracic spine, and right shoulder. Left cervical and shoulder symptoms are reproduced with resisted testing when the cervical spine is extended, the side is bent to the left, or the spine is rotated left. Specific manual muscle testing (isometric; (5/5 is WNL) of the upper extremities is WNL (5/5).

Sensory Integrity

Increased sensitivity to light touch and pinprick is noted in the left C6 dermatome.

Reflex Integrity

Hyperreflexia (3+) is noted for the left brachioradialis DTR. The biceps brachialis, triceps, and abductor digiti minimi are equal (2+) bilaterally. The SHR test result is negative. Hoffmann's sign shows a positive result on the left.

Pain

Palpation

Mild tenderness, without reproduction of significant shoulder pain, is noted in the left upper trapezius, left middle trapezius, left rhomboids, and right infraspinatus muscle belly. Palpation of the lymph nodes (sternocleidomastoid, supraclavicular, and axillary) is normal. Palpation of the abdomen indicates rigidity and exquisite tenderness in the right upper abdominal quadrant. No joint effusion or soft tissue edema is noted. Palpation of her upper extremity pulses is deferred because her symptoms and medical screening questionnaire do not indicate the possibility of cardiovascular disease.

Special Tests

Musculoskeletal System	Test
Cervical spine (positive tests; none of the rib provocational tests reproduce right shoulder pain)	Cervical quadrant test in extension left: left cervical and left shoulder pain with "tingling" in the left hand (see Fig. 5-19) Compression testing of cervical spine in extension only: left cervical and left shoulder pain only (see Fig. 5-15) Cervical quadrant test in flexion right: left cervical and left shoulder pain only Valsalva's maneuver: left shoulder pain
Cervical spine (negative tests)	None
Shoulder right (positive tests)	None
Shoulder right (negative tests)	Distraction and compression of the glenohumeral joint Hawkins' impingement sign Load and shift test (anterior and posterior instability) Distraction and compression of the acromioclavicular joint O'Brien's test (SLAP) Crank test (labrum) Empty can test (supraspinatus tendon) Speed's test (biceps tendon)
Thoracic spine (positive tests)	None
Thoracic spine (negative tests)	Segmental joint mobility and provocation testing (prone posterior-anterior glides) (see Fig. 5-22) Thoracic quadrant tests
Ribs (positive test; none of the rib provocational tests reproduce right shoulder pain)	Mobility and provocation testing: left first rib tender and hypomobile (see Fig. 5-25) CRLF test: hypomobile on the left (see Fig. 5-26) Coughing: left cervical and left shoulder pain
Ribs (negative tests)	Mobility and provocation testing of ribs R2 to R5 anteriorly (see Fig. 5-25) Lateral compression testing of the middle and lower ribs (supine) Deep inhalation

Joint Integrity and Mobility

Cervical Spine

Tests are deferred to save time. Previous portions of the evaluation have not implicated the cervical spine as a source of the right shoulder pain.

Continued

CASE STUDY 13-5—cont'd

Shoulder (Right)
- Glenohumeral: Hypomobile, mild in all directions, with muscle guarding and no pain
- Sternoclavicular: Hypomobile, mild in distraction and inferior glide, with no pain
- Acromioclavicular: Normal in all directions, with no pain
- Scapulothoracic: Normal in all directions, with no pain

Thoracic Spine
Tests are deferred to save time. The rationale is the same as noted for the cervical spine.

Ribs
The patient has rib hypomobility, mild for the left first rib, with muscle guarding.

Neuromuscular System
Alex has no gross gait, locomotion, or balance disorders.

Imaging Studies
- Cervical (2004): A review of the films reveals the following: mild DDD at C3-4 and C4-5 and moderate DDD at the C5-6 and C6-7 levels with mild posterior vertebral osteophytes. Facet DJD at same levels and degrees noted in the previous sentence. Moderate foraminal stenosis at left C5-6 and mild stenosis at left C4-5. A loss of the normal cervical spine lordosis is observed. Incidentally noted is an incomplete ponticulus ponticus on the posterior arch of the atlas.
- Shoulder, right (2008): A review of the films reveals the following: normal shoulder with a type I acromion.

Diagnosis
Alex's right shoulder symptoms do not appear to be musculoskeletal in origin. Although mild chronic joint dysfunction is noted in the right shoulder girdle, this patient's signs and symptoms are inconsistent with an active orthopedic problem of the right shoulder. The cervical and thoracic spine and ribs do not appear to be a source of her right shoulder symptoms. Of concern is the patient's history of diabetes, hepatitis, fever, shoulder pain associated with greasy meals (lunch), and the exquisite tenderness in the right upper abdominal quadrant. The left shoulder and hand symptoms are thought to be secondary to mild and chronic left cervical radiculopathy (Musculoskeletal Pattern F: Impaired joint mobility, motor function, muscle performance, ROM, and reflex integrity associated with spinal disorders).

Pain
The primary pain generator in this case appears not to be musculoskeletal in origin.

Strain
The biomechanical strains that may be exacerbating Alex's pain and dysfunction are her chronic neck and left upper extremity symptoms and the restricted mobility in her thoracic spine. The physiologic strains that may be exacerbating her pain and dysfunction are diet (excessive caffeine, red meat, shellfish, and dairy) and signs of possible gastrointestinal disease.

Brain
Because she has had chronic neck and left upper extremity symptoms and the physical examination of her right shoulder is mostly negative, Alex is likely to have a component of central sensitization aggravating her right shoulder symptoms, especially if her symptoms cannot be attributed to a visceral disease or medical condition. Although she does not exhibit any overt signs of fear, anger, or frustration, Alex is under a lot of stress at work and is working long hours. The patient may benefit from a referral for pain and stress management.

Prognosis
Prognosis is uncertain and depends on the presence of visceral disease and whether the visceral disease is comorbid or the primary generator of her symptoms.

Intervention
Alex is referred back to her primary care physician to rule out any gastrointestinal problems. Cholecystitis secondary to gallstones is diagnosed in the patient. Her gastrointestinal symptoms and right shoulder pain are reduced approximately 50% on a controlled diet. The right shoulder blade pain does not disappear, however, until after a cholecystectomy. She continues to report chronic neck and left upper extremity symptoms, but she is not referred back for physical therapy to address these symptoms.

SUMMARY

The best way to determine whether the patient's symptoms may be caused by visceral disease is first to eliminate all possible musculoskeletal tissue as a source of the symptoms. This process requires skill, confidence, and experience in performing a thorough history and comprehensive physical evaluation. If the physical therapist cannot reproduce the patient's symptoms or has difficulty identifying a tissue in lesion, or if the patient does not respond to treatment, then ruling out a visceral pathologic condition becomes imperative. A patient who is referred to physical therapy with an orthopedic diagnosis, but who demonstrates signs and symptoms of visceral disease, can be saved from severe morbidity—and sometimes death—by early referral to the appropriate level of medical care. Of course, many physical therapy patients have known comorbid visceral disease (i.e., both orthopedic and visceral problems). A positive musculoskeletal examination does not eliminate the possibility of an unrelated viscus injury or disease. Comorbid visceral disease is important to identify because it most likely puts a strain on the healing and rehabilitation of the orthopedic injury or impairment and should therefore changing the normal plan of care and prognosis accordingly.

ACKNOWLEDGMENTS

Gray wishes to thank Ola Grimsby and Jim Rivard for their contributions and support.

REFERENCES

1. Massey BF Jr: 2002 APTA presidential address: what's all the fuss about direct access? *Phys Ther* 82:1120, 2002.
2. Boissonnault WG, Koopmeiners MB: Medical history profile: orthopaedic physical therapy outpatients, *J Orthop Sports Phys Ther* 20:2, 1994.
3. Payne R: Cancer pain: anatomy, physiology, and pharmacology, *Cancer* 63:2266, 1989.
4. Boissonnault WG, Bass C: Pathological origins of trunk and neck pain: pelvic and abdominal visceral disorders, *J Orthop Sports Phys Ther* 12:192, 1990.
5. Procacci P, Maresca M: Clinical aspects of visceral pain, *Funct Neurol* 4:19, 1989.
6. Cervero F: Mechanisms of acute visceral pain, *Br Med Bull* 47:549, 1991.
7. Gebhart G, Ness T: Central mechanisms of visceral pain, *Can J Physiol Pharmacol* 69:627, 1991.
8. Lynn R: Mechanisms of esophageal pain, *Am J Med* 92:11S, 1992.
9. Cousins M: Introduction to acute and chronic pain: implications for neural blockade. In Cousins M, Bridenbaugh P, editors: *Neural blockade in clinical anesthesia and management of pain*, Philadelphia, 1988, Lippincott.
10. Raj P: Prognostic and therapeutic local anesthetic block. In Cousins M, Bridenbaugh P, editors: *Neural blockade in clinical anesthesia and management of pain*, Philadelphia, 1988, Lippincott.
11. Ruch T: Visceral sensation and referred pain. In Fulton J, editor: *Textbook of physiology*, Philadelphia, 1949, Saunders.
12. Galea MP: Neuroanatomy of the nociceptive system. In Strong J, Unruh AM, Wright A, et al, editors: *Pain: a textbook for therapists*, New York, 2002, Churchill Livingstone.
13. Lewit K: The contribution of clinical observation to neurobiological mechanisms in manipulative therapy. In Korr IM, editor: *The neurobiologic mechanisms in manipulative therapy*, New York, 1978, Plenum.
14. Patterson M: A model mechanism for spinal segmental facilitation, *J Am Osteopath Assoc* 76:62, 1976.
15. Goodman CC, Snyder TEK: Introduction to differential screening in physical therapy. In *Differential diagnosis in physical therapy*, ed 2, Philadelphia, 1995, Saunders.
16. Boissonnault WG, Janos SC: Screening for medical disease: physical therapy assessment and treatment principles. In Boissonnault WG, editor: *Examination in physical therapy practice: screening for medical disease*, ed 2, New York, 1995, Churchill Livingstone.
17. Koopmeiners MB: Screening for gastrointestinal system disease. In Boissonnault WG, editor: *Examination in physical therapy practice: screening for medical disease*, ed 2, New York, 1995, Churchill Livingstone.
18. Abramson DI, Miller DS: Clinical and laboratory tests of arterial circulation. In *Vascular problems in musculoskeletal disorders of the limbs*, New York, 1981, Springer.
19. Michel TH, Downing J: Screening for cardiovascular system disease. In Boissonnault WG, editor: *Examination in physical therapy practice: screening for medical disease*, ed 2, New York, 1995, Churchill Livingstone.
20. Natkin E, Harrington G, Mandel M: Anginal pain referred to the teeth: report of a case, *Oral Surg* 40:678, 1975.
21. Henry J, Montuschi E: Cardiac pain referred to site of previously experienced somatic pain, *Br Med J* 9:1605, 1978.
22. Grieve G: Clinical features. In *Common vertebral joint problems*, New York, 1981, Churchill Livingstone.
23. Lewis T, Kellgren J: Observations relating to referred pain, visceromotor reflexes and other associated phenomena, *Clin Sci* 4:47, 1939.
24. Cyriax J: Referred pain. In *Textbook of orthopaedic medicine: diagnosis of soft tissue lesions*, ed 8, London, 1982, Bailliere Tindall.
25. Laurberg S, Sorensen K: Cervical dorsal root ganglion cells with collaterals to both shoulder skin and the diaphragm: a fluorescent double labeling study in the rat—a model for referred pain? *Brain Res* 331:160, 1985.
26. Bahr R, Blumberg H, Janig W: Do dichotomizing afferent fibers exist which supply visceral organs as well as somatic structures? A contribution to the problem of referred pain, *Neurosci Lett* 24:25, 1981.
27. Doran F: The sites to which pain is referred from the common bile duct in man and its implication for the theory of referred pain, *Br J Surg* 54:599, 1967.
28. Hobbs S, Chandler M, Bolser D, et al: Segmental organization of visceral and somatic input onto C3-T6 spinothalamic tract cells of the monkey, *J Neurophysiol* 68:1575, 1992.
29. Bolser D, Hobbs S, Chandler M, et al: Convergence of phrenic and cardiopulmonary spinal afferent information on cervical and thoracic spinothalamic tract neurons in the monkey: implications for referred pain from the diaphragm and the heart, *J Neurophysiol* 65:1042, 1991.
30. Campbell S: Referred shoulder pain: an elusive diagnosis, *Postgrad Med* 73:193, 1983.
31. Calliet R: Visceral referred pain. In *Shoulder pain*, ed 3, Philadelphia, 1981, Davis.
32. Leland J: Visceral aspects of shoulder pain, *Bull Hosp Jt Dis* 14:71, 1953.
33. Capps J: *An experimental and clinical study of pain in the pleura, pericardium, and peritoneum*, New York, 1932, Macmillan.
34. Bateman J: Applied physiology of the shoulder and neck. In *The shoulder and neck*, Philadelphia, 1978, Saunders.
35. Walsh RM, Sadowski GE: Systemic disease mimicking musculoskeletal dysfunction: a case report involving referred shoulder pain, *J Orthop Sports Phys Ther* 31(12):696, 2001.
36. Boissonnault W, Bass C: Pathological origins of trunk and neck pain: disorders of the cardiovascular and pulmonary system, *J Orthop Sports Phys Ther* 12:208, 1990.
37. Williams PL, Warwick R, Dyson M, et al, editors: Myology. In *Gray's anatomy*, ed 37, New York, 1989, Churchill Livingstone.
38. Angel J, Sims C, O'Brien W, et al: Postcoital pneumoperitoneum, *Obstet Gynecol* 71:1039, 1988.
39. Christiansen W, Danzl D, McGee H: Pneumoperitoneum following vaginal insufflation and coitus, *Ann Emerg Med* 9:480, 1980.
40. Rucker C, Miller R, Nov H: Pneumoperitoneum secondary to perforated appendicitis: a report of two cases and a review of the literature, *Am J Surg* 33:188, 1967.

41. Lozman H, Newman A: Spontaneous pneumoperitoneum occurring during postpartum exercises in the knee chest position, *Am J Obstet Gynecol* 72:903, 1956.
42. Aronson M, Nelson P: Fatal air embolism in pregnancy resulting from an unusual sex act, *Obstet Gynecol* 30:127, 1967.
43. Quigley J, Gaspar I: Fatal air embolism on the eighth day of puerperium, *Am J Obstet Gynecol* 32:1054, 1936.
44. Goodman CC, Snyder TEK: Overview of gastrointestinal signs and symptoms. In *Differential diagnosis in physical therapy*, ed 2, Philadelphia, 1995, Saunders.
45. Sarli L, Costi R, Sansebastiano G, et al: Prospective randomized trial of low-pressure pneumoperitoneum for reduction of shoulder-tip pain following laparoscopy, *Br J Surg* 87(9):1161–1165, 2000.
46. Vargo M, Flood K: Pancoast's tumor presenting as cervical radiculopathy, *Arch Phys Med Rehabil* 71:606, 1990.
47. Welch WC, Erhard R, Clyde B, et al: Systemic malignancy presenting as neck and shoulder pain, *Arch Phys Med Rehabil* 75:918, 1994.
48. Kovach SG, Huslig EL: Shoulder pain and Pancoast's tumor: a diagnostic dilemma, *J Manipulative Physiol Ther* 7:25, 1984.
49. Goodman CC, Snyder TEK: Overview of pulmonary signs and symptoms. In *Differential diagnosis in physical therapy*, ed 2, Philadelphia, 1995, Saunders.
50. Loeb S: *Professional guide to signs and symptoms*, Springhouse, Pa, 1993, Springhouse.
51. Arnall D, Ryan M: Screening for pulmonary system disease. In Boissonnault WG, editor: *Examination in physical therapy practice: screening for medical disease*, ed 2, New York, 1995, Churchill Livingstone.
52. Niethammer JG, Hubner KF, Buonocore E: Pulmonary embolism: how V/Q scanning helps in diagnosis, *Postgrad Med* 87:263, 1990.
53. Boissonnault W, Bass C: Pathological origins of trunk and neck pain: diseases of the musculoskeletal system, *J Orthop Sports Phys Ther* 12:216, 1990.
54. Netter FH: Diseases and pathology. In *The Ciba collection of medical illustrations: respiratory system*, ed 2, West Caldwell, NJ, 1980, Ciba-Geigy.
55. Coventry MB: Problem of painful shoulder, *JAMA* 151:177, 1953.
56. Ammons W: Cardiopulmonary sympathetic afferent input to lower thoracic spinal neurons, *Brain Res* 529:149, 1990.
57. Nevens F, Janssens J, Piessens J, et al: Prospective study on prevalence of esophageal chest pain in patients referred on an elective basis to a cardiac unit for suspected myocardial ischemia, *Dig Dis Sci* 36:229, 1991.
58. Lagerqvist B, Sylven C, Beermann B: Intracoronary adenosine causes angina pectoris like pain: an inquiry into the nature of visceral pain, *Cardiovasc Res* 24:609, 1990.
59. Askey JM: The syndrome of painful disability of the shoulder and hand complicating coronary occlusion, *Am Heart J* 22:1, 1941.
60. Goodman CC, Snyder TEK: Overview of cardiovascular signs and symptoms. In *Differential diagnosis in physical therapy*, ed 2, Philadelphia, 1995, Saunders.
61. Churchill M, Geraci J, Hunder G: Musculoskeletal manifestations of bacterial endocarditis, *Ann Intern Med* 87:754, 1977.
62. Hunder G: When musculoskeletal symptoms point to endocarditis, *J Musculoskelet Med* 9:33, 1992.
63. Abramson DI, Miller DS: Clinical entities with both vascular and orthopedic components. In *Vascular problems in musculoskeletal disorders of the limbs*, New York, 1981, Springer.
64. Wilgis EFS: Compression syndromes of the shoulder girdle and arm. In *Vascular injuries and diseases of the upper limb*, Boston, 1983, Little, Brown.
65. Wilgis EFS: Diagnosis. In *Vascular injuries and diseases of the upper limb*, Boston, 1983, Little, Brown.
66. Rohrer MJ: Vascular problems. In Pappas AM, editor: *Upper extremity injuries in the athlete*, New York, 1995, Churchill Livingstone.
67. Abramson DI, Miller DS: Vascular complications of musculoskeletal disorders produced by trauma. In *Vascular problems in musculoskeletal disorders of the limbs*, New York, 1981, Springer.
68. O'Leary MR, Smith MS, Druy EM: Diagnostic and therapeutic approach to axillary-subclavian vein thrombosis, *Ann Emerg Med* 16:889, 1987.
69. Jiha JG, Laurito CE, Rosenquist RW: Subclavian vein compression and thrombosis presenting as upper extremity pain, *Anesth Analg* 85:225, 1997.
70. Goodman CC, Snyder TEK: Overview of hepatic and biliary signs and symptoms. In *Differential diagnosis in physical therapy*, ed 2, Philadelphia, 1995, Saunders.
71. Goodman CC, Snyder TEK: Overview of renal and urologic signs and symptoms. In *Differential diagnosis in physical therapy*, ed 2, Philadelphia, 1995, Saunders.
72. Davidson R, Lewis E, Daehler D, et al: Perinephrenic abscess and chronic low back pain, *J Fam Pract* 15:1059, 1982.
73. Swarbrick E, Hegarty J, Bat L, et al: Site of pain from the irritable bowel, *Lancet* 2:443, 1980.
74. Cervero F: Neurophysiology of gastrointestinal pain, *Baillieres Clin Gastroenterol* 2:183, 1988.

PART 4
TREATMENT APPROACHES

CHAPTER 14

Robert A. Donatelli
and Timothy J. McMahon

Manual Therapy Techniques

The primary goals of the clinician are to optimize function, decrease pain, restore proper mechanics, facilitate healing, and assist regeneration of tissue. Manual therapy has been demonstrated clinically to be an important part of rehabilitation and of assessment of restricted joint movement. Clinical application of manual techniques is based on an understanding of joint mechanics, tissue histology, and muscle function. Notable advancement has been made in describing the benefits of passive movement by such researchers as Frank, Akeson, Woo, Mathews, Amiel, and Peacock.[1-3] With this knowledge, the clinician can apply manual therapy techniques during critical stages of wound healing to influence the extensibility of scar tissue, reduce the development of restrictive adhesions, and provide foundations of neuromuscular mechanisms to restore homeostasis.[1] Through an understanding of the effects of immobilization and soft tissue healing constraints, criteria for phases of manual therapy techniques can be established.

This chapter focuses on manual therapy for the shoulder complex from a basic science and problem-solving approach. Manual therapy is discussed in relation to soft tissue and joint mobilization and muscle reeducation. Various manual therapy techniques are described. Management of the shoulder patient is discussed from a perspective of protective versus nonprotective injuries. Evidence-based practice is presented for manual therapy for the shoulder.

Normal joint function includes a dynamic combination of arthrokinematics (intimate mechanics of joint surfaces), osteokinematics (the movement of bones), muscle function, fascial extensibility, and neurobiomechanics (see Chapter 6). Dysfunction and pain of the shoulder can result from altered function of any or all of these systems. A detailed sequential evaluation that hypothesizes particular impairments dictates which particular manual therapy strategy is appropriate. Please refer to Chapter 4 for shoulder evaluation procedures. Clearing the cervical and thoracic spine and brachial plexus is reviewed in Chapters 5 and 8. The manual techniques discussed in this chapter focus on the shoulder complex.

DEFINITIONS

Several terms must be defined when discussing manual therapy. Articulation, oscillation, distractions, manipulation, and mobilization all describe specialized types of passive movement.

Manual therapy is defined in the *Guide to Physical Therapy Practice* as "skilled hand movements intended to improve tissue extensibility; increase range of motion; induce relaxation; mobilize or manipulate soft tissue and joints; modulate pain; and reduce soft tissue swelling, inflammation, or restriction."[4]

Articulatory techniques are derived from the osteopathic literature. They are defined as passive movement applied in a smooth rhythmic fashion to stretch contracted muscles, ligaments, and capsules gradually.[5] They include gentle techniques designed to stretch the joint in each of the planes of movement inherent to the joint.[5] The force used during articular techniques is usually a prolonged stretch into the restriction or tissue limitation.

Oscillatory techniques were best defined by Maitland,[6] who described oscillations as passive movements to the joint, which can be a small or large amplitude and applied anywhere in a range of movement, and which can be performed while the joint surfaces are held distracted or compressed. The four grades of oscillation are as follows: grade I is a small-amplitude movement performed at the beginning of a range; grade II is a large-amplitude movement performed within the range, but not reaching the limit of the range; grade III is a large-amplitude movement up to the limit of a range; and grade IV is a small-amplitude movement performed at the limit of a range.[6] Grades I and II are used primarily for neurophysiologic effects and do not engage detectable resistance. Grades III and IV are designed to initiate mechanical changes in the tissue and do engage tissue resistance.

Distraction is defined as "separation of surfaces of a joint by extension without injury or dislocation of the parts."[7] Distraction techniques are designed to separate the joint surface attempting to stress the capsule.

Manipulation is defined by *Dorland's Illustrated Medical Dictionary* as "skillful or dextrous treatment by the hand. In physical therapy, the forceful passive movement of a joint beyond its active limit of motion."[8] Maitland[6] described two manipulative procedures. Manipulation is a sudden movement or thrust, of small amplitude, performed at a speed that renders the patient powerless to prevent it. Manipulation under anesthesia is a medical procedure used to restore normal joint movement by breaking adhesions.

Mobilization is defined as "the making of a fixed or ankylosed part movable, or restoration of motion to a joint."[7] To the clinician, mobilization is passive movement that is designed to improve soft tissue and joint mobility. It can include oscillations, articulations, distractions, and thrust techniques.

Mobilization, in this chapter, is defined as a specialized passive movement, attempting to restore the arthrokinematics and osteokinematics of joint movement. Mobilization includes articulations, oscillations, distractions, and thrust techniques. The techniques are built on active and passive joint mechanics and are directed at the periarticular structures that have become restricted secondary to trauma and immobilization. These same techniques can be effective tools in assessment of specific joint impairments.

Soft tissue mobilization (STM), for the purposes of this chapter, is as defined by Johnson: "STM is the treatment of soft tissue with consideration of layers and depth by initially evaluating and treating superficially proceeding to bony prominence, muscle, tendon, and ligament."[9]

Mobilization techniques can be performed as physiologic movements or accessory movements. *Physiologic movements* are movements of the humerus in the body planes (e.g., flexion, extension, abduction, adduction, and external and internal rotation). *Accessory movements* are movements of the humerus within the joint that include roll, spin, glide, slide, distractions, and oscillations.

EVIDENCE-BASED PRACTICE

Several studies to date have investigated the efficacy of manual therapy interventions for shoulder dysfunction. Some studies have focused on physiologic parameters in response to particular mobilization techniques,[10-12] whereas others have focused on randomized controlled studies[13-19] comparing physical therapy with other traditional treatment approaches.

The highest level of evidence to support the use of an intervention is provided by controlled randomized studies. Systematic reviews of randomized clinical trials before 1996 showed that studies had sample sizes that were too small and study designs too poor to make any conclusions about the effectiveness of physical therapy for patients with shoulder soft tissue disorders.[14]

Some studies compared the effectiveness of alternative methods of treatment with physical therapy for treatment of painful stiff shoulders. A randomized study by Van der Windt et al[16] investigated corticosteroid injections versus physical therapy for treatment of painful stiff shoulders. Primary outcome measures were the patient's main complaint and the pain and shoulder disability questionnaire. Early results indicated significant improvement in all outcomes for the corticosteroid-treated group over the physical therapy group. The difference between the groups at weeks 26 and 52 was small, however. In a follow-up of 76% of the participants in the original study, investigators found that as many as half the patients experienced recurrent complaints across groups.[15] The study concluded that in the long term, no significant differences existed between the treatment groups.

More recent randomized clinical trials demonstrated the effectiveness of manual therapy for shoulder disorders. A randomized clinical study by Bang and Deyle[17] compared the effectiveness of supervised exercise for shoulder impingement syndrome with and without manual therapy intervention. The subjects in the manual therapy group received joint mobilization and STM to the involved shoulder complex and the involved upper quarter, based on a clarifying examination. The study used pain (assessed by the Visual Analog Scale for function and brake tests), isometric strength tests, and the functional assessment questionnaire to determine the effectiveness of interventions. Participants were assessed after 2 months of treatment. Results of the study demonstrated a decrease in pain and an increase in function for both groups, but the manual therapy intervention group had significantly greater improvement.[17] Strength was also significantly improved in the manual therapy group, but not in the supervised strengthening group.

In a similar study, investigators compared the effect of comprehensive treatment (hot packs, active range of motion [AROM], physiologic stretching, muscle strengthening, STM, and patient education) with and without joint mobilization in patients with primary impingement syndrome.[18] The results of the study indicated improvements in 24-hour pain measurements and in subacromial compression test results, but no significant differences in ROM and function were reported.

Several investigations looked at specific effects of joint mobilization on ROM measures and periarticular structures. A study using cadavers demonstrated that end-range mobilization techniques were more effective in improving glenohumeral abduction ROM than those techniques performed in the middle of the range.[10] Vermeulen et al[12] demonstrated, in a multi-subject case report, that the end-range mobilization techniques in patients with adhesive capsulitis resulted in increases in passive ROM (PROM) and AROM and in the arthrographic assessment of joint capacity. These changes were still present during follow-up 9 months later.

Vermeulen et al[13] published a more recent study comparing high-grade and low-grade mobilization techniques in the management of patients with adhesive capsulitis. The study demonstrated that the high-grade mobilization technique showed a statistically significant difference in trend between both groups over a total follow-up of 12 months for external rotation, shoulder rating questionnaire, and shoulder disability questionnaire. The *high-grade mobilization technique* used mobilization techniques that were Maitland grades III and IV, and the *low-grade mobilization technique* used techniques that were Maitland grades I and II.[6]

Johnson et al[19] demonstrated that a posteriorly directed joint mobilization technique was more effective than an anteriorly directed mobilization technique for improving external rotation ROM in subjects with adhesive capsulitis. Both groups had a significant decrease in pain.[19] In the foregoing study, Kaltenborn grade III mobilizations, which apply force "after the slack of the joint has been taken up," were used to stretch tissues crossing the joint. The end-range position of the mobilization was held for at least 1 minute. Each stretch mobilization was repeated so that a total of 15 minutes of sustained stretch was performed at each treatment session.

Gamze et al[20] studied 46 patients who were randomly assigned to one of the following three groups: group 1 received ice application and exercise and joint mobilization with STM ($n = 19$), group 2 received ice application and exercise with supervision ($n = 14$), and group 3 received ice application and a home exercise program ($n = 13$). The results demonstrated that, after 12 sessions of joint mobilization and STM techniques and exercise ROM in flexion, abduction, and external rotation in the manual therapy group, patients with shoulder impingement syndrome improved significantly, whereas ROM in the exercise group did not improve.[20] Overall, manual physical therapy applied by experienced physical therapists combined with supervised exercise in a brief clinical trial was better than exercise alone for patients diagnosed with impingement syndrome.

In another study, Gamze et al[21] demonstrated better outcomes with manual therapy in a prospective, randomized clinical comparison of the effectiveness of two physical therapy treatment approaches for impingement syndrome. The first approach consisted of joint mobilization and STM techniques, and the second was a self-training program. Group 1 was instructed in an AROM, stretching, and strengthening exercise program, including rotator cuff muscles, rhomboids, levator scapulae, and serratus anterior, with an elastic band at home at least 7 times a week for 10 to 15 minutes. Group 2 received a prescription for 12 sessions of joint mobilization and STM techniques, ice application, stretching and strengthening exercise programs, and patient education in clinic 3 times per week. Manual physical therapy applied by experienced physical therapists combined with supervised exercise in a brief clinical trial is better than exercise alone for increasing strength, decreasing pain, and improving function in patients with shoulder impingement syndrome.

Further randomized controlled studies comparing treatment methods for different shoulder impairment classifications are needed to guide clinical decision making, improve outcomes, and reduce use of inefficient costly treatment.

EFFECTS OF PASSIVE MOVEMENT ON SCAR TISSUE: INDICATIONS AND CONTRAINDICATIONS FOR MOBILIZATION

Research indicates that mobilization is most effective in reversing the changes that occur in connective tissue following immobilization.[1] Mobilization must be carefully analyzed after trauma or surgery. When is it safe to apply stress to scar tissue? How much stress should be applied to the scar to promote remodeling? In what direction should stress be applied? These important questions must be answered before the clinician can determine the indications for mobilization of scar tissue. Indications for mobilization are discussed in regard to protective and nonprotective categories of shoulder injuries.

One study investigated the effect of PROM versus immobilization on surgically repaired rotator cuff tendons in 65 rats.[19] The study demonstrated that immediate postoperative passive motion was found to be detrimental to passive shoulder mechanics. The investigators speculated that passive motion results in increased scar formation in the subacromial space and therefore leads to decreased mobility and greater joint stiffness. The immobilization group allowed tendon to bone healing that prevented increased scar formation. The study emphasized that the immobilization period lasted only 2 weeks. The two mobilization groups were started on passive movement immediately. The arc of motion consisted of motion in both internal and external rotation from the neutral position. In humans, the movement was analogous to rotation at 0° of forward flexion in group 1 and 90° of abduction in group 2. In the early mobilization groups at both 2 and 6 weeks after the repair, internal ROM was significantly decreased, whereas external ROM was not. No differences between the groups in terms of collagen organization or mechanical properties were reported.

The foregoing study showed that early mobilization of flexor tendon repairs was beneficial in increasing ROM by preventing adhesions within the sheath.[20,21] Because the rotator cuff tendon does not have a sheath, and the repair is tendon to bone, early mobilization has beneficial effects. Specific adaptations to the demands imposed may depend on the periarticular structural properties that are stressed.

ROLE OF MOBILIZATION

The mobilization techniques are assumed to induce various beneficial effects. The neurophysiologic effect is based on the stimulation of peripheral mechanoreceptors and the inhibition of nociceptors. The biomechanical effect is a result of forces directed to the joint resistance within the limitations of the patient's tolerance. The primary roles of joint mobilization are to restore joint mobility and to facilitate proper biomechanics of involved structures.

The neurophysiologic effect is based on the stimulation of peripheral mechanoreceptors and the inhibition of nociceptors (pain fibers). Nociceptors are unmyelinated nerve fibers, which have a higher threshold of stimulation than mechanoreceptors.[22,23] Evidence indicates that stimulation of peripheral mechanoreceptors blocks the transmission of pain to the central nervous system.[22] Wyke[22] postulated that this phenomenon is the result of a direct release of inhibitory transmitters within the basal spinal nucleus that inhibits the onward flow of incoming nociceptive afferent activity. Joint mobilization is one method of enhancing the frequency of discharge from the mechanoreceptors, thereby diminishing the intensity of many types of pain.

The biomechanical effect of joint mobilization is focused on the direct tension of periarticular tissue to prevent complications resulting from immobilization and trauma. The lack of stress to connective tissue results in changes in normal joint mobility. The periarticular tissue and muscles surrounding the joint demonstrate significant changes after periods of immobilization. Frank et al[1] and Akeson et al[3] substantiated a decrease in water and glycosaminoglycans (GAG, the fibrous tissue lubricant), an increase in fatty fibrous infiltrates (which may form adhesions as they mature into scar), an increase in abnormally placed collagen cross-links (which may contribute to the inhibition of collagen fiber gliding), and the loss of fiber orientation within ligaments (a loss that significantly reduces their strength). Passive movement or stress to the tissue can help to prevent these changes by maintaining tissue homeostasis.[2] The exact mechanisms of prevention are uncertain.

Contraindications

We can understand contraindications to joint mobilization by becoming aware of the common abuses of passive movement. The abuses of passive movement can be broken down into two categories: creating an excessive trauma to the tissue and causing undesirable or abnormal mobility.[1] Improper techniques, such as extreme force, poor direction of stress, and excessive velocity, may result in serious secondary injury. In addition, mobilization to joints that are moving normally or that are hypermobile can create or increase joint instability.

Ultimately, selection of a specific technique determines the contraindications. For example, the very gentle grade I oscillations, as described by Maitland, rarely have contraindications. These techniques are mainly used to block pain. They are of small amplitude and controlled velocity. In contrast, manipulative techniques have many contraindications. Haldeman[24] described the following conditions as major contraindications to thrust techniques: arthritides, dislocation, hypermobility, recent trauma, bone weakness and destructive disease, circulatory disturbances, neurologic dysfunction, and infectious disease.

Principles of Joint Mobilization Techniques: Specificity of Manual Techniques

Manual therapy techniques are designed to restore intimate joint mechanics. Several general principles should be remembered during application of the techniques.

Hand Position

The mobilization hand should be placed as close as possible to the joint surface, and the forces applied should be tangent to the joint and directed at the restricted periarticular tissue. The stabilization hand counteracts the movement of the mobilizing hand by applying an equal but opposite force, or by supporting or preventing movement at surrounding joints. Excessive tension in the therapist's hands during joint mobilization can cause the patient to guard against the mobilization.

Direction of Movement

The direction of movement of mobilization should take into account the mechanics of the joint mobilized, the arthrokinematic and osteokinematic impairments of the dysfunction, and the current reactivity of the involved tissue. However, the major consideration should be moving the humeral head into the restriction or into the barrier. A study that investigated the presence of the cytocontractile protein vimentin in the connective tissue of patients with adhesive capsulitis demonstrated that contracture resulted from selective involvement of the anterior capsule. The rotator cuff interval, the coracohumeral ligament, and the axillary fold were noted to be the specific areas in the anterior capsule that demonstrated the greatest amount of vimentin. The study showed that fibroplasia, heavy production of type III collagen fibers, involved the entire joint capsule.[25] The clinical implication of this study is that manual therapy for patients with adhesive capsulitis must focus on the coracohumeral ligament, rotator cuff interval, and axillary fold areas of the anterior capsule. No evidence of contracture of the posterior capsule was reported. Specificity of the direction of imposed demand may result in more successful outcomes of manual therapy.

The direction of forces to the joint is also determined based on the desired response. Neuromuscular relaxation and pain modulation effects will be appreciated if the direction of force is opposite the pain. Biomechanical effects will be appreciated if forces are directed toward resistance, but to the patient's tolerance. The resistance represents the direction of capsular or joint limitation. Movement into the restriction is an attempt to make mechanical changes within the capsule and the surrounding tissue. The mechanical changes may include breaking up of adhesions, realignment of collagen, and increasing fiber glide. Certain movements stress specific parts of the capsule. For example, arthrogram studies demonstrated that external rotation of the glenohumeral joint stresses the anterior recess of the capsule.[26]

Body Mechanics

Proper body mechanics are essential in application of mobilization techniques. The therapist is able to impart the desired direction and force of movement when working from a position of stability. The therapist should stand close to the area being mobilized and use weight shifting through legs and trunk to assist movement in the vector of mobilization. The therapist's hands and arms should be positioned to act as fulcrums and levers to fine-tune mobilization.

Duration and Amplitude

Several animal model studies used different loads and loading time to determine the most effective technique for obtaining permanent elongation of collagenous tissue. The studies used rat tendons under varied loads to demonstrate the elongation of tissue. A high-load, short-duration treatment (105 to 165*g* for 5 minutes) was compared with a low-load, long-duration treatment (5*g* for 15 minutes).[27,28] The results indicated that a low-load, long-duration stretch was more effective in obtaining permanent elongation of the tissue. In humans, Bonutti et al[29] determined that the optimal method to obtain plastic deformation and reestablish ROM is static progressive stretch. One to two 30-minute sessions per day of static progressive stretch for 1 to 3 months produced an overall average increase in motion of elbow contractures of 69%, with excellent compliance by the patients.

As previously noted, the use of low-load prolonged stretch with heat to facilitate plastic deformation of shoulder capsular restrictions is advocated. The patient must be in a subacute stage of reactivity, and the stretch is to the patient's tolerance. Heat used in conjunction with the stretch has been found to be more effective than stretch alone.[30,31] The patient's shoulder is placed in the plane of the scapula (POS) with a wedge. The stretch is performed by using Thera-Band resistance to assist with positioning or the use of a hand weight and gravity to stretch periarticular structures. Duration of stretch can be gradually progressed from 10 to 30 minutes.

Little research has been performed on joint mobilization to determine the optimum duration of oscillation. Often the duration is determined by the change desired by the therapist. For example, glenohumeral joint mobilization of grades I or II performed to facilitate neuromuscular relaxation can be continued until muscle guarding is reduced and ROM increases.

Joint Position and End-Range Mobilization Combined with Low-Load Stretch: Specificity of Low-Load Stretch and Manual Therapy Techniques in Shoulder Postures

Several studies in the literature indicated that soft tissue structures surrounding the glenohumeral joint become taut or lax depending on the posture of the joint. Turkel et al[32] demonstrated that no single structure stabilizes the glenohumeral joint in all positions, and the position and tightness of the anterior structures vary with abduction and external rotation. For example, at 90° of passive abduction and external rotation, the inferior glenohumeral ligament is the most stabilizing. Therefore, positioning a patient with tightness of the inferior glenohumeral ligament in 90° of abduction and external rotation is a specific stretch to that tissue. Anterior glides may be more effective if they are initiated into the end of range while the patient is in the foregoing position (Fig. 14-1). At 0° of abduction, the most stabilizing structures for the glenohumeral joint are the subscapularis muscle and tendon. Therefore, positioning the patient at 0° of abduction with external rotation is a specific stretch to the subscapularis tendon and muscle (Fig. 14-2).

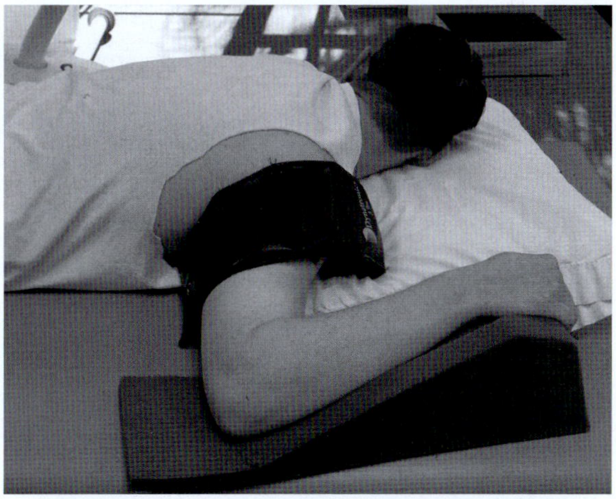

Figure 14-1 Prone left shoulder at 90° abduction with external rotation on a wedge.

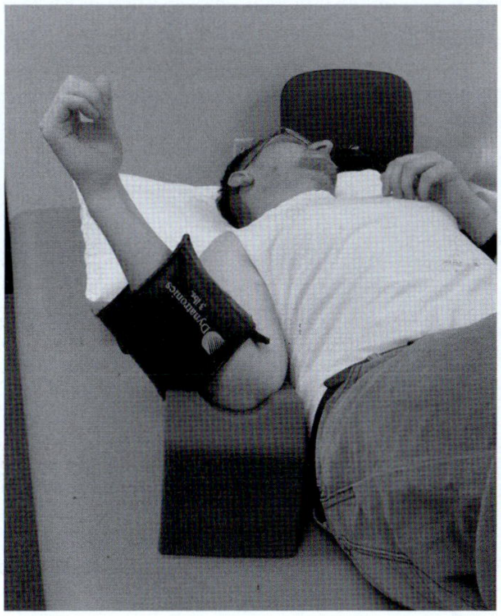

Figure 14-2 Supine at 0° of abduction external rotation on a 30° wedge (plane of the scapula).

At 45° of abduction and external rotation, the subscapularis, middle glenohumeral ligament, and anterior superior fibers of the inferior glenohumeral ligament are the most stabilizing to the joint. Therefore, positioning the patient at 45° of abduction with passive external rotation is specific to stretching the anterior middle and inferior capsule (Fig. 14-3).

Specific techniques for the posterior capsule can be enhanced by the results of a study that investigated the strain measurements within the posterior capsule with the specific position of internal rotation.[33]

Using cadaver specimens, investigators attached a force transducer to the superior, middle, and inferior fibers of the posterior capsule. An in vivo position was used to demonstrate the most significant strain positions of the posterior capsule in vitro. Passive internal rotation at 30° of abduction in the POS (anterior to the frontal plane 30°) demonstrated statically significant strain values for the upper and middle fibers of the posterior capsule (Fig. 14-4). A position of 60° of abduction with passive internal rotation provided a significant increase in strain values on the posterior capsule in general (Fig. 14-5). A position of

30° of extension with passive internal rotation provided a significant increase in strain values on the on the inferior fibers of the posterior capsule (Fig. 14-6). A position of 90° of flexion, adduction, and internal rotation demonstrated a significant increase in strain values for the posterior capsule in general (Fig. 14-7).

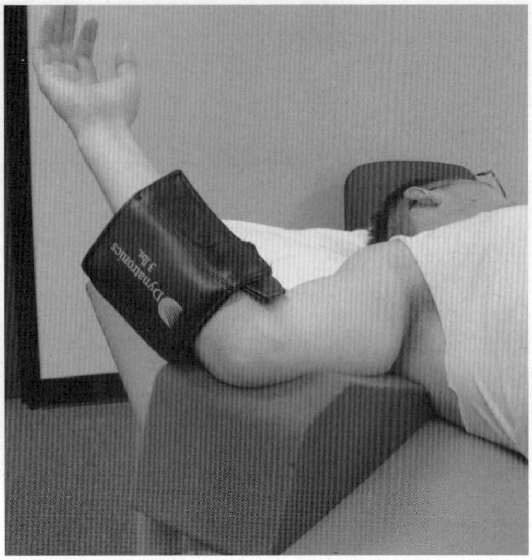

Figure 14-3 45° of abduction with passive external rotation would be specific to stretching to the anterior middle and inferior capsule.

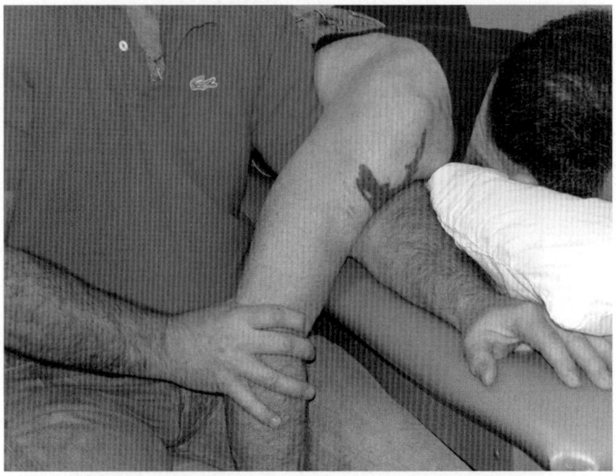

Figure 14-4 Posterior tilt of the humeral head using the forearm as a fulcrum.

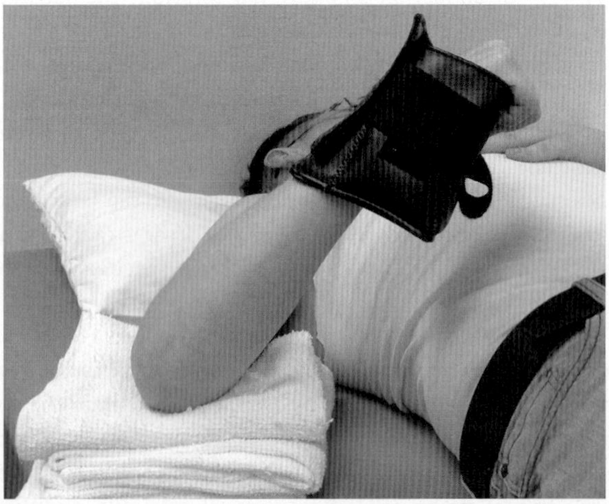

Figure 14-5 60° of abduction with passive internal rotation provides a significant increase in strain values on the posterior capsule in general.

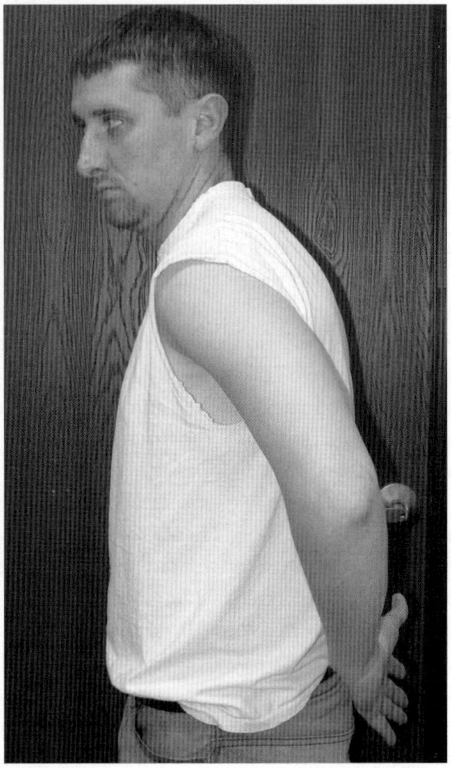

Figure 14-6 30° of extension with passive internal rotation provided significant increase in strain values on the inferior fibers of the posterior capsule.

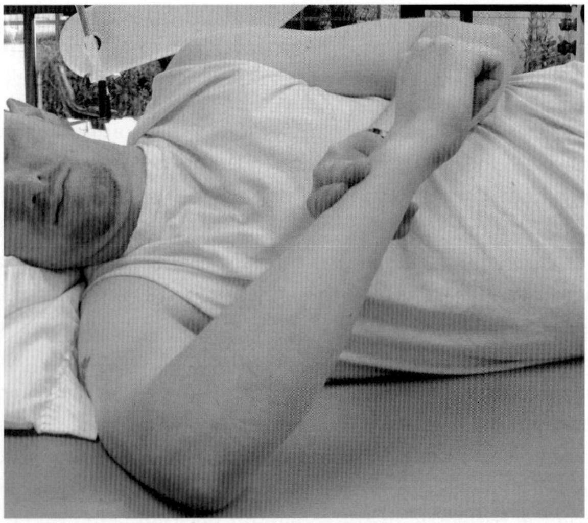

Figure 14-7 At 90° of flexion, adduction and internal rotation demonstrated a significant increase in strain values for the posterior capsule in general.

CASE STUDY 1

The *Guide to Physical Therapist Practice* describes the preferred practice patterns for protective shoulder injuries under Practice Pattern 4I—Impaired Joint Mobility, Motor Function, Muscle Performance, and Range of Motion Associated with Bony or Soft Tissue Surgery.[4] *Protective injuries* result from surgery or trauma, with substantial soft tissue (muscle, ligament, tendon, capsule) damage or repair. Examples of protective injuries include anterior capsular shift, Bankart's repair, rotator cuff repair, and shoulder dislocation. Rehabilitation for patients with protective injuries is divided into six phases: maximum protection, protected mobilization, moderate protection, late moderate protection, minimum protection, and return to function. This case study illustrates the concepts of phased rehabilitation in a patient with a protective shoulder injury.

Examination

History

A 16-year-old female basketball player is referred for postoperative rehabilitation of a right rotator cuff repair involving the supraspinatus. The tendon demonstrates a 2-cm full-thickness tear. The procedure performed was arthroscopic repair. Before surgery, the patient had pain and limited elevation activities for the last 2 years. Functional limitations include weakness and instability, especially with basketball activities, and difficulty sleeping on the affected side. Additional past medical history includes previous hydrocortisone injection and anti-inflammatory medications, with little change in symptoms. The patient had stiffness, weakness, and some mild pain 2 weeks after the operation.

Systems Review

Integumentary System

Hypermobility of wrist, knee, elbow bilaterally, and left shoulder joints is evident.

Musculoskeletal System

Palpable tenderness and trigger points are noted on the subscapularis, serratus anterior, levator scapulae, pectoralis minor, and lower portions of longus colli muscles.

The patient has scapular gliding along the pectoralis major and minor tightness, as well as excessive mobility of the scapula in an anterior direction.

Test and Measures

Posture

The patient's posture is slightly elevated and protracted. The right scapula and right upper extremity are held in slight internal rotation.

Range of Motion

Table 14-1 shows ROM measurements.

Table 14-1 Protective Injury Case Study 1: Summarization of Range-of-Motion Measurements

		Weeks Postoperative				
		2	4	6	8	16
PROM (degrees)	Flexion	80	130	140	165	176
	Abduction	58	90	102	160	170
	External rotation, neutral position	−5	14	25	45	64
	External rotation, 45° abduction position	−10	18	30	53	75
	External rotation, 90° abduction position	NT	NT	38	56	80
	Internal rotation, 45° abduction position	43	63	63	65	70
	Extension	NT	NT	60	69	78
AROM (degrees)	Flexion	NT	NT	125	160	170
	Scaption	NT	NT	130	165	175

AROM, active range of motion; NT, not tested; PROM, passive range of motion.

Evaluation

This adolescent female athlete has a protective shoulder injury and prior surgical repair of the supraspinatus tendon. The patient is currently in the protective mobilization phase. She appears to have anterior pectoral tightness and middle trapezius stretch weakness.

Phase 1: Maximum Protection Phase

1 to 14 Days after the Wound

Intervention

The patient is immobilized in a sling postoperatively for the first 10 to 14 days. Active-assistive ROM (AAROM) and PROM are in the following protected ranges: internal and external rotation at 45° of abduction in the POS (30° anterior to the frontal plane) to be started 2 weeks postoperatively. Ice and rest for the arm are advised for pain reduction. Appropriate modalities, such as low-level laser therapy, to promote healing can be initiated within the first 3 to 5 postoperative days.

Immobilization of the rotator cuff repair for a 2-week period is initiated to protect the tendon to bone repair, thus preventing increased scar tissue formation that would result in restrictions of joint mobility.[19]

Continued

CASE STUDY 1—cont'd

Rationale

Immobilization during the first 3 to 5 days is critical to allow the inflammatory and proliferation stages to proceed. The inflammatory stage begins 1 hour after the wound and continues for 72 hours, during which time vasodilatation, edema, and phagocytosis of debris in and around the wound are occurring.[19] The matrix and cellular proliferative stage begins 24 hours after the wound and is characterized by endothelial capillary buds, with fibroblasts synthesizing the extracellular matrix.[19,20] The scar is still quite cellular, with the presence of macrophages, mast cells, and fibroblasts. Little to no motion should occur during the first 3 to 5 days, to protect the newly forming network of capillaries.[2] Excessive motion too early can result in a prolonged inflammatory stage and excessive scarring. Heat should also be avoided secondary to vascular stress on capillary budding. Ice can be used to control swelling and pain.

Gentle stress to the tissue is initiated by day 12 to 14 after the wound. The fibroblastic stage of healing has already begun with presence of fibroblasts in the wound.[19,20] Gentle early motion, such as with grades I and II joint mobilization and PROM in protected positions, helps to facilitate alignment of newly formed collagen fibers, aid muscle relaxation, and prevent adhesion formation. In protective injuries with surgical involvement, it is helpful to have an operative report to inform the therapist of the specific tissues involved in the procedure. For this case study, the supraspinatus was the primary involvement.

Phase 2: Protected Mobilization

14 Days to 3 Weeks

Intervention

Continued grade I and II joint mobilization are progressing toward grade III and IV mobilization by 3 weeks. Scapular gliding is passive and active assistive. PROM and AAROM are performed in protected positions, as described for the previous phase. Low-load prolonged stretch is performed with heat during the stretch into external rotation. Low load means no pain, and a gentle stretching sensation is desirable. (See Table 14-1 for current ROM measures.)

Rationale

The goals of this phase are to promote a functional scar and to attempt to decrease other compensatory or contributing dysfunctions. Early mobilization is critical in affecting scar tissue length, glide, and tensile strength. As the inflammatory phase ends, the fibroplasia stage of healing has already begun. The production of scar tissue begins on the fourth day of wound healing and increases rapidly during the first 3 weeks.[2,34] Peacock[2] substantiated this peak production of scar tissue by the increased quantities of hydroxyproline. Hydroxyproline is a byproduct of collagen synthesis.[2,35] Collagen production begins and continues to increase for up to 6 weeks.[2,19,20]

The newly synthesized collagen fibrils are weak against tensile force. Intramolecular and intermolecular cross-linking of collagen develops,[6] and it is designed to resist tensile forces.[2,35] The first peak in tensile strength occurs around the 21st day after the wound.[2]

Gentle mobilization techniques can be effective during early fibroplasia because of the immaturity of the collagen tissue. Arem and Madden[36] demonstrated that, after 14 weeks of scar maturation, elongation of scar was no longer possible. In contrast, the 3-week-old scar was substantially lengthened when it was subject to the same tension.[36] Peacock[2] hypothesized that the mechanism by which the length of the scar is increased becomes critical for the restoration of the gliding mechanism. Stretching, or an increase in length of the scar, is a result of straightening or reorientation of the collagen fibers, without a change in their dimensions.[2] For this to occur, the collagen fibers must glide on each other. The gliding mechanism is hampered in unstressed scar tissue by the development of abnormally placed cross-links and a random orientation of the newly synthesized collagen fibrils.[34] Early gentle passive motion starting around the 14th day and progressing to the 21st day facilitates the development of tissue tensile strength by helping align newly synthesized collagen. Additionally, improved tensile strength allows for early AROM in the next phase.

Phase 3: Moderate Protection Phase

3 to 6 Weeks

Reexamination

Continued muscle guarding of subscapularis is noted. The serratus anterior, longus colli, and scalene muscles show little to no tenderness. The patient reports decreasing soreness and pain in the glenohumeral joint at rest. Sutures have been removed, and superficial closure is complete. The patient continues with anterior chest muscle tightness and decreased scapular excursion. (See Table 14-1 for PROM measurements.)

Intervention

Intervention includes PROM stretching and physiologic oscillations to 30° of external rotation in neutral and 45° abducted positions, joint mobilization of the glenohumeral joint with grades III and IV in a posterior-anterior direction, and gentle anterior-posterior capsule stretching. Continued low-load prolonged stretch into external rotation is performed with heat during the stretch. Muscle reeducation is initiated with proprioceptive neuromuscular facilitation (PNF) and scapular techniques with active, eccentric, and concentric patterns (primarily posterior elevation and depression). Gentle AAROM and AROM are initiated, but the combination of external rotation and abduction continues to be avoided. At 5 weeks, isometrics are initiated in the POS (30° anterior to frontal plane) for internal and external rotation, horizontal abduction prone, and extension.

CASE STUDY 1—cont'd

Rationale

The moderate protection phase allows for more AAROM progressing toward AROM by the fourth week. Collagen production continues to be high until the sixth week.[2,19,20] The goal of rehabilitation at this stage is to facilitate extensibility of newly synthesized collagen further, to realign randomly oriented collagen, and to enhance fiber glide between collagen fibers. Tensile strength has reached its first peak, thus allowing gentle AROM as early as 3 weeks[2] in protected positions (rotation before elevation, especially in contractile component injuries).

An additional goal of rehabilitation in this phase is to prevent muscle atrophy, inhibition, and the effects of immobilization. PNF scapular patterns with a progression toward resisted patterns during this phase foster activation and restoration of scapular muscle activity and provide dynamic proximal stability. Progressive isometric exercises in protected positions can be used at approximately 5 weeks by the patient at home or work to stimulate inhibited muscle and provide dynamic tension to healing soft tissue.

Phase 4: Late Moderate Protection

6 to 12 Weeks

Reexamination

Scapular mobility is within normal limits (see Table 14-1 for ROM measurements).

Intervention

At 6 to 8 weeks, PROM stretching is performed, with an emphasis on external ROM in the POS and the 45° abducted position. PNF scapular patterns are continued, to work on any areas of weakness. AROM PNF patterns for upper extremity are initiated with some resistance in weak aspects of the pattern. Active scapular stabilization and movement patterns incorporate closed kinetic chain exercises.

At 8 to 12 weeks, AROM exercises are begun in unrestricted ROM (no loading of joint in external rotation and abduction). Progressive resistive exercises (PREs) in protected ROM are performed, with an emphasis on rotator cuff strengthening progressing to overhead exercises. Submaximal isokinetic internal and external rotation is performed in the POS (limited external rotation to 45°).

Rationale

At 6 weeks, collagen production tapers off. The maturation or remodeling phase of healing begins at approximately 3 weeks and continues for up to 12 to 18 months.[19] Maximizing scar extensibility is essential because, by 14 weeks, scar deformability may be greatly decreased.[35] Strengthening is emphasized more during this phase.

Some strengthening has already begun, by using PNF scapular patterning to reestablish balance of function of the parascapular muscles in the previous phase. During the first 2 to 3 weeks of this phase, active and reactive scapular stabilization activities are initiated. These exercises help to restore force couples around the scapula and usually involve some cocontraction or synergy patterns of the rotator cuff. During the last 3 to 4 weeks of this phase, emphasis shifts toward strengthening the rotator cuff throughout the full range of movement. Through the progressions described, proximal stability and force couples are established before distal force couples. Low-level weights or Thera-Band resistance for this case study for internal and external rotation affects healing of the subscapularis tendon and enhance dynamic glenohumeral joint stability.

Phase 5: Minimal Protection

12 to 16 Weeks

Reevaluation

The patient demonstrates some elevation of the scapula during the late elevation phase. Excessive scapular elevation is increased with resistance. Activities of daily living (ADLs) are within normal limits. No pain is reported with most activities and exercises. (See Table 14-1 for ROM measurements.)

Intervention

Intervention involves continued progression of weights and repetitions of the previous phase of exercises. Chest pass throwing against a Plyotrampoline is performed with a 2.5-lb ball. STM is performed to the apparent remaining fascial restrictions along the inferior clavicle, followed by manual and PRE strengthening of the lower trapezius and serratus anterior. PNF resistive patterns are performed close to end-range abduction and external rotation.

Rationale

Multiple repetitions in unrestricted ROM continue to provide stress to the maturing scar. Manual techniques during this phase are used to fine-tune function further and to clear any remaining restrictions. Neuromuscular control at end-range abduction and external rotation is essential to help protect capsular reconstruction and return to sport.

Phase 6: Return to Function

More Than 16 Weeks

Reevaluation: Tests and Measures

Hand-held dynamometer testing shows the ratio of external to internal rotators at 81% and 20% stronger than uninvolved side.

Intervention

The patient begins progressive basketball shooting and drill activities at 18 weeks. She is instructed not to begin team play until 22 weeks postoperatively. The patient is discharged at 18 weeks with an extensive program of rotator cuff strengthening and scapular stabilization exercises.

Rationale

The return to function phase usually begins at approximately 16 weeks if the elements of movement are free of

Continued

CASE STUDY 1—cont'd

abnormal patterns and pain. This phase happens sooner based on the patient's response, the specific trauma, and the required level of function. Exercises are more functionally based, and maximal efforts are used. Isokinetic testing of rotator cuff muscles informs the therapist of any deficits, in particular internal-to-external ratios that may indicate an increased hazard for return to function. Currently, reimbursement issues and managed care policies may not allow physical therapists to observe a patient completely through all phases of rehabilitation. Proper education of progressive activities and appropriate time frames for return to full function need to be outlined for patients with limited follow-up.

In summary, protective shoulder injuries can be safely progressed through a phased program of rehabilitation based on stages of soft tissue healing. Table 14-2 summarizes the various stages. Manual therapy techniques used at specific stages of healing can enhance the strength and extensibility of scar tissue, reestablish force couples, and restore functional movement patterns.

Table 14-2 Summarization of Phases of Rehabilitation for Protective Shoulder Injuries

Phases	Maximum Protection	Protected Mobilization	Moderate Protection	Late Moderate Protection	Minimum Protection	Return to Function
Time	1–10 days	10 days–3 wk	3–6 wk	6–12 wk	12–16 wk	+16 wk
Stage of healing	Inflammatory, proliferative early fibroplasia	Early fibroplasia	Fibroplasia, maturation	Maturation	Maturation	Maturation
Goals	Protect newly formed scar	Facilitate functional scar, aligning new collagen fibers; clear spinal and rib dysfunction	Enhance tensile strength of scar	Stress scar; restore force couples; proximal, distal	Same as previous phase; progressively increase strength rotator cuff, parascapular muscles	Return to function
Manual therapy techniques	7–10 days after wound, grades 1 and 2 joint mobilizations	Joint mobilizations grades 1 and 2 progress to 3, 4; STM surrounding tissue; PNF scapular patterns; protected PROM	As previous, STM to suture, scapular release techniques; PNF scapular patterns	Scapular release techniques; PNF UE patterns; low-load prolonged stretch	PNF UE patterns with significant resistance; low-load prolonged stretch if needed	As needed for any deficits
Other therapeutic interventions	Position education; anti-inflammatory modalities; ice	Home program of PROM in protected ranges	Codman's exercises, T-bar, Swiss ball, foam roller; AAROM and AROM exercises	Isokinetics in protected ROM submaximally; active scapular stabilization exercises; PREs	Same as previous, increasing effort and ROM; Plyoball throwing	Progressive return to sport drills, light recreational activities

AAROM, active-assistive range of motion; AROM, active range of motion; PNF, proprioceptive neuromuscular facilitation; PREs, progressive resistive exercises, PROM, passive range of motion; STM, soft tissue mobilization; UE, upper extremity.

CASE STUDY 2

The *Guide to Physical Therapist Practice* describes the preferred practice patterns for nonprotective shoulder injuries under Preferred Practice Patterns 4 B, C, D, E, and G.[4] *Nonprotective shoulder injuries* are primarily shoulder dysfunctions that have no significant soft tissue healing constraints. Examples of nonprotective injuries include postacromioplasty status, prolonged immobilization, adhesive capsulitis, and impingement syndromes. These patients frequently have pain, stiffness, and limited function. This case study illustrates the concepts of rehabilitation for a patient with a nonprotective injury.

CASE STUDY 2—cont'd

Examination

History

A 46-year-old female homemaker has left shoulder pain and stiffness. The patient was referred 5 days after arthroscopic surgery and closed manipulation. She began having pain and stiffness several months before, possibly caused by overworking in her yard. Her left shoulder became increasingly stiff and painful in the 5 to 6 weeks before surgery. The diagnosis given was adhesive capsulitis. Her past medical history includes "stiff neck" 2 to 3 years ago. Her subjective functional complaint is that she is unable to reach overhead or to fasten her bra. She has moderate difficulty with dressing and placing her hand behind her back, and with washing the opposite axilla.

Systems Review

Musculoskeletal System

The patient has the following tenderness and muscle spasm: posterior cervical spine C1-2; anterior cervical spine along longus colli muscles at C5-6 on the left; posterior aspects of left ribs 2 to 4, the left subscapularis, supraspinatus, infraspinatus, teres minor, and levator scapulae. All other systems are unremarkable.

Test and Measures

Posture

The left scapula is protracted and downwardly rotated, and with winging. She has slight forward head position with increased tone of the sternocleidomastoid muscle bilaterally.

Range of Motion

Table 14-3 shows the patient's initial shoulder ROM measurements. Upper quarter screening shows extension and side bending on the left of the cervical spine limited by 50% and painful actively and passively with overpressure.

Table 14-3 Nonprotective Injury Case Study 2: Summarization of Range-of-Motion Measurements

	Time	Initial	2 Wk	4 Wk	6 Wk	10 Wk
PROM (degrees)	Flexion	102	112	140	150	174
	Abduction	70	80	120	150	170
	External rotation, neutral position	−20	5	30	36	62
	External rotation, 45° abduction position	10	20	45	56	70
	External rotation, 90° abduction position	NT	NT	40	46	75
	Internal rotation, 45° abduction position	52	54	52	53	71
	Hyperextension	48	50	53	53	71
AROM (degrees)	Scaption	70	90	112	132	155

AROM, active range of motion; NT, not tested; PROM, passive range of motion.

Special Tests

Capsular testing reveals restricted motion in all directions.

Evaluation

The patient has a nonprotective shoulder injury. She has adhesive capsulitis with strong muscle guarding and possible adaptive shortening of subscapularis. Currently, she is unable to assess capsular restrictions fully secondary to muscle guarding of rotator cuff and subscapularis muscles.

Initial Phase

Intervention

Indirect techniques, such as STM, are used on the cervical, rib, and shoulder musculature. PROM stretching to tolerance is performed in external and internal rotation. Pain-free joint mobilizations of grades II and III to the glenohumeral joint are performed. The patient is instructed in positioning comfort for the left shoulder and cervical spine.

Rationale

The initial phase of rehabilitation for nonprotective injuries primarily focuses on anti-inflammatory modalities, grade II and III joint mobilization, and education. Patients often perform habitual patterns of movement that maintain their current state of dysfunction. Correction, modification, or cessation of predisposing activities is essential. Goals of rehabilitation during this phase are to reduce inflammation and pain, to restore proximal stability to the spine, to promote scapular muscle activity, and to avoid painful positions. Clearing spinal and rib dysfunctions that contribute to or are source problems for shoulder signs and symptoms is essential during this phase for an optimal functional outcome.

Intermediate Phase

Reevaluation

By the third treatment, the patient reports decreased soreness of the left shoulder at rest. The patient still is experiencing pain with reaching and overhead activities. Pain and stiffness of cervical spine are decreased, but shoulder ROM remains restricted. She continues to have an abnormal position of the left scapula. (See Table 14-3 for ROM measurements.)

Intervention

The patient continues PROM stretching and joint mobilization as previously. She is started on a low-load prolonged stretch into external rotation with heat in the POS by using Thera-Band and a 1-lb weight initially for 10 minutes progressing to 20 minutes during a series of four to five treatment sessions. PROM with isokinetics is initiated for internal and external rotation in the POS in the available ROM. Scapular release techniques are used to mobilize fascial restrictions within the subscapularis, serratus anterior, and levator scapulae. Joint mobilization techniques are used to address facet joint irritation at C5-6 and suboccipitally. PNF scapular

Continued

CASE STUDY 2—cont'd

patterns progress from passive to resistive movements, with an emphasis on posterior depression.

Rationale

The intermediate phase of rehabilitation begins when the patient's reactivity allows for more aggressive progression of techniques. The goals of this phase are to maximize ROM of all components of shoulder movement and to normalize force couples of the scapula and glenohumeral joint. Emphasis is placed on restoring rotation at the glenohumeral joint and then on elevation.

Traditional manual therapy techniques used to treat limited shoulder ROM have followed the arthrokinematic movements of joint surfaces occurring at the glenohumeral. Kaltenborn[37] determined the appropriate method of applying a gliding mobilization technique by the convex-concave rule. For example, sliding of the convex humeral head on a concave glenoid surface occurs in the opposite direction of the humerus. Therefore, during elevation of the shoulder, the humeral head is sliding inferiorly as the bone moves superiorly. However, data are now available that challenge the concave-convex rule of arthrokinematic motion.

Poppen and Walker[38] reported a movement of the humeral head in a superior and inferior direction during elevation of the shoulder. Howell et al[39] demonstrated translatory motion of the head of the humerus to be opposite of that predicted by the concave-convex rule. Only patients with instability had demonstrated translation in the direction predicted by the concave-convex rule.[39] Soft tissue tension of the capsular and ligament components, rather than joint surface geometry, may be a greater determinant of the arthrokinematics of the glenohumeral joint.

The type and frequency of force used to mobilize depend on the implicated tissue. In this case study, the implicated tissues of restriction are the anterior and inferior capsule, the glenohumeral ligaments, and the subscapularis. The use of low-load prolonged stretch is advocated, in addition to oscillation techniques, for more substantial soft tissue restrictions. Connective tissue structures such as ligaments, tendons, and capsules respond to mechanical stress in a time-dependent or viscoelastic manner.[40-43] *Viscoelasticity* is a mechanical property of materials that describes the tendency of a substance to deform at a constant rate. The rate of deformation does not depend on the speed of the external force applied. If the amount of deformation does not exceed the elastic range, the structure can return to the original resting length after the load is removed. If loading is continued into the plastic range, beyond the yield point, failure of the tissue will occur. Failure is thought to be a function of breaking of intermolecular cross-links, rather than rupture of the collagen tissue.[44]

If a permanent increase in ROM is a goal of treatment, then manual therapy should be aimed at producing plastic deformation. Taylor et al[45] showed an increased risk of tissue trauma and injury with rapid stretch rates. Rapidly applied forces may cause material to react in a stiff, brittle fashion, with consequent tissue tearing. Gradually applied loads may lead tissue to respond in a more yielding manner with plastic deformation. When the tissue is held under a constant external load and at a constant length, force relaxation occurs.[46]

In addition to increasing extensibility of glenohumeral capsular and ligamentous structures, muscle extensibility must also be addressed. Clinically, the subscapularis is commonly restricted in shoulder dysfunction. The subscapularis is the most stabilizing factor during external rotation of the glenohumeral joint in 0° of abduction.[38] Additionally, most patients tend to guard or immobilize a painful shoulder by adducting and internally rotating the glenohumeral joint, thus shortening the subscapularis.

During prolonged immobilization and dysfunction, such as in adhesive capsulitis, the subscapularis may acclimate to a shortened position. Muscles respond to immobilization by degeneration of myofilaments, changes in sarcomere alignment and configuration, decreases in mitochondria, and a decreased ability to generate tension.[47] Muscles acclimate to immobilization in a shortened position by losing sarcomeres. Tabary et al[48] found that muscles immobilized in a shortened position for 4 weeks had a 40% decrease in total sarcomeres and displayed an increased resistance to passive movement. Muscles immobilized in a lengthened position had 20% more sarcomeres and demonstrated no change in resistance to passive motion.

Functionally, limited subscapularis extensibility may affect functional elevation. Otis et al[49] reported the importance of restoring rotation to the glenohumeral joint to facilitate elevation. These investigators demonstrated that the contribution of the infraspinatus moment arm to abduction is enhanced with internal rotation, whereas that of the subscapularis is enhanced with external rotation.[49] Low-load prolonged stretch and rotational exercises in the POS in this case study are an attempt to reverse the effects of immobility, thus increasing the extensibility and strength of the subscapularis. Restrictions of the subscapularis also tend to affect parascapular muscles secondary to the altered scapulohumeral rhythm.

Scapular release techniques and STM (described later in this chapter and in Chapter 10) can be used to release fascial restrictions that develop as a result of abnormal movement patterns. In this particular case, the patient had excessive protraction and downward rotation of the scapula with myofascial trigger points in the levator scapulae, serratus anterior, and pectoralis minor. Warwick and Williams[50] reported a possible fusion of the serratus anterior and levator scapulae by their fascial connection. Excessive tone of pectoralis minor effectively depresses the scapula and restricts the scapular rotation necessary for proper elevation. Furthermore, the serratus anterior and levator scapulae work as a force couple to

CASE STUDY 2—cont'd

rotate the scapula. Increasing the extensibility of the fascia of these three muscles would allow proper functioning of parascapular force couples during elevation.

Return to Function Phase

Reevaluation

All ADLs are performed without pain, and the patient has started working in the yard without limitations. The patient has no cervical pain, but ROM of the cervical spine is three-fourths normal with side bending on the right and left. (See Table 14-3 for 10-week ROM measurements.)

Intervention

The patient is instructed in exercise progressions for the next 2 months, with an emphasis on rotator cuff and parascapular muscle exercises. She is allowed to progress back to swimming and gardening activities to tolerance.

Rationale

Once ROM and strength are optimized, a home program is finalized to facilitate physiologic changes (e.g., increased sarcomeres and remodeling of periarticular tissue) further. In the competitive and industrial athlete, form, technique, and training error corrections are essential to prevent recurrence of dysfunction.

In summary, rehabilitation of nonprotective injuries depends on the implicated tissue or systems in dysfunction or restriction. Table 14-4 summarizes the phases of rehabilitation. Glenohumeral joint arthrokinematics may be strongly influenced by periarticular tissue extensibility and muscle function, rather than by pure joint geometry. Manual techniques must comply with the type of tissue or system response desired. Continual reassessment of subjective, functional, and objective measures assists the therapist in evaluating treatment effectiveness.

Table 14-4 Summary of Phased Rehabilitation for Nonprotective Shoulder Injuries

Phases	Initial	Intermediate	Return to Function
Signs and symptoms (reactivity)	Pain at rest; difficulty sleeping; pain before resistance	No pain at rest; pain with resistance; moderate reactivity; limited rotation and elevation; weakness of rotator cuff or parascapular muscles	ROM maximized; functional movement pain free; muscle imbalances resolving
Goals	Decrease pain	Restore rotation ROM and strength of parascapular muscles and rotator cuff	Return to function
Manual therapy techniques	Grades 1 and 2 joint mobilizations	Grades 3 and 4 joint mobilizations; STM; scapular release techniques; PNF scapular and UE patterns; low-load prolonged stretch	Fine-tuning of functional patterns with PNF
Other therapeutic interventions	Anti-inflammatory modalities; positioning and activity education	Heat with stretch; isokinetic and isotonics working rotation before elevation in POS; isometrics; AAROM with T bars, Swiss balls, foam rollers; glenohumeral joint and scapular taping techniques	Home program, correction of technique and training errors

AAROM, active-assistive range of motion; PNF, proprioceptive neuromuscular facilitation; POS, plane of the scapula; ROM, range of motion; STM, soft tissue mobilization; UE, upper extremity.

GLENOHUMERAL JOINT TECHNIQUES

Inferior Glide of the Humerus

Patient Position

The patient is supine, with the involved extremity close to the edge of the table. A strap may be used to stabilize the scapula. The extremity is abducted to the desired range.

Therapist Position

With the therapist facing the lateral aspect of the patient's upper arm the therapist's cephalad hand web space is placed on the patient's superior glenohumeral inferior to the acromion. The assisting hand supports the weight of the patient's arm by holding the distal upper arm superior to the epicondyles and bracing the patient's arm against the therapist. The assisting hand or arm can also impart distractive force and change amount of rotation. The mobilizing hand glides the head of the humerus inferiorly and attempts to stress the axillary pouch or inferior portion of the glenohumeral capsule.

Inferior Glide of the Humerus with Passive External Rotation

Patient Position

The patient's position is prone, with the shoulder over the edge of the treatment table.

Therapist Position

The therapist holds the patient's humerus in external rotation while providing an inferior-posterior glide to the humeral head (Fig. 14-8). Oscillations or prolonged stretch can be used with this technique.

Longitudinal Distraction: Inferior Glide of the Humerus

Patient Position

The patient is supine, with the involved extremity as close as possible to the edge of the table.

Therapist Position

The therapist is facing the joint, with the inner hand up into the patient's axilla and pressing against the scapuloglenoid (Fig. 14-9). The outer mobilizing hand grips the epicondyles of the patient's humerus and imparts a distractive force that stresses the inferior capsule. To increase the efficiency of the pull, the therapist can shift weight and rotate the body slightly away from the patient. A prolonged stretch is often effective with this technique.

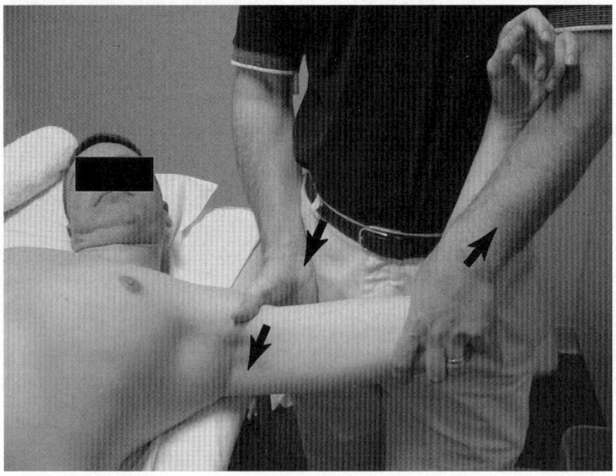

Figure 14-8 Inferior glide of the humerus with passive external rotation.

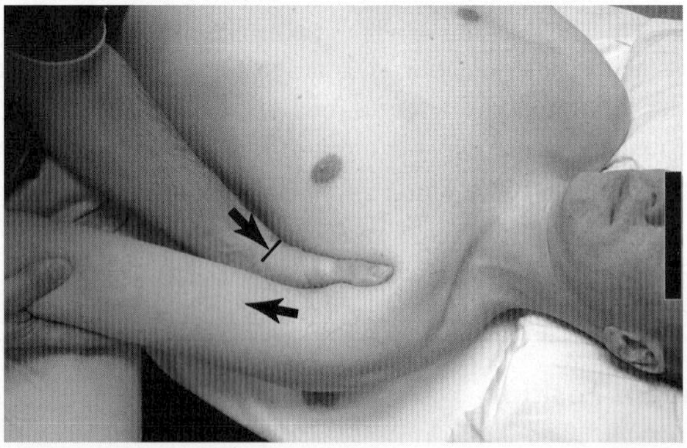

Figure 14-9 Longitudinal distraction: inferior glide of the humerus.

Posterior Glide of the Humerus

Patient Position

The patient is supine, with the arm slightly abducted and flexed into the POS and resting on the therapist's thigh.

Therapist Position

The therapist is sitting on the treatment table at a 45° turn from the sagittal plane. The mobilizing hand is placed on the patient's anterior humeral head, with a wedge or rolled towel under the lateral scapula (Fig. 14-10). The assisting hand supports the patient's distal extremity to facilitate relaxation. The mobilization is directed posteriorly along the plane of the glenoid. This technique is useful for reactive shoulders with posterior capsule tightness.

Posterior Glide of the Humerus

Patient Position

The patient is supine, with the involved shoulder flexed 90° and horizontally adducted to first tissue resistance.

Therapist Position

The therapist is on the opposite side of patient's shoulder. The mobilizing hand is on the same side as the involved shoulder. The therapist cups patient's elbow in the mobilizing hand and assists mobilization with therapist's sternum. The assisting hand stabilizes the scapula under the patient. Mobilization movement is along 35° of glenoid tilt. The level of flexion

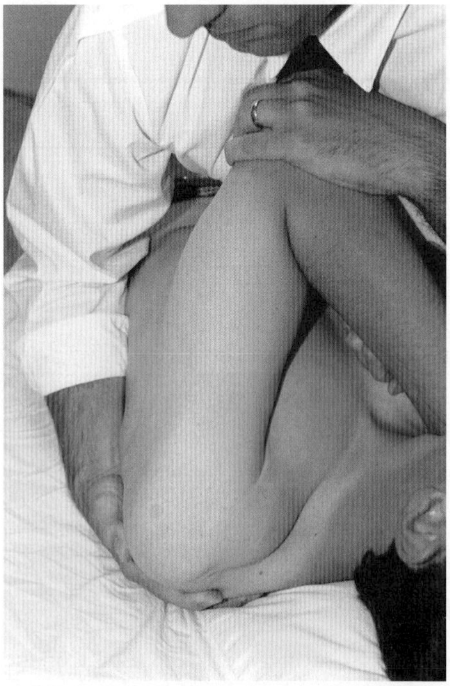

Figure 14-10 Posterior glide of the humerus.

can be changed to work the most restricted part of the capsule. This technique is useful in patients with subacute and chronic posterior capsule tightness.

Posterior Glide of the Humeral Head in Side Lying

Patient Position

Patient is positioned in side lying, with the involved shoulder facing upward.

Therapist Position

With the therapist facing the patient, the therapist's cephalad hand contacts the patient's proximal humerus, and the caudal hand holds the involved extremity by the elbow (Fig. 14-11). The mobilization is a force couple motion, with the proximal hand providing the primary mobilizing force in an anterior-posterior direction while the caudal hand provides a slight circumduction motion, usually opposite that of the proximal hand.

Posterior Glide Using a Fulcrum Technique

Patient Position

The patient is prone, with the shoulder near the edge of the treatment table.

Therapist Position

The therapist positions his or her left forearm under the patient's anterior humeral head. The therapist's right hand is on the patient's forearm and provides a distraction and adduction force. At the same time the force is initiated, the therapist lifts the patient's humeral head by using his or her left forearm as a lever.

Lateral Distraction of the Humerus

Patient Position

The patient is supine, close to the edge of the table, with the involved extremity flexed at the elbow and glenohumeral joint. The extremity rests on the therapist's shoulder. A strap and the table stabilize the scapula.

Therapist Position

The therapist is facing laterally, and both hands grasp the patient's humerus as close as possible to the joint. The therapist should assess which vector of movement is most severely restricted by starting laterally with mobilization and proceeding caudally. To improve delivery of oscillation or stretch, the therapist should align his or her trunk along the vector of mobilization.

Anterior Glide of the Head of the Humerus

Patient Position

The patient is prone, with the involved extremity as close as possible to the edge of the table. The head of the humerus must be off the table. A wedge or towel roll is placed just medial to the joint line under the coracoid process. The extremity is abducted and flexed into the POS.

Therapist Position

The therapist is distal to the patient's abducted shoulder facing cephalad (Fig. 14-12). The outer hand applies slight distractive force while the inner mobilizing hand glides the head of the patient's humerus anteriorly, thereby stressing the anterior capsule. The tendon of the subscapularis is also stressed with this technique. Mobilization can be fine-tuned by changing the angle of the anterior force to the most severely restricted area.

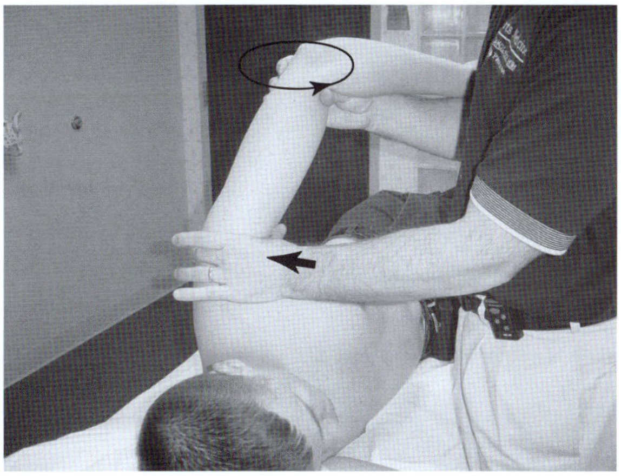

Figure 14-11 Posterior glide of the humeral head in side lying.

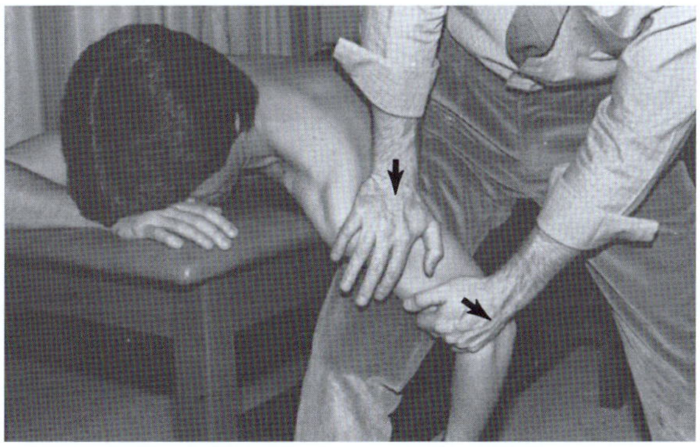

Figure 14-12 Anterior glide of the head of the humerus.

Anterior-Posterior Glide of the Head of the Humerus

Patient Position

The patient is prone, with the involved extremity over the edge of the table abducted to the desired range. A strap may be used to stabilize the scapula.

Therapist Position

The therapist is facing laterally in a sitting position, with the forearm of the patient's involved extremity held between the therapist's knees (Fig. 14-13). Both hands grasp the head of the patient's humerus and apply anterior-posterior movement to oscillate the head of the humerus. Grades I and II are mainly used with this technique, to stimulate mechanoreceptor activity.

Anterior-Posterior Glide of the Head of the Humerus

Patient Position

The patient is supine, with the involved extremity supported by the table. A towel roll, pillow, or wedge is placed under the patient's elbow to hold the arm in the POS.

Therapist Position

The therapist is facing laterally in a sitting position (Fig. 14-14). The fingertips hold the head of the humerus while a gentle up-and-down movement is applied. This technique is used with grade I and II oscillations.

External Rotation of the Humerus

Patient Position

The patient is supine, with the involved extremity supported by the table. The arm is held in the POS.

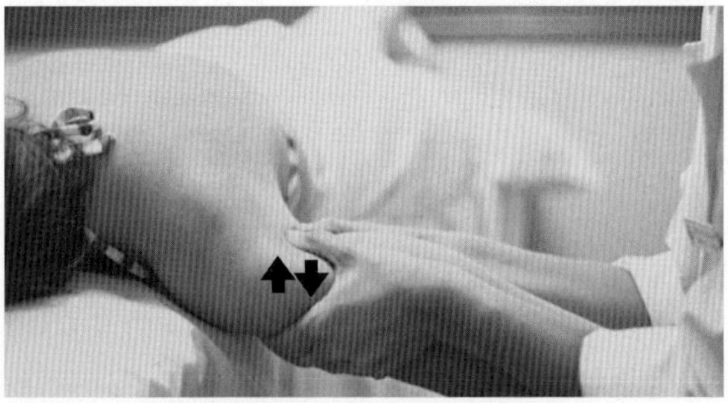

Figure 14-13 Prone anterior-posterior glide of the head of the humerus.

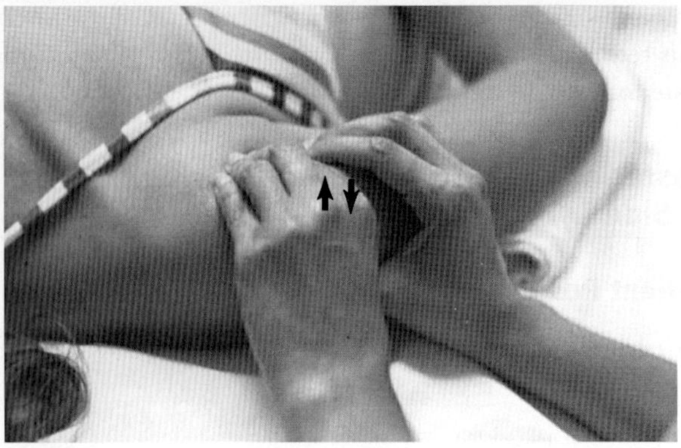

Figure 14-14 Supine anterior-posterior glide of the head of the humerus.

Therapist Position

The therapist is facing laterally, with the caudal mobilizing hand grasping the patient's distal humerus and the heel of the cephalad mobilizing hand over the lateral aspect of the head of the humerus (Fig. 14-15). Force is applied through both hands. The caudal hand rotates the patient's humerus externally and provides long-axis distraction while the cephalad hand pushes the head of the humerus in a posterior direction.

External Rotation, Abduction, and Inferior Glide of the Humerus

Position

The patient is supine, with the involved extremity supported by the table. The arm is abducted in the POS.

Therapist Position

The therapist is facing laterally, with the caudal hand holding the patient's distal humerus and the heel of the cephalad hand over the head of the humerus (Fig. 14-16). The caudal hand abducts the patient's arm and externally rotates the humerus while maintaining the POS. The cephalad hand simultaneously

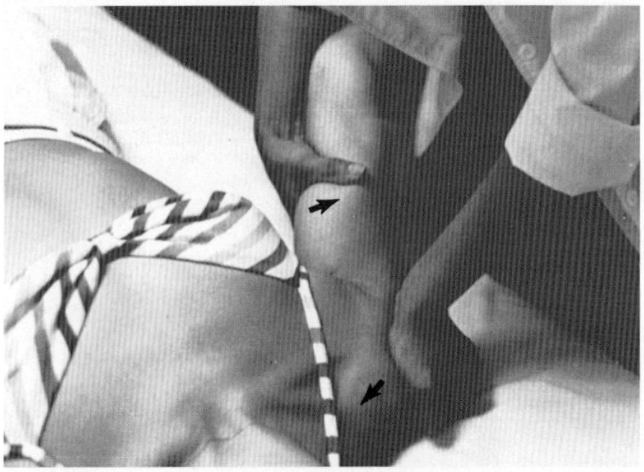

Figure 14-15 Supine external rotation of the humerus.

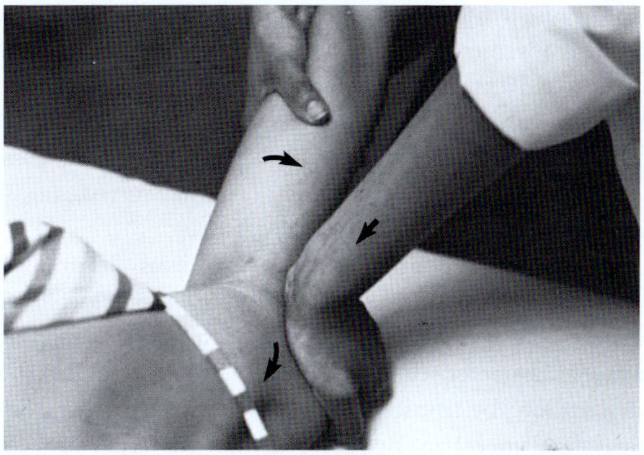

Figure 14-16 Supine external rotation, abduction, and inferior glide of the humerus.

pushes the head of the patient's humerus into external rotation and slight inferior glide. The force can be oscillated or thrusted, or it can be a prolonged stretch.

STERNOCLAVICULAR AND ACROMIOCLAVICULAR TECHNIQUES

Superior Glide of the Sternoclavicular Joint

Patient Position

The patient is supine, with the involved extremity close to the edge of the table.

Therapist Position

The therapist is facing cranially (Fig. 14-17). The volar surface left thumb pad is placed over the inferior surface of the most medial aspect of the clavicle. The right thumb reinforces the dorsal aspect of the left thumb. Both thumbs mobilize the clavicle superiorly. Graded oscillations are most successful with this technique.

Inferior-Posterior Glide of the Sternoclavicular Joint

Patient Position

The patient is supine, with the head supported on a pillow. The patient's cervical spine side is bent toward and rotated away from the involved side 20° to 30°.

Therapist Position

The therapist is at the head of the patient and uses thumb pad or pisiform contact on the most medial portion of the patient's clavicle (Fig. 14-18). Mobilization is performed in an inferior-posterior-lateral direction parallel to the joint line. Elevating the involved shoulder to a position of restriction and then performing mobilization of the sternoclavicular joint may assist the rotational component of clavicle motion joint.

Anterior Glide of the Acromioclavicular Joint

Patient Position

The patient is supine, at a diagonal to allow the involved acromioclavicular joint to be over the edge of the table.

Therapist Position

Mobilizing force is performed with both thumbs (dorsal surfaces together) (Fig. 14-19). The therapist places the distal tips of the thumbs posteriorly to the most lateral edge of the patient's clavicle. Both thumbs push the clavicle anteriorly. Graded oscillations are mainly used with this technique.

Gapping of the Acromioclavicular Joint

Patient Position

The patient is sitting close to the edge of the table.

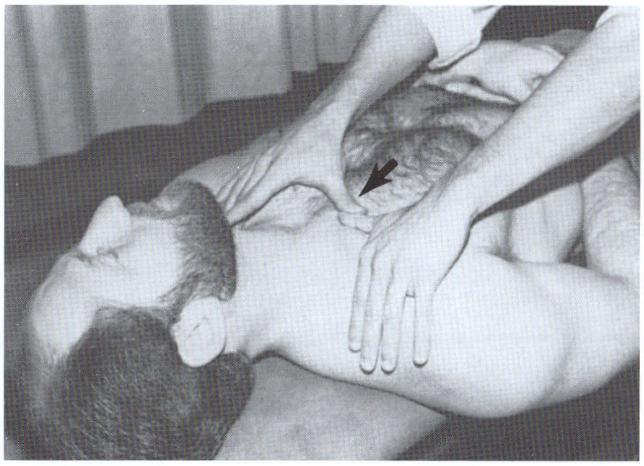

Figure 14-17 Superior glide of the sternoclavicular joint.

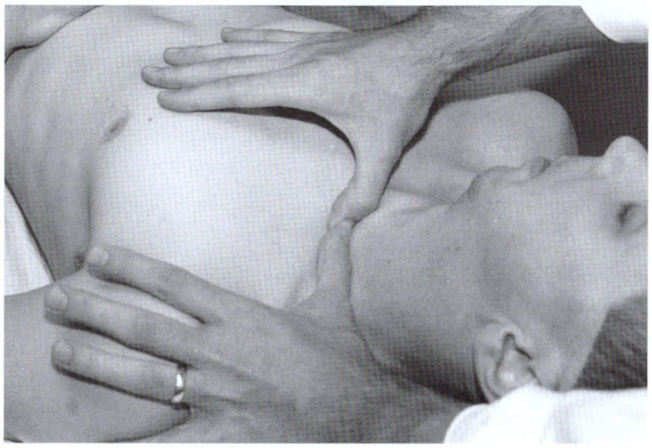

Figure 14-18 Inferior-posterior glide of the sternoclavicular joint.

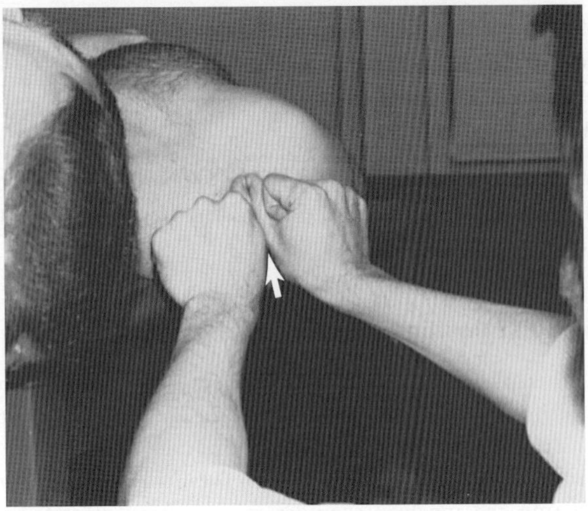

Figure 14-19 Anterior glide of the acromioclavicular joint.

Therapist Position

The therapist is facing laterally, with the heel of the left hand over the spine of the patient's scapula and the thenar eminence to the right hand over the distal clavicle (Fig. 14-20). The force is applied simultaneously. Both hands push the bones in opposite directions, to obtain a general stretch to the capsular structures of the acromioclavicular joint. Oscillations or a prolonged stretch are used with this technique.

SOFT TISSUE MOBILIZATION AND SCAPULOTHORACIC RELEASE TECHNIQUES

Soft tissue mobilization, for the purposes of this chapter, is as defined by Johnson: "STM is the treatment of soft tissue with consideration of layers and depth by initially evaluating and treating superficially, proceeding to bony prominence, muscle, tendon, ligament, etc."[9] The goals of STM in the patient are similar to those of joint mobilization: development of functional scar tissue, elongation of collagen tissue, increase in GAGs, and facilitation of lymphatic drainage.[33]

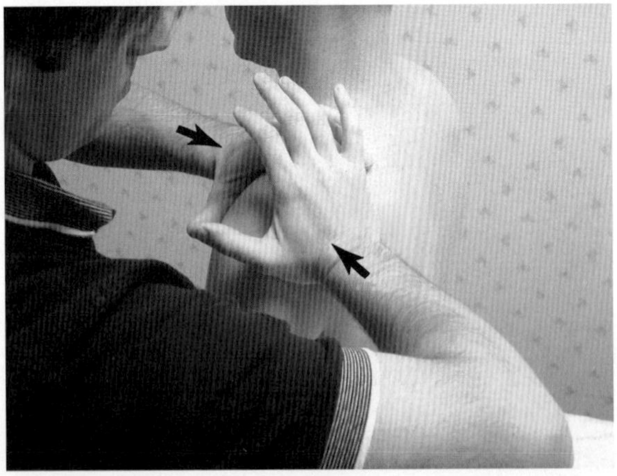

Figure 14-20 Gapping of the acromioclavicular joint.

In overuse syndromes, trauma, postsurgical conditions, and abnormal movement patterns of the shoulder, areas of tenderness and restricted extensibility of connective tissue may develop. Adhesions within the fascia may reduce the muscle's ability to broaden during contraction and to lengthen during passive elongation.[33] Abnormal compensations may occur, possibly leading to breakdown of compensating tissue.

Within the shoulder complex, several areas are important to evaluate for fascial restrictions. Scapulothoracic releasing techniques are also described because of the musculotendinous and fascial characteristics of this articulation. The following is a description by muscle or space between structures to evaluate and mobilize. Box 14-1 defines the types of techniques referred to in the figure legends.

Subscapularis

Patient Position

The patient is supine, with the shoulder abducted to tolerance.

Therapist Position

The therapist is facing the patient's axilla with the mobilizing fingers on the muscle belly of the subscapularis (Fig. 14-21). Parallel mobilization or perpendicular strumming or direct

BOX 14-1 Treatment Hand Techniques

- *Sustained pressure:* Pressure applied directly to restricted tissue at the desired depth and direction of maximal restriction
- *Direct oscillations:* Repeated oscillations on and off a restriction with uptake of slack as restriction resolves
- *Perpendicular mobilization:* Direct oscillations or sustained pressure techniques performed perpendicular to muscle fiber or soft tissue play
- *Parallel mobilization:* Pressure applied longitudinally to restrictions along the edge of the muscle belly or along bony contours
- *Perpendicular (transverse) strumming:* Repeated rhythmic deformations of a muscle belly to improve muscle play and reduce tone

Modified from Johnson GS: Soft tissue mobilization. In Donatelli R, Wooden MJ, editors: *Orthopaedic physical therapy,* New York, 1994, Churchill Livingstone.

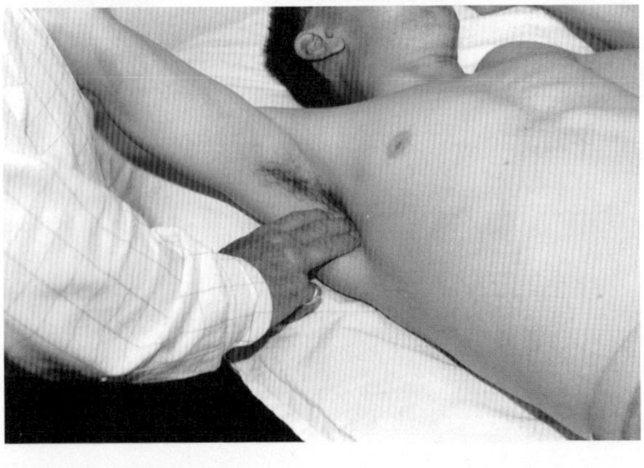

Figure 14-21 Subscapularis palpation.

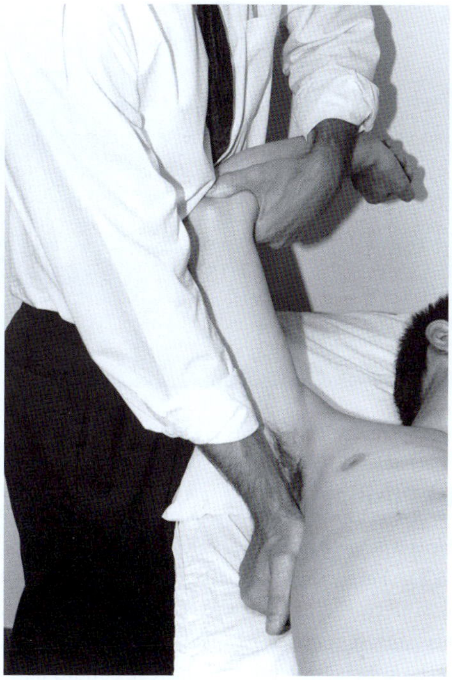

Figure 14-22 Subscapularis arc stretch.

oscillation may be used. Assistive techniques include sustaining pressure while elevating and adducting the shoulder (see Fig. 14-22).

Subscapularis Arc Stretch

Patient Position

The patient is supine.

Therapist Position

The therapist's cephalad hand simultaneously elevates, externally rotates, and distracts the involved shoulder while the caudal hand (thenar side) stabilizes the lateral border of the scapula (Fig. 14-22). Both movements occur simultaneously, in a slightly arcing fashion.

Side-Lying Subscapularis, Teres Major Tilt Stretch

Patient Position

The patient is side lying facing the therapist with hips flexed to approximately 45° for stability.

Therapist Position

With the therapist facing the patient, the therapist's caudal hand and upper extremity skin lock on the inferior border of the patient's scapula (Fig 14-23). The therapist's cephalad hand and upper extremity wrap around the patient's humerus,

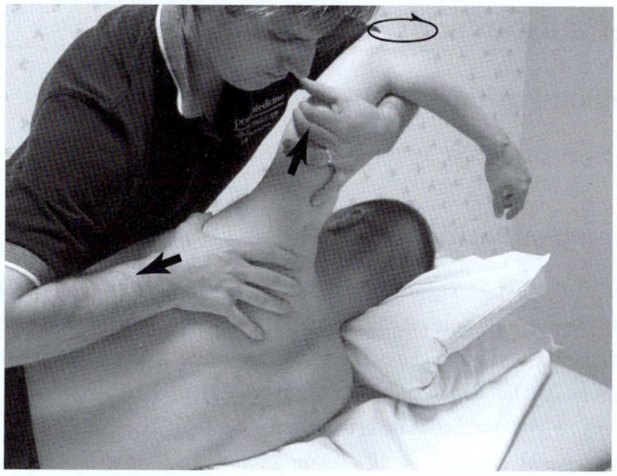

Figure 14-23 Side-lying subscapularis, teres major tilt stretch.

and the therapist's elbow and proximal arm control the amount of external rotation. The forces from the therapist's upper extremities are in opposite directions, or one hand can stabilize and one can be the primary mobilizer. This technique can also be used with contraction-relaxation stretching to increase contractile component extensibility.

Pectoralis Minor

Patient Position

The patient is supine or side lying, with the arm slightly abducted and flexed.

Therapist Position

The therapist's mobilizing fingers glide along in a superficial vector along ribs 3 to 5 lateral to medial underneath the pectoralis major (Fig. 14-24). Often, the pectoralis minor is bound down and tender in shoulder dysfunction. STM techniques used are direct oscillation, sustained pressure, and perpendicular and parallel deformations. Assistive techniques include inhalation and contraction-relaxation with shoulder protraction.

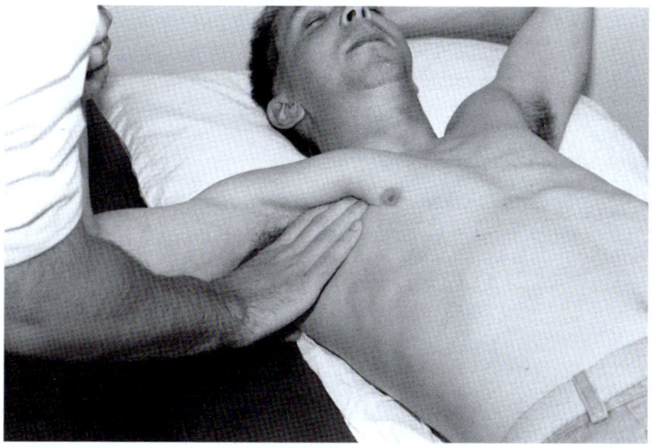

Figure 14-24 Pectoralis minor.

Serratus Anterior: Upper Portion

Patient Position

The patient is side lying, with involved side upward.

Therapist Position

The therapist is standing posterior to the patient's shoulder. The caudal hand elevates the scapula in a cephalad and anterior direction off the rib cage (Fig. 14-25). The therapist can use the fingers of the top hand to roll over and palpate the superior fibers of the serratus anterior that attach to the patient's first and second ribs, as well as the fascial attachments between the levator scapulae and serratus anterior.[50] STM techniques are sustained pressure and direct oscillation. Assistive techniques include resistive PNF, diagonal contraction-relaxation, and deep breath.

Serratus Anterior: Lower Portion

Patient Position

The patient is side lying.

Therapist Position

The therapist places the mobilizing fingers along an interspace of ribs 2 to 8 on interdigitations of serratus anterior (Fig. 14-26). STM techniques used are parallel techniques along rib contours medially to laterally or laterally to medially. Assistive techniques include deep breath, contraction-relaxation with scapular depression, and rotation of the thoracic spine to the same side. Restrictions may be evident in patients with a previous history of rib fracture or abdominal surgery.

Inferior Clavicle

Patient Position

The patient is supine, with the involved extremity supported by a pillow.

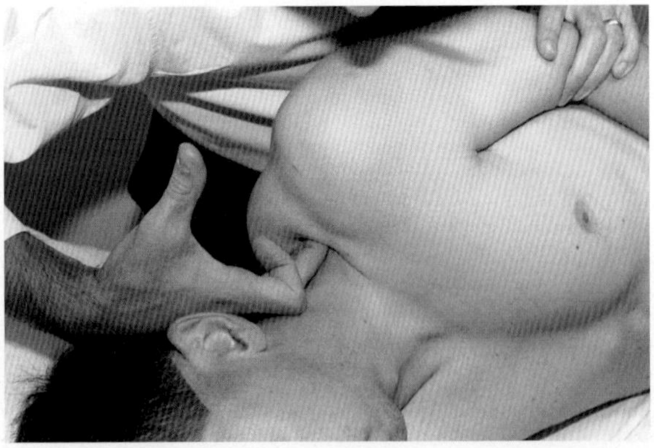

Figure 14-25 Serratus anterior: upper portion.

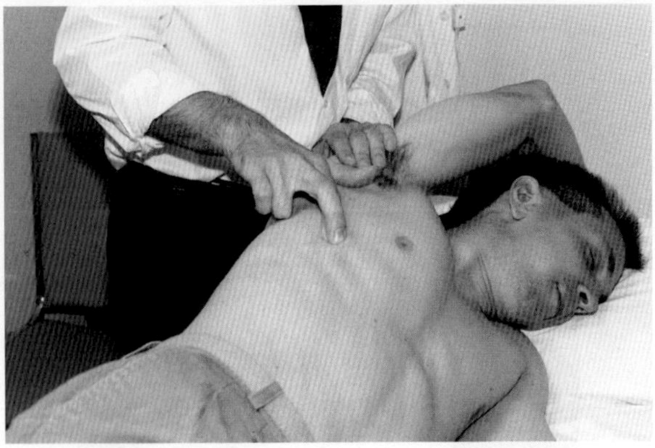

Figure 14-26 Serratus anterior: lower portion.

Therapist Position

The therapist is on the same side as the involved shoulder (Fig. 14-27). Palpating medially to laterally or vice versa along the inferior clavicle, the therapist looks for fascial restrictions and tenderness, especially at the costoclavicular ligament, the subclavius muscle, and the conoid and trapezoid ligaments. This region is important to evaluate and treat in shoulder patients who have a protracted and externally rotated scapula with adaptive shortening of the anterior chest musculature.

Scapular Distraction

Patient Position

The patient is side lying close to the edge of the table, with the involved extremity accessible to the therapist. A pillow may be placed against the patient's chest to provide anterior support.

Therapist Position

In Figure 14-28A, the binder illustrates the tilting aspect of the scapula before the therapist attempts to lift the scapula off the thoracic wall. Figure 14-28B shows the tilting of the scapula. The therapist is facing the patient, with the

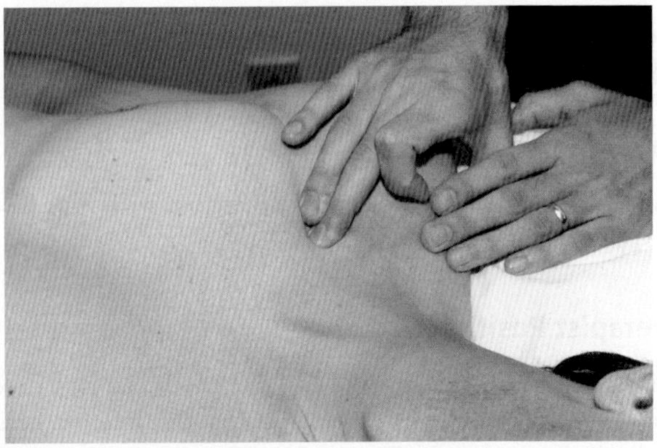

Figure 14-27 Inferior clavicle.

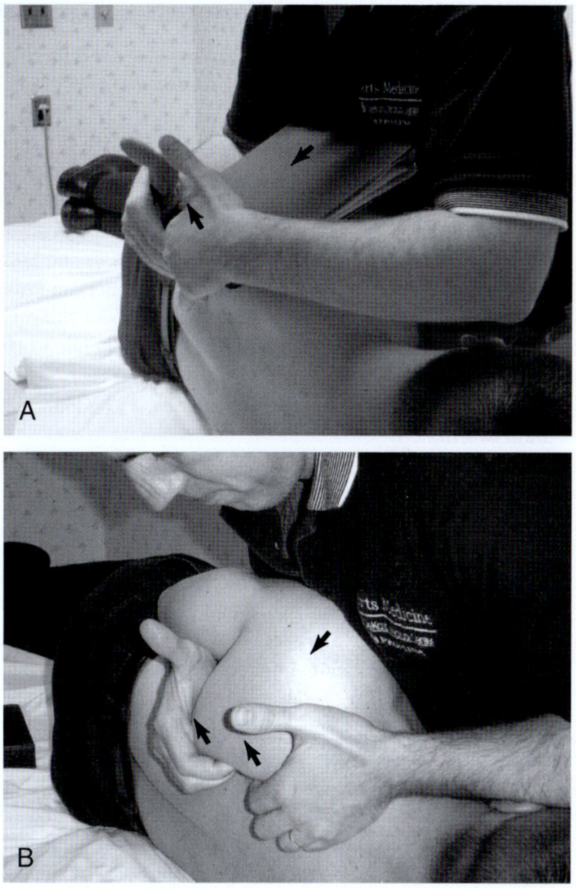

Figure 14-28 Scapular distraction: tilt. **A,** Tilt technique demonstrated with a note book. **B,** Force through the chest of the therapists to allow the fingers to get under the edge of the notebook (vertebral border of the scapula).

caudal hand underneath the inferior angle of the patient's scapula and the cephalad hand grasping the vertebral border of the scapula. The therapist's anterior sternum is the third contact point assisting the scapular tilt. Both hands tilt the scapula away from the thoracic wall along with the distraction of the scapula when the therapist leans backward.

Scapular Distraction: Posterior Approach

Patient Position

The patient is side lying as previously, but closer to the posterior edge of the table.

Therapist Position

The therapist is posterior to the patient, with the therapist's hips in perpendicular orientation to the patient's trunk (Fig. 14-29). The therapist's adjacent leg is on the treatment table, with the knee bent and placed along the patient's mid-thoracic spine. The outer mobilizing hand grasps the vertebral border of the patient's scapula. The inner hand supports the patient's anterior glenohumeral joint. Once hand placement is achieved, the therapist leans backward, thus distracting the scapula away from the thoracic wall. Sustained stretch is most effective with this technique.

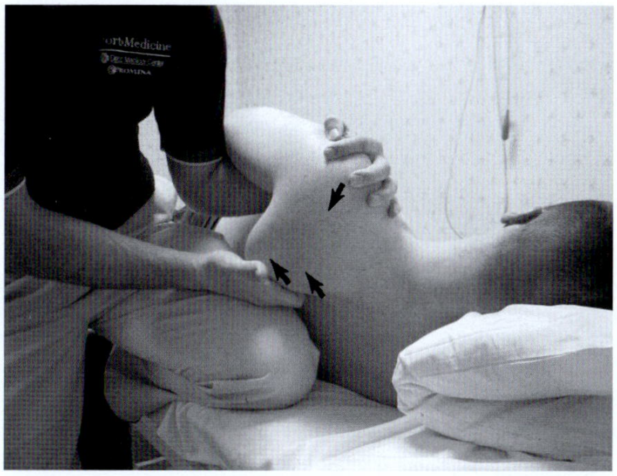

Figure 14-29 Scapular distraction, posterior approach.

Scapular External Rotation

Patient Position

The patient is side lying, with the involved extremity accessible to the therapist.

Therapist Position

The therapist is facing the patient, with the caudal hand under the patient's extremity through the axillary area (Fig. 14-30). The cephalad hand grasps the superior aspect of the patient's scapula while the caudal hand grasps the inferior angle. The force is applied simultaneously, thus producing external rotation of the scapula. This demonstrates external rotation of the scapula with soft tissue technique by using the therapist's elbow to mobilize the upper trapezius and levator scapulae. Assistive techniques include having the patient actively rotate cervical spine toward and away from involved side and spray and stretch to the upper trapezius trigger points.

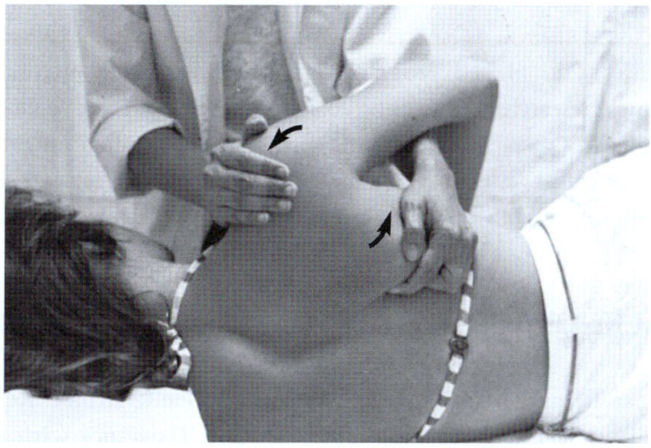

Figure 14-30 Scapular external rotation.

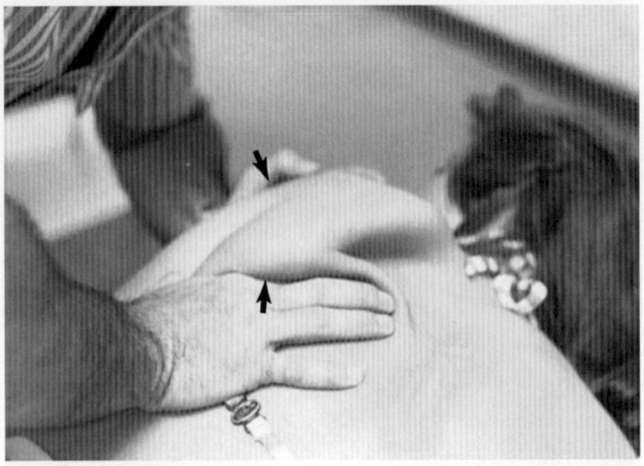

Figure 14-31 Scapular distraction, prone.

Scapular Distraction: Prone

Patient Position

The patient is prone, with the involved extremity supported by the table.

Therapist Position

The therapist is facing cephalad, with the outer hand under the head of the patient's humerus and the adjacent mobilizing hand web space under the inferior angle of the scapula (Fig. 14-31). The forces are applied simultaneously. The outer hand lifts the patient's glenohumeral joint while the adjacent hand lifts the inferior angle of the scapula.

SUMMARY

Rehabilitation of shoulder injuries using manual techniques is based on an understanding of the following: the stages of soft tissue healing; normal and abnormal arthrokinematics and osteokinematics of the shoulder complex; the effects of biomechanical stress on various tissues; and muscle function. The application of manual techniques for the shoulder depends on a thorough sequential examination and continuous reevaluation. Indications and contraindications for mobilization are based on an understanding of the histologic features of immobilized and traumatized tissue. Clinical management of shoulder injuries is discussed from a perspective of protective versus nonprotective injuries, and phased programs of rehabilitation are presented. Clinical research is beginning to demonstrate the positive effects of manual therapy in patients with shoulder dysfunction, but further studies must be conducted, and traditional concepts and techniques should comply with current and future discoveries.

ACKNOWLEDGMENTS

Donatelli and McMahon would like to thank Aimee Reiss, MPT, and David Ciganek, ATC, for their assistance with the manual technique pictures.

REFERENCES

1. Frank C, Akeson WH, Woo S, et al: Physiology and therapeutic value of passive joint motion, *Clin Orthop Relat Res* 185:113, 1984.
2. Peacock EE Jr : *Wound repair*, ed 3, Philadelphia, 1984, Saunders.
3. Akeson WH, Amiel D, Woo SLY: Immobility effects on synovial joints: the pathomechanics of joint contracture, *Biorheology* 17:95, 1980.
4. American Physical Therapy Association: *Guide to physical therapist practice*, ed 2, Alexandria, Va, 2001, American Physical Therapy Association.
5. Stoddard A: *Manual of osteopathic technique*, London, 1959, Hutchinson.
6. Maitland GD: *Peripheral manipulation*, London, 1970, Butterworth.
7. Clayton L, editor: *Taber's cyclopedic medical dictionary*, Philadelphia, 1977, Davis.
8. Friel J, editor: *Dorland's illustrated medical dictionary*, ed 25, Philadelphia, 1974, Saunders.
9. Johnson GS: Course notes, functional orthopedic I, Institute for Physical Art, San Francisco, March 1991.
10. Hsu AT, Ho L, Ho S, et al: Joint position during anterior-posterior glide mobilization: its effect on glenohumeral abduction range of motion, *Arch Phys Med Rehabil* 81(2):210–214, 2000.
11. Mao CY, Jaw WC, Cheng HC: Frozen shoulder: correlation between the response to physical therapy and follow-up shoulder arthrography, *Arch Phys Med Rehabil* 78(8):857–859, 1997.
12. Vermuelen HM, Obermann WR, Burger BJ, et al: End range mobilization techniques in adhesive capsulitis of the shoulder joint: a multiple-subject case report, *Phys Ther* 80(12):1204–1213, 2000.
13. Vermuelen HM, Rozing PM, Obermann SC, et al: Comparison of high-grade and low-grade mobilization techniques in the management of adhesive capsulitis of the shoulder: randomized controlled trial, *J Am Phys Ther* 86:355–368, 2006.
14. Van der Heijden GJ, van der Windt DA, de Winter AF: Physiotherapy for patients with soft tissue shoulder disorders: a systematic review of randomized clinical trials, *BMJ* 315:25–30, 1997.
15. Winters JC, Jorritsma W, Groenier KH, et al: Treatment of shoulder complaints in general practice: long term results of a randomized, single blind study comparing physio-therapy, manipulation, and corticosteroid injection, *BMJ* 318:1395–1396, 1999.
16. Van der Windt DA, Koes BW, Deville W, et al: Effectiveness of corticosteroid injections versus physiotherapy for treatment of painful stiff shoulder in primary care: randomized trial, *BMJ* 317:1292–1296, 1998.
17. Bang MD, Deyle GD: Comparison of supervised exercise with and without manual physical therapy for patients with shoulder impingement syndrome, *J Orthop Sports Phys Ther* 30(3):126–137, 2000.
18. Conroy DE, Hayes KW: The effect of joint mobilization as a component of comprehensive treatment for primary shoulder impingement syndrome, *J Orthop Sports Phys Ther* 28(1):3–14, 1998.
19. Johnson A, Godges J, Zimmerman G, et al: The effect of anterior versus posterior glide joint mobilization on external rotation range of motion in patients with shoulder adhesive capsulitis, *J Orthop Sports Phys Ther* 37(3):88–99, 2007.
20. Gamze S, Baltaci B, Gul, et al: Manual therapy versus exercises in patients with shoulder impingement syndrome, *Med Sci Sports Exerc* 41(5 Suppl 1):41–42, 2009.

21. Gamze S, Gul B, Baran Y: Comparison of interventions with and without manual physical therapy for patients with shoulder impingement syndrome: a prospective, randomized clinical trial, *Med Sci Sports Exerc* 37(Suppl 5):S200, 2005.
22. Wyke BD: The neurology of joints, *Ann R Coll Surg Engl* 41:25, 1966.
23. Wyke BD: Neurological aspects of pain therapy: a review of some current concepts. In Swerdlow M, editor: *The therapy of pain*, Lancaster, UK, 1981, MTP Press.
24. Haldeman S: *Modern developments in the principles and practice of chiropractic*, East Norwalk, Conn, 1980, Appleton-Century-Crofts.
25. Hans U, Pascal B: Primary frozen shoulder global capsular stiffness versus localized contracture, *Clin Orthop Relat Res* 456:79–84, 2006.
26. Kummel BM: Spectrum of lesion of the anterior capsule mechanism of the shoulder, *Am J Sports Med* 7:111, 1979.
27. Warren CG, Lehman JF, Koblanski NJ: Elongation of rat tail tendon: effects of load and temperature, *Arch Phys Med Rehabil* 52:465, 1971.
28. Warren CG, Lehman JF, Koblanski NJ: Heat and stretch tech-procedure: an evaluation using rat tail tendon, *Arch Phys Med Rehabil* 57:122, 1976.
29. Bonutti PM, Windau JE, Ables BA, et al: Static progressive stretch to reestablish elbow range of motion, *Clin Orthop Relat Res* 303:128, 1994.
30. Lehman JF, Masock AJ, Warren CG, et al: Effects of therapeutic temperatures on tendon extensibility, *Arch Phys Med Rehabil* 51:481, 1970.
31. Lentell G, Hetherington T, Eagn J, et al: The use of thermal agents to influence the effectiveness of a low load prolonged stretch, *Orthop Sports Phys Ther* 17:200, 1992.
32. Turkel SJ, Panio MW, Marshall JL, et al: Stabilizing mechanisms preventing anterior dislocation of glenohumeral joint, *J Bone Joint Surg Am* 63:1208, 1981.
33. Johnson GS: Soft tissue mobilization. In Donatelli R, Wooden MJ, editors: *Orthopaedic physical therapy*, New York, 1994, Churchill Livingstone.
34. Kelly M, Madden JW: Hand surgery and wound healing. In Wolfort FG, editor: *Acute hand injuries: a multispecialty approach*, Boston, 1980, Little, Brown.
35. Cohen KI, McCoy BJ, Diegelmann RF: An update on wound healing, *Ann Plast Surg* 3:264, 1979.
36. Arem AJ, Madden JW: Effects of stress on healing wounds: intermittent noncyclical tension, *J Surg Res* 20:93, 1976.
37. Kaltenborn FM: *Mobilization of the extremity joints*, Oslo, 1980, Olaf Norris Bokhandel.
38. Poppen NK, Walker PS: Normal and abnormal motion of the shoulder, *J Bone Joint Surg Am* 58:195, 1976.
39. Howell SM, Galinat BJ, Renzi AJ, et al: Normal and abnormal mechanics of the glenohumeral joint in the horizontal plane, *J Bone Joint Surg Am* 70:227, 1988.
40. Vidik A: On the rheology and morphology of soft collagenous tissue, *J Anat* 105:184, 1969.
41. Reigger LL: Mechanical properties of bone. In Davis GJ, Gould JA, editors: *Orthopaedic and sports physical therapy*, St. Louis, 1985, Mosby.
42. Betsch DF, Bauer E: Structure and mechanical properties of rat tail tendon, *Biorheology* 17:84, 1980.
43. Butler DL, Grood ES, Noyes FR, et al: Biomechanics of ligament and tendons, *Exerc Sport Sci Rev* 6:126, 1979.
44. Hirsh G: Tensile properties during tendon healing, *Acta Orthop Scand* 153:1, 1974.
45. Taylor DC, Dalton JD, Seaber AV, et al: Viscoelastic properties of musculotendon units: the biomechanical effects of stretching, *Am J Sports Med* 18:300, 1990.
46. Van Brocklin JD, Follis DG: A study of the mechanical behavior of toe extensor tendons under applied stress, *Arch Phys Med* 46:369, 1965.
47. Cooper RR: Alterations during immobilization and regeneration of skeletal muscle in cats, *J Bone Joint Surg Am* 54:919, 1972.
48. Tabary JC, Tabary C, Tardieu C, et al: Physiological and structural changes on the cat soleus muscle due to immobilization at different lengths by plaster casts, *J Physiol* 224:231, 1972.
49. Otis JC, Jiang CC, Wickiewicz TL, et al: Changes in the movement arms of the rotator cuff and deltoid muscles with abduction and rotation, *J Bone Joint Surg Am* 76:667, 1994.
50. Warwick R, Williams P, editors: *Gray's anatomy*, British ed 35, Philadelphia, 1973, Saunders.

CHAPTER

15

Richard A. Ekstrom
and Roy W. Osborn

Muscle Length Testing and Electromyographic Evidence for Manual Strength Testing and Exercises for the Shoulder

The shoulder girdle is composed of complex connections relying not only on static stability from bone and ligamentous structures, but also on the dynamic stability provided by a highly organized series of muscle actions. Normal shoulder function depends on coordinated muscular action in the presence of a normal joint.

The examination of the patient with a shoulder problem typically includes manual muscle testing and muscle length assessment. The plan of care may incorporate strengthening, stretching, or neuromuscular control exercises or the use of physical agents. The primary focus of this chapter is to present an overview of shoulder muscle length assessment, manual muscle testing, and strengthening exercises that may be used for rehabilitation of the shoulder.

MUSCLE LENGTH

Because of their ability to change length, skeletal muscles can create movement. Each skeletal muscle has an ideal resting length, which correlates with its ability to generate force during contraction.[1] The optimal muscle length of the agonist and antagonist permits a full range of joint motion to occur. Several factors can create a change in this ideal length and can result in decreased muscle excursion. Trauma to the muscle or to the connective tissue can lead to extensive formation of scar tissue or myositis ossificans. Changes in the length of a bone because of trauma, injury to a motor nerve, surgical procedures, and prolonged immobilization can lead to muscle length changes. In addition, investigators have shown that muscle length can change as a result of postural habits that may put the muscle in either a prolonged shortened or lengthened position.[2-4] Stretching exercises have been shown to lead to muscle lengthening by the addition of sarcomeres.[4,5] Muscle shortening or lengthening can affect the function of either the agonist or the antagonist, or both, and consequently can change the movement or stabilization available at the joints on which these muscles act. Therefore, as clinicians attempt to develop appropriate intervention programs for patients with shoulder problems, recognition of muscle length imbalances may be important.

Assessment of the resting position of the scapula and movement patterns requires close scrutiny of the axioscapular, axiohumeral, and scapulohumeral musculature because of their direct and indirect influence on scapular position. The *axioscapular muscles* are the trapezius, levator scapulae, rhomboid major and minor, pectoralis minor, and serratus anterior muscles, all of which can have a direct effect on the scapular position in relation to the thoracic wall. The *axiohumeral muscles* are the pectoralis major and latissimus dorsi, which have an indirect influence on scapular position and a direct effect on humeral position within the glenohumeral joint. The *scapulohumeral muscles* are the rotator cuff and teres major muscles. Structural conditions such as scoliosis and kyphosis must also be accounted for because of their effect on the scapular position on the chest wall.

Axioscapular Muscles

The axioscapular muscles have their origin on the axial skeleton (skull, vertebrae, pelvis, sternum, and ribs) with their insertion on the scapula. These muscles are responsible for positioning and stabilizing the scapula to permit upper limb movements such as reaching, grasping, and lifting. The resting position of the scapula has received considerable attention.[3,4,6-9] The medial scapular border should be approximately 3 inches from the spine and essentially parallel to the spinous processes.[4,6,9] The position of the clavicle can provide guidance related to the amount of elevation or depression of the scapula. The acromioclavicular joint should be slightly higher than the sternoclavicular joint.[4] Sahrmann[4] believes that most patients with shoulder pain develop the condition as a result of movement impairment of the scapula that disrupts the relationship between the humeral head and the glenoid fossa. Resting scapular position may also cause lengthening or shortening of axioscapular muscles that also can affect shoulder function.

Trapezius

Concentric contraction of the upper trapezius muscle with the spine fixed creates elevation of the scapula through its attachment to the distal clavicle and acromion. If the scapula is fixed or the ipsilateral upper extremity load is heavy, the trapezius muscle can create ipsilateral rotation and side bending of the cervical spine. The middle fibers of the trapezius muscle adduct the scapula with concentric contraction or assist the rhomboid muscles with control of scapular abduction during eccentric contraction. The lower fibers of the trapezius muscle depress and adduct the scapula with concentric contraction. When combined with concentric contraction of the upper trapezius and serratus anterior muscles, a force couple is produced, causing scapular upward rotation.[10]

If an individual performs repetitive, unilateral carrying of heavy loads or other habitual activities with the upper trapezius muscles in a lengthened position, the muscle can lengthen, resulting in scapular downward rotation at rest.[4] The patient's appearance is that of a long, sloping shoulder (Fig. 15-1). This position of downward rotation of the scapula may contribute to shoulder dysfunction in part because of a change in the length-tension curve for the upper trapezius and serratus anterior muscles that causes weakness of these muscles in the shortened position. This alteration may also change the resting position of the glenohumeral joint. Because of the downward rotation position of the scapula at rest, the scapula must upwardly rotate an increased amount to achieve shoulder elevation. Inadequate scapular upward rotation may lead to impingement problems of the shoulder.[4]

Excessive scapular abduction is also a common postural fault when subjects have a forward head and rounded shoulder posture. This posture may lead to lengthening of the trapezius and rhomboids with shortening of the serratus anterior. This lengthened state may cause weakness in these muscles when they are placed in a shortened position.[6]

Levator Scapulae

Concentric contraction of the levator scapulae muscle with the spine fixed causes elevation, adduction, and downward rotation of the scapulae.[4] According to Sahrmann,[4] this muscle is a synergist with the upper trapezius for scapular elevation and adduction, but an antagonist for scapular rotation. Shortness of this muscle may elevate the medial portion of the scapula, but not the acromial end, thus producing downward rotation of the scapula. Differentiating between shortness of the levator scapulae and rhomboid muscles (scapula adducted and downwardly rotated) versus upper trapezius muscle lengthening (scapula abducted and downwardly rotated) is believed to be extremely important in the design of a corrective therapeutic intervention program.[4]

Rhomboid Major and Minor

The rhomboid muscles work with the middle trapezius muscle during concentric contraction to retract the scapula and with the levator scapulae and pectoralis minor muscles to create downward scapular rotation. Shortening or tightness of the rhomboid muscles can position the scapula closer to the spinous processes (Fig. 15-2) and may result in downward rotation of the scapula. Figure 15-3 demonstrates restricted scapular upward rotation as a result of rhomboid muscle shortness. Normally, the inferior angle of the scapula should reach the midaxillary line during full shoulder flexion.[4]

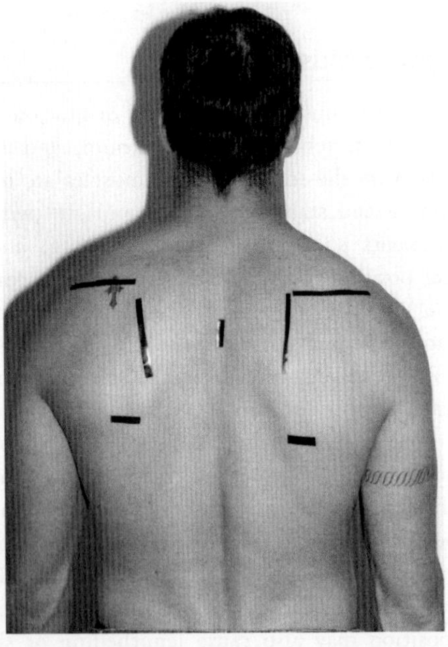

Figure 15-1 Subject in relaxed stance demonstrating an abducted scapula with a lengthened upper trapezius muscle.

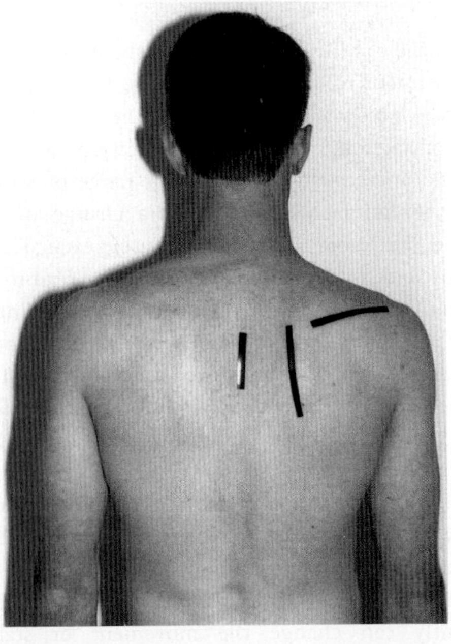

Figure 15-2 Subject in relaxed stance demonstrating an abducted scapular position.

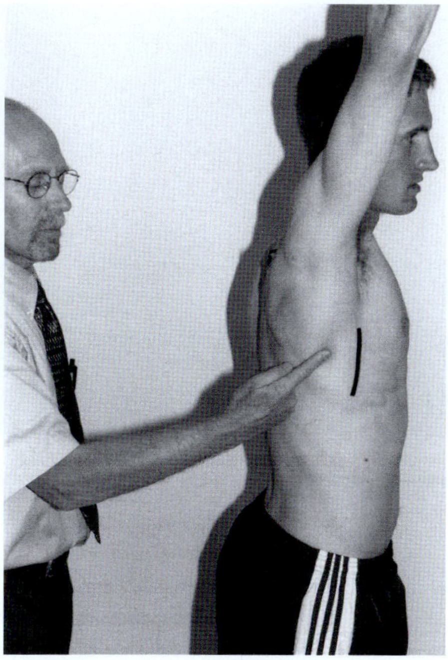

Figure 15-3 Subject with restricted upward rotation of the scapula.

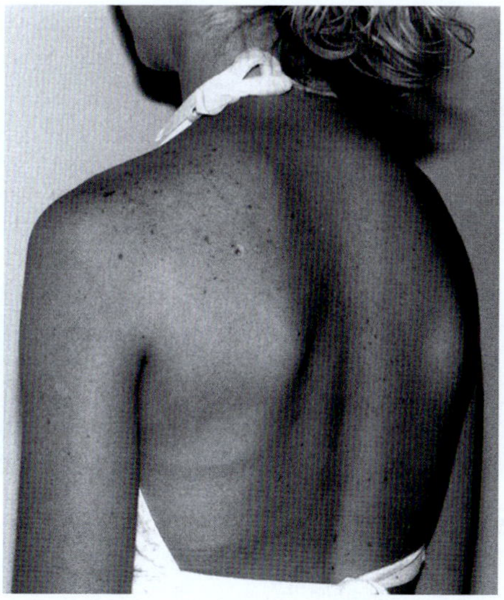

Figure 15-4 Subject in relaxed stance demonstrating prominence of the inferior angle of the scapula because of a shortening of the pectoralis minor muscle.

Serratus Anterior

Concentric contraction of the serratus anterior muscle causes scapular abduction and protraction and upward rotation of the scapula. When the scapula is habitually abducted, this muscle may undergo shortening together with the pectoralis minor muscle (see Fig. 15-1). Conversely, when the rhomboid and levator scapulae muscles are short, the serratus anterior muscle is placed in an elongated position together with the pectoralis minor muscle. If the serratus anterior is elongated, a change in the length-tension curve may result in weakness of this muscle in its shortened position during flexion or abduction of the shoulder.

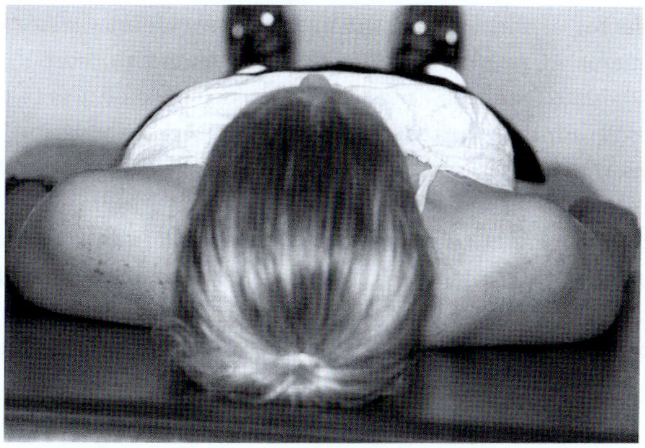

Figure 15-5 Supine resting position that demonstrates shortening of the pectoralis minor muscles. The posterior angle of the acromion is more than 1 inch off the table.

Pectoralis Minor

The pectoralis minor muscle can assist the serratus anterior muscle in protracting the scapula during a concentric contraction. In addition, it creates scapular downward rotation when concentric contraction is combined with the levator scapulae and rhomboid muscles.[11] Tightness of this muscle can create a forward "tipping" of the scapula, which may be noted as a prominence of the inferior angle of the scapula (Fig. 15-4).

Shortening of the pectoralis minor muscle may be combined with shortening of the serratus anterior muscle in an individual with an abducted scapular position at rest. Shortening of the pectoralis minor muscle may impede the upward rotation of the scapula during elevation of the arm and may limit shoulder flexion range of motion. When the patient with a short pectoralis minor is in the supine position, it is apparent that the acromion process is elevated off the table to a greater degree than normal (Fig. 15-5). Sahrmann recommended that the lateral angle of the spine of the scapula should be no more than 1 inch off the table.[4] However, this distance changes significantly in subjects of differing body build. Pressure over the anterior shoulder in the area of the coracoid process stretches this muscle. Muraki et al[12] found that maximum stretch is placed on the pectoralis minor when the shoulder is first flexed to 30°. Then an upward force is placed through the shaft of the humerus to elevate and retract the scapula. In Figure 15-6, the shoulder is placed in approximately 30° of flexion, and then the scapula is fully retracted as stretch is applied by posteriorly tilting the scapula. The patient with tightness in this muscle should describe a "pull" in the anterior chest in line with the muscle fibers when stretched.

Axiohumeral Muscles

The axiohumeral muscles originate on the axial skeleton and have their insertion on the humerus. These muscles have a direct effect on the glenohumeral joint and an indirect effect on the scapular position because of their proximal attachments on the humerus.

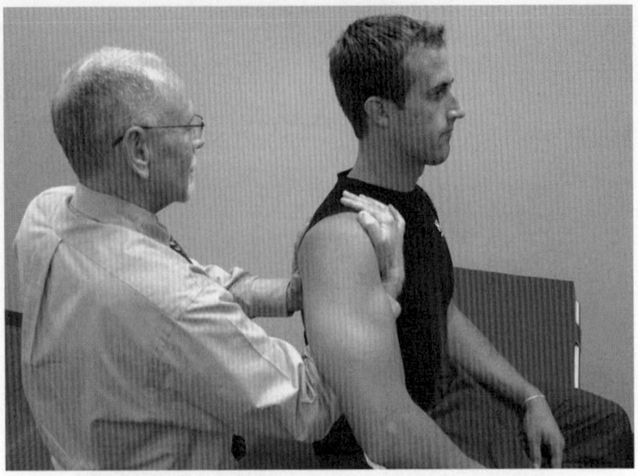

Figure 15-6 Technique for testing the length of and stretching the pectoralis muscle: shoulder flexion to 30° and then retraction and posterior tilting of the scapula.

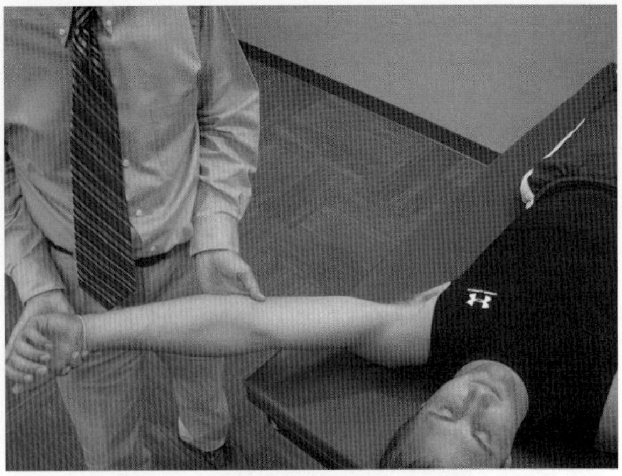

Figure 15-8 Assessment of pectoralis major (sternocostal portion) muscle length.

Pectoralis Major

The pectoralis major muscle is a powerful medial rotator and adductor of the arm. Shortness of this muscle may place the humerus in an internally rotated posture and the scapula in an abducted position. (Fig. 15-7) In addition, shortness of this muscle limits the extent of shoulder horizontal abduction. To assess the length of the sternocostal head of this muscle, the subject should be lying supine with the arm at 155° of abduction and in lateral rotation (Fig. 15-8).[4] In this position, the subject's arm should be able to make contact with the table surface. The subject in Figure 15-8 demonstrates shortness of the sternocostal fibers of the pectoralis major muscle because the upper arm is unable to make contact with the table. Careful observation of the anterior chest wall may also detect elevation of the ipsilateral side of the chest as the upper limb reaches its end range of elevation. This tightness is commonly found in subjects who demonstrate an abducted (protracted) scapula and a medially rotated humerus (see Fig. 15-7).

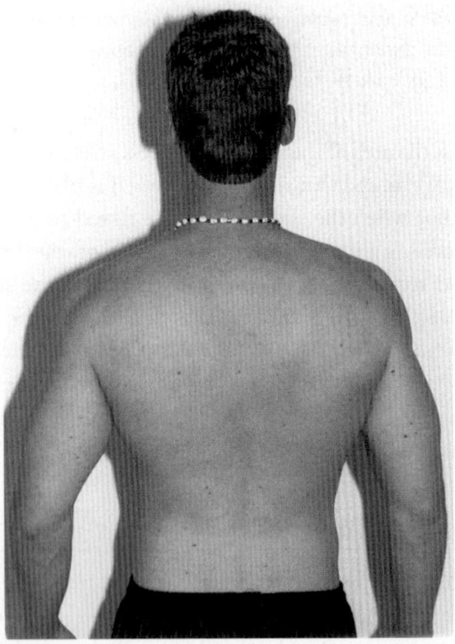

Figure 15-7 Subject in a relaxed stance demonstrating an abducted scapula with shoulder internal rotation.

Latissimus Dorsi

The latissimus dorsi muscle is capable of performing adduction, medial rotation, and extension of the humerus. To assess the length of this muscle, the subject is positioned supine with the hips and knees flexed to flatten the lumbar spine. The subject then raises the arm into shoulder flexion and maintains lateral rotation of the humerus while the therapist observes restricted passive elevation and possible compensatory movement in the lower spine[4] (Fig. 15-9). In a subject with shortening of the latissimus dorsi muscle, shoulder flexion is limited, the rib cage will moves anteriorly, and the lumbar spine may elevate off the table as the muscle becomes taut. This muscle is capable of indirectly influencing scapular position because of its attachment to the humerus.

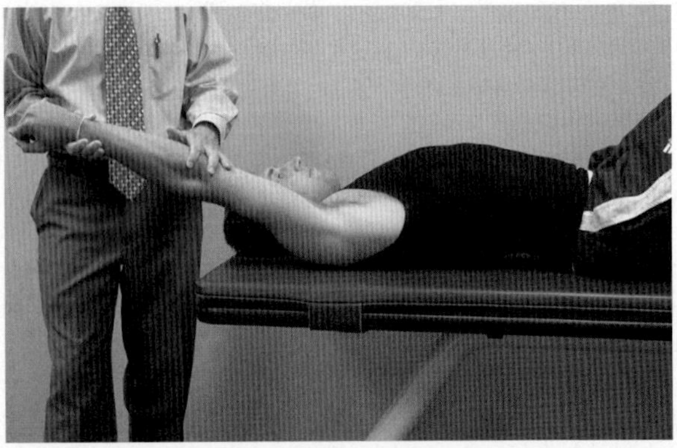

Figure 15-9 Assessment of latissimus dorsi muscle length.

Scapulohumeral Muscles

The scapulohumeral muscles have their origin on the scapula and insertion on the humerus. They consist of the supraspinatus, infraspinatus, teres minor, subscapularis, and teres major muscles. The supraspinatus, infraspinatus, teres minor, and subscapularis comprise the rotator cuff muscles of the shoulder. The rotator cuff muscles center the humeral head in the glenoid fossa and provide the "fine tuning" or "steering" necessary for performing various upper limb tasks.

Subscapularis

When contracting concentrically, the subscapularis muscle is a medial rotator of the humerus. This muscle also functions to center the humeral head in the glenoid fossa and acts as a humeral head depressor with the other rotator cuff muscles during overhead activities. To assess the length of the subscapularis muscle, the subject is positioned supine with the elbow held against the trunk while the humerus is rotated into lateral rotation (Fig. 15-10). Performing this motion bilaterally permits the examiner to compare the two extremities quickly. In addition, tightness of the subscapularis muscle prevents dissociation of the humerus from the scapula during the final 40° of elevation. The lack of dissociation of the humerus from the scapula causes abduction of the scapula or protrusion of the inferior angle beyond the lateral wall of the trunk.

Infraspinatus and Teres Minor

Concentric contraction of the infraspinatus and teres minor muscles produces lateral rotation of the humerus. Cocontraction of the external rotators and subscapularis muscle results in depression and centering of the humeral head in the glenoid fossa during overhead activities. Shortness of the infraspinatus and teres minor muscles results in a decrease in medial rotation of the humerus. Muscle length assessment for these muscles can be performed with a single motion.

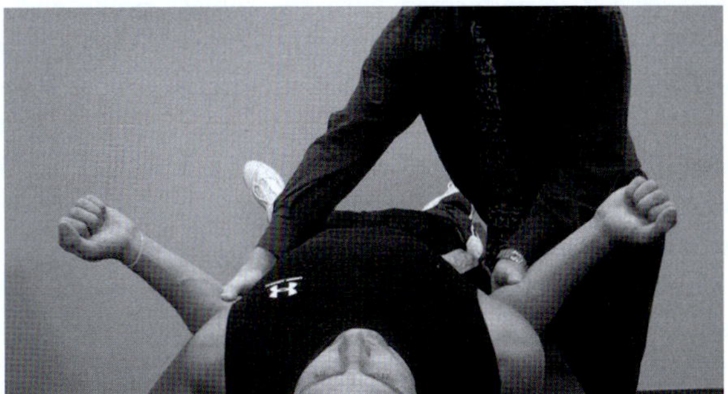

Figure 15-10 Assessment of subscapularis muscle length.

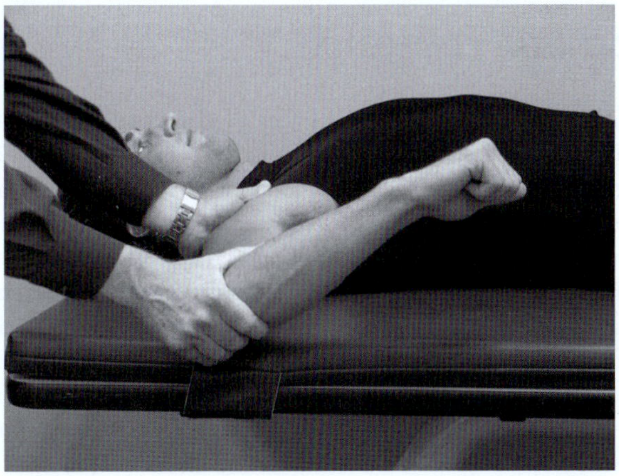

Figure 15-11 Assessment of the posterior joint capsule and infraspinatus and teres minor muscle length.

The subject is positioned supine with the humerus abducted 90° and the elbow positioned at 90° of flexion (Fig. 15-11). The examiner stabilizes the scapula by pushing posteriorly on the head of the humerus with one hand while the other hand rotates the subject's arm into medial rotation. When the examiner feels the scapula elevate off the table or feels tissue tension increase during medial rotation, end range has been reached. Figure 15-11 shows a subject with shortness of the infraspinatus and teres minor muscles assessed using this method. Normal medial rotation is approximately 70° when the arm is abducted to 90°.[4] Restriction in medial rotation can also be caused by capsular tightness of the glenohumeral joint.

Teres Major

Concentric contraction of the teres major can produce medial rotation, adduction, or extension of the shoulder. To assess the length of the teres major muscle, the subject is positioned supine so the table can assist with stabilization of the scapula. The subject performs shoulder flexion, as is also performed with the latissimus dorsi muscle length test (see Fig. 15-9). The examiner observes the amount of shoulder flexion achieved and the position of the inferior angle of the scapula. If the inferior angle of the scapula protrudes more than half an inch beyond the lateral wall of the trunk (excessive scapular abduction), a short teres major muscle is suspected.[4] To verify, the examiner has the subject return his or her arm to the starting position and repeat the shoulder flexion motion while the examiner stabilizes the inferior angle of the scapula at the lateral chest wall to prevent excessive scapular abduction. If the subject has less shoulder flexion compared with the previous attempt, the teres major muscle is further implicated. To confirm the shortening of the teres major muscle more definitively, the examiner instructs the subject to rotate the shoulder medially and maintain the position of shoulder flexion with the scapula stabilized. If the subject is able to gain additional shoulder flexion, the teres major is most likely shortened.[4]

GENERAL COMMENTS

During the observation component of the examination for a patient with a shoulder problem, it is helpful to determine the degree of medial or lateral rotation of the humerus while the patient is in an upright, relaxed, standing position. To assess the direction of shoulder rotation, the therapist stands behind the subject and observes the position of the olecranon process of the elbow.[4] In a subject with scapular abduction (protraction) coupled with medial rotation of the shoulder, the olecranon process appears more lateral in position, as shown in Figure 15-7. The therapist should then correct the scapular position and reassess the position of the olecranon process.[4]

Although the aforementioned techniques are valuable for identifying muscles having a change in length, the clinician should be aware that joint capsular tissue can also be shortened concurrently with muscles. The clinician is advised to assess capsular mobility, to ensure optimal intervention planning that addresses both muscle and capsular length changes.

MANUAL MUSCLE TESTING

Manual muscle testing is an integral part of the physical examination of the shoulder and provides information that is useful in the management of shoulder ailments. Several textbooks have been published on manual muscle testing techniques.[6,13-16] To become proficient at manual muscle testing, a clinician must practice and must be meticulous with patient positioning and stabilization.

Manual muscle testing positions have been generally based on anatomic knowledge of muscle origins and insertions, and expected muscle action. Analysis by electromyography (EMG) has been used in studies to quantify the muscle activity during manual muscle testing and exercises.[17-24] Ideally, a muscle test would create maximum amplitude on EMG for the muscle being tested, with minimal activity in the synergistic muscles. When available, this discussion includes published data from EMG that are pertinent to manual muscle testing.

Investigators have demonstrated that the intratester and intertester reliability of manual muscle testing is high for identifying a grade of strength when rated on a numeric scale.[25-27] However, manual muscle testing remains problematic because muscle strength can vary widely within muscle grades.[28,29] Many times, considerable weakness must be present before it can be detected. In large muscle groups, patients with up to a 50% loss of absolute force when compared with the normal extremity, as measured by dynamometry, are often rated as normal using manual muscle testing.[28,30,31] Agre and Rodriquez[32] found that muscles producing forces as low as 8% compared with the opposite normal limb were graded as good (4/5) during a manual muscle test. Other investigators found that dynamometer measurements detected increases in strength over time, with no change in manual muscle test scores.[33,34] Because manual muscle testing does not provide precise objective measurements of strength deficits, the use of a hand-held dynamometer during manual muscle testing of the shoulder is recommended.

Dynamometry data can provide objective measurements of strength (force) when comparing extremities or as a measure of progress in strengthening during rehabilitation. Most studies found high levels of intratester reliability in hand-held dynamometer testing.[34-38] An examiner inexperienced with hand-held dynamometer use may want to perform muscle testing with and without the dynamometer. When the dynamometer is interposed between the examiner and the subject, it may reduce the sensitivity of the examiner.

Another consideration is that the isometric hold during manual muscle testing should be held for at least 4 seconds to allow for maximum tension development.[39] A longer hold may reveal weakness not detectable with a 1- to 2-second hold.

Testing a muscle in both a shortened position and a lengthened position may be important because the length of the muscle at the time of the examination can affect the force produced by the muscle. A muscle held in a chronically lengthened position as the result of postural habits or other reasons may test weak in a shortened position, but it may be strong in a more lengthened position.[4] This result reflects a change in the normal length-tension curve. Other muscles may be weak at any point in the range of motion because of disuse atrophy. Whether the muscle is tested in a shortened position or a lengthened position, the clinician is provided with valuable information when developing a corrective strengthening program.

STRENGTH TESTING

Supraspinatus

Jobe and Moynes[40] recommended that the supraspinatus muscle be tested with the shoulder internally rotated and abducted to 90° in the plane of the scapula ("empty can" or Jobe position). Worrell et al[41] compared the Jobe position with the position recommended by Blackburn et al.[42] The *Blackburn test* is performed with the subject prone and the shoulder abducted 100° and laterally rotated with the thumb up. These investigators found that significantly more activity on EMG was produced when the supraspinatus muscle was tested in the Blackburn position. Similar studies did not find a significant difference in activity on EMG in the supraspinatus muscle when the two positions were compared.[24,43]

Other EMG studies compared muscle tests with the shoulder at 90° of abduction in the plane of the scapula with either external rotation (Fig. 15-12) or internal rotation.[17,43,44] No study found a significant difference in the muscle activity of the supraspinatus muscle when the two positions were compared. However, these researchers recommended using the test with lateral rotation (thumb-up or "full can" position) because this is a position in which less subacromial impingement, and therefore less pain, is expected.

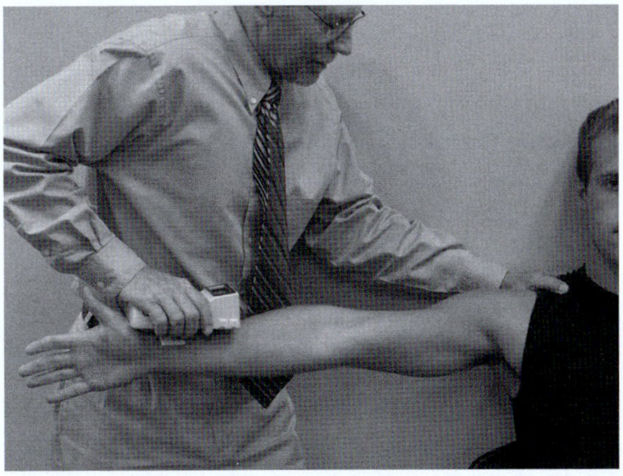

Figure 15-12 Manual muscle test for the supraspinatus in the "full can" position.

Itoi et al[45] verified that less pain is produced in the full can position compared with the empty can (thumb-down) position when supraspinatus tendon tears are tested in patients. Therefore, testing the supraspinatus muscle in the full can position is recommended.

Determining specific supraspinatus muscle weakness may not be possible because the deltoid muscle is always active with the supraspinatus muscle. Weakness detected with this muscle test often results from pain production that inhibits muscle contraction. Weakness in the absence of pain necessitates a differential diagnosis between a neurologic source and muscle or tendon rupture.

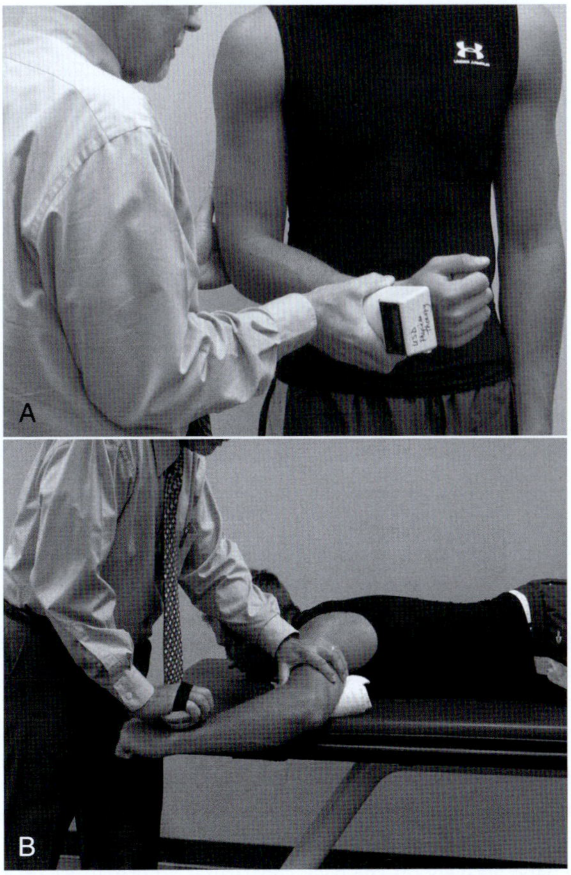

Figure 15-13 Manual muscle test for the infraspinatus and teres minor. **A,** Test with shoulder in 0° of abduction and medially rotated approximately 45°. **B,** Test with shoulder at the end range of shoulder lateral rotation with 90° of abduction.

Infraspinatus and Teres Minor

Most EMG studies demonstrated no significant difference in the muscle activity of the infraspinatus when shoulder lateral rotation was performed concentrically during exercises or isometrically during muscle tests at 0°, 45°, or 90° of shoulder abduction.[17,21,23,44] However, Reinold et al[46] found a significant increase in infraspinatus activity when subjects exercise in the side-lying position with 0° of shoulder abduction as compared with the 90° abducted position. Investigators found that the infraspinatus muscle activity is best isolated from the supraspinatus and posterior deltoid muscles with the shoulder in 0° of abduction and medially rotated approximately 45° (Fig. 15-13A).[17] The lateral rotator muscles should be tested in this position and at the end range of shoulder lateral rotation with 90° of abduction (see Fig. 15-13B). In the second position, the glenohumeral joint is less stable and requires more activity from posterior deltoid and other rotator cuff muscles.[17]

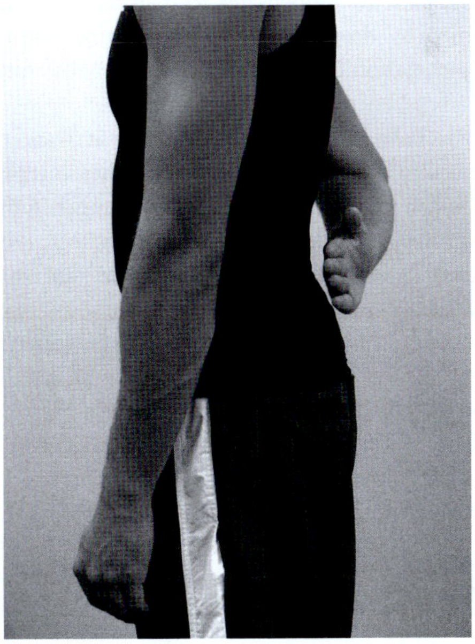

Figure 15-14 Muscle test for the subscapularis using the Gerber lift-off test.

Subscapularis

Greis et al[19] and Kelly et al[17] found that the activity on EMG of the subscapularis muscle is maximal and best isolated from the other shoulder internal rotators by the *Gerber lift-off test* (Fig. 15-14).[47] This muscle test is performed by raising the

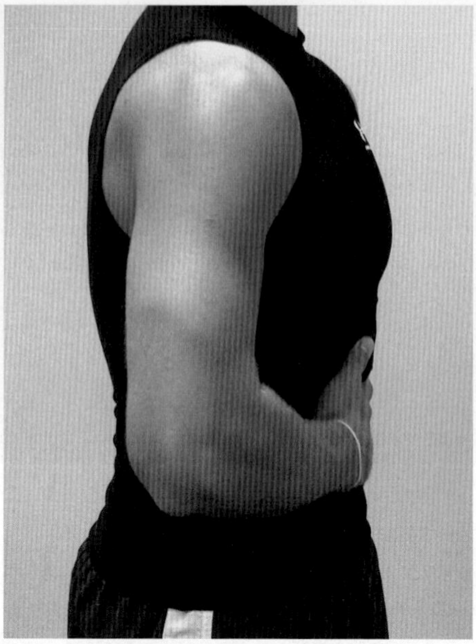

Figure 15-15 Muscle test for the subscapularis using the belly-press test.

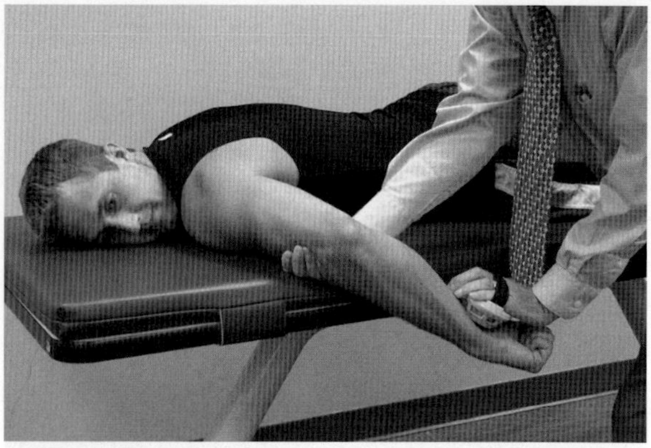

Figure 15-16 Manual muscle test for the shoulder internal rotator muscles with the arm in abduction.

dorsum of the hand off the midlumbar area by maintaining or increasing internal rotation of the humerus and increasing extension of the shoulder. The ability to lift the dorsum of the hand actively off the back constitutes a normal lift-off test result. This test can be performed only if the patient has adequate internal range of motion and the position is not painful.

An alternative to the lift-off test is the *belly-press test*.[48,49] This test is performed by pressing the palm into the abdomen by internally rotating the shoulder while keeping the elbow in the frontal plane (Fig. 15-15). A positive sign for weakness is when the patient compensates to maintain pressure against the abdomen by dropping the elbow behind the trunk and extending the shoulder, rather than internally rotating the shoulder.

Both the belly-press and lift-off tests activate the upper and lower subscapularis more than all other internal rotator muscles.[48] The belly-press activates the upper subscapularis muscle significantly more than the lift-off test, whereas the lift-off test produces greater activity in the lower subscapularis.

The shoulder internal rotators should be tested with the shoulder at 90° of abduction for patients unable to assume the Gerber lift-off test position (Fig. 15-16). With this test, a high level of subscapularis muscle activity still occurs, coupled with increased activity in the pectoralis major and latissimus dorsi muscles, compared with the lift-off test.[17]

Deltoid

Kendall et al[6] described testing for the anterior and posterior deltoid with the patient in the sitting position. The anterior deltoid muscle is tested with the shoulder abducted in the plane of the scapula to 90° and with the humerus in slight lateral rotation. The posterior deltoid muscle is tested with the shoulder in abduction to 90° with slight horizontal abduction and medial rotation. By analysis on EMG, Brandell and Wilkinson[18] found Kendall's tests for the anterior and middle deltoid muscles to be quite selective. Reinold et al[43] demonstrated significantly greater middle deltoid activity in the empty can position and greater posterior deltoid activity in the prone full can position described by Blackburn et al.[42]

Horizontal abduction of the shoulder with external rotation also elicits high levels of muscle activity in both the middle and posterior deltoid muscles.[18] Shoulder hypertension (hyperextension, not hypertension) isolates the posterior deltoid from the anterior and middle deltoid muscles, but not from the latissimus dorsi muscle.[18] These positions may also be considered for testing deltoid strength.

Pectoralis Major

Muscle tests for the sternocostal and clavicular parts of the pectoralis major muscle are pictured in Figure 15-17.[6] For the sternocostal part, the arm is brought toward the opposite hip, and for the clavicular part, the arm is taken toward the nose as resistance is isometrically applied.

Latissimus Dorsi, Teres Major, and Posterior Deltoid

The latissimus dorsi, teres major, and posterior deltoid muscles can be tested as a unit using a *generic shoulder extension test* (Fig. 15-18).[13] The shoulder is extended with full internal rotation.

Upper Trapezius

The upper trapezius muscle can be tested with the *shoulder shrug muscle test* (Fig. 15-19A).[6] Ekstrom et al[50] found the greatest activity in the upper trapezius with a slight modification of this test. These investigators added abduction

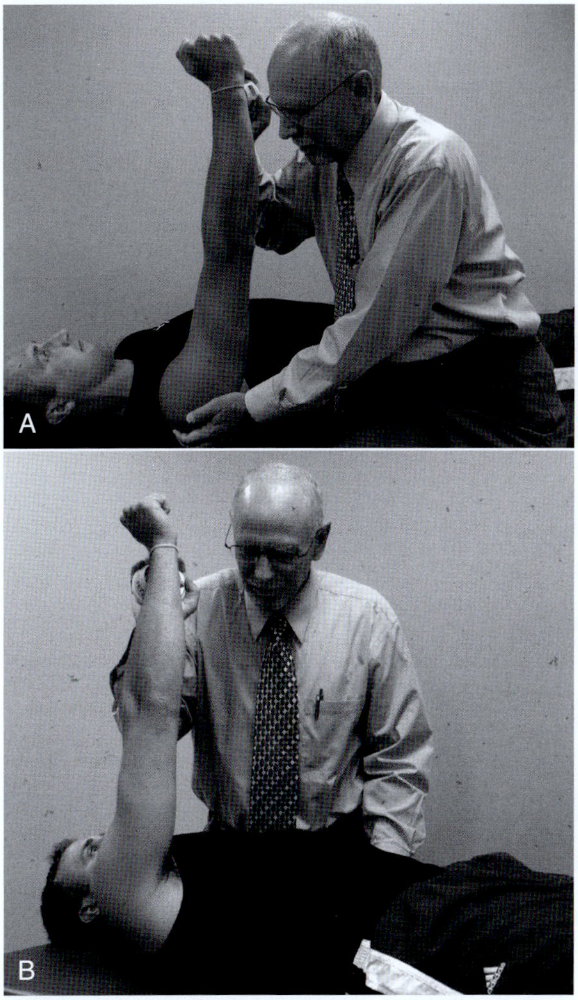

Figure 15-17 A, Muscle test for the pectoralis major. **A,** Test for the sternocostal part of the muscle. **B,** Test for the clavicular part of the muscle.

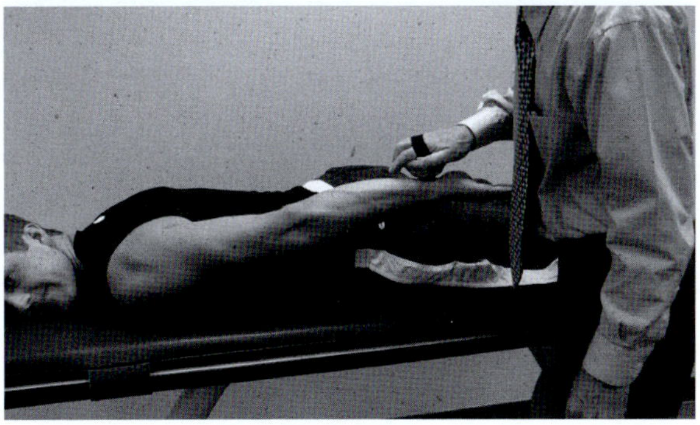

Figure 15-18 Muscle test for the latissimus dorsi, teres major, and posterior deltoid.

of the shoulder to 90° and then applied resistance simultaneously above the elbow and to the head. However, this test may not be very discriminatory for the upper trapezius muscle because a high level of activity in the levator scapulae muscle also occurs during scapular elevation.[51]

The upper trapezius muscle can also be tested along with the middle trapezius and lower trapezius muscles by using a horizontal abduction muscle test (see Fig. 15-19B) or a test with the arm raised above the head in line with the lower trapezius muscle fibers (see Fig. 15-19C).[18] Both tests create high levels of activity on EMG in all parts of the trapezius muscle.[18]

Middle Trapezius

The middle trapezius muscle can be tested with horizontal abduction with the shoulder in lateral rotation (see Fig. 15-19B).[6,50] Analysis on EMG demonstrated that this test produces not only maximum activity in the middle trapezius muscle, but also high levels of activity in the upper and lower trapezius muscles.[18] Therefore, this test allows all parts of the trapezius muscle to be tested as a unit.

Lower Trapezius

Maximum activation of the lower trapezius muscle is achieved through a muscle test with the arm raised overhead in line with the lower trapezius muscle fibers (see Fig. 15-19C).[17,50] This test also produces high levels of activity on EMG in the upper and middle trapezius muscles. Therefore, it is another method that can be used for testing all parts of the trapezius muscle.[18]

Serratus Anterior

Kendall et al[6] recommended the muscle test as shown in Figure 15-20 for testing the serratus anterior muscle. Ekstrom et al[50] demonstrated significantly more activity on EMG in the serratus anterior muscle when it was tested in this position as compared with a supine-scapular protraction test. In this test, the shoulder is flexed or abducted in the plane of the scapula to 125°. The scapula is upwardly rotated as a result of this position, and the examiner tries to derotate the scapula by applying simultaneous pressure downward on the arm and at the inferior angle of the scapula.

Rhomboid Major and Minor

The recommended test for the rhomboid major and minor muscles is shown in Figure 15-21.[6] No evidence on EMG exists to verify whether this is the optimal test. In this test, the examiner tries to derotate the scapula from a downwardly rotated position.

MUSCLE STRENGTHENING

In general terms, *muscle strength* can be defined as the ability of the skeletal muscle to develop force to provide stability and mobility for the musculoskeletal system.[1] In more specific terms, muscular strength is the greatest measurable force that can be exerted by a muscle or muscle group to overcome resistance during a single, maximal effort.[52,53]

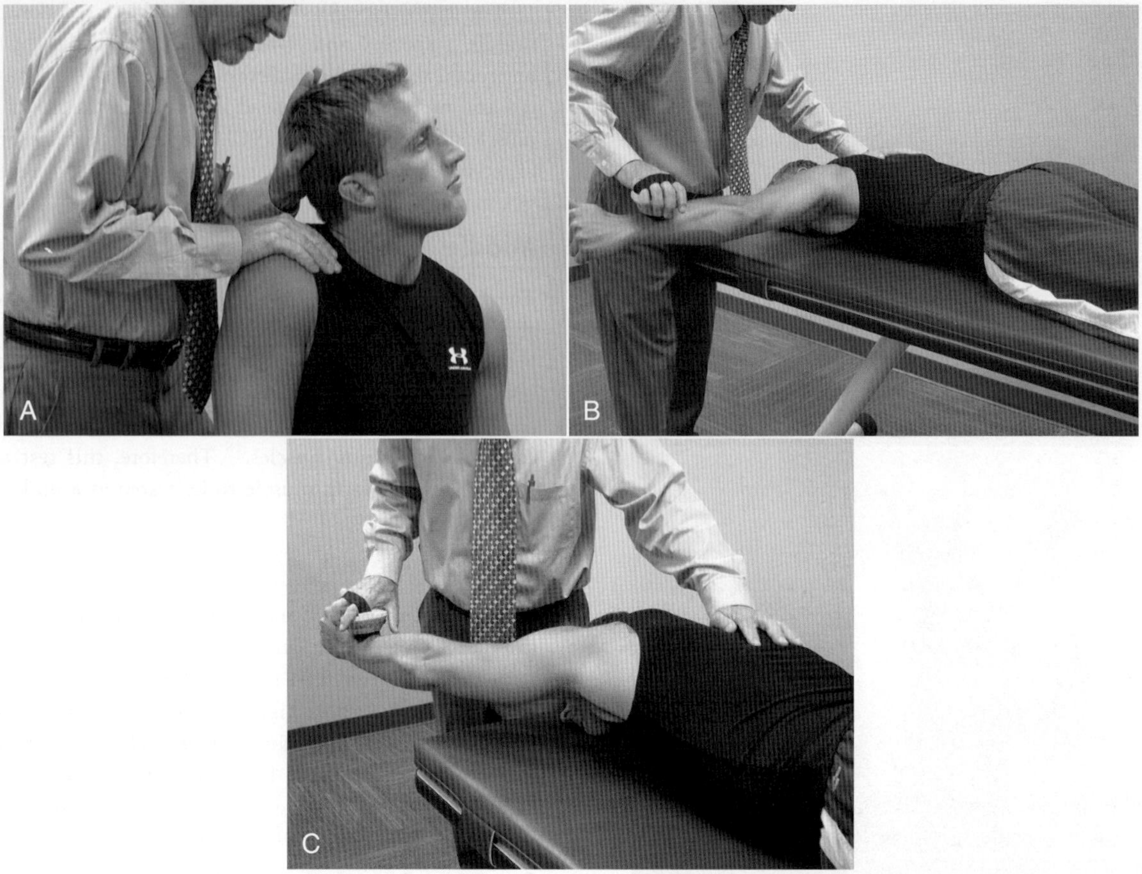

Figure 15-19 Muscle testing for the trapezius. **A,** Upper trapezius. **B,** Middle trapezius. **C,** Lower trapezius.

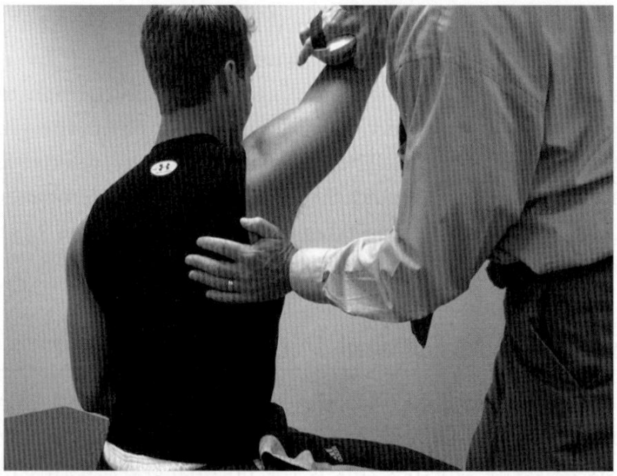

Figure 15-20 Muscle test for the serratus anterior.

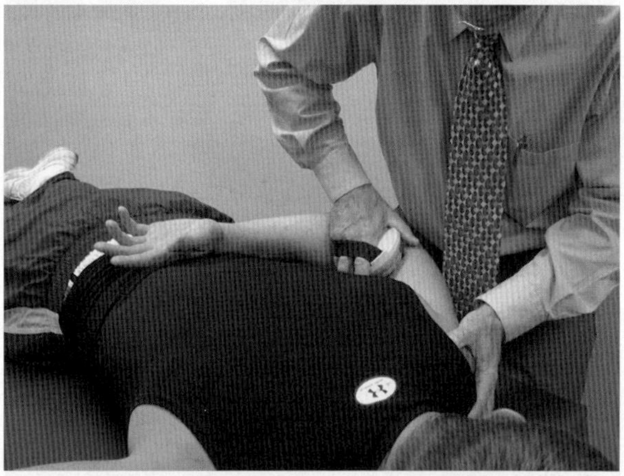

Figure 15-21 Muscle test for the rhomboids.

Strengthening activities are common components of comprehensive intervention programs for patients with shoulder abnormalities.[40,54-58] For a muscle to gain strength, the resistance applied must exceed the metabolic capacity of the muscle.[59] A recommended strengthening program is performed with 1 to 3 sets of heavy resistance exercise in the range of 6 to 12 repetition maximum (RM).[60-62]

Typically, clinicians develop intervention plans for individuals who require a combination of strength and endurance to perform activities of daily living or job-related functions. *Muscular endurance* refers to the ability of a muscle to perform a repetitive activity (or activities) for a prolonged period against a load or resistance.[63] An example of an endurance activity is when an assembly line worker repetitively performs an activity over a long period or is required to hold a static position for an extended period. In some circumstances, a worker may perform the same repetitive motions 150 to 200 times or more per day. When designing a rehabilitation program for an individual working under these conditions, endurance activities (high repetition, low resistance) for the upper limb, and possibly the trunk musculature, may be a high priority. In this example, as many as 3 to 5 sets of 40 to 50 or more repetitions may be used, employing a low level of resistance.

In the next section, various strengthening exercises for the shoulder are described, and the evidence on EMG for muscle action that occurs with each exercise is discussed.

Shoulder Girdle and Glenohumeral Joint Strengthening Exercises

A rehabilitation program for the shoulder should include not only exercises for muscles controlling the glenohumeral joint, but also exercises for strengthening the scapular muscles. Scapular control is important as a foundation on which the glenohumeral joint can function in a normal manner.[4]

Normal scapulohumeral rhythm must be maintained during elevation of the upper extremity. In other words, during full elevation of the shoulder through approximately 180°, the scapula should upwardly rotate approximately 60° while the humerus flexes or abducts approximately 120°. This movement requires good coordinated function of the rotator cuff and deltoid muscles at the glenohumeral joint and scapular control by the serratus anterior and trapezius muscles. The following information provides evidence for exercises that may be used for strengthening the various muscles of the shoulder girdle and glenohumeral joint. Of special interest to many clinicians is how best to activate the muscles of the rotator cuff. The shoulder complex does not work in isolation; trunk position and strength may also influence any shoulder exercise program.

Military Press

Several investigators performed EMG studies to evaluate the muscle activation levels during the *military press exercise* (Fig. 15-22).[20,64-66] The anterior and middle deltoid, supraspinatus, upper trapezius, and serratus anterior muscles have been shown to be highly activated with EMG signal amplitudes of 62% maximal voluntary isometric contraction (MVIC) or greater.[20,64,65] Townsend et al[65] demonstrated high levels of supraspinatus muscle activity of 80% MVIC even during exercise of moderate intensity.

Horizontal Bench Press, Incline Press, and Decline Press

Barnett et al[64] compared pectoralis major, anterior deltoid, and triceps brachii muscle activity during all three exercises. They found maximum activity in the sternocostal head of the pectoralis major during the horizontal bench press and maximum activity in the clavicular head of the pectoralis major during an *incline press* (Fig. 15-23), especially with a narrower hand grip. Hand spacing did not affect the muscle activity of the sternocostal head of the pectoralis major.

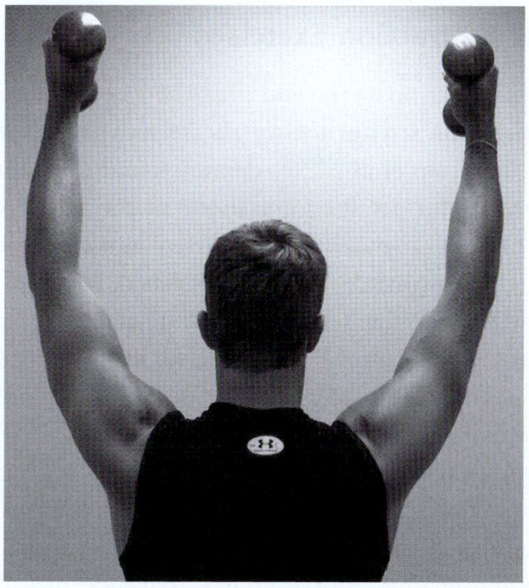

Figure 15-22 Military press exercise.

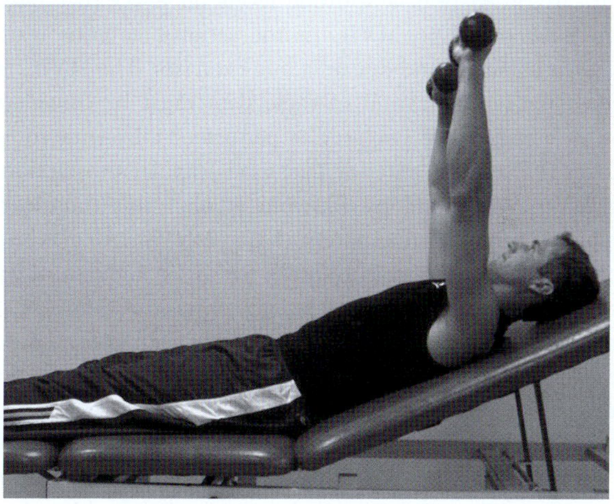

Figure 15-23 Incline press exercise.

Glass and Armstrong[67] compared just the incline (30°) and decline (−15°) bench press positions and found greater activity in the sternocostal part of the pectoralis major during the decline position, but no significant difference in the clavicular head during the two exercises.

The anterior deltoid activity increased during the incline press. Welsch et al[68] recorded peak levels of muscle activity in the pectoralis major and anterior deltoid of 56% MVIC during a horizontal barbell bench press exercise performed at 6 RM. The triceps brachii muscle activity was greatest during the horizontal bench press. Narrow hand spacing increased triceps brachii activity as compared with a wider hand grip.[64]

Because the difference in muscle activity among the decline, incline, and horizontal bench press is not great, any position can be used during rehabilitation. Progressing from a horizontal bench press to increasing levels of an incline press is a good method of gradually progressing to overhead activities.

Scapular Protraction Exercises

Shoulder protraction at the end phase of a bench press exercise is often used for strengthening the serratus anterior muscle. However, Ekstrom et al[50,69,70] demonstrated that this exercise is not optimal for producing activity in the serratus anterior muscle. During a maximally resisted muscle test in this position, the amplitude on EMG reached levels of only 54 ± 27% MVIC in the serratus anterior, and an exercise performed at 5 RM intensity produced amplitude levels on EMG of 62 ± 19% MVIC. The serratus anterior muscle reaches maximum amplitude levels on EMG only when upward rotation of the scapula is resisted.

Other scapular protraction exercises for serratus anterior strengthening, such as the forward punch, serratus anterior punch, and dynamic hug exercises, have been studied.[71,72] Hintermeister et al[71] found that the forward punch exercise performed with moderate resistance produced amplitudes on EMG of 49% MVIC in the serratus anterior muscle. Decker et al[72] recorded peak amplitude levels on EMG that ranged from 94% to 109% MVIC in the serratus anterior during the serratus punch and dynamic hug exercises. The MVIC performed for normalization of these data must be considered. The authors of these two studies performed a baseline muscle test for the serratus anterior that used scapular protraction as the MVIC. As found by Ekstrom et al,[50] this muscle test produced only approximately 54% MVIC. A maximum muscle test for the serratus anterior must include an upward rotation component of the scapula, such as in the muscle test proposed by Kendall et al.[6] Taking this into consideration, these exercises are not optimal for strengthening the serratus anterior, but they may be used as low-level exercises early in a rehabilitation program.

The *push-up plus exercise* performed with full scapular protraction (Fig. 15-24) was shown to produce high levels of muscle activity in the serratus anterior muscle.[69,73] Ekstrom et al[69] found that this exercise produced amplitude on EMG of 78 ± 24% MVIC. Lear and Gross[73] found that increased resistance could be added to the serratus anterior during this exercise when the feet were elevated onto a stool or chair. The reason that this exercise may produce greater muscle activity in the serratus anterior than straight protraction exercises is that the thoracic spine goes into kyphosis (ribs pulled posteriorly), which produces upward rotation of the scapula in relationship to the rib cage.

Decker et al[72] recorded nearly maximum muscle activity in the upper subscapularis, supraspinatus, and infraspinatus during the push-up plus exercise. These investigators also demonstrated peak amplitudes in the subscapularis muscle of 49.8% MVIC during the forward punch exercise and 94.1% MVIC during the dynamic hug exercise. Therefore, these exercises may be of value in strengthening and retraining the rotator cuff.

Abduction in the Scapular Plane and Other Humeral Elevation Exercises

The scapular plane is generally approximately 30° to 45° anterior from the frontal plane in individuals and is considered the best functional position of the humerus when abduction exercises are performed. The most active muscles are the glenohumeral joint elevators and the scapular upward rotators. The primary glenohumeral joint elevators are considered to be the deltoid and supraspinatus muscles, and the scapular upward rotators are the serratus anterior and trapezius muscles. The rotator cuff muscles must keep the humeral head centered in the glenoid fossa during this exercise. All the foregoing muscles maintain normal scapulohumeral rhythm.

Abduction in the plane of the scapula should be performed with moderate lateral rotation (thumb-up position) of the shoulder, to minimize the possibility of impingement (Fig. 15-25).[43] The muscle activity of the supraspinatus during exercises in the plane of the scapula with external rotation (full can) and internal rotation (empty can) positions were compared, and no significant difference in muscle activity was found between the two exercises.[43,44,74] However, Reinold et al[43] recorded significantly less deltoid activity during the full can exercise, so they concluded that this may be the optimal position to recruit the supraspinatus for rehabilitation and testing. During low-intensity scaption exercises in the full can position, Townsend et al[65] recorded

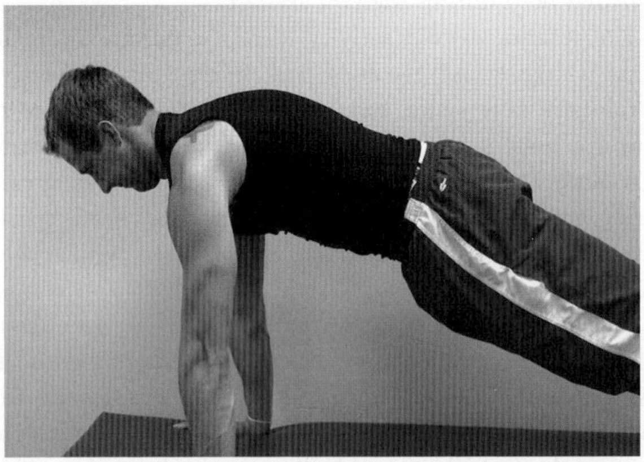

Figure 15-24 Push-up plus exercise for the serratus anterior muscle.

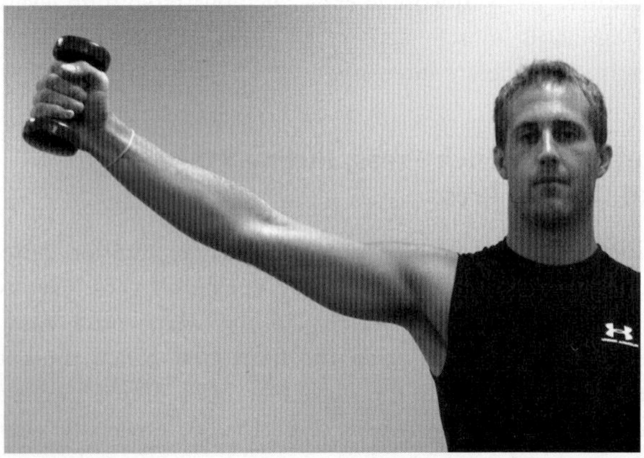

Figure 15-25 "Full can" exercise in the plane of the scapula.

muscle activity levels in the supraspinatus and infraspinatus ranging from 62% to 64% MVIC and muscle activity in the anterior and middle deltoid muscles ranging from 71% to 72% MVIC. Alpert et al[75] recorded comparable activity in the supraspinatus and infraspinatus but significantly lower levels of muscle activity in the teres minor during this exercise. These investigators recorded high levels of muscle activity in the anterior and middle deltoid, but relatively low levels of activity in the posterior deltoid.

Investigators demonstrated increasing activity of both the trapezius and the serratus anterior muscles from the beginning range to the end range of shoulder abduction.[20,70,76,77] Ekstrom et al[70] found that abduction in the plane of the scapula greater than 120° performed at 5 RM intensity produced 96 ± 24% MVIC in the serratus anterior muscle.

This finding agreed with that of Moseley et al,[20] who reported maximum activation of the serratus anterior between 120° and 150° of elevation. This finding is not surprising because approximately two thirds of the serratus anterior muscle has its insertion at the inferior angle of the scapula, and it acts as an upward rotator of the scapula. This exercise may be tolerated by some patients with shoulder problems if the midrange of abduction is avoided, to help minimize impingement and a painful arc of movement at the glenohumeral joint.

Hardwick et al[77] studied the wall slide exercise at more than 90° of flexion and found it to produce comparable amplitude on EMG in the serratus anterior muscle as compared with shoulder abduction in the plane of the scapula. Resistance can be increased by pushing the ulnar border of the forearms against the wall as the hands slide upward (Fig. 15-26). For some patients, this shoulder elevation exercise may be easier to perform because of the support on the wall, which allows for assistance in control of the exercise.

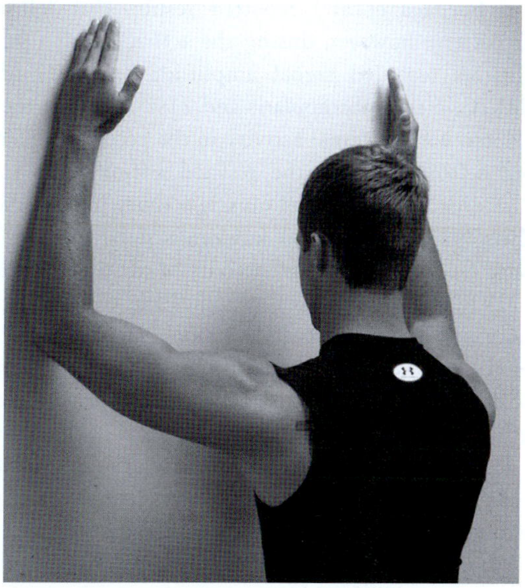

Figure 15-26 Wall slide exercise for the serratus anterior.

Shoulder External Rotation Exercises

External rotation of the shoulder activates the posterior deltoid, infraspinatus, supraspinatus, teres minor, and scapular retractor and depressor muscles.[44] Shoulder external rotation exercises can be performed with a patient in a variety of positions including side lying with 0° of shoulder abduction (Fig. 15-27A), prone with the shoulder abducted to 90° (see Fig. 15-27B), or in varying degrees of abduction in either the plane of the scapula or the frontal plane with the subject in either a sitting or a standing position (see Fig. 15-27C).

Reinold et al[46] demonstrated a trend toward greater activation of the infraspinatus and teres minor muscles with external rotation at 0° of abduction with subjects positioned in the side-lying position as compared with external rotation with the shoulder at 90° of abduction when subjects were prone. However, these investigators did not find a statistical difference in the activity of these muscles when external rotation was performed in five different positions at a 10 RM intensity. Myers et al[78] also failed to find a significant difference in the activation of these muscles when they were exercised with external rotation at 0° or 90° of shoulder abduction. The supraspinatus is activated to approximately the same levels as the infraspinatus and teres minor during external rotation exercises.[44] The posterior deltoid was more active during external rotation at 90° of abduction in both the prone and standing positions when compared with 0° of abduction when side lying.[46]

During isokinetic testing, Greenfield et al[79] determined that subjects could produce significantly more torque in external rotation with the shoulder abducted to 45° in the plane of the scapula as compared with the frontal plane. Investigators also demonstrated that prone external rotation with the shoulder abducted to 90° is a good exercise for activating the lower trapezius muscle (see Fig. 15-27B).[70,80] During external rotation performed at 5 RM intensity, the activity in the lower trapezius muscle was 79% MVIC.[70] This exercise causes maximum depression of the scapula and tends to isolate lower trapezius activity from the middle and upper trapezius.[23,70]

Shoulder Internal Rotation Exercises

The internal rotation muscles of the shoulder are the subscapularis, pectoralis major, latissimus dorsi, teres major, and anterior deltoid. Shoulder internal rotation can be performed with the subject in various positions including 0° of abduction (Fig. 15-28A), 90° of abduction (see Fig. 15-28B), and at any angle in between those two positions. It can be performed in the frontal plane, the plane of the scapula, or in varying degrees of shoulder flexion. Kronberg et al[66] found the greatest amount of muscle activity in the subscapularis, pectoralis major, and latissimus dorsi when the shoulder was internally rotated at 0° of abduction. However, as the shoulder was abducted to 90°, the subscapularis muscle activity remained quite high, with a decrease of pectoralis major muscle activity.

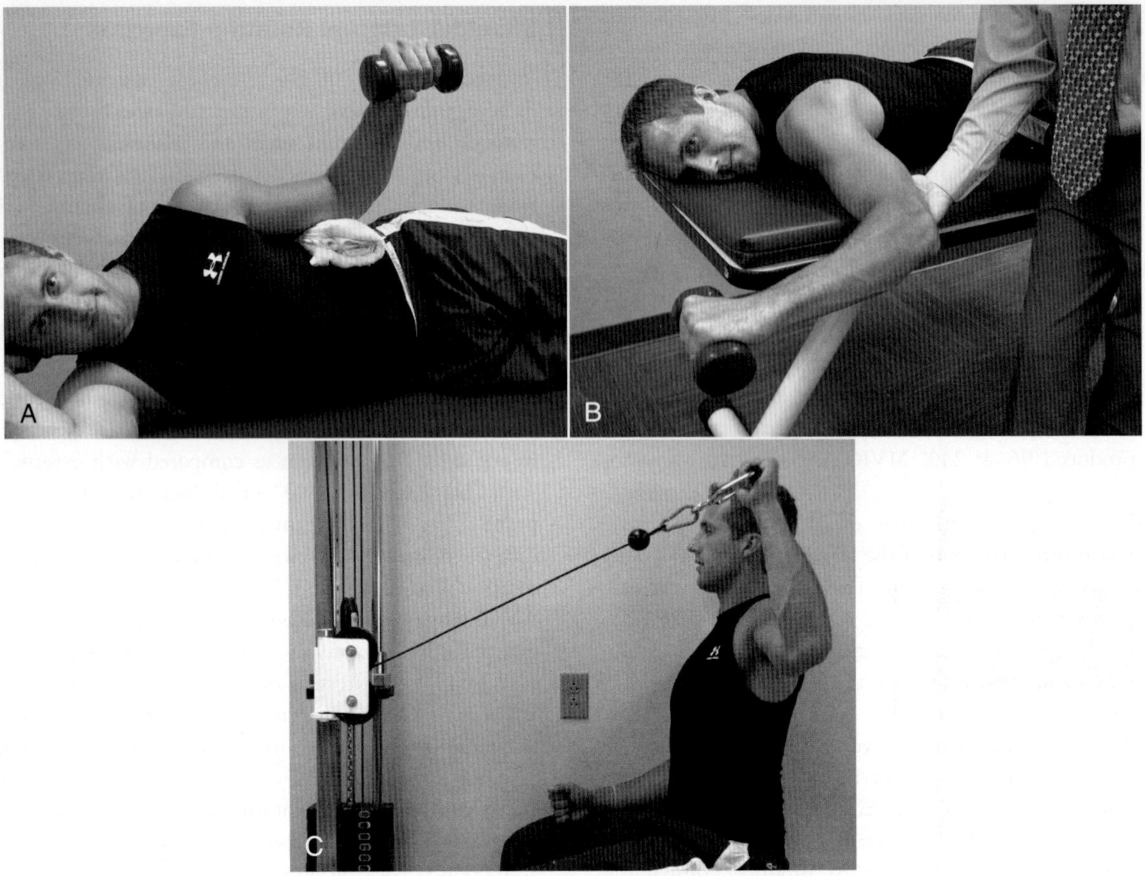

Figure 15-27 Shoulder external rotation. **A,** In the side-lying position. **B,** In the prone position. **C,** Using a pulley system.

Suenaga et al[81] performed maximum isometric contractions of the internal rotator muscles during several positions of the shoulder. These investigators demonstrated slightly greater signal amplitude on EMG (96% MVIC) of the subscapularis when it was abducted to 90° as compared with the 0° abducted position. These investigators also found that the pectoralis major muscle activity greatly decreased at 90° of abduction, but the latissimus dorsi activity decreased only slightly. Anterior deltoid activity was relatively low during all the internal rotation exercises. Decker et al[82] performed tubing exercises at 10 RM intensity and found a trend toward higher peak signal amplitude levels on EMG in the upper subscapularis muscle at 90° of abduction (91% MVIC) as compared with abduction at 45° (87% MVIC) and 0° of shoulder abduction (84% MVIC), but the values were not significantly different. Myers et al[78] also failed to find a significant difference in the subscapularis activity in the two positions when tubing resistance exercises were performed.

Greis et al[83] studied the Gerber lift-off test. During this test, the subject places his or her hand behind the back in the midlumbar area, and then the subject is asked to lift the hand away from the back (see Fig. 15-14). These investigators concluded that the subscapularis is primarily responsible for performing this motion because this test requires internal rotation at end range. They recorded peak signal amplitudes on EMG in the subscapularis of 78% MVIC during the active test and of 100% MVIC during a resisted test. During the active and resisted tests, the muscle activity in the pectoralis major ranged from 3% to 3.8% MVIC, compared with 15% and 33% MVIC for the teres major and 12% and 38% MVIC for the latissimus dorsi.

Tokish et al[48] found similar results during the active lift-off test. Suenaga et al[81] reported results that followed a similar pattern; however, during the active lift-off test, these investigators recorded signal amplitude on EMG of only 45% MVIC in the subscapularis and 21% MVIC in the latissimus dorsi, with minimal activity in the pectoralis major and anterior deltoid. During the resisted lift-off test, Suenaga et al[81] recorded high levels of muscle activity in both the subscapularis (91% MVIC) and latissimus dorsi (73% MVIC). They also recorded fairly high activity of the posterior deltoid (50% MVIC), a finding possibly indicating that they applied resistance not only to internal rotation, but also to shoulder extension. *Resisted shoulder extension with internal rotation,* as shown in Figure 15-29, is a recommended method to strengthen the subscapularis if an individual has the available range of motion to perform the exercise. The recommended angle of pull is in line with the scapular plane, with emphasis on the internal rotation component of the movement.

Tokish et al[48] also studied the belly-press test for subscapularis muscle activity. This test is performed by having the subject press the hand against the belly while keeping the

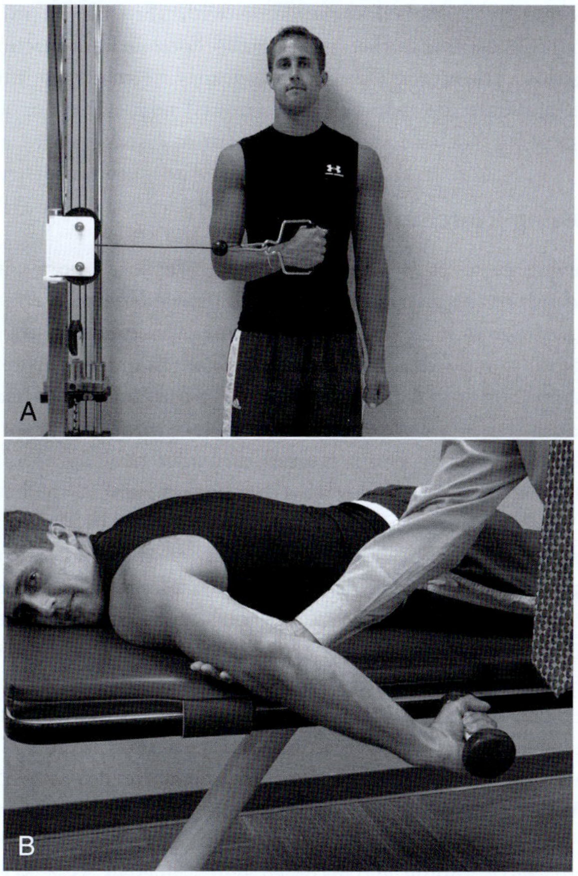

Figure 15-28 Shoulder internal rotation. **A,** Using a pulley system. **B,** In the prone position.

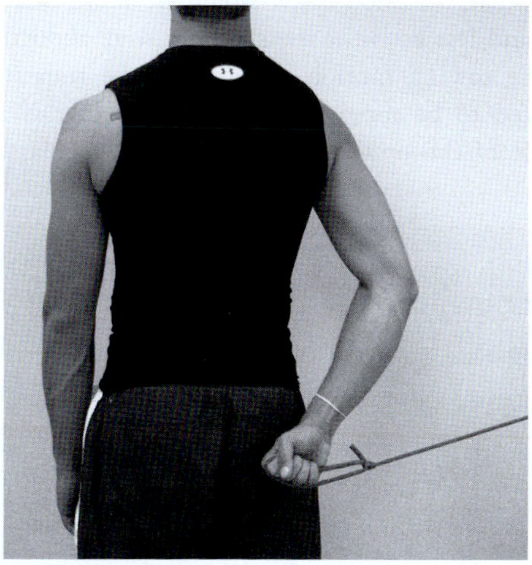

Figure 15-29 Arm pull behind the back with shoulder extension and internal rotation for subscapularis strengthening.

elbow in the frontal plane, to create resisted internal rotation of the shoulder (see Fig. 15-15). This test produced greater activity in the upper subscapularis than did the active lift-off test (86% MVIC versus 57% MVIC), but less activity in the lower subscapularis (59% MVIC versus 80% MVIC).

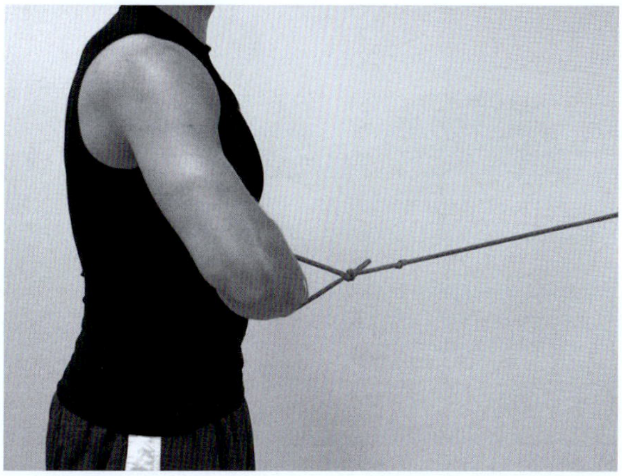

Figure 15-30 Internal rotation exercise for the subscapularis with the elbow kept in the frontal plane.

The test produced activity of less than 23% MVIC in all the other internal rotators. A *resisted belly-press motion* (Fig. 15-30) should be considered for appropriate patients. The patient should maintain the elbow in the frontal plane, with emphasis on internal rotation motion at the shoulder, while minimizing elbow motion and shoulder extension.

Prone Shoulder Horizontal Abduction Exercise at 90°, 100°, and 135° of Abduction

Shoulder horizontal abduction exercises with the subject in the prone position are often performed for strengthening the trapezius, rhomboids, posterior deltoid, and infraspinatus muscles. Very high levels of amplitudes on EMG, ranging from 66% to 108% MVIC, have been recorded in the three parts of the trapezius during these exercises.[66,70] The activity of the middle trapezius is slightly higher than that of the upper of lower trapezius when this exercise is performed at 90° of abduction (Fig. 15-31A).[70] When it is performed at 135° of abduction with the thumb-up position, maximum activity occurs in both the middle and lower trapezius muscles (see Fig. 15-31B).[70]

Townsend et al[65] and Reinold et al[46] recorded very high levels of activity in the posterior and middle deltoid when the shoulder was horizontally abducted with either internal or external rotation. The amount of abduction during the test varied from 90° to 100°.

Townsend et al[65] also recorded peak signal amplitudes on EMG of 88% MVIC in the infraspinatus muscle when the shoulder was horizontally abducted with external rotation, but Reinold et al[46] recorded values of only 39% and 44% MVIC in the infraspinatus and teres minor muscles, respectively. However, Reinold et al[46] recorded very high levels of muscle activity in the supraspinatus (82% MVIC) during horizontal abduction. Some discrepancy exists between the findings of these two studies, and it may result from the 10° difference of abduction in which the exercise was performed. The Blackburn prone position for muscle testing the supraspinatus is also performed with the shoulder abducted to 100°, and it has been

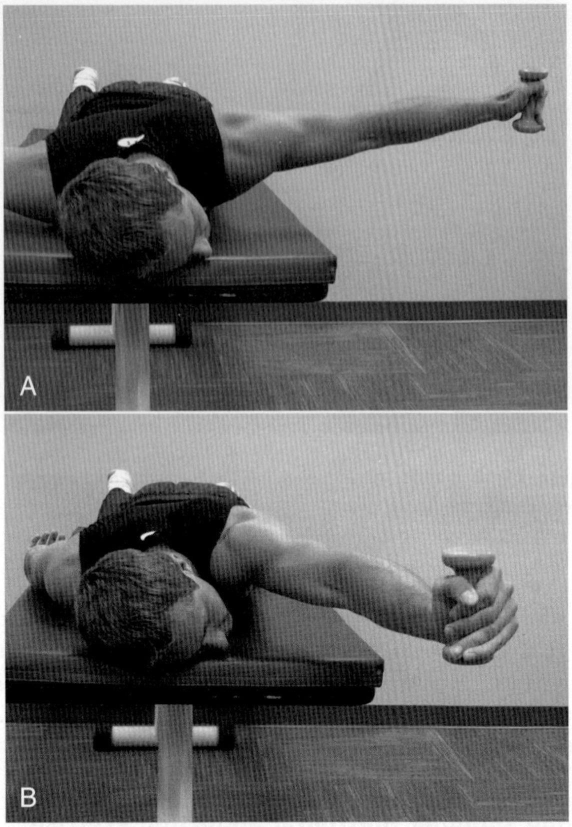

Figure 15-31 Prone shoulder horizontal abduction exercise. **A,** At 90° of abduction. **B,** At 135° of abduction.

shown to activate the supraspinatus to levels that are not significantly different when compared with a muscle test at 90° of abduction in the plane of the scapula while the subject is sitting.[43] Therefore, horizontal abduction exercises appear to be good exercises for strengthening and training of the rotator cuff.

Investigators demonstrated less activity in the trapezius when horizontal abduction was performed with the shoulder internally rotated as compared with the externally rotated position.[50] When the shoulder is internally rotated, the scapula elevates, so one can speculate that activity of the rhomboid and levator scapula muscles is increased.

Dumbbell Fly Exercise

The *dumbbell fly exercise* is performed by horizontally adducting the shoulders with dumbbells in the hands while lying in the supine position. Welsch et al[68] compared the muscle activity of the pectoralis major and anterior deltoid muscles during the dumbbell fly exercise and barbell bench press performed at 6 RM. These investigators did not find any significant difference in the peak signal amplitudes on EMG of the muscles when the two exercises were compared. However, the time of activation during the dumbbell fly exercise was slightly less when compared with the barbell bench press.

Ferreira et al[84] found increased muscle activity in both the clavicular head of the pectoralis major and the anterior deltoid during the dumbbell fly exercise with the subject in an inclined position, rather than in the horizontal or declined position. The reason for this finding may be that these muscles not only are working as horizontal adductors, but also must work as elevators of the humerus to resist gravity.

Rowing Exercise

Rowing exercises are usually performed to help improve the strength of the scapular adductors and shoulder extensor muscles. *Bilateral or unilateral rowing* can be performed with the subject in a sitting or standing position and using a pulley system (Fig. 15-32) or elastic tubing for resistance. Conversely, these exercises can be performed unilaterally with the subject in the prone position and the upper extremity hanging over the side of a treatment table with a dumbbell weight in the hand.

Several studies evaluated unilateral rowing in the prone position.[20,65,70] The humerus is usually moderately abducted approximately 30° during this exercise. Moseley et al[20] performed this exercise with low intensity and recorded peak muscle activity in the upper trapezius of 112% MVIC, middle trapezius of 59% MVIC, lower trapezius of 67% MVIC, and rhomboids of 56% MVIC. Ekstrom et al[70] performed the prone unilateral row at 5 RM intensity and recorded 63% MVIC in the upper trapezius, 79% in the middle trapezius, and 45% MVIC in the lower trapezius. Myers et al[78] evaluated the unilateral row in standing subjects with moderate resistance from elastic tubing and recorded peak values of 51% MVIC in the lower trapezius and 59% MVIC in the rhomboids.

When rowing exercises are performed with the shoulder in minimal abduction, the scapula downwardly rotates as the shoulder is extended during the rowing motion. One can then speculate that the rhomboids would be more active in this position and less active if the shoulder were abducted to 90° during the rowing motion. Conversely, the trapezius would be expected to be more active as the shoulder is abducted, as a result of the upward rotation of the scapula. This may

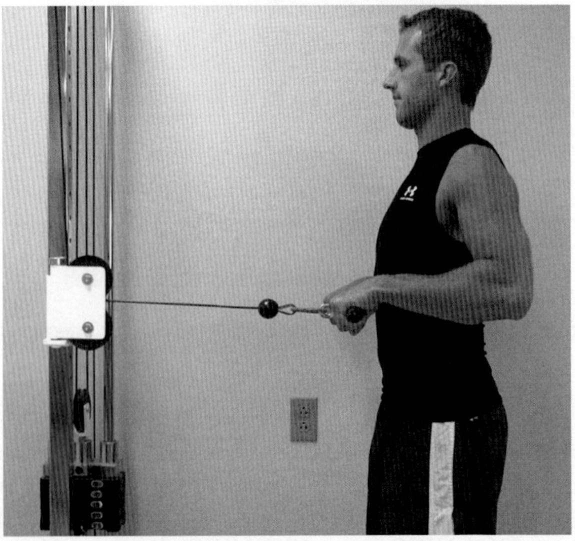

Figure 15-32 Rowing exercise.

be the case because investigators demonstrated that the trapezius is more active during horizontal abduction of the shoulder than during rowing.[70]

Other shoulder muscles that are active during rowing exercises are the posterior deltoid, latissimus dorsi, teres major, and teres minor. Townsend et al[65] recorded very high levels of muscle activity in the posterior deltoid (88% MVIC), and Myers et al[78] recorded muscle activity of 40% MVIC in the latissimus dorsi and very high activity in the teres minor of 109% MVIC.

Shoulder Shrug

The *shoulder shrug exercise* is performed to strengthen the scapular elevators, which are the levator scapulae and upper trapezius muscles. These muscles have been shown to be highly activated during this exercise.[20,71] With some patients, it may be desirable to try to isolate upper trapezius activation from levator scapulae muscle activity. Because the upper trapezius is an upward rotator of the scapula and the levator scapulae is a downward rotator, one may be able to isolate upper trapezius muscle activity better if shoulder shrugging is performed with the scapula upwardly rotated. The military press (see Fig. 15-22) or the *wall slide exercise with the arms overhead* (Fig. 15-33A), as described by Sahrmann,[4] is appropriate for strengthening the upper trapezius muscle. During the wall slide exercise, the subject strongly elevates the scapula as the hands slide up the wall. Dumbbell weights can be held in the hands to increase the resistance.

When the shoulder shrug is performed against resistance with the shoulder adducted (see Fig. 15-33B), all the rotator cuff muscles are activated to a moderate degree, to help prevent inferior subluxation of the humerus.[71] The shrug therefore can be considered a low-level exercise for the rotator cuff musculature.

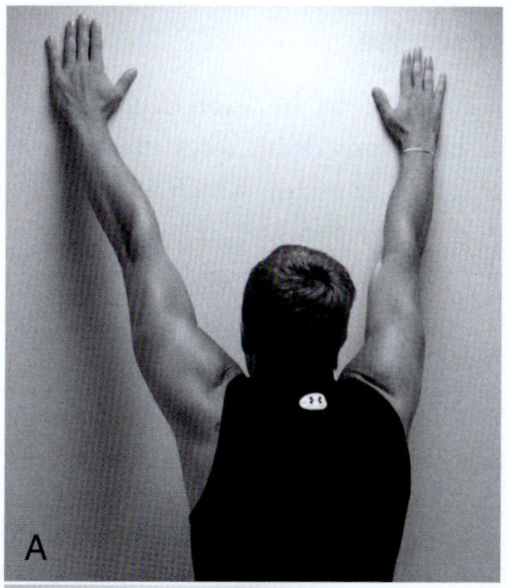

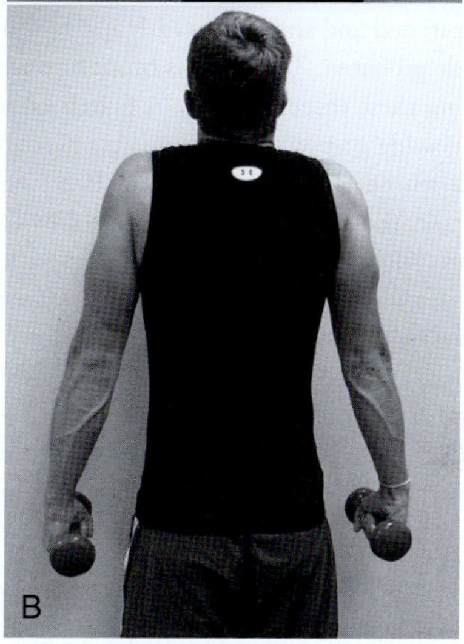

Figure 15-33 Shoulder shrug. **A,** During wall slide. **B,** Performed against resistance.

Press-Up Exercise

The *press-up exercise* is performed in the sitting position by pressing down with the upper extremities to lift the buttock off a bench or table (Fig. 15-34). A high level of muscle activity has been demonstrated in the pectoralis major (84% MVIC) and minor (89% MVIC) muscles during the press-up exercise, with lesser muscle activity in the latissimus dorsi (55% MVIC).[20,65] This exercise also activates the scapular stabilizing muscles to a lesser degree.

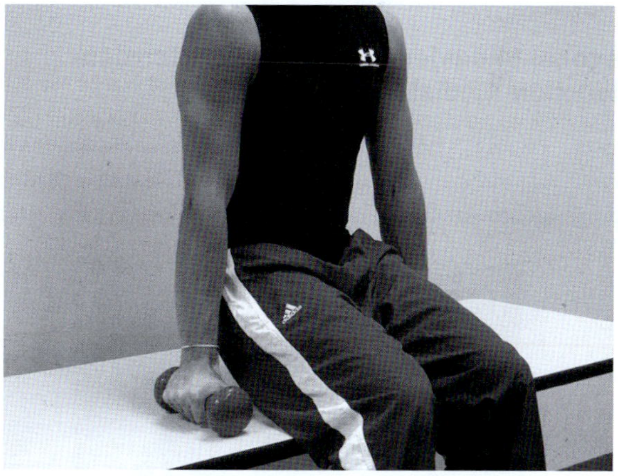

Figure 15-34 Press-up exercise.

Push-Up Exercise

The muscles thought to be highly activated during the *push-up exercise* are the pectoralis major, anterior deltoid, and triceps brachii. Cogley et al[85] studied the muscle activity of the pectoralis major and triceps brachii during a push-up exercise with the hand positions at shoulder width, wider than shoulder width, and closer than shoulder width apart. For the triceps brachii, the mean signal amplitudes on EMG ranged from 99% to 109% MVIC with the narrow base hand position producing significantly greater signal amplitudes in the triceps brachii when compared with the wide base. The results for the pectoralis major were similar, with the signal amplitudes on EMG ranging from 83% to 101% MVIC. Therefore, to increase muscle activity in both these muscle groups, the hand spacing should be narrowed.

Pull-Down Exercise

The muscles thought to be exercised with the *pull-down exercise* are the latissimus dorsi, teres major, pectoralis major, and posterior deltoid muscles, which are the primary adductors or extensors of the shoulder. The pull-down exercise can be performed with shoulder adduction, extension, or a combination of both, depending on the hand grip and position of the arms during the exercise (Fig. 15-35).

Signorile et al[86] performed an analysis on EMG of the muscles already mentioned in addition to the long head of the triceps brachii during pull-down exercises with the hands in four different positions. The hand positions included hands close together in neutral pronation and supination, grip with the hands supinated and shoulder width apart, and a wide grip with the hands pronated. The bar was brought down in front of the head during these three exercises. A fourth exercise was performed with a wide grip with the hands pronated with the bar pulled down behind the head. A narrow hand grip promotes extension of the shoulder during the pull-down, and a wide grip promotes more shoulder adduction during the pull-down. All the exercises were performed at 10 RM intensity.

These investigators found that the pull-down anterior to the head with a wide grip produced significantly greater activity in the latissimus dorsi when compared with the other three exercises.[86] The pull-down close grip exercise tended to produce greater muscle activity in the pectoralis major and posterior deltoid than did the other grip positions, but the difference was not significant. No significant difference was reported for the teres major with any of the grips. It appears that no reason exists to perform pull-downs behind the head for any of these muscles. However, this exercise could be beneficial for other muscles that were not analyzed, such as the scapular retractor muscles.

Diagonal Shoulder Exercise with Extension-Adduction-Medial Rotation

Decker et al[87] performed the *extension-adduction-internal rotation diagonal exercise* (Fig. 15-36) at 10 RM and used elastic tubing for resistance. This exercise produced peak signal amplitudes on EMG of 104% MVIC for the pectoralis major, 98% MVIC for the upper subscapularis, 76% MVIC for the supraspinatus, and 49% MVIC for the latissimus dorsi muscles. Because the exercise direction is in line with the sternocostal head of the pectoralis major, it is an excellent exercise for the development of this muscle, as well as for general activation of the rotator cuff.

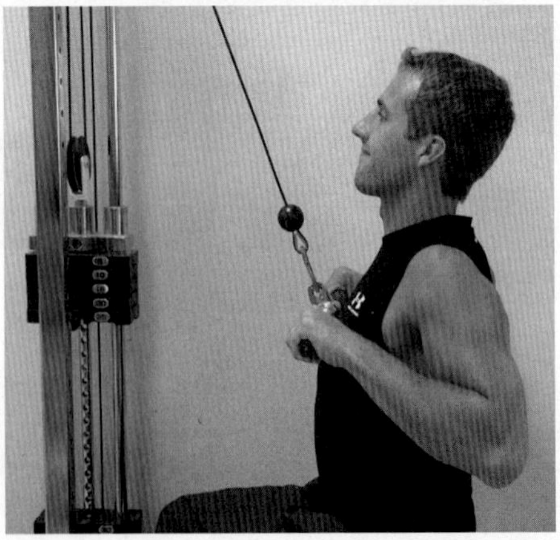

Figure 15-35 Pull-down exercise.

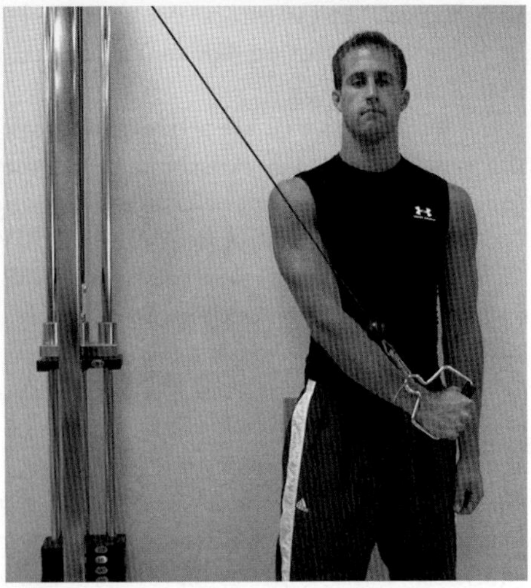

Figure 15-36 Diagonal exercise with extension-adduction-internal rotation.

Diagonal Shoulder Exercise with Flexion-Adduction-Lateral Rotation

The *flexion-adduction-lateral rotation diagonal exercise pattern* (Fig. 15-37) highly activates the anterior and middle parts of the deltoid and the pectoralis major (clavicular head) muscle.[88] Maximal activation of the serratus anterior muscle occurs at 100% MVIC.[70] This exercise requires maximum protraction and upward rotation of the scapula. When the scapula is fully protracted, the trapezius activity tends to

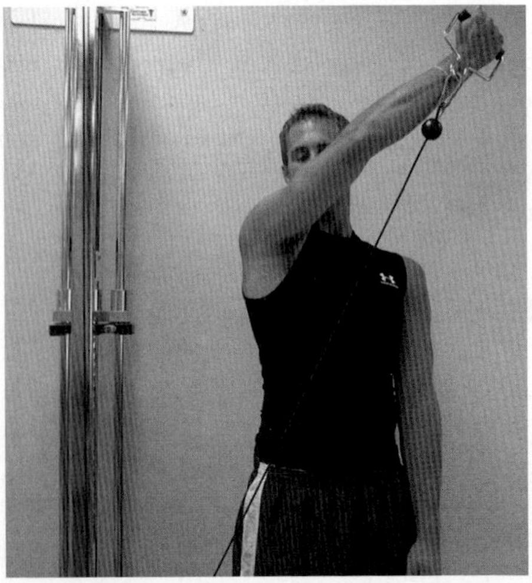

Figure 15-37 Diagonal exercise with flexion-adduction-external rotation.

decrease during shoulder elevation and thus transfers more of the load for upward rotation to the serratus anterior muscle.

Upper Extremity Weight-Bearing Exercises

Uhl et al[89] studied muscle activity of the infraspinatus, supraspinatus, anterior deltoid, posterior deltoid, and pectoralis major muscles during progressive weight bearing through the upper extremity. The progressive weight-bearing exercises were as follows: kneeling with weight on hands, quadruped position, quadruped with one-arm lift, quadruped with arm and lower extremity lift, push-up, push-up with feet elevated, and push-up position with weight on only one upper extremity with the elbow straight. Muscle activity during the easiest to most difficult exercise ranged from 2% to 29% MVIC in the supraspinatus, 4% to 86% MVIC in the infraspinatus, 2% to 46% MVIC in the anterior deltoid, 4% to 74% MVIC in the posterior deltoid, and 7% to 44% MVIC in the pectoralis major. The one-arm support in the push-up position substantially increased the activity on EMG as compared with other exercises, especially in the infraspinatus and posterior deltoid.

REFERENCES

1. Harms-Ringdahl K, editor: *Muscle strength*, New York, 1993, Churchill Livingstone.
2. Prentice WE, Voight ML, editors: *Techniques in musculoskeletal rehabilitation*, New York, 2001, McGraw-Hill.
3. Tovin BJ, Greenfield BH: In *Evaluation and treatment of the shoulder: an integration of the guide to physical therapist practice*, Philadelphia, 2001, Davis.
4. Sahrmann SA: *Diagnosis and treatment of movement impairment syndromes*, St. Louis, 2002, Mosby.
5. Guyton AC: *Textbook of medical physiology*, Philadelphia, 1991, Saunders.
6. Kendall FP, McCreary EK, Provance PG: *Muscles, testing and function*, ed 4, Baltimore, 1993, Williams & Wilkins.
7. Hoppenfeld S: *Physical examination of the spine and extremities*, New York, 1976, Appleton-Century-Crofts.
8. Donatelli RA, Wooden MJ, editors: *Orthopaedic physical therapy*, ed 4, St. Louis, 2010, Churchill Livingstone Elsevier.
9. Sobush DC, Simoneau GC, Dietz KE, et al: The Lennie test for measuring scapular position in healthy young adult females: a reliability and validity study, *J Orthop Sport Phys Ther* 23:39, 1996.
10. Norkin CC, Levangie PK: *Joint structure and function*, ed 3, Philadelphia, 2001, Davis.
11. Williams PL, Warwick R, Dyson M, et al: In *Gray's anatomy*, ed 37, New York, 1989, Churchill Livingstone.
12. Muraki T, Mitsuhiro A, Izumi T, et al: Lengthening of the pectoralis minor muscle during passive shoulder motions and stretching techniques: a cadaveric biomechanical study, *Phys Ther* 89:333, 2009.
13. Hislop HJ, Montgomery J: *Muscle testing, techniques of manual examination*, ed 7, Philadelphia, 2002, Saunders.
14. Palmer ML, Epler M: *Clinical assessment procedures in physical therapy*, Philadelphia, 1990, Lippincott.
15. Reese NB: *Muscles and sensory testing*, Philadelphia, 1999, Saunders.
16. Clarkson HM: *Musculoskeletal assessment, joint range of motion and manual muscle strength*, Philadelphia, 1989, Lippincott Williams & Wilkins.
17. Kelly BT, Kadramas WR, Speer KP: The manual muscle examination for rotator cuff strength: an electromyographic investigation, *Am J Sports Med* 24:581, 1996.
18. Brandell BR, Wilkinson DA: An electromyographic study of manual testing procedures for the trapezius and deltoid muscles, *Physiother Can* 43:33, 1991.
19. Greis PE, Kuhn JE, Schultheis J, et al: Validation of the lift-off test and analysis of subscapularis activity during maximal internal rotation, *Am J Sports Med* 24:589, 1996.
20. Moseley JB, Jobe FW, Pink M, et al: EMG analysis of the scapular muscles during a shoulder rehabilitation program, *Am J Sports Med* 20:28, 1992.
21. Kronberg M, Németh G, Broström L: Muscle activity and coordination in the normal shoulder: an electromyographic study, *Clin Orthop Relat Res* 257:76, 1990.
22. Townsend H, Jobe FW, Pink M, et al: Electromyographic analysis of the glenohumeral muscles during a baseball rehabilitation program, *Am J Sports Med* 19:264, 1991.
23. Ballantyne BT, O'Hare SJ, Paschall JL, et al: Electromyographic activity of selected shoulder muscles in commonly used therapeutic exercises, *Phys Ther* 73:668, 1993.
24. Malanga GA, Jenp YN, Growney ES, et al: EMG analysis of shoulder positioning in testing and strengthening the supraspinatus, *Med Sci Sports Exerc* 28:661, 1996.
25. Lilienfeld AM, Jacobs M, Willis M: A study of the reproducibility of muscle testing and certain other aspects of muscle scoring, *Phys Ther Rev* 34:279, 1954.
26. Silver M, McElroy A, Morrow L, et al: Further standardization of manual muscle test for clinical study: applied in chronic renal disease, *Phys Ther* 50:1456, 1970.
27. Florence JM, Pandya S, King WM, et al: Clinical trials in Duchenne dystrophy: standardization and reliability of evaluating procedures, *Phys Ther* 64:41, 1984.
28. Beasley WC: Influence of method on estimates of normal knee extensor force among normal and post-polio children, *Phys Ther Rev* 36:21, 1956.
29. Aitkens S, Lord J, Bernauer E, et al: Relationship of manual muscle testing to objective strength measurements, *Muscle Nerve* 12:173, 1989.
30. Watkins MP, Harris BA, Kozlowski BA: Isokinetic testing in patients with hemiparesis: a pilot study, *Phys Ther* 64:184, 1984.
31. Krebs DE: Isokinetic, electrophysiologic, and clinical function relationships following tourniquet-aided knee arthrotomy, *Phys Ther* 69:803, 1989.
32. Agre JC, Rodriquez AA: Validity of manual muscle testing in post-polio subjects with good or normal strength, *Arch Phys Med Rehabil* 70(Suppl):A17, 1989.
33. Schwartz S, Cohen ME, Herbison GJ, et al: Relationship between two measures of upper extremity strength: manual muscle test compared to hand-held myometry, *Arch Phys Med Rehabil* 73:1063, 1992.
34. Hayes KW, Falconer J: Reliability of hand-held dynamometry and its relationship with manual muscle testing in patients with osteoarthritis in the knee, *J Orthop Sports Phys Ther* 16:145, 1992.
35. Bohannon RW: Test-retest reliability of hand held dynamometry during a single session strength assessment, *Phys Ther* 66:206, 1986.
36. Byl NN, Richards S, Asturias J: Intrarater and interrater reliability of strength measurements of the biceps and deltoid using a hand-held dynamometer, *J Orthop Sports Phys Ther* 9:339, 1988.

37. Donatelli R, Ellenbecker TS, Ekedahl SR, et al: Assessment of shoulder strength in professional baseball pitchers, *J Orthop Sports Phys Ther* 30:544, 2000.
38. Wadsworth CT, Krishnan R, Sear M, et al: Intrarater reliability of manual muscle testing and hand-held dynamometric muscle testing, *Phys Ther* 67:1342, 1987.
39. Caldwell LS, Chaffin DB, Dukes-Dobos FN, et al: A proposed standard procedure for static muscle strength testing, *Am Ind Hyg Assoc J* 35:201, 1974.
40. Jobe FW, Moynes DR: Delineation of diagnosis criteria and a rehabilitation program for rotator cuff injuries, *Am J Sports Med* 10:336, 1982.
41. Worrell TW, Corey BJ, York SL, et al: An analysis of supraspinatus EMG activity and shoulder isometric force development, *Med Sci Sports Exerc* 24:744, 1992.
42. Blackburn TA, McLeod WD, White B, et al: EMG analysis of posterior rotator cuff exercise, *J Athl Train* 25:40, 1990.
43. Reinold MM, Macrina LC, Wild KE, et al: Electromyographic analysis of the supraspinatus and deltoid muscles during 3 common rehabilitation exercises, *J Athl Train* 42:464, 2007.
44. Boettcher CE, Ginn KA, Cathers I: Standard maximum isometric voluntary contraction tests for normalizing shoulder muscle EMG, *J Orthop Res* 26:1591, 2008.
45. Itoi E, Kido T, Sano A, et al: Which is more useful, the "full can test" or the "empty can test" in detecting the torn supraspinatus tendon? *Am J Sports Med* 27:65, 1999.
46. Reinold MM, Wilk KE, Fleisig GS, et al: Electromyographic analysis of the rotator cuff and deltoid musculature during common shoulder external rotation exercises, *J Orthop Sports Phys Ther* 34:385, 2004.
47. Gerber C, Krushell RJ: Isolated rupture of the tendon of the subscapularis muscle: clinical features in 16 cases, *J Bone Joint Surg Br* 73:389, 1991.
48. Tokish JM, Decker MJ, Ellis HB, et al: The belly-press test for the physical examination of the subscapularis muscle: electromyographic validation and comparison to the lift-off test, *J Shoulder Elbow Surg* 12:427, 2003.
49. Gerber C, Hersche O, Farron A: Isolated rupture of the subscapularis tendon: results of operative repair, *J Bone Joint Surg Am* 78:1015, 1996.
50. Ekstrom RA, Soderberg GL, Donatelli RA: Normalization procedures using maximum voluntary isometric contractions for the serratus anterior and trapezius muscles during surface EMG analysis, *J Electromyogr Kinesiol* 15:418, 2005.
51. De Freitas V, Vitti M, Furlani J: Electromyographic study of levator scapulae and rhomboideus major muscles in movements of the shoulder and arm, *Electromyogr Clin Neurophysiol* 20:205, 1980.
52. American Physical Therapy Association: *Guide to physical therapist practice*, ed 2, Alexandria, Va, 2001, American Physical Therapy Association.
53. Hageman PA, Sorensen TA: Eccentric isokinetics. In Albert M, editor: *Eccentric muscle training in sports and orthopaedics*, ed 2, New York, 1995, Churchill Livingstone.
54. Matsen FA, Arntz CT: Subacromial impingement. In Rockwood CA, Matsen FA, editors: *The shoulder*, Philadelphia, 1990, Saunders.
55. Jobe FW: Superior glenoid impingement, *Clin Orthop Relat Res* 330:98, 1996.
56. Kamkar A, Irrgang JJ, Whitney SL: Nonoperative management of secondary shoulder impingement syndrome, *J Orthop Sports Phys Ther* 17:212, 1993.
57. Ellenbecker TS, Derscheid GL: Rehabilitation of overuse injuries of the shoulder, *Clin Sports Med* 8:583, 1989.
58. Reinold MM, Escamilla R, Wilk KE: Current concepts in the scientific and clinical rationale behind exercises for glenohumeral and scapulothoracic musculature, *J Orthop Sports Phys Ther* 39:105, 2009.
59. American College of Sports Medicine: *ACSM's guidelines for exercise testing and prescription*, ed 6, Philadelphia, 2000, Lippincott Williams & Wilkins.
60. Fleck SJ, Kraemer WJ: *Designing resistance training programs*, ed 2, Champaign, Ill, 1997, Human Kinetics.
61. Prentice WE: Restoring muscular strength, endurance, and power. In Prentice WE, editor: *Rehabilitation techniques in sports medicine*, ed 3, Boston, 1999, WCB/McGraw-Hill.
62. Stone WJ, Coulter SP: Strength/endurance effects from three resistance training protocols with women, *J Strength Cond Res* 8:231, 1994.
63. Prentice WE: Impaired muscle performance: regaining muscular strength and endurance. In Prentice WE, Voight MI, editors: *Techniques in musculoskeletal rehabilitation*, Boston, 2001, McGraw-Hill.
64. Barnett C, Kippers V, Turner P: Effects of variations of the bench press exercise on the EMG activity of five shoulder muscles, *J Strength Cond Res* 9:222, 1995.
65. Townsend H, Jobe FW, Pink M, et al: Electromyographic analysis of the glenohumeral muscles during a baseball rehabilitation program, *Am J Sports Med* 19:264, 1991.
66. Kronberg M, Nemeth G, Brostrom LA: Muscle activity and coordination in the normal shoulder: an electromyographic study, *Clin Orthop Relat Res* 257:76, 1990.
67. Glass SC, Armstrong T: Electromyographic activity of the pectoralis muscle during incline and decline bench presses, *J Strength Cond Res* 11:163, 1997.
68. Welsch EA, Bird M, Mayhew JL: Electromyographic activity of the pectoralis major and anterior deltoid muscles during three upper-body lifts, *J Strength Cond Res* 19:449, 2005.
69. Ekstrom RA, Bifulco KM, Lopau CJ, et al: Comparing the function of the upper and lower parts of the serratus anterior muscle using surface electromyography, *J Orthop Sports Phys Ther* 34:235, 2004.
70. Ekstrom RA, Donatelli RA, Soderberg GL: Surface electromyographic analysis of exercises for the trapezius and serratus anterior muscles, *J Orthop Sports Phys Ther* 33:247, 2003.
71. Hintermeister RA, Lange GW, Schultheis JM, et al: Electromyographic activity and applied load during shoulder rehabilitation exercises using elastic resistance, *Am J Sports Med* 26:210, 1998.
72. Decker MJ, Hintermeister RA, Faber KJ, et al: Serratus anterior muscle activity during selected rehabilitation exercises, *Am J Sports Med* 27:784, 1999.
73. Lear LJ, Gross MT: An electromyographic analysis of the scapular stabilizing synergists during a push-up progression, *J Orthop Sports Phys Ther* 28:146, 1999.
74. Kelly B, Kadrmas W, Speer K: The manual muscle examination for rotator cuff strength: an electromyographic investigation, *Am J Sports Med* 24:581, 1996.
75. Alpert SW, Pink MM, Jobe FW, et al: Electromyographic analysis of deltoid and rotator cuff function under varying loads and speeds, *J Shoulder Elbow Surg* 9:47, 2000.
76. Guazzelli Filho J, de Freitas V, Furlani J: Electromyographic study of the trapezius muscle in free movements of the shoulder, *Electromyogr Clin Neurophysiol* 34:279, 1994.

77. Hardwick DH, Beebe JA, McDonnell MK, et al: A comparison of serratus anterior muscle activation during a wall slide exercise and other traditional exercises, *J Orthop Sports Phys Ther* 36:903, 2006.
78. Myers JB, Pasquale MR, Laudner KG, et al: On-the-field resistance-tubing exercises for throwers: an electromyographic analysis, *J Athl Train* 40:15, 2005.
79. Greenfield BH, Donatelli R, Wooden MJ, et al: Isokinetic evaluation of shoulder rotational strength between the plane of scapula and the frontal plane, *Am J Sports Med* 18:124, 1990.
80. Ballantyne B, O'Hare S, Paschall J, et al: Electromyographic activity of selected shoulder muscles in commonly used therapeutic exercises, *Phys Ther* 73:668, 1993.
81. Suenaga N, Minami A, Fujisawa H: Electromyographic analysis of internal rotational motion of the shoulder in various arm positions, *J Shoulder Elbow Surg* 12:501, 2003.
82. Decker MJ, Tokish JM, Ellis HB, et al: Subscapularis muscle activity during selected rehabilitation exercises, *Am J Sports Med* 31:126, 2003.
83. Greis PE, Kuhn JE, Schultheis J, et al: Validation of the lift-off test and analysis of subscapularis activity during maximal internal rotation: paper presented at the 21st annual meeting of the AOSSM, Toronto, Ontario, Canada, July 1995, *Am J Sports Med* 24:589, 1996.
84. Ferriera MI, Büll ML, Vitti M: Electromyographic validation of basic exercises for physical conditioning programmes. IV. Analysis of the deltoid muscle (anterior portion) and pectoralis major muscle (clavicular portion) in frontal-lateral cross, dumbbells exercises, *Electromyogr Clin Neurophysiol* 43:67, 2003.
85. Cogley RM, Archambault TA, Fibeger JF, et al: Comparison of muscle activation using various hand positions during the push-up exercise, *J Strength Cond Res* 19:628, 2005.
86. Signorile JF, Zink AJ, Szwed SP: A comparative electromyographical investigation of muscle utilization patterns using various hand positions during the late pull-down, *J Strength Cond Res* 16:539, 2002.
87. Decker M, Tokish J, Ellis H, et al: Subscapularis muscle activity during selected rehabilitation exercises, *Am J Sports Med* 31:126, 2003.
88. Ekholm J, Arborelius UP, Hillered L, et al: Shoulder muscle EMG and resisting moment during diagonal exercise movements resisted by weight-and-pulley-circuit, *Scand J Rehabil Med* 10:179, 1978.
89. Uhl T, Carver T, Mattacola C, et al: Shoulder musculature activation during upper extremity weight-bearing exercise, *J Orthop Sports Phys Ther* 33:109, 2003.

CHAPTER

16

Johnson McEvoy
and Jan Dommerholt

Myofascial Trigger Points of the Shoulder

Shoulder problems are common, with a 1-year prevalence ranging from 4.7% to 46.7% and a lifetime prevalence of 6.7% to 66.7%.[1] Many different structures give rise to shoulder pain, including the structures in the subacromial space, such as the subacromial bursa, the rotator cuff, and the long head of biceps,[2,3] and are presented in various chapters of this book. Muscle and specifically myofascial trigger points (MTrPs), have been recognized to refer pain to the shoulder region and may be a source of peripheral nociceptive input that gives rise to sensitization and pain. MTrP referral patterns have been published for the shoulder region.[4-6]

Often, little attention is paid to MTrPs as a primary or secondary pain source. Instead, emphasis is placed only on muscle mechanical properties such as length and strength.[7,8] The tendency in manual therapy is to consider muscle pain as secondary to joint or nerve dysfunctions. A study of cervical joint dysfunction and MTrPs demonstrated a correlation between the presence of MTrPs in the upper trapezius and C3 and C4 dysfunctions; however, a cause-and-effect relationship was not established.[9] Clinicians should assess both joints and examine muscles for MTrPs and treat accordingly.[9] Interest in MTrPs has increased, as evidenced by a growth in research with more Medline citations in the last decade than in the previous two decades combined.[8] An orthopedic manual therapy text and popular sports medicine texts have included MTrPs in differential diagnosis and management strategies.[8,10,11] Leading pain management textbooks include chapters on myofascial pain.[12,13] A survey of physician members of the American Pain Society showed overwhelming agreement that myofascial pain is a distinct clinical entity.[14]

This chapter focuses on MTrPs, including the philosophical framework, palpation technique, and treatment options with reference to other soft tissue procedures. Selected treatment techniques are presented as examples. Readers are encouraged to seek further information through cited references. Furthermore, in shoulder rehabilitation, a comprehensive orthopedic physical therapy evaluation is imperative. Clinicians should be guided by fundamental physical therapy principles, research, clinical reasoning, and patient goals. The aim of this chapter, and of other chapters of this book, is to assist clinicians in developing a more comprehensive approach to shoulder rehabilitation. Inclusion of MTrPs in the assessment and management of shoulder pain and dysfunction does not necessarily replace other techniques and approaches, but it does add an important dimension to the management plan.

TRIGGER POINTS

A *myofascial trigger point* is defined as a hyperirritable spot in skeletal muscle, which is associated with a hypersensitive palpable nodule in a taut band.[4] When compressed, a MTrP may give rise to characteristic referred pain, tenderness, motor dysfunction, and autonomic phenomena.[4] MTrPs have been described as active or latent. *Active MTrPs* are associated with spontaneous pain complaints, whereas *latent MTrPs* are clinically dormant and are painful only when palpated or needled.[4] Another feature of MTrPs is the *local twitch response* (LTR), which is a sudden contraction of muscle fibers within a taut band elicited by a snapping palpation or with insertion of a needle into the MTrP.[4] The minimum criterion for identification of an active MTrP is exquisite spot tenderness of a nodule in a taut band, which, when adequately palpated, gives rise to the patient's recognition of the current pain complaint. A latent MTrP, due to its lack of relationship to spontaneous pain, is defined as exquisite spot tenderness of a nodule in a taut band (Box 16-1).[15,16]

Typical referral pain patterns for several shoulder muscles are presented in Figure 16-1. The "X" indicates only potential MTrP locations and should be considered as a general guideline. Accurate palpation, using the recommended criteria, is the key to identifying MTrPs in an individual muscle, and the examiner must realize that any one muscle may have multiple MTrPs. Often, MTrPs do not lie in their own referral patterns. Commonly, MTrPs will refer distally inferring that often the muscle responsible for the pain will be located proximal to the pain pattern.[17,18]

MTrPs were described as far back as the 16th century by French physician Guillaume de Baillou (1538–1616), who used the term *muscular rheumatism* to describe what is now

BOX 16-1 Recommended Criteria for the Identification of a Myofascial Trigger Point

- Taut band palpable (where muscle is accessible)
- Exquisite spot tenderness of a nodule in a taut band
- Patient recognition of current pain complaint by pressure on the tender nodule (identifies an active trigger point)

recognized as myofascial pain.[19] Many other clinicians have described trigger points; however, Travell and Simons are considered the authoritative sources.[20] Travell (1901–1997) was initially trained in cardiology and subsequently became interested in referred pain from palpation of taut bands in skeletal muscles.[21] As a side note, Travell became the personal physician to Presidents Kennedy and Johnson and was the first female White House physician.[21] Later in her career, she collaborated with Dr. David Simons (1922–2010), a physiatrist, and they coauthored the widely distributed trigger point manuals.[4,22,23] Several other noted textbooks on myofascial pain and MTrPs have been published.[5,19,24,25]

The prevalence of myofascial pain has been reported in various populations, but the prevalence in the general population is unknown.[4] Investigators reported that between 84% and 93% of patients in pain management centers had myofascial pain.[26,27] Thirty percent of patients presenting with pain in a primary care general medical clinic had myofascial pain, thus making myofascial pain the largest single diagnostic pain group.[28] Furthermore, patients with upper body pain were more likely to have myofascial pain than pain located elsewhere.[28] In older adults with low back pain, MTrPs were identified in 96% of symptomatic subjects versus 10% of controls.[29] MTrPs were identified in 93.9% of patients with migraine compared with 29% of control subjects.[30] Myofascial pain has been described by various clinical specialties in selected patient groups.

With regard to the shoulder, patients with a medical diagnosis of rotator cuff tendinopathy ($n = 58$) lasting more than 6 weeks and less than 18 months were reported to have MTrPs in the supraspinatus (88%), infraspinatus (62%), teres

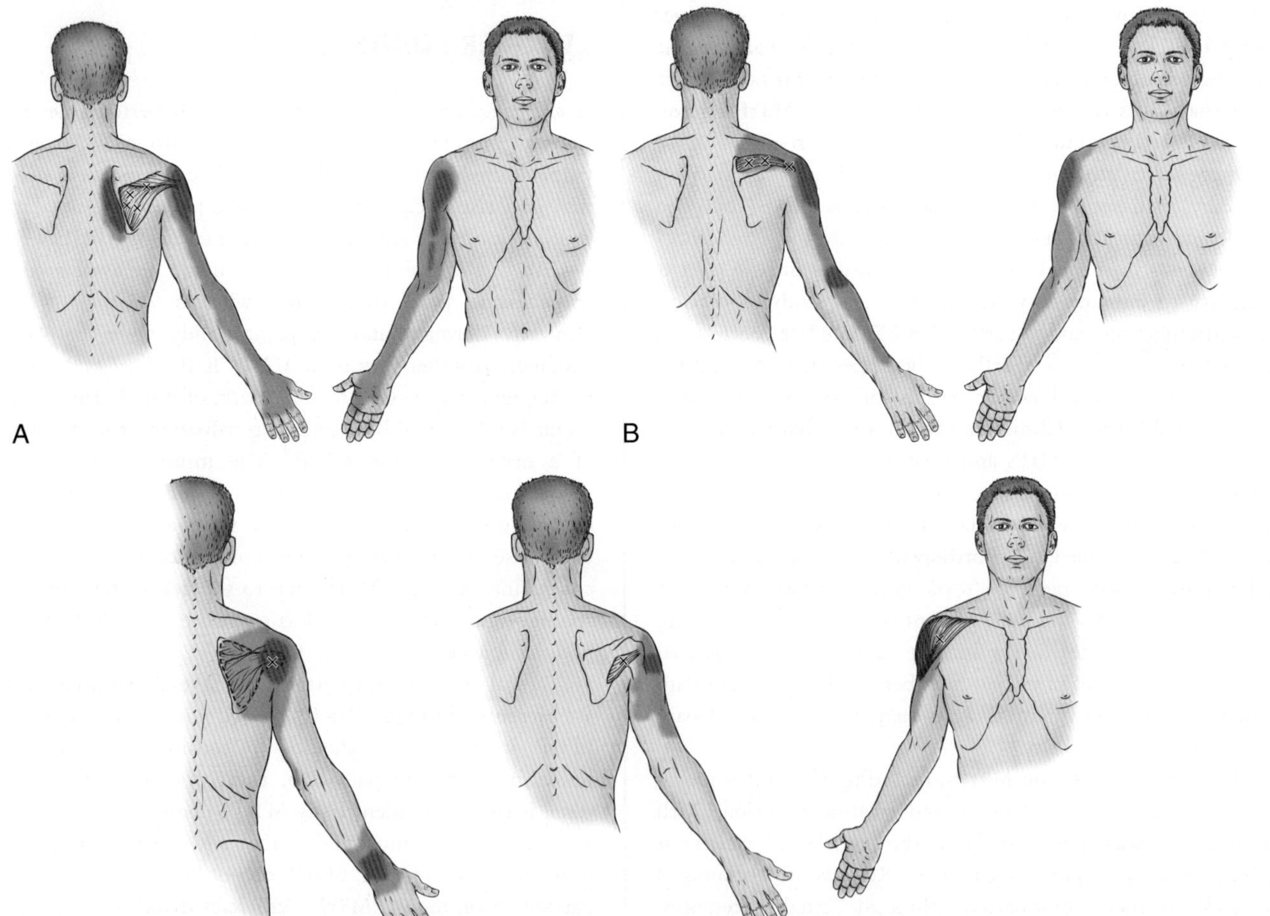

Figure 16-1 Myofascial trigger points and their corresponding referral zones: **A,** infraspinatus; **B,** supraspinatus; **C,** subscapularis; **D,** teres minor; **E,** anterior deltoid;

(continued)

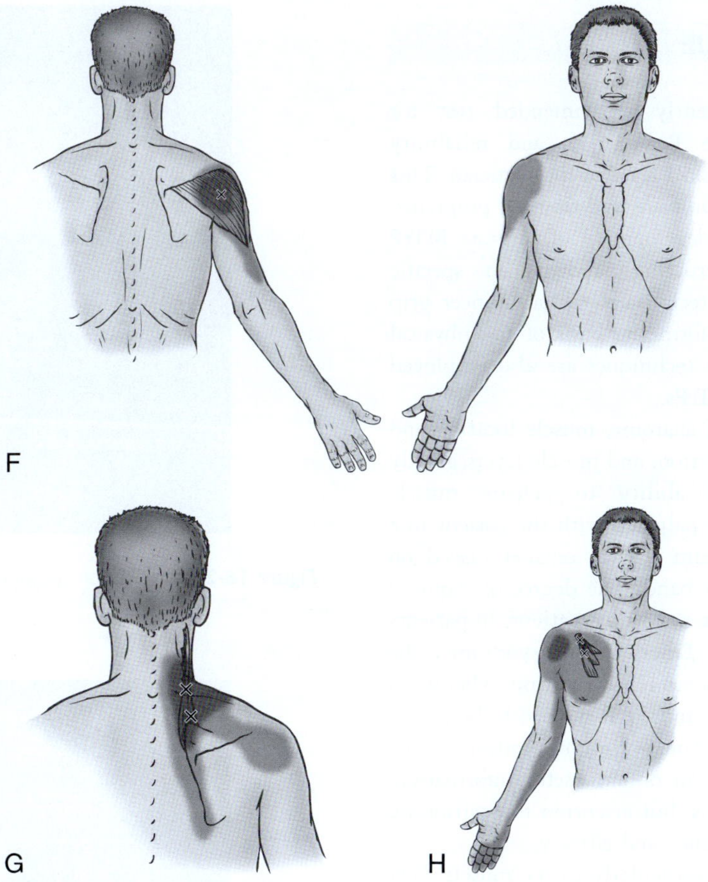

Figure 16-1 Cont'd F, posterior deltoid; **G,** levator scapulae; **H,** pectoralis minor. (From Muscolino JE: *The muscle and bone palpation manual: with trigger points, referral patterns, and stretching,* St. Louis, 2009, Mosby.)

minor (20.7%), and subscapularis (5.2%) muscles.[31] Patients with shoulder impingement had a greater number of active MTrPs in the supraspinatus (67%), infraspinatus (42%), and subscapularis (42%) when compared with normal control subjects.[32] Patients demonstrated widespread pressure hypersensitivity and the presence of active MTrPs that, when examined, could reproduce the recognized pain complaint.[32] A study of patients with chronic unilateral nontraumatic shoulder pain ($n = 72$), conducted in a Dutch physical therapy practice, identified active MTrPs in all subjects with the following prevalence: infraspinatus (78%); upper trapezius (58%); middle trapezius (43%); anterior, middle, and posterior deltoid (47%, 50%, 44%, respectively); and teres minor (47%) muscles.[33] Brukner and Khan[10] considered MTrPs to be among the most common causes of shoulder pain from a sports medicine perspective and recommended assessing for MTrPs in the clinical setting.

PALPATION RELIABILITY

Currently, no gold standard diagnostic imaging or laboratory test exists for MTrPs, and clinicians must rely on the history and physical examination findings for the diagnosis of myofascial pain.[34] Because of the reliance on physical examination, adequate intrarater and interrater palpation reliability for the identification of MTrPs is important in construct validity.[16]

Nine published studies addressed MTrP palpation interrater[2,15,35-40] and intrarater[31] reliability of various subjects and muscles. Palpation reliability studies were systematically reviewed by McEvoy and Huijbregts,[16] who used the *Data Extraction and Quality Scoring Form for Reliability Studies of Spinal Palpation.*[41] The review concluded that MTrPs can be reliably identified in certain muscles, but a caveat to these findings is that reliability depends on a high level of rater expertise, training, and consensus discussion on technique.[16] Furthermore, location of MTrPs by palpation in the upper trapezius was found to be highly reliable when a three-dimensional infrared camera was used for assessment.[40]

With regard to the shoulder, Bron et al[2] and Gerwin et al[15] examined muscles relating to the shoulder, and interrater reliability was supported in both studies for all muscles tested, including the infraspinatus, posterior deltoid, biceps brachii, trapezius, and latissimus dorsi muscles. Al-Shenqiti and Oldham[31] studied the rotator cuff muscles, infraspinatus, supraspinatus, teres minor, and subscapularis, and intrarater reliability was supported with kappa values of 0.85, 0.86, 0.88, and 0.79, respectively.

PALPATION TECHNIQUE

Palpation is the only currently recommended test for identification of MTrPs (see Box 16-1), and reliability depends on the expertise and skill level of the clinician. This finding has implications for clinicians and training programs, which should emphasize the development of accurate MTrP palpation skills before instructing students in specific treatment options. Palpation techniques include pincer grip and flat palpation, and they form the basis of the physical examination technique. These techniques are also employed as a mode of treatment for MTrPs.

An in-depth knowledge of anatomy, muscle location and attachments, muscle fiber direction, and muscle layers greatly enhances the accuracy and ability to palpate muscle adequately. Muscles should be palpated with the patient in a relaxed position, with optimum passive tension placed on the muscle to expose the taut band. The degree of required tension or slack depends on the individual patient. In patients with hypermobility, such as Ehlers-Danlos syndrome, the muscle often must be put in a stretched position, whereas in other, less mobile patients, the muscle may need to be placed in a more relaxed position. The optimum position is the position where the clinician can obtain useful information. This statement may be obvious, but attention to positioning is important for clinical efficiency and efficacy.

The clinician palpates perpendicularly to the muscle fiber direction to identify the taut band. During the examination, the muscle is palpated with enough compression to induce local tenderness. Eliciting referred pain is not always necessary, but if that is desired, the MTrP may need to be compressed for at least 15 seconds because it may take some time for the referred pain to arise. Some muscles present palpation challenges, given that these muscles may not be accessible. Consider, for example, the difference between flat palpation of the accessible infraspinatus muscle and limited palpation of the less accessible subscapularis muscle.[4,22,23]

- Flat palpation: Finger or thumb pressure is applied directly to the muscle perpendicular to the muscle fiber direction while the muscle fibers are compressed against the underlying tissue or bone (Fig. 16-2). An example is palpation of the infraspinatus and teres minor flat against the scapula.
- Pincer palpation: A pincer grip is employed between the clinician's fingers and thumb, essentially again perpendicular to the muscle fiber direction. The muscle fibers are rolled in the grasp to allow examination of the tissues (Fig. 16-3). For example, the pincer grip palpation is used to palpate MTrPs in the upper trapezius muscle and the axillary portions of the pectoralis major and latissimus dorsi muscles.

PATHOGENESIS

The *integrated hypothesis* (IH) of trigger point formation was introduced by Travell and Simons as a theoretical framework for MTrP development.[4,8] The IH is an evidence-informed combination of electrodiagnostic, clinical, and histopathologic studies, and it has been updated several times in light of new research evidence (Fig. 16-4).[7,34,42-44]

Muscle is the largest collective organ in the human body, and through its synergistic relationship with the nervous system, it executes complex movements of the body. Muscle architecture is made up of fascicles of fibers, which, in turn, are composed of myofibrils.[45,46] The basic unit of the myofibril is the sarcomere, which lies between the Z-lines and is a multiple-protein complex composed of actin and myosin and stabilized by nebulin and titin.[45,46]

The *sliding filament theory* describes the interaction of actin and myosin in molecular cross-bridging, with subsequent shortening of the sarcomere, as a basis for muscle contraction.[45,46] Ultimately, this process is modulated by

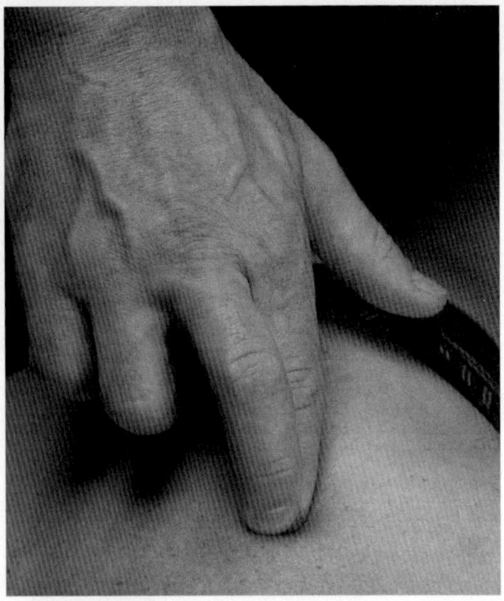

Figure 16-2 Flat palpation. (Courtesy of Myopain Seminars ©2010.)

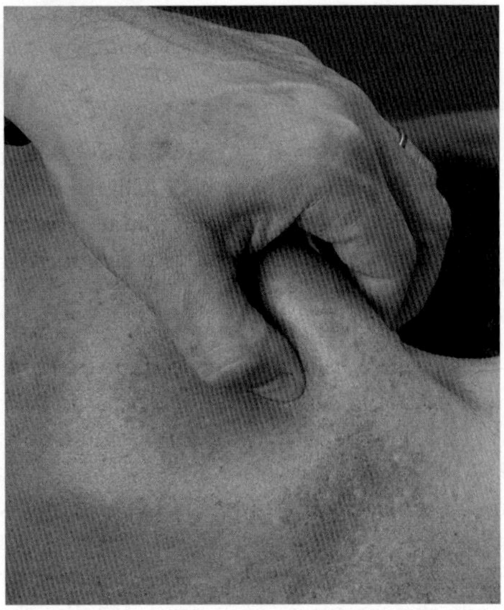

Figure 16-3 Pincer palpation. (Courtesy of Myopain Seminars ©2010.)

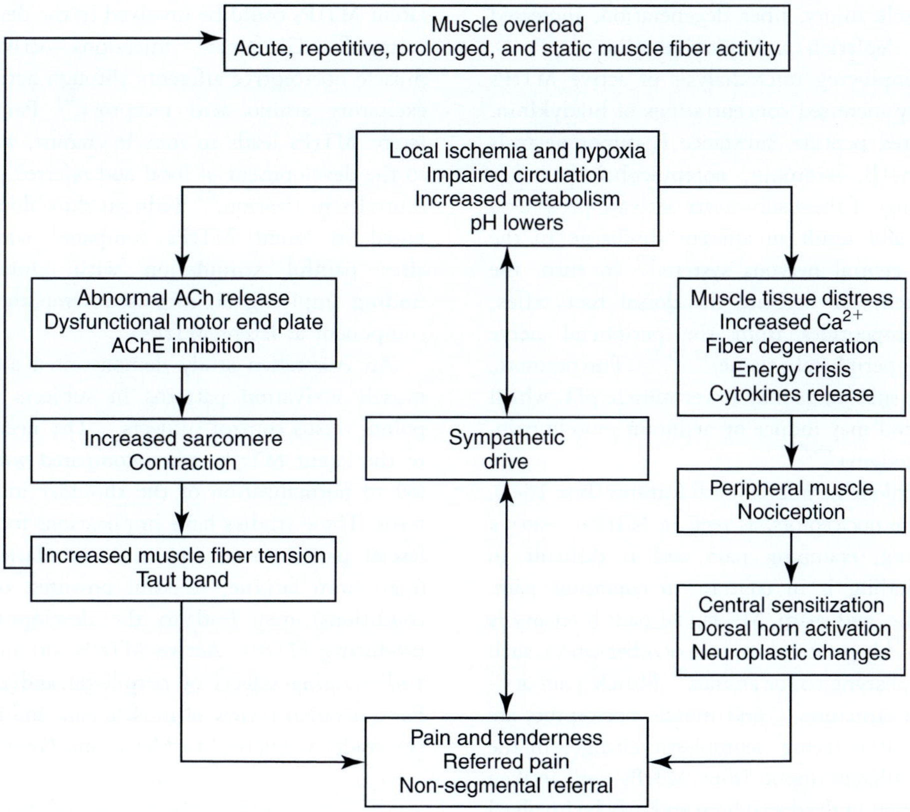

Figure 16-4 Integrated hypothesis of trigger point formation. (Courtesy of Myopain Seminars ©2010.)

the motor neuron at the neuromuscular junction. When an impulse travels along the motor neuron, it depolarizes the membrane, with subsequent release of acetylcholine (ACh) neurotransmitter from the presynaptic boutons into the synaptic cleft. ACh binds to a postsynaptic receptor with depolarization of the membrane and the rise of a miniature end-plate potential (MEPP). When sufficient MEPPs occur, an action potential is propagated, which travels through the T-tubules and thus releases calcium (Ca^{2+}) from the sarcoplasmic reticulum. This process, in turn, stimulates the molecular cross-bridges and closing of the actin and myosin filaments involved in muscle contraction. At the neuromuscular junction, ACh is hydrolyzed by acetylcholinesterase (AChE) into acetate and choline and is recycled into the nerve terminal. ACh release is modulated by motor nerve activity and by the concentration of AChE. Reduction of AChE would result in excess of ACh in the synaptic cleft, with subsequent up-regulation of postsynaptic MEPPs and maintenance of muscle contraction. In essence, this process is very complex.[8,45-47]

The IH postulates that multiple muscle fiber end plates release, or sustain increased concentration of ACh with resultant continued sarcomere contraction without electrogenic activation of the motor end plate.[34] In support of this, electromyographic (EMG) studies have demonstrated that motor end-plate noise is more prevalent in MTrPs than in areas outside this zone.[48-52] The excess ACh results in increased and sustained localized fiber tension. Multiple contraction knots, with areas of sarcomere shortening, have been visualized under light microscopic examination of canine MTrP biopsies.[53] Microscopic studies of MTrPs in cadavers demonstrated split, ragged, and thickened muscle fibers with type II muscle fiber atrophy.[54,55] Another study, conducted with electron microscopy, reported areas of alternatively shortened and lengthened sarcomeres in biopsies of MTrPs.[56] In a rat study, experimentally increased release of ACh from end plates resulted in muscle fiber damage that may be a precursor for MTrP formation.[57] A more recent study, using stimulated single-fiber EMG, demonstrated neuroaxonal degeneration and neuromuscular transmission disorders in MTrPs.[58] Sarcoplasmic reticulum dysfunction of the calcium pump has also been postulated to play a role in MTrP formation.[34]

An adequate number of dysfunctional motor end plates does produce a palpable taut band.[34] in vivo imaging of MTrPs with magnetic resonance and ultrasound elastography visualized the taut band as an area of increased stiffness.[59-61] Adequately trained clinicians are able to locate taut bands reliably, with accuracy that approaches the physical dimensions of the fingertips.[40] These studies support construct validity for the MTrP taut band phenomena.

Acute, repetitive, or prolonged muscle fiber contraction increases local metabolic demand, which may lead to ischemia and hypoxia.[62,63] Active MTrPs demonstrate a highly resistive vascular bed under Doppler imaging within the stiffened region.[61] Muscle ischemia has been shown to activate muscle nociceptors, with resulting pain.[47,64,65] This tissue distress results in local muscle injury, fiber degeneration, increased Ca^{2+} release, energy depletion, and cytokine release.[47]

A novel study employing microdialysis of active MTrPs reported significantly increased concentrations of bradykinin, calcitonin gene–related peptide, substance P, tumor necrosis factor-α, interleukin-1β, serotonin, norepinephrine, and a lowered pH.[66-68] Many of these substances activate peripheral muscle nociceptors and result in afferent discharge to the dorsal horn of the central nervous system.[69] In turn, the central nervous system can activate the dorsal root reflex, which releases neuropeptides from the peripheral nerve terminal into the peripheral tissue.[47,70-72] Furthermore, release of sensitizing substances may lower muscle pH, which may inhibit AChE and may induce or maintain muscle pain, hyperalgesia, and allodynia.[66,67,73]

Muscle pain has unique neurobiological features (Box 16-2). Stimulation of muscle nociceptors, as seen in MTrPs, causes a poorly defined aching, cramping pain and is difficult to localize.[47,74] This finding is in contrast to cutaneous pain, which is local, specific, and sharp. Myofascial pain intensity is comparable to, or possibly greater than, pain of other causes, such as arthritis, cystitis, pharyngitis, or angina.[28] Muscle pain activates unique cortical structures,[75] and muscle nociceptors are particularly effective at inducing neuroplastic changes in the dorsal horn.[76] The afferent input from MTrPs can awaken previously silent neurons in the dorsal horn and may be involved in the spread or referral of muscle pain extrasegmentally.[77,78] Muscle pain can be inhibited strongly by descending pain modulating pathways.[79-81] This finding has implications for management of MTrPs and may explain why muscle pain responds to a broad base of treatments. Furthermore, educating the patient on muscle pain may assist in modulating pain through cognitive pathways.

Active MTrPs have received most attention because of their role in spontaneous pain elicitation; however, interest in latent MTrPs has increased. Activation of latent MTrPs provokes active MTrPs and subsequent pain, under certain circumstances. Subjects with latent MTrPs in the medial gastrocnemius muscle presented with nociceptive hypersensitivity at these latent MTrPs.[82] In another study, muscle cramps were induced in nearly 93% of the subjects following glutamate injections into latent MTrPs, but not in non-MTrP areas, a finding suggesting that appropriately stimulated latent MTrPs could be involved in the development of muscle cramps.[83] Glutamate injections activate small-diameter muscle nociceptive afferents through activation of peripheral excitatory amino acid receptors.[84] Painful stimulation of latent MTrPs leads to muscle cramps, which can contribute to the development of local and referred pain and widespread central sensitization.[85] Reduced skin blood flow response was noted in latent MTrPs compared with non-MTrP areas after painful stimulation with glutamate injection, a finding implying an increased sympathetic vasoconstriction component at latent MTrPs.[86]

An Australian study demonstrated alteration of shoulder muscle activation patterns in subjects with latent trigger points versus control subjects.[87] Dry needling and stretching to the latent MTrPs, when compared with sham ultrasound, led to normalization of the shoulder muscle activation patterns. These studies have implications for patients with myofascial pain because intrinsic stimulation of latent MTrPs (e.g., from fatigue, stressful postures, or certain metabolic conditions) may lead to the development of active pain producing MTrPs. Active MTrPs, in turn, may lead to the wide-ranging effects of peripheral and central sensitization. For a detailed review of muscle pain and central sensitization, the reader is referred to Mense and Gerwin[47] and Sluka.[69]

BOX 16-2 Muscle Pain Characteristics

- Muscle pain causes a poorly defined, aching, cramping type of pain that is difficult to localize.
- MTrP pain intensity is comparable to pain from other causes.
- Muscle pain stimulates unique cortical structures.
- Muscle nociceptors are particularly effective at inducing neuroplastic changes in the dorsal horn.
- MTrPs may refer pain extrasegmentally.
- Muscle pain can be inhibited significantly by descending pain modulating pathways.

MTrP, myofascial trigger point.

ETIOLOGY AND PERPETUATING FACTORS

MTrPs have several potential causes, including low-level muscle contractions, uneven intramuscular pressure distribution, alterations in blood flow, direct trauma, unaccustomed eccentric contractions, eccentric contractions in unconditioned muscle, and maximal or submaximal concentric contractions.[4,7] Skeletal muscle fatigue can lead to an alteration in normal function of the neuromuscular pathway, with a subsequent increase in concentration of ACh and consequences as outlined by the IH.

From a clinical perspective, several proposed factors are relevant to the development of MTrPs. Simons et al[4] identified mechanical, nutritional, metabolic, and psychological precipitating and perpetuating factors. To develop optimum treatment and a suitable plan of care, physical therapists must become aware of these precipitating, predisposing, and perpetuating factors.[4] Some of these factors may lie outside the direct scope of physical therapy, but awareness helps to direct patients to the appropriate health care provider, including a physician or psychologist.[7] Examples of perpetuating factors include the following:

- Mechanical: postural dysfunctions, including forward head posture, excessive thoracic kyphosis, scoliosis, leg length inequalities, pelvic torsion, joint hypermobility, ergonomic habits, poor body mechanics[4,7,88]
- Physiologic: poor sleep hygiene and non-restorative sleep; fatigue; general fitness, conditioning, and coordination, among others[4,7,88,89]
- Medical: hypothyroidism, systemic lupus erythematosus, Lyme disease, ehrlichiosis, candidiasis, interstitial cystitis,

irritable bowel syndrome, and parasitic disease, among others[4,7,88,89]

- Nutritional and metabolic: deficiencies or insufficiencies of vitamin B_1, B_6, B_{12}, C, and D, folic acid, and ferritin, magnesium, and zinc[4,7,88,89]
- Psychological: stress and tension, emotional state, fear avoidance, psychological disorders, mental illness, genetics, patient beliefs, and addictions, among others[4,7,88,89]

MANAGEMENT STRATEGIES

The development of a suitable plan of care for shoulder pain and dysfunction is based on clinical assessment and includes the patient's history, as well as subjective and objective factors. Clinicians should always remain aware of possible differential diagnoses. Shoulder pain may arise from local or referred phenomena, including orthopedic and visceral structures. In relation to the shoulder, a pain profile should be carried out to include the location of pain, the type of pain, the intensity and frequency, aggravating and relieving factors and irritability, and the behavior of complaint. The use of pain drawings may be helpful for assessment and documentation. The history and development of the presenting complaint are important to review. It is essential to examine the patient's lifestyle, including sports, occupation, and hobbies, among others. Recognizing whether the complaint started insidiously or was precipitated by trauma or overuse assists in the differential diagnosis, such as fracture, rotator cuff derangement, or impingement syndrome, and also helps to identify the mechanism of injury. A medical history, medication usage, and a red flag questionnaire should be routinely obtained, to raise the suspicion of possible visceral somatic disease, such as cardiac disease or Pancoast's tumor, etc. In this regard, red flag questions should be part of the routine assessment.[90] For example, the incidence of shoulder adhesive capsulitis in patients with diabetes mellitus is estimated to be two to four times higher than in the general population; adhesive capsulitis affects approximately 20% of persons with diabetes.[91] Chapter 13 reviews visceral referred pain to the shoulder region.

Objectively, the patient should be assessed by an orthopedic physical therapy evaluation, as detailed in other chapters of this book. Attention should be paid to the joints of the shoulder, including the glenohumeral and scapular-thoracic articulations. The neck, thorax, elbow, and hand require screening for differential diagnosis and dysfunction. Key elements of assessment may include the following: observation; static and dynamic postural assessment; and movement testing, including active and passive range of motion and accessory joint mobility. Pain provocation and special tests are essential to the examination process. Of significant importance to muscle and MTrPs are the assessment of muscle length, end feel, and strength and muscle pain provocation tests, including MTrP palpation.

Accessible muscles suspected of harboring MTrPs are skillfully palpated using flat palpation and pincer grip techniques, as previously outlined. These techniques are valuable because they often elicit the patient's pain, a feature of obvious clinical importance. Palpation of muscles for MTrPs usually occurs at the end of the objective orthopedic assessment. This timing reduces the possibility that MTrP palpation-induced pain provocation, or indeed pain relief, will interfere with interpretation of orthopedic tests. Nonetheless, it may be beneficial to treat the MTrP with manual trigger point compression release (TPCR) and to ascertain the effects on the objective findings because the results of the painful arc or impingement tests, for example, often improve. Maitland[92] recommended a test-treat-retest strategy to assess the effects of manual therapy, and this strategy can be adapted to MTrP interventions. From the subjective and objective evaluation, suspicion should be raised about which muscles are potentially involved in the patient's clinical profile.

The most common clinically relevant shoulder muscles that may present with MTrPs are the infraspinatus, supraspinatus, subscapularis, teres minor, trapezius, levator scapulae, latissimus dorsi, and deltoid muscles. Clinicians should not limit themselves to assessing only common muscles, however, but should also remain cognizant of the potential for other muscle involvement (Box 16-3).

BOX 16-3 Common Muscles Involved in Anterior and Posterior Shoulder Pain*

Anterior Shoulder Pain	*Posterior Shoulder Pain*
Infraspinatus	Deltoid
Deltoid	Levator scapulae
Scalene	Supraspinatus
Supraspinatus	Teres major
Pectoralis major	Teres minor
Pectoralis minor	Subscapularis
Biceps brachii	Triceps brachii
Latissimus dorsi	Trapezius

*This is not an exhaustive list. Shoulder muscles may cause pain into the upper arm, forearm, and hand. Refer to Simons, Travell, and Simons[4] and Dejung et al[5] for further information.

REVIEW OF TREATMENT OPTIONS

Treatment options for MTrPs include the following: noninvasive manual therapies; invasive needling therapies; modality-based therapies; exercise therapy; and medical, pharmacologic, and psychological therapies (Fig. 16-5). The main emphases of this section are on TPCR, massage technique, spray and stretch (S&S), invasive needling, modalities, stretch and strengthening, education, and attention to perpetuating factors. This chapter does not cover medical, pharmacologic, injection therapy, or psychological therapies, although the lack of discussion here does not imply that these approaches are not important. Therapeutic options must be considered in relation to the updated IH of trigger point

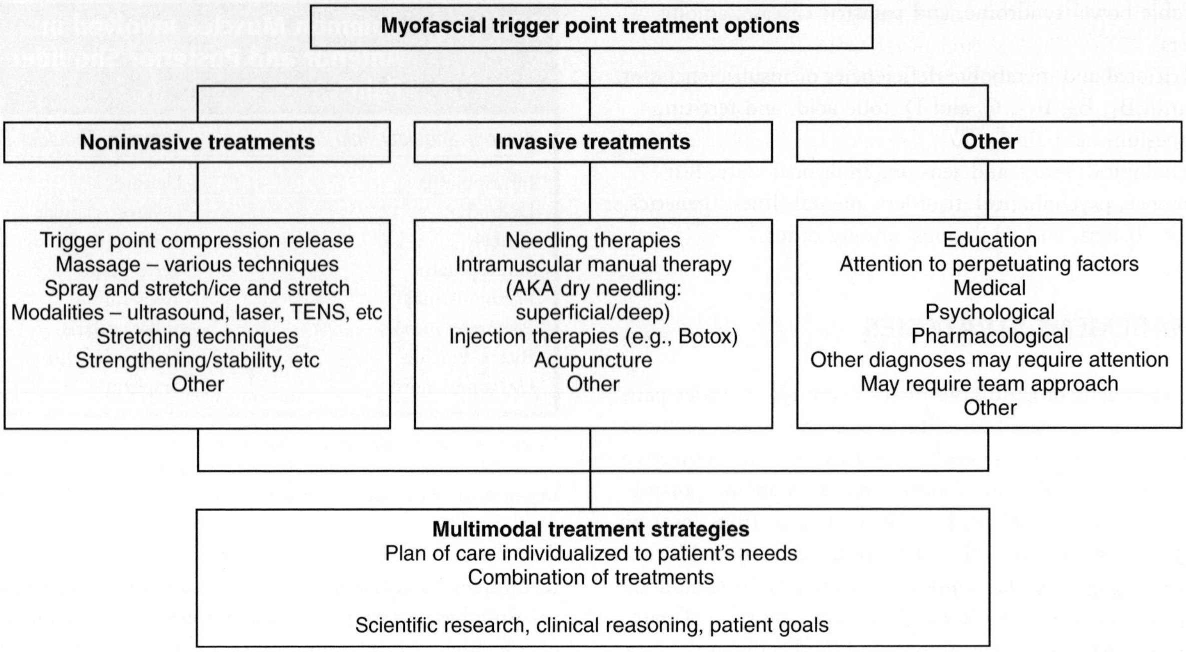

Figure 16-5 Treatment options for myofascial trigger points. (Courtesy of Myopain Seminars ©2010.)

formation and the way in which an individual treatment may affect the mechanisms that lead to the development of the taut band, pain, and sensitization (see Fig. 16-4). A systematic review of noninvasive MTrP treatment has been published,[93,94] as has another publication discussing manual therapies and modalities.[8] Several articles have been published on invasive needling therapies and current practice reviews.[95,96]

TREATMENT TECHNIQUES

The techniques included in this section are examples of treatment options. They are not intended to be comprehensive. Clinicians should refer to other chapters of this book for relevant anatomy, biomechanics, pathomechanics, and manual therapy techniques. Further training, including practical skills, may be required, and clinicians should limit themselves to techniques included in their professional scope of practice. Treatment of musculoskeletal pain with soft tissue techniques should be based on appropriate assessment and development of a plan of care. Clinicians should remain cognizant of treatment contraindications, precautions, and safety issues. Therapists should ensure good body mechanics and avoid prolonged repetitive movements, to reduce the risk of occupational injury and overuse.

Noninvasive Manual Therapies

Noninvasive manual therapies include a plethora of techniques, including TPCR,[4,22] massage,[4,97] myofascial release (MFR),[98-100] S&S,[4,22,101] postisometric relaxation,[102-104] muscle energy technique,[105] neuromuscular technique and therapy,[106,107] manual medicine,[108,109] occipital release and retraction extension,[110] strain counterstrain,[111] and a home program of TPCR,[112] and coupled with sustained stretch.[113] A case study employing Kinesio Taping for MTrPs in the anterior and medial deltoid muscle reported improvement in shoulder range of motion, pain, and function, notwithstanding the limitations of a case study.[114] Traditionally, the most common noninvasive methods used in the treatment of myofascial pain are TPCR, massage techniques, and S&S.

Trigger Point Compression Release and Massage

TPCR was previously known as *ischemic compression*. TPCR is usually considered the primary manual therapy technique for MTrPs and has been described for the majority of muscles.[4,5,22,23] TPCR is believed to compress the contractured sarcomeres when perpendicular pressure is applied to the MTrP, thus leading to longitudinal elongation of the sarcomere.[115] No research has been published to support this hypothesis. Also likely is a reflex neural component that may, in part, offer some understanding of the technique.

With regard to the shoulder, the muscle to be treated is positioned for best access and comfort for the patient. The muscle is placed, when appropriate, in a position of optimal resting tension, to expose the taut band for adequate palpation relative to the surrounding muscle tissue. The clinician should be cognizant of the regional practical anatomy, including the muscle attachments, fiber direction, muscle layers, and surrounding anatomic landmarks. Precautions should be noted to avoid inappropriate stretching, compression, or occlusion of neurovascular structures such as the brachial plexus and subclavian artery.

When the patient is appropriately positioned, the MTrP is located by palpating transverse to the muscle fiber direction of the accessible shoulder muscle. Some muscles have challenging accessibility and make palpation difficult. As an example, the clinician should compare the accessibility to palpation of the supraspinatus or subscapularis with that of the infraspinatus or deltoid. Palpating transverse to the muscle fibers allows optimum exposure of the taut band relative to the surrounding muscle fibers and assists in identification of the tender nodule on the taut band. When the MTrP is identified, it is compressed with the clinician's finger or thumb by flat palpation or a pincer grip. The compression intensity can be in the region of 7/10 on the patient's reported pain scale, and this compression is held until a reduction in discomfort is experienced by the patient; this change may take 20 to 60 seconds or longer.[116] This compression may also be delivered either at low pressure below the patient's pain threshold for a prolonged period (90 seconds) or at high pressure for a shorter duration (30 seconds).[117] The immediate reduction in MTrP sensitivity from TPCR is evidenced by an increase in pain pressure threshold (PPT), and it is not caused by a reduction of palpation pressure by the clinician.[116]

Similar effects were noted for TPCR and transverse friction massage, as described by Cyriax, for MTrPs with a similar reduction in Visual Analog Scale (VAS) score and increase in PPT for both treatments.[118] In clinical practice, it would be judicious to titer the treatment to the individual patient's ability to tolerate manual treatments.

Self induced TPCR to the upper back, with a plastic self-release device, was effective in reducing MTrP irritability.[112] Similarly, a home program of TPCR and stretching was effective in diminishing MTrP sensitivity and pain intensity in individuals with neck and upper back pain.[113] Clearly, it is important to consider education on a home program of self-directed treatment.

Trigger Point Compression Release: Infraspinatus and Teres Minor (Fig. 16-6)

Rationale This technique targets one of the most common muscles in the shoulder region (infraspinatus) that develops MTrPs. The referred pain pattern is expansive and may include the shoulder, forearm, and hand. The infraspinatus muscle is flat, thin, and relatively expansive. To assess the infraspinatus muscle and its neighboring teres minor, the therapist palpates all over the infraspinatus fossa on the posterior scapula.

Patient Position The patient is sitting, side lying (side up), or prone. The shoulder is positioned to place optimum tension on the muscle for MTrP palpation.

Therapist Position The therapist stands behind the patient.

Procedure The infraspinatus muscle is palpated by flat palpation perpendicular to the muscle fiber direction against the infraspinous fossa. In the upper portion, the fibers run in a direction similar to that of the spine of the scapula and more obliquely in the outer lower portion. The clinician assesses the muscle for taut bands with spot tenderness to identify MTrPs.

The procedure is similar for the teres minor. The muscle is located on the lateral aspect of the infraspinous fossa and runs in an oblique direction to the posterior shoulder inserting into the greater tubercle of the humerus

Trigger Point Compression Release: Supraspinatus (Fig. 16-7)

Rationale Palpation of supraspinatus is difficult because of its depth and its position under the trapezius. However, the supraspinatus is an important muscle to be able to identify.

Patient Position The patient is sitting or side lying (side up). The shoulder is positioned to place optimum tension on the muscle for MTrP palpation.

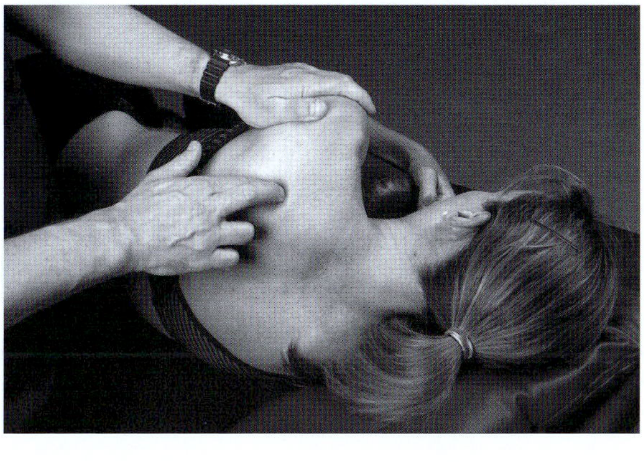

Figure 16-6 Trigger point compression release: infraspinatus and teres minor. (Courtesy of Myopain Seminars ©2010.)

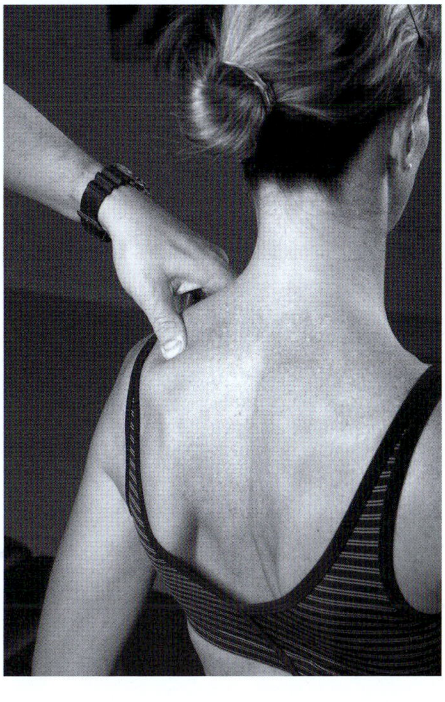

Figure 16-7 Trigger point compression release: supraspinatus. (Courtesy of Myopain Seminars ©2010.)

Therapist Position The therapist stands behind the patient.

Procedure The spine of the scapula and the medial angle are located by palpation; between and below lies the supraspinous fossa. The supraspinatus is palpated through the more superficial trapezius by flat palpation directly into the fossa, by assessing along the length of the muscle. This procedure is challenging, and a taut band is not usually palpable. The clinician assesses for local tenderness and referred pain and for the patient's response to treatment with compression. Caution should be exercised in the lateral portion because of potential, but unlikely, suprascapular nerve compression.

Trigger Point Compression Release: Subscapularis (Fig. 16-8)

Rationale The subscapularis is an important muscle for stabilization of the shoulder, but because of its subscapular position, it is often ignored in palpation. Patients with weakness seen on Gerber's lift-off test or with restricted external rotation, especially neutral, should be assessed for myofascial pain of the subscapularis muscle.

Patient Position The patient is supine, with the arm abducted and laterally rotated, with a degree of shoulder girdle protraction. The shoulder is positioned to place optimum resting tension on the muscle for MTrP palpation, and support may be given by the clinician's non-palpating hand and arm. This position may vary for each individual, and the clinician should seek to adapt this technique to suit the patient's presentation. Caution should be exercised when treating persons with unstable or hypermobile shoulders.

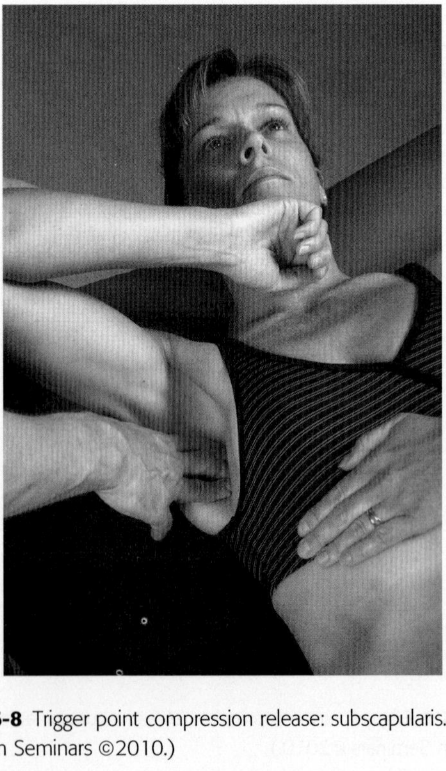

Figure 16-8 Trigger point compression release: subscapularis. (Courtesy of Myopain Seminars ©2010.)

Therapist Position The therapist is in front of the treated side.

Procedure The therapist gently places his or her hand into the patient's lower axilla between the ribs and the bulk of the latissimus dorsi laterally. The therapist then advances gently toward the subscapularis muscle lying against the accessible and lateral part of the subscapular fossa. The muscle is compressed while the therapist looks for localized tenderness and potential referred pain elicitation. Testing and treatment are performed along the accessible length of the muscle. The clinician assesses whether compression changes shoulder external rotation or pain and strength as seen on Gerber's lift-off test. Caution needs to be noted with regard to the axillary neurovascular bundle superiorly.

Trigger Point Compression Release: Upper Trapezius (Fig. 16-9)

Rationale This technique targets the upper trapezius muscle. This is not to say that the lower or middle trapezius is less important, and all parts of the trapezius should be routinely palpated for MTrPs. The trapezius is important for stability of the scapula, and its contribution to shoulder dysfunction should not be underestimated. The upper portion can be palpated using pincer grip, with anterior and posterior access. The middle and lower portions are usually palpated by flat palpation.

Patient Position Sitting and side lying (side up) are the usual preferred positions. The scapula is positioned to place optimum passive tension on the muscle for MTrP palpation.

Therapist Position The therapist is behind the patient.

Procedure The upper trapezius muscle is palpated by pincer grip. The fiber direction runs in an oblique direction upward from the acromion and the spine of the scapula toward the posterior occiput and cervical spine. The clinician assesses the muscle for taut bands with spot tenderness to identify MTrPs along its length from lateral to medial attachments. This muscle is tender to palpation, and the therapist must avoid being aggressive by titrating the palpation pressure.

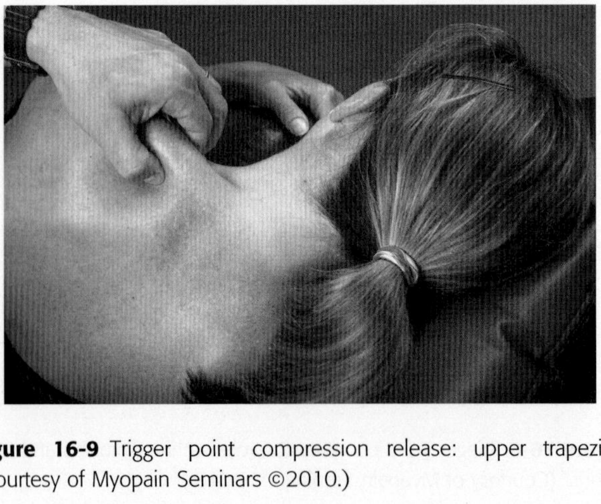

Figure 16-9 Trigger point compression release: upper trapezius. (Courtesy of Myopain Seminars ©2010.)

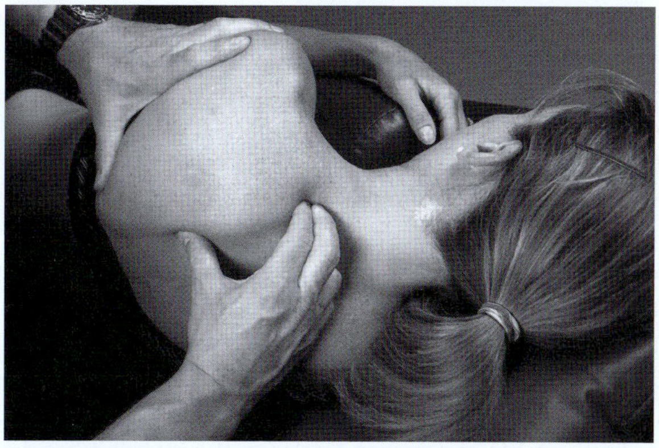

Figure 16-10 Trigger point compression release: levator scapulae. (Courtesy of Myopain Seminars ©2010.)

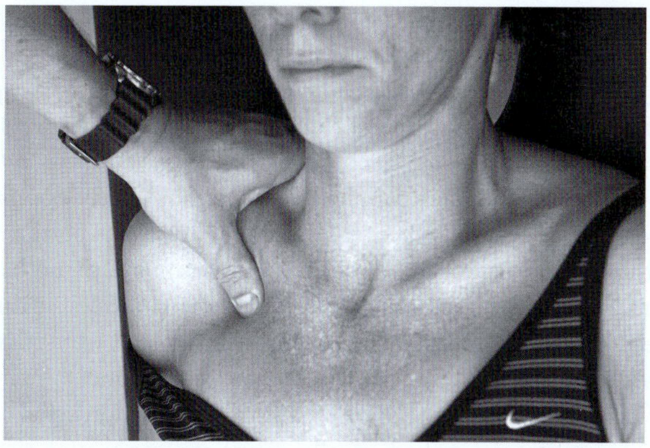

Figure 16-11 Trigger point compression release: pectoralis minor. (Courtesy of Myopain Seminars ©2010.)

Trigger Point Compression Release: Levator Scapulae (Fig. 16-10)

Rationale The levator scapulae is an important muscle in relation to MTrP referral pain at the angle of the neck and along the medial aspect of the scapula. Often, the levator scapulae is a facilitated muscle with high tone and may predispose the scapula to downward rotation, with a resultant effect on the subacromial space. Therefore, it is an important muscle to assess and treat for scapular thoracic and glenohumeral joint dysfunctions. Often, patients also present with shortness of the pectoralis minor in conjunction with levator scapulae dysfunction.

Patient Position The patient is side lying (side up). A pillow is placed to support the patient's head, to optimize the position and tension on the levator scapulae. The shoulder girdle can be elevated or depressed to optimize passive tension.

Therapist Position The therapist is behind the patient.

Procedure The medial angle and upper medial border of the scapula by are located by palpation, and the scapular attachment of the levator scapulae muscle is identified. The inferior part of the muscle can be palpated under the trapezius muscle, especially if it is placed in optimum tension. The muscle is palpated along its length in a transverse fashion from the scapula toward the transverse processes of C1 to C4. The therapist palpates for tenderness, tension, and referred pain.

Trigger Point Compression Release: Pectoralis Minor (Fig. 16-11)

Rationale The action of the pectoralis minor in protracting the scapula as part of postural syndromes and the effect of this muscle on the subacromial space make it an important focus for MTrP release. Often, patients also present with shortness of the levator scapulae in conjunction with pectoralis minor dysfunction.

Patient Position The patient is supine. The patient's hand is placed on the abdomen or is positioned in a degree of abduction with the arm supported to ensure that the pectoral muscles are relaxed. The shoulder girdle can be elevated or depressed, to optimize passive tension on the pectoralis minor.

Therapist Position The therapist is in front of the treated side.

Procedure The coracoid process is located by palpation. From here, at an oblique angle, the pectoralis minor descends medially and inferiorly toward its insertions at the third, fourth, and fifth ribs. The clinician palpates the muscle by flat palpation through the overlying pectoralis major. Here the pectoralis minor can be palpated as a thin, firm muscle. The therapist then assesses for tension, tenderness, and elicited referred pain and compresses for treatment. Caution should be noted with regard to the axillary artery and brachial plexus, which lie inferior to the coracoid process and deep to the upper part of the pectoralis minor muscle.

Massage Therapy

Massage therapy, a traditional keystone of physical therapy, evolved in several European countries in the 19th century.[119-121] In relation to MTrPs, different massage techniques have been proposed, and a potential mechanism of action on MTrPs has been offered.[4,115] The main aim of massage can be considered, similar to TPCR, to lengthen the taut band and increase the local circulation. Massage techniques include kneading, rolling, friction, and stripping strokes along or across the taut band.[97,120,122] Massage strokes may be helpful to assess the localized tissue stiffness characteristics and to aid the clinician in honing in on tender nodules and the taut band of MTrPs. In essence, massage therapy can be used as a dynamic assessment and treatment tool.

In a review of massage therapy for chronic nonspecific low back pain, specific manual massage techniques, such as acupressure, outperformed less specific techniques such as Swedish massage.[123] This finding has implications for the choice of techniques employed to treat MTrPs of the shoulder, and it indicates the importance of specific localization in manual techniques. In practical terms, a combination of

TPCR, massage therapy, and myofascial manipulation (MFM) techniques is suggested as a mainstay of manual therapy.

The muscles of the subscapularis, supraspinatus, infraspinatus, and teres minor blend through their fascial and tendon attachments with the glenohumeral capsule and are often implicated in shoulder pain and dysfunction. Cyriax popularized *friction massage,* which is a common treatment option for pain and scar tissue and is also used to stimulate tissue healing, especially for tendons.[124,125] Other techniques include the Graston technique, an instrument-assisted soft tissue mobilization method.[126-128] These techniques aim to influence connective tissue mobility and stimulation by employing forces applied usually across the connective tissue fibers.[129] Clinical evidence for friction massage in tendinitis is limited, and future research is needed.[130-132] However, friction massage remains a popular treatment option, often based on clinical observation. Techniques for the rotator cuff tendons are included later in this chapter.

Massage Technique: Posterior Scapular Region (Fig. 16-12)

Rationale Massage techniques may be beneficial for certain pain conditions, especially when these techniques are more specifically directed. Massage is also valuable for assessing the quality and tonal elastic properties of connective tissues and for assessing pain response to pressure. MTrPs can be identified and located for treatment. Areas of restrictions can be identified. Massage is a dynamic process in which assessment and treatment are often carried out simultaneously. The value of massage technique should not be underestimated. Massage can be combined with TPCR or MFM techniques.

Patient Position The patient is supine, with the shoulder maintained in a comfortable position, or the patient can be side lying, with the arm and shoulder supported.

Therapist Position The therapist is on the treated side, maintaining good body mechanics.

Procedure The therapist can assess the postscapular region by using various massage strokes, including effleurage and kneading parallel and perpendicular to the muscle fiber directions. Therapists should remain cognizant of muscle fiber direction and muscle layers from superficial to deep. Here the therapist can readily assess the latissimus dorsi, trapezius, rhomboids, levator scapulae, infraspinatus, teres minor, teres major, deltoid, triceps, and lateral part of the serratus anterior (usually best access in side lying) muscles. When MTrPs are identified, the direct technique can be applied using TPCR. This treatment can be interspersed with soft tissue massage, such as effleurage and kneading from the center of the trigger point away in both directions. Friction massage can be used to treat MTrPs; however, TPCR may be more tolerable. Friction massage can be introduced to areas of significant restrictions and tenderness as appropriate and titrated to suit the individual patient. Massage is usually well tolerated and should be of an intensity tailored to the patient. Caution should be exercised in patients with allodynia.

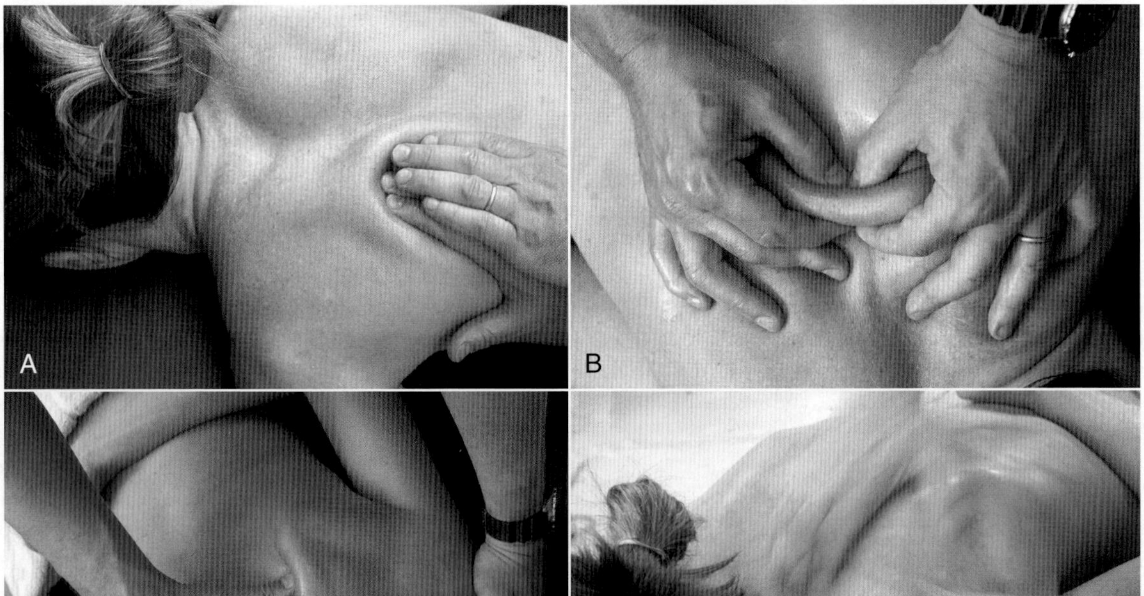

Figure 16-12 A to **D,** Massage technique: posterior scapular region. (Courtesy of Myopain Seminars ©2010.)

Massage techniques can also be applied to the lateral and anterior chest areas to incorporate treatment to muscles such as the pectoralis major, pectoralis minor, anterior deltoid, and biceps. Appropriate draping is important.

Friction Massage: Rotator Cuff (Fig. 16-13)

Rationale This treatment is used to relieve pain and to stimulate tendon healing.

Patient Position The patient is sitting supported for the subscapularis and supraspinatus muscles and is sitting or prone for the infraspinatus and teres minor muscles.

Therapist Position The therapist stands behind the patient on the treated side. For the friction massage technique, the therapist supports the index finger by crossing the middle finger over it.

Procedure The tendon to be treated is located by functional testing and is positioned to offer best exposure. The therapist contacts the tendon with the reinforced finger and moves transversely across the tendon to ensure that the fingers move with the patient's skin as one, to prevent skin friction burn, blistering, and bruising. No oil is used, and the patient's skin should be dry. Usually, local tissue anesthesia occurs within 2 to 3 minutes, and caution should be exercised if this does not occur or if the treatment appears to aggravate the condition. The friction treatment generally lasts up to 10 minutes or longer, and treatment frequency may vary from one to three times per week. Contraindications include, but

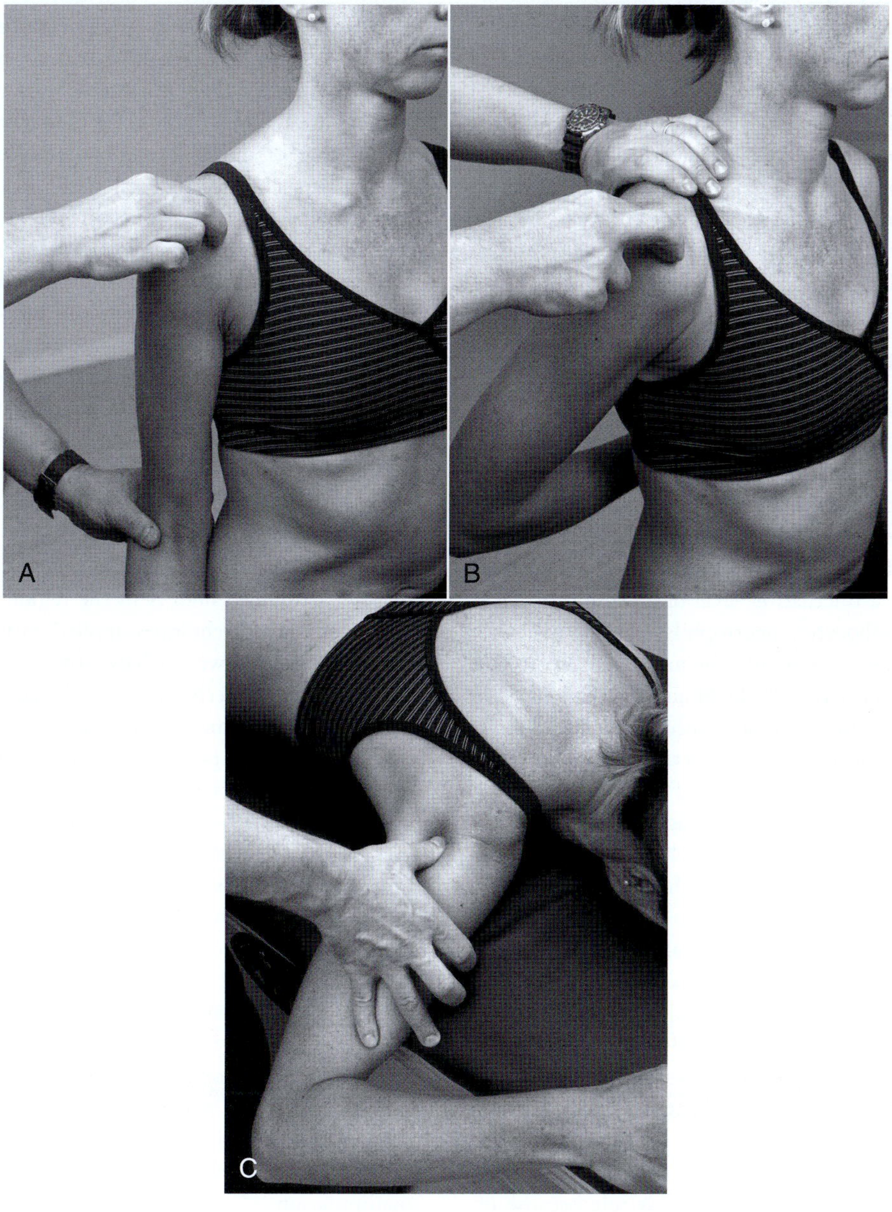

Figure 16-13 A to **C,** Friction massage: rotator cuff. (Courtesy of Myopain Seminars ©2010.)

are not limited to, acute injuries, infections, hematoma, and skin conditions, and special caution is needed in patients with poor circulation or diabetes or in patients who take blood thinning medication.

- Subscapularis: The patient's arm is in neutral, supported with some external rotation to rotate the lesser tubercle laterally to access the tendon. The tendon lies medial to the lesser tubercle and lateral and somewhat inferior to the coracoid process. Friction is carried out in a superior-inferior direction.
- Supraspinatus: The patient's arm is in extension, adduction, and internal rotation. The tendon inserts into the superior aspect of the greater tubercle of the humerus, which is located just inferior to the anterior-lateral acromion. Friction is carried out transversely across the tendon in an inferior-medial–superior-lateral direction.
- Infraspinatus and teres minor: The patient is prone, with the arm off the edge of the bed and supported. The spine of the scapula and the infraspinous fossa are identified from where the infraspinatus muscle arises. From here, the therapist tracks the muscle up to its insertion to the greater tubercle of the humerus at the posterior shoulder. The tendon of the infraspinatus lies superior to that of the teres minor, and both are covered in the posterior shoulder region by the posterior deltoid. Palpation through the relaxed posterior deltoid friction is delivered in an almost superior-inferior direction.

Myofascial Manipulation

The word *fascia* is derived from the Latin word for "band" and refers to sheets of dense fibrous connective tissue that envelop body structures. Fascia plays an essential role in human structure, movement, function, and defense.[133] Connective tissue is made up of specific cells and extracellular matrix (ECM), including fibroblasts, adipocytes, and mesenchymal stem cells, as well as a fluctuating level of defense cells such as macrophages, lymphocytes, neutrophils, eosinophils, and mast cells.[133] Fibroblasts are usually the most abundant cells; they synthesize the majority of the ECM and therefore play an essential role in the maintenance of connective tissue.[133]

Myofibroblasts are specialized contractile fibroblasts that have been reported to function in wound contraction[134] and are present in fascial tissues.[135,136] Fibroblastic activity is influenced by injury, mechanical stress, steroid hormone levels, and dietary content.[133] The ECM consists of the extracellular substances, namely, insoluble protein fibrils, including collagen and elastin, and soluble proteoglycans, and it functions to oppose stresses of movement and gravity while also maintaining structure and shape.[133] The collagen and elastin components of the ECM resist mainly tensile forces, whereas proteoglycans oppose primarily compressive forces.[133]

Fascia is richly innervated by mechanoreceptors with a sympathetic nerve supply.[135-141] Schleip et al[142] proposed that fascia has a neurosensory transducer function and may be in an advantageous position to fulfill this role because of its position farther from the axis of movement compared with joint ligaments. Furthermore, fascia assists in load transfer among the spine, pelvis, legs, and arms and acts as an integrated functional stability system.[143,144] The anatomy of the pectoral and upper limb myofascial complex has been described in detail, and investigators have linked its importance to force transmission between the upper and lower extremities.[145-149] Myofascial expansions show a similarity to MTrP referral patterns, and this is an area for further investigation.[145] This similarity has implications for treatment of the shoulder region and suggests the importance of the interdependence of parts of the kinetic chain. For example, one should consider the interactions among the lower extremity, hip, pelvis spine, trunk, shoulder, and upper limb during javelin throwing or baseball pitching.

Numerous descriptions of soft tissue techniques for the treatment of myofascia,[150] including MFR,[98-100] Rolfing,[151] MFM,[152] fascial manipulation (FM),[148,150] and neuromuscular technique[153] have been published. Fascia is responsive to mechanical load and demonstrates plastic properties.[135,136,140,141,154] The so-called tissue release, felt by the clinician during MFM, MFR, or FM, is purportedly the result of mechanical stress induced by the technique.[141] In addition, stimulation of mechanoreceptors reduces sympathetic tonus and induces changes in local tissue viscosity, which may in part explain the release phenomenon.[141] Such benefits may influence myofascial proprioception and nociception and may assist in addressing postural syndromes, such as protracted shoulders and forward head postures.

In practical terms, MFM should be directed at primary short and tight myofascial tissues in a slow and melting manner, to induce a parasympathetic state and to avoid myotatic stretch reflexes.[140] Attention should also be given to the antagonistic muscles of the related joint.[140] The techniques may involve manual stretching, by taking up the slack around a restriction, engaging the barrier, and holding until a release is experienced, which may take a few seconds to a half a minute or longer.[99,104] In MFR, sustained hold is in the region of 90 to 120 seconds or longer.[98] FM techniques applied to fascial densities in the low back was shown to halve the pain in a mean time of 3.24 minutes.[129] Techniques may be augmented by limb pulling or trunk rotations.[99] Local manual techniques, such as skin rolling, folding, or pressing, may be employed for local areas of restriction.[104] In essence, MFM is a skilled technique whereby the clinician is assessing and treating interactively during the process. Needle therapies and acupuncture may affect fascia because needle manipulation techniques have been shown to induce extensive fibroblast spreading.[155,156]

Common areas of shoulder restriction include the anterior pectoral myofascial structures, including the pectoralis minor, and the posterior neck region, involving the levator scapulae. Clinicians should consider the shoulder myofascial complex and continuity in relation to the whole kinetic chain.

FM technique apparently restores impeded gliding of collagen and elastic fibers within the ground substance by exploiting heat generated from the friction of deep manipulation.[129] The effectiveness of FM in reducing shoulder pain was shown in a cohort of 28 patients. The FM consisted of deep kneading of muscular fascia at specific points along myofascial sequences.[150] Examples of techniques are presented in this section, and additional techniques for the shoulder complex are offered elsewhere in this book. Donatelli popularized a clinically useful scapular distraction technique (see Chapter 14).

Traditionally, the main focus of MFM, MFR, and FM has been on the myofascial complex and not directly on MTrPs, and to what extent these techniques benefit patients with MTrPs is unknown.[4] It is possible that MFM, MFR, and FM have both direct and indirect effects on MTrPs. Interest in fascia has increased, as evidenced by the international Fascia Research Congresses. Despite this development, many questions remain unanswered. For example, what is the role of perimysium in the formation of MTrPs, given its role in muscle contractibility? Does MTrP dry needling stimulate connective tissue or muscle fibroblasts, and does that contribute to the immediate reduction in pain following needling procedures.[157]

Myofascial Manipulation: Scapular–Thoracic Soft Tissue Mobilization (Fig. 16-14)

Rationale This general technique mobilizes the soft tissue components of the scapula-thoracic articulation. The position for this procedure allows a dynamic mobilization technique. The therapist can access passive restrictions in scapular movement and can use the position to mobilize and stretch scapular and thoracic soft tissue.

Patient Position The patient is side lying, treated side upward. The patient's arm should be comfortably positioned on a pillow.

Therapist Position The therapist stands facing the patient. The therapist's upper hand cups the acromion, and the lower hand acts as the dynamic mobilizer.

Procedure The scapula can be moved and dynamically assessed and mobilized in its planes of movement or in combinations of these movements: elevation, depression, protraction, retraction, lateral rotation, medial rotation, upward rotation, downward rotation, and anterior and posterior tipping. This procedure can be very beneficial in improving dynamic mobility around the scapula thoracic joint. It can also help to identify potential restrictions in myofascia and to identify areas for more localized soft tissue therapy such as TPCR or intramuscular manual therapy (IMT).

Myofascial Manipulation: Pectoralis Minor Release (Fig. 16-15)

Rationale This specific soft tissue technique assists in releasing the pectoralis minor and superficial anterior chest fascia. It is a popular technique for addressing a tight pectoralis minor muscle, as seen in the Janda crossed syndrome of the shoulder girdle. When this muscle is found to be tight, it is important to assess the levator scapulae also.

Patient Position The patient is supine, with the arm by the side and the hand on the chest.

Therapist Position The therapist stands at the head of the patient. One of the therapist's hands is placed on the patient's hand that is resting on the chest. The therapist's other hand isolates the coracoid process.

Procedure A suitable force is applied to distance the clinician's hands, which are near for applying a force along the superficial anterior chest fascia and pectoralis minor. The therapist holds with low force and waits until a release is felt, which may take 30 seconds to several minutes. This technique can be adapted for pectoralis major, clavicular, sternal, and costal sections by applying forces along the fiber direction with a similar technique.

Myofascial Manipulation: Scapular-Cervical Mobilization (Fig. 16-16)

Rationale The relationship of the cervical spine with the shoulder should not be overlooked. It is always wise to screen the neck for dysfunction. The trapezius and levator scapulae muscles have an important role in elevating the scapula. The levator scapulae may also act as a downward rotator, however, and therefore when facilitated may affect scapular-thoracic and glenohumeral joint motion.

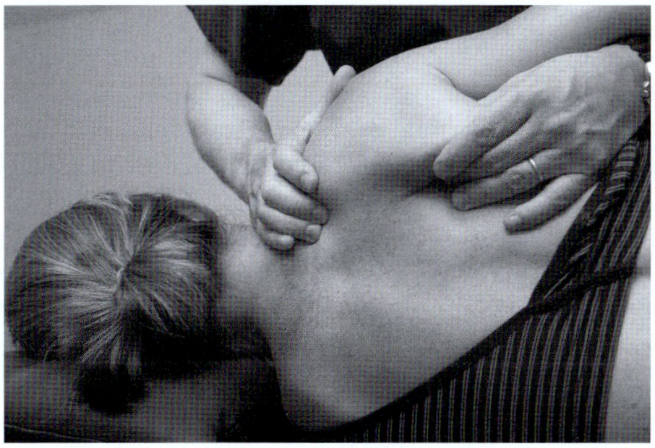

Figure 16-14 Myofascial manipulation: scapular–thoracic soft tissue mobilization. (Courtesy of Myopain Seminars ©2010.)

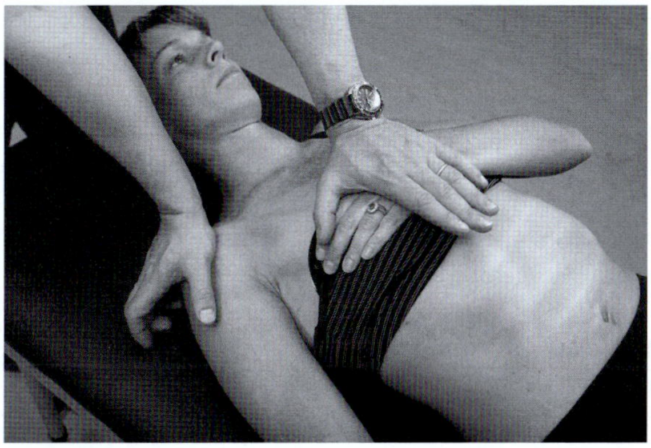

Figure 16-15 Myofascial manipulation: pectoralis minor release. (Courtesy of Myopain Seminars ©2010.)

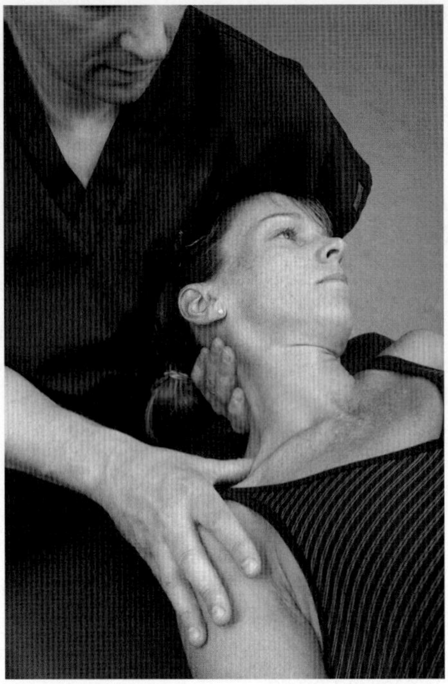

Figure 16-16 Myofascial manipulation: scapular-cervical mobilization. (Courtesy of Myopain Seminars ©2010.)

Patient Position The patient is supine, with hands resting on the abdomen.

Therapist Position The therapist is standing or seated directly at the head of the patient. One of the therapist's hands cradles the patient's cervical spine at the occiput, with the patient's head resting on the forearm of the therapist. The therapist's other hand is placed on the superior aspect of the shoulder joint at the acromion.

Procedure The patient relaxes, and the clinician gently and slowly assesses the quality of passive movement of the neck with combinations of side flexion, forward flexion, and rotation. This dynamic procedure assesses for restrictions or tension. At these points, the patient is gently stretched by using both clinician sensitivity and patient feedback. The therapist's opposite hand can depress the acromion. This technique helps to stretch the posterior lateral neck structures, particularly the upper trapezius and levator scapulae. The therapist holds with low force and waits until a release is felt, which may take 30 seconds to several minutes. This maneuver can be combined with TPCR of the upper trapezius and levator scapulae. Caution should be exercised with this technique in patients with suspected or confirmed acute or chronic discogenic, arthrogenic, and neurogenic diagnoses.

Myofascial Manipulation: Anterior Lateral Fascial Elongation (Fig. 16-17)

Rationale This technique insists in releasing the superficial anterior fascia. This fascia can often be restricted in patients with rounded shoulder, kyphosis, protracted shoulder girdle postures, and a tight sternal-xiphoid-symphyseal line.

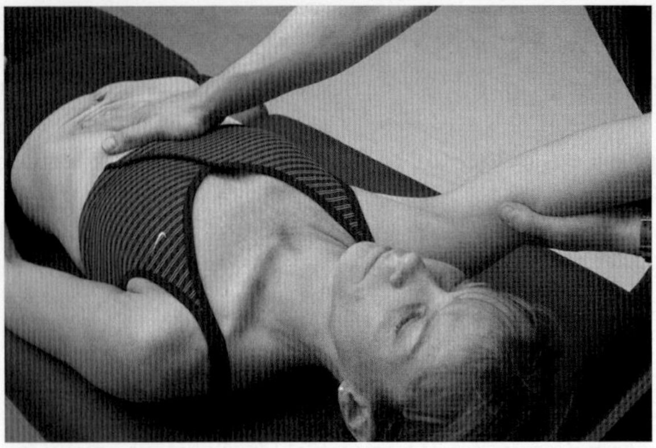

Figure 16-17 Myofascial manipulation: anterior lateral fascial elongation. (Courtesy of Myopain Seminars ©2010.)

Patient Position The patient is supine, with the shoulder elevated to the appropriate angle to engage the restriction.

Therapist Position The therapist is on the treated side and supports the patient's arm while applying gentle traction to the limb. The therapist's opposite hand is placed appropriately on the patient's lower ribs below the breast line.

Procedure The therapist applies a suitable traction force to the patient's arm while applying a simultaneous force caudally on the lower chest in the direction of the palpated restrictions. This dynamic process alters and adjusts forces to meet the changing fascial limitations. The therapist holds with low force and waits until a release is felt, which may take 30 seconds to several minutes. This technique can also be carried out with pelvic rotation, to alter the forces on the anterior fascial slings and muscles.

Spray and Stretch

The S&S technique was a foundation of the Travell and Simons approach to the management of MTrPs,[4,22,23] and it was initially described by Dr. Hans Kraus in 1941.[158] A vapocoolant spray, such as ethyl chloride, fluoromethane, or a combination of pentafluoropropane and tetrafluoroethane, is sprayed directly on the skin over the muscle and referral zone of the MTrP in several sweeps as the muscle is stretched. This procedure is repeated approximately three times; thereafter, the skin should be rewarmed with a hot pack.[4] The technique may produce an afferent sensory barrage, which may inhibit local muscle contraction by affecting the efferent neuromuscular activity and permitting more beneficial stretching of the target muscle.[4] In place of S&S, ice and stretch (I&S) have been employed, in which ice held in an insulated cup is passed over the skin. Vapocoolants can be expensive and hazardous, and they threaten the environment by ozone depletion or greenhouse gas effects. No published research has compared S&S with I&S. In myofascial pain, S&S and I&S are used to reduce pain and to increase range of motion. They may be the most effective noninvasive methods for inactivation of acute MTrPs.[4]

One study supported the use of S&S over stretch alone in increasing hip flexion range of motion.[101] S&S had a positive effect on the VAS score and PPT in patients with neck pain.[159] S&S had immediate positive effects on PPT and was more effective when combined with deep pressure massage than were a hot pack and ultrasound.[160] In a multimodal trial, S&S were more effective when combined with other modalities than a hot pack and active range of motion.[117] A more recent study compared S&S with S&S and skin rewarming with a moist heat pack on MTrPs in the upper trapezius.[161] Adding skin rewarming improved VAS scores and cervical range of motion, but not the PPT of MTrPs.[161] A case study describing S&S for myofascial pain of the posterior shoulder reported significant pain relief with treatment to the subscapularis, among other muscles, coupled with stretching of tight pectoral muscles and attention to posture in a 59-year-old dentist.[162]

S&S can be a valuable technique for treatment of shoulder muscles. Nevertheless, I&S is preferred over S&S for the safety and environmental reasons noted earlier.

Ice and Stretch: Latissimus dorsi in the Side-Lying Position (Fig. 16-18)

Rationale The bulk of the latissimus dorsi, with its large expanse from the hip to the shoulder, makes it an excellent candidate for I&S.

Patient Position The patient is side lying, with the arm elevated above the head (side up), or the patient is supine, crook lying, with arm elevation.

Therapist Position The therapist stands at the head of the patient and holds the patient's humerus.

Procedure Ice is passed along the skin overlying the latissimus dorsi and along the posterior (medial and lateral) aspect of the arm, in sweeps, as the therapist pushes the humerus down to stretch the latissimus dorsi. To increase the stretch, a foam roll may be placed under the opposite side of the rib-ilium space to augment side flexion and to increase the stretch on the latissimus dorsi. This muscle can also be treated when the patient is supine, and in this position it allows a combination of muscles to be treated, including the pectoralis minor, pectoralis major, and subscapularis, combined with the latissimus dorsi.

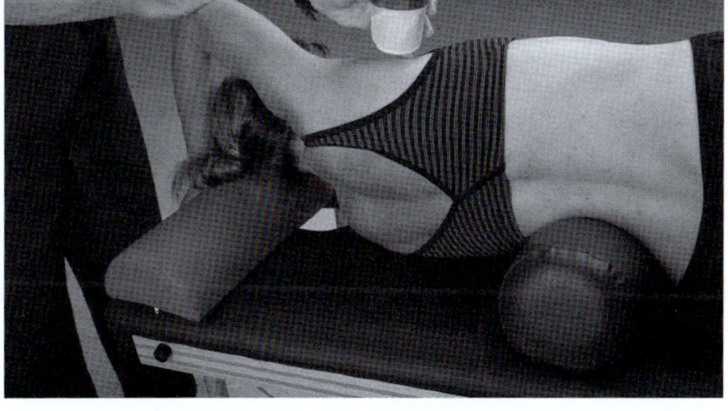

Figure 16-18 Ice & stretch: latissimus dorsi, side-lying position. (Courtesy of Myopain Seminars ©2010.)

Trigger Point Intramuscular Manual Therapy/Dry Needling

Trigger point IMT, also known as trigger point dry needling (TrP-DN), is an invasive therapy in which an acupuncture needle is inserted into the skin, fascia, and muscle to treat MTrPs.[95] Different needling techniques and models are available, including trigger point, radiculopathy, and spinal segmental sensitization models.[21,95,96,163-166] The two main MTrP needling techniques are superficial dry needling (SDN) and deep dry needling (TrP-DN). SDN usually entails inserting a needle into the skin or fascia overlying a trigger point, and was popularized by Dr. Peter Baldry in the early 1980s as a safer approach to needling certain more difficult muscles such as the scalene muscles.[95,166] In contrast, during TrP-DN, the needle is inserted directly into the MTrP, and the main aim is to elicit LTRs, which occur during dynamic needle penetration of the MTrP. The reproduction of LTRs during needling therapy is essential and is associated with improved outcomes; direct needling of MTrPs appears to be an effective treatment for pain.[167,168] Historically, TrP-DN developed from Travell's trigger point injection technique, in which local anesthetic was injected into the MTrP while the hypodermic needle was moved through the muscle to elicit LTRs.[21] Investigators proposed, and later supported, that the therapeutic effect was likely related to the mechanical movement of the needle and the elicitation of LTRs, as opposed to the anesthetic or fluid effect.[21,167-169]

The exact mechanism of action of TrP-DN on myofascial pain is not known, but investigators have reported that TrP-DN reduced nociceptive chemical concentrations in the vicinity of active MTrPs.[66,67] In an animal study, TrP-DN was effective at diminishing spontaneous electrical activity (end-plate noise) when LTRs were elicited.[170] Other modes of action of analgesia have been proposed from experimental animal studies including recovery of circulation[171] and descending pain inhibitory system.[172,173]

A meta-analysis of MTrP needling therapies supported the use of this approach in the treatment of pain, but this analysis could not conclude efficacy beyond placebo, mainly because of the difficulty of placebo needling design.[168] A Cochrane database systematic review supported the use of TrP-DN for chronic low back pain, especially when combined with other treatments.[174] TrP-DN was reported to offer pain relief and improvement in quality of life in older patients with osteoarthritic knee pain,[175] neck pain,[176] and low back pain,[177] when compared with acupuncture.

In patients with bilateral shoulder pain, with active MTrPs in the infraspinatus muscles, TrP-DN of the infraspinatus muscle increased active and passive range-of-shoulder internal rotation and PPT of MTrPs and reduced pain, compared with the control side.[178] In addition, TrP-DN of a primary MTrP (infraspinatus) inhibited the activity in satellite MTrPs (situated in the referral zone of primary MTrP) in the anterior deltoid and extensor carpi radialis longus muscles.[178] In another study, TrP-DN, as part of a rehabilitation program, was reported to be superior to standard rehabilitation alone in the treatment of hemiparetic shoulder pain syndrome.[179] The TrP-DN group demonstrated significant decreases in the severity and frequency of perceived pain, reduced use of analgesic medications, more normal sleep patterns, and increased compliance with the rehabilitation program.[179] TrP-DN of the extensor carpi radialis longus muscle reduced pain intensity, increased the pressure threshold in the ipsilateral trapezius muscle, and increased cervical spine range of motion in patients with active MTrPs in the upper trapezius.[180]

Three case studies of shoulder impingement in tennis and racquetball players who were treated with TrP-DN and stretching to the subscapularis muscle described successful treatment and return to painless function.[181] A more recent case study series described the treatment of four female international volleyball players who received TrP-DN to the infraspinatus (4), teres minor (4), and anterior deltoid (2) muscles, with improvement in verbal pain score and range of motion of the shoulder after treatment.[182] One session of TrP-DN to the supraspinatus evoked short-term segmental antinociceptive effects in the C5 segment when compared with a control group.[183] Latent MTrPs affected muscle activation patterns of the shoulder, as measured by EMG, when compared with control subjects, and TrP-DN and stretching restored the muscle activation to normal.[87] This finding has clinical implications because the aim of shoulder rehabilitation is often to improve and normalize glenohumeral and scapular function.

TrP-DN requires fundamental skills and training for safe and efficient practice. Clinicians should seek suitable training, should ensure that TrP-DN falls within their scope of practice, and should follow local laws and insurance policies.

Trigger Point Intramuscular Manual Therapy/Dry Needling: Infraspinatus (Fig. 16-19)

Rationale The infraspinatus is one of the most common muscles of the shoulder to harbor active MTrPs. The muscle is easily accessible and responds well to trigger point IMT.

Patient Position The patient is prone or side lying, with the arm positioned optimally to expose the MTrP for palpation.

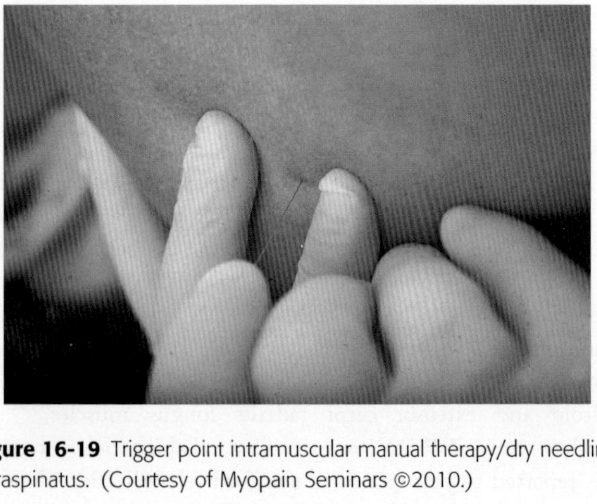

Figure 16-19 Trigger point intramuscular manual therapy/dry needling: infraspinatus. (Courtesy of Myopain Seminars ©2010.)

Therapist Position The therapist can stand or sit behind the patient.

Procedure The medial and lateral borders of the scapula and the spine of the scapula are identified by palpation. Next, the infraspinatus muscle is palpated for MTrPs, and the palpating hand locates the taut band. Landmarks are checked again, and the needle is inserted into the MTrP and is moved in and out of the muscle with the aim of eliciting LTRs. During needling, the needle is drawn back to the fascia and is redirected into the muscle at a new angle. Depending on the patient's tolerance, needling is continued until LTRs are reduced or eradicated. The needle is removed and disposed of appropriately, and hemostasis is applied for 30 seconds or as needed. The muscle is then put through gentle stretching or range of motion after needling as appropriate. The main caution here is to protect the lung and prevent pneumothorax.

This procedure is carried out with universal precautions and sterile single-use disposable needles only. Dry needling should be performed only by a licensed health care practitioner who has been adequately trained and who is permitted by local laws to practice dry needling within the state or jurisdiction.

Trigger Point Intramuscular Manual Therapy/Dry Needling: Lateral Subscapularis (Position 1) (Fig. 16-20)

Rationale The subscapularis muscle is not readily accessible. The IMT technique can allow access to parts of this muscle that are not accessible manually.

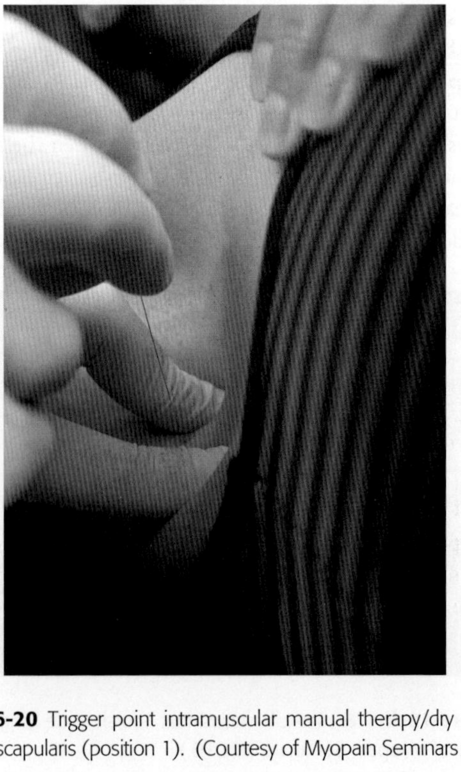

Figure 16-20 Trigger point intramuscular manual therapy/dry needling: lateral subscapularis (position 1). (Courtesy of Myopain Seminars ©2010.)

Patient Position The patient is supine, with the arm abducted and laterally rotated with a degree of shoulder girdle protraction. The shoulder is positioned to place optimum resting tension on the muscle for MTrP palpation, and support may be given by the clinician's non-palpating hand and arm. This position may vary for each individual, and the clinician should seek to adapt this technique to suit the patient's presentation. Caution should be exercised with persons with unstable or hypermobile shoulders.

Therapist Position The therapist sits or stands in front of the treated side.

Procedure The palpating hand is placed flat against the lateral border of the scapula, with fingertips resting against the patient's ribs. The needle is inserted perpendicular to the scapula between the palpating fingers and parallel to the ribs. The needle is not directed toward the ribs. The needle is advanced slowly to elicit LTRs in the subscapularis muscle. Again, treatment is set to the tolerance of the patient, and hemostasis is applied after treatment. The muscle is put through gentle stretching or range of motion after needling as appropriate. The main caution here is to protect the lung and prevent pneumothorax.

Trigger Point Intramuscular Manual Therapy/Dry Needling: Medial Subscapularis, Lateral Aspect of the Rhomboids, and Medial Serratus Anterior (Position 2) (Fig. 16-21)

Rationale The subscapularis is not readily accessible. The IMT technique can allow access to parts of this muscle that are not accessible manually.

Patient Position The patient is in the prone position, with the hand behind the back in the hammerlock position, with the elbow supported. This position assists to wing the scapula and to raise the medial border to allow access to the subscapularis between the scapula and the thorax.

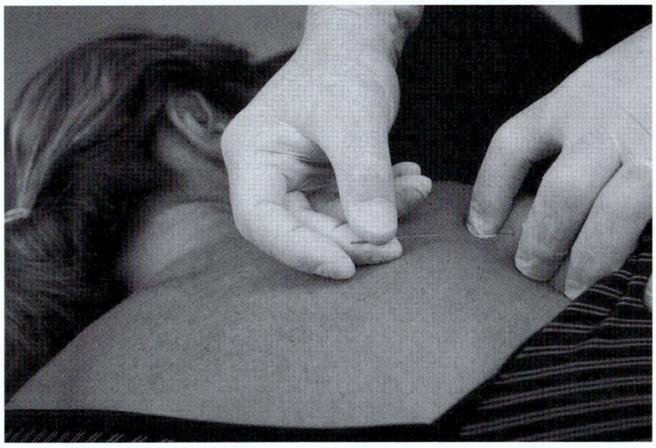

Figure 16-21 Trigger point intramuscular manual therapy/dry needling: medial subscapularis, lateral aspect of the rhomboids, and medial serratus anterior (position 2). (Courtesy of Myopain Seminars ©2010.)

Therapist Position The therapist is standing on the treated side.

Procedure The palpating hand raises the medial border of the scapula away from the thorax to accentuate the subscapular-thoracic space. The needle is inserted toward the subscapular fossa, parallel to the ribs. The needle is never directed toward the ribs or lung. From here, the medial subscapularis, the lateral aspect of the rhomboids, and the medial serratus anterior muscle can be accessed. Again, needling is carried out to elicit LTRs within the patient's tolerance. The muscles are put through gentle stretching or range of motion after needling as appropriate. The main caution here is to protect the lung and prevent pneumothorax.

The procedure is carried out with universal precautions and sterile single-use disposable needles only. Dry needling should be performed only by a licensed health care practitioner who has been adequately trained and who is permitted by local laws to practice dry needling within the state or jurisdiction.

Modality-Based Physical Therapies

Many different types of modality-based physical therapies have been recommended in the treatment of MTrPs. These include ultrasound, laser, transcutaneous electrical nerve stimulation (TENS), interferential current (IFC), and shock waves.[4,8,93,94,184]

Ultrasound

Evidence for therapeutic ultrasound in the management of MTrPs is conflicting.[8,93,94] A study exploring the immediate antinociceptive effect of ultrasound on MTrP sensitivity reported a significant but short-term increase in PPT after 5 minutes of 1 W/cm^2, 100% (1 MHz), with no change noted in the control group (5 minutes of 0.1W/cm^2, 100% 1 MHz),[185] a finding suggesting dose specificity. Another study showed that ultrasound to shoulder MTrPs had a short-term neurosegmental antinociceptive effect and, as such, may be beneficial to decrease pain sensitivity temporarily.[186] The clinical applicability is however, limited by the short-term effect. Both phonophoresis and ultrasound were equally effective over placebo in treating neck MTrPs, in reducing pain, and in improving neck disability index scores.[187] A high-power pain threshold (HPPT) static continuous ultrasound technique offered greater pain reduction in active MTrPs of the trapezius over conventional motion-based ultrasound (VAS changes, 8.32 to 3.32 versus 8.48 to 7.72, respectively), with significantly fewer treatment sessions in the HPPT ultrasound group.[188] Clinicians are advised to use caution with this technique, however, because a rapid rise in tissue temperature may cause a burn.

Since 2001, there has been an interest in low-intensity pulsed ultrasound (LIPUS), which comprises the static delivery of very low-dose pulsed ultrasound (e.g., in the range of 30 mW/cm^2 for up to 20 minutes) to soft tissue and bone structures. Initial research was generally encouraging.[189] LIPUS has been reported to influence healing positively in rat tendons during the granulation phase only,[190] mouse muscle laceration,[191] rat articular cartilage,[192] and human bone fractures.[193] Further research on the role of LIPUS in the treatment of MTrPs and soft tissue structures, such as the rotator cuff, is warranted.

Ultrasound therapy may be useful in the treatment of acute MTrP pain and soft tissue structures of the shoulder or as supportive treatment to manual invasive and noninvasive treatments. Further clinical research is needed to ascertain the role of ultrasound and LIPUS in musculoskeletal conditions.

Laser

Several studies reported a positive effect of low-intensity laser for MTrPs when compared with placebo laser treatment.[194-201] Several different types of laser were tested, including gallium arsenide, helium-neon, and infrared diode. Overall, laser therapy is effective for the short-term management of MTrPs,[8,93,94] and it has the advantages of being safe, well tolerated, accessible, and noninvasive.[201,202] Laser is a good choice as a direct treatment for MTrPs; however, clinicians should be able to palpate for MTrPs to ensure correct location of the laser beam.

Transcutaneous Electrical Nerve Stimulation and Interferential Current

TENS is the most commonly researched electrotherapy modality for MTrPs.[117,203-208] Most research has examined the immediate effects of TENS and has concluded that TENS has a short-term effect; one trial reported significant improvement in pain and PPT of MTrPs at 3-month follow-up.[204] High-frequency, high-intensity TENS with 100-Hz and 250-μs stimulation was the most valuable of four tested TENS combinations in attenuating MTrP pain, but it had no effect on MTrP PPT.[206] A multiprotocol study reported that TENS or IFC, in conjunction with other manual or physical treatments, was more effective in reducing MTrP pain.[117] Clinicians should consider TENS or IFC as supportive treatment to manual invasive and noninvasive treatments.

Shock Wave Therapy

A shock wave is a compression wave with a high peak pressure and a short life cycle that, in medicine, is usually generated by electrohydraulic, electromagnetic, or piezoelectric emitter machines.[209] Shock wave therapy (SWT) was originally employed in medicine for the treatment of calcific deposits such as renal stones.[209] Since then, shock waves have been used for various musculoskeletal conditions of tendon, plantar fascia, and bone. SWT has been used in the treatment of shoulder conditions including calcific tendinitis and tendinosis,[210,211] as well as supraspinatus tendon syndrome.[212,213]

More recently, interest has been shown in the use of shock waves for muscle. Research on SWT in the treatment of MTrPs is limited; however, one preliminary study demonstrated that active MTrPs could be identified by causing the familiar referred pain from muscles that are usually difficult to access by palpation.[214] Furthermore, focused extracorporeal SWT to MTrPs in athletes with acute or chronic shoulder pain improved isokinetic force production and overall performance and reduced pain.[215]

SWT may prove particularly beneficial in addressing the peripheral-central sensitization aspects of MTrPs, as proposed in the updated IH of MTrP formation. Animal research concluded that the application of extracorporeal SWT led to a significant decrease in the mean number of neurons immunoreactive for substance P within the dorsal root ganglion of L5 in rabbits exposed to high-energy shock waves to the ventral side of the distal femur, whereas no such change was seen in the contralateral untreated side.[216] Furthermore, selective loss of unmyelinated nerve fibers after extracorporeal shock waves was reported in a rabbit model, a finding that may, in part, explain the reduction in pain by partial denervation of sensory nerves.[217] Research on the role of SWT in MTrPs is warranted, but among the limitations of SWT are availability and cost, which need to be taken into account when comparing SWT with other modalities and treatments.

Radial Shock Wave Therapy: Rotator Cuff (Fig. 16-22)

Rationale Radial SWT is used for the treatment of pain, stimulation of tendon, and osteotendinous junction healing or for the treatment of calcific tendinopathy of the shoulder.

Patient Position For the anterior lateral shoulder, the patient is in the long-sitting position on the treatment table, with the back supported, or is supine. For the posterior shoulder, the side-lying or prone position is preferred.

Therapist Position The therapist sits or stands on the treated side.

Procedure The area to be treated is identified, and it may include the subscapularis, supraspinatus, infraspinatus, and teres minor tendon insertion zones. This area may also include the long head of the biceps. The arm is placed in the optimum position to expose the area to be treated, which may include some degree of external rotation for the subscapularis or extension, adduction, and internal rotation for the supraspinatus. The radial shockwave head is placed on the area to be treated with ultrasound gel. Shock waves are delivered at the required dosage (e.g., 1.6-bar, 10-Hz, 2000 shock waves), as deemed appropriate. The shock wave head is moved to locate the most tender area, based on patient biofeedback. MTrPs can be treated in a similar fashion using radial shock wave.

Stretching and Strengthening

Therapeutic exercise programs are central to the practice of physical therapy and focus on the prevention and rehabilitation of movement dysfunction.[218] The focus here is

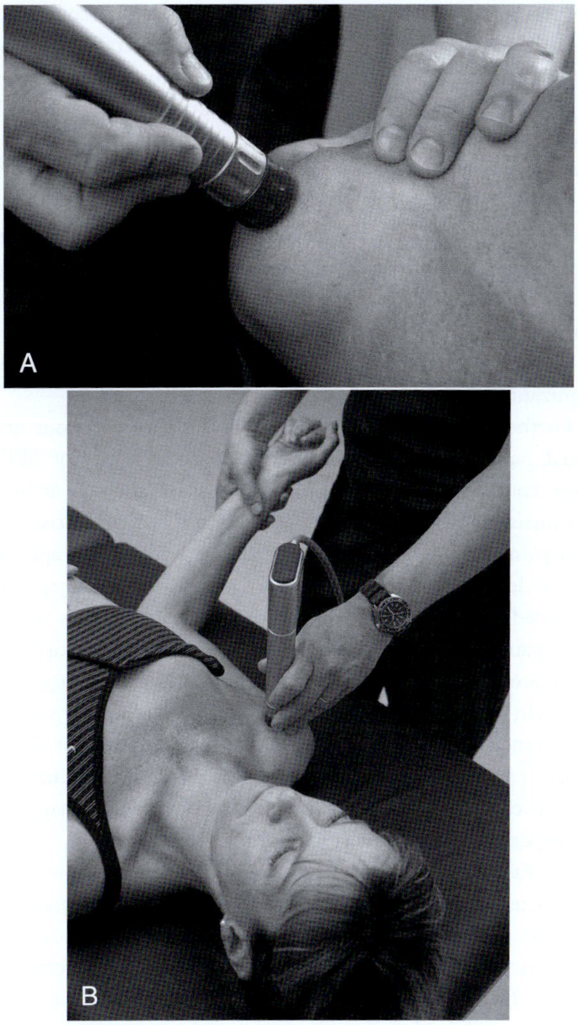

Figure 16-22 A and B, Radial shock wave therapy: rotator cuff. (Courtesy of Myopain Seminars ©2010.)

on stretching and strengthening as related to the treatment of myofascial pain. Patients with chronic pain may benefit from exercise-induced hypoalgesia, which may be mediated by opioid and nonopioid mechanisms.[219]

The IH proposes the taut band to result from contractured sarcomeres, and based on this premise, the main rationales of treatment include stretching and regaining length of the associated muscle.[4] Care should be taken to avoid overzealous, inappropriate, or aggressive stretching because stretching may possibly be a precipitating or perpetuating factor in MTrPs in some patients. Care should be taken with stretching alone because one study suggested that stretching may have an adverse effect on MTrP sensitivity.[220]

A muscle stretching program should be prescriptive and based on the individual needs and assessment of muscles for MTrPs, muscle length, and end feel. Myofascia may manifest with neuromuscular, viscoelastic, or connective tissue alterations.[221,222] Muscle length influences the length-tension relationship, and stretching therefore may have a negative impact on muscle strength and force production.[222,223] This concept should be considered when exercise programs and stretching regimens are designed. For muscle length assessment, refer to Chapter 15, Sahrmann[222] and Kendal et al.[224]

Posture is considered an important influence on MTrPs, and Travell and Simons placed significant emphasis on it.[4] Alterations in shoulder girdle posture may include rounded shoulders, thoracic hyperkyphosis, and forward head posture.[224] The *Janda upper crossed syndrome* describes a common clinical postural pattern: short muscles are the pectoralis major and minor, latissimus dorsi, levator scapulae, and upper trapezius; long muscles are the serratus anterior and the upper, middle, and lower trapezius.[221] Posture may influence the function of the shoulder and play a role in movement dysfunction, for example, by altering the subacromial space.[225,226]

Patients with episodic tension-type headache have greater forward head posture and numbers of MTrPs in the trapezius, sternocleidomastoid, and temporalis muscles when compared with healthy controls.[227] Similar trends have been shown in patient with unilateral migrane.[228] High visual stress induced during seated computer activity was shown to provoke MTrP sensitivity and changes in EMG.[229] A further study reported MTrP development after 1 hour of continuous typing.[230]

When indicated, static stretching should be carried out with gentle, non-painful action aiming to stretch the target muscles with good form. Recommended static stretching parameters are 15 to 30 seconds with three to five repetitions.[11,223,231] Clinicians should consider a preparatory technique such as TPCR, IMT, moist heat, or stretching as part of the S&S or I&S technique. Stretching can be augmented by methods such as postisometric relaxation, contraction and relaxation, active isolated stretching, or muscle energy technique.[4,102,103,108,221,232] Specific muscle stretches were presented by Travell and Simons.[4,23] Specifically for shoulder mechanics, maintaining internal and external range of shoulder motion appears to be of particular importance; the sleeper stretch for the posterior capsule and a subscapularis and anterior glenohumeral capsular stretch are presented elsewhere in this book (see Chapter 14).

Special caution should be noted with persons with hypermobility syndrome or a history of joint subluxations or dislocation, to avoid inappropriate stretching.[233] The estimated prevalence of hypermobility in the general population has been reported to be 4% to 7%, it is 9.5% in ballet dancers, and it is 11.7% in high school students; hypermobility is more common in girls and women than in boys and men.[233-236] In a cohort of patients with myofascial neck pain, 18.5% had benign joint hypermobility syndrome.[237] The Beighton score identifies persons with hypermobility and is commonly used in sports medicine, orthopedics, and rheumatology.[233,238]

Little research on strengthening in the treatment of MTrPs has been published. In considering the IH and MTrP research, it is reasonable that zealous strengthening may provoke active MTrPs or may turn latent MTrPs into active MTrPs. Muscles with active MTrPs are under metabolic stress, and further loading may lead to aggravation of the MTrP. Caution should be exercised in the early stage of rehabilitation of persons with MTrPs, and the degree of progression with strengthening should be titrated to suit the individual patient. The demands for a deconditioned, sedentary male smoker vary greatly from the needs of a professional athlete. The treatment strategy should address MTrPs to reduce pain, restore normal muscle length, and ensure proper biomechanical orientation of myofascial elements, followed by stretching and strengthening of the affected muscle.[239] The potential for improvement with strengthening, however, should not be overlooked because muscle weakness may be a predisposing, precipitating, or perpetuating factor in the reactivation of latent MTrPs. Improving fatigue resistance, strength, and stability should be the main aim of treatment. The ability of skeletal muscle to tolerate repeated activity partially depends on individual variation and on the magnitude and repetition of the force.[240]

Research into the potential role of eccentric exercise in the treatment of MTrPs is lacking and is an area for future attention. Maintaining adequate strength in the scapular thoracic stabilizing muscles, such as the trapezius, the serratus anterior, and the rotator cuff muscles, is vital. Muscle balance ratios for the shoulder have been presented, including ratios between the internal and external rotators of 66% for both fast and slow isokinetic torque arm speed in normal subjects,[241] as well as for professional baseball pitchers.[242] Muscle strengthening for the shoulder based on evidence from EMG is summarized in Chapter 15 and elsewhere,[11,243,244] including evidence specifically for the shoulder.[245-247]

CLINICAL IMPLICATIONS FOR THE PHYSICAL THERAPY MANAGEMENT OF MYOFASCIAL TRIGGER POINTS

Considering the multisystemic nature of musculoskeletal pain, evidence supports the greater efficacy of multimodal therapies,[248] and this also applies to the management of MTrPs.[117] In clinical practice, it may be helpful to employ several types of treatment approaches, including manual therapy, TPCR and massage, I&S, stretching, hot packs, electrophysical agents, and dry needling techniques. These treatments are best carried out in a graded progressive manner within the tolerance of the patient. The clinician usually employs several forms of treatment and should keep the IH in mind when choosing treatments combined with the available evidence.

Treatments can be painful and noxious because of MTrP hyperalgesia or allodynia. Clinicians should remain aware of the potential for immediate pain or post-treatment soreness, which can be present for several days. Patients should be warned and educated about the potential for post-treatment soreness. It is important to titer the treatment to suit the individual patient and circumstances. The *peak-end rule*[249] recognizes patients' memories of painful medical treatments may affect their decisions about future treatments. Redelmeier and Kahneman[249] reported that patients' judgments of total pain were strongly correlated with the peak intensity of the pain and with the intensity of pain recorded during the last 3 minutes of the procedure. In a study of patients undergoing colonoscopy in which half of the patients randomly received a less painful end to the procedure, the results demonstrated improved perception and a willingness to undergo future colonoscopy in the patients who received the less painful conclusion.[250] This finding has implications for clinicians treating patients with myofascial pain and suggests that treatments should be designed to control the peak intensity of the pain and to make the final part of the treatment more pleasurable, for instance, by the application of a hot pack. For example, TPCR may be delivered in low pressure, below the patient's pain threshold for a prolonged period of perhaps 90 seconds, as opposed to high pressure for a shorter duration of maybe 30 seconds,[117] thus being cognizant of the peak-end rule.

Furthermore, clinicians should educate patients about myofascial pain because patients may not be as aware of MTrPs when compared with other pain diagnoses such as arthritis, tendinitis, or bursitis. A study examining patients' satisfaction with pain treatment showed that patients with MTrPs appeared to have less accurate beliefs regarding their pain symptoms and expressed more dissatisfaction with physicians' efforts to treat their pain when compared with patients with neurologic or rheumatologic disorders.[251] This finding has implications for the plan of care and treatment design and underpins the importance of patient education. Being able to provoke the patient's pain by skilled palpation is often very valuable in the patient's understanding of MTrPs, no more perhaps than the experience of a positive straight leg raise test.[13]

Additionally, it is important to pay attention to predisposing, precipitating, and perpetuating factors. Success of treatment often lies in the identification and modification of these factors within the framework of the biopsychosocial model. Boyling and Jull[248] proposed consideration of the biopsychosocial model, patient-centered outcomes, including physical impairment and functioning, assessing the responsiveness of treatment, and taking into consideration patient's values, experiences, and opinions of treatments. Evidence-informed practice requires the conversion of scientific evidence into clinical practice with the integration of best available evidence, clinical experience, reasoning, and judgment in a patient goal–oriented manner.[252] Management of patients with MTrPs requires these attributes and a series of skill sets in combination, to achieve a meaningful and often lasting impact on patient's pain and function.

A team approach may be required to develop a multifactorial plan of care, which may include physicians, physical therapists, anesthesiologists, psychologists, and clinical social workers, among others. When patients are not improving, they should be reassessed, and differential diagnoses should be reconsidered with a review by the primary physician or coordinating pain management specialist.

SUMMARY

Myofascial pain of the shoulder is prevalent and is commonly found in patients with shoulder pain and dysfunction. Interest in MTrPs has increased as research has expanded. Myofascial pain is currently best summarized by the updated IH.

Currently, no gold standard clinical test exists for MTrPs. Palpation reliability is supported for certain muscles in adequately skilled and trained clinicians, a finding that stresses the importance of training.

Many shoulder muscles provoke myofascial pain, most commonly the infraspinatus, supraspinatus, subscapularis, teres minor, trapezius, levator scapulae, pectoralis minor and major, latissimus dorsi, and deltoid muscles. Clinicians are encouraged to examine patients routinely for MTrPs as part of the regular shoulder assessment.

Myofascial pain may be subject to recurrence or chronicity as a result of perpetuating factors, including mechanical, physiologic, medical, and psychological issues. Attention to these factors is important in multimodal care. Many treatments have been described for MTrPs, and these include TPCR, massage techniques, S&S, and needling therapies. Multimodal therapy for myofascial pain is likely to yield improved results, especially when it is combined with education and correction of perpetuating factors.

REFERENCES

1. Luime JJ, Koes BW, Hendriksen IJ, et al: Prevalence and incidence of shoulder pain in the general population: a systematic review, *Scand J Rheumatol* 33(2):73–81, 2004.
2. Bron C, Wensing M, Franssen JLM, et al: Interobserver reliability of palpation of myofascial trigger points in shoulder muscles, *J Man Manip Ther* 15(4):203–215, 2007.
3. Brukner P, Khan K, Kibler W, et al: Shoulder pain. In Brukner P, Khan K, editors: *Clinical sports medicine*, ed 3, London, 2009, McGraw-Hill.
4. Simons DG, Travell JG, Simons LS: *Travell and Simons' myofascial pain and dysfunction: the trigger point manual*, ed 2, Baltimore, 1999, Williams & Wilkins.
5. Dejung B, Gröbli C, Colla F, et al: *Triggerpunkttherapie*, Bern, 2003, Hans Huber.
6. Travell JG, Rinzler SH: The myofascial genesis of pain, *Postgrad Med* 11:425–434, 1952.
7. Dommerholt J, Bron C, Franssen JLM: Myofascial trigger points: an evidence-informed review, *J Man Manip Ther* 14 (4):203–221, 2006.
8. Dommerholt J, McEvoy J: Myofascial trigger point approach. In Wise C, editor: *Orthopaedic manual physical therapy: from art to evidence*, Philadelphia, 2011, Davis.
9. Fernández de las Peñas C, Fernández Carnero J, Miangolarra-Page JC: Musculoskeletal disorders in mechanical neck pain: myofascial trigger points versus cervical joint dysfunction, *J Musculoskelet Pain* 13(1):27–35, 2005.
10. Brukner P, Khan K: *Clinical sports medicine*, ed 3 rev, Sydney, 2010, McGraw-Hill.
11. Houglum PA: *Therapeutic exercise for musculoskeletal injuries*, ed 2, Champaign, Ill, 2005, Human Kinetics.
12. Dommerholt J, Shah JP: Myofascial pain syndrome. In Ballantyne JCRJ, Fishman SM, editors: *Bonica's management of pain*, Baltimore, 2010, Lippincott Williams & Williams, pp 450–471.
13. Gerwin RD, Dommerholt J: Treatment of myofascial pain syndromes. In Boswell MV, Cole BE, editors: *Weiner's pain management: a practical guide for clinicians*, Boca Raton, Fla, 2006, CRC, pp 477–492.
14. Harden RN, Bruehl SP, Gass S, et al: Signs and symptoms of the myofascial pain syndrome: a national survey of pain management providers, *Clin J Pain* 16(1):64–72, 2000.
15. Gerwin RD, Shannon S, Hong CZ, et al: Interrater reliability in myofascial trigger point examination, *Pain* 69(1–2):65–73, 1997.
16. McEvoy J, Huijbregts P: Reliability of myofascial trigger point palpation: a systematic review. In Dommerholt J, Huijbregts P, editors: *Myofascial trigger points: pathophysiology and evidenced-informed diagnosis and management*, Sudbury, 2011, Jones and Bartlett.
17. Escobar PL, Ballesteros J: Teres minor. Source of symptoms resembling ulnar neuropathy or C8 radiculopathy, *Am J Phys Med Rehabil* 67(3):120–122, 1988.
18. Facco E, Ceccherelli F: Myofascial pain mimicking radicular syndromes, *Acta Neurochir Suppl* 92:147–150, 2005.
19. Baldry PE: *Myofascial pain and fibromyalgia syndromes*, Edinburgh, 2001, Churchill Livingstone.
20. Tough EA, White AR, Richards S, et al: Variability of criteria used to diagnose myofascial trigger point pain syndrome: evidence from a review of the literature, *Clin J Pain* 23 (3):278–286, 2007.
21. Travell J: *Office hours: day and night. The autobiography of Janet Travell, M.D.*, New York, 1968, World.
22. Travell JG, Simons DG: *Myofascial pain and dysfunction: the trigger point manual*, Baltimore, 1983, Williams & Wilkins.
23. Travell JG, Simons DG: *Myofascial pain and dysfunction: the trigger point manual*, (vol 1), Baltimore, 1992, Williams & Wilkins.
24. Rachlin ES, Rachlin IS: *Myofascial pain and fibromyalgia: trigger point management*, St. Louis, 2002, Mosby.
25. Dommerholt J, Huijbregts P: *Myofascial trigger points: pathophysiology and evidence-informed diagnosis and management*, Sudbury, Mass, 2011, Jones and Bartlett.
26. Fishbain DA, Goldberg M, Steele R, et al: DSM-III diagnoses of patients with myofascial pain syndrome (fibrositis), *Arch Phys Med Rehabil* 70(6):433–438, 1989.
27. Gerwin R: A study of 96 subjects examined both for fibromyalgia and myofascial pain [abstract], *J Musculoskelet Pain* 3(Suppl 1):121, 1995.
28. Skootsky SA, Jaeger B, Oye RK: Prevalence of myofascial pain in general internal medicine practice, *West J Med* 151:157–160, 1989.
29. Weiner DK, Sakamoto S, Perera S, et al: Chronic low back pain in older adults: prevalence, reliability, and validity of physical examination findings, *J Am Geriatr Soc* 54 (1):11–20, 2006.
30. Calandre EP, Hidalgo J, Garcia-Leiva JM, et al: Trigger point evaluation in migraine patients: an indication of peripheral sensitization linked to migraine predisposition? *Eur J Neurol* 13(3):244–249, 2006.
31. Al-Shenqiti AM, Oldham JA: Test-retest reliability of myofascial trigger point detection in patients with rotator cuff tendonitis, *Clin Rehabil* 19(5):482–487, 2005.
32. Hidalgo-Lozano A, Fernandez-de-las-Penas C, Alonso-Blanco C, et al: Muscle trigger points and pressure pain hyperalgesia in the shoulder muscles in patients with unilateral shoulder impingement: a blinded, controlled study, *Exp Brain Res* 202(4):915–925, 2010.
33. Bron C, Dommerholt J, Stegenga B, et al: High prevalence of myofascial trigger points in patients with shoulder pain, submitted for publication.

34. Simons DG: Review of enigmatic MTrPs as a common cause of enigmatic musculoskeletal pain and dysfunction, *J Electromyogr Kinesiol* 14:95–107, 2004.
35. Wolfe F, Simons DG, Fricton J, et al: The fibromyalgia and myofascial pain syndromes: a preliminary study of tender points and trigger points in persons with fibromyalgia, myofascial pain syndrome and no disease, *J Rheumatol* 19(6): 944–951, 1992.
36. Nice DA, Riddle DL, Lamb RL, et al: Intertester reliability of judgments of the presence of trigger points in patients with low back pain, *Arch Phys Med Rehabil* 73(10):893–898, 1992.
37. Njoo KH, Van der Does E: The occurrence and inter-rater reliability of myofascial trigger points in the quadratus lumborum and gluteus medius: a prospective study in non-specific low back pain patients and controls in general practice, *Pain* 58(3):317–323, 1994.
38. Lew PC, Lewis J, Story I: Inter-therapist reliability in locating latent myofascial trigger points using palpation, *Man Ther* 2(2):87–90, 1997.
39. Hsieh CY, Hong CZ, Adams AH, et al: Interexaminer reliability of the palpation of trigger points in the trunk and lower limb muscles, *Arch Phys Med Rehabil* 81(3):258–264, 2000.
40. Sciotti VM, Mittak VL, DiMarco L, et al: Clinical precision of myofascial trigger point location in the trapezius muscle, *Pain* 93(3):259–266, 2001.
41. Seffinger MA, Najm WI, Mishra SI, et al: Reliability of spinal palpation for diagnosis of back and neck pain: a systematic review of the literature, *Spine* 29(19):E413–E425, 2004.
42. Gerwin RD, Dommerholt J, Shah JP: An expansion of Simons' integrated hypothesis of trigger point formation, *Curr Pain Headache Rep* 8(6):468–475, 2004.
43. McPartland JM, Simons DG: Myofascial trigger points: translating molecular theory into manual therapy, *J Man Manip Ther* 14(4):232–239, 2006.
44. McPartland JM: Travell trigger points: molecular and osteopathic perspectives, *J Am Osteopath Assoc* 104(6):244–249, 2004.
45. MacIntosh BR, Gardiner PF, McComas AJ: *Skeletal muscle: form and function*, ed 2, Champaign, Ill, 2005, Human Kinetics.
46. Jones D, Round JM, de Haan A: *Skeletal muscle from molecules to movement: a textbook of muscle physiotherapy for sport, exercise, physiotherapy and medicine*, Edinburgh, 2004, Churchill Livingstone.
47. Mense S, Gerwin RD: *Muscle pain: understanding the mechanisms*, Berlin, 2010, Springer.
48. Simons DG, Hong C-Z, Simons LS: Nature of myofascial trigger points, active loci [abstract], *J Musculoskelet Pain* 3 (Suppl 1):62, 1995.
49. Simons DG, Hong C-Z, Simons LS: Endplate potentials are common to midfiber myofascial trigger points, *Am J Phys Med Rehabil* 81(3):212–222, 2002.
50. Simons DG, Hong C-Z, Simons L: Prevalence of spontaneous electrical activity at trigger spots and control sites in rabbit muscle, *J Musculoskelet Pain* 3:35–48, 1995.
51. Couppé C, Midttun A, Hilden J, et al: Spontaneous needle electromyographic activity in myofascial trigger points in the infraspinatus muscle: a blinded assessment, *J Musculoskelet Pain* 9(3):7–17, 2001.
52. Macgregor J, Graf von Schweinitz D: Needle electromyographic activity of myofascial trigger points and control sites in equine cleidobrachialis muscle: an observational study, *Acupunct Med* 24(2):61–70, 2006.
53. Simons DG, Stolov WC: Microscopic features and transient contraction of palpable bands in canine muscle, *Am J Phys Med* 55(2):65–88, 1976.
54. Reitinger A, Radner H, Tilscher H, et al: Morphologische Untersuchung an Triggerpunkten, *Manuelle Medizin* 34:256–262, 1996.
55. Windisch A, Reitinger A, Traxler H, et al: Morphology and histochemistry of myogelosis, *Clin Anat* 12(4):266–271, 1999.
56. Pongratz D: Neuere Ergebnisse zur Pathogenese myofaszialer Schmerzsyndrom, *Nervenheilkunde* 21(1):35–37, 2002.
57. Mense S, Simons DG, Hoheisel U, et al: Lesions of rat skeletal muscle after local block of acetylcholinesterase and neuromuscular stimulation, *J Appl Physiol* 94(6):2494–2501, 2003.
58. Chang CW, Chen YR, Chang KF: Evidence of neuroaxonal degeneration in myofascial pain syndrome: a study of neuromuscular jitter by axonal microstimulation, *Eur J Pain* 12(8):1026–1030, 2008.
59. Chen Q, Bensamoun S, Basford JR, et al: Identification and quantification of myofascial taut bands with magnetic resonance elastography, *Arch Phys Med Rehabil* 88(12):1658–1661, 2007.
60. Chen Q, Basford J, An KN: Ability of magnetic resonance elastography to assess taut bands, *Clin Biomech (Bristol, Avon)* 23(5):623–629, 2008.
61. Sikdar S, Shah JP, Gebreab T, et al: Novel applications of ultrasound technology to visualize and characterize myofascial trigger points and surrounding soft tissue, *Arch Phys Med Rehabil* 90(11):1829–1838, 2009.
62. Strobel ES, Krapf M, Suckfull M, et al: Tissue oxygen measurement and 31P magnetic resonance spectroscopy in patients with muscle tension and fibromyalgia, *Rheumatol Int* 16(5):175–180, 1997.
63. Brückle W, Sückfull M, Fleckenstein W, et al: Gewebe-pO2-Messung in der verspannten Rückenmuskulatur (m. erector spinae), *Z Rheumatol* 49:208–216, 1990.
64. Graven-Nielsen T, Mense S: The peripheral apparatus of muscle pain: evidence from animal and human studies, *Clin J Pain* 17(1):2–10, 2001.
65. Mense S, Stahnke M: Responses in muscle afferent fibres of slow conduction velocity to contractions and ischaemia in the cat, *J Physiol* 342:383–397, 1983.
66. Shah JP, Danoff JV, Desai MJ, et al: Biochemicals associated with pain and inflammation are elevated in sites near to and remote from active myofascial trigger points, *Arch Phys Med Rehabil* 89(1):16–23, 2008.
67. Shah JP, Phillips TM, Danoff JV, et al: An in-vivo microanalytical technique for measuring the local biochemical milieu of human skeletal muscle, *J Appl Physiol* 99:1980–1987, 2005.
68. Shah JP, Gilliams EA: Uncovering the biochemical milieu of myofascial trigger points using in vivo microdialysis: an application of muscle pain concepts to myofascial pain syndrome, *J Bodyw Mov Ther* 12(4):371–384, 2008.
69. Sluka K, editor: *Mechanisms and management of pain for the physical therapist*, Seattle, 2009, IASP Press.
70. Rees H, Sluka KA, Lu Y, et al: Dorsal root reflexes in articular afferents occur bilaterally in a chronic model of arthritis in rats, *J Neurophysiol* 76(6):4190–4193, 1997.
71. Sluka KA, Rees H, Westlund KN, et al: Fiber types contributing to dorsal root reflexes induced by joint inflammation in cats and monkeys, *J Neurophysiol* 74(3):981–989, 1995.
72. Rees H, Sluka KA, Westlund KN, et al: Do dorsal root reflexes augment peripheral inflammation? *Neuroreport* 5(7): 821–824, 1994.

73. Sluka KA, Kalra A, Moore SA: Unilateral intramuscular injections of acidic saline produce a bilateral, long-lasting hyperalgesia, *Muscle Nerve* 24(1):37–46, 2001.
74. Mense S: Algesic agents exciting muscle nociceptors, *Exp Brain Res* 196(1):89–100, 2009.
75. Svensson P, Minoshima S, Beydoun A, et al: Cerebral processing of acute skin and muscle pain in humans, *J Neurophysiol* 78(1):450–460, 1997.
76. Wall PD, Woolf CJ: Muscle but not cutaneous C-afferent input produces prolonged increases in the excitability of the flexion reflex in the rat, *J Physiol* 356:443–458, 1984.
77. Hoheisel U, Koch K, Mense S: Functional reorganization in the rat dorsal horn during an experimental myositis, *Pain* 59(1):111–118, 1994.
78. Hoheisel U, Mense S, Simons D, et al: Appearance of new receptive fields in rat dorsal horn neurons following noxious stimulation of skeletal muscle: a model for referral of muscle pain? *Neurosci Lett* 153:9–12, 1993.
79. Mense S: Descending antinociception and fibromyalgia, *Z Rheumatol* 57(Suppl 2):23–26, 1998.
80. Mense S: Neurobiological concepts of fibromyalgia: the possible role of descending spinal tracts, *Scand J Rheumatol Suppl* 113:24–29, 2000.
81. Mense S: The pathogenesis of muscle pain, *Curr Pain Headache Rep* 7(6):419–425, 2003.
82. Li LT, Ge HY, Yue SW, et al: Nociceptive and non-nociceptive hypersensitivity at latent myofascial trigger points, *Clin J Pain* 25(2):132–137, 2009.
83. Ge HY, Zhang Y, Boudreau S, et al: Induction of muscle cramps by nociceptive stimulation of latent myofascial trigger points, *Exp Brain Res* 187(4):623–629, 2008.
84. Cairns BE, Gambarota G, Svensson P, et al: Glutamate-induced sensitization of rat masseter muscle fibers, *Neuroscience* 109(2):389–399, 2002.
85. Xu YM, Ge HY, Arendt-Nielsen L: Sustained nociceptive mechanical stimulation of latent myofascial trigger point induces central sensitization in healthy subjects, *J Pain* May 5 [Epub ahead of print].
86. Zhang Y, Ge HY, Yue SW, et al: Attenuated skin blood flow response to nociceptive stimulation of latent myofascial trigger points, *Arch Phys Med Rehabil* 90(2):325–332, 2009.
87. Lucas KR, Polus BI, Rich PS: Latent myofascial trigger points: their effect on muscle activation and movement efficiency, *J Bodyw Mov Ther* 8:160–166, 2004.
88. Dommerholt J, Bron C, Franssen JLM: Myofascial trigger points: an evidence-informed review. In Dommerholt J, Huijbregts P, editors: *Myofascial trigger points: pathophysiology and evidence-informed diagnosis and management*, Sudbury, Mass, 2011, Jones and Bartlett.
89. Gerwin RD: A review of myofascial pain and fibromyalgia: factors that promote their persistence, *Acupunct Med* 23 (3):121–134, 2005.
90. Boissonnault WG: *Primary care for the physical therapist: examination and triage*, ed 2, St. Louis, 2010, Saunders Elsevier.
91. Tighe CB, Oakley WS Jr, : The prevalence of a diabetic condition and adhesive capsulitis of the shoulder, *South Med J* 101(6):591–595, 2008.
92. Maitland GD: *Vertebral manipulation*, Oxford, 1986, Butterworth Heinemann.
93. Rickards LD: The effectiveness of non-invasive treatments for active myofascial trigger point pain: a systematic review of the literature, *Int J Osteopath Med* 9(4):120–136, 2006.
94. Rickards LD: The effectiveness of non-invasive treatments for active myofascial trigger point pain: a systematic review. In Dommerholt J, Huijbregts P, editors: *Myofascial trigger points: pathophysiology and evidence-informed diagnosis and management*, Sudbury, Mass, 2009, Jones and Bartlett.
95. Dommerholt J, Mayoral O, Gröbli C: Trigger point dry needling, *J Man Manip Ther* 14(4):E70–E87, 2006.
96. Resteghini P: Myofascial trigger points: pathophsyiology and treatment with dry needling, *J Orthop Med* 28(2):60–68, 2006.
97. Clay JH, Pounds DM: *Basic clinical massage therapy: integrating anatomy and treatment*, Philadelphia, 2003, Lippincott Williams & Wilkins.
98. Barnes J: *Myofascial release: the search for excellence*, 1990, self-published.
99. Manheim CJ: *The myofascial release manual*, ed 4, Thorofare, NJ, 2008, Slack.
100. Barnes J: Myofascial release. In Hammer WI, editor: *Functional soft tissue examination and treatment by manual methods: new perspectives*, ed 2, Gaithersburg, Md, 1999, Aspen.
101. Kostopoulos D, Rizopoulos K: Effect of topical aerosol skin refrigerant (spray and stretch technique) on passive and active stretching, *J Bodyw Mov Ther* 12(2):96–104, 2008.
102. Lewit K, Simons DG: Myofascial pain: relief by post-isometric relaxation, *Arch Phys Med Rehabil* 65(8):452–456, 1984.
103. Lewit K: Postisometric relaxation in combination with other methods of muscular facilitation and inhibition, *Manuelle Medizin* 2:101–104, 1988.
104. Lewit K: *Manipulative therapy in rehabilitation of the locomotor system*, Oxford, 1999, Butterworth Heinemann.
105. Chaitow L, Crenshaw KBS: *Muscle energy techniques*, ed 3, Edinburgh, 2006, Churchill Livingstone.
106. Chaitow L, DeLany J: Neuromuscular techniques in orthopedics, *Tech Orthop* 18(1):74–86, 2003.
107. Chaitow L, DeLany J, Dowling DJ: *Modern neuromuscular techniques*, ed 2, Edinburgh, 2003, Churchill Livingstone.
108. Greenman PE: *Principles of manual medicine*, ed 3, Philadelphia, 2003, Lippincott Williams & Wilkins.
109. Ferguson LW, Gerwin R: *Clinical mastery in the treatment of myofascial pain*, Philadelphia, 2005, Lippincott Williams & Wilkins.
110. Hanten WP, Barrett M, Gillespie-Plesko M, et al: Effects of active head retraction with retraction/extension and occipital release on the pressure pain threshold of cervical and scapular trigger points, *Physiother Theory Pract* 13:285–291, 1997.
111. Dardzinski JA, Ostrov BE, Hamann LS: Myofascial pain unresponsive to standard treatment: successful use of a strain and counterstrain technique with physical therapy, *J Clin Rheumatol* 6(4):169–174, 2000.
112. Gulick DT, Palombaro K, Lattanzi JB: Effect of ischemic pressure using a Backnobber II device on discomfort associated with myofascial trigger points, *J Bodyw Mov Ther* in press.
113. Hanten WP, Olsen SL, Butts NL, et al: Effectiveness of a home program of ischemic pressure followed by sustained stretch for treatment of myofascial trigger points, *Phys Ther* 80(10):997–1003, 2000.
114. Garcia-Muro F, Rodriguez-Fernandez AL, Herrero-de-Lucas A: Treatment of myofascial pain in the shoulder with Kinesio taping: a case report, *Man Ther* 15(3):292–295, 2010.
115. Simons DG: Understanding effective treatments of myofascial trigger points, *J Bodyw Mov Ther* 6(2):81–88, 2002.

116. Fryer G, Hodgson L: The effect of manual pressure release on myofascial trigger points in the upper trapezius muscle, *J Bodyw Mov Ther* 9(4):248–255, 2005.
117. Hou CR, Tsai LC, Cheng KF, et al: Immediate effects of various physical therapeutic modalities on cervical myofascial pain and trigger-point sensitivity, *Arch Phys Med Rehabil* 83 (10):1406–1414, 2002.
118. Fernández-de-las-Peñas C, Alonso-Blanco C, Fernández-Carnero J, et al: The immediate effect of ischemic compression technique and transverse friction massage on tenderness of active and latent myofascial trigger points: a pilot study, *J Bodyw Mov Ther* 10(1):3–9, 2006.
119. Terlouw TJ: Roots of physical medicine, physical therapy, and mechanotherapy in the Netherlands in the 19th century: a disputed area within the healthcare domain, *J Man Manip Ther* 15(2):E23–E41, 2007.
120. Holey EA, Cook EM: *Evidence-based therapeutic massage: a practical guide for therapists*, Edinburgh, 2003, Churchill Livingstone.
121. Barclay J: *In good hands: the history of the Chartered Society of Physiotherapy 1894–1994*, Oxford, 1994, Butterworth Heinemann.
122. Beck MF: *Theory and practice of therapeutic massage*, ed 4, South Melbourne, Australia, 2006, Thomson Delmar Learning.
123. Furlan AD, Imamura M, Dryden T, et al: Massage for low back pain: an updated systematic review within the framework of the Cochrane Back Review Group, *Spine* 34(16):1669–1684, 2009.
124. Hammer WI: *Functional soft tissue examination and treatment by manual methods: new perspectives*, ed 2, Gaithersburg, Md, 1999, Aspen.
125. Cyriax J, Coldham M: *Textbook of orthopaedic medicine, vol 2: Treatment by manipulation, massage and injection*, ed 11, London, 1984, Bailliere Tindall.
126. Crothers A, Walker B, French SD: Spinal manipulative therapy versus Graston technique in the treatment of non-specific thoracic spine pain: design of a randomised controlled trial, *Chiropr Osteopat* 16:12, 2008.
127. Hammer WI, Pfefer MT: Treatment of a case of subacute lumbar compartment syndrome using the Graston technique, *J Manipulative Physiol Ther* 28(3):199–204, 2005.
128. Hammer WI: The effect of mechanical load on degenerated soft tissue, *J Bodyw Mov Ther* 12(3):246–256, 2008.
129. Borgini E, Stecco A, Day JA, et al: How much time is required to modify a fascial fibrosis? *J Bodyw Mov Ther* 14 (4):318–325, 2010.
130. Brosseau L, Casimiro L, Milne S, et al: Deep transverse friction massage for treating tendinitis, *Cochrane Database Syst Rev* (1) CD003528, 2002.
131. Weerapong P, Hume PA, Kolt GS: The mechanisms of massage and effects on performance, muscle recovery and injury prevention, *Sports Med* 35(3):235–256, 2005.
132. Pfefer MT, Cooper SR, Uhl NL: Chiropractic management of tendinopathy: a literature synthesis, *J Manipulative Physiol Ther* 32(1):41–52, 2009.
133. Gray H, Bannister LH, Berry MM, et al, editors: *Gray's anatomy: the anatomical basis of medicine and surgery*, ed 38, Edinburgh, 1995, Churchill Livingstone.
134. Gabbiani G, Ryan GB, Lamelin JP, et al: Human smooth muscle autoantibody. Its identification as antiactin antibody and a study of its binding to "nonmuscular" cells, *Am J Pathol* 72(3):473–488, 1973.
135. Schleip R, Naylor IL, Ursu D, et al: Passive muscle stiffness may be influenced by active contractility of intramuscular connective tissue, *Med Hypotheses* 66(1):66–71, 2006.
136. Schleip R, Klingler W, Lehmann-Horn F: Active fascial contractility: fascia may be able to contract in a smooth muscle-like manner and thereby influence musculoskeletal dynamics, *Med Hypotheses* 65(2):273–277, 2005.
137. Vshivtseva VV, Lesova LD: [Features of the innervation of fascia and their microcirculatory bed in the rat], *Arkh Anat Gistol Embriol* 88(5):16–22, 1985.
138. Sakada S: Mechanoreceptors in fascia, periosteum and periodontal ligament, *Bull Tokyo Med Dent Univ* 21(Suppl):11–13, 1974.
139. Tanaka S, Ito T: Histochemical demonstration of adrenergic fibers in the fascia periosteum and retinaculum, *Clin Orthop Relat Res* 126:276–281, 1977.
140. Schleip R: Fascial plasticity: a new neurobiological explanation. Part 2, *J Bodyw Mov Ther* 7(2):104–116, 2003.
141. Schleip R: Fascial plasticity: a new neurobiological explanation: Part 1, *J Bodyw Mov Ther* 7(1):11–19, 2003.
142. Schleip R, Vleeming A, Lehmann-Horn F, et al: Concerning "A hypothesis of chronic back pain: ligament subfailure injuries lead to muscle control dysfunction" (M. Panjabi) [letter], *Eur Spine J* 16(10):1733–1735, 2007 author reply 1736.
143. Vleeming A, Pool-Goudzwaard AL, Stoeckart R, et al: The posterior layer of the thoracolumbar fascia: its function in load transfer from spine to legs, *Spine* 20(7):753–758, 1995.
144. Vleeming A, Stoeckart R: The role of the pelvis in coupling the spine and the legs: a clinical-anatomical perspective on pelvic stability. In Vleeming A, Mooney V, Stoeckart R, editors: *Movement, stability and lumbopelvic pain: integration of research and therapy*, ed 2, Edinburgh, 2007, Churchill Livingstone.
145. Stecco A, Macchi V, Stecco C, et al: Anatomical study of myofascial continuity in the anterior region of the upper limb, *J Bodyw Mov Ther* 13(1):53–62, 2009.
146. Stecco A, Masiero S, Macchi V, et al: The pectoral fascia: anatomical and histological study, *J Bodyw Mov Ther* 13 (3):255–261, 2009.
147. Stecco C, Porzionato A, Lancerotto L, et al: Histological study of the deep fasciae of the limbs, *J Bodyw Mov Ther* 12 (3):225–230, 2008.
148. Stecco L: *Fascial manipulation for muscuskeletal pain*, Padua, Italy, 2004, Piccin.
149. Myers TW: *Anatomy trains: myofascial meridians for manual and movement therapists*, ed 2, New York, 2009, Elsevier.
150. Day JA, Stecco C, Stecco A: Application of Fascial Manipulation© technique in chronic shoulder pain: anatomical basis and clinical implications, *J Bodyw Mov Ther* 13 (2):128–135, 2009.
151. Rolf IP: *Rolfing: reestablishing the natural alignment and structural integration of the human body for vitality and well-being*, Rochester, Vt, 1989, Healing Arts Press.
152. Cantu RI, Grodin AJ: *Myofascial manipulation: theory and clinical application*, ed 2, Austin, Tex, 2006, Pro-Ed.
153. Chaitow L, DeLany J: *Clinical applications of neuromuscular technique*, Edinburgh, 2000, Churchill Livingstone.
154. Chaudhry H, Huang C-Y, Schleip R, et al: Viscoelastic behavior of human fasciae under extension in manual therapy, *J Bodyw Mov Ther* 11(2):159–167, 2007.
155. Langevin HM, Bouffard NA, Badger GJ, et al: Subcutaneous tissue fibroblast cytoskeletal remodeling induced by acupuncture: evidence for a mechanotransduction-based mechanism, *J Cell Physiol* 207(3):767–774, 2006.

156. Langevin HM, Bouffard NA, Churchill DL, et al: Connective tissue fibroblast response to acupuncture: dose-dependent effect of bidirectional needle rotation, *J Altern Complement Med* 13(3):355–360, 2007.
157. Dommerholt J: Trigger point therapy. In Schleip R, Finley RT, Chaitow L, et al, editors: *Fascia in manual and movement therapies*, Edinburgh, in press, Churchill Livingstone.
158. Kraus H: The use of surface anaesthesia in the treatment of painful motion, *J Am Med Assoc* 116:2582–2583, 1941.
159. Jaeger B, Reeves JL: Quantification of changes in myofascial trigger point sensitivity with the pressure algometer following passive stretch, *Pain* 27:203–210, 1986.
160. Hong C-Z, Chen Y-C, Pon CH, et al: Immediate effects of various physical medicine modalities on pain threshold of the active myofascial trigger points, *J Musculoskelet Pain* 1 (2):37–53, 1993.
161. Bahadir C, Dayan VY, Ocak F, et al: Efficacy of immediate rewarming with moist heat after conventional vapocoolant spray therapy in myofascial pain syndrome, *J Musculoskelet Pain* 18(2):147–152, 2010.
162. Nielsen AJ: Case study: myofascial pain of the posterior shoulder relieved by spray and stretch, *J Orthop Sports Phys Ther* 3(1):21–26, 1981.
163. Fischer A: New injection techniques for treatment of musculoskeletal pain. In Rachlin ES, Rachlin IS, editors: *Myofascial pain and fibromyalgia: trigger point management*, ed 2, St. Louis, 2002, Mosby.
164. Gunn CC: *The Gunn approach to the treatment of chronic pain*, ed 2, New York, 1997, Churchill Livingstone.
165. Travell J: Basis for the multiple uses of local block of somatic trigger areas (procaine infiltration and ethyl chloride spray), *Miss Valley Med J* 71:13–22, 1949.
166. Baldry PE: *Acupuncture, trigger points and musculoskeletal pain*, Edinburgh, 2005, Churchill Livingstone.
167. Hong CZ: Lidocaine injection versus dry needling to myofascial trigger point: the importance of the local twitch response, *Am J Phys Med Rehabil* 73(4):256–263, 1994.
168. Cummings TM, White AR: Needling therapies in the management of myofascial trigger point pain: a systematic review, *Arch Phys Med Rehabil* 82(7):986–992, 2001.
169. Lewit K: The needle effect in the relief of myofascial pain, *Pain* 6:83–90, 1979.
170. Chen JT, Chung KC, Hou CR, et al: Inhibitory effect of dry needling on the spontaneous electrical activity recorded from myofascial trigger spots of rabbit skeletal muscle, *Am J Phys Med Rehabil* 80(10):729–735, 2001.
171. Takeshige C, Sato M: Comparisons of pain relief mechanisms between needling to the muscle, static magnetic field, external qigong and needling to the acupuncture point, *Acupunct Electrother Res* 21(2):119–131, 1996.
172. Takeshige C, Sato T, Mera T, et al: Descending pain inhibitory system involved in acupuncture analgesia, *Brain Res Bull* 29(5):617–634, 1992.
173. Takeshige C, Kobori M, Hishida F, et al: Analgesia inhibitory system involvement in nonacupuncture point-stimulation-produced analgesia, *Brain Res Bull* 28(3):379–391, 1992.
174. Furlan A, Tulder M, Cherkin D, et al: Acupuncture and dry-needling for low back pain, *Cochrane Database Syst Rev* (1) CD001351, 2005.
175. Itoh K, Hirota S, Katsumi Y, et al: Trigger point acupuncture for treatment of knee osteoarthritis–a preliminary RCT for a pragmatic trial, *Acupunct Med* 26(1):17–26, 2008.
176. Itoh K, Katsumi Y, Hirota S, et al: Randomised trial of trigger point acupuncture compared with other acupuncture for treatment of chronic neck pain, *Complement Ther Med* 15 (3):172–179, 2007.
177. Itoh K, Katsumi Y, Kitakoji H: Trigger point acupuncture treatment of chronic low back pain in elderly patients: a blinded RCT, *Acupunct Med* 22(4):170–177, 2004.
178. Hsieh YL, Kao MJ, Kuan TS, et al: Dry needling to a key myofascial trigger point may reduce the irritability of satellite MTrPs, *Am J Phys Med Rehabil* 86(5):397–403, 2007.
179. Dilorenzo L, Traballesi M, Morelli D, et al: Hemiparetic shoulder pain syndrome treated with deep dry needling during early rehabilitation: a prospective, open-label, randomized investigation, *J Musculoskelet Pain* 12(2):25–34, 2004.
180. Tsai CT, Hsieh LF, Kuan TS, et al: Remote effects of dry needling on the irritability of the myofascial trigger point in the upper trapezius muscle, *Am J Phys Med Rehabil* 89 (2):133–140, 2010.
181. Ingber RS: Shoulder impingement in tennis/racquetball players treated with subscapularis myofascial treatments, *Arch Phys Med Rehabil* 81(5):679–682, 2000.
182. Osborne NJ, Gatt IT: Management of shoulder injuries using dry needling in elite volleyball players, *Acupunct Med* 28 (1):42–45, 2010.
183. Srbely JZ, Dickey JP, Lee D, et al: Dry needle stimulation of myofascial trigger points evokes segmental anti-nociceptive effects, *J Rehabil Med* 42(5):463–468, 2010.
184. Kahn J: Electrical modalities in the treatment of myofascial conditions. In Rachlin ES, Rachlin IS, editors: *Myofascial pain and fibromyalgia, trigger point management*, St. Louis, 2002, Mosby.
185. Srbely JZ, Dickey JP: Randomized controlled study of the antinociceptive effect of ultrasound on trigger point sensitivity: novel applications in myofascial therapy? *Clin Rehabil* 21(5):411–417, 2007.
186. Srbely JZ, Dickey JP, Lowerison M, et al: Stimulation of myofascial trigger points with ultrasound induces segmental antinociceptive effects: a randomized controlled study, *Pain* 139 (2):260–266, 2008.
187. Ay S, Dogan SK, Evcik D, et al: Comparison the efficacy of phonophoresis and ultrasound therapy in myofascial pain syndrome, *Rheumatol Int* 2010 Mar 31 [Epub ahead of print].
188. Majlesi J, Unalan H: High-power pain threshold ultrasound technique in the treatment of active myofascial trigger points: a randomized, double-blind, case-control study, *Arch Phys Med Rehabil* 85(5):833–836, 2004.
189. Khanna A, Nelmes RT, Gougoulias N, et al: The effects of LIPUS on soft-tissue healing: a review of literature, *Br Med Bull* 89:169–182, 2009.
190. Fu SC, Hung LK, Shum WT, et al: In vivo low-intensity pulsed ultrasound (LIPUS) following tendon injury promotes repair during granulation but suppresses decorin and biglycan expression during remodeling, *J Orthop Sports Phys Ther* 40 (7):422–429, 2010.
191. Chan YS, Hsu KY, Kuo CH, et al: Using low-intensity pulsed ultrasound to improve muscle healing after laceration injury: an in vitro and in vivo study, *Ultrasound Med Biol* 36(5): 743–751, 2010.
192. Naito K, Watari T, Muta T, et al: Low-intensity pulsed ultrasound (LIPUS) increases the articular cartilage type II collagen in a rat osteoarthritis model, *J Orthop Res* 28(3): 361–369, 2010.

193. Watanabe Y, Matsushita T, Bhandari M, et al: Ultrasound for fracture healing: current evidence, *J Orthop Trauma* 24(Suppl 1): S56–S61, 2010.
194. Ilbuldu E, Cakmak A, Disci R, et al: Comparison of laser, dry needling, and placebo laser treatments in myofascial pain syndrome, *Photomed Laser Surg* 22(4):306–311, 2004.
195. Altan L, Bingol U, Aykac M, et al: Investigation of the effect of GaAs laser therapy on cervical myofascial pain syndrome, *Rheumatol Int* 25(1):23–27, 2005.
196. Ceccherelli F, Altafini L, Lo Castro G, et al: Diode laser in cervical myofascial pain: a double-blind study versus placebo, *Clin J Pain* 5(4):301–304, 1989.
197. Gur A, Sarac AJ, Cevik R, et al: Efficacy of 904 nm gallium arsenide low level laser therapy in the management of chronic myofascial pain in the neck: a double-blind and randomize-controlled trial, *Lasers Surg Med* 35(3):229–235, 2004.
198. Hakguder A, Birtane M, Gurcan S, et al: Efficacy of low level laser therapy in myofascial pain syndrome: an algometric and thermographic evaluation, *Lasers Surg Med* 33(5):339–343, 2003.
199. Snyder-Mackler L, Barry AJ, Perkins AI, et al: Effects of helium-neon laser irradiation on skin resistance and pain in patients with trigger points in the neck or back, *Phys Ther* 69(5):336–341, 1989.
200. Dundar U, Evcik D, Samli F, et al: The effect of gallium arsenide aluminum laser therapy in the management of cervical myofascial pain syndrome: a double blind, placebo-controlled study, *Clin Rheumatol* 26(6):930–934, 2007.
201. Simunovic Z, Trobonjaca T, Trobonjaca Z: Treatment of medial and lateral epicondylitis—tennis and golfer's elbow—with low level laser therapy: a multicenter double blind, placebo-controlled clinical study on 324 patients, *J Clin Laser Med Surg* 16(3):145–151, 1998.
202. Simunovic Z: Low level laser therapy with trigger points technique: a clinical study on 243 patients, *J Clin Laser Med Surg* 14(4):163–167, 1996.
203. Hsueh TC, Cheng PT, Kuan TS, et al: The immediate effectiveness of electrical nerve stimulation and electrical muscle stimulation on myofascial trigger points, *Am J Phys Med Rehabil* 76(6):471–476, 1997.
204. Ardiç F, Sarhus M, Topuz O: Comparison of two different techniques of electrotherapy on myofascial pain, *J Back Musculoskelet Rehabil* 16:11–16, 2002.
205. Farina S, Casarotto M, Benelle M, et al: A randomized controlled study on the effect of two different treatments (FREMS AND TENS) in myofascial pain syndrome, *Eura Medicophys* 40(4):293–301, 2004.
206. Graff-Radford SB, Reeves JL, Baker RL, et al: Effects of transcutaneous electrical nerve stimulation on myofascial pain and trigger point sensitivity, *Pain* 37(1):1–5, 1989.
207. Lee JC, Lin DT, Hong C-Z: The effectiveness of simultaneous thermotherapy with ultrasound and electrotherapy with combined AC and DC current on the immediate pain relief of myofascial trigger points, *J Musculoskelet Pain* 5(1):81–90, 1997.
208. Smania N, Corato E, Fiaschi A, et al: Repetitive magnetic stimulation: a novel therapeutic approach for myofascial pain syndrome, *J Neurol* 252(3):307–314, 2005.
209. Coombs RE, Zhou SS, Schaden WE, editors: *Musculoskeletal shockwave therapy*, London, 2000, Greenwich Medical Media.
210. Pleiner J, Crevenna R, Langenberger H, et al: Extracorporeal shockwave treatment is effective in calcific tendonitis of the shoulder: a randomized controlled trial, *Wien Klin Wochenschr* 116(15–16):536–541, 2004.
211. Daecke W, Kusnierczak D, Loew M: Long-term effects of extracorporeal shockwave therapy in chronic calcific tendinitis of the shoulder, *J Shoulder Elbow Surg* 11(5):476–480, 2002.
212. Gross MW, Sattler A, Haake M, et al: [The effectiveness of radiation treatment in comparison with extracorporeal shock-wave therapy (ESWT) in supraspinatus tendon syndrome], *Strahlenther Onkol* 178(6):314–320, 2002.
213. Haake M, Sattler A, Gross MW, et al: [Comparison of extracorporeal shockwave therapy (ESWT) with roentgen irradiation in supraspinatus tendon syndrome: a prospective randomized single-blind parallel group comparison], *Z Orthop Ihre Grenzgeb* 139(5):397–402, 2001.
214. Bauermeister W: The diagnosis and treatment of myofascial trigger points using shockwaves. In Abstracts from the Sixth World Congress on Myofascial Pain and Fibromyalgia, Munich, Germany, July 18–22, 2004: myopain 2004 [abstract], *J Musculoskelet Pain* 12(Suppl 9):13, 2004.
215. Müller-Ehrenberg H, Thorwesten L: Improvement of sports-related shoulder pain after treatment of trigger points using focused extracorporeal shock wave therapy regarding static and dynamic force development, pain relief and sensomotoric performance [abstract], *J Musculoskelet Pain* 15(Suppl 13):33, 2007.
216. Hausdorf J, Lemmens MA, Kaplan S, et al: Extracorporeal shockwave application to the distal femur of rabbits diminishes the number of neurons immunoreactive for substance P in dorsal root ganglia L5, *Brain Res* 1207:96–101, 2008.
217. Hausdorf J, Lemmens MA, Heck KD, et al: Selective loss of unmyelinated nerve fibers after extracorporeal shockwave application to the musculoskeletal system, *Neuroscience* 155 (1):138–144, 2008.
218. Kendall FP: Kendall urges a return to basics, *PT Bulletin Online* 3(23), 2002.
219. Hoeger Bement M: Exercise-induced hypoalgesia: an evidenced-based review. In Sluka K, editor: *Mechanisms and management of pain for the physical therapist*, Seattle, 2009, IASP Press.
220. Edwards J, Knowles N: Superficial dry needling and active stretching in the treatment of myofascial pain: a randomised controlled trial, *Acupunct Med* 21(3):80–86, 2003.
221. Chaitow L, Liebenson C: *Muscle energy techniques*, ed 2, Edinburgh, 2001, Churchill Livingstone.
222. Sahrmann S: *Diagnosis and treatment of movement impairment syndromes*, St. Louis, 2002, Mosby.
223. Weerapong P, Hume PA, Kolt GS: Stretching: mechanisms and benefits for sport performance and injury prevention, *Phys Ther Rev* 9(4):189–206, 2004.
224. Kendall F, Kendall McCreary E, Provance P, et al: *Muscles: testing and function with posture and pain*, ed 5, Baltimore, 2005, Lippincott Williams & Wilkins.
225. Gumina S, Di Giorgio G, Postacchini F, et al: Subacromial space in adult patients with thoracic hyperkyphosis and in healthy volunteers, *Chir Organi Mov* 91(2):93–96, 2008.
226. Solem-Bertoft E, Thuomas KA, Westerberg CE: The influence of scapular retraction and protraction on the width of the subacromial space: an MRI study, *Clin Orthop Relat Res* 296:99–103, 1993.
227. Fernandez-de-Las-Penas C, Cuadrado ML, Pareja JA: Myofascial trigger points, neck mobility, and forward head posture in episodic tension-type headache, *Headache* 47(5):662–672, 2007.

228. Fernandez-de-Las-Penas C, Cuadrado ML, Pareja JA: Myofascial trigger points, neck mobility and forward head posture in unilateral migraine, *Cephalalgia* 26(9):1061–1070, 2006.
229. Treaster D, Marras WS, Burr D, et al: Myofascial trigger point development from visual and postural stressors during computer work, *J Electromyogr Kinesiol* 16(2):115–124, 2006.
230. Hoyle JA, Marras WS, Sheedy JE, et al: Effects of postural and visual stressors on myofascial trigger point development and motor unit rotation during computer work, *J Electromyogr Kinesiol* 2010 Jun 25 [Epub ahead of print].
231. Taylor DC, Dalton JD Jr, Seaber AV, et al: Viscoelastic properties of muscle-tendon units: the biomechanical effects of stretching, *Am J Sports Med* 18(3):300–309, 1990.
232. Mattes AL: *Active isolated stretching*, Sarasota, Fla, 1995, AL Mattes (2932 Lexington Street, Sarasota, Fla 34231-6118).
233. Alter MJ: *Science of flexibility*, ed 2, Champaign, Ill, 1996, Human Kinetics.
234. Hakim A, Grahame R: Joint hypermobility, *Best Pract Res Clin Rheumatol* 17(6):989–1004, 2003.
235. Seckin U, Tur BS, Yilmaz O, et al: The prevalence of joint hypermobility among high school students, *Rheumatol Int* 25 (4):260–263, 2005.
236. Klemp P, Stevens JE, Isaacs S: A hypermobility study in ballet dancers, *J Rheumatol* 11(5):692–696, 1984.
237. Sahin N, Karatas O, Ozkaya M, et al: Demographics features, clinical findings and functional status in a group of subjects with cervical myofascial pain syndrome, *Agri* 20(3):14–19, 2008.
238. Beighton P, Solomon L, Soskolne CL: Articular mobility in an African population, *Ann Rheum Dis* 32(5):413–418, 1973.
239. Wheeler AH: Myofascial pain disorders: theory to therapy, *Drugs* 64(1):45–62, 2004.
240. Stauber WT: Factors involved in strain-induced injury in skeletal muscles and outcomes of prolonged exposures, *J Electromyogr Kinesiol* 14(1):61–70, 2004.
241. Ivey FM Jr, Calhoun JH, Rusche K, et al: Isokinetic testing of shoulder strength: normal values, *Arch Phys Med Rehabil* 66 (6):384–386, 1985.
242. Ellenbecker TS, Mattalino AJ: Concentric isokinetic shoulder internal and external rotation strength in professional baseball pitchers, *J Orthop Sports Phys Ther* 25(5):323–328, 1997.
243. Donatelli R: *Sports-specific rehabilitation*, St. Louis, 2006, Churchill Livingstone.
244. Kraemer WJ, Ratamess NA: Fundamentals of resistance training: progression and exercise prescription, *Med Sci Sports Exerc* 36(4):674–688, 2004.
245. Dimond D, Donatelli R, Morimatsu K: *The bare minimum: the Donatelli shoulder method. Assessment and treatment*, 2009, D Dimond.
246. Reinold M, Escamilla R, Wilk K: Current concepts in the scientific and clinical rationale behind exercises for glenohumeral and scapulothoracic musculature, *J Orthop Sports Phys Ther* 39(2):105–117, 2009.
247. McEvoy J, O'Sullivan K, Bron C: Therapeutic exercises for the shoulder region. In Fernandez-de-las Penas C, Cleland JA, Huijbregts P, editors: *Neck and arm pain syndromes: evidence-informed screening, diagnosis, and management in manual therapy*, St. Louis, 2011, Churchill Livingstone Elsevier.
248. Boyling JD, Jull GA: The future scope of manual therapy. In Boyling JD, Grieve GPM, Jull GA, editors: *Grieve's modern manual therapy: the vertebral column*, ed 3, Edinburgh, 2004, Churchill Livingstone.
249. Redelmeier DA, Kahneman D: Patients' memories of painful medical treatments: real-time and retrospective evaluations of two minimally invasive procedures, *Pain* 66(1):3–8, 1996.
250. Redelmeier DA, Katz J, Kahneman D: Memories of colonoscopy: a randomized trial, *Pain* 104(1–2):187–194, 2003.
251. Roth RS, Horowitz K, Bachman JE: Chronic myofascial pain: knowledge of diagnosis and satisfaction with treatment, *Arch Phys Med Rehabil* 79(8):966–970, 1998.
252. Cicerone KD: Evidence-based practice and the limits of rational rehabilitation, *Arch Phys Med Rehabil* 86(6): 1073–1074, 2005.

CHAPTER

17

Donn Dimond and
Robert A. Donatelli

Strength Training Concepts

Strengthening is an important part of any patient's rehabilitation. To strengthen and progress a patient optimally, numerous variables need to be considered. The therapist must consider the type of exercise and its frequency, intensity, and duration. All these variables determine the success of any strengthening program. The therapist must also understand the physiologic and neural adaptations that occur within the muscle and how long it takes to make these changes. Can we convert muscle fiber types with strength training? Should eccentric, concentric, or isometric exercises be used or a combination of all three? Is it necessary to periodize the patient's strength training, and will it result in significant changes in muscle strength? How does the therapist incorporate neuromuscular exercises into a strengthening program? Answers to these questions are essential to professionals responsible for prescribing resistance exercise for improvement of a patient's way of life, be it on the field of play or their everyday function.

Simply stated, *strength* is the ability of the muscle to exert a maximum force at a specified velocity.[1] *Power* is defined as the force exerted multiplied by the velocity of movement.[1] Muscular power is a function of both strength and speed of movement. *Endurance* is the ability to sustain an activity for extended periods of time.[1] Local muscle endurance is best described as the ability to resist muscular fatigue.[1] Dimond and Donatelli believe that a good strength base, a foundation of muscular power, and muscular endurance are important to reestablishing function and improving performance.

In today's therapy environment, much emphasis is placed on functional exercises. Unfortunately, most of the exercises considered as functional seem to be performed in a weight-bearing position with significant muscular cocontraction. In fact, strengthening exercises have been labeled as nonfunctional because they are performed in the open kinetic chain (OKC). For the purposes of this chapter, a *functional exercise* is defined as an exercise specific to the muscle groups that are important to the activity the patient wishes to resume; sufficient resistance, repetitions, and sets are used to stimulate the muscle to adapt by increasing strength. Several studies demonstrated that when OKC exercises were used to strengthen the glenohumeral rotators, significant gains were made both in the velocity of a baseball during a pitch and in the velocity of a tennis ball in a tennis serve.[2,3] Therefore, strength training the rotators of the glenohumeral joint by moving the shoulder into internal and external rotation in an OKC position is a functional exercise. Another study found that by strength training subjects aged between 60 and 83 years of age with weight machines, the subjects were able to decrease the amount of time it took them to climb a flight stairs.[4] Finally, another study found that combining OKC exercise with functional exercise had better outcomes than just functional exercise by itself in patients who had undergone anterior cruciate ligament reconstruction.[5]

This chapter begins by describing the different types of muscle action. Neural adaptations at both at the local level and within the central nervous system as a result of strength training are discussed. Muscle cellular adaptations, including fiber conversion, change in sarcomeres, and hypertrophy versus hyperplasia are also discussed, as are mechanical muscle changes secondary to strength training, as well as connective tissue changes. The discussion of hormonal and metabolic changes is followed by a description of the effects of aging on muscle and exercise adaptations in older persons. Gender differences and muscle changes are also considered. Finally, time frames for developing strength gains in addition to the amount of resistance, sets, and repetitions needed to make these changes are examined. Understanding the cellular and molecular adaptations of skeletal muscle in response to strength training is important to provide the framework to improve performance in the athlete and the health and quality of life of the general population with or without chronic diseases.

TYPES OF MUSCLE ACTIONS

The three main muscle strengthening actions are eccentric, concentric, and isometric. Simply stated, an *eccentric action* occurs whenever an opposing force acting on a muscle exceeds the force produced by that muscle.[6] This causes the muscle to lengthen while it is being activated. Eccentric actions are characterized by their ability to achieve high muscle forces, an enhancement of the tissue damage that is associated with muscle soreness, and perhaps require unique control strategies.[7] Eccentric actions are used frequently throughout everyday life and especially in athletic competition. A common human movement strategy is to combine concentric and eccentric actions into a sequence called the *stretch-shorten cycle*.[7] This cycle typically involves a small-amplitude, moderate-velocity to high-velocity eccentric contraction that is followed by a concentric contraction.[7] Eccentric contractions are mechanically efficient and can attenuate impact forces and maximize performance.[7]

The second type of action is a *concentric contraction*. A concentric contraction occurs when the force produced by the muscle exceeds the external force or load.[6] This contraction causes the muscle to shorten and is the latter action of the stretch-shorten cycle. This cycle, as pointed out earlier, happens in most day-to-day activities and occurs without specialized training.[6] Enoka[6] considered that, by performing a concentric contraction only without an eccentric action, muscle performance would be decreased.

The last type of muscle action is called an *isometric action*. Isometric strengthening occurs when the force generated by muscle and the external force are the same, and no lengthening or shortening of the muscle occurs. Isometric strengthening has been shown to be very joint-angle specific and has minimal carryover to other joint angles. There is only a 20° carryover either way from where the muscle was trained, although one study did show greater carryover throughout the entire range when the muscle is trained isometrically in the lengthened position.[8]

NEURAL ADAPTATIONS

The first signs of muscle adaptation to strengthening exercises are neural adaptations. Several studies demonstrated that early strength gains induced by resistance training are primarily the result of modifications of the nervous system. These modifications can be both at the local level and at the central nervous system level. Moritani and deVries,[9] in a landmark study, found that "neural factors" accounted for the significant improvements observed during the first 4 weeks of an 8-week resistance-training program. Staron et al[10] demonstrated that only after 6 weeks of training was significant muscle fiber hypertrophy detected. The neural adaptations elicited by resistance training include decreased cocontraction of antagonists and expansion in the dimensions of the neuromuscular junction, findings indicating greater content of presynaptic neurotransmitter and postsynaptic receptors.[11-13] Greater synchronicity of the discharge of motor units after strength training has also been reported.[14] Aagaard et al[15] suggested that increases in motor neuronal output induced by strength training caused increased central motor drive, elevated motor neuron excitability, and reduced presynaptic inhibition. Lagerquist et al[16] found similar increases in strength in both the trained and untrained soleus muscle of subjects who were trained for 5 weeks. Based on these results, the investigators concluded that the increase in strength of the untrained limb may be caused by supraspinal mechanisms. They also went on to suggest that the increased force production of the trained limb versus the untrained limb may result from a synergistic effect of the increased somatosensory stimuli and descending supraspinal commands. Another study found that the cross-education effect may be partly controlled by adaptations in the sensorimotor cortex and the temporal lobe.[17] In fact, one article recommended incorporating motor learning theory and imagined contractions with strength training.[18]

Eccentric contractions have been found to induce greater cross-education effects than concentric and isometric muscle actions. Zhou[19] found increases of 5% to 35% in force production for the untrained limb during both isometric and concentric muscle actions, whereas Hortobagyi[20] found increases as high as 104% during eccentric muscle action in the untrained limb.

Views are conflicting on the relative contribution of neural versus muscle adaptation with strength training lasting longer than 2 to 3 months. Deschenes and Kraemer[1] indicated that, with prolonged resistance training, the degree of muscle hypertrophy is limited and that significant hypertrophic responses can occur within a finite period lasting no more than 12 months. A secondary neural adaptation explains the continued strength gains with prolonged resistance training. The secondary phase of neural adaptations takes place between the 6th and 12th months. In contrast, Shoepe et al[21] demonstrated substantial muscle hypertrophy as a result of several years of resistance training, when compared with a group of sedentary individuals.

CELLULAR ADAPTATIONS

Muscles are made up of hundreds of thousands of muscle cells, which are also referred to *muscle fibers*. These muscle fibers are made up, in part, of hundreds of myofibrils that extend along the length of the muscle fibers. The *myofibrils* are composed of two types of protein filaments: thick filaments and thin filaments. A *sarcomere* is the small structural unit that makes up the myofibril and contains both the thick and thin filaments. When a muscle contracts, the sarcomeres shorten. Thick filaments are made up of a contractile protein called *myosin*. Thin filaments are made up of three different contractile proteins called *actin, tropomyosin,* and *troponin*. The turnover rate of these muscle proteins is among the slowest in the body. Within skeletal muscle synthesis, growth of contractile proteins lags behind that of other proteins such as mitochondria and sarcoplasmic reticulum.[22,23] The synthesis and accretion of contractile proteins account for the hypertrophy that occurs with resistance training. This hypertrophy is evident mostly within the intracellular myofibrils (25% to 35%), in addition to hypertrophy within the whole muscle (5% to 8%).[1,24]

The human body has different types of muscle fibers: type I, type IIa, and type IIx (used to be referred as type IIb). Any muscle can have the following hybrids of these fiber types: type I/IIa, type IIa/IIx, and type I/IIa/IIx.[25] Type I fibers tend to have a slower contraction time, high resistance to fatigue, and low force production. Type IIa have a fast contraction time, intermediate resistance to fatigue, and high force production. Type IIx have a very fast contraction time, low resistance to fatigue, and very high force production.

Muscle Fiber Type: Specific Adaptations

Malisoux et al[25] found that 8 weeks of training involving stretch-shorten cycle exercises increased single-fiber diameter, peak force, and shortening velocity and led to enhanced fiber power. All these changes were seen in type I, IIa, and IIa/IIx fibers. In addition, peak power was improved in type IIa fibers.

Investigators have documented clearly that a prolonged program of resistance training brings about fiber type conversion with the muscle. The most common finding is an increase in the percentage of type IIa fibers with a decrease in the percentage of type IIb (type IIx) fibers.[26-28] As soon as a type IIb (IIx) muscle fiber is stimulated, it appears to start a process of transformation toward type IIa, by changing the quality of proteins and expressing different types and amounts of myosin adenosine triphosphatase (mATPase).[29] Following a resistance training program, very few type IIb (IIx) fibers remain, a situation that is reversed during detraining. However, when resistance training is starting again, the conversion from type IIb (IIx) to type IIa is quicker. Although resistance training promotes hypertrophy in all three major muscle fiber types in humans—I, IIa, and IIb (IIx) —the amount of hypertrophy differs with each fiber type. Based on examination of pretraining to post-training muscle samples, investigators established that muscle hypertrophy is greatest in the type IIa fibers, followed by the type IIb (IIx), with type I fibers demonstrating the least amount of hypertrophy.[10,26-28,30]

Change in Sarcomeres

Besides fiber type adaptations at the cellular level, other structural signs of muscle damage are present. Electron microscopy has been shown that sarcomeres become out of register, Z-line streaming is evident, regions of overextended sarcomeres are present, and regional disorganization of the myofilaments and t-tubule damage occur.[31] Evidence indicates an increase in sarcomeres after bouts of eccentric exercise.[32] In fact, one study found an 11% increase in sarcomere number after eccentric loading.[31]

HYPERTROPHY VERSUS HYPERPLASIA

Resistance exercise is a potent stimulus to increase the size of muscle. For a muscle to become larger, it must either increase in cross-sectional area (CSA; hypertrophy) or raise the number of muscle fibers (hyperplasia). Investigators generally believe that the number of muscle fibers is innate and does not change during life.[33] In contrast, several researchers reported muscle is capable of increasing its size as a result of an increase in fiber number.[34,35] The exact mechanism responsible for muscle hypertrophy is uncertain, although several theories have been expressed in the literature. Skeletal muscles are capable of remodeling under various conditions. The activation of myogenic stem cells within the muscle is one of the most important events during skeletal muscle remodeling.[35] The muscle (myogenic) stem cells remain dormant under the basement of the myofibers, and on stimulation these stem cells differentiate into satellite cells to form myofibers.[35] The muscle or myogenic stem cells start to generate, by a series of cell divisions, daughter cells that become satellite cells. Evidence suggests that strength training induces a significant increase in satellite cell content in skeletal muscle. Evidence also suggests that strength training down-regulates the expression of myostatin, which is responsible for inhibiting satellite cell activation.[36] Because the myonuclei in mature muscle fibers are not able to divide, investigators have suggested that the incorporation of satellite cell nuclei into muscle fibers results in the maintenance of a constant nuclear-to-cytoplasmic ratio. Therefore, new muscle fibers are formed following strength training. When resistance or endurance exercises promote satellite cell proliferation and when differentiation can be detected in injured fibers and in fibers with no discernible damage, muscle hyperplasia occurs in human skeletal muscle.[34,35,37,38]

Force developed by the myofilaments (actin and myosin) may stimulate the uptake of amino acids and thus result in muscle tissue growth.[39] Heavy forces encountered during resistance training lead to disruption in the Z-lines. The disorganization after disruption of the Z-disks may cause the myofibril to split and grow back to full size.[40] Furthermore, the disruption and rebuilding of the muscle result in an increase in the connective tissue surrounding the muscle fibers.

In summary, as a result of strength training exercises, physiologic adaptations of muscle lead to an increase in strength. These adaptations include hypertrophy (within the first 6 to 8 weeks), hyperplasia, hormonal changes, increase in the connective tissue surrounding the muscle fibers, disruption of the myofilaments, and neuromuscular changes (within the first 2 weeks of training). In addition, metabolic adaptations occur within the muscle fiber that increase the ability of the muscle to generate adenosine triphosphate (ATP) for anaerobic metabolism. Anaerobic metabolism requires that the muscle increase phosphocreatine and glycogen stores, increase the enzyme creatine phosphokinase that breaks down phosphocreatine, and augment the rate-limiting enzyme phosphofructokinase of glycolysis.

MECHANICAL CHANGES IN PASSIVE AND DYNAMIC MUSCLE STIFFNESS

At the mechanical level, evidence of increases in dynamic and passive muscle stiffness is present.[41] Whitehead et al[32] stated that the rise in passive muscle tension depends on the length range over which the muscle is worked. With biceps brachii eccentric loading, the muscle sense organs and the body's ability to sense joint position have shown both an increase and a decrease in the flexed position. This finding seems to depend on whether a muscle spindle injury (which increases the flexed position) is actually present, with high-intensity strengthening, or whether sarcomere disruption (which decreases the flexed position) has occurred.[7] Mechanically, one sees signs of a shift in the muscle's optimum length toward a longer muscle length, a decrease in active tension, an increase in passive tension, and muscle swelling and soreness.[31] This muscle swelling and soreness leads to delayed-onset muscle soreness, which is thought to be purely mechanical and not an inflammatory response.[41]

CONNECTIVE TISSUE CHANGES

Not only do changes occur in the muscles and their respective cells, but changes also take place in the tendons. Tendons in trained individuals are different from those in untrained individuals. Data in humans show that the larger CSA of the trained tendon results in lower stress on the tendon during maximal isometric contractions in trained compared with untrained individuals and provides a more injury-resistant tendon.[42] Ying et al[43] found that the Achilles tendons of individuals with a history of physical activity had a larger CSA than in their sedentary counterparts. An adaptive response that results in the increased net synthesis of type I collagen in the peritendinous tissue around the Achilles tendon was found to take place after 4 weeks of training.[44] Type I collagen fibers are thicker than the other collagen fibers. Although an initial increase in type I collagen occurs, this does not transfer over to an immediate increase in the CSA of a nonpathologic tendon. Nonpathologic tendons appear to need a prolonged training effect to have an increase in the CSA. One study found that the CSA was increased by 20% to 30% in long distance runners versus untrained subjects.[45] Another study, however, showed no increase in CSA after just 6 months of recreational running.[46]

When an injury process is present, however, the response to resistance training within the tendon to its normal state is quicker. With eccentric training in patients with Achilles tendinosis, Ohberg et al[47] showed an actual decrease in the pathologic Achilles tendon width along with decreased pain in a 12-week period. Because most of the foregoing studies used isotonic or concentric resistance training as their mode of exercise, it would be interesting to see what type of changes would take place using eccentric resistance training in healthy subjects and whether Achilles tendon CSA and maximal strain would increase more quickly with eccentric loading versus concentric or isotonic contractions.

With a chronic overload injury to a tendon, up-regulation of type I and type III collagen occurs, with a preference for type III.[42] Type III collagen is thinner than type I and has been shown to be more prevalent in rupture sites in the Achilles tendon than at other areas in the same tendon.[42] Training can increase type I collagen production and can improve patients' overall symptoms of tendinopathy and may also decrease the chances of acute tendon rupture.[42]

In summary, resistance training not only changes the muscles but also has an effect on the connective tissue. The connective tissue can increase in size and strength, features that may help to decrease the incidence of injury. However, the length of this training in healthy subjects is still in question. By eccentrically loading a pathologic tendon, one can improve a patient's symptoms and normalize the tendon's size within 12 weeks.

HORMONAL RESPONSES

Resistance training has been shown to elicit a significant acute hormonal response, which is more critical to tissue growth and remodeling than chronic changes in resting hormonal concentrations. Concentrations of anabolic steroids such as testosterone and the growth hormone (GH) have been shown to elevate during 15 to 30 minutes of exercise using high volume, moderate to high intensity, short rest periods, and stressing of a large muscle mass when compared with low-volume, high-intensity protocols using long rest intervals.[47]

Although single bouts of exercise can cause a significant acute rise in serum total and free testosterone concentrations in male subjects, no significant rise in female subjects occurs regardless of age.[48] Other anabolic hormones such as insulin and insulin-like growth factor-I (IGF-I) are critical to skeletal muscle growth. Blood glucose and amino acid levels regulate insulin. However, following resistance exercise, elevations in circulating IGF-I have been reported, presumably in response to GH-stimulated secretion.[47] A significant rise in GH occurs regardless of sex, but not in older women.[48]

AGING AND MUSCLE CHANGES

Professional athletes increasingly performing longer and longer. Demographic data clearly illustrate that, overall, the population of the United States is growing older. Aging causes a loss of functional capacity resulting from a decrease in muscle mass (sarcopenia).[49] Approximately one third of the total muscle mass is lost between 30 and 80 years of age.[50] This decrease in muscle loss is primarily as a result of selective loss and remodeling of motor units. By the seventh decade of life, some muscles may have only half the number of motor units and 75% of the total number of fibers compared with muscles of young adults.[51] The type II fibers appear to be the most severely affected, gradually decreasing in both size and number with advancing age. Loss of fiber begins at approximately 25 years of age and accelerates thereafter.[52] However, it appears that training can both reverse aging atrophy and maintain fiber type distributions in older individuals similar to those found in young persons. Several studies determined that strength improvements in older persons are coupled with cellular and whole muscle hypertrophy.[11,53-55] Moreover, muscle hypertrophy responses to resistance training have been found to be indistinguishable between young and older people.[11,56]

Research has suggested that power (high-velocity) training is more effective than strength training in improving physical function in community-dwelling adults.[57] Another study found that using 80% of one repetition maximum (1 RM) for the resistance was the most effective way to achieve simultaneous improvements in muscle strength, power, and endurance in older adults.[58] Another study found that power training increased balance over a nontraining group, especially using a load of 20% 1 RM.[59]

Although in general 2 to 3 sets of strength training are most beneficial, some studies found that, in older individuals, a single set of exercises was sufficient to enhance muscle function and physical performance significantly (chair rise, 6-meter backward walk, 400-meter walk, and stair climbing test), although gains in muscle strength and endurance were greater in the 3-set group.[60] Another study found that regardless of the intensity (high, 80% 1 RM; low, 50% 1 RM) improvements in strength, endurance, and stair climbing time were significant by doing 1 set of 12 repetitions.[61] In addition, older individuals who supplemented their exercise regimen with creatine had a greater increase in fat-free mass and total body mass as compared with the placebo group with strength training.[62] The following recommendations for strength training variables are beneficial to use in older persons as well as in young athletes or patients:

- Strength training repetitions: 6 to 12
- Multiple sets: 2 to 3
- At least 2 days per week and a maximum of 3 days per week of strength training
- 90 seconds to 2 minutes of rest between sets
- Training of the large muscle groups before the smaller muscle groups

The choice of the exercises should be based on an evaluation of muscle strength and the muscles that are important to the type of activity the patient wishes to resume. The greater the intensity of the activity the patient wishes to return to, the more intense the rehabilitation or training should be.

GENDER DIFFERENCES AND MUSCLE CHANGES

Sex differences are apparent in muscle cross-sectional examination before and after training; type IIa fibers are the largest in men, whereas type I fibers are the largest in women.[63] Furthermore, Staron et al[26] demonstrated, with heavy resistance training, that the conversion of type IIb (IIx) fibers to type IIa fibers occurred at 2 weeks in female subjects and at 4 weeks in male subjects.

One study found that, by measuring muscle quality (maximal force production per unit of muscle mass) after 9 weeks of strength training, young women (20 to 30 years old) had significantly greater gains than did young men, old men, and old women.[64] In fact, after 30 weeks of detraining, the young women still had greater muscle quality than did the other three groups. In another study that looked at muscle volume in response to strength training in both old and young men and women, however, young men were the only subjects who were able to maintain their gain in muscle volume after 31 weeks of detraining.[65]

Differences also appear to exist in relation to eccentric strength across genders and the life span. Investigators found that concentric peak torque decreased more with age than did eccentric peak torque for both men and women.[66] Another study found that women tended to preserve muscle quality better with age for eccentric peak torque.[67] In addition, older women seemed to have an enhanced capacity, approximately a decade longer, to store elastic energy than did age-matched men and younger men and women.[67]

TYPES OF MUSCLE ACTION ADAPTATIONS

Eccentric Strengthening

After a bout of eccentric exercise, an adaptation takes place. This adaptation can be called the *repeated bout effect*. When one performs an eccentric bout of exercise, a repeated bout effect adaptation protects the muscle against further damage from subsequent eccentric bouts.[41] This adaptation can help to improve performance and help to prevent injury. With eccentric strengthening and the foregoing adaptations come increases in strength, in CSA, and in neural activation.[68] Along with muscle adaptation, investigators have discussed possible tendon adaptations. With biceps brachii eccentric loading, the muscle sense organs and the body's ability to sense joint position both show an increase and a decrease in the flexed position. This finding seems to depend on whether a muscle spindle injury (increase flexed position) is actually present or whether only sarcomere disruption (decreased flexed position) has occurred, with muscle spindle injury resulting from high-intensity strengthening.[7] An increased signal from a muscle spindle has been shown with heavy eccentric strengthening, whereas no studies have provided evidence of more significant neural adaptation with concentric strengthening.

Typically, eccentric contractions can generate two to three times more force than a concentric contraction.[69] This finding led some investigators to believe that by training somebody eccentrically, that person will have a greater capability of overloading the muscle to a greater extent and enhancing muscle mass, strength, and power when compared with concentric strengthening.[69] This generalization may seem fair but may be too simple.

Many studies have shown an increase, decrease, or no change in functional performance, concentric strength, and eccentric strength after eccentric training.[70-81] The outcomes noted earlier can be attributed to different training protocols and methods of assessment.[70] Current research has shown that eccentric training is more effective than concentric training for developing eccentric strength and that concentric strengthening is more effective for developing concentric strength.[71]

The specificity of training is another application of the *specific adaptations to imposed demands principle* (SAID).

The degree of that strength gain is relative to the volume and intensity and velocity of the eccentric exercise. In most studies, the load used was appropriate to induce failure in the muscle. The actual volume does vary, but one study supported the use of low-volume eccentric exercise.[81] Another study found that when compared with high-intensity eccentric training, low-intensity eccentric training had the same amount of muscle damage but without the large drop in muscle performance.[82] Based on these two studies, one may not need to use a high-intensity and high-volume model for eccentric strength gains. Other research has shown that to obtain the greatest hypertrophy and strength gains, one needs to work eccentrically 180° per second over the range.[83] This study was performed with isokinetic equipment, however, so the carryover to isotonic exercise is unknown.

Concentric Strengthening

As discussed earlier, neural, contractile, and muscle fiber type adaptations occur with strength training. Most athletes use a combination of eccentric, concentric, and isometric contractions. Because of the need to control a load when returning it to the starting position, most strengthening studies have used a combination of eccentric and concentric actions. As previously noted, the stretch-shorten cycle is initiated by an eccentric action followed by a concentric contraction, whereas an eccentric contraction can happen by itself. Because of this characteristic, anytime a person works isotonically, he or she is working eccentrically even if concentrating on the shortening contraction. In the real world, it is almost impossible to work only concentrically. That is what makes it so difficult to discuss the adaptations of concentric-only contractions. What follows is an attempt to discuss concentric strengthening adaptations. The changes associated with concentric strength training are poorly understood.[84]

Concentric-only strengthening does not produce as much exercise-induced muscle injury as does eccentric strengthening.[85] In fact, more muscle damage is produced when a muscle is loaded eccentrically than if it were loaded eccentrically and concentrically, regardless whether this was done alternately or separated.[86] Whereas eccentric strengthening carryover seems to be very specific to intensity, mode, and velocity of training, concentric strengthening may be more general with its carryover. In one study, investigators found that velocity-specific concentric-only strengthening resulted in increased peak torques higher and lower than the training velocity.[87] Another study, however, found that concentric training was less mode and speed specific than was corresponding eccentric training.[88]

Isometric Strengthening

The question exists about what type of adaptations the muscle will undergo with isometric strengthening. One study reported that this adaptation depends on the type of rate of contraction. Progressive contractions produced modification of the nervous system at the peripheral level, whereas ballistic contractions affected the muscle's contractile properties.[89] Another study found that increased isometric strength may result from factors associated with hypertrophy, independent of neural adaptations.[90]

CLINICAL APPLICATION

How does a clinician apply the foregoing information to a clinical situation? First, clinicians must integrate eccentric strengthening into practice. It needs to be more than just lowering the weight after a concentric contraction. Based on current research, clinicians know that to rehabilitate a patient for functional tasks or to train an athlete, the patient must perform eccentric movements. In the definition of a stretch-shorten cycle, an eccentric contraction is a low-amplitude and moderate-velocity to high-velocity contraction. Therefore, eccentric movements must be faster than concentric contractions. Eccentric isotonic training must produce forces two to three times greater than its concentric counterpart to have the proper intensity. This does not necessarily mean to double or triple the isotonic load. Force that is generated during an exercise depends on the amount of resistance used, and the greater the resistance, the slower the speed. (Force equals mass times acceleration). Because an eccentric action should be happening at a greater speed, the clinician may need only to increase the load by 20% to 30% if the limb is moving twice as fast as the concentric contraction. The clinician must allow a rest period longer than 48 hours. Clinicians must work with patients in a specific eccentric manner to obtain maximum gains from their rehabilitation and performance training. How to do that safely and effectively in a controlled clinical setting isotonically is the first question that needs to be answered.

What injuries or muscle groups would benefit the most from eccentric strengthening? Several studies discussed the use of eccentric strengthening in treating patients with Achilles tendinosis, patellar tendinopathy, iliotibial band syndrome in runners, and chronic isolated posterior cruciate ligament injury in knees.[91-95] Although these studies focused on the lower extremities, they can be carried over to the upper extremities. MacLean et al[94] demonstrated, in knees with a posterior cruciate ligament deficit, a significantly decreased eccentric-to-concentric ratio compared with the contralateral hamstring. In the study by Mafi et al,[91] more patients with chronic Achilles tendinosis had a better overall satisfaction and decreased pain with eccentric strengthening training than with concentric strengthening training. Another study, by Young et al,[95] showed that eccentric training with a decline squat protocol was superior to a traditional eccentric protocol, with decreased pain and improved sporting function in elite volleyball players over 12 months who had suffered patellar tendinopathy. Ohberg et al[47] showed, with eccentric training in patients with Achilles tendinosis, an actual decrease in Achilles tendon width along with decreased pain. These studies indicate that eccentric strengthening should be a definite part of any tendinopathy treatment.

Other applications may include using eccentric actions and loading on muscle groups that primarily work concentrically but that have been immobilized. An example is a patient who has undergone anterior cruciate ligament repair. If the knee has been braced and the quadriceps group has been in a shortened position, muscular atrophy will occur, along with a decrease in the number of sarcomeres. This remolding can occur within the first 5 days of immobilization.[7] If clinicians eccentrically load the quadriceps group properly in the open chain, sarcomere lengthening will occur, along with an increase in the actual number of sarcomeres. This adaptation will help to speed up the return of good quadriceps eccentric action and possibly the concentric contraction as well. With the eccentric loading of the tibia in the open chain position, the tibia will be gliding posteriorly, and this will eliminate any anterior shear force on the anterior cruciate ligament. With a concentric open chain quadriceps contraction, the force generated is an anterior shear.

When working with patients and athletes, clinicians must consider the specific function of a muscle in relation to that athlete's sport. Rojas et al[96] found that, in female softball players, the biceps brachii activity during the windmill pitch is higher than during an overhand throw and is most active during the 9-o'clock and follow-through phases of the pitch. The investigators concluded that the repetitive eccentric biceps contractions may help to explain the high incidence of anterior shoulder pain clinically observed in elite windmill pitchers. Therefore, to help decrease this incidence, it would be beneficial to train the biceps brachii eccentrically, to allow it adapt and attenuate the eccentric force being generated by the windmill pitch.[96] Another muscle that would benefit from eccentric loading is the subscapularis. One study[97] found that decreased subscapularis muscle strength in the position simulating the late cocking phase of throwing motion resulted in increased maximum external rotation and also increased glenohumeral contact pressure. If the clinician is able to strengthen the subscapularis eccentrically in the 90/90 position, this may prove to be beneficial to pitchers. Escamilla and Andrews[98] reviewed the literature and found that, during throwing (including during the baseball pitch, the American football throw, the windmill softball pitch, the volleyball serve and spike, and the tennis serve and volley), high rotator cuff muscle activity is generated to help resist the high shoulder distractive forces of approximately 80% to 120% of body weight during the arm cocking and deceleration phases.[98] To help resist this distractive force, the posterior rotator cuff and scapular rotators need to strengthen eccentrically.

The same is true for a baseball pitcher, who by eccentrically training the rotator cuff muscles may be able to adapt to higher eccentric forces and therefore decrease his or her chances of suffering a deceleration injury. To gain these benefits from eccentric training, however, the patient would most likely need to be trained very specifically by training the same muscle groups with the same intensity as needed for the sport. One study showed a decrease in the occurrence of hamstring strain injuries in elite soccer players after eccentric overload training.[99]

Examples of when not to use an eccentric loading action are, obviously, during the initial rehabilitation after a tendon repair, and in the initial stages of muscle healing. Because the force generated by an eccentric action can be two to three times greater than a concentric contraction, failure may be generated at the repair site or at the site of tissue injury. For example, if a patient underwent supraspinatus tendon repair just 2 weeks earlier, eccentric loading should be avoided. However, if the same patient is working on active assistive range of motion with wall walks and at the top of the exercise starts to lower the arm without assistance from the wall, the patient will eccentrically load that tendon and may rerupture the tendon repair. Because concentric loading generates less force, it may be more beneficial when working with a repaired tendon to use concentric-only strengthening initially when the tissue has healed enough to withstand an external load.

Isometric contractions seem to be most beneficial when they are used to increase the endurance of those muscles that function as spinal stabilizers.[100] This approach helps to maintain low but continuous activation of the paraspinal and abdominal wall muscles that function as stabilizers.[101] According to research, isometric contractions lend themselves to more of a neural than a contractile adaptation.[101]

EXERCISE VARIABLES

To achieve the physiologic adaptations described earlier, several variables must be considered. The variables that need to be carefully planned for in the development of an exercise program include the choice of exercise, the order of the exercises, the number of sets, the number of repetitions, the intensity of the exercise, the duration of rest between sets and exercises, and the frequency of the training.

The type of exercise should be specific to the specific muscle deficits revealed in the initial evaluation. Furthermore, the type of exercises should be specific to the muscle groups that are important to improving the performance of the athlete. For example, in the overhead-throwing athlete, the external rotators, infraspinatus and teres minor, provide a breaking action in the deceleration of the shoulder. Eccentric loading to the external rotators is a specific exercise to strengthen the external rotators, and eccentric activity of the external rotators is specific to the movement pattern and exercise performed by the athlete in competition. Furthermore, high-speed eccentric loading is very damaging to the muscle. Increasing the eccentric strength of the external rotators provides greater protection of the muscle from damage. This concept is discussed in more detail later in this chapter.

The order of the exercises performed by the athlete typically involves performance of large muscle group exercises before smaller muscle group exercises. Because the metabolic demand is greater for large muscle group exercises, exercises that recruit more than one muscle group, such as closed kinetic chain exercises, should be performed before isolation exercises.[29]

Once again, debate exists in the literature regarding the number of sets and the frequency of strength training. For the athlete, the number of sets within a workout is directly related to the individual training goals. Multiple-set programs optimize the development of strength and local muscular endurance.[102] Gains in strength occur more rapidly with multiple-set programs compared with single-set protocols.[103] Single-set exercise programs may be effective for individuals who are untrained or those just beginning a resistance training program. One-set workouts are also useful for maintenance programs. Furthermore, strength changes over a short-term training period and nonperiodized multiple-set programs may not be different between one, two, or three sets of 10 to 12 RM.[104] However, when a single-set protocol was compared with multiple-set periodized programs, significantly superior results were observed with the multiple-set periodized programs that lasted more than 1 month.[105] Gotshalk et al[105] demonstrated higher volumes of total work produced significantly greater increases in circulating anabolic hormones during the recovery phase following multi-set heavy resistance exercise protocols.

McLester et al[106] demonstrated that training 1 day per week was an effective means of increasing strength, even in experienced recreational weight lifters. However, this study reported superior results with training 3 days per week when compared with 1 day per week when the total volume of the exercise was held constant.

Advanced training frequency varies considerably. Hoffman et al[107] demonstrated that football players training 4 to 5 days per week achieved better results that those who trained either 3 or 6 days per week. Frequencies as high as 18 sessions per week have been reported in Olympic weight lifters.[108,109]

The intensity of the exercise or the amount of resistance used for a specific exercise is the most important variable in resistance training. The most common method of determining the amount of resistance used in a strength training program is the maximal load that can be lifted a given number of repetitions within a single set. The greatest effects on strength measures or maximal power outputs are achieved when the strength training repetitions range between 6 and 12.[29] In other words, the maximum weight that can be lifted 6 times and 6 times only is the amount of resistance to start with in the program. Sets and repetitions are added at subsequent workouts until 3 sets of 12 repetitions are reached. After reaching the foregoing repetitions and the goal is set, the repetitions are reduced down to 8, and additional weight is added, allowing only 8 repetitions. Investigators have demonstrated that once 15 repetitions are achieved with a specific weight, the muscle will no longer continue to improve in strength. However, lighter loads allowing 15 to 20 repetitions are very effective for increasing absolute local muscle endurance.[110,111]

Maximizing power requires a good strength base. Given that both force and time components are relevant to maximizing power, training to increase muscle power requires two general loading strategies. First, heavy resistance training recruits high-threshold fast-twitch muscle fibers that are needed for strength. The second strategy is to incorporate lighter loads, and depending on the exercise this may encompass 30% to 60% of 1 RM.[112,113] Weight training for power has been referred to as *explosive strength training*. Paavolainen et al[113] demonstrated that explosive strength training was able to improve 5-km running time by improving running economy and muscle power, although a large volume of endurance training was performed concomitantly. The maximum amount of resistance used in the explosive strength training exercises was 40% of 1 RM. When performing explosive weight training exercises, the athlete moves as fast as possible throughout the range of motion; the result is that the athlete loses contact with the ground in an explosive squat or loses contact with the bar in a bench press. During a traditional bench press and a squat weight training exercises performed at an explosive velocity, one study showed that 40% to 60% of 1 RM and 50% to 70% of 1 RM, respectively, may be most beneficial in the development of power.[114,115]

The final variable that is important to muscle adaptation from strength training is the time intervals between sets. The rest interval depends on the intensity of the training. For example, investigators have shown that acute force and power production may be compromised by short rest periods of 60 seconds or less.[116] Longitudinal studies have shown that greater strength increases result from long rest periods between sets, 2 to 3 minutes versus 30 to 40 seconds.[117,118]

To make progressive, efficient, and major strength gains in the athlete, one must apply numerous concepts. The patient must be worked specifically toward his or her goal, whether it is strength, hypertrophy, power, or endurance in the context of his or her life or sport. At the same time, the patient must vary the strengthening program with periodization if he or she will be training for extended periods. The basic concept of periodization is changing the intensity, velocity, and volume as needed. The clinician must also consider the type of muscle action (eccentric, concentric, and isometric) and the amount of focus that action will require to help the athlete in his or her sport. When rehabilitating or training a patient, the following exercise variables are recommended:

- Strength training repetitions are as follows: 8 to 12 repetitions for strength and hypertrophy, 4 to 6 repetitions for power, and 12 to 15 repetitions for endurance.
- Multiple sets are indicated for all types of strengthening.
- At least 2 days of strength training per week should be included.
- Rest periods are as follows: 1 to 2 minutes for smaller muscle groups and 2 to 3 minutes for larger muscle groups.
- Start with multiple joint exercise and finish with single joint exercises.
- Intensity starts with 8 RM for strength and 10 RM for hypertrophy, 6 RM for power at either high or moderate velocity, and 15 RM for muscular endurance.
- Velocity can be slow, moderate, or fast, depending on specific goals.
- Eccentric strengthening must be focused on for the deceleration muscles, and eccentric and concentric exercises together are needed for the acceleration muscles.
- Anytime a patient is strength training for more than 4 weeks, the program needs to periodize.
- The choice of exercises should be based on an evaluation of muscle strength and the muscles that are important to the patient's type of activity. As previously noted, the greater the intensity of the activity the patient participates in, the more intense the strength training should be.

GLENOHUMERAL AND SCAPULAR ROTATOR STRENGTHENING EXERCISES

One-Arm Row

This exercise is best performed on a bench. Make sure that you form a stable base with the nonworking arm and the leg on that same side. Keep the back flat, and do not hunch over the weight (Fig. 17-1A). As you lift the weight up, squeeze the shoulder blade toward the middle of your back (Fig. 17-1B).When lowering the weight, make sure that it is under control, and do not just let it fall down.

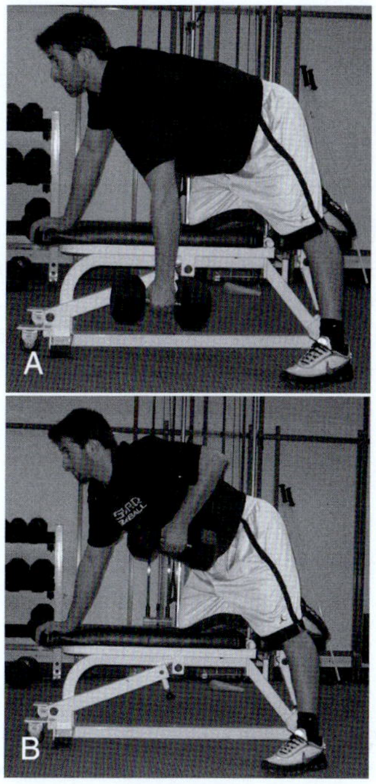

Figure 17-1

Bench and Reach

Some controversy exists about whether a baseball player should do an exercise like this, but this exercise is very important to the development of the serratus anterior muscle. This particular muscle is one of the most important muscles in a baseball athlete, especially the pitcher.
This exercise begins with the weight at the shoulders (think of that position as the base of the triangle) (Fig. 17-2A) and finishes with the weight at the top with the shoulder blades off the bench (the top of the triangle) (Fig. 17-2B). Again, make sure to lower the weight under control.

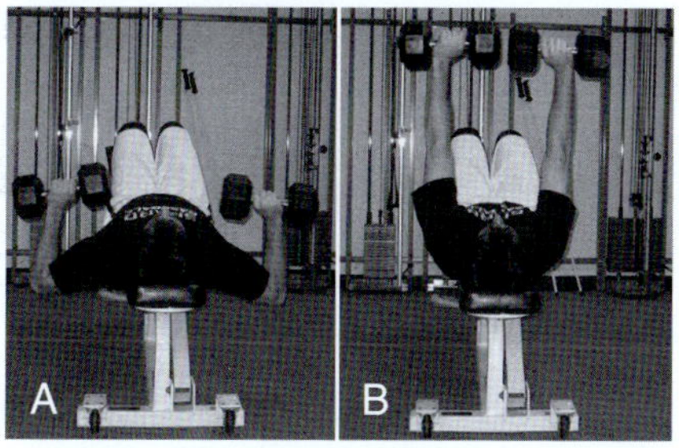

Figure 17-2

Dynamic Hug

For this exercise, face away from the pulleys, which should be spaced slightly wider than shoulder width (Fig. 17-3A). Keep your arms slightly lower than your shoulder (60° elevation). Press forward, like you are hugging a tree (Fig. 17-3B). Return to the starting position under control.

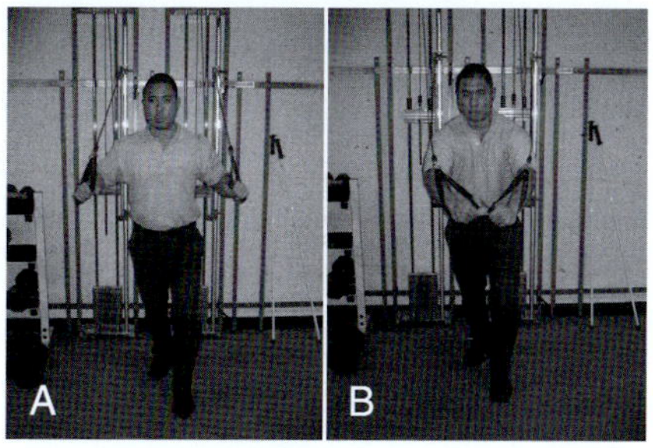

Figure 17-3

Lateral Pull-down

Place your hands a little farther out than shoulder width (Fig. 17-4A). Lean back slightly. Pull the bar down to your chest (never to the back of your neck) (Fig. 17-4B). Control the bar back to its return position.

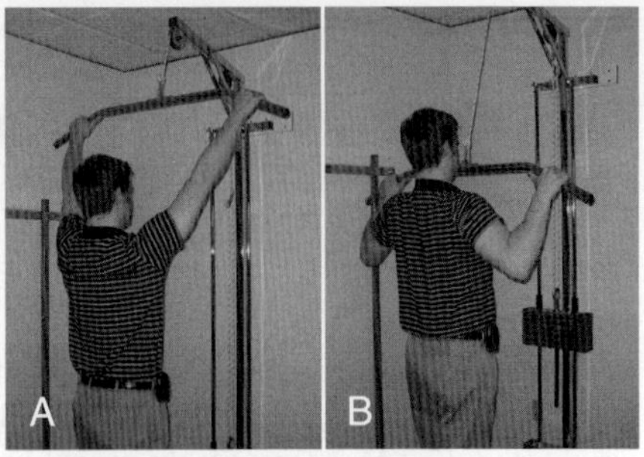

Figure 17-4

Lower Trap Lift

This exercise is probably the hardest one to do with proper form. Just as with the one-arm row, you want to form a stable base on the bench. Start with the arm draped down to the side with the elbow bent (Fig. 17-5A). As you raise the arm up, pretend that you have a plate of glass that your forearm is resting on to keep the elbow and wrist level (Fig. 17-5B).

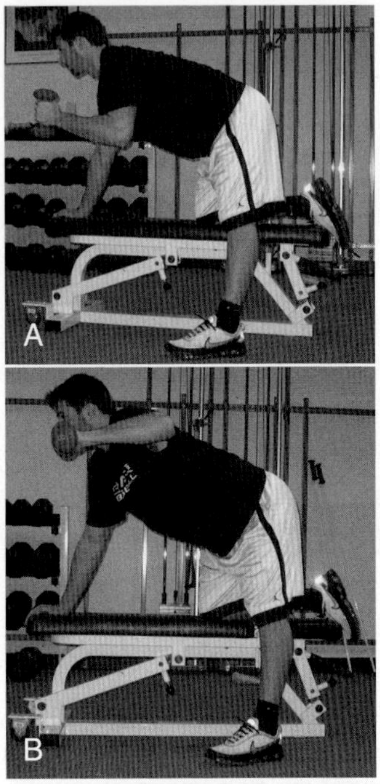

Figure 17-5

Midtrap Lift

This exercise works the stabilizer muscles in the back. It also helps to control the deceleration of the arm. Make sure that your thumb is turned up (Fig. 17-6A) and that you are squeezing your shoulder blade toward your backbone as you lift the weight (Fig. 17-6B).

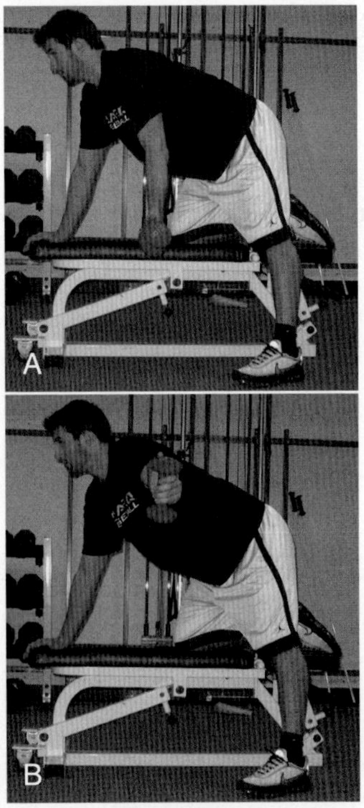

Figure 17-6

Shoulder External Rotation on Bent Knee

This exercise works both the infraspinatus and supraspinatus. Start off with the weight at knee height (Fig. 17-7A) and rotate your arm up toward the ceiling (Fig. 17-7B). Make sure that the elbow does not straighten.

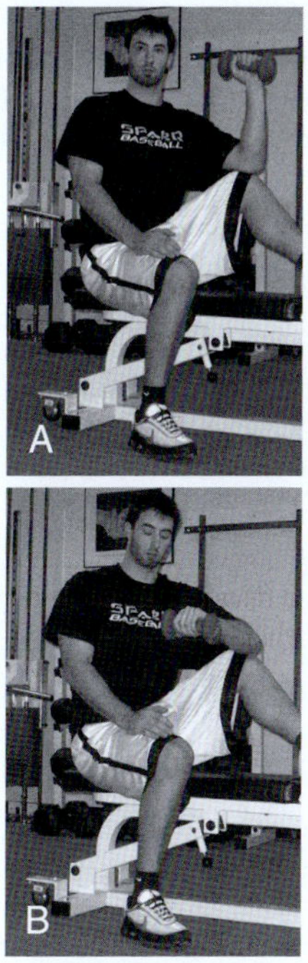

Figure 17-7

Subscapular Lift

Lie on your stomach with your pitching arm on top of your back (Fig. 17-8A). While keeping the elbow bent, lift your entire arm up toward the ceiling (Fig. 17-8B). Start with no weight on this one; it is a hard exercise.

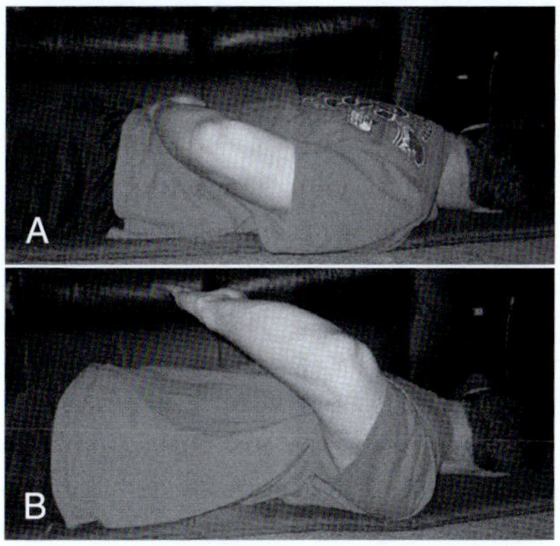

Figure 17-8

Serratus Anterior Lift

While standing, hold a weight out in front of you as shown, slightly above parallel (Fig. 17-9A). Keeping the thumb up, raise the weight up, above your head (Fig. 17-9B). Lower the weight to starting position and repeat.

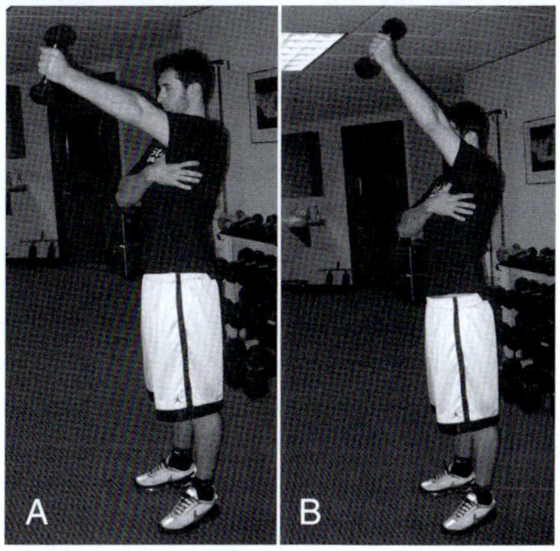

Figure 17-9

Biceps Curl

The biceps muscle is the most important stabilizer for the shoulder in the overhead athlete. We like the two variations shown. The first one is done at shoulder height (Fig. 17-10A), and the second one (Fig. 17-10B) is done while standing on one or two legs.

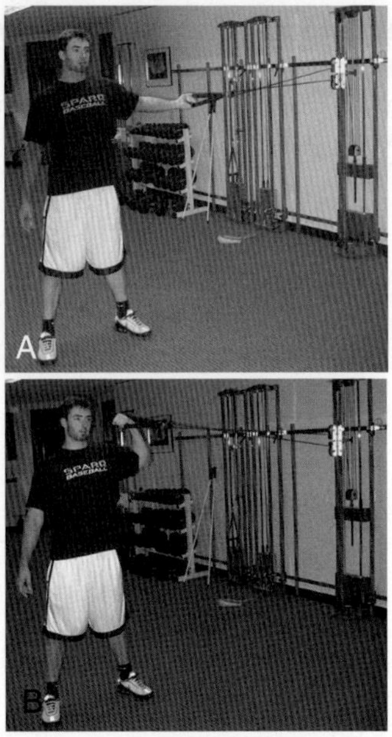

Figure 17-10

Triceps Extension

This exercise works to strengthen the back of the arm and to help protect the elbow along with the biceps curls (see Fig. 17-10). We prefer this exercise because it really isolates the triceps without putting additional stress on the shoulder, as do some other triceps exercises. It is important to keep your elbow close to your trunk when doing this exercise so that you are not cheating and using other muscles (Fig. 17-11A and B).

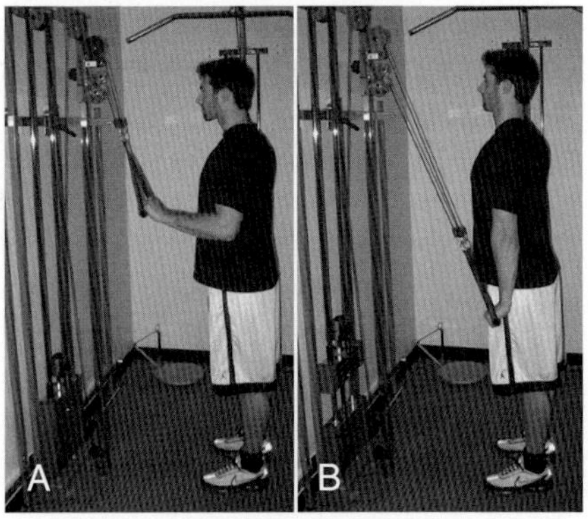

Figure 17-11

REFERENCES

1. Deschenes M, Kraemer W: Performance and physiologic adaptations to resistance training, *Am J Phys Med Rehabil* 81 (11):3–16, 2002.
2. Monte M, Cohen D, Campbell K, et al: Isokinetic concentric versus eccentric training of shoulder rotators with functional evaluation of performance enhancement in elite tennis players, *Am J Sports Med* 22(4):513–517, 1994.
3. Wooden M, Greenfield B, Johanson M, et al: Effects of strength training on throwing velocity and shoulder muscle performance in teenage baseball players, *J Orthop Sports Phys Ther* 15(5):223–227, 1992.
4. Vincent KR, Braith RW, Feldman RA, et al: Resistance exercise and physical performance in adults aged 60 to 83, *J Am Geriatr Soc* 50(6):1100–1107, 2002.
5. Mikkelsen C, Werner S, Eriksson E: Closed kinetic chain alone compared to combined open and closed kinetic chain exercises for quadriceps strengthening after anterior cruciate ligament reconstruction with respect to return to sports: a prospective matched follow-up study, *Knee Surg Sports Traumatol Arthrosc* 8(6):337–342, 2000.
6. Enoka RM: Eccentric contractions require unique activation strategies by the nervous system, *J Appl Physiol* 81 (6):2339–2346, 1996.
7. Proske U, Morgan DL: Muscle damage from eccentric exercise: mechanism, mechanical signs, adaptation and clinical applications, *J Physiol* 537(2):333–345, 2001.
8. Bandy WD, Hanten WP: Changes in torque and electromyography activity of the quadriceps femoris muscles following isometric training, *Phys Ther* 73(7):455–465, 1993.
9. Moritani T, deVries H: Neural factors versus hypertrophy in the time course of muscle strength gain, *Am J Phys Med* 58:115–130, 1979.
10. Staron RS, Leonardi MJ, Karapondo DL: Strength and skeletal muscle adaptations in heavy-resistance-trained women after detraining and retraining, *J Appl Physiol* 70:631–640, 1991.

11. Hakkinen K, Alen M, Kallimen M: Neuromuscular adaptation during prolonged strength training, detraining, and re-strength-training in middle-aged and elderly people, *Eur J Appl Physiol* 83:51–62, 2000.
12. Hakkinen K, Kallimen M, Izquierdo M: Changes in agonist-antagonist EMG, muscle CSA, and force during strength training in middle aged and older people, *J Appl Physiol* 84:1249–1341, 1998.
13. Dechenes MR, Judelson DA, Kraemer WJ: Effects of resistance training on neuromuscular junction morphology, *Muscle Nerve* 23:1576–1581, 2000.
14. Milner-Brown H, Stein R, Lee R: Synchronization of human motor units: possible roles of exercise and supraspinal reflexes, *Electroencephalogr Clin Neurophysiol* 38:245–254, 1975.
15. Aagaard P, Simonsen E, Andersen J, et al: Neural adaptations to resistance training: changes evoked in V-wave and H-reflex responses, *J Appl Physiol* 92:2309–2318, 2002.
16. Laqerquist O, Zehr E, Docherty D: Increased spinal reflex excitability is not associated with neural plasticity underlying the cross education effect, *J Appl Physiol* 100:83–90, 2006.
17. Farthing J, Borowsky R, Chilibeck P, et al: Neuro-physiological adaptations associated with cross-education of strength, *J Sci Med Sport* 8:255–263, 2005.
18. Gabriel D, Kamen G, Frost G: Neural adaptations to resistive exercises: mechanisms and recommendations for training practices, *Sports Med* 37:1–14, 2007.
19. Zhou S: Chronic neural adaptations to unilateral exercise: mechanisms of cross education, *Exerc Sport Sci Rev* 28:177–184, 2000.
20. Hortobagyi TK: Cross education and the human central nervous system, *IEEE Eng Med Biol Mag* 24:22–28, 2005.
21. Shoepe T, Stelzer J, Garner D, et al: Functional adaptability of muscle fibers to long-term resistance exercise, *Med Sci Sports Exerc* 35(6):944–951, 2003.
22. Balogopal P, Rooyacker O, Adey D: Effects of aging on in vivo synthesis of skeletal muscle myosin heavy-chain and sarcoplasmic protein in humans, *Am J Physiol* 273:E790–E800, 1997.
23. Rooyackers O, Adey D, Ades P: Effect of age on in vivo rates of mitochondrial protein synthesis in human skeletal muscle, *Proc Natl Acad Sci U S A* 93:15364–15369, 1996.
24. McCall G, Byrnes W, Fleck S: Acute and chronic hormonal responses to resistance training designed to promote muscle hypertrophy, *Can J Appl Physiol* 24:96–107, 1999.
25. Malisoux L, Francaux M, Nielens H, et al: Stretch-shortening cycle exercises: an effective training paradigm to enhance power output of human single muscle fibers, *J Appl Physiol* 100:771–779, 2006.
26. Staron RS, Karapondo DL, Kraemer WJ: Skeletal muscle adaptations in heavy resistance training in men and women, *J Appl Physiol* 76:1247–1255, 1994.
27. Kraemer W, Patton J, Gordon S: Compatibility of high intensity strength and endurance training on hormonal and skeletal muscle adaptations, *J Appl Physiol* 78:976–989, 1995.
28. Volek J, Duncan N, Mazzetti S: Performance and muscle fiber adaptations to creatine supplementation and heavy resistance training, *Med Sci Sports Exerc* 31:1147–1156, 1999.
29. Kraemer W, Duncan N, Volek J: Resistance training and elite athletes: adaptations and program considerations, *J Orthop Sports Phys Ther* 28(2):110–119, 1998.
30. Johnson T, Klueber K: Skeletal muscle following tonic overload: functional and structural analysis, *Med Sci Sports Exerc* 23:49–55, 1991.
31. Yu JG, Malm C, Thornell: Eccentric contractions leading to DOMS do not cause loss of desmin nor fibre necrosis in human muscle, *Histochem Cell Biol* 118(1):29–34, 2002.
32. Whitehead NP, Morgan DL, Gregory JE, et al: Rises in whole muscle passive tension of mammalian muscle after eccentric contractions at different lengths, *J Appl Physiol* 95:1224–1234, 2003.
33. Malina R: Growth of muscle tissue and muscle mass. In Faulkner F, Tanner J, editors: *Human growth: a comprehensive treatise*, vol 2, New York, 1986, Plenum, pp 77–99.
34. Larsson L, Tesch P: Motor unit fiber density in extremely hypertrophied skeletal muscle in men: muscle electro-physiological signs of fiber hyperplasia, *Eur J Appl Physiol* 55:130–136, 1986.
35. Yan Z: Skeletal muscle adaptation and cell cycle regulation, *Exerc Sport Sci Rev* 2801:24–26, 2000.
36. Kim J, Cross J, Bamman M: Impact of resistance loading on myostatin expression and cell cycle regulation in young and older men and women, *J Appl Physiol* 101:53–59, 2006.
37. Irintchev A, Wernig A: Muscle damage and repair in voluntarily running mice: strain and muscle differences, *Cell Tissue Res* 249:509–521, 1987.
38. Rosenblatt JD, Parry DJ: Adaptation of rat extensor digitorum longus muscle to gamma irradiation and overlaid, *Pflugers Arch* 423:255–264, 1993.
39. Goldberg A, Etlinger J, Goldspink D, et al: Mechanisms of work-induced hypertrophy of skeletal muscle, *Med Sci Sports* 7:248–261, 1975.
40. Goldspink G: Changes in striated muscle fibers during contraction and growth with particular reference to myofibril splinting, *J Cell Sci* 9:123–127, 1971.
41. McHugh MP: Recent advances in the understanding of the repeated bout effect: the protective effect against muscle damage from a single bout of eccentric exercise, *Scand J Med Sci Sports* 13(2):88–97, 2003.
42. Kjaer M: Role of extracellular matrix in adaptation of tendon and skeletal muscle to mechanical loading, *Physiol Rev* 84:649–698, 2004.
43. Ying M, Yeung E, Li B, et al: Sonographic evaluation of the size of Achilles tendon: the effect of exercise and dominance of the ankle, *Ultrasound Med Biol* 29:637–642, 2003.
44. Langberg H, Rosendal L, Kjaer M: Training induced changes in peritendinous type I collagen turnover determined by microdialysis in humans, *J Physiol* 534:297–302, 2001.
45. Rosager S, Aagaard P, Dyhre-Poulsen P, et al: Load displacement properties of the human triceps surae aponeurosis and tendon in runners and non-runners, *Scand J Med Sci Sports* 12:90–98, 2002.
46. Magnusson SP, Hansen P, Kjaer M: Tendon properties in relation to muscular activity and physical training, *Scand J Med Sci Sports* 13:211–233, 2003.
47. Kadi F: Adaptation of human skeletal muscle to training and anabolic steroids, *Acta Physiol Scand Suppl* 168:4–53, 2000.
48. Hakkinen K, Pakarinen A, Kraemer W, et al: Basal concentrations and acute response of serum hormones and strength development during heavy resistance training in middle aged and elderly men and women, *Scand J Rheumatol* 34:309–314, 2005.
49. Tzanoff S, Norris A: Effects of muscle mass decrease on age related BMR changes, *J Appl Physiol* 43:1001–1006, 1977.
50. Doherty T, Vandrervoot A, Taylor A, et al: Effects of motor unit losses on strength in older men and women, *J Appl Physiol* 74:868–874, 1993.

51. Larrson L, Sjodin B, Karlsson J: Histochemical and biochemical changes in human skeletal muscle with age in sedentary males, age 22-65 years, *Acta Physiol Scand* 103:31–39, 1978.
52. Fromtera W, Meredith C, O'Reilly K, et al: Strength conditioning in older men: skeletal muscle hypertrophy and improved function, *J Appl Physiol* 64:1038–1044, 1988.
53. Taafe D, Marcus R: Dynamic muscle strength alterations to detraining and retraining in elderly men, *Clin Physiol* 17:311–324, 1997.
54. Esmarck B, Anderson J, Olsen S, et al: Timing of post-exercise protein intake is important for muscle hypertrophy with resistance training in elderly humans, *J Physiol* 535:301–311, 2001.
55. Newton R, Hakkinen K, Hakkinen A, et al: Mixed-methods of resistance training increases power and strength of young and older men, *Med Sci Sports Exerc* 34:1376–11375, 2002.
56. Lindstedt SL, Reich TE, Keim P, et al: Do muscles function as adaptable locomotor springs? *J Exp Biol* 205:2211–2216, 2002.
57. Miszko T, Cress M, Slade J, et al: Effect of strength and power training in physical function in community dwelling older adults, *J Gerontol A Biol Sci Med Sci* 58:171–175, 2003.
58. de Vos N, Singh N, Ross D, et al: Optimal load for increasing muscle power during explosive resistance training in older adults, *J Gerontol A Biol Sci Med Sci* 60:638–647, 2005.
59. Orr R, de Vos N, Singh N, et al: Power training improves balance in healthy older adults, *Clin Physiol Funct Imaging* 26:305–313, 2006.
60. Galvao D, Taaffe D: Resistance exercise dosage in older adults: single versus multiset effects on physical performance and body composition, *J Am Geriatr Soc* 53:2090–2097, 2005.
61. Vincent K, Braith R, Feldman R, et al: Resistance exercise and physical performance in adults aged 60 to 83, *J Am Geriatr Soc* 50:1100–1107, 2002.
62. Brose A, Parise G, Tarnopolsky M: Creatine supplementation enhances isometric strength and body composition improvements following strength exercise training in older adults, *J Am Geriatr Soc* 53:2090–2097, 2005.
63. Staron R, Hagerman F, Hikida R: Fiber type composition of the vastus lateralis muscle of young men and women, *J Histochem Cytochem* 48:623–629, 2000.
64. Ivey F, Tracy B, Lemmer J, et al: Effects of strength training and detraining on muscle quality: age and gender comparisons, *Scand J Med Sci Sports* 14:16–23, 2004.
65. Ivey F, Roth S, Ferrell R, et al: Effects of age, gender, and myostatin genotype on the hypertropic response to heavy resistance strength training, *J Appl Physiol* 86:195–201, 1999.
66. Porter MM, Myint A, Kramer JF, et al: Concentric and eccentric knee extension strength in older and younger men and women, *Can J Appl Physiol* 20(4):429–439, 1995.
67. Lindle RS, Metter EJ, Lynch NA, et al: Age and gender comparisons of muscle strength in 654 women and men aged 20–93 yr, *J Appl Physiol* 83(5):1581–1587, 1997.
68. Higbie EJ, Cureton KJ, Warren GL III, , et al: Effects of concentric and eccentric training on muscle strength, cross-sectional, and neural activation, *J Appl Physiol* 81:2173–2181, 1996.
69. LeStayo PC, Woolf JM, Lewek MD, et al: Eccentric muscle contractions: their contribution to injury, prevention, rehabilitation, and sport, *J Orthop Sports Phys Ther* 33:557–571, 2003.
70. Tomberlin JP, Basford JR, Schwen EE, et al: Comparative study of is kinetic eccentric and concentric quadriceps training, *J Orthop Sports Phys Ther* 14:31–36, 1991.
71. Colliander EB, Tesch PA: Effects of eccentric and concentric muscle actions in resistance training, *Acta Physiol Scand* 140:31–39, 1990.
72. Komi P, Buskirk ER: Effect of eccentric and concentric muscle conditioning on tension and electrical activity of human muscle, *Ergonomics* 15:417–434, 1972.
73. Colliander EB, Tesch PA: Responses to eccentric and concentric resistance training in females and males, *Acta Physiol Scand* 141:149–156, 1990.
74. Jones DA, Rutherford OM: Human muscle strength training: the effects of three different regimes and the nature of the resultant changes, *J Physiol* 391:1–11, 1987.
75. Dudley GA, Tesch PA, Miller BJ, et al: Importance of eccentric actions in performance adaptations to resistance training, *Aviat Space Environ Med* 62:543–550, 1991.
76. Johnson BL, Adamczyk JW, Tennoe KO, et al: A comparison of concentric and eccentric muscle training, *Med Sci Sports Exerc* 8:35–38, 1976.
77. Duncan PW, Chandler JM, Cavanaugh DK, et al: Mode and speed specificity of eccentric and concentric exercise training, *J Orthop Sports Phys Ther* 11:70–75, 1989.
78. Johnson BL: Eccentric vs concentric muscle training for strength development, *Med Sci Sports Exerc* 4:111–115, 1972.
79. Ellenbecker TS, Davies GJ, Rowinski MJ: Concentric versus eccentric isokinetic strengthening of the rotator cuff: objective data versus functional tests, *Am J Sports Med* 16:64–69, 1988.
80. Hortobagyi T, Katch FI: Role of concentric force in limiting improvement in muscular strength, *J Appl Physiol* 68:650–658, 1990.
81. Paddon-Jones D, Abernethy PJ: Acute adaptation to low volume eccentric exercise, *Med Sci Sports Exerc* 33(7): 1213–1219, 2001.
82. Paschalis V, Koutedakis Y, Jamurtas AZ, et al: Equal volumes of high and low intensity of eccentric exercise in relation to muscle damage and performance, *J Strength Cond Res* 19 (1):184–188, 2005.
83. Farthing JP, Chilibeck PD: The effects of eccentric and concentric training at different velocities on muscle hypertrophy, *Eur J Appl Physiol* 89(6):578–586, 2003.
84. Weir JP, Housch DJ, Housch TJ, et al: The effect of unilateral concentric weight training and detraining on joint angle specificity, cross training, and the bilateral deficit, *J Orthop Sports Phys Ther* 25(4):264–270, 1997.
85. Clarkson PM, Hubal MJ: Exercise-induced muscle damage in humans, *Am J Phys Med Rehabil* 81(11 Suppl):S52–S69, 2002.
86. Nosaka K, Lavender AP, Newton MJ: Effect of alternating eccentric and concentric versus separated eccentric and concentric actions on muscle damage. In *Annual meeting abstracts: A-25: athlete care: treatment and prevention*. Indianapolis, 2-5 June 2004.
87. Housch DJ, Housch TJ: The effects of unilateral velocity-specific concentric strength training, *J Orthop Sports Phys Ther* 17(5):252–256, 1993.
88. Seger JY, Thorsteensson A: Effects of eccentric versus concentric training in thigh muscle strength and EMG, *Int J Sports Med* 26(1):45–52, 2005.
89. Maffiuletti NA, Martin A: Progressive versus rapid rate of contraction during 7 wk of isometric resistance training, *Med Sci Sports Exerc* 33(7):1120–1127, 2001.
90. Ebersole KT, Housch TJ, Johnson GO, et al: Mechanomyographic and electromyographic responses to unilateral isometric training, *J Strength Cond Res* 16(2):192–201, 2001.

91. Mafi N, Lorentzon R, Alfredson H: Superior short term results with eccentric calf muscle training compared to concentric training in a randomized prospective multicenter study on patients with chronic Achilles tendinosis, *Knee Surg Sports Traumatol Arthrosc* 9(1):42–47, 2001.
92. Peers KH, Lysens RJ: Patellar tendinopathy in athletes: current diagnostic and therapeutic recommendations, *Sports Med* 35(1):71–87, 2005.
93. Fredericson M, Wolf C: Iliotibial band syndrome in runners: innovations in treatment, *Sports Med* 35(5):451–459, 2005.
94. MacLean CL, Taunton JE, Clement DB, et al: Eccentric and concentric isokinetic moment characteristics in the quadriceps and hamstrings of the chronic isolated posterior cruciate ligament injured knee, *Br J Sports Med* 33:405–408, 1999.
95. Young MA, Cook JL, Purdam CR, et al: Eccentric decline squat protocol offers superior results at 12 months compared with traditional eccentric protocol for patellar tendinopathy in volleyball players, *Br J Sports Med* 39(2):102–105, 2005.
96. Rojas IL, Provencher MT, Bhatia S, et al: Biceps activity during windmill softball pitching: injury implications and comparison with overhand throwing, *Am J Sports Med* 37 (3):558–565, 2009.
97. Mihata T, Gates J, McGarry MH, et al: Effect of rotator cuff muscle imbalance on forceful internal impingement and peel-back of the superior labrum: a cadaveric study, *Am J Sports Med* 37(11):2222–2227, 2009.
98. Escamilla RF, Andrews JR: Shoulder muscle recruitment patterns and related biomechanics during upper extremity sports, *Sports Med* 39(7):569–590, 2009.
99. Askling C, Karlsson J, Thorstensson A: Hamstring injury occurrence in elite soccer players after preseason strength training with eccentric overload, *Scand J Med Sci Sports* 13 (4):244–250, 2003.
100. Biering-Sorensen F: Physical measurements as risk indicators for low back trouble over a one year period, *Spine* 9:106–119, 1984.
101. McGill S: *Low back disorders: evidence based prevention and rehabilitation*, Champaign, Ill, 2000, Human Kinetics.
102. McDouagh M, Davies C: Adaptive response of mammalian skeletal muscle to exercise with high loads, *Eur J Appl Physiol* 52:139–155, 1984.
103. Baker J, Cooper S: Strength and body composition: single versus triple set resistance training programmes, *Med Sci Sports Exerc* 36(5 Suppl):S53, 2004.
104. Fleck S, Kraemer W: *Designing resistance training programs*, ed 2, Champaign, Ill, 1997, Human Kinetics.
105. Gotshalk L, Loebel C, Nindi B, et al: Hormonal responses of multiset versus single set heavy resistance exercise protocols, *Can J Appl Physiol* 22(3):244–255, 1997.
106. McLester J, Bishop P, Guilliams M: Comparison of 1 day and 3 day per week of equal-volume resistance training in experienced subjects, *J Strength Cond Res* 14(3):273–281, 2000.
107. Hoffman J, Kraemer W, Fry A, et al: The effects of self-selection for frequency of training in a winter conditioning program for football, *J Appl Sport Sci Res* 3:76–82, 1990.
108. Kraemer W, Ratamess N: Fundamentals of resistance training: progression and exercise prescription, *Med Sci Sports Exerc* 36:674–688, 2004.
109. Campos G, Luecke H, Wendeln, et al: Muscular adaptations in response to three different resistance-training regimes: specificity of repetition maximum training zones, *Eur J Appl Physiol* 88:50–60, 2002.
110. Stone W, Coulter S: Strength/endurance effects from three resistance-training protocols with women, *J Strength Cond Res* 8:231–234, 1994.
111. Wilson G, Newton R, Murphy A, et al: The optimal training load for the development of dynamic athletic performance, *Med Sci Sports Exerc* 25:1279–1286, 1993.
112. Baker D, Nance S, Moore M: The load that maximizes the average mechanical power output during jump squats in power-trained athletes, *J Strength Cond Res* 15:92–97, 2001.
113. Paavolainen L, Hakkinen K, Hamalainen I, et al: Explosive-strength training improves 5km running time by improving running economy and muscle power, *J Appl Physiol* 86:1527–1533, 1999.
114. Siegel J, Gilders R, Staron R, et al: Human muscle power output during upper and lower body exercises, *J Strength Cond Res* 16:173–178, 2002.
115. Kraemer W: A series of studies: the physiological basis for strength training in American football: fact over philosophy, *J Strength Cond Res* 11:131–142, 1997.
116. Pincivero D, Lephart S, Karunakara R: Effects of rest interval on Isokinetic strength and functional performance after short-term high intensity training, *Br J Sports Med* 31:229–234, 1997.
117. Robinson J, Stone M, Johnson C, et al: Effects of different weight training exercise/rest intervals on strength, power, and high intensity exercise endurance, *J Strength Cond Res* 9:216–221, 1995.
118. Evans W, Campbell W: Sarcopenia and age related changes in body composition and functional capacity, *J Nutr* 123:465–468, 1993.

PART 5
SURGICAL CONSIDERATIONS

CHAPTER 18

Joseph S. Wilkes

Rotator Cuff Repairs

The causes of rotator cuff tears vary and depend on the age of the patient and on the precipitating activity. Rotator cuff tears may be traumatic or degenerative. Because of their locations, the supraspinatus, primarily, and the infraspinatus, secondarily, are the most frequently torn muscles of the rotator cuff (Fig. 18-1). The prevalence of rotator cuff tears in cadavers varies depending on the study from 7% to 37%.[1-3] Rotator cuff tears 15 mm or smaller are frequently asymptomatic, and the percentage of the population with tears is greater with advancing age.[4] Painful tears seem to be associated with ischemia in the tendon or instability associated with the tear that can produce additional disorders such as labral tears, biceps injury, coracoid impingement, and degenerative joint changes.[4,5] Asymptomatic tears have a tendency to progress very slowly, whereas painful tears become larger if they are not treated.[4] Nonoperative treatment with therapy or simple coracoacromial decompression may stabilize these lesions, but some of them progress at a fast rate and remain painful.[5] These painful shoulders are at risk for becoming difficult to repair and may develop arthropathy.[6]

ETIOLOGY

The relationship between the impingement syndrome and rotator cuff disorders, including tears, is well known.[7] Impingement occurs when the coracoacromial arch causes mechanical irritation of the tendon because of narrowing of the subacromial bursal space from either bony encroachment, such as from spur formation or abnormalities of the acromion, or enlargement of the tendon, such as from tendinitis and inflammation (Fig. 18-2).[8,9]

Impingement is not the only cause of rotator cuff tears. Eccentric overload of the rotator cuff muscles that results in overuse and fatigue can cause failure of the tendon fibers of the rotator cuff and is probably the most common cause of tears in young, athletic patients.[10] Fiber failure can also result from chronic tendinitis, including eccentric overload patterns of the rotator cuff that cause tears of the undersurface of the cuff by creating repetitive deceleration stresses (Fig. 18-3). Injuries to the rotator cuff interval or the superior aspect of the capsule and the coracohumeral ligament add strain to the rotator cuff, because the rotator cuff then becomes a primary stabilizer, and can precipitate fiber failure.[11-13] Another cause of rotator cuff lesions is shoulder dislocation. Primary anterior shoulder dislocation is the cause of rotator cuff tears in up to 60% of patients, and glenohumeral instability can cause fraying of either the upper or lower surface of the cuff, depending on whether impingement, known as *secondary impingement,* or overload-type force is placed on the rotator cuff.[14-20]

Acute tears of the rotator cuff can result from extrinsic overload, such as when a great force is applied to the abducted arm while the rotator cuff is active. Another example of extrinsic overload is a situation in which a person is forced to catch himself or herself during a fall by reaching overhead and placing a large distraction force on the arm. These mechanisms can injure the capsule and other muscles of the shoulder.[21]

Internal impingement in abduction activities can injure the supraspinatus and subscapularis muscles.[22,23] Additionally, coracoid impingement syndrome may result from rotator interval lesions and can cause rotator cuff and biceps fraying.[24]

Other causes of rotator cuff tears are calcific tendinitis (Fig. 18-4),[25] tumors,[26] and degenerative changes of the acromioclavicular joint that produce inferior spurs (Fig. 18-5).[27] Tears in older patients primarily result from coracoacromial arch abrasion.[28-30] Rotator cuff tears that occur in patients less than 40 years old could be related to genetics.[31]

How the rotator cuff tear develops depends on the pattern of the abnormal forces applied to the rotator cuff. Patients with primary impingement have fraying of the upper surface of the rotator cuff that subsequently leads to rotator cuff tears and tendon ruptures (Fig. 18-6). The subscapularis also can be involved in the impingement syndrome, and its integrity

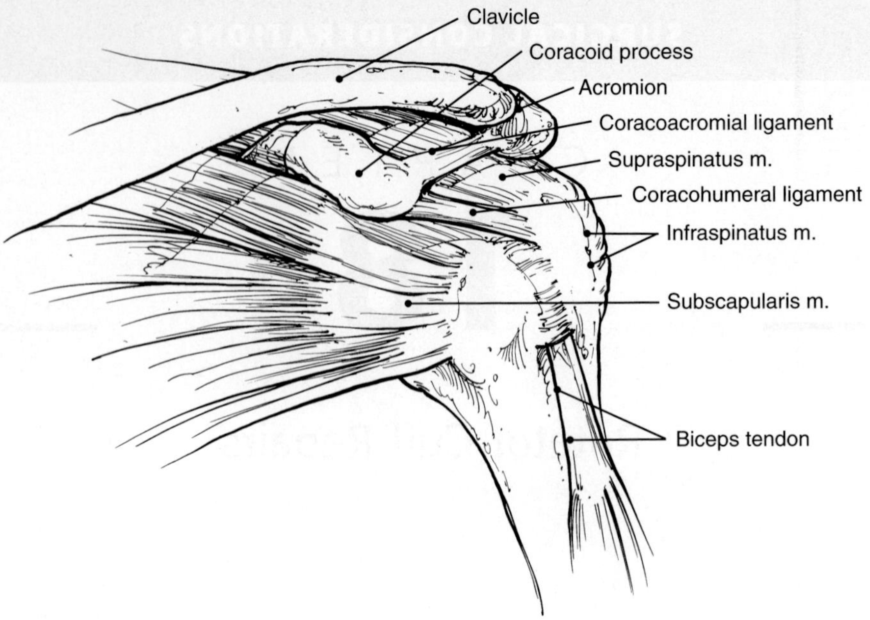

Figure 18-1 Anterior-superior view of the shoulder shows the relationship of the osseous structures with the rotator cuff and the coracoacromial arch.

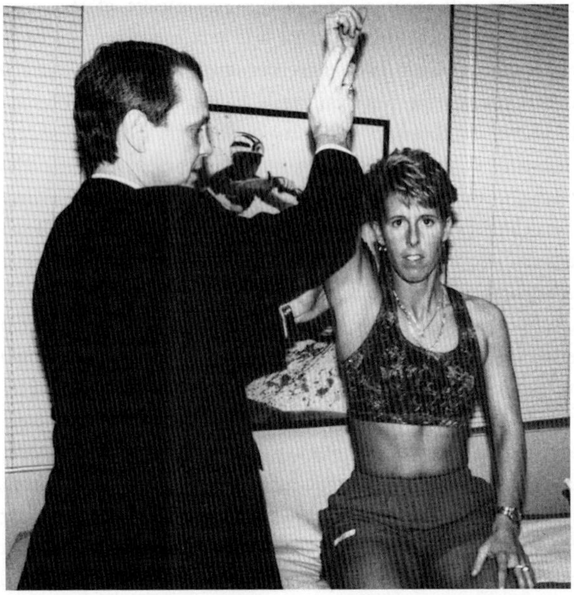

Figure 18-2 The pain of impingement is reproduced with the arm in the fully abducted and flexed position.

should be evaluated.[32] In a reconstruction procedure, the subscapularis should be used cautiously because secondary impingement causes the same type of wear pattern.

DIAGNOSIS

The diagnosis of a rotator cuff tear can be difficult because the signs and symptoms are similar to those of acute rotator cuff tendinitis. The clinical history and physical examination are

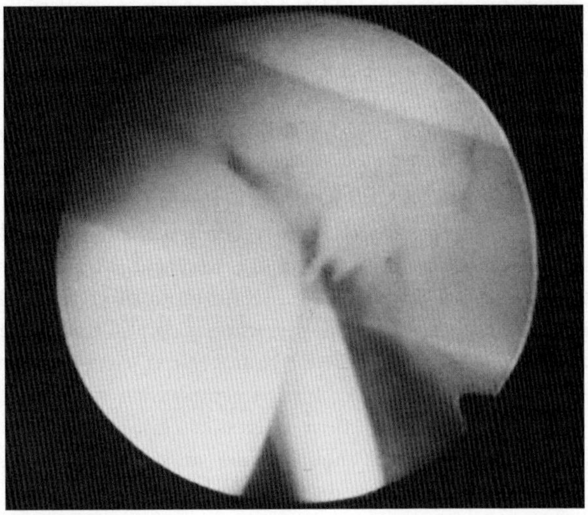

Figure 18-3 Arthroscopic view of the inferior surface of the rotator cuff shows fraying of the undersurface.

the most important components in making the diagnosis.[33] As part of the initial examination of a patient with a shoulder problem, plain radiographs are obtained and frequently show sclerotic or cystic changes in the area of the greater tuberosity, findings that may indicate advanced rotator cuff disease. If symptoms persist after a trial of nonoperative treatment, further noninvasive evaluation should be undertaken to determine the status of the rotator cuff.

Diagnostic Imaging Techniques

In addition to plain radiography, two main imaging methods are used to confirm the presence, location, and size of a defect in the rotator cuff. For many years, the arthrogram was the

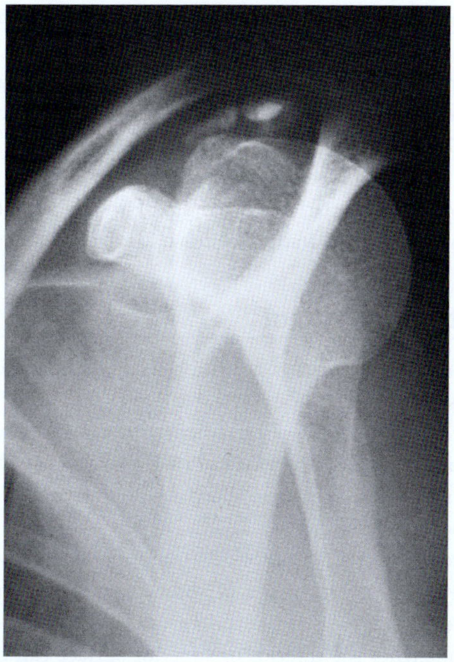

Figure 18-4 Calcific deposit within the supraspinatus tendon.

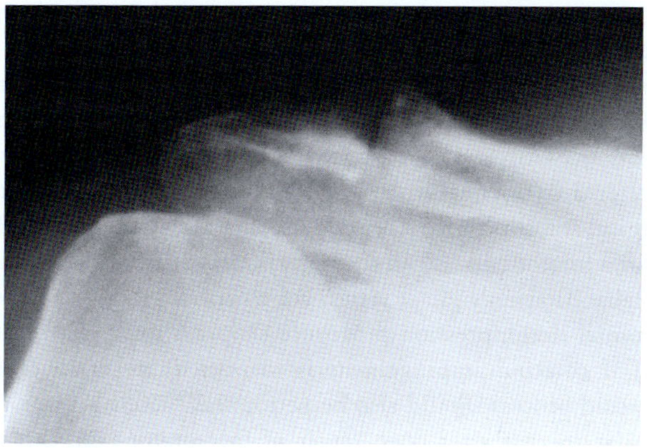

Figure 18-5 Osteoarthritis of the acromioclavicular joint. An inferior spur is impinging on the rotator cuff.

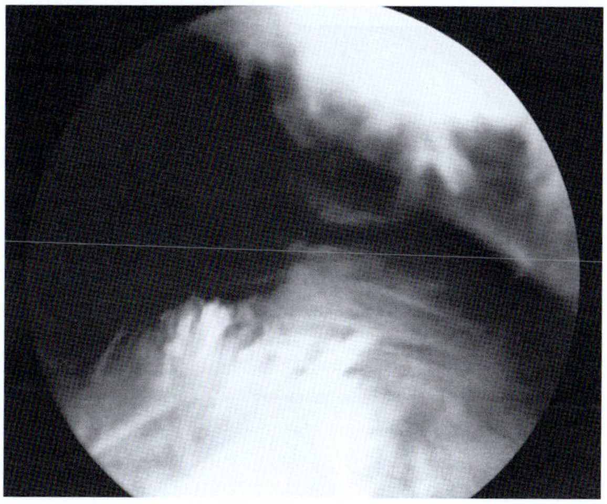

Figure 18-6 Arthroscopic subacromial view shows fraying of the rotator cuff (grade II).

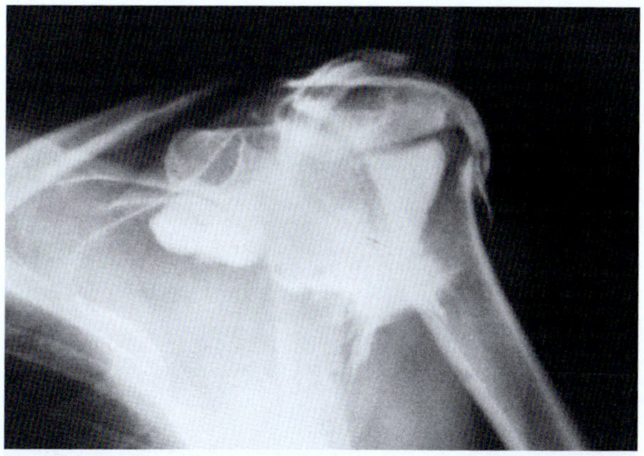

Figure 18-7 Arthrogram of the shoulder with dye extravasation into the subacromial bursa indicates a tear of the rotator cuff.

standard for documenting a rotator cuff tear (Fig. 18-7).[34] An arthrogram is produced by using radiography after radiographic dye is injected into the glenohumeral joint. Extravasation of dye into the area of the subacromial bursa suggests a rupture. Arthrograms are extremely sensitive for full-thickness rotator cuff tears, with greater than 90% sensitivity and specificity,[35,36] an accuracy of 98% to 99%, and an 8% incidence of false-negative results.[37] However, arthrograms usually cannot provide information about incomplete tears, tears on the superior surface, or advanced rotator cuff tendon disease. Ultrasonography is noninvasive and has approximately the same accuracy as the arthrogram.[38]

Magnetic resonance imaging (MRI) has become well established in the evaluation of the rotator cuff tear. With this technology, the sensitivity and specificity are greater than 90% for all tears in most studies.[38] MRI can detect not only the presence of full-thickness tears, but also the presence of partial tears, their size, and their location with a high degree of accuracy (Fig. 18-8).[37,39]

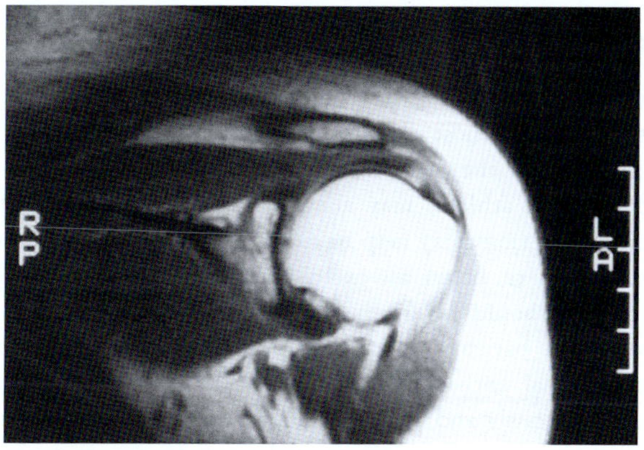

Figure 18-8 Magnetic resonance imaging of the supraspinatus showing the compact space under the coracoacromial area and an abnormal signal in the supraspinatus tendon that indicates a tear.

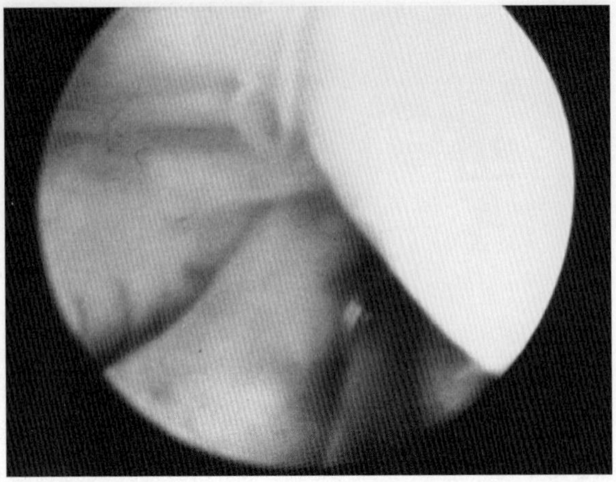

Figure 18-9 Arthroscopic view of the glenohumeral joint shows the undersurface of the supraspinatus portion of the rotator cuff.

Arthroscopic Evaluation

When rehabilitation methods do not relieve a patient's symptoms, surgery may be helpful.[40,41] Arthroscopy also can play an important role in evaluating the rotator cuff for tears. Both the inferior and superior surfaces of the rotator cuff along with the biceps tendon can be seen arthroscopically. The rotator cuff can be palpated with arthroscopic instruments to determine its integrity (Fig. 18-9) and to differentiate partial-thickness and full-thickness tears from chronic tendinitis. Arthroscopy also can help detect instabilities that may be associated with rotator cuff disorders. During the arthroscopic examination, the integrity of the anterior labrum and inferior glenohumeral ligament should be assessed, and the shoulder joint should be examined for instability. SLAP (*s*uperior *l*abrum *a*nterior to *p*osterior) lesions of the labrum can indicate glenohumeral dysfunction.[42]

TREATMENT

Nonoperative Treatment

Initially, a trial of nonoperative treatment should be prescribed for most rotator cuff problems. Reduction or elimination of the precipitating activities or modification of technique in athletes may alleviate pain and allow healing. Steroid injections may help to reduce inflammation and allow the patient to begin an exercise program. However, these injections should be given infrequently and should not be given to patients with complete rotator cuff tears. Nonsteroidal anti-inflammatory drugs (NSAIDs) should be used judiciously and under the supervision of a physician.

Exercises to reduce inflammation and to restore range of motion of the shoulder should be prescribed for each patient on an individual basis. The communication between the patient and those who are treating him or her is extremely important during any exercise program for rotator cuff disease.

If symptoms persist, imaging studies as noted earlier can help to establish whether, in fact, a tear in the rotator cuff exists. Once a tear has been identified, surgical repair is usually recommended. Nonoperative treatment can be continued in some patients with small incomplete tears and in patients with irreparable rotator cuffs.[5,40,43]

Operative Treatment

The indication for surgical treatment is a documented partial-thickness or full-thickness rotator cuff tear that has not responded to nonoperative treatment and produces symptoms that interfere with the patient's normal functioning. However, acute, symptomatic tears in relatively young people probably should be repaired early.[44,45]

Arthroscopic evaluation of the rotator cuff can be combined with the surgical treatment of most tears. Partial-thickness tears of less than 50% of the thickness of the rotator cuff with fraying on either the inferior or superior surface can be treated with débridement of the involved portion of the tendon (Fig. 18-10).[46,47] The débridement allows for freshening of the injured portion of the rotator cuff and thus stimulates a healing response. The remaining fibers hold the cuff in position to heal, and a postoperative program to protect the cuff during this healing phase should be instituted. Certainly, a patient with a more advanced partial-thickness tear that is greater than or equal to 50% of the torn fibers should undergo surgical stabilization of the rotator cuff and should be treated as if for a rotator cuff tear in the postoperative period with regard to rehabilitation and activities. For a superior lesion, a coracoacromial decompression procedure should also be performed, and if coracoid impingement is identified, resection of the coracoid process should also be performed.[48] Rehabilitation is similar to that after open repair of the rotator cuff, but the program is slightly accelerated. The rehabilitation period in these patients can be shortened because they have intact fibers

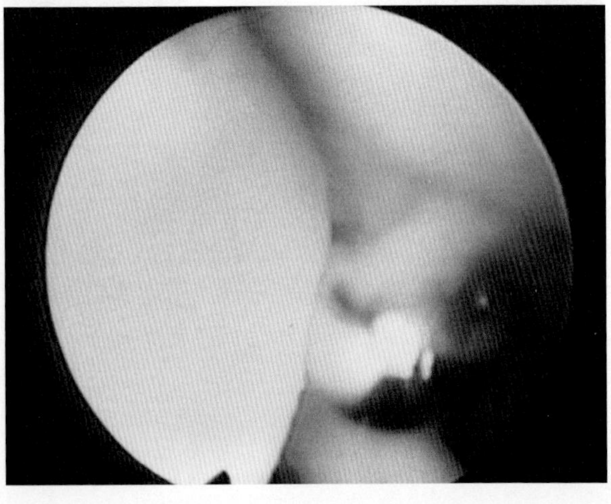

Figure 18-10 Arthroscopic view of the glenohumeral joint with an arthroscopic motorized blade trimming the frayed rotator cuff ends.

remaining to protect the integrity of the rotator cuff. The results with this method are initially very good, but long-term results vary.[49,50]

During the arthroscopic evaluation, the intra-articular portion of the biceps tendon should be examined for injuries associated with rotator cuff lesions. Frequently, débridement or tenodesis of the long head of the biceps muscle is indicated when patients have a rotator cuff tear. Instability and labral abnormalities also can be evaluated at this time.

Some partial-thickness tears should be repaired to prevent progression,[51] and repair should be considered for all small full-thickness tears.[52] An arthroscopically assisted method has been developed for the repair of most rotator cuff tears. The same principles of repair are used in the arthroscopically assisted method as in an open repair. Under arthroscopic visualization, the greater tuberosity in the area of the involved tendon is burred down to a bleeding bony trough. Next, using an intra-articular suturing technique, the surgeon passes sutures through suture anchors in the greater tuberosity, and the rotator cuff is attached to the bone by tightening the suture. Side-to-side suture repair is used for larger tears (Fig. 18-11).[53-58]

Some lesions must be repaired by an open technique. Muscle retraction, poor tissue quality, and weak bones are indications for open repair. Tears are repaired through a superior-lateral incision of the surgeon's choice (Fig. 18-12).

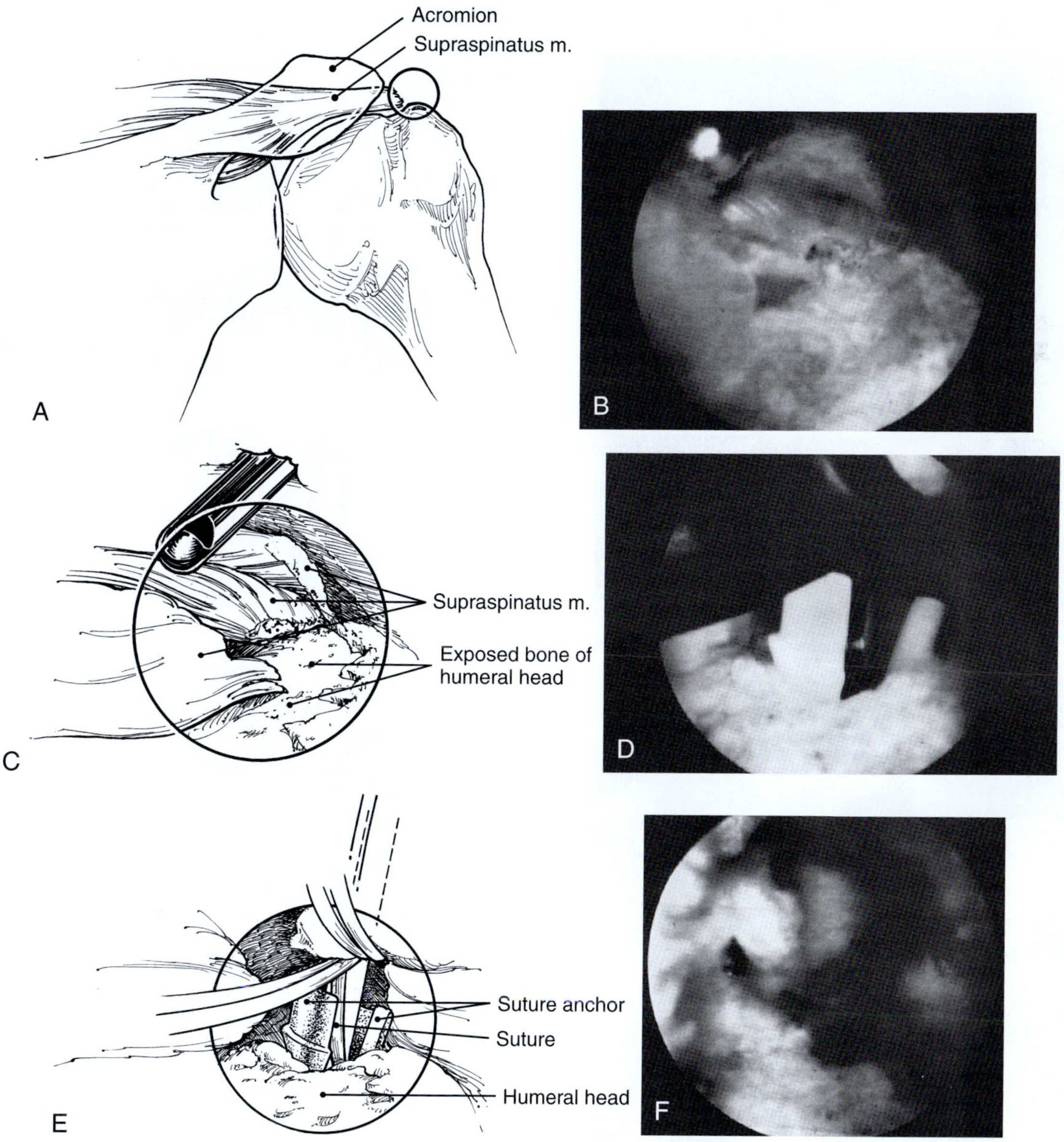

Figure 18-11 **A,** Arthroscopically assisted repair of a rotator cuff tear. The arthroscopic portal is in the subacromial bursa. **B,** Arthroscopic view from the subacromial bursa of a tear of the rotator cuff. **C,** Rupture of the tendinous insertion of the supraspinatus at its attachment to the humeral head. **D,** Arthroscopic view of the greater tuberosity after preparation for rotator cuff repair. **E,** Sutures are passed through suture anchors in the greater tuberosity. **F,** Arthroscopic view of the repaired rotator cuff.

(continued)

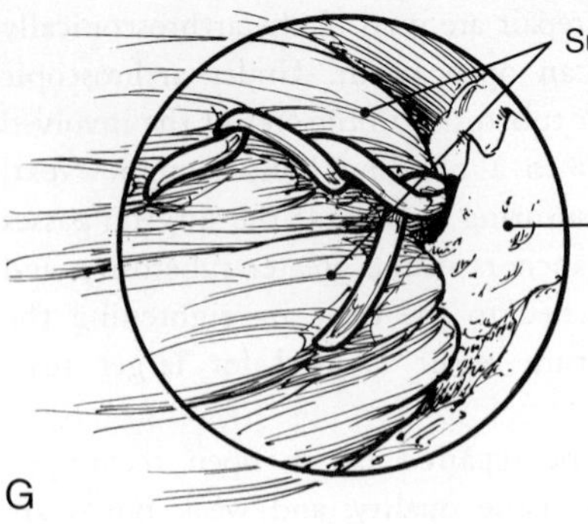

Figure 18-11 Cont'd G, Supraspinatus tendon is sutured to the humeral head.

Exposure of the rotator cuff tear is facilitated by coracoacromial decompression. Small tears can generally be débrided and advanced to the bony bed without problems (see Fig. 18-12B and C). Medium-sized and large tears frequently need moderate mobilization of the muscle bellies by tension to obtain good repair to the bony bed, or a V-Y repair can be done (Fig. 18-13). Massive rotator cuff repairs require extensive mobilization of the muscle bellies and perhaps of the surrounding muscles, particularly of the subscapularis or infraspinatus, to allow coverage of the humeral head. In these patients, the biceps tendon usually is damaged severely or ruptured, and tenodesis can be performed at the bicipital groove (Fig. 18-14).[27,59-61]

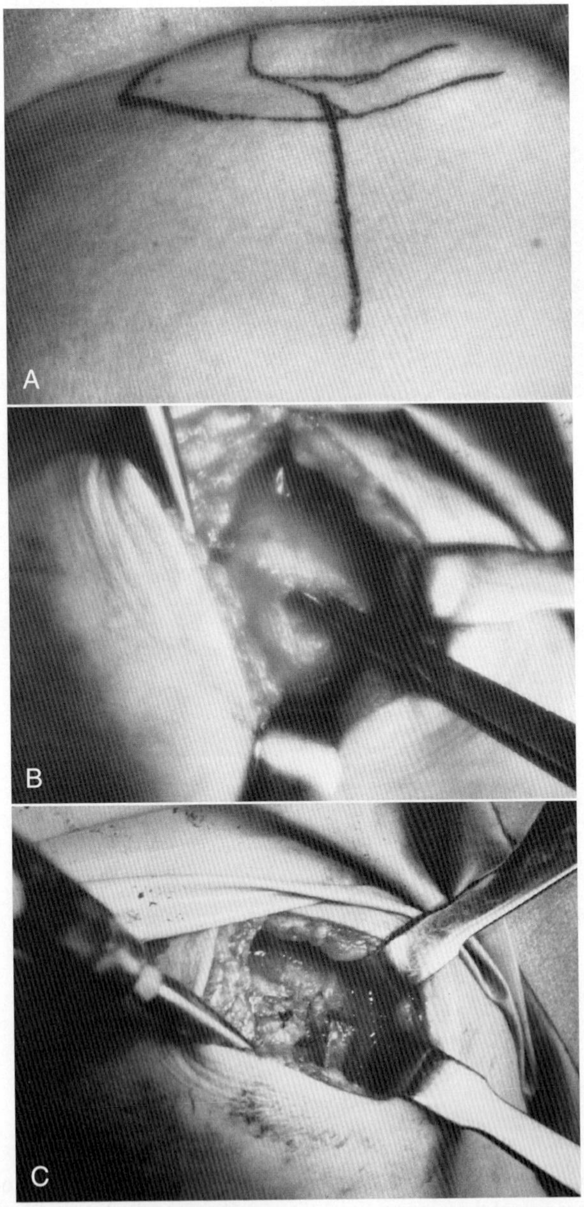

Figure 18-12 A, The acromion and clavicle are outlined for the intended superior-lateral incision. **B,** Small tear exposed with the open technique. **C,** Small tear repaired by open technique.

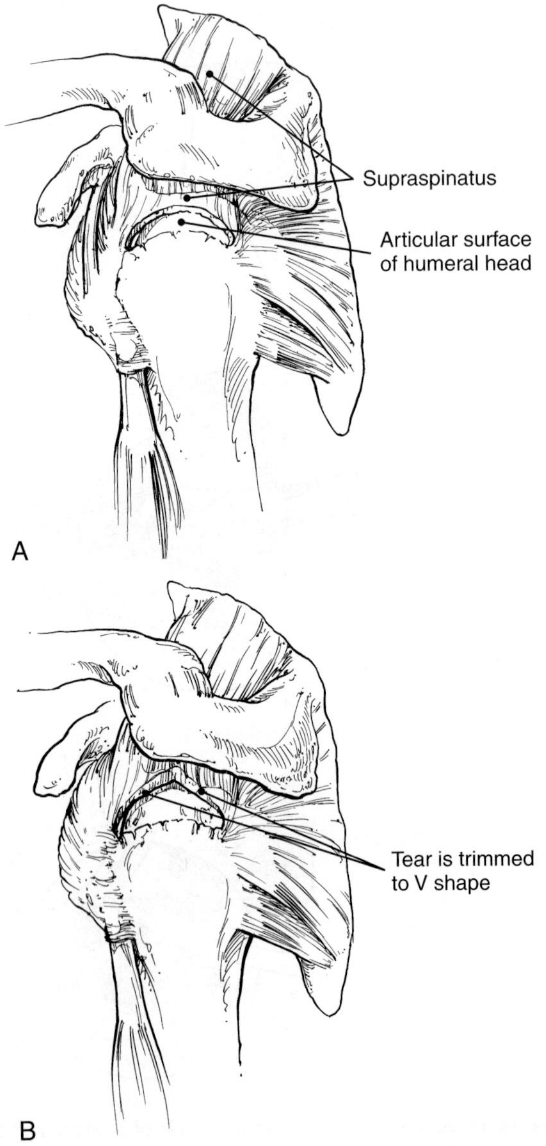

Figure 18-13 A, Medium to large tear with supraspinatus muscle retraction. **B,** Tear is trimmed and cut into a V shape.

(continued)

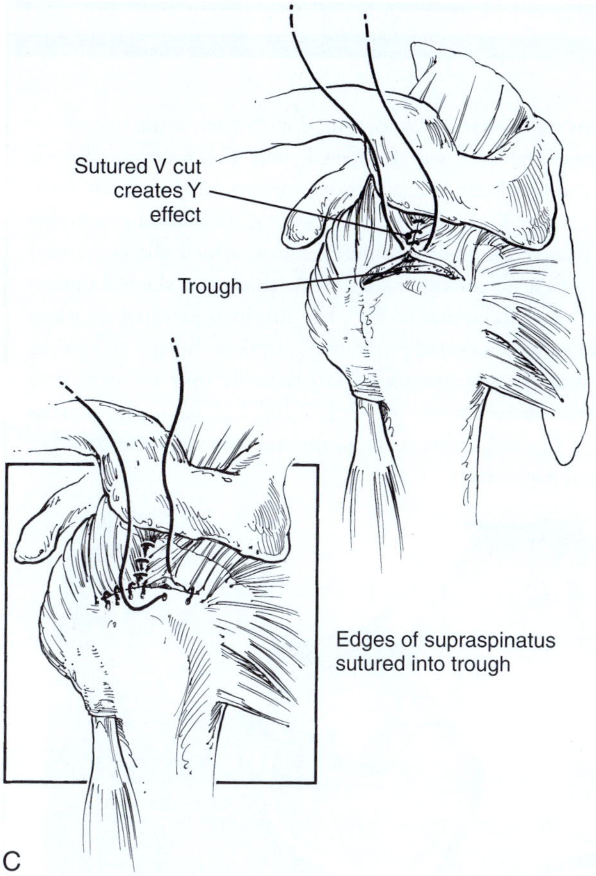

Figure 18-13 Cont'd C, V-Y closure of the tear. The edges of the V cut are reapposed along the direction of the muscle fibers. The edges of the supraspinatus are buried in a bony trough in the humeral head.

Surgical treatment of irreparable rotator cuff tears depends on the level of symptoms and function. For low-demand individuals with fair function but significant pain, arthroscopic débridement may give good results. In patients who need greater function or who have unrelieved pain, an attempt at surgical repair or reconstruction can be beneficial. For those with severe loss of function and significant pain, joint replacement may be considered with possibly a reverse total shoulder.[43,62]

RESULTS

The results of rotator cuff repair are variable and seem to have a direct relationship with the patient's age and the severity of the tear.[63,64] Although investigators have shown that repair of rotator cuff tears results in a significant increase in function for all patients, the degree of patient satisfaction with the repair depends on the size of the tear, associated pathologic conditions, and the age of the patient. Patients older than 65 years have a less favorable outcome than those younger than 65 years of age, although symptomatic patients of any age with complete rotator cuff tears have at least partial relief of their symptoms after a successful rotator cuff repair.[65-74] Appropriate postoperative care is the key to a satisfactory result after successful surgical repair. Immobilization or active rest, with passive range of motion for an appropriate length of time (see Chapter 15 for recommendations on length of immobilization) for the type of lesion, and repair followed by progressive mobilization and general and specific strengthening programs lead to more acceptable results.[75-78]

Recurring tears of the rotator cuff, especially in older patients, are complex and can require extensive reconstruction if they are symptomatic. Mobilization of the infraspinatus and subscapularis muscles, along with muscle transfers, has been described.[79-81] Rotator cuff arthropathy has been reported in association with long-term rotator cuff dysfunction.[82]

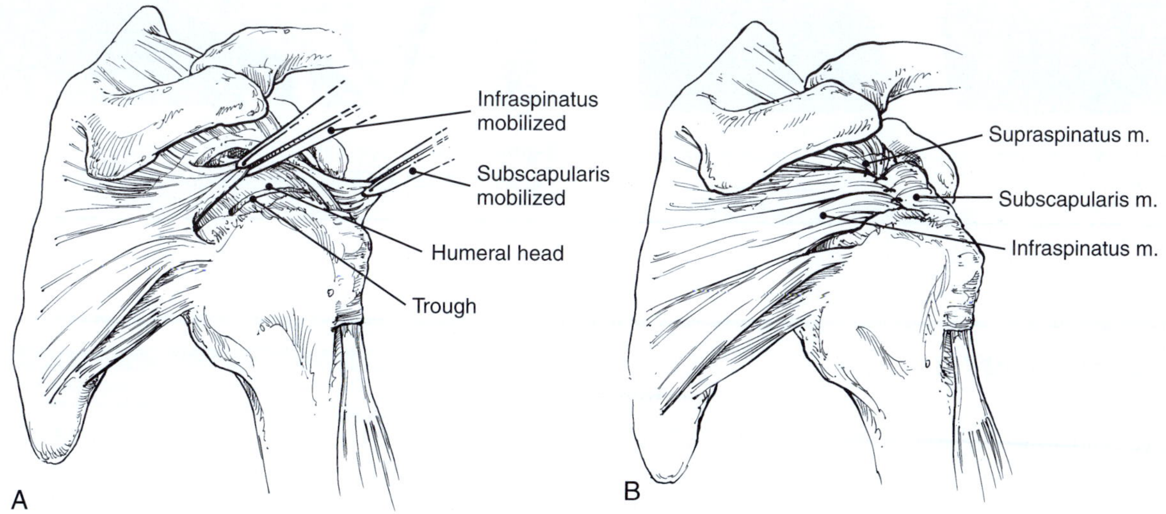

Figure 18-14 A, Massive tear of the rotator cuff with the "bald head" appearance of the humeral head. Mobilization of the infraspinatus and subscapularis and elevation of the supraspinatus muscle body to repair the rotator cuff. **B,** Repaired massive tear after muscle mobilization.

CASE STUDY 1

A 46-year-old woman is a volleyball coach for a local college. She has participated in volleyball as an athlete and a coach for more than 20 years. She noted increasing pain and discomfort in her right shoulder. She was treated with NSAIDs and physical therapy, without relief. An MRI scan was performed for continued symptoms, which showed an abnormal supraspinatus tendon with probable rotator cuff tear. During the initial examination by the orthopedic surgeon, the patient had full range-of-shoulder motion, but she had a positive impingement sign and some weakness on abduction at 90°. She had no instability, and her neurovascular examination was intact. Radiographic examination showed normal bony structures and joint spaces. A review of the MRI scan showed a grossly abnormal tendon and a probable tear in the supraspinatus muscle of the rotator cuff. She was scheduled for arthroscopic examination of the shoulder.

At surgery, diagnostic arthroscopy showed an intact biceps tendon and articular surfaces. She had a separation of the anterior-superior labrum, but the inferior labrum was intact, with no evidence of instability. When its inferior surface was viewed, the rotator cuff tendon was found to be abnormal and to have a tear (Fig. 18-15). It was abnormal over a fairly large area, and it was thought that open repair was necessary. Therefore, an open incision in the anterior-lateral aspect of the shoulder was made to expose the rotator cuff, and a 2-cm superior tear was identified with some retraction of the tendon. The area was freshened, and the rotator cuff was repaired to a bony bed with advancement of the tendon back to the bone (Fig. 18-16). After surgery, she started pendulum and passive range-of-motion exercises, which she continued for the first 4 weeks after surgery. At that time, she had flexion to 90° and abduction to 60°, but minimal external rotation. She began a structured program of physical therapy at 4 weeks after surgery and progressed satisfactorily over the next 6 to 8 weeks to full range of motion and full strength. At that point, 3 months after surgery, she was allowed to resume her normal activities.

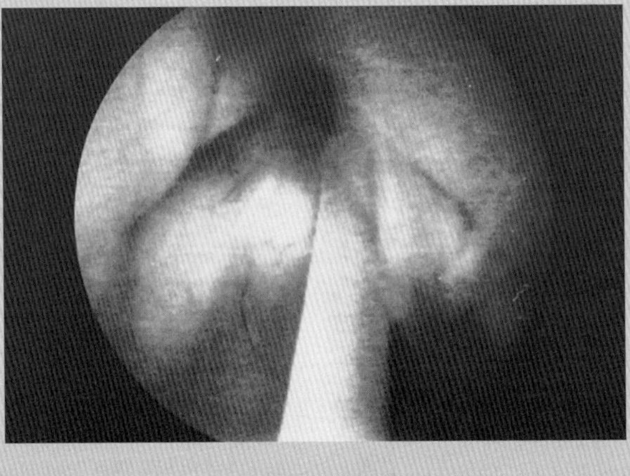

Figure 18-15 Arthroscopic view of the inferior surface of the rotator cuff tear in Case Study 1.

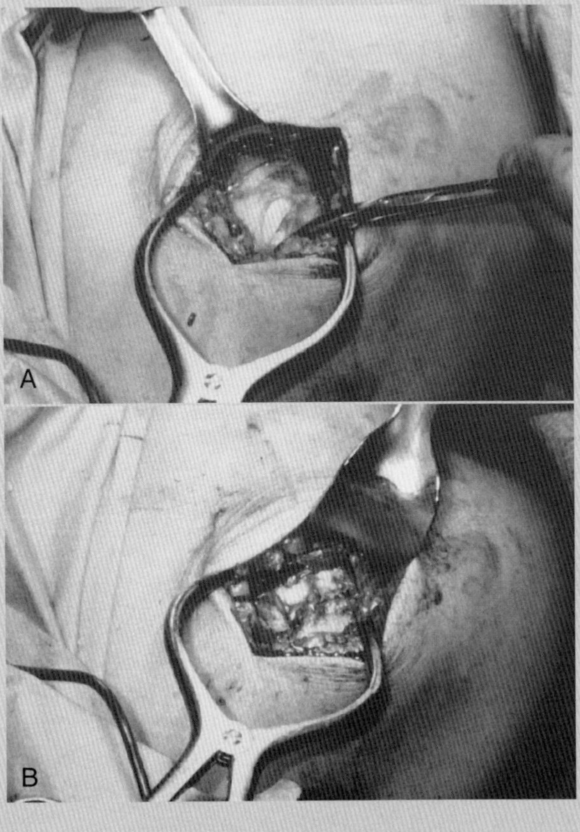

Figure 18-16 **A,** Appearance of the rotator cuff tear in Case Study 1 after exposure by open technique. **B,** Repaired rotator cuff in Case Study 1.

CASE STUDY 2

A 48-year-old man was seen in the orthopedic surgeon's office with insidious right shoulder pain but without a known precipitating injury. He had pain in the 60°-to-120° arc of motion and some pain on forced abduction at 90°. However, he had good strength, no instability, and full range of motion. He began a trial of physical therapy and NSAIDs, which allowed him to improve slightly.

He returned in 6 months with recurrent pain in the shoulder. His physical examination was essentially unchanged at that time. An MRI scan showed a probable

CASE STUDY 2—cont'd

rotator cuff tear. The patient underwent arthroscopic evaluation and was found to have no evidence of instability and an intact labrum. However, he had fraying of the undersurface of the rotator cuff and some fraying of the articular side of the subscapularis on the superior aspect (Fig. 18-17A). Examination with the arthroscope in the subacromial bursa showed a 1-cm tear of the rotator cuff without retraction. The tear extended through approximately 80% of the supraspinatus tendon (see Fig. 18-17B), which was slightly pulled away from the bone. After subacromial decompression, the bony bed on the greater tuberosity was freshened with a motorized arthroscopic blade through a third portal lateral to the acromion. Two sutures were placed through the supraspinatus tendon, and after two holes were drilled in the greater tuberosity, the sutures were anchored into the bone with plastic suture anchors. With the shoulder in the abducted position, the sutures were tied digitally, thus pulling the rotator cuff tendon back down to the bony bed (Fig. 18-18).

After surgery, the patient was started on full passive range-of-motion exercises. By 6 weeks, he had achieved full range of motion and had started strengthening exercises. By 10 weeks, he had excellent range of motion and was gaining strength with relief of postoperative pain. He was started on an increased exercise program.

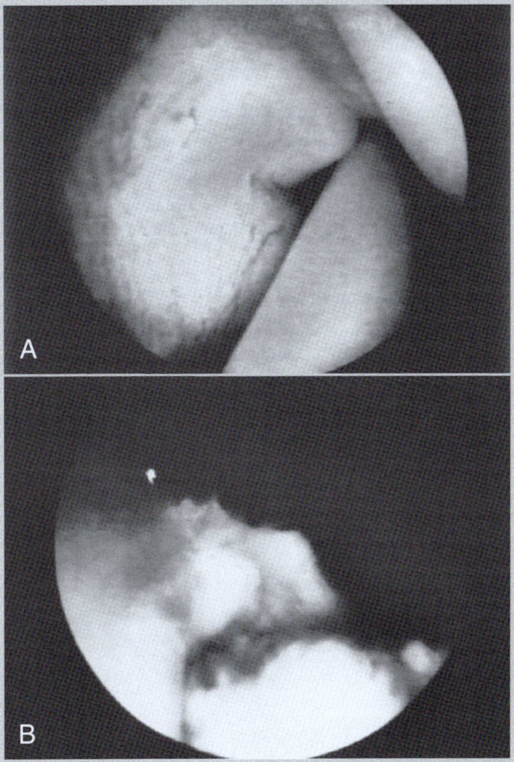

Figure 18-17 A, Arthroscopic view of the undersurface of the rotator cuff in Case Study 2. **B,** Arthroscopic subacromial view of the superior surface of the rotator cuff showing an incomplete tear of the rotator cuff in Case Study 2.

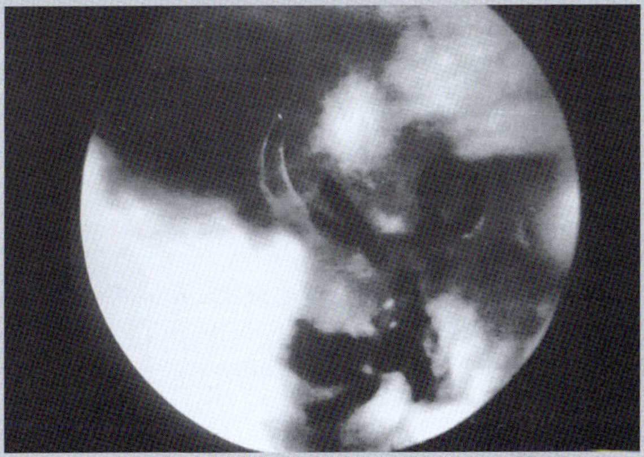

Figure 18-18 Arthroscopic subacromial view of the repaired rotator cuff in Case Study 2.

CASE STUDY 3

Initial History

A 55-year-old, right-hand dominant man presented with pain in his right shoulder that had been present for approximately 2 months fairly constantly. He had previously had occasional episodes of pain, especially after vigorous exertion, that lasted for a few hours to a couple of days. He had also had occasional episodes of numbness and tingling radiating down the right arm and a known history of cervical disk disease. His occupation as a concession vender requires some vigorous activity with lifting, carrying, and some overhead activities.

He complained that his present pain was different from his previous cervical disease. The pain was centered over the superior-lateral aspect of the shoulder and was obvious with shoulder activities. Activities that required abduction and overhead use of the arm resulted in feelings of weakness and pain.

The episodes of pain had increased in frequency and intensity, and over the last 2 months they had become constant and were interfering with work and sleep. He

Continued

CASE STUDY 3—cont'd

had tried NSAIDs and a home exercise program, without success.

Examination

He had no observable abnormalities on visual inspection except prominence of the acromioclavicular joint. No significant atrophy was noted. He was able to raise his arm in a full range of motion. His strength was good to manual testing on flexion, adduction, and internal rotation but was slightly weak in abduction and external rotation. He had tenderness over the greater tuberosity and in the bicipital groove. He had positive results of Neer's and Hawkin's tests and a negative Speed test result. No evidence of laxity, instability, or labral disease was noted. Results of neurovascular testing were normal, and all other motor functions were intact.

Initial Imaging

Radiographs of the shoulder were obtained in three views and revealed the humeral and glenoid structures to be intact. Some degeneration at the acromioclavicular joint was evident.

Working Diagnosis

The diagnosis was rotator cuff tendinitis, acute and subacute, with a possibility of a cuff tear.

Initial Treatment

He was started on a conservative program of NSAIDs and physical therapy with modalities to help with inflammation and rehabilitation of the rotator cuff.

Follow-up

The therapy program caused increased pain and disuse of the arm and was discontinued. An MRI scan was prescribed.

Additional Imaging

The MRI scan revealed an 8 × 4.5 cm rotator cuff tear involving both the supraspinatus and infraspinatus and additionally showed hypertrophy and spurring of the acromioclavicular joint.

Surgery

The patient was counseled on treatment options, with the recommendation for surgery to repair the torn rotator cuff. He was agreeable and was taken to surgery, where he underwent arthroscopy of the right shoulder. Findings included a separated and frayed superior labrum and an intact biceps tendon and articular surfaces. No evidence of instability was noted. He had a large tear of the rotator cuff involving the supraspinatus and the infraspinatus, with only mild retraction of the tendon. The tear exhibited both transverse and longitudinal components. The subscapularis was intact.

The repair included excision of the subacromial bursal tissue and subacromial decompression, acromioplasty, and excision of the distal clavicle. The cuff was repaired with a combination of side-to-side sutures in the longitudinal component with a double-row technique using suture anchors and fiber tape sutures (Fig. 18-19). The frayed labrum was trimmed but did not require repair.

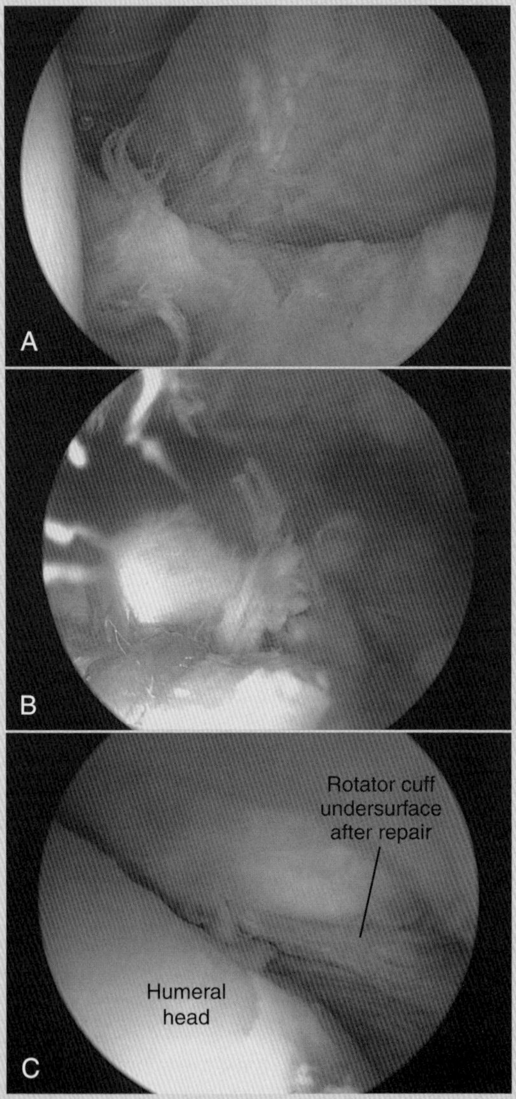

Figure 18-19 Large rotator cuff tear with mild retraction in Case Study 3. **A,** The acromion is visible from inside the glenohumeral joint through the defect in the cuff. **B,** Subacromial view after repair. The greater tuberosity and position of the suture anchors are shown, as well as one of the side-to-side sutures. **C,** View of the rotator cuff from inside the joint after repair showing good approximation to the greater tuberosity.

CASE STUDY 3—cont'd

Initial postoperative care consisted of an abduction pillow sling for most activities and sleeping. He was allowed to start range of motion of the hand, wrist, and elbow. He was also provided with a shoulder continuous passive motion device, with a goal of 80° of abduction and 30° of external rotation at the end of 4 weeks. He was then referred for physical therapy.

Rehabilitation

Evaluation (4 Weeks Postoperatively)

- Range of motion
  - Hand-wrist-elbow: normal
  - Shoulder
  - Flexion: 55°
  - Abduction (passive): 52°
  - External rotation: 48°
  - Internal rotation and extension: sacrum
- Strength: hand and elbow intact to gentle pressure
- Testing: shoulder not tested
- Sensation: intact
- Edema: mild swelling in the elbow

Treatment Goals

- Protect the repair.
- Increase functional use for activities of daily living (ADLs).
- Return to normal range of motion.
- Recover strength.
- Eliminate edema.

Treatment

4 to 8 weeks Postoperatively

1. Use heat for loosening the shoulder stiffness.
2. Perform exercises: active-assisted and passive range of motion to the patient's tolerance in the supine position; pendulum exercises and continued range of motion of the hand, wrist, and elbow; and scapular retraction activities.
3. At 6 weeks, start active range of motion and very light rotator cuff rehabilitation exercises.
4. Use postexercise icing.
5. Have the patient perform ADLs with the uninvolved arm, with very gentle use of the operative arm.

8 to 12 Weeks Postoperatively

1. Range of motion measures flexion 82°, abduction 72°, and external rotation 58°.
2. Wean the patient from the abduction pillow splint.
3. Promote aggressive active range of motion and moderate-level strengthening of the rotator cuff muscles.
4. Ensure joint mobilization.
5. Use aggressive scapulothoracic mobilization and strengthening.
6. Use modalities for inflammation control.
7. Have the patient use the operative arm for light activities.

12 to 16 Weeks Postoperatively

1. Range of motion measures flexion 175°, abduction 160°, and external rotation 75°.
2. Use specific stretching activities to address remaining stiffness.
3. Use specific exercises to address residual weakness.
4. Start an activity-specific program (i.e., sports training).
5. Continue icing and NSAIDs if needed.

16+ Weeks Postoperatively

1. Range of motion is normal.
2. Design the program to address residual deficits in motion, strength, and kinetics. Start all activities and progress to the patient's previous functioning level over 4 to 8 weeks.

REFERENCES

1. Lehman C, Cuomo F, Kummer FJ, et al: The incidence of full thickness rotator cuff tears in a large cadaveric population, *Bull Hosp Jt Dis* 54:30–31, 1995.
2. Tempelhof S, Rupp S, Seil R: Age-related prevalence of rotator cuff tears in asymptomatic shoulders, *J Shoulder Elbow Surg* 8:296–299, 1999.
3. Moosmayer S, Smith HJ, Tang R, et al: Prevalence and characteristics of asymptomatic tears of the rotator cuff: an ultrasonographic and clinical study, *J Bone Joint Surg Br* 91:196–200, 2009.
4. Teefey A, Yamaguchi K, Ditsios K, et al: The demographic and morphological features of rotator cuff disease: a comparison of asymptomatic and symptomatic shoulders, *J Bone Joint Surg Am* 88:1699–1704, 2006.
5. Budoff JE, Nirschl RP, Guidi EJ: Current concepts review: débridement of partial-thickness tears of the rotator cuff without acromioplasty long-term follow-up and review of the literature, *J Bone Joint Surg Am* 80(5):734–748, 1998.
6. Jensen KL, Williams GR Jr, Russell J, et al: Current concepts review: rotator cuff tear arthropathy, *J Bone Joint Surg Am* 81 (9):1312–1314, 1999.
7. Neer CS II: Anterior acromioplasty for the chronic impingement syndrome in the shoulder: a preliminary report, *J Bone Joint Surg Am* 54:41, 1972.
8. Nash HL: Rotator cuff damage: re-examining the causes and treatments, *Phys Sportsmed* 16:129, 1988.
9. Bigliani LU, Ticker JB, Flatow EL, et al: The relationship of acromial architecture to rotator cuff disease, *Clin Sports Med* 10(4):823–838, 1991.
10. Fowler PJ: Shoulder injuries in the mature athlete, *Adv Sports Med Fitness* 1:225, 1988.
11. Jost B, Koch PP, Gerber CG: Anatomy and functional aspects of the rotator interval, *J Shoulder Elbow Surg* 9(4):336–341, 2000.
12. Hatakeyama Y, Itoi E, Urayama M, et al: Effect of superior capsule and coracohumeral ligament release on strain in the repaired rotator cuff tendon: a cadaveric study, *Am J Sports Med* 29(5):633–640, 2001.

13. Lee S-B, Kim K-J, O'Driscoll S, et al: Dynamic glenohumeral stability provided by the rotator cuff muscles in the mid-range and end-range of motion, *J Bone Joint Surg Am* 82:849–857, 2000.
14. Berbig R, Weishaupt D, Prim J, et al: Primary anterior shoulder dislocation and rotator cuff tears, *J Shoulder Elbow Surg* 8 (3):220–225, 1999.
15. Stayner LR, Cummings J, Andersen J, et al: Shoulder dislocations in patients older than 40 years of age, *Orthop Clin North Am* 31(2):231–239, 2000.
16. Pevny T, Hunter RE, Freeman JR: Primary traumatic anterior shoulder dislocation in patients 40 years of age and older, *Arthroscopy* 14(3):289–294, 1998.
17. Taylor DC, Arciero RA: Pathologic changes associated with shoulder dislocations: arthroscopic and physical examination findings in first-time, traumatic anterior dislocations, *Am J Sports Med* 25(3):306–311, 1997.
18. Savoie FH, Field LD, Atchinson S: Anterior superior instability with rotator cuff tearing: SLAC lesion, *Orthop Clin North Am* 32(3):457–461, 2001.
19. Gartsman GM, Hammerman SM: Superior labrum, anterior and posterior lesions: when and how to treat them, *Clin Sports Med* 19(1):115–124, 2000.
20. Morgan CD, Burkhart SS, Palmeri M, et al: Type II SLAP lesions: three subtypes and their relationships to superior instability and rotator cuff tears, *Arthroscopy* 14(6):553–565, 1998.
21. Namdari S, Henn RF III, Green A: Traumatic anterosuperior rotator cuff tears: the outcome of open surgical repair, *J Bone Joint Surg Am* 90:1906–1913, 2008.
22. Edelson G, Teitz C: Internal impingement in the shoulder, *J Shoulder Elbow Surg* 9(4):308–315, 2000.
23. Meister K: Internal impingement in the shoulder of the overhand athlete: pathophysiology, diagnosis, and treatment, *Am J Orthop* 29(6):433–438, 2000.
24. Paulson MM, Watnik NF, Dines DM: Coracoid impingement syndrome, rotator interval reconstruction, and biceps tenodesis in the overhead athlete, *Orthop Clin North Am* 32(3):485–493, 2001.
25. Hsu HC, Wu JJ, Jim YF, et al: Calcific tendinitis and rotator cuff tearing: a clinical and radiographic study, *J Shoulder Elbow Surg* 3:159, 1994.
26. Fallon PJ, Hollinshead RM: Solitary osteochondroma of the distal clavicle causing a full-thickness rotator cuff tear, *J Shoulder Elbow Surg* 3:266, 1994.
27. Bigliani LU, Rodosky MW: Techniques in repair of large rotator cuff tears, *Tech Orthop* 9:133, 1994.
28. Brewer BJ: Aging of the rotator cuff, *Am J Sports Med* 7 (2):102–110, 1979.
29. Cuomo F, Kummer FJ, Zuckerman JD, et al: The influence of acromioclavicular joint morphology on rotator cuff tears, *J Shoulder Elbow Surg* 7(6):555–559, 1998.
30. Brown JN, Roberts SNJ, Hayes MG, et al: Shoulder pathology associated with symptomatic acromioclavicular joint degeneration, *J Shoulder Elbow Surg* 9(3):173–176, 2000.
31. Tashjian RZ, Farnham JM, Albright FS, et al: Evidence for an inherited predisposition contributing to the risk for rotator cuff disease, *J Bone Joint Surg Am* 91:1136–1142, 2009.
32. Travis RD, Burkhead WZ Jr, Doane R: Technique for repair of the subscapularis tendon, *Orthop Clin North Am* 32 (3):495–500, 2001.
33. Hawkins RJ, Mohtadi N: Rotator cuff problems in athletes. In DeLee JC, Drez DD Jr, editors: *Orthopaedic sports medicine: principles and practice*, Philadelphia, 1995, Saunders.
34. Brems J: Rotator cuff tear: evaluation and treatment, *Orthopedics* 11(1):69–81, 1988.
35. Iannotti JP, editor: *Rotator cuff disorders: evaluation and treatment*, Park Ridge, Ill, 1991, American Academy of Orthopaedic Surgeons.
36. Mink JH, Harris E, Rappaport M: Rotator cuff tears: evaluation using double-contrast shoulder arthrography, *Radiology* 157(3):621–623, 1985.
37. Hawkins RJ, Misamore GW, Hobeika PE: Surgery for full-thickness rotator cuff tears, *J Bone Joint Surg Am* 67 (9):1349–1355, 1985.
38. Burk DL Jr, Karasick D, Kurtz AB, et al: Rotator cuff tears: prospective comparison of MR imaging with arthrography, sonography and surgery, *AJR Am J Roentgenol* 153(1):87–92, 1989.
39. Snyder SJ: Rotator cuff lesions: acute and chronic, *Clin Sports Med* 10(3):595–614, 1991.
40. Brox JI, Gjengedal E, Uppheim G, et al: Arthroscopic surgery versus supervised exercises in patients with rotator cuff disease (stage II impingement syndrome): a prospective, randomized, controlled study in 125 patients with a 2¼-year follow-up, *J Shoulder Elbow Surg* 8(2):102–111, 1999.
41. McKee MD, Yoo DJ: The effect of surgery for rotator cuff disease on general health status: results of a prospective trial, *J Bone Joint Surg Am* 82(7):970–979, 2000.
42. Bey MJ, Elders GJ, Huston LJ, et al: The mechanism of creation of superior labrum, anterior, and posterior lesions in a dynamic biomechanical model of the shoulder: the role of inferior subluxation, *J Shoulder Elbow Surg* 7(4):397–401, 1998.
43. Dines DM, Moynihan DP, Dines JS, et al: Irreparable rotator cuff tears: what to do and when to do it. The surgeon's dilemma, *J Bone Joint Surg Am* 88:2294–2302, 2006.
44. Hawkins RJ, Mohtadi N: Rotator cuff problems in athletes. In DeLee JC, Drez DD, editors: *Orthopaedic sports medicine: principles and practice*, Philadelphia, 1994, Saunders.
45. Gartsman GM: Arthroscopic management of rotator cuff disease, *J Am Acad Orthop Surg* 6(4):259–266, 1998.
46. Payne LZ, Altchek DW, Craig EV, et al: Arthroscopic treatment of partial rotator cuff tears in young athletes: a preliminary report, *Am J Sports Med* 25(3):299–305, 1997.
47. Budoff JE, Nirschl RP, Guidi EJ: Débridement of partial thickness tears of the rotator cuff without acromioplasty: long-term follow-up and review of the literature, *J Bone Joint Surg Am* 80(5):733–748, 1998.
48. Warner JJ, Higgins L, Parsons IM, et al: Diagnosis and treatment of anterosuperior rotator cuff tears, *J Shoulder Elbow Surg* 10:37–46, 2001.
49. Hyvonen P, Lohi S, Jalovaara P: Open acromioplasty does not prevent the progression of an impingement syndrome to a tear: nine-year follow-up of 96 cases, *J Bone Joint Surg Br* 80 (5):813–816, 1998.
50. Hoe-Hansen CE, Palm L, Norlin R: The influence of cuff pathology on shoulder function after arthroscopic subacromial decompression: a 3- and 6-year follow-up study, *J Shoulder Elbow Surg* 8(6):585–589, 1999.
51. Weber SC: Arthroscopic débridement and acromioplasty versus mini-open repair in the treatment of significant partial-thickness rotator cuff tears, *Arthroscopy* 15(2):126–131, 1999.
52. Gartsman GM: Arthroscopic rotator cuff repair, *Clin Orthop Relat Res* 390:95–106, 2001.
53. Yamaguchi K, Ball CM, Galatz LM: Arthroscopic rotator cuff repair: transition from mini-open to all-arthroscopic, *Clin Orthop Relat Res* 390:83–94, 2001.

54. Gartsman GM: All arthroscopic rotator cuff repairs, *Orthop Clin North Am* 32(3):501–510, 2001.
55. Burkhart SS: Arthroscopic treatment of massive rotator cuff tears, *Clin Orthop Relat Res* 390:107–118, 2001.
56. Ma CB, MacGillivray JD, Clabeaux J, et al: biomechanical evaluation of arthroscopic rotator cuff stitches, *J Bone Joint Surg Am* 86:1211–1216, 2004.
57. Huijsmans PE, Pritchard MP, Berghs BM, et al: Arthroscopic rotator cuff repair with double-row fixation, *J Bone Joint Surg Am* 89:1248–1257, 2007.
58. Ma CB, Comerford L, Wilson J, et al: Compared with single-row fixation biomechanical evaluation of arthroscopic rotator cuff repairs: double-row, *J Bone Joint Surg Am* 88:403–410, 2006.
59. Ellman H, Hanker G, Bayer M: Repair of the rotator cuff: end-result study of factors influencing reconstruction, *J Bone Joint Surg Am* 68(8):1136–1144, 1986.
60. Neviaser JS, Neviaser RJ, Neviaser TJ: The repair of chronic massive ruptures of the rotator cuff of the shoulder by use of a freeze-dried rotator cuff, *J Bone Joint Surg Am* 60(5):681–684, 1978.
61. Packer NP, Calvert PT, Bayley JI, et al: Operative treatment of chronic ruptures of the rotator cuff of the shoulder, *J Bone Joint Surg Br* 65(2):171–175, 1983.
62. Moursy M, Forstner R, Koller H, et al: Latissimus dorsi tendon transfer for irreparable rotator cuff tears: a modified technique to improve tendon transfer integrity, *J Bone Joint Surg Am* 91:1924–1931, 2009.
63. Hattrup SJ: Rotator cuff repair: relevance of patient age, *J Shoulder Elbow Surg* 4(2):95–100, 1995.
64. Burkhart SS, Danaceau SM, Pearce CE: Arthroscopic rotator cuff repair: analysis of results by tear size and by repair technique: margin convergence versus direct tendon-to-bone repair, *Arthroscopy* 17(9):905–912, 2001.
65. Adamson GJ, Tibone JE: Ten-year assessment of primary rotator cuff repairs, *J Shoulder Elbow Surg* 2:57, 1993.
66. Wilson F, Hinov V, Adams G: Arthroscopic repair of full-thickness tears of the rotator cuff: 2-14-year follow-up, *Arthroscopy* 18(2):136–144, 2002.
67. Habernek H, Schmid L, Frauenschuh E: Five year results of rotator cuff repair, *Br J Sports Med* 33(6):430–433, 1999.
68. Gerber C, Fuchs B, Hodler J: The results of repair of massive tears of the rotator cuff, *J Bone Joint Surg Am* 82(4):505–515, 2000.
69. Rokito AS, Cuomo F, Gallagher MA, et al: Long-term functional outcome of repair of large and massive chronic tears of the rotator cuff, *J Bone Joint Surg Am* 81(7):991–997, 1999.
70. Worland RL, Arredondo J, Angles F, et al: Repair of massive rotator cuff tears in patients older than 70 years, *J Shoulder Elbow Surg* 8(1):26–30, 1999.
71. Grondel RJ, Savoie FH 3rd, Field LD: Rotator cuff repairs in patients 62 years of age or older, *J Shoulder Elbow Surg* 10 (2):97–99, 2001.
72. Yel M, Shankwiler JA, Noonan JE, et al: Results of decompression and rotator cuff repair in patients 65 years old and older: 6- to 14-year follow-up, *Am J Orthop* 30(4):347–352, 2001.
73. Galatz LM, Griggs S, Cameron BD, et al: Prospective longitudinal analysis of postoperative shoulder function: a ten-year follow-up study of full-thickness rotator cuff tears, *J Bone Joint Surg Am* 83(7):1052–1056, 2001.
74. O'Holleran JD, Kocher MS, Horan MP, et al: Determinants of patient satisfaction with outcome after rotator cuff surgery, *J Bone Joint Surg Am* 87:121–126, 2005.
75. O'Holleran JD, Kocher MS, Horan MP, et al: Open, mini-open, and all-arthroscopic rotator cuff repair surgery: indications and implications for rehabilitation, *J Orthop Sports Phys Ther* 39(2):81–89, 2009.
76. Lafosse L, Brzoska R, Toussaint B, et al: The outcome and structural integrity of arthroscopic rotator cuff repair with use of the double-row suture anchor technique: surgical technique, *J Bone Joint Surg Am* 90:275–286, 2008.
77. Katz LM, Hsu S, Miller S, et al: Poor outcomes after SLAP repair: descriptive analysis and prognosis, *Arthroscopy* 25 (8):849–855, 2009.
78. Huberty DP, Schoolfield JD, Brady PC, et al: Incidence and treatment of postoperative stiffness following arthroscopic rotator cuff repair, *Arthroscopy* 25(8):880–890, 2009.
79. Djurasovic M, Marra G, Arroyo JS, et al: Revision rotator cuff repair: factors influencing results, *J Bone Joint Surg Am* 83 (12):1849–1855, 2001.
80. Warner JJP, Parsons IM 4th: Latissimus dorsi tendon transfer: a comparative analysis of primary and salvage reconstruction of massive, irreparable rotator cuff tears, *J Shoulder Elbow Surg* 10(6):514–521, 2001.
81. Schoierer O, Herzberg G, Berthonnaud E, et al: Anatomical basis of latissimus dorsi and teres major transfers in rotator cuff tear surgery with particular reference to the neurovascular pedicles, *Surg Radiol Anat* 23(2):75–80, 2001.
82. Jensen KL, Williams GR, Russell IJ, et al: Rotator cuff tear arthropathy, *J Bone Joint Surg Am* 81(9):1312–1324, 1999.

CHAPTER

19

Randa A. Bascharon
and Robert C. Manske

Surgical Approach to Shoulder Instabilities

The shoulder is a unique joint in that it is the most mobile joint in the human body.[1] This mobility renders the shoulder inherently unstable. The shoulder's unconstrained characteristics predispose it to deviant joint mobility leading to instability. This instability increases the shoulder's vulnerability to dysfunction and makes it one of the most frequently dislocated joints in the body. Shoulder instability is not always pathologic, however, and it can manifest in several forms, including simple congenital laxity, acquired laxity, multidirectional laxity, symptomatic repetitive or chronic subluxations, and acute or chronic dislocations. *Glenohumeral instability* is defined as excessive symptomatic translation of the humeral head relative to the glenoid when stress is applied.[2]

The goal of this chapter is to provide an algorithmic overview of shoulder instability while discussing the fundamental differences among the various pathologic presentations of instability. Unfortunately, a common misunderstanding is that shoulder laxity and instability are of equivalent stature. A significant amount of capsular laxity is present in the normal shoulder, and this characteristic makes differentiation of normal from pathologic very difficult. Furthermore, overall laxity, often described as generalized ligamentous laxity, is found bilaterally and is asymptomatic.[3] A thorough outline of normal shoulder anatomy and biomechanics helps to clarify the foundational principles of shoulder stability.

Implications that lead to disruption of normal shoulder functioning are reviewed. Next, contributing factors that lead to the development of shoulder instability are described. This discussion is followed by an explanation of the pathophysiology of shoulder instability.

Comprehensively, the spectrum of shoulder instabilities is discussed, including principles of assessment and evaluation of the unstable shoulder. Furthermore, a step-by-step characterization of the differences among the shoulder instability patterns is provided. Once shoulder instabilities are identified, a systematic decision-making process for proper treatment is outlined. This knowledge, which is essential for successful clinical outcomes, will help to clarify the vagueness often associated with unstable shoulder conditions.

SHOULDER ANATOMY

Understanding normal shoulder anatomy is necessary to grasp the contributors to instability. Furthermore, comprehending the interplay between normal anatomic relationships and shoulder biomechanics is important to identify accurately the factors influencing shoulder stability. Shoulder mobility is a continuum from often subtle microsubluxation to more obvious gross dislocations.[3]

Anatomic factors influencing shoulder joint stability can be grouped into static stabilizers and active stabilizers. The principal static mechanisms include the ligamentous restraints of the glenohumeral joint, the glenoid labrum, and negative intra-articular pressure. Active stabilization is provided by the surrounding muscles, primarily the rotator cuff. Surprisingly, the bony anatomy of the shoulder joint does not provide intrinsic stability; only one fourth of the humeral head contacts the glenoid at any given time.[4] Despite its small size, the glenoid fossa can remain in the most stable position in relation to the humeral head during movement. It has the unique capacity to recoil when a sudden force is applied to the shoulder joint. This ability lessens the impact on the shoulder as the scapula slides along the chest wall.

Shoulder Stabilizers

Static (Passive) Shoulder Stabilizers

Glenohumeral Ligaments

The glenohumeral ligaments are the primary static stabilizers that offer passive shoulder girdle stabilization. All four ligaments have a stabilizing role. Three ligaments are located anteriorly, and they reinforce the ventral joint capsule. This reinforcement is necessary because the anterior shoulder capsule itself offers little inherent stability. It is thin and lax, with little resistance to excess motion. The anterior joint capsule is more of a conglomeration of the inferior, middle, and superior glenohumeral ligaments, which are all fused with the labral attachment to the glenoid rim (Fig. 19-1).[5]

Additional passive stabilization is aided by receptors in the shoulder capsule that provide proprioceptive feedback.

The principal static stabilizer of the shoulder is the inferior glenohumeral complex. It has earned its role as the primary passive stabilizer of the shoulder for several reasons. First, in comparison with the other glenohumeral ligaments, the inferior glenohumeral ligament complex covers a larger surface area, spanning from the 2-o'clock position anteriorly to the 8- to 9-o'clock position posteriorly. Second, the characteristic design of this complex, in conjunction with its anatomic positioning, allows stabilization in multiple planes. Appropriately, it has been described as a "hammock" because of its mobility patterns and thick anterior and posterior bands with a thin axillary pouch.[5] Much like a swinging hammock, the inferior glenohumeral ligament slides anteriorly and superiorly when the shoulder is externally rotated. This movement causes tightening of the anterior band and fanning out of the posterior band. When internally rotated, the band swings posteriorly and inferiorly, thus causing the opposite to occur: the posterior band tightens, and the anterior band fans.

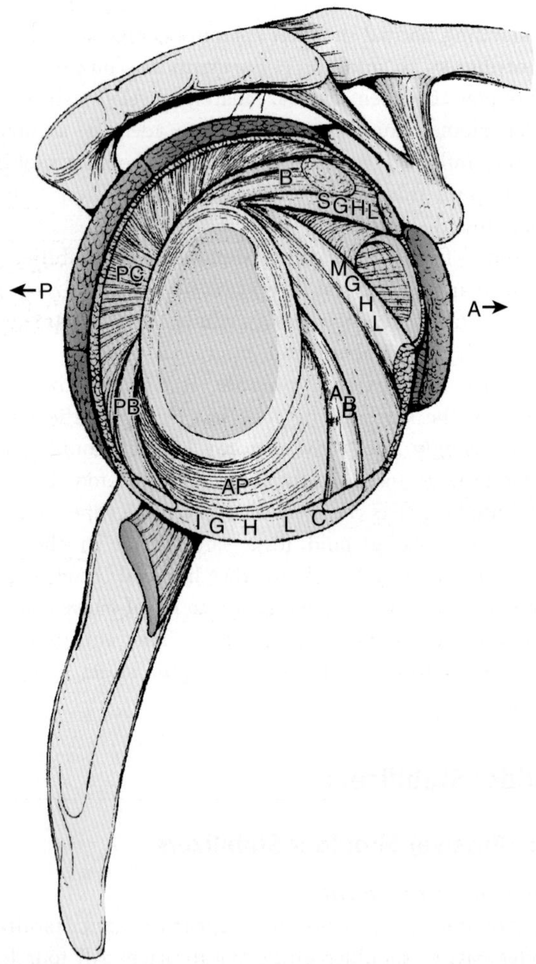

Figure 19-1 Anatomic depiction of the glenohumeral ligaments and inferior glenohumeral ligament complex (IGHLC). A, anterior; AB, anterior band; AP, axillary pouch; B, biceps tendon; MGHL, middle glenohumeral ligament; P, posterior; PB, posterior band; PC, posterior capsule; SGHL, superior glenohumeral ligament. (From O'Brien SJ, Voos JE, Neviaser AS, et al: Developmental Anatomy of the Shoulder and Anatomy of the Glenohumeral Joint. In Rockwood Jr CA, Matsen III FA, Wirth MA, et al. (Eds): *The Shoulder*, ed 4, Philadelphia, 2009, Saunders.)

Assisting the inferior glenohumeral ligament in stabilization during external rotation, the middle glenohumeral ligament limits external rotation when the arm is in the lower and middle ranges of abduction. When the arm is in 90° of abduction, the middle glenohumeral ligament has little influence on external rotation, and it offers no stability during internal rotation.

The superior glenohumeral ligament is the primary restraint to the inferior humeral subluxation when the arm is in 90° of abduction. The superior band is the primary stabilizer to anterior and posterior stress at 0° of abduction. Furthermore, the superior glenohumeral ligament is part of the rotator cuff interval. The significance of this relationship was noted by Harryman et al,[6] who discovered that when the rotator cuff interval was tightened, posterior inferior translation decreased.

Similar to the superior glenohumeral ligament, the anterior-inferior band of the glenohumeral ligament complex stabilizes the shoulder during anterior and posterior stresses. The difference is that the anterior-inferior band of the glenohumeral ligament complex functions in this capacity when the shoulder is abducted at 45° or more, whereas the superior glenohumeral ligament primarily stabilizes anterior and posterior stress when the arm is not abducted. The anterior band of the inferior glenohumeral ligament aids with rollback of the humeral head in the glenoid and is a constraint at the extremes of shoulder motion.

The supporting ligament structures described earlier surround the glenoid in a circular fashion. Seamlessly, the static structures fan from the periphery of glenoid, beginning with the labrum. The glenoid labrum is a fibrous structure that attaches to the rim of the glenoid. A fibrocartilaginous transition zone stretches from the articular cartilage of the glenoid to the fibers of the labral tissue. Attached to the labrum are the glenohumeral ligaments and the capsular conglomeration. Specifically, the superior glenoid labrum serves as a point of attachment for the superior glenohumeral ligament, the middle glenohumeral ligament, and the posterior-superior capsule. Integral to the glenoid labrum is the insertion of the tendon of the long head of the biceps. This tendon inserts on the superior aspect of the joint and blends to become indistinguishable from the posterior glenoid labrum. The biceps tendon has been identified to have several significant shoulder stabilizing effects.

Glenoid Labrum

Not only is the glenoid labrum a point of attachment for the biceps tendon and supporting shoulder ligaments, but also it provides its own important contributions to the stability of the shoulder. According to Howell and Galinat,[4] the labrum deepens the flat glenoid fossa by 50%, a finding that is significant considering that the glenoid does not provide inherent stability for the humeral head.[4] When this concavity of the glenoid and labral complex is lost, its stabilizing effect can be reduced by 20%.[7] This significance is also highlighted by studies showing that the intact labrum provides 75% of the vertical and 67% of the horizontal humeral head contact area.[8] When the labrum is intact, an apparent bumper effect allows stabilization of the humeral head within the glenoid. This effect appears to be more important in the superior-inferior direction than in the anterior-posterior direction. Furthermore, Matsen et al[9] suggested that the labrum may serve as a "chock block" to prevent excessive humeral head rollback.

The glenoid labrum has a close relationship with the biceps tendon, which attaches at the superior portion of the labrum. The biceps tendon enters in the joint through the rotator interval, to insert onto the supraglenoid tubercle. This tendon insertion begins approximately 5 mm medially from the superior edge of the glenoid. The superior labrum does not always attach firmly to this region of the glenoid. A small synovial recess may exist beneath the superior labrum and may create a predisposition to certain patterns of superior labral tears. Furthermore, differences in the biceps insertion can have implications for the type of superior disease that develops. Another factor contributing to the vulnerability of this region is the diminished vascularity of the superior and anterior-superior labrum. This region of diminished vascularity may contribute to delayed or incomplete healing after injury and higher rates of treatment failure after surgical repair.

Negative Intra-articular Pressure

Negative intra-articular pressure can provide a passive stabilizing effect to the glenohumeral joint. Negative intra-articular pressure creates cohesion between the humeral head and the glenoid fossa that has a passive static stabilizing benefit. Even though negative intra-articular pressure supplies only a small amount of stability (up to 20 to 30 lb), Speer's cadaver studies[10] showed that as long as the joint is not vented, muscle activity is not required to hold the shoulder together.

Active (Dynamic) Stabilizers of the Shoulder Joint

Statically, the labrum and the capsular ligamentous complex offer stabilization of the shoulder, whereas active stabilization comes from the muscles surrounding the joint. The rotator cuff muscles provide compressive stabilization by intrinsic muscle forces. The principal extrinsic muscular forces originate from the deltoid. The action of the deltoid produces primarily vertical shear force that displaces the humeral head superiorly.

Detailed research demonstrated that shoulder stability is a balanced synchronicity between the static and dynamic stabilizers of the joint. Disruption of either of these stabilizers not only results in instability but also inevitably causes damage to these supports. Glousman et al[11] showed that synchronous eccentric deceleration and concentric contraction of the rotator cuff and biceps tendon are necessary for humeral stability during middle ranges of humeral motion. This stability is afforded by dynamic compression. *Dynamic compression* refers to the ability of the rotator cuff musculature to supply a compressive effect to the humeral head during shoulder movements. Several force couples help to maintain this stability. The first is the force couple created by active contractions of the rotator cuff itself. The inferiorly directed force couples of the rotator cuff muscles not only cause compression of the humeral head but also create rotation on the fossa.[12,13] Fatigue of the rotator cuff from overuse or incompetent ligament support can result in less than optimal synchronicity that leads to further damage.

This concept of synchronous mobility for shoulder stability applies to the relationship of the scapula and the glenoid.[14] Lippit et al[7] confirmed the importance of dynamic balance for appropriate positioning of the glenoid articular surface so that the joint reaction force produced is compressive, rather than shear. When the synchronous function of the scapular stabilizers (serratus anterior, trapezius, latissimus dorsi, rhomboids, and levator scapulae) is normal, the scapula and the glenoid articular structures are maintained in the most stable functional position.[7] Therefore, the importance of scapular stabilizer and rotator cuff strengthening in patients who participate in upper extremity–dominant sports must be acknowledged.

Shoulder Biomechanics

Key elements of shoulder anatomy and biomechanical function are important in understanding shoulder stability. Biomechanical studies demonstrated the structural importance of the biceps tendon–superior labrum complex to the glenohumeral joint. Furthermore, disruption of this complex has detrimental effects on the overall stability of the shoulder joint.

The shoulder stabilizing effects of the biceps tendon occur through multiple modalities. This tendon compresses the glenohumeral joint and places tension on periligamentous fibers. The biceps tendon acts as an anterior-superior barrier. In this role, the biceps tendon places the joint into a position that secondarily tightens the ligamentous structures. Electromyography demonstrates that, during the overhead throwing motion, high activity is seen in the biceps during the late cocking phase. In this phase, the shoulder is in extreme abduction and external rotation. Even higher biceps electromyography activity is found in pitchers with known shoulder instability as compared with normal control subjects.

The stabilizing function of the biceps tendon and its relationship with rotator cuff disease was studied by Warner et al,[15] who demonstrated the importance of the biceps tendon in superior stability of the glenohumeral joint. Patients with biceps tendon rupture have a 2- to 6-mm increase in superior translation of the humeral head when the arm is abducted in the scapular plane.

Pagnani and Dome[16] investigated translations of the glenohumeral joint with and without detachment of the biceps tendon–superior labrum complex. Significant increases of humeral superior-inferior and anterior-posterior translation in shoulders with superior labrum anterior to posterior (SLAP) lesions were identified when the arm was in the abducted position. To delineate the role of the biceps tendon–superior labrum complex further, these investigators created SLAP lesions. However, because these simulated SLAP lesions did not involve detachment of the biceps insertion, no increased translations of the humeral head were observed.[16]

Rodosky et al[17] studied superior labral complex interplay. The short and long head of the biceps contributed to torsional rigidity of the shoulder in abduction and external rotation. The biceps seemed to support the function of the inferior glenohumeral ligament in the abducted and externally rotated position. When the biceps tendon was detached in a SLAP lesion, the torsional rigidity of the joint was decreased, and an increased strain was placed on the inferior glenohumeral ligament.[17]

PATHOGENESIS OF SHOULDER INSTABILITY

At its simplest, shoulder instability is a clinical syndrome that occurs when shoulder laxity produces symptoms.[18] The pathogenesis of shoulder instability consists of the chain of events leading to changes in structure and function of the shoulder that ultimately create loss of stability. Often, the transition from a normal to a deviant capsulolabral complex becomes implicit in shoulder instability. Nevertheless, classification of shoulder instability is based on multiple factors. To simplify these factors, shoulder instability can be represented by the five Ds: direction, degree, duration, other determinants, and medical disorders contributing to shoulder instability (Table 19-1).

The direction of instability is a common descriptor for shoulder instability. This categorization identifies the instability as unidirectional, bidirectional, or multidirectional. The degree of instability categorizes the amount of translation of the humeral head from the glenoid. It can be referred to either as *subluxation,* which is partial separation of the humeral head from the glenoid, or *dislocation,* which is a complete separation of the humeral head from the glenoid concavity. The duration of symptoms should be recorded as acute, subacute, chronic (humeral head has remained dislocated for more than 6 weeks), or recurrent. Other determinants

Table 19-1 The Five Ds of Shoulder Instability Classification

Classification	Subclassification	Pearls
Direction	Anterior	Accounts for 97% of recurrent dislocations Results from a fall or anterior force to the arm when in an abducted and externally rotated position
	Posterior	Posterior force with arm forward elevated and adducted 3% of recurrent dislocations
	Inferior	Inferior rare
	Superior	Superior rare and often secondary to severe rotator cuff insufficiency
Degree	Subluxation	Partial translation of the humeral head from the glenoid fossa
	Dislocation	Complete translation beyond the glenoid rim of the humeral head from the glenoid fossa
Duration	Acute	Less than 3 weeks
	Subacute	3–6 weeks
	Chronic	6 weeks or longer
	Recurrent	Can cause secondary deficiencies
Other determinants	Trauma	
	Macrotrauma	Anterior Posterior
	Microtrauma	Usually acquired secondary to microinstability Associated with rotator cuff tendinosis/dysfunction
	Atraumatic	Multidirectional instability Present with severe pain and not overt instability
	Age	Recurrent dislocations: more than 90% in patients younger than 20 years and 10% in patient older than 40 years Dislocation uncommon in patients more than 40 years old Associated rotator cuff tears: 30% in those older than 40 years and 80% in those older than 60 years Greater tuberosity fractures more prevalent in those more than 40 years old
	Voluntary	People with posterior instability learn to dislocate their shoulders through selective muscular contractions; some do it for secondary gain Surgical treatment often not successful
Disorders	Seizures	Nonoperative treatment should be initial approach
	Neuromuscular disorders	
	Collagen disorders	Ehlers-Danlos syndrome, Marfan's syndrome Extensive supervised conservative treatment Abnormal tissue stretching and recurrent dislocations can contribute to higher rates of surgical failures

of shoulder instability include the trauma that resulted in instability, the patient's age, and induced dislocation such as in the voluntary dislocator. Disease entities such as seizures, neuromuscular disorders, collagen deficiencies, and congenital disorders also serve as categories of shoulder instability.

Changes in the shoulder's normal anatomic mechanisms and physical functions cause specific underlying abnormalities leading to instability. Furthermore, multiple physiologic dysfunctions cause recurrent instability, and this instability is not isolated to one pathologic lesion. The pathophysiology is multifactorial and distinctive, based on direction and the level of traumatic overlay. Table 19-2 is an overview of the pathophysiology of shoulder instability.

Recurrent Shoulder Instability

Recurrent shoulder instability is a result of both primary and secondary deficiencies of the static and dynamic stabilizers of the shoulder. Instability occurs when the mechanisms of these stabilizers are out of balance. Primary deficiencies are those contributing to the onset of instability. However, repeated instability can cause secondary deficiencies contributing to further subluxation and recurrent dislocations.

Table 19-2 Pathophysiology of Shoulder Instability

Type of Shoulder Instability	Pathophysiology		Discussion
Anterior	Traumatic soft tissue deficiency	Bankart's lesions	Detachment of the labrum from the anterior-inferior glenoid, seen in 100% of younger patients and in 75% of those older than 50 years Passive restraints and concavity compression lost Glenoid depth decreased by 50% IGHL detached in 85% of traumatic anterior dislocation and considered a major pathoanatomic factor; usually seen in younger patients Detachment of the anterior-inferior labrum and capsule from glenoid doubles anterior translation Plastic deformation of the capsule
		Anterior labral ligamentous lesion (ALPSA)	Anterior IGHL, labrum and anterior scapular periosteum stripped and displaced in a sleeve-type fashion medially on the glenoid neck Seen in acute and chronic dislocations
		Superior labral extensions	Caused by traction on the upper extremity and throwing motions, both of which produce eccentric traction of the biceps anchor May also be caused by torsional peel-back of the posterior superior labrum during cocking phase of throwing Decreased vascularity and age increase likelihood of labral tears Multiple tear types exist and can be associated with rotator cuff or biceps disease SLAP lesion: superior labrum anterior posterior lesion involving the superior labrum and extending into the attachment of the biceps tendon SLAC lesion: anterior superior labrum lesion in which the anterior supraspinatus can have partial or complete tear causing various amounts of instability; can be caused by acute or chronic trauma
		Humeral avulsion of glenohumeral ligament (HAGL)	Lateral detachment of the IGHL from the humeral neck. Occurs from continued forced abduction at 95°–105° with impaction tears to the capsule
	Traumatic bone deficiency	Humeral bone deficiency	Hill-Sachs lesion: an impaction fracture to the posterior-superior humeral head when it is impacted against the anterior rim of the glenoid during dislocation Located in the posterior-superior portion of humeral head Engaging Hill-Sachs lesion: catches and locks the humeral head in a functional position; instability results from the defect engaging the glenoid rim in the functional arc of motion at 90° of abduction and external rotation Nonengaging Hill-Sachs lesion: can cause catching when the arm is in a nonfunctional position; abduction of less than 70°
		Glenoid bone deficiency	Impression or avulsion fractures can occur Glenoid rim fractures occur in anterior and posterior dislocations If more than 20% of the glenoid is involved, risk for recurrent instability exists

Continued

Table 19-2 Pathophysiology of Shoulder Instability—cont'd

Type of Shoulder Instability	Pathophysiology	Discussion
Posterior	Trauma	Not a high rate of recurrence
		Bony architecture disrupted if glenoid rim fracture occurs, causing changes in glenoid version
	Repetitive microtrauma	Higher rate of recurrent subluxations
		Usually from repetitive overuse such as in overhead sports, weight lifting, football linemen
		Direction of instability patterns should be evaluated carefully
	Atraumatic disorder	Voluntary subluxation seen in this category
		Horizontal adduction and internal rotation resulting from psychologic issues or secondary gain
		In abduction, selective use of internal rotators to sublux the shoulder posterior
		Congenital dysplasia of the glenoid can cause inadequate glenoid version
Multidirectional	Laxity	Subtly laxity in both shoulders not uncommon
		Repetitive overhead activities may play a role leading to gradual stretching of the restraining structures
		Distinction between laxity and instability crucial
	Lesions of the rotator interval	Enlarged rotator interval contributing to increased amounts of humeral head translations

IGHL, inferior glenohumeral ligament; SLAC, Superior labrum anterior cuff; SLAP, Superior labrum anterior to posterior.

Previously, investigators thought that one essential pathologic lesion was responsible for recurrent shoulder subluxation or dislocation. Historically, detachment of the labrum from the anterior rim of the glenoid cavity was considered the sole source of shoulder instability.[9] Bankart's classic article identified two types of primary lesions that occur with acute dislocations. The first type generally occurs in the anterior and inferior direction when the humeral head is forced through the weakest part of the capsule (Fig. 19-2). This is generally between the lower border of the subscapularis and long head of the triceps muscle. In the second type, the humeral head is forced anteriorly, thus tearing the fibrocartilaginous labrum from the entire anterior half of the glenoid rim and tearing the capsule and periosteum from the anterior surface of the neck of the scapula. This results in the humeral head anteriorly displaced out of the glenoid cavity. This traumatic detachment of the glenoid labrum is now known as Bankart lesion. Rowe and Sakellarides[19] found Bankart's lesions in 85% of recurrent dislocations and in 64% of recurrent shoulder subluxations. Additionally, when investigated, it was found that 84% of previously failed surgical stabilization procedures were in patients who had Bankart lesions.[19]

Most investigators today agree that a Bankart lesion is the most commonly observed pathologic lesion in recurrent subluxation or dislocation of the shoulder. However, contemporary research has reinforced that several vital primary and secondary pathologic lesions are responsible for recurrent shoulder instability. These lesions can be both soft tissue and bony.[20] These deficiencies collectively are fundamental to continued shoulder instability. In most cases, one individual shoulder lesion is not the sole cause of shoulder instability.

Recurrent instability can cause secondary deficiencies that further contribute to an unstable shoulder. This disorder is exemplified by resultant stretching of the anterior capsule and subscapularis tendon, fraying and degeneration of the glenoid labrum, and erosion of the anterior glenoid rim. In addition, secondary trauma to the rotator cuff and biceps tendon can lead to rotator cuff dysfunction. Rowe and Sakellarides[19] found that excessive laxity of the shoulder capsule was also a cause of instability of the shoulder joint. These investigators found excessive laxity in 28% of traumatic recurrent dislocations, in 26% of transient subluxations, and in 86% of previous surgical failures.[19] Plastic deformation of the capsuloligamentous complex can cause excessive laxity, or this condition can be caused by a congenital collagen deficiency.

Plastic deformation can result from an isolated macrotraumatic event or repetitive microtrauma causing injury to the capsuloligamentous complex. Warren et al[21] found that structural damage to the capsular structures occurred in a circular pattern. The *circle concept* is based on cadaveric studies demonstrating that humeral dislocation did not occur unless both the anterior and posterior capsular structures were disrupted.[21] Through an arthroscopic study of anterior shoulder dislocations, Baker et al[22] delineated the capsuloligamentous complex failure patterns. These investigators found that 62% were disruptions of the capsuloligamentous insertion into the glenoid neck, and 38% of the acute injuries were intrasubstance ligamentous failures.[22]

A multitude of research performed in throwing athletes provides further evidence that recurrent instability is multifactorial.

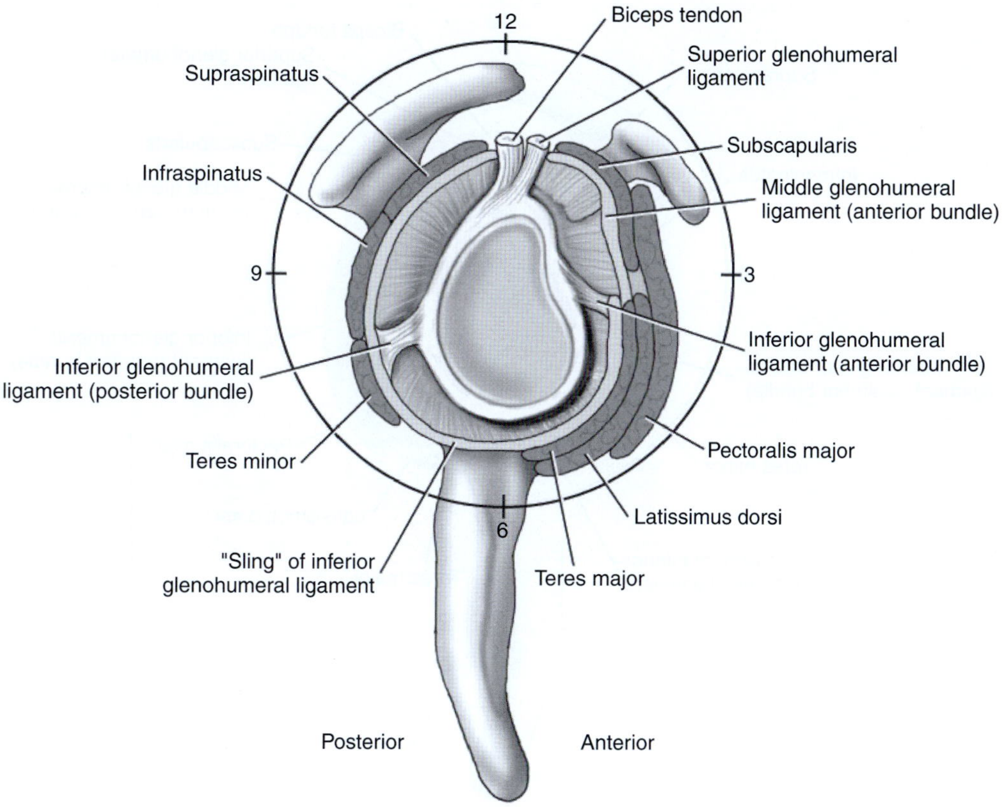

Figure 19-2 Bankart lesion. (From Magee DJ: *Orthopedic physical assessment,* ed 5, Philadelphia, 2007, Saunders.)

Both pathoanatomic and biomechanical deficiencies can contribute to shoulder instability. The throwing athlete is at risk for repetitive microtrauma leading to instability as a result of continued injury to the capsuloligamentous complex. Burkhart and Morgan[20] and other investigators presented a unified concept of the disabled throwing shoulder through research of the pathoanatomic features resulting in deficient biomechanics. Previously, investigators thought that shoulder instability in the throwing athlete originated from microinstability. However, Burkhart and Morgan[20] theorized that a posterior-inferior capsular contracture leading to a SLAP lesion could be the critical factor (Fig. 19-3). This contracture first causes a glenohumeral internal rotation deficit (Fig. 19-4). This deficit worsens over time. The contracture of the posterior-inferior glenohumeral ligament causes angulation instead of translation of the humeral head in a posterior-superior direction during the cocking phase of the throw. This, in turn, allows excessive external rotation resulting from the posterior-superior shift of the center of rotation of the humeral head. In conjunction with this movement is a loss of the normal buttress or cam effect of the inferior humeral head across the inferior glenohumeral ligament that functionally loosens this ligament.[20] This change, in turn, permits even more external rotation and creates further alteration of throwing biomechanics (see Chapter 3).

This "hyperexternal" rotation, along with an alteration in the direction of pull of the biceps tendon at 90° of abduction, and the torsional posteriorly and superiorly centered forces change the biomechanics during the cocking phase of the throw. Ultimately, this change can cause a peel-back mechanism of the biceps tendon–superior labrum complex that leads to a SLAP lesion.[20] This mechanism typically leads to SLAP lesions that are more posterior than anterior. Unfortunately, this process is magnified by further external rotation and a posterior-superior shift that occurs once the superior labrum is unstable. Furthermore, this intricate cascade leading to the peel-back mechanism can cause excessive twisting of the posterior-superior rotator cuff fibers and eventual failure of the articular side and anterior ligament fiber.[20]

Humeral head impaction fractures and glenoid rim fractures are produced following anterior dislocation and are contributors to recurrent instability. The posterior-superior humeral head is impacted against the rim of the anterior glenoid during the dislocation process. These impression fractures are known as *Hill-Sachs lesions.* Normally, these lesions are created by the position of the arm when the dislocation occurs. They can be either engaging or nonengaging, depending on whether the humeral head catches and locks the humeral head in a functional position (engaging) or a nonfunctional position (nonengaging). Burkhart and De Beer[23] described that instability results from the Hill-Sachs lesion when the defect engages the glenoid rim in the functional arc of motion, which is 90° of abduction and external rotation. Similarly, the instability that occurs when the arm is abducted less than 70° (nonfunctional position) results when the humeral defect engages the glenoid rim.[23]

Glenoid rim fractures can occur during anterior or posterior dislocations and can result in recurrent instability

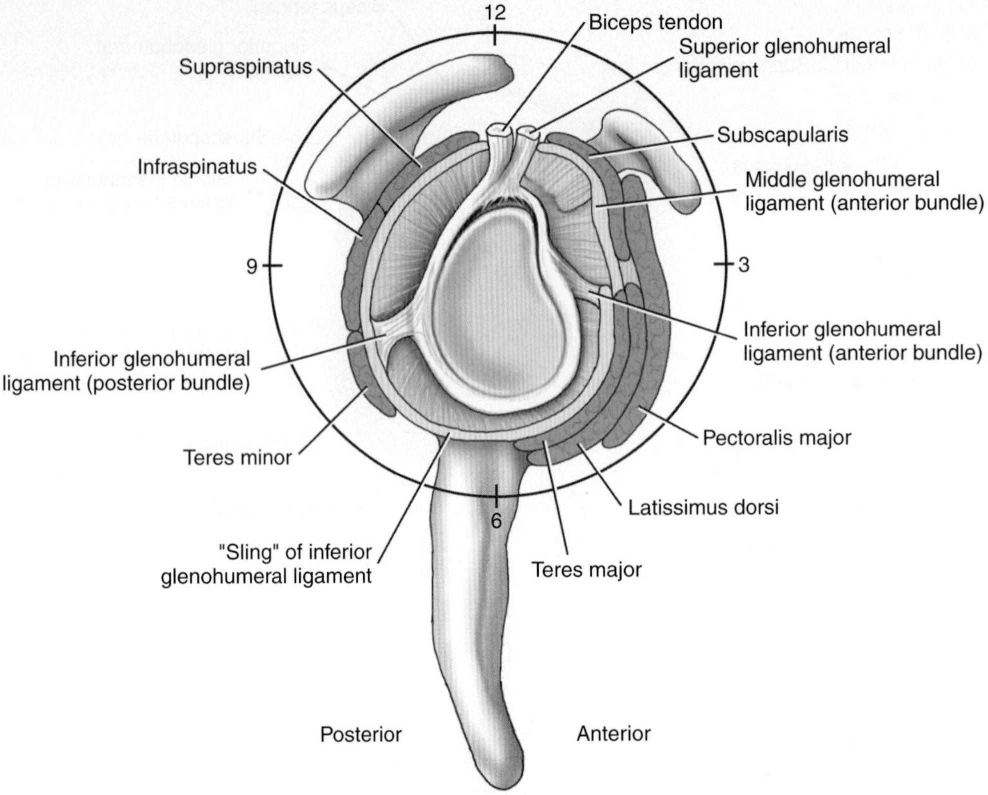

Figure 19-3 SLAP lesion. (From Magee DJ: *Orthopedic physical assessment,* ed 5, Philadelphia, 2007, Saunders.)

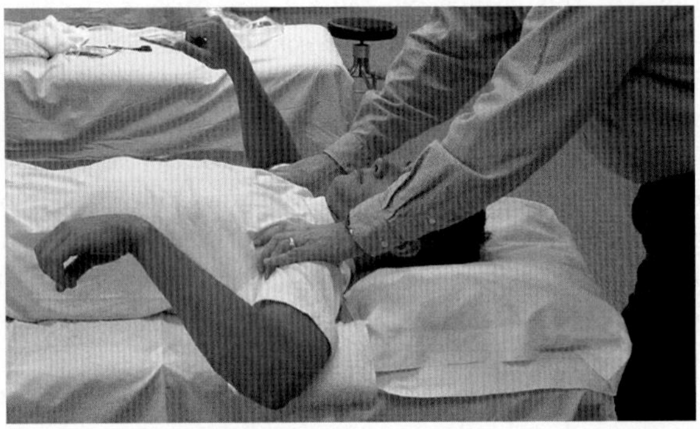

Figure 19-4 Glenohumeral internal rotation deficit (GIRD). (From Manske RC: Postsurgical Orthopedic Sports Rehabilitation: *Knee & Shoulder,. St. Louis, 207, Mosby.*)

if the lesion involves more than 20% of the glenoid. The compression Bankart lesion is secondary to compression of the anterior-inferior bony articulation of the glenoid by the humeral head. Normal anatomy of the glenoid is represented by a pear shape, with the inferior portion of the glenoid typically resembling a true circle. Repeated episodes of instability create the "inverted pear" lesion.

Recurrent posterior instability and subluxation are far more likely to result from microtrauma than from recurrent posterior macrotraumatic dislocations. These instability patterns can be unidirectional, bidirectional, or multidirectional. Several overuse and microtraumatic injuries result in the posterior instability often seen in sports that involve repetitive movement patterns, especially in the overhead position. Weight lifting during bench press and blocking techniques of offensive linemen can lead to microtraumatic injuries causing recurrent instability.

Multidirectional instability (MDI) is also influenced by the repetitive microtrauma of overhead activities. Usually, gradual stretching of the restraining structures occurs in an individual who also has subtle congenital laxity. This process eventually can transform asymptomatic laxity into symptomatic instability.

Increased understanding of shoulder pathophysiology has led to an improved delineation of rotator interval lesions and the role of these lesions in MDI. The rotator interval is anatomically described as a triangular space with the apex centered at the transverse humeral ligament over the biceps sulcus. It is a section of the glenohumeral joint capsule and is bordered superiorly by the anterior margin of the supraspinatus tendon. Inferiorly, it is bordered by the superior aspect of the subscapularis tendon. The rotator interval is strengthened by the coracohumeral ligament and the superior glenohumeral ligament. An enlarged rotator interval contributes to humeral head translation and plays a significant role in posterior stability of the shoulder joint.

HISTORY AND PHYSICAL EXAMINATION OF THE UNSTABLE SHOULDER

Because shoulder instability has many causes, correct diagnosis and identification of possible primary and secondary deficiencies contributing to recurrent instability are imperative to devising an appropriate treatment plan. Diagnosis begins with a detailed yet focused history of the instability episode. Often, the information on the initial episode of instability is the key to determining the direction of the pathologic process. A thorough history should define the direction of the dislocation, the age of the patient, and the magnitude and frequency of the dislocation or subluxation of the shoulder.

The direction and type of instability are often identified by the position of the arm when symptoms occur. In complete dislocations, the ease of relocation helps to differentiate between subluxation and dislocations associated with generalized ligamentous laxity. Clues to the type of disorder can be gathered by asking about the location of the pain. A differential diagnosis of the shoulder disease should be formulated, and a thorough review of systems should be conducted to identify other medical conditions that may be contributing to the shoulder disorder. Additionally, it is imperative to listen for "red flags," as described by Stith et al.[24] When performing the systems review, the clinician must be aware of conditions related to diseases outside of the scope of the physical therapist's practice.[25]

Physical examination of the shoulder should always be performed using a systematic approach, to avoid overlooking concurrent diseases. Both shoulders should always be carefully examined. Palpation of the shoulder helps to define the location of the pain and provides useful information on pathoanatomy (Table 19-3). Thorough assessment of motion, laxity, and stability should be performed regardless of the type of instability. Strength testing should include testing of the rotator cuff, deltoid, and serratus anterior for scapular winging. Several specialty tests for the shoulder that are listed in Table 19-4 should be used during examination of shoulder instability.[26,27]

Table 19-3 Palpation in the Diagnosis of Shoulder Disorders

Location of Shoulder Pain	Pathologic Process Present
Anterior lateral deltoid	Supraspinatus tendon injury
Posterior joint line	Posterior labrum or infraspinatus injury
Anterior joint line	Capsulolabral tear Biceps tendon injury
Coracoid	Subscapularis tendon injury Pectoralis minor strain Coracohumeral ligament sprain
Posterior pain	Posterior instability
Diffuse pain	Multidirectional instability, posterior instability, osseous lesions, and fractures of the shoulder girdle
Referred pain proximal and distal to the shoulder	Cervical radiculopathy Nerve lesions

DIAGNOSTIC IMAGING IN THE EVALUATION OF SHOULDER INSTABILITY

Imaging studies may be helpful in delineating anatomic and pathologic factors in shoulder instability. Radiographs, computed tomography scans, and magnetic resonance imaging (MRI) all have their role in the diagnosis of shoulder instability (Table 19-5).

DECISION-MAKING PROCESS FOR TREATMENT OF SHOULDER INSTABILITY

The decision-making process for appropriate treatment is challenging. Several questions are key to making the appropriate treatment plan that will provide the patient with optimal results and will minimize recurrence or complications. The decision-making process is nothing short of algorithmic.

The simplified classification system devised by Matsen et al[9] exemplifies the type of decision-making process that is necessary to approach instability of the shoulder. Matsen coined two iconic acronyms that differentiate the treatment process between traumatic and atraumatic shoulder instability. *TUBS* stands for treatment of shoulder instability caused by macrotrauma (*T*raumatic, *U*nidirectional *B*ankart *S*urgery), and *AMBRII* represents the other spectrum of shoulder instability (*A*traumatic, *M*ultidirectional, *B*ilateral, *R*ehabilitation, *I*nferior capsular shift, and *I*nterval closure).

The complexity of an appropriate diagnosis of shoulder instability is often problematic when designing the treatment protocol algorithm. The most common errors are incorrect diagnosis and failure to address primary and secondary deficiencies causing the instability. The questions provided in the next section are important for correctly diagnosing shoulder disorders. Subsequently, additional questions identify other factors to consider in devising an optimal treatment course.

Defining the Diagnosis

- Is the shoulder pain related to a pathologic process from the shoulder itself?
  - If so, does the shoulder demonstrate instability, or is the pain generated from a different shoulder pathologic source?
- If shoulder instability is determined, do the history and physical examination provide clues to the following?
  - Direction
  - Magnitude
  - Frequency
- Are the following contributing factors to the patient's symptoms?
  - Patient's age
  - Activity level
- What information does the diagnostic workup provide that will influence the ultimate treatment course? Does evidence indicate bone lesions or soft tissue injury that

Table 19-4 Tests in the Examination of Shoulder Instability

Shoulder Instability Examination	Procedure	Information Provided
Shift and load test	The patient is placed in the supine position. The test is done by placing one hand along the edge of the scapula to stabilize it and grasping the humeral head with the other hand. To test for anterior instability: The patient's shoulder is abducted to 70° and is forward flexed to 45° to 50° while axially loading by applying a slight compressive force. Posterior instability: The shoulder is examined by forward flexing the arm to 90° with 20° to 30° of adduction with a posteriorly directed force to the arm. The amount of anterior and posterior translation of the humeral head in the glenoid is observed with the arm abducted 0°.	Easy subluxation of the shoulder indicates loss of the glenoid concavity. This finding indicates the need for surgical treatment.
Sulcus test	The patient's arm is in 0° (Fig. 19-5) and 45° of abduction. This test is done by pulling distally on the extremity and observing for a sulcus or dimple between the humeral head and the acromion that does not reduce with 45° external rotation. The distance between the humeral head and acromion should be graded from 0 to 3 with the arm in 0° and 45° of abduction.	Subluxation at 0° of abduction is more indicative of laxity at the rotator interval. Subluxation at 45° indicates laxity of the inferior glenohumeral ligament complex. 1+: subluxation less than 1 cm 2+: 1 to 2 cm of subluxation 3+: more than 2 cm of inferior subluxation
Apprehension test[26]	Anterior apprehension is evaluated with the shoulder in 90° of abduction and the elbow in 90° of flexion, with a slight external rotation force applied to the extremity as anterior stress is applied to the humerus. Control of the proximal humerus should be maintained during any of the apprehension or stress tests to prevent dislocation during these procedures.	This test produces an apprehension reaction in a patient who has anterior instability.
Relocation test	An anterior force is applied to the proximal humerus in an attempt to center the humeral head.	A positive test results occurs when the patient has decreased anterior shoulder pain or decreased apprehension.
Posterior clunk test	The arm is placed in 90° and is abducted. It is brought to a forward flexed, internally rotated position while posterior stress is applied to the elbow. The clunk is felt as the humeral head subluxes posteriorly, thus producing pain or a feeling of subluxation in an unstable shoulder (Fig. 19-6).	Posterior instability can be evaluated with a posterior clunk test.
Shoulder Lachman's test	This test is performed with the patient supine and the extremity in various degrees of abduction and external rotation in the plane of the scapula. When examining the patient's right shoulder, the examiner's left hand is used to grasp the proximal humerus while the right hand is used to hold the elbow lightly. Anterior stress is applied to the proximal humerus by using the left hand, and the amount of translation and the end point are evaluated. The amount of instability is graded from 0 to 4.	Grade 1 indicates translation greater than the opposite uninvolved extremity. Grade 2 means that the humeral head slips up to the rim of the glenoid. Grade 3 means that it slips over the labrum but then spontaneously relocates. Grade 4 indicates dislocation.
O'Brien's test[27]	The patient is placed in the upright position. The shoulder is placed in 90° of elevation and is adducted. A resisted upward force with the forearm fully pronated and supinated is applied.	Increased pain in the pronated position indicates a SLAP lesion. Pain in both positions indicates acromioclavicular disease.

SLAP, superior labrum anterior to posterior.

diagnostically will aid in the decision to pursue a specific surgical procedure?
- What is the appropriate classification of the shoulder instability?

Defining the Treatment Course

- What is the direction of instability?
  - Anterior
  - Posterior
  - Multidirectional
- Is this a primary dislocation or a recurrent instability?
- What is the cause of the instability?
  - Macrotraumatic
  - Microtraumatic
  - Acquired or atraumatic
- Is this patient a candidate for conservative treatment?
  - If so, does this include immobilization or protective bracing?
  - Does the patient require rehabilitation, and what are the goals of the rehabilitation plan to support the end goal of treating the shoulder instability?

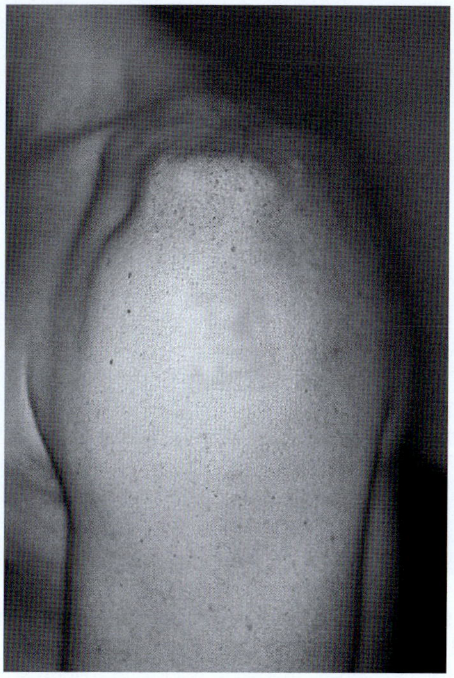

Figure 19-5 Sulcus sign. (From Miller MD, Howard RF, Plancher KD: *Surgical atlas of sports medicine*, Philadelphia, 2003, Saunders.)

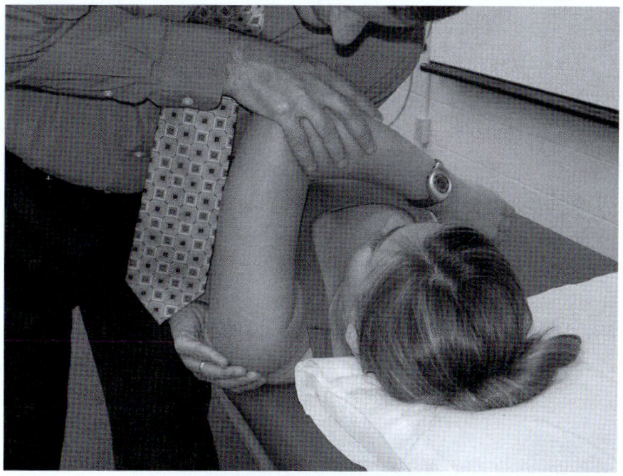

Figure 19-6 Posterior glide test.

- Is the patient a candidate for primary operative intervention instead of a conservative treatment course? What are the surgical treatment options and why?
  - Is the patient a candidate for an arthroscopic or open surgical procedure?
- If the patient has recurrent instability, is he or she responding to conservative treatment options?
  - If not, what are the contributing factors?
  - Does the patient require surgical intervention? If surgery is required, what is the appropriate procedure, and should it be open or arthroscopic?
- If surgical intervention is necessary, what is the postoperative care?

Table 19-5 Diagnostic Imaging to Evaluate Shoulder Instability

Imaging Study	Diagnostic Value
Radiographs	Allows evaluation of shoulder anatomy to rule out fractures of the shoulder girdle
Anterior-posterior view of the arm in slight internal rotation (Fig. 19-7)	Helps to identify fracture of the greater tuberosity
True scapular anterior posterior radiograph	Permits evaluation of glenoid fossa fracture
West Point axillary view (Fig. 19-8)	Used to assess bony avulsions of the attachment of the IGHL, bony Bankart's lesions, or anterior-inferior glenoid deficiency
Stryker notch view	Can quantify and evaluate Hill-Sachs lesion
Computed tomography (CT) (Fig. 19-9)	Can be an accurate means of determining glenoid version and overall glenoid morphology and can reconstruct glenoid anatomy in three dimensions Can aid in preoperative planning
Magnetic resonance imaging (MRI) (Fig. 19-10)	Used for assessment of associated disease Contrast enhancement improves ability to detect labral tears, rotator cuff tears, and articular cartilage lesions

IGHL, inferior glenohumeral ligament.

- What are the defining criteria for the following (conservative and surgical)?
  - Duration of immobilization
  - Rehabilitation protocol
  - Timeline for return to sport, labor, or high-risk activities

DECISION-MAKING PROCESS FOR CONSERVATIVE TREATMENT OF SHOULDER INSTABILITY

Regardless of the instability pattern, appropriate diagnosis is paramount to determining the appropriate treatment plan. A conservative approach is warranted as an initial course of action pending the history, physical examination, and diagnostic workup. The patient with a primary traumatic anterior shoulder dislocation that requires reduction is often treated conservatively with immobilization and subsequent rehabilitation. The position of a patient with initial dislocation has come under scrutiny. Historically, the arm was positioned in adduction and internal rotation. Itoi et al,[28,29] however, performed cadaveric and MRI studies on live humans

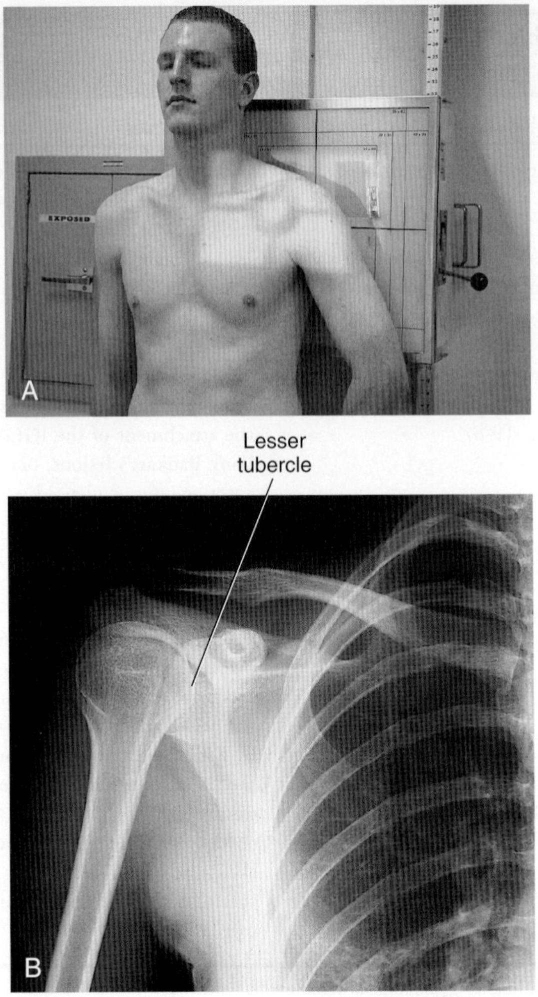

Figure 19-7 The position for taking an AP view of the shoulder with the arm internally rotated to allow visualization of the proximal humerus at approximately a 90-degree different angle than the standard AP view with external rotation. (From Long BW, Frank ED, Erlich RA: *Radiography essentials for limited practice,* ed 2, 2006, Saunders.)

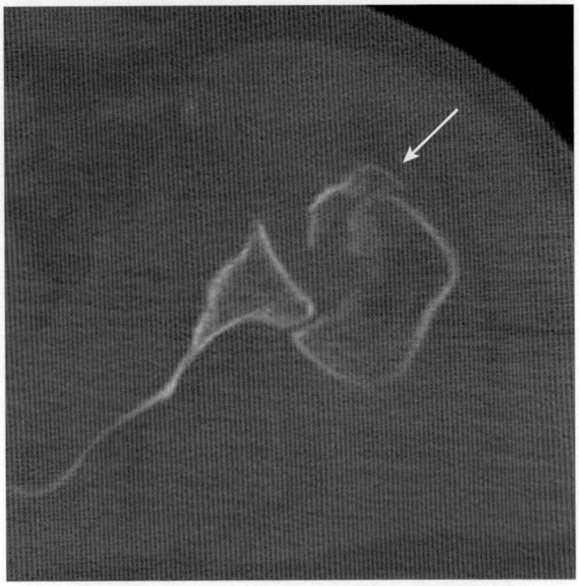

Figure 19-9 Posterior shoulder dislocation as shown in an axial computed tomography (CT) scan. Fracture of the lesser tuberosity (*arrow*) may accompany posterior dislocation. (From Schwartz ML, Thornton DD. Diagnostic Imaging of the Shoulder Complex. In Wilk KE, Reinold MM, Andrews JR: *The Athlete's Shoulder*, ed 2, Philadelphia, 2008, Churchill Livingstone.)

and demonstrated that placing the shoulder in slight external rotation may create a better coaptation of Bankart's lesion. Itoi et al[29] reported that in those immobilized with external rotation, the redislocation rate was 0%, whereas 82% of the patients had returned to sports. This increased healing rate may be in part the result of improved soft tissue contact. Miller et al,[30] using an electronic force sensor, found increased contact force with external rotation of the shoulder following acute dislocation.

Controversy exists because other investigators have not been able to report outcomes nearly as favorable as those of as Itoi et al[29] in attempts to immobilize acute dislocations in external rotation. Finestone et al[31] examined 51 patients

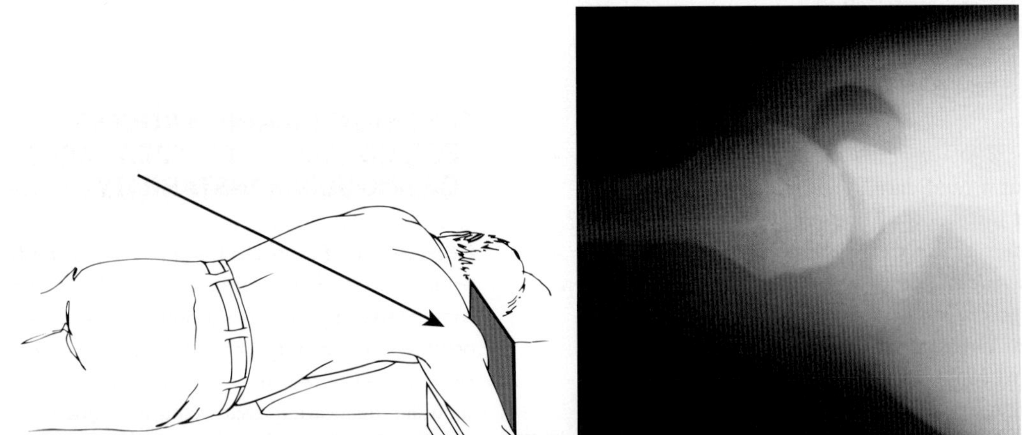

Figure 19-8 A, Patient position necessary to take a West Point view of the shoulder. (From Browner B, Jupiter J, Trafton P: *Skeletal trauma: basic science, management, and reconstruction*, ed 3, 2003, Saunders.) **B,** The result of a West Point view of the glenohumeral joint. Note the acromion superior to the glenoid and the coracoid process, which is inferior to the glenoid in this view. (From Swain J: *Diagnostic Imaging for Physical Therapists*, St. Louis, 2009, Saunders.)

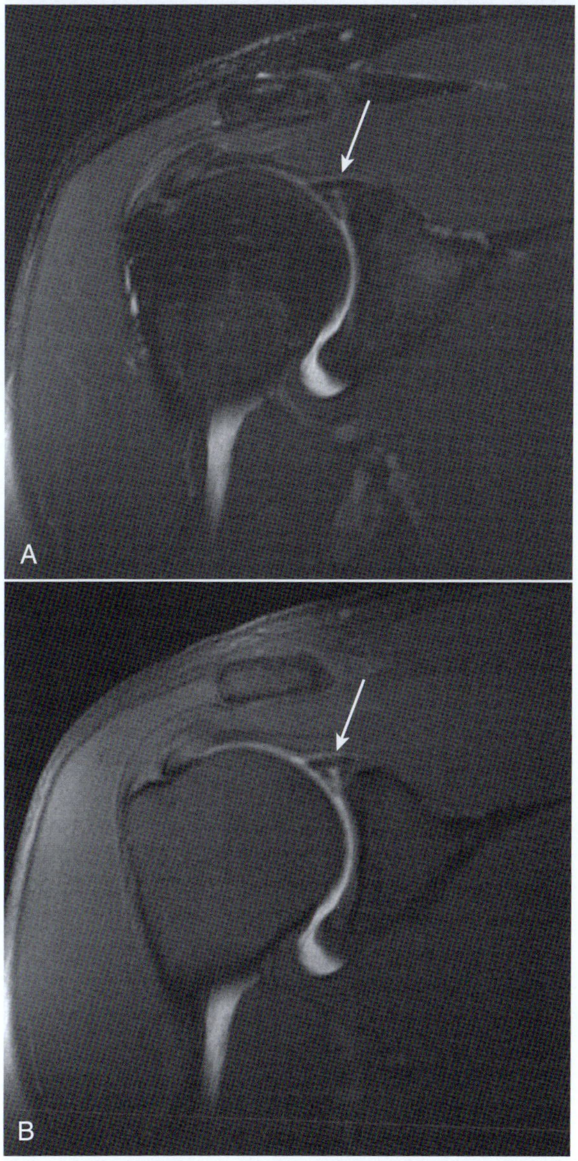

Figure 19-10 Superior labral anterior-posterior (SLAP) lesion. **A,** Coronal T2 fat-suppressed image. A linear high signal extends into the substance of the superior labrum (*arrow*). **B,** Coronal T1 fat-suppressed magnetic resonance arthrogram. Intra-articular contrast extends into the superior labral tear (*arrow*), increasing its conspicuity. (From Schwartz ML, Thornton DD: Diagnostic Imaging of the Shoulder Complex. In Wilk KE, Reinold MM, Andrews JR: *The Athlete's Shoulder,* ed 2, Philadelphia, 2008, Churchill Livingstone.)

who were randomly placed into either a group treated by shoulder immobilization in internal rotation or a group treated by immobilization in external rotation. At a follow-up of 33.4 months, 37% of patients in the internal rotation group and 42% of patients in the external rotation group had sustained a further dislocation. Tanaka et al[32] followed up 15 active male patients with primary dislocation who were treated with immediate immobilization into external rotation. Eleven of the shoulders had continued nonoperative treatment after 3 weeks of immobilization, and 7 had recurrent dislocations within 2 years of follow-up. Because of inconsistencies among studies, further study is definitely warranted.

Posterior instability and MDI are always initially treated conservatively. Conversely, surgical intervention is often the treatment of choice for recurrent anterior instability, bony Bankart lesions, or avulsion fractures. Furthermore, if initial attempts at conservative measures fail in patients with posterior instability or MDI, surgical intervention then becomes significant.

Initial conservative treatment for anterior instability is nonoperative.[33] Early conservative treatment for instability includes patient education and activity modification to decrease pain and inflammation.[34] Normalization of the rotator cuff and the return of scapular force couples are first priorities during early rehabilitation. Return of these force couples helps to enhance dynamic shoulder stabilization. This requires early and diligent dynamic and neuromuscular control of the scapular and rotator cuff muscles.[35]

Among the instability patterns, anterior instability is the only exception to an initial conservative approach. Typically, this disorder occurs in a young individual with anterior macrotraumatic primary instability. Although a conservative approach is still often the first course of action, a more aggressive approach has been adopted. This newer approach has resulted from the high recurrence rates of this condition after the first incidence and has led many investigators to advocate consideration of surgical intervention much earlier in the treatment strategy. A patient who is less than 25 years old, who is involved in high-risk activities, and who is a first-time anterior dislocator is a prime candidate for initial operative intervention. Results of studies support operative intervention because of the significant decrease in the redislocation rate after acute surgical stabilization. Those young, high-risk patients with MRI-documented Bankart lesions have a higher than 50% recurrence rate with nonoperative intervention. Nonoperative therapy is not discouraged; however, surgery is recommended if the patient has evidence of recurrent subluxations or repeated dislocation. Surgical intervention prevents further damage to the joint and less capsular attenuation.

In-season athletes who suffer from anterior dislocation can be managed with physical therapy and bracing. However, the risk of further damage to the shoulder is an ongoing concern. Buss et al[36] studied the outcome of physical therapy and bracing for 30 in-season athletes who had acute or recurrent anterior dislocation. These investigators reported an average of 1.4 instability episodes per athlete per season. Approximately half of these patients underwent anterior stabilization after the season was over.

The first line of treatment for posterior instability and MDI is nonsurgical. The key to successful conservative rehabilitation for treatment of posterior instability and MDI lies in an accurate diagnosis of the given instability pattern.[37] The exception to initial conservative management is the patient with recurrent posterior dislocation, who is less likely to respond to a therapy regimen. Recurrent posterior dislocations are rare, however, and should not be mistaken for posterior MDIs. Commonly, the patient with recurrent posterior subluxation, which is atraumatic as a result of repetitive microtrauma, responds well to rehabilitation. Similarly, patients with MDI often respond to a conservative treatment protocol. The underlying goal with MDI is to maintain mobility while limiting excessive translation of the glenohumeral joint. Nevertheless, in the patient with posterior instability or MDI, the emphasis is placed on strengthening the dynamic stabilizers of the rotator cuff, including the posterior cuff muscles, the infraspinatus, and teres minor. Additionally, deltoid strengthening and scapulothoracic stabilization exercises are important.

Neuromuscular control is the subconscious integration of sensory information processed by the central nervous system that results in controlled motor patterns.[38] Early in rehabilitation, neuromuscular control is gained through manual rhythmic stabilization drills performed for the shoulder, rotator cuff, and scapular stabilizers. These neuromuscular control exercises can be done with the patient in a comfortable position by alternating isometrics with the arm in the scapular plane at approximately 45° of abduction and alternating submaximal contractions of the internal and external shoulder rotators (Fig. 19-11A). The balance position can also be used in which the shoulder is flexed approximately 90° while the patient is lying supine (Fig. 19-11B). In this position, contraction of the deltoid muscle becomes a synergistic stabilizer through its compressive effect. Often, the presenting complaint in both these instabilities is scapular winging. Treatment of scapular dyskinesis and restoration of scapulothoracic motion are imperative for success with both these instabilities. Closed kinetic chain upper extremity exercises are usually well tolerated because they approximate the glenohumeral joint (Fig. 19-11C). Both rotator cuff and scapular muscles contract to stabilize the shoulder during closed kinetic chain activities.

Once the patient is able to tolerate more advanced exercises, dumbbells and bands can be used for increasing resistance demands. Dumbbell progressive resistance exercise programs should be incorporated to place greater stress on the shoulder in gradual increments. However, because the rotator cuff and scapular muscles are generally small, only slight increments are needed. Increasing the load by 1 lb is often sufficient to prevent exacerbation of the injury to the shoulder and surrounding structures. Because these patients typically have poor rotator cuff and scapular control, the emphasis should be on exercises such as scapular plane elevation, rowing motions, side-lying external rotation, and prone progressions such as horizontal abduction at 90° (Fig. 19-12A), prone extension (Fig. 19-12B), and prone horizontal abduction at 120° (Fig. 19-12C). These exercises use the posterior cuff muscles, the rhomboids, the middle and lower trapezius, and the serratus anterior. These isotonic exercises should be of sufficient quantity to cause fatigue of these muscles. This approach is generally done through lower load and higher repetition because these are not powerful prime movers but rather smaller, endurance-type muscles of the shoulder.

Once the patient has adequate rotator cuff and scapular control, is able to maintain stability, and has normalized range of motion (ROM), plyometric-type high-demand exercises may be attempted if these types of higher-level activities are needed for sports, recreation, or work activities. Plyometric exercises using weighted balls (Fig. 19-13) or wall push-ups can be attempted. These exercises are performed to increase strength, power, and endurance, in the hope of allowing the patient to transition back to full functional status.

Surgical stabilization is considered for recurrent posterior traumatic instability and for persistent atraumatic posterior instability not improved with conservative treatment. The indication for surgical stabilization for patients with MDI is persistent instability that continues despite concentrated rehabilitation and activity modification.

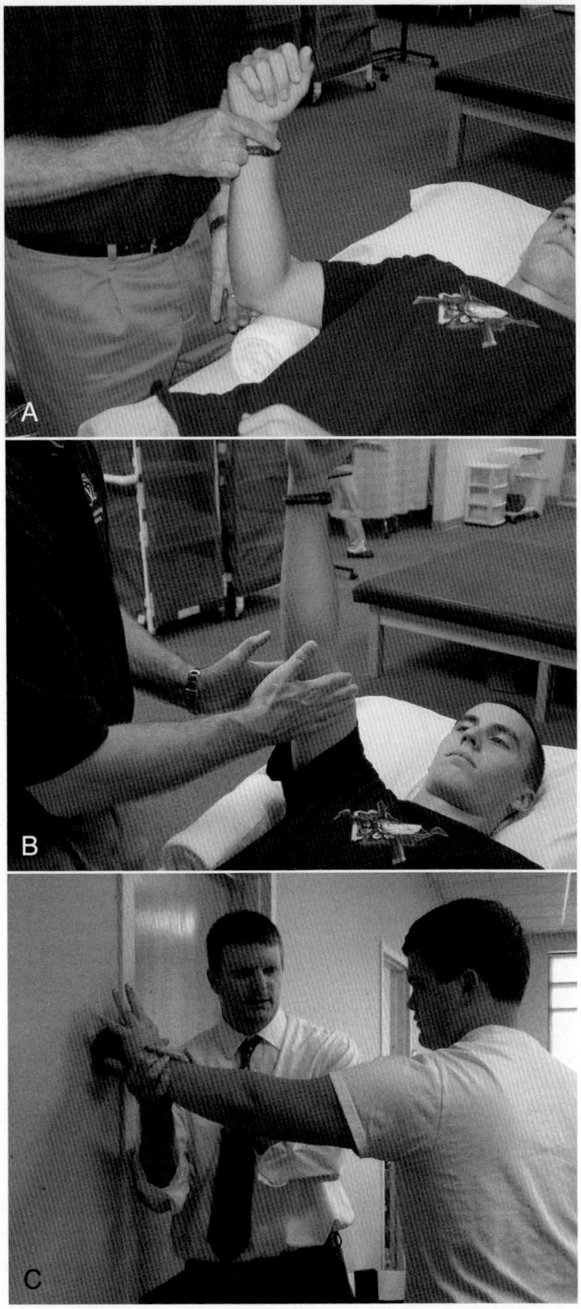

Figure 19-11 Rhythmic stabilization drills. **A,** Internal rotation, external rotation isometrics. **B,** Balance position isometrics. **C,** Closed kinetic chain isometrics.

SURGICAL INTERVENTION FOR SHOULDER INSTABILITY

Regardless of the instability pattern, an algorithmic thought process should be used in making the decision to recommend surgical intervention. Surgery becomes a treatment option for

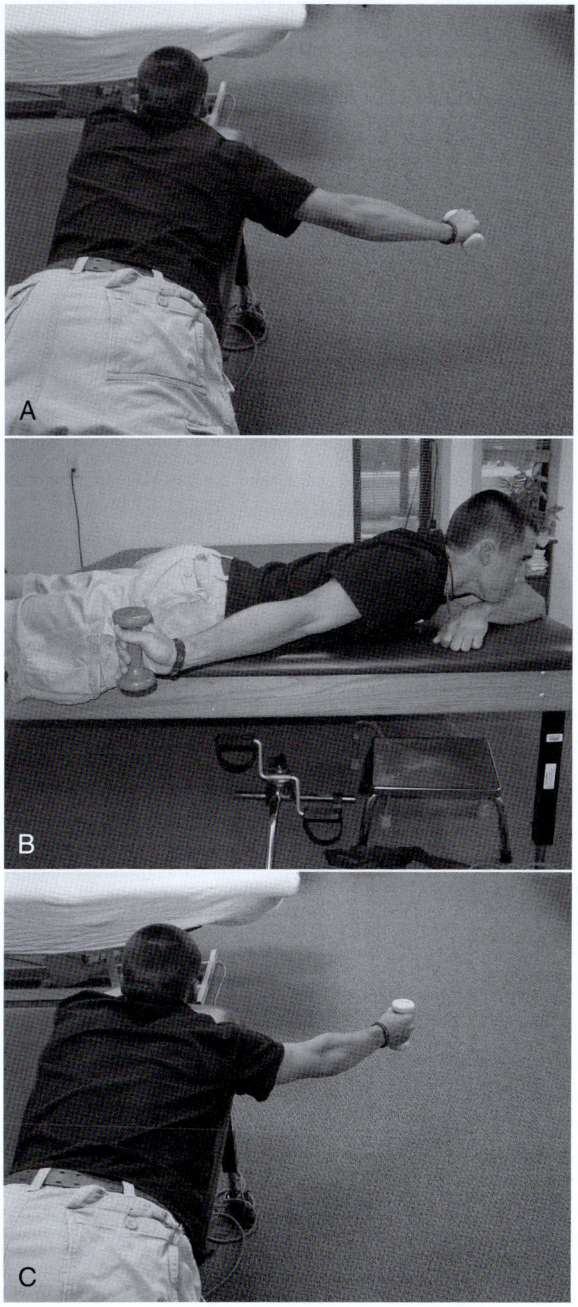

Figure 19-12 Dumbbell progressive resistance exercises. **A,** Horizontal abduction at 90 degrees. **B,** Prone extension. **C,** Prone horizontal abduction at 120 degrees.

recurrent instability in patients in whom conservative treatment options have failed and in patients with traumatic dislocations, such as patients with primary anterior shoulder dislocations. Determination of the appropriate surgical indications, contraindications, and risk factors is based on a combination of history, physical examination, and preoperative imaging.

Once surgical intervention is deemed necessary, the next critical decision is appropriate selection of the surgical stabilization procedure. A correct decision often requires examination of the patient under anesthesia. Unfortunately, the importance of information gained by this examination is

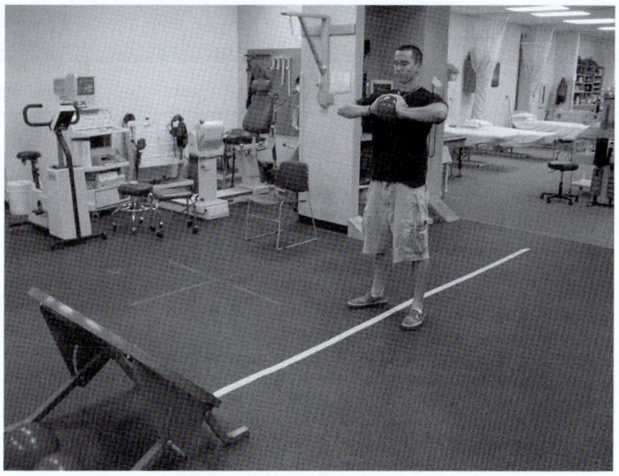

Figure 19-13 Plyometrics.

often underestimated, and all too often this vital step is bypassed. Details of the surgical repair should be predicated on evaluation of the pathoanatomic features and the correlation with the instability pattern. The type of repair and the order and direction of repair are based on simple anatomic principles. The pathologic lesion should be defined, and a surgical procedure should be performed that provides the best anatomic correction (Table 19-6).

POSTOPERATIVE MANAGEMENT FOR SHOULDER INSTABILITY

Anterior Instability Stabilization

The postoperative management of the patient with isolated anterior instability has several goals, foremost among them being maintenance of anterior-inferior stability. An additional goal is the restoration of adequate motion, specifically external rotation. A successful return to sports or physical activities of daily living requires adequate respect for the biologic healing response of the repaired and imbricated tissue. Immediate postoperative immobilization in abduction orthosis is common after arthroscopic repair.

Rehabilitation following arthroscopic Bankart's reconstruction and superior labral repair includes the progression of ROM and strength. This progression is predicated on physiologic healing limitations. Most postoperative protocols allow for early passive ROM, active-assistive ROM, active ROM, and glenohumeral joint mobilization as needed. Few limitations in the initial ROM are typically recommended unless capsular plication or concomitant procedures were performed. Avoidance of 90° of abduction and limited external rotation are advised in the first 6 weeks after surgery. No aggressive attempts at active ROM or passive end-range stretching are recommended, to protect the repairs.

Bankart's repairs require early protected ROM, and this is one of the most specific recommendations followed in the initial 4 to 6 weeks of the postoperative period. External rotation is limited, to minimize tensile stress to the

Table 19-6 Surgical Procedures for Shoulder Instability

	Shoulder Instability	Surgical Procedure	Pearls
Anterior	Macrotraumatic or microtraumatic pathologic condition with plastic ligamentous deformation in association with glenolabral damage	Modified Bankart procedure preferred, open or arthroscopic, using suture anchors	Primary arthroscopic anterior stabilization routinely is performed for recurrent anterior instability, uncomplicated revision surgery, and high-risk first-time dislocators.
	Microtraumatic lesions with subtle anterior instability shown by relocation test and no significant associated labral damage	Arthroscopic capsular imbrication procedure preferred	Contraindications to arthroscopic repair include a Hill-Sachs lesion involving greater than 20% to 30% of the articular surface that engages the glenoid rim with the arm in a position of abduction and external rotation and a bony abnormality such as glenoid rim defect greater than 25% of the articular surface. Multiple dislocations are a relative contraindication to arthroscopic repair.
Posterior	Posterior instability with mild to moderate inferior instability	Posterior imbrication procedure	Surgery is not recommended in patients with atraumatic type of posterior instability, unless they have frequent and significant disability and conservative treatment has failed. The dislocation must not be habitual, and the patient must be emotionally stable.
	Recurrent posterior dislocation in association with large reverse Hill-Sachs lesion	Modified McLaughlin's procedure Special procedures indicated with bony deficiency of 25% or more of the glenoid In the acute setting, bone defect may be secured open or arthroscopically to restore bony stability	
	Recurrent instability	Autogenous bone generally required to recreate the glenoid surface Laterjet procedure and tricortical iliac bone graft common procedures for restoring the glenoid surface Rarely, posterior bone block procedure necessary to stabilize posterior dislocations	
	Multidirectional instability (AMBRII lesions)	Lateral capsular shift	The capsular shift technique is recommended for atraumatic multidirectional instability in a patient who is not a throwing or overhead athlete. For an overhead athlete with recurrent posterior subluxation, a muscle-splitting technique with medial shift is preferred.
	Excessive anterior or posterior translation coupled with a positive sulcus sign of 2+ to 3+	Anterior or posterior capsulorrhaphy based on direction of translation with attention to closure of the rotator interval (necessary to help eliminate inferior laxity at 0° of abduction)	
	Multidirectional instability with anterior, posterior, and inferior laxity	Pancapsular plication with capsular shift from the 7-o'clock position posterior to anterior and closure of the rotator cuff interval	

AMBRII, atraumatic, multidirectional, bilateral, rehabilitation, inferior capsular shift, and interval closure.

anterior-inferior aspect of the repaired labrum. However, specific ROM positions of external rotation in a position of abduction can specifically limit stress to the anterior-inferior joint capsule and labrum. Studies have shown that, after the first 45° of external rotation, a significant rise in the tension of the anterior capsule occurs. The position of abduction used during passive external rotation ROM is critical. During 90° of abduction, the inferior glenohumeral ligament is the primary restraint to anterior translation. This position can place great stress on the capsule where Bankart's repair has occurred. Passive external rotation in the first 30° of abduction places more specific tensile loading near the superior glenohumeral ligament and superior capsular structures, away from the repair site.

Significant evidence points to the importance of rotator cuff and scapular stabilization after superior labral repair, to return to normal arthrokinematics of the glenohumeral joint. The return of dynamic stabilization of the rotator cuff and scapula is an important element in rehabilitation following superior labral repair.

In the early postoperative phases of arthroscopic repair, Codman's exercises can be started immediately. Active-assisted

ROM exercises, external rotation from 0° to 30°, and elevation in the plane of the scapula in the prone position from 0° to 70° are also begun at this time. This regimen can be maintained for the first 6 weeks. From weeks 6 to 12, active-assisted ROM and active ROM exercises are started, to gain full motion. No strengthening exercise or any type of repetitive exercise is started until after full ROM has been established. Early resistance exercises with aggressive early postoperative rehabilitation do not appear to offer substantial advantages and can compromise the repair. Strengthening is begun once the patient has full, painless, active ROM. Strengthening is begun at 12 weeks, with sports-specific exercises started at 16 to 20 weeks. Final contact athletic training is started between 20 and 24 weeks postoperatively.

For open surgical stabilization procedures, during weeks 0 to 4, the arm is immobilized. Pendulum and ROM exercises are begun. From 4 to 8 weeks, passive ROM and active-assisted shoulder ROM is performed. During this period, external rotation limited to 45°. Rotator cuff strengthening with the arm at low abduction angles is started before any active forward elevation is initiated. From 8 to 12 weeks, deltoid isometric exercises are started with the arm in low abduction angles. Abduction is slowly increased during rotator cuff and deltoid strengthening exercises. In addition, scapular strengthening and horizontal abduction in prone exercises are also begun. From 12 to 18 weeks, restoration of terminal external rotation is achieved. Proprioceptive neuromuscular feedback patterns are used, and plyometric exercises as well as sports-specific motions using a pulley, wand, or manual resistance are begun. After 18 weeks, conventional weight training is begun, and rehabilitation is oriented toward a return to sports. Full contact sports are instituted when abduction and external rotation strength are symmetrical on manual muscle testing.

Postoperative management after arthroscopic or open stabilization surgery is critical and must be individualized, based on the type of surgical procedure performed and the quality of the repaired tissue. Usually, the patient has a period of immobilization of the shoulder in a sling for 4 weeks after a labral repair and for up to 6 weeks for capsular plication. If a subscapularis takedown was performed for an open repair, this is generally protected for 4 weeks. Pendulum exercises and passive forward elevation in the plane of the scapula to 90° are allowed immediately. Passive external rotation is permitted to 0°, along with joint translation mobilization techniques into the barrier. Active ROM is allowed after the sling immobilization is discontinued. Terminal passive stretching exercises are delayed until 8 to 10 weeks after surgery. Once ROM is nearly full, strengthening is started. Return to sport is generally delayed until 4 months after surgery, when the patient has gained full ROM and nearly full strength.

The following are some rehabilitation and return-to-play guidelines after shoulder surgery. Rehabilitation after shoulder surgery is divided into four phases. Phase 1 consists of primary healing of capsulolabral tissue with of sling immobilization, active-assistive ROM or passive ROM exercise, joint translation mobilization, and isometrics. Phase 2 spans weeks 6 to 12 and involves gaining full ROM. Phase 3 involves strengthening of the shoulder, including dynamic strengthening. From 4 to 8 months after surgery, the patient returns to sport-specific rehabilitation; he or she returns to sport when ROM and strength are nearly normal.

General Principles

Depending on the characteristics of the type of shoulder instability, patients are more likely than not to receive a course of nonoperative treatment in the form of rehabilitation. After acute dislocation, the immobilization phase often transitions into rehabilitation. For the patient with recurrent shoulder instability that inevitably may require surgical stabilization, rehabilitation becomes a vital factor in postoperative management. In addition to surgical stabilization, postoperative rehabilitation is also critical for the continued restoration of the synchrony of the static and dynamic shoulder stabilizers. General guidelines can be provided, although rehabilitation programs differ in their details according to the procedure performed.

The underlying principle of shoulder instability rehabilitation is to restore functional motion, strength and stability. The ultimate goal of rehabilitation is a successful return to activities of daily living, work, or sports. For the rehabilitation to be successful, however, appropriate recognition of the shoulder disease that caused the instability is important. Furthermore, the success or failure of the rehabilitation protocol highly depends on the correct diagnosis.

Rehabilitation goals include motion and strengthening parameters that are contingent on the diagnosis or the surgical procedure performed (see Table 19-6). Modalities and appropriate pain control are catalysts for staying on course with the rehabilitation protocol. Once most discomfort is controlled, early motion in pain-free ranges can be initiated. Each type of instability has its parameters for immobilization and appropriate timing of ROM initiation, as outlined in Tables 19-7 to 19-10. Early in the postoperative course, muscle strengthening should begin with closed chain exercises. Additionally, in the early phases of shoulder strengthening, the scapular stabilizers must also be included. In later rehabilitation phases, proprioceptive neuromuscular facilitation (PNF) exercises provide specific sensory inputs to facilitate a specific movement pattern or exercise. As a result, PNF exercises have been found to enhance recovery.

Although not often considered a modality for the upper extremity, aquatic physical therapy can provide a protected environment for the soft tissues while early motion is begun. When used strategically, and in the appropriate time frame, the incorporation of aquatic physical therapy can have tremendous benefits. These benefits are provided by the buoyancy effect of water for the upper extremity. This buoyancy decreases the weight of the arm to one eighth of its original weight at 90° of abduction or forward flexion. Therefore, less stress is placed on the soft tissues than during active exercises.[39]

Table 19-7 Rehabilitation after Anterior Capsulolabral Reconstruction

General Guidelines

- Restoration of shoulder motion is critical for successful athletic performance.
- Efforts at motion restoration should be controlled so that the repair is not compromised.
- Resisted exercise may begin as early as the third postoperative week, with surgeon approval.
- Somatosensory training is important to enhance successful sport performance.
- Supervised physical therapy takes 3 to 6 months.

Activities of Daily Living Progression

- Bathing or showering without the splint is allowed after suture removal.
- Overhead activities are limited until ROM is restored.

Phase I: Immediate Postoperative Phase (Day 1–Week 3)	Goals	Decrease pain and inflammation Increase pain-free ROM while protecting repair Preserve elbow, wrist, and hand strength and ROM Preserve or enhance cardiovascular endurance Educate patient
	Restrictions	Splint use for 1–2 wk (waking hours ± sleeping)
	Therapeutic exercises	Pain-free flexion and abduction PROM one or two times per day Pain-free IR and ER in scapular plane with surgeon approval Upper body cycle for PROM or AAROM Rhythmic stabilization for scapular muscles Submaximal isometrics Abduction Extension Flexion IR and ER (in neutral) Arm curls Arm extensions Ball, putty, or sponge squeezes Resisted wrist flexion, extension, radial deviation, ulnar deviation, supination, pronation Trunk muscle strengthening (sport-specific if possible) Total leg strengthening (sport-specific if possible) Cardiovascular endurance training (sport-specific if possible)
	Concerns	Unremitting pain Markedly restricted glenohumeral joint mobility Excessive glenohumeral joint mobility
Phase II: Intermediate Postoperative Phase (Weeks 3–12)	Goals	Eliminate pain Regain full pain-free ROM while protecting repair Increase strength of GH and ST musculature Improve proprioception Increase elbow, wrist, and hand strength Preserve or enhance cardiovascular endurance
	Therapeutic exercises	Upper body cycle or rowing machine warmup Pain-free self-ROM (e.g., wand exercises) one or two times per day Manual joint mobilization techniques as needed (protect anterior capsule) Posterior cuff stretching (e.g., IR, horizontal adduction) Pectoralis minor stretching as needed (protect anterior capsule) Isotonics and isokinetics progressing (per healing and symptoms) from submaximal to maximal effort Flexion Scaption ("full-can") IR and ER progression from 0°–90° of elevation in scapular and/or frontal planes; limit rotation ROM Horizontal abduction (in prone or with reverse-fly machine); limit to scapular or frontal plane Rows Push-ups with a "plus" Press-ups

Table 19-7 Rehabilitation after Anterior Capsulolabral Reconstruction—cont'd

		Plyometrics beginning approximately week 10 Position replication activities (e.g., dart throwing, bean bag toss) Continue with arm, leg, torso exercise (sport-specific) Sport-specific cardiovascular exercise (e.g., upper body cycle, rowing machine)
	Concerns	Lack of full ROM by 8–10 weeks Excessive joint mobility Significant weakness by week 12
Phase III: Advanced Strengthening (Weeks 12–16)	Criteria to advance to phase III	Full, pain-free AROM and PROM Minimal pain with activity and exercise Satisfactory stability (per surgeon) Strength 70% or more of contralateral side
	Goals	Fully eliminate pain Regain full pain-free ROM Increase strength of GH and ST musculature Improve proprioception Increase elbow, wrist, and hand strength Preserve or enhance cardiovascular endurance
	Therapeutic exercises	Progress intensity per symptoms Exercise selection should be based on deficits identified by strength testing Eccentrics for posterior musculature and biceps brachii Progress plyometrics Position replication activities Anticipatory muscle activation exercises and activities Arm, leg, and torso strengthening as needed Cardiovascular exercise
	Concerns	Pain with resistance training other than acute or delayed-onset muscle soreness Excessive joint mobility
Phase IV: Return to Activity (Week 16+)	Criteria to advance to phase IV	Strength 85% or more of contralateral side
	Goals	Return to full, pain-free activity, including athletics
	Therapeutic exercise	Sport-specific training
	Concerns	Considerable lingering pain or instability with sports-specific training

AAROM, active-assistive range of motion; AROM; active range of motion; ER, external rotation; GH, glenohumeral; IR, internal rotation; PROM, passive range of motion; ROM, range of motion; ST, scapulothoracic.
Modified from Manske RC: *Postsurgical orthopedic sports rehabilitation: knee and shoulder,* St. Louis, 2007, Mosby.

Table 19-8 Rehabilitation Guidelines for Bankart Repair

Phase I: Early Protective Phase (0–5 Weeks)	Goals	Protect surgical procedure Educate patient regarding procedure and therapeutic progression Regulate pain and control inflammation Initiate ROM exercises and dynamic stabilization Perform neuromuscular re-education of external rotators and ST muscles
	Treatment plan (0–3 weeks)	Sling immobilization for 2–4 wk Gripping exercises Elbow, wrist, and hand ROM Pendulum exercises (weighted and unweighted) PROM to AAROM IR and ER proprioception training (controlled range) Initiate gentle alternating isometrics for IR and ER in 0° of abduction to scapular plane Initiate passive forward flexion to 90° Initiate scapular mobility

Continued

Table 19-8 Rehabilitation Guidelines for Bankart Repair—cont'd

	Treatment plan (3–5 weeks)	ROM progression Forward flexion to 110°–130° ER in scapular plane to 35° (position set at time of surgery) IR in scapular plane to 60° Progress submaximal alternating isometrics for IR and ER in scapular plane Initiate scapular strengthening Manual scapular retraction Resisted band retraction No shoulder extension past trunk Deltoid isometrics in all directions Biceps and triceps strengthening Initiate light band work for IR and ER
	Milestones for progression	Forward flexion to 110° Abduction to 110° ER in scapular plane to 35° IR in scapular plane to 60° Tolerance of submaximal isometrics Knowledge of home care and contraindications Normalized mobility of related joints (acromioclavicular, sternoclavicular, ST)
Phase II: Intermediate Phase (5–8 Weeks)	Goals (general)	Normalize arthrokinematics Achieve gains in neuromuscular control Normalize posterior shoulder flexibility
	Treatment plan	ROM progression Forward flexion to 150°–165° ER in scapular plane to 65° Full IR in scapular plane Initiate joint mobilizations as necessary Initiate posterior capsular stretching Progress strengthening IR and ER band in scapular plane Side-lying ER Full can (no weight if substitution patterns) Clockwise/counterclockwise ball against wall Initiate PNF patterns in available range Body blade at neutral or rhythmic stabilization
	Milestones for progression	Forward flexion to 150°–165° ER in scapular plane to 65° Full IR in scapular plane Symmetric posterior capsule mobility Progressing isotonic strength with IR and ER in available range
Phase III: Strengthening Phase (8–14 Weeks)	Goals (general)	Normalize ROM Progress strength Normalize scapulothoracic motion and strength Perform overhead activities without pain
	Treatment plan	ROM progression; initiate stretching IR and ER at 90° of GH abduction Achieve movement within 10° of full AROM in all planes Progression of scapular retractors and stabilizers Prone program; lower trapezoids, middle trapezoids, rhomboids Lower Trapezius; scapular depression Progress strengthening Challenging rhythmic stabilization Upper body ergometer: forward and retrograde Bilateral ball against wall; progress with perturbation Initiate isokinetic IR and ER in scapular plane Initiate IR and ER at 90° of GH abduction

Table 19-8 Rehabilitation Guidelines for Bankart Repair—cont'd

		Isotonic strengthening; flexion, abduction
		Closed kinetic chain therapeutic exercise
	Milestones for progression	Within 10° of full AROM in scapular plane
		IR and ER less than 50% deficit
		Less than 30% strength deficits; primary shoulder muscles and scapular stabilizers
Phase IV: Advanced Strengthening Phase (14–24 Weeks)	Goals (general)	Achieve pain-free full ROM
		Improve muscular endurance
		Improve dynamic stability
	Treatment plan	Maintain flexibility
		Progress strengthening
		Advanced CKC therapeutic exercise
		Wall push-ups; with and without ball
		Continue with overhead strengthening
		Continue with isokinetic IR and ER strengthening at 90° of GH abduction
		Advance isotonic strengthening
		Advance rhythmic stabilization training in various ranges and positions
		Initiate plyometric strengthening
		Chest passes
		Trunk twists
		Overhead passes
		90°/90° single-arm plyometrics
	Milestones for progression	Strength deficits <20% for IR and ER at 90° of GH abduction
		Less than 20% strength deficits throughout
Phase V: Return to Activity Phase (4–6 Months)	Goals (general)	Pain-free full ROM
		Normalized strength
		Return to sport or activity program
	Treatment plan	Continue isokinetic training
		Continue with stability training
		Advance plyometric training
		Continue with CKC therapeutic exercise
	Milestones for activity	Strength deficits less than 10% throughout
		Normalized CKC testing
		Completion of return to sport or activity program

AAROM, active-assistive range of motion; AROM; active range of motion; CKC, closed chain kinetic; ER, external rotation; GH, glenohumeral; IR, internal rotation; PNF, proprioceptive neuromuscular facilitation; PROM, passive range of motion; ROM, range of motion; ST, scapulothoracic.
Modified from Manske RC: *Postsurgical orthopedic sports rehabilitation: knee and shoulder,* St. Louis, 2007, Mosby.

Table 19-9 Multidirectional Instability: Capsular Shift Procedures Guidelines

Phase I: Immediate Postoperative Phase (Weeks 1–3)	Goals	Promote healing: reduce pain and inflammation
		Forward flexion to 90°
		ER to 30°
	Treatment	Immobilizer
		Elbow and wrist AROM
		Gripping exercises
		AAROM: forward flexion (scapular plane)
		AAROM: ER
		Scapular isometrics
		Pain-free, submaximal deltoid isometrics
		Modalities as needed
	Criteria for advancement	ER to 30°
		Forward flexion to 90°
		Minimal pain or inflammation

Continued

Table 19-9 Multidirectional Instability: Capsular Shift Procedures Guidelines—cont'd

Phase II: Intermediate Phase (Weeks 3–8)	Goals	Continue to promote healing Begin to restore scapular and rotator cuff strength Continue to restore forward flexion and ER
	Treatment (weeks 3–6)	Discharge immobilizer per physician Wand exercises for forward flexion and ER Pulleys (if 110° forward flexion) Progress scapula strengthening (begin manual and closed chain)
	Treatment (weeks 6–8)	Pain-free, submaximal IR and ER isometrics Progress to scapular isotonics Progress to IR and ER isotonics Initiate latissimus strengthening Initiate biceps strengthening Hydrotherapy (if required) Initiate humeral head control exercises Initiate scapular plane elevation (with adequate scapular and rotator cuff strength) Modalities as needed
	Criteria for advancement	Minimal pain and inflammation Forward flexion to 160° ER to 75° IR and ER strength 5−/5
Phase III: Advanced Strengthening Phase (Weeks 8–12)	Goals	Restore full ROM Restore normal scapulohumeral rhythm Upper extremity strength 5/5 Restore normal flexibility
	Treatment	Continue AAROM: forward flexion and ER Begin AAROM for IR Continue aggressive scapula strengthening Progress strengthening for the rotator cuff, deltoid, biceps, and latissimus (incorporate eccentric training) Begin proprioceptive neuromuscular training patterns Progress humeral head control drills Progress IR and ER to 90°/90° position if required Use full upper extremity flexibility program Begin isokinetic training Modalities as needed
	Criteria for advancement	Full shoulder ROM Upper extremity strength 5/5 Normal upper extremity flexibility No pain or inflammation
Phase IV: Return to Activity Phase (Weeks 12–16)	Goals	Restore normal neuromuscular function Maintain strength and flexibility to meet the demands of functional activity Prevent reinjury
	Treatment	Isokinetic testing Continue full upper extremity strengthening and flexibility program Activity-specific plyometric program Address trunk and lower extremity needs Endurance training Sport- or activity-specific program Home exercise program
	Criteria for discharge	Pain-free Independent home exercise program Independent sport- or activity-specific program

AAROM, active-assistive range of motion; AROM; active range of motion; ER, external rotation; IR, internal rotation; ROM, range of motion.
Modified from Manske RC: *Postsurgical orthopedic sports rehabilitation: knee and shoulder,* St. Louis, 2007, Mosby.

Table 19-10 Rehabilitation Program after Thermal-Assisted Capsulorrhaphy for Patients with Acquired Laxity

Phase I: Protection Phase (Day 1–Week 6)	Goals	Allow soft tissue healing
		Diminish pain and inflammation
		Initiate protected motion
		Retard muscular atrophy
	Treatment (weeks 0–2)	Sling use for 7–10 days
		Sleep in sling/brace for 14 days
	Exercises (weeks 0–2)	Hand gripping exercises
		Elbow and wrist ROM exercises
		AROM cervical spine
		PROM and AAROM shoulder exercises
		Elevation to 75°–90° (flexion to 70° week 1, flexion to 90° by week 2)
		IR in scapular plane at 30°–45° of abduction (45° by 2 weeks)
		ER in scapular plane at 30° to 45° of abduction (25° by 2 weeks)
		NO aggressive stretching
		Rope and pulley (shoulder flexion) AAROM
		Cryotherapy to control pain (before and after treatment)
		Submaximal isometrics (ER, IR, abduction, flexion, extension)
		Rhythmic stabilization exercises at 7 days
		Proprioception and neuromuscular control drills
	Exercises (weeks 3–4)	Shoulder ROM exercises (PROM, AAROM, AROM)
		Elevation to 125°–135°
		IR, in scapular plane, full motion (60°–65°)
		ER, in scapular plane 45° by week 4
		At week 4, begin ER and IR at 90° of abduction
		ER at 90° of abduction to 45°–50°
		No extension
		NO aggressive stretching
		Shoulder strengthening exercises
		AROM program (begin at week 3)
		Initiate LIGHT isotonic program (use 1 lb at week 4)
		ER and IR exercise tubing (0° of abduction)
		Continue dynamic stabilization drills
		Scapular strengthening exercises
		Biceps/triceps strengthening
		Proprioceptive neuromuscular facilitation D2 flexion/extension manual resistance (limited ROM)
		Emphasize ER strengthening and scapular musculature
		Continue use of cryotherapy and modalities to control pain
	Exercises (weeks 5–6)	Continue all exercises listed above
		Progress ROM to the following
		Elevation to 160° degrees by week 6
		ER at 90° of abduction (75°–80°) by 6 weeks
		IR at 90° degrees of abduction (60°–65°) by 6 weeks
		Initiate Thrower's Ten Program (strengthening)
		Continue emphasis on ER and scapular muscles
Phase II: Intermediate Phase (Weeks 7–12)	Goals	Restore full ROM (week 8)
		Restore functional ROM (weeks 10–11)
		Normalize arthrokinematics
		Improve dynamic stability, muscular strength
	Exercises (weeks 7–8)	Progress shoulder ROM to the following
		Elevation to 180°
		ER at 90 degrees of abduction to 90°–100° by week 8
		IR at 90 degrees of abduction to 60°–65° by week 8
		Continue stretching program
		May become more aggressive with ROM progression and stretching
		May perform joint mobilization techniques
		Strengthening exercises
		Continue Thrower's Ten Program

Continued

Table 19-10 Rehabilitation Program after Thermal-Assisted Capsulorrhaphy for Patients with Acquired Laxity—cont'd

		Continue manual resistance, dynamic stabilization drills Rhythmic stabilization drills Initiate plyometrics (two-hand drills)
	Exercises (weeks 9–12)	Progress shoulder ROM to the overhead athlete's demands Gradual progression from weeks 9–12 Continue stretching into ER ER at 90° of abduction to 110°–115° by weeks 10–12 Continue stretching program for posterior structures (IR, horizontal adduction) Strengthening exercises Progress isotonic program Continue Thrower's Ten Program May initiate more aggressive strengthening Push-ups Bench press (do NOT allow arm below body) Latissimus pull-downs (IN FRONT of body) Single-hand plyometrics throwing (initiate 14–18 days following the introduction of two-hand plyometrics) Plyoball wall drills
Phase III: Advanced Activity and Strengthening Phase (Weeks 12-25)	Goals	Improve strength, power, and endurance Enhance neuromuscular control Functional activities
	Criteria to enter phase III	1. Full ROM 2. No pain or tenderness 3. Muscular strength 80% of contralateral side
	Exercises (weeks 12–16)	Continue all stretching exercises Self-performed capsular stretches, AROM, passive stretching Continue all strengthening exercises Thrower's Ten Program Progress isotonics Plyometrics Two-hand drills progress to one-hand drills Throwing into plyoback 1-lb ball (week 13) Neuromuscular control/dynamic stabilization drills
	Exercises (weeks 16–22)	Initiate interval sport program (e.g., throwing, tennis, swimming) at week 16 Progress all exercises listed above May resume normal training program Continue specific strengthening exercises Progress interval program (throwing program to phase II) at weeks 22–23
	Exercises (week 22)	Progress to phase II interval throwing program or sport-specific training Continue isotonic strengthening Continue flexibility and ROM Continue plyometrics
Phase IV: Return to Activity Phase (Week 26 and Beyond)	Goals	Gradual return to unrestricted activities Maintain static and dynamic stability of shoulder joint
	Criteria to enter phase IV	1. Full functional ROM 2. No pain or tenderness 3. Satisfactory muscular strength (isokinetic test) 4. Satisfactory clinical examination
	Exercises	Continue maintenance for ROM (stretching) Continue strengthening exercises (Thrower's Ten Program) Gradual return to competition Progress throwing program to game situations at months 6–7

AAROM, active-assistive range of motion; AROM; active range of motion; ER, external rotation; IR, internal rotation; PROM, passive range of motion; ROM, range of motion.

Modified from Manske RC: *Postsurgical orthopedic sports rehabilitation: knee and shoulder,* St. Louis, 2007, Mosby.

Posterior Instability Stabilization

Patients with long-standing shoulder instability that has not been addressed with adequate rehabilitation frequently have dysfunctional scapulothoracic articulations, a finding underlining the importance of rehabilitation for the postoperative patient.

Any surgical procedure for posterior instability seeks to reduce excessive laxity in the posterior capsule. These patients should avoid stress to this area in the early phases of recovery. As with any other surgical procedure, early passive ROM is highly beneficial to enhance circulation within the joint to promote healing.[40] In most cases, the patient's shoulder should be placed in a sling to protect the joint from excessive internal rotation.

Physical therapy should begin within 1 week of surgery. The patient should have supervised rehabilitation and an independent home fitness program (Table 19-11).

Multidirectional Instability Stabilization

The current postoperative stabilization protocol for MDI involves approximately 6 weeks of immobilization, to allow soft tissue healing. The patient is allowed to perform only elbow and hand ROM. These restrictions are usually in place for a minimum of 3 weeks and sometimes for up to 6 weeks postoperatively.[40] After the initial immobilization, the patient begins gentle supine passive ROM exercises. Isometric exercises for the rotator cuff and scapular stabilizers are instituted as soon as possible, to limit muscle atrophy. Occasionally, because of the intimate relationship between the rotator cuff muscles and the shoulder capsule, isometrics for the cuff may be delayed initially for approximately 4 weeks. Once gentle shoulder motion is allowed, wand exercises to tolerance are introduced. Flexion and internal rotation are increased beginning on postoperative week 2. External rotation is mobilized to neutral and then is increased 10° per week. The reason for the slow progression of external rotation ROM is either the anterior component of the stabilization procedure or the subscapularis, which may have been taken down to have adequate visualization of the procedure. Abduction is allowed to 45° and then is increased 10° per week after 6 weeks.

Beginning at 6 weeks, a gradual progressive strengthening program is initiated. This strengthening protocol includes the rotator cuff and scapulothoracic musculature. In open surgery, the subscapularis is detached and is subsequently repaired. It is paramount that the subscapularis is appropriately protected in the initial phases of rehabilitation. To protect the repair, internal rotation strengthening should not be instituted until 6 weeks postoperatively. Additionally, early attempts to gain aggressive external rotation should be limited in these patients until adequate soft tissue healing of the subscapularis has occurred.

The immobilization period lasts for up to 6 weeks. After the sixth postoperative week, gentle ROM and joint mobilization programs that assist ROM to return to within normal limits can commence. Exercises should begin with gentle isometrics in a safe range, to allow continued repair

Table 19-11 Postoperative Rehabilitation for Patients with Posterior Instability

Weeks	Goals	Program
1–3	Encourage gradual return of motion	Passive motion with active-assisted motion in the scapular plane
		Motion limited in internal rotation to maximum of 30°
		External rotation based on patient tolerance
		Pendulum exercises
		Submaximal, pain-free isometrics in all planes
3–6		Strengthening with neutral tubing
		Prone horizontal adduction exercises with a limit of 45°
		Unlimited internal rotation (avoid extremes of motion)
		Scapular stabilization
		Rhythmic stabilization in PNF patterns
		Immobilization to end between weeks 4 and 6 (depends on degree of capsular laxity and extend of procedure)
6–12	Full range of motion with normal arthrokinematics without pain	Strengthening increased using upper extremity ergometer
		Posterior capsular stretching (titrated depending on degree of original laxity and current internal rotation contracture)
		Increase dynamic stabilization exercises
12+		Plyometrics program
		Gradual return to sport (specific and functional drills)
		Evaluation of readiness to return to activity
		Return to contact sport at ± 4 months, full unrestricted throwing at ± 6 months

PNF, proprioceptive neuromuscular facilitation.

Modified from Guanche CA: Posterior and multidirectional instability of the shoulder. In Schepsis AA, Busconi BD, editors: *Sports medicine,* Philadelphia, 2006, Lippincott Williams & Wilkins.

protection. Over the course of the next 6 weeks, these exercises can include both band and light dumbbell-type progressive resistive exercises. Eccentric exercise programs and PNF techniques are not generally started before the 8-week time frame. Approximately 12 to 16 weeks postoperatively, sports such as swimming can begin, and the patient may also start an interval throwing program. A gradual return to unrestricted activities is allowed at 4 to 6 months.

Rehabilitation Errors

In the post-traumatic or postoperative setting, a fine balance exists between waiting too long to start ROM and interrupting the soft tissue repair. Nevertheless, the decision-making process is contingent on the direction of instability and on the type of stabilization procedure performed. For example, after arthroscopic and open anterior reconstructions in unidirectional traumatic instability, the rehabilitation goals are almost paradoxical in that a graduated increase in motion is warranted to avoid stiffness of the shoulder, whereas limited motion will help to protect the capsular reconstruction and the accompanying subscapularis repair. Conversely, following an open capsular shift for MDI, stiffness is rarely a concern. Hence, if active motion is started too early, recurrent instability can result. For this reason, most investigators agree that patients with atraumatic MDI should have shoulder immobilization for a minimum of 6 to 8 weeks postoperatively. Investigators have postulated that previous arthroscopic failures for anterior stability occurred because of early motion and cyclic stress that caused fatigue of the plication stitches and, ultimately, failure of the repair.

SUMMARY

Shoulder instability has many parameters to consider, all of which ultimately affect the final treatment plan and prognosis. The intent of this chapter is to give a comprehensive overview of shoulder instability. The intricacy and complexity of the shoulder require a thorough understanding of factors leading to an unstable shoulder. Recognition of the pathogenesis and pathologic features of shoulder instability is critical to the decisions required to evaluate and manage appropriately the diverse array of instability patterns found in the shoulder.

REFERENCES

1. Wilk KE, Arrigo CA, Andrews JR: Current concepts: the stabilizing structures of the glenohumeral joint, *J Orthop Sports Phys Ther* 25(6):364–379, 1997.
2. Ellenbecker TS: *Clinical examination of the shoulder*, Philadelphia, 2004, Saunders.
3. Davies GJ, Wilk K, Ellenbecker T, et al: *Current concepts of orthopaedic physical therapy*, ed 2, *The shoulder: physical therapy patient management utilizing current evidence,* LaCrosse, Wis, 2006, Orthopaedic Section, American Physical Therapy Association.
4. Howell SM, Galinat BJ: The glenoid-labral socket: a constrained articular surface, *Clin Orthop Relat Res* 243:122–125, 1989.
5. O'Brien SJ, Schwartz RS, Warren RF, et al: Capsular restraints to anterior-posterior motion of the abducted shoulder: a biomechanical study, *J Shoulder Elbow Surg* 4(4):298–308, 1995.
6. Harryman D, Sidles J, Harris S, et al: The role of the rotator interval capsule in passive motion and stability of the shoulder, *J Bone Joint Surg Am* 74:53–66, 1992.
7. Lippit SB, Harris SL, Harryman DTII, et al: Diagnosis and management of AMBRI syndrome techniques, *Tech Orthop* 6:61–73, 1991.
8. Perry J: Anatomy and biomechanics of the shoulder in throwing, swimming, gymnastics, and tennis, *Clin Sports Med* 2:247–251, 1983.
9. Matsen FA, Thomas SC, Rockwood CA, et al: Glenohumeral instability. In Rockwood CA, Matsen FA, editors: *The shoulder*, vol 2, ed 2, Philadelphia, 1990, Saunders, pp 633–639.
10. Speer K: Anatomy and pathomechanics of shoulder instability, *Clin Sports Med* 14:751–760, 1995.
11. Glousman R, Jobe F, Tibone J, et al: Dynamic electromyographic analysis of the throwing shoulder with glenohumeral instability, *J Bone Joint Surg Am* 70:220–226, 1988.
12. Inman VT, Saunders DM, Abbott LC: Observations on the function of the shoulder joint, *J Bone Joint Surg Br* 26:1–30, 1944.
13. Speer KP, Garret WE: Muscular control of motion and stability about the pectoral girdle. In Matsen FA, Fu Hawkins RJ, editors: *The shoulder: a balance of mobility and stability*, Rosemont, Ill, 1993, American Academy of Orthopaedic Surgeons, pp 162–164.
14. Rowe CR: Acute and recurrent anterior dislocations of the shoulder, *Orthop Clin North Am* 11(2):253–270, 1980.
15. Warner JJ, Deng XH, Warren RF, et al: Static capsuloligamentous restraints to superior-inferior translation of the glenohumeral joint, *Am J Sports Med* 20(6):675–685, 1992.
16. Pagnani MJ, Dome DC: Surgical treatment of traumatic anterior shoulder instability in American football players, *J Bone Joint Surg Am* 84(5):711–715, 2002.
17. Rodosky MW, Harner CD, Fu FH: The role of the long head of the biceps muscle and superior glenoid labrum in anterior stability of the shoulder, *Am J Sports Med* 22:121–130, 1994.
18. Walton J, Paxinos A, Tzannes A, et al: The unstable shoulder in the adolescent athlete, *Am J Sports Med* 30:758–767, 2002.
19. Rowe CR, Sakellarides HT: Factors related to recurrence of anterior dislocation of the shoulder, *Clin Orthop Relat Res* 20:40, 1961.
20. Burkhart SS, Morgan CD: The peel-back mechanism: its role in producing and extending posterior type II SLAP lesions and its effect on SLAP repair and rehabilitation, *Arthroscopy* 14:637–640, 1998.
21. Warren RF, Kornblatt IB, Marchard R: Static factors affecting shoulder stability, *Orthop Trans* 8:89, 1984.
22. Baker CL, Uribe JW, Whitman C: Arthroscopic evaluation of acute initial anterior shoulder dislocations, *Am J Sports Med* 18:25–28, 1990.
23. Burkhart SS, De Beer JF: Traumatic glenohumeral bone defects and their relationship to failure of arthroscopic Bankart repairs: significance of the inverted-pear glenoid and the humeral engaging Hill-Sachs lesion, *Arthroscopy* 16(7):677–694, 2000.
24. Stith JS, Sahrmann SA, Dixon KK, et al: Curriculum to prepare diagnosticians in physical therapy, *J Phys Ther Educ* 9(2): 46–53, 1995.

25. Manske RC, Stovak M: Preoperative and postsurgical musculoskeletal examination of the shoulder. In Manske RC, editor: *Postsurgical orthopedic sports rehabilitation: knee and shoulder*, St. Louis, 2006, Mosby.
26. Tan CK, Guisasola I, Machani B, et al: Arthroscopic stabilization of the shoulder: a prospective randomized study of absorbable versus nonabsorbable suture anchors, *Arthroscopy* 22(7):716–720, 2006.
27. O'Brien SJ, Pagnani MJ, Fealy S, et al: The active compression test: a new and effective test for diagnosing labral tears and acromioclavicular joint abnormality, *Am J Sports Med* 26:610–613, 1998.
28. Itoi E, Hatakeyama Y, Urayama M, et al: Position of immobilization after dislocation of the glenohumeral joint: a cadaveric study, *J Bone Joint Surg Am* 81:385–390, 1999.
29. Itoi E, Hatakeyama Y, Kido T, et al: A new method of immobilization after traumatic anterior dislocation of the shoulder: a preliminary study, *J Shoulder Elbow Surg* 12:413–415, 2003.
30. Miller BS, Sonnabend DH, Jatrick C, et al: Should acute anterior dislocations of the shoulder be immobilized in external rotation? A cadaveric study, *J Shoulder Elbow Surg* 13:589–592, 2004.
31. Finestone A, Milgrom C, Radeva-Petrova DR, et al: Bracing in external rotation for traumatic anterior dislocation of the shoulder, *J Bone Joint Surg Am* 91(7):918–921, 2009.
32. Tanaka Y, Okamura K, Imai T: Effectiveness of external rotation immobilization in highly active young men with traumatic primary anterior shoulder dislocation or subluxation, *Orthopedics* 33(9):670, 2010.
33. Neer CS, Foster CR: Inferior capsular shift for involuntary inferior and multidirectional instabilities of the shoulder: a preliminary report, *J Bone Joint Surg Am* 62:897–908, 1980.
34. Ellenbecker TS, Manske RC, Kelley M: *The shoulder: physical therapy management utilizing current evidence*, LaCrosse, Wis, 2011, Orthopaedic Section, American Physical Therapy Association.
35. Davies GJ, Manske RC, Schulte R, et al: Rehabilitation of macro-instability. In Ellenbecker TS, editor: *Shoulder rehabilitation: nonoperative treatment*, New York, 2006, Thieme.
36. Buss DD, Lynch GP, Meyer CP, et al: Nonoperative management for in-season athletes with anterior shoulder instability, *Am J Sports Med* 32(6):1430–1433, 2004.
37. Austin JC, Hasan SS, Heckmann TP, et al: Posterior shoulder instability. In Wilk KE, Reinold MM, Andrews JR, editors: *The athlete's shoulder*, ed 2, Philadelphia, 2009, Churchill Livingstone Elsevier.
38. Williams GN, Chmielewski T, Rudolph K, et al: Dynamic knee stability: current theory and implications for clinicians and scientists, *J Orthop Sports Phys Ther* 31:546–566, 2001.
39. Thein JW, Brody LT: Aquatic-based rehabilitation and training for the elite athlete, *J Orthop Sports Phys Ther* 27:1, 32–42, 1998.
40. Guanche CA: Posterior and multidirectional instability of the shoulder. In Schepsis AA, Busconi BD, editors: *Sports medicine*, Philadelphia, 2006, Lippincott Williams & Wilkins.

CHAPTER

20

Xavier A. Duralde,
Scott D. Pennington,
and Douglas M. Murray

Total Shoulder Replacements

Shoulder arthroplasty can often result in seemingly miraculous improvement in both pain and function for the patient with glenohumeral joint arthritis.[1] The earliest reported arthroplasty of the shoulder was performed in 1892 by a French surgeon, J.E. Pean,[2] who inserted a shoulder replacement made of platinum and rubber into a young man afflicted with tuberculous arthritis. This prosthesis unfortunately required removal for sepsis in the early postoperative period. The modern era of shoulder arthroplasty was pioneered by Dr. Charles S. Neer II,[3] who initially developed shoulder hemiarthroplasty for the treatment of severe proximal humeral fractures in the early 1950s. Neer's shoulder prosthesis was redesigned in 1973 and has remained the prototype for all subsequent successful variations in shoulder arthroplasty design (Fig. 20-1).[4] In contrast to arthroplasty of the hip and knee, shoulder replacement remains a more rarely performed procedure. The average shoulder specialist performs this operation approximately 40 times per year, and the average general orthopedic surgeon performs this procedure only once per year. Advances in knowledge of shoulder anatomy and kinematics and a clearer understanding of shoulder injuries have led to notable improvements in the design of the latest generation of shoulder prostheses. Improvements in modularity and design have improved the surgeon's ability to duplicate the patient's native anatomy more closely and to perform complex reconstructions for arthritic conditions. More recently, the reverse total shoulder arthroplasty has become available in the United States, and it provides a nonanatomic solution for patients whose arthritic conditions or fracture configurations were previously considered beyond surgical treatment.[5,6]

This chapter discusses the clinical evaluation of patients afflicted with arthritis of the glenohumeral joint and the distinguishing features of each of the various arthritic processes, along with their respective implications in terms of surgical technique, postoperative rehabilitation, and overall prognosis. Although glenohumeral joint arthroplasty is very reliable in terms of pain relief, the functional outcome is related to the diagnosis. Modification in postoperative rehabilitation is required, depending not only on bony anatomy but also on the condition of the surrounding soft tissue.

The indications for shoulder arthroplasty have been expanding steadily since its first use in proximal humerus fractures. Currently, the most common indications for shoulder arthroplasty are osteoarthritis,[7] avascular necrosis,[8] cuff tear arthropathy,[5,9,10] acute fractures,[11,12] and post-traumatic arthritis.[13]

CLINICAL CONSIDERATIONS

History

Patients who are candidates for shoulder arthroplasty must undergo a thorough evaluation before consideration of surgery.[14] This evaluation should include a history of the onset and progression of shoulder pain, a detailed medical history, a physical examination, and a radiographic evaluation. From a medical standpoint, the patient's condition must be adequate to tolerate anesthesia and surgery. Certain medical conditions, such as rheumatoid arthritis, affect not only the bones but also the soft tissue around the glenohumeral joint and influence surgical technique and rehabilitation. Patients with osteonecrosis and humeral head collapse are often receiving high doses of steroids, which can also have substantial detrimental effects on the surrounding soft tissue of the shoulder. Careful evaluation of other body systems, including the heart, lungs, and immune system, is a critical part of the patient evaluation before shoulder arthroplasty.

Other important historical considerations include the patient's age, hand dominance, work and recreational activities, socioeconomic and educational background, and family history. The patient's ability to participate in postoperative rehabilitation in terms of both motivational level and understanding is crucial to the success of this procedure.

The primary indication for prosthetic replacement of the glenohumeral joint is pain.[4] This is true with prosthetic replacement of any joint in the body. Commonly, patients report progression of pain over several years. Typical complaints include night pain and pain at rest, work, or recreational sports. Shoulder pain can have multiple causes. Other causes of shoulder pain, including neurologic, cervical,

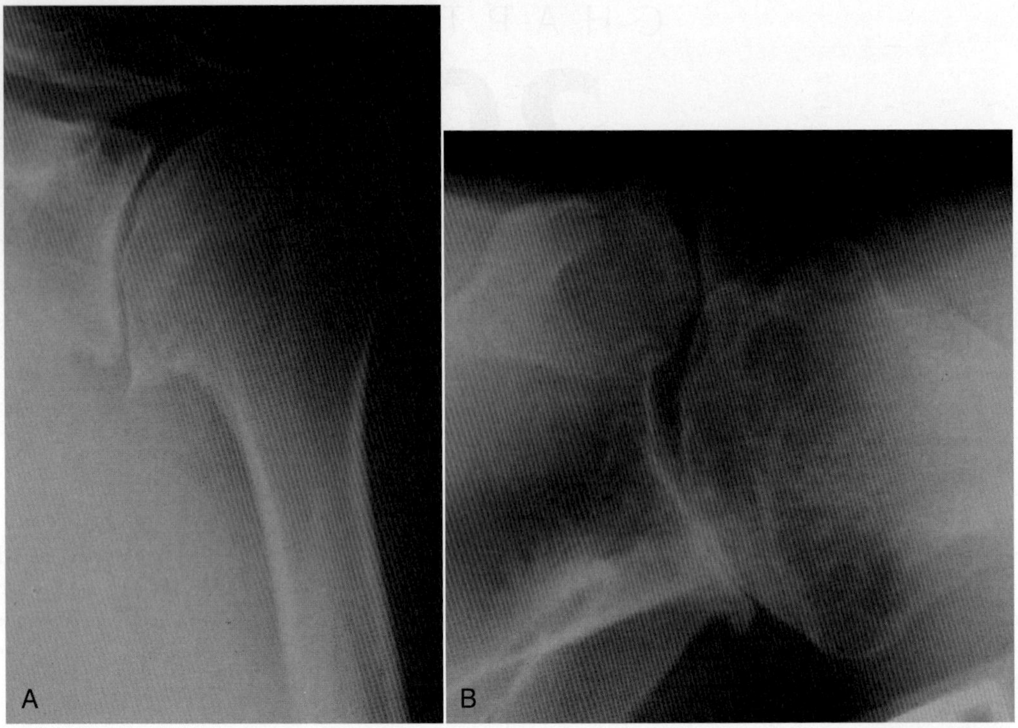

Figure 20-1 Anteroposterior (**A**) and axillary (**B**) radiographic views of glenohumeral joint osteoarthritis. Notice the hypertrophic osteophytes on the humeral head, bone-on-bone contact between the head and glenoid, and posterior subluxation of the humeral head on the glenoid.

thoracic, and abdominal sources, should all be investigated and excluded. In addition, multiple structures surrounding the glenohumeral joint, including the rotator cuff and acromioclavicular joint, can be sources of pain, especially in patients with rheumatoid disease. These sources of pain should be excluded before shoulder arthroplasty is considered.[15] Pain characteristics, such as location, character, frequency, duration, and radiation, are important to evaluate before surgery.

Limitation of shoulder function and motion should be considered only secondarily as an indication for shoulder replacement. It is highly unusual to recommend and perform shoulder arthroplasty in the absence of severe pain. Although most patients do note a significant improvement in range of motion (ROM) and function, the primary indication for conventional shoulder arthroplasty remains pain. Improvement in function and ROM is more limited in patients with associated soft tissue injury, severe bone loss, scarring, or nerve or muscle injury. Pain is also a primary indication for reverse total shoulder arthroplasty, although this prosthesis is able to provide forward flexion to patients with "pseudoparalysis," a painless inability to forward flex the arm secondary to a massive, irreparable rotator cuff tear.

Physical Examination

Following a careful general physical examination, a thorough evaluation of both shoulders is required, to include active ROM (AROM) and passive ROM (PROM), strength, tenderness, and crepitus. ROM is generally restricted both actively and passively, and active elevation is characterized by substitution and exaggerated scapulothoracic motion. Limitation of external rotation is very sensitive in determining the degree of glenohumeral restriction in an arthritic shoulder.[4] Glenohumeral arthritis is differentiated from adhesive capsulitis radiographically; patients with adhesive capsulitis typically have normal radiographs. Patients with severe weakness, such as those with massive rotator cuff tears, have limitation in active motion but not passive motion.

Tenderness can be elicited in the arthritic shoulder by palpation of the posterior joint line. The tuberosity is typically not tender in the absence of rotator cuff disease. Pain may be elicited throughout the ROM. Crepitation in the glenohumeral joint can be elicited with both AROM and PROM of the shoulder, and often a ratcheting motion is visible during active motion of the glenohumeral joint.

A patient's strength postoperatively is critical in terms of functional improvement following shoulder arthroplasty. A standardized five-point muscle grading system allows the surgeon to compare preoperative and postoperative strength.[14] Patients with long-standing glenohumeral arthritis typically display muscle atrophy and weakness, as well as pain inhibition to resistive testing. Nerve injury and rotator cuff disruption must be identified preoperatively because these disorders will affect both operative technique and postoperative rehabilitation. Strength is usually tested by resisted forward elevation (anterior deltoid and supraspinatus), external rotation (infraspinatus and teres minor), and abdominal compression testing (subscapularis).

Osteoarthritis

Osteoarthritis of the glenohumeral joint is the most common indication for total shoulder arthroplasty.[4] Although it occurs only one tenth as often as osteoarthritis of the hip and knee, glenohumeral joint osteoarthritis usually affects patients approximately 10 years earlier, and total shoulder arthroplasty is commonly performed on patients in their early 50s. Pathologically, signs of osteoarthritis include loss of the glenohumeral articular space, large rimming, osteophytes of the humeral neck, and peripheral glenoid spurring (Fig. 20-2). Posterior glenoid erosion with posterior subluxation is common, and loose bodies are typically seen. Anterior capsular contractures, combined with posterior capsular stretching, often result in an appearance of anterior flattening of the shoulder on clinical examination. The rotator cuff is intact in 90% to 95% of cases.[16] Biceps tears, when they do occur, are secondary to osteophytes in the proximal humerus. Bone quality in glenohumeral osteoarthritis is excellent and typically supports both humeral and glenoid prostheses well.

Surgical technique for total shoulder arthroplasty in an osteoarthritic patient begins with excision of the rimming osteophytes around the humeral head. This method decreases the quantity of bony tissue within the capsule and aids in the recuperation of motion following surgery. Resection of these osteophytes can be challenging at the time of surgery because the demarcation between normal bone and osteophyte is not as clear-cut as one would expect based on preoperative radiographs. Glenoid version must also be restored, to recenter the humeral head. This objective can be achieved either through contouring of the anterior glenoid rim or, more rarely, bone grafting posteriorly.[4] Failure to do this may lead to posterior instability of the shoulder. Successful total shoulder arthroplasty depends not only on restoration of the articular surfaces, but also on soft tissue balancing. Anterior soft tissue contractures, including the subscapularis, must be released, and the posterior capsule may require plication to restore posterior stability. Reestablishment of proper resting tension for both the rotator cuff and deltoid myofascial sleeves is critical to the restoration of strength following surgery. These two elements are determined by proper size selection and orientation of the humeral and glenoid components. The growing trend among shoulder specialists is to perform tenodesis of the biceps tendon during total shoulder replacement, to prevent future complications with this structure following surgery. In rare cases of concomitant impingement syndrome, acromioplasty may be desirable.

In general, the results of total shoulder arthroplasty have been superior to those of humeral head replacement alone for osteoarthritis, in terms of both motion and pain.[17,18] Patients who undergo humeral head replacement alone for osteoarthritis do not realize the full benefit of the procedure for approximately 1 year postoperatively, whereas patients with total shoulder arthroplasty often report that the arthritic-type pain disappears by the first postoperative day. The most common intraoperative complication of total shoulder replacement in osteoarthritis remains fracture of the humerus, which has been reported in up to 5% of cases.[19] This complication typically requires some

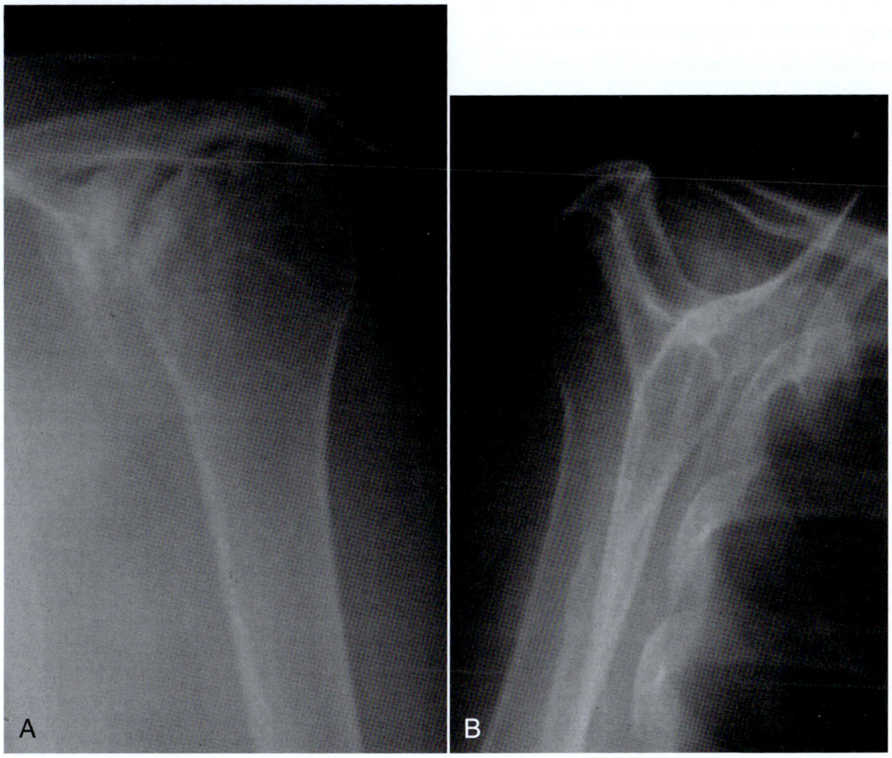

Figure 20-2 Anteroposterior (**A**) and scapular (**B**) lateral radiographs of rheumatoid arthritis of the glenohumeral joint. Note the severe bone loss, erosions in the humeral head, and centralization because of loss of glenoid bone stock.

type of internal fixation at the time of the initial surgical procedure and may result in increased blood loss and inflammation postoperatively.

These special surgical considerations in the treatment of osteoarthritis by total shoulder arthroplasty have implications for postoperative rehabilitation. The only muscle released during this procedure is the subscapularis, which requires protection postoperatively by limiting passive external rotation and avoiding resisted internal rotation for at least 6 weeks until this muscle has healed. Some surgeons prefer lesser tuberosity osteotomy to subscapularis tenotomy and thus may allow more passive external rotation and resisted internal rotation at 4 weeks, based on the faster rate of bone-to-bone healing than tendon-to-tendon healing. Active elevation, however, can be started on the first day after the operation. Capsular releases require the immediate institution of stretching exercises in the midrange to maintain flexibility. Patients with severe posterior wear and capsular stretching may have a tendency to posterior subluxation in the early postoperative period. In this situation, the surgeon may request that exercises be done in the upright position and the arm be elevated more in the plane of abduction than flexion, to prevent stress on the posterior shoulder capsule in the early postoperative period until adequate scarring has occurred.

Patients with glenohumeral joint osteoarthritis are ideal candidates for total shoulder arthroplasty and have the best prognosis of all patients who undergo this procedure. Good to excellent results are typically found in more than 90% of patients.[1,7] Active forward elevation ranges, on average, between 130° and 145° in reported series, and external rotation typically averages approximately 40°.[20] Significant improvements in activities of daily living (ADLs) and shoulder function are reported routinely from multiple centers around the world.[1,7]

Rheumatoid Arthritis

Rheumatoid arthritis is a progressive, systemic disease that affects not only the joint surfaces but also the muscles, ligaments, tendons, and bone itself. Approximately 80% of patients with rheumatoid arthritis have involvement of their shoulder joint, and treatment of rheumatoid arthritis of the shoulder is often hampered by associated upper extremity involvement of the elbow, wrist, and fingers.[21] Rheumatoid arthritis occurs in a variety of fashions. Dr. Neer described three clinical varieties of rheumatoid arthritis involving the shoulder: dry, wet, and resorptive forms.[22] The dry form resembles osteoarthritis with sclerosis, rimming osteophytes, and loss of the joint space. This condition is sometimes referred to as *mixed arthritis*. Contractures may be noted in this form of rheumatoid arthritis, but they are rare in all other forms. In the dry form, bone quality is typically good, although severe erosion is noted at the articular surfaces. The wet and resorptive forms of rheumatoid arthritis are characterized by severe bone loss, bone erosion secondary to pannus formation, and central glenoid wear with medial migration of the humeral head (Fig. 20-3). These patients often have a marked synovial hypertrophy in both the glenohumeral joint and subdeltoid bursa, which will require excision at the time of surgery. Rotator cuff tears are present in approximately 30% to 40% of patients with rheumatoid arthritis, in marked contrast to osteoarthritis. Bone destruction and osteoporosis are also much more common in rheumatoid arthritis. Medical treatment for patients with rheumatoid arthritis often includes high-dose steroid treatment, which also affects soft tissue surrounding the joints.

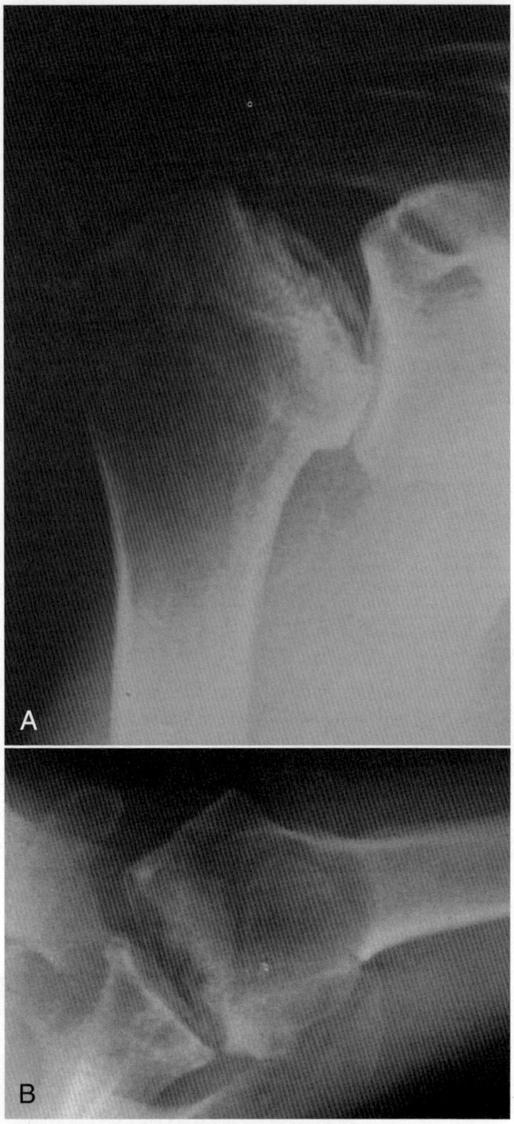

Figure 20-3 Anteroposterior (**A**) and axillary (**B**) lateral radiographs of a patient with avascular necrosis of the humeral head. Notice the subchondral collapse and crescent sign indicative of subchondral fracture.

During surgery, great care must be taken to avoid fracture to the bone, which is much more osteoporotic than in osteoarthritis. In some cases, rotator cuff repair is possible and can be performed simultaneously with shoulder arthroplasty. A glenoid prosthesis is placed only when adequate bone stock is available and an intact or easily repairable rotator cuff is found at the time of surgery. Soft tissue contractures, which are so typical of osteoarthritis, are rarely a problem in rheumatoid arthritis, and balancing of soft tissue does play as important a role as it does in osteoarthritis. Occasionally, in patients with large rotator cuff tears, humeral head replacement alone is preferred, to prevent early glenoid loosening because of superior migration of the humerus and subsequent eccentric loading of the superior glenoid. (The superior migration happens anyway. If the glenoid prosthesis is left out, it cannot break loose.) This eccentric glenoid loading has been referred to as the "rocking horse glenoid" in the orthopedic literature.[23] In cases of severe bone loss, erosion, and centralization of the humeral head, arthroplasty is still indicated for pain relief, although functional improvement is much more limited in these patients.

Postoperatively, rehabilitation for arthroplasty in the patient with rheumatoid arthritis progresses at a much slower pace. Therapy must be modified to protect the rotator cuff repair, if applicable. In patients with severe tissue loss, a "limited goals" program may be instituted to regain function from "eyes to the thighs." Patients who have humeral head replacement alone may have more pain in the early postoperative period than reported following total shoulder arthroplasty. Excessive force should be avoided during stretching exercises. Patients with rheumatoid arthritis may be weaker overall, with more limited goals obtained in function and AROM. Nonambulatory patients should be restricted from active transfers for approximately 4 to 6 months after this operation. It is critical to avoid aggravation of other affected joints in both the upper and lower extremities during rehabilitation of the shoulder. Pain relief following shoulder arthroplasty in rheumatoid arthritis is reported in more than 90% of patients.[24] Functional results are more limited and are more dependent on the quality of the bone and soft tissue surrounding the shoulder joint. Most patients obtain a good or acceptable functional result, but deterioration of results is noted in time because of progression of the disease in the soft tissue. Average active forward elevation has been reported postoperatively between 75° and 100°, with external rotation averaging between 30° and 45°. Average function postoperatively is approximately 70% of normal for an age-matched group.[24] Glenoid loosening has been reported postoperatively in more than 40% of patients.[21]

Arthritis of Dislocation

The term *arthritis of dislocation* refers to glenohumeral joint arthritis after instability repair. This disorder is characterized by altered joint anatomy and biomechanics typically resulting from an internal rotation contracture following instability repair. This form of arthritis is most commonly seen following nonanatomic repairs and usually occurs in patients less than 45 years old.[25] Contracture of the anterior structures, including the subscapularis and anterior capsule, is typically encountered. Hardware may also complicate the surgical approach. This problem can follow unidirectional repairs in patients with multidirectional instability. Patients may have posterior subluxation of the shoulder, as seen in osteoarthritis, with internal rotation contractures and progressive posterior glenoid wear. The pathoanatomy in this process is similar to that of osteoarthritis, but it is complicated by postoperative anterior contractures, hardware, and the high demands of this patient group because of their young age.

At surgery, special attention is directed toward release of anterior capsular contractures. The subscapularis may require lengthening, and soft tissue must be balanced with anterior capsular releases and posterior capsular imbrication. Hardware is usually removed if it is in the way of prosthetic placement, and glenoid version must be corrected as in osteoarthritis. Because this form of arthritis typically occurs in younger age groups, humeral head replacement may be selected by the surgeon to prevent progressive glenoid loosening because of high demands placed on the shoulder. This approach may result in less complete pain relief than reported with total shoulder replacement, especially in the early postoperative period.[17,18]

The results of arthroplasty for arthritis of dislocation are inferior to those of arthroplasty for osteoarthritis.[25] Average forward elevation following this procedure is approximately 120°, with external rotation of approximately 40°. Patients in some series regained only 60% of normal shoulder function following arthroplasty for arthritis of dislocation.[26]

Avascular Necrosis

Avascular necrosis of the humeral head occurs secondary to an acute vascular insult to the proximal humerus. This disorder results in collapse and irregularity of the humeral head, with subsequent loss of bony support for the articular cartilage (Fig. 20-4).[8,27] The articular cartilage is not primarily affected but becomes disrupted following collapse of the bone of the humeral head. If the disease is allowed to progress, the glenoid becomes secondarily arthritic by articulating against this irregular humeral head. Avascular necrosis has been separated into four stages.[8] Stage III is defined by collapse of the humeral head. Stage IV occurs when the glenoid becomes involved. Arthroplasty is indicated for these last two stages. The most common identified cause of avascular necrosis of the humeral head is corticosteroid use. Other causes include trauma, sickle cell anemia, Gaucher's disease, alcohol abuse, and caisson disease. Some cases can be idiopathic. The rotator cuff is usually normal in these patients. Stage IV avascular necrosis is also characterized by capsular contractures, which are typically not present during stage III.

The surgical management of stage III avascular necrosis includes humeral head replacement alone. By definition, the glenoid is normal at this stage and does not require replacement. Capsular contractures tend to be minimal. Once avascular necrosis has progressed to stage IV, total shoulder replacement is indicated. Capsular releases are typically required at this stage.

Postoperatively, physical therapy can progress in a relatively aggressive fashion. These patients are often younger, with good soft tissue quality, and can tolerate rapid progress. Patients must be examined for systemic disease, which may affect other joints and soft tissue. Involvement of other musculoskeletal structures requires modification of the rehabilitation program.

Overall prognosis in this patient group is good, with average forward elevation of approximately 130° and external rotation of 80°. These patients tend to regain approximately 75% of normal shoulder function.[27]

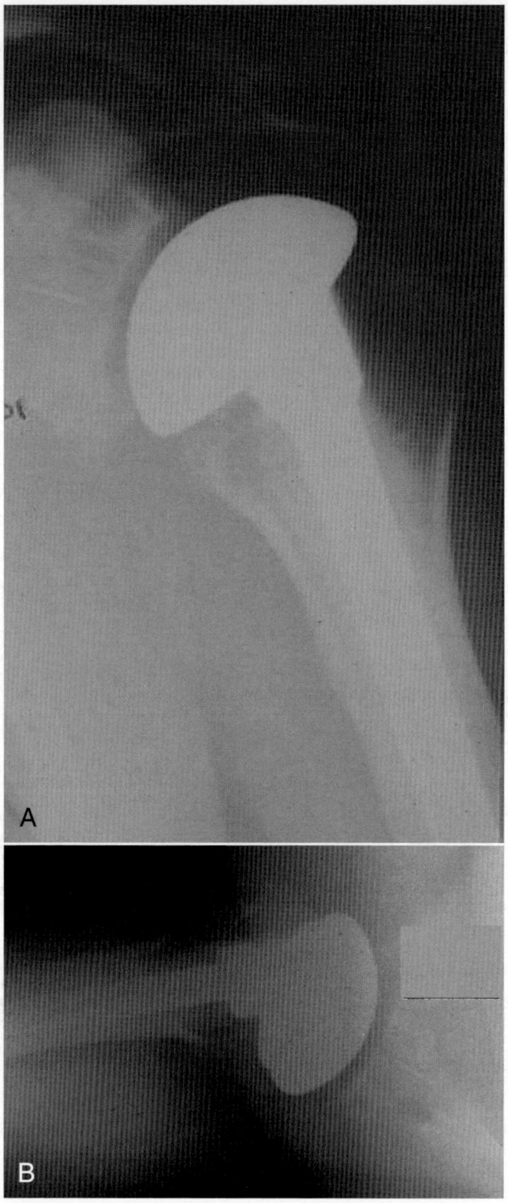

Figure 20-4 Anteroposterior (**A**) and axillary (**B**) lateral radiographs of a total shoulder replacement. The normal anatomic relationships have been reestablished by the humeral head and glenoid prostheses. The variety of stem sizes and humeral head sizes in third-generation prostheses allows the surgeon to customize the prosthesis to each individual patient.

Cuff Tear Arthropathy

Cuff tear arthropathy is a challenging problem for both the surgeon and the therapist. It is characterized by severe destruction of the glenohumeral joint, humeral head collapse, and a massive, irreparable rotator cuff tear. This process is more common in patients who are more than 70 years old and is seen more frequently in women than in men. Cuff tear arthropathy is characterized radiographically by a high-riding humeral head that causes superior glenoid and undersurface acromial wear, called *acetabularization,* because the rotator cuff is no long interposed between the humeral head and the acromion. The greater tuberosity wears away from the proximal humerus, thus leading to rounding of the humeral head in a process that has been similarly been described as *femoralization.* Patients have gross instability of the shoulder because of the massive tear, a large effusion, and severe weakness.

Before 2006, surgical options for patients with rotator cuff arthropathy were limited.[10] Historically, conventional constrained prostheses were used to compensate for rotator cuff deficiency. Outcomes were generally poor, however, with respect to both function and pain.[10,28] Humeral head replacement led to adequate pain relief in 80% to 90% of patients, but functional use was "limited goals" below shoulder level. A new era in shoulder surgery was pioneered by Dr. Paul Grammont in France in the late 1980s.[29] He developed a successful reverse total shoulder arthroplasty, in which a hemisphere is implanted on the glenoid, and the humeral head is replaced with a cup, such that the ball-and-socket configuration is reversed. This nonanatomic design lengthens the deltoid and medializes the center of rotation, thus obviating the need for a rotator cuff to produce a compressive force on the humeral head to permit forward flexion. The deltoid lever arm is doubled, and deltoid muscle fibers that were medial to the center of rotation in a normal shoulder are lateral to the center of rotation after reverse total shoulder arthroplasty and therefore can used for abduction and elevation.[5,30,31]

Reverse total shoulder arthroplasty can be performed through a superior approach or a deltopectoral approach. The superior approach has the advantages of preserving the remains of the subscapularis and having little or no risk of postoperative instability. Visualization of the glenoid and scapular neck may be poor, and suboptimal placement of the components can lead to loosening. Further, this approach requires disruption of the deltoid, the muscle on which the entire function of the reverse total shoulder relies. The deltopectoral approach preserves more active external rotation but has an increased risk of instability because the subscapularis must be detached. Because the function of the reverse total shoulder depends on the increased lever arm of the deltoid, tensioning this muscle intraoperatively is a critical part of the surgical procedure. An intact teres minor muscle is critical for postoperative active external rotation, and many surgeons perform a concomitant latissimus dorsi transfer if the teres minor is incompetent and the patient preoperatively has an external rotation lag sign.[32]

Although the reverse total shoulder has been used since the 1980s in Europe, scant literature is available on a preferred rehabilitation protocol.[33] Generally, rehabilitation after reverse total shoulder focuses on joint protection and deltoid function. For 12 weeks, patients "should always be able to visualize their elbow regardless of what they are doing," thereby avoiding the adduction, external rotation, and extension dislocation position. Gradual flexion in the scapular plate is begun passively immediately after primary reverse total shoulder arthroplasty and is increased to a limit of 90° during the initial stages of soft tissue healing. Passive external rotation to 30° is allowed unless the patient had a concomitant subscapularis repair. Pure abduction is initially avoided, as is internal rotation ROM for the first 6 weeks.

Except during therapy and bathing, patients use a sling for up to 6 weeks, especially if the superior approach is used or in cases of revision surgery. Deltoid and periscapular isometrics help to restore initial deltoid function. After 3 weeks, passive forward flexion may progress to 120° and passive external rotation to 45°. At 6 weeks, passive internal rotation is begun in the protected position of 60° of abduction to avoid dislocation, and passive forward flexion is allowed to the patient's tolerance. Active-assisted ROM and AROM begin at week 6, initially supine with the scapula stabilized. Internal rotation and external rotation isometrics are begun at week 8. Resistive exercises are generally begun at 12 weeks. Because the quality and quantity of both bone and soft tissue can vary greatly among reverse total shoulder arthroplasties, communication with the surgeon is critical to determine a patient's ideal time to begin ROM activities. See Category D Rehabilitation of Reverse Shoulder arthroplasty.

A multicenter French study of 484 reverse total shoulder arthroplasties performed for massive rotator cuff tears and cuff tear arthropathy demonstrated an improved elevation from 71° to 130°, and at 52 months postoperatively, 90% of patients were satisfied or very satisfied with their shoulder.[5] Although the reverse total shoulder arthroplasty can have profound clinical effects on both ROM and pain, the complication rate is 3 times that of conventional shoulder arthroplasty; complications include fracture, loosening, infection, scapular notching, and instability. Instability with reverse total shoulder arthroplasty depends on surgical technique (it has not be documented after reverse total shoulder arthroplasty done by the superior approach). It most often occurs as a patient pushes off from a seated position or attempts to tuck in his or her shirt. Both radiographic and clinical results deteriorate in time (approximately 8 years), so many surgeons reserve this salvage procedure for older patients.[5]

Acute Fractures

Shoulder arthroplasty is indicated for four-part fractures, humeral head split fractures, and three-part fractures in older patients.[34,35] The greater and lesser tuberosities are typically displaced from the shaft and humeral head. At the time of surgery, hemorrhage and inflammation from trauma are present, and these fractures may also be further complicated by axillary nerve damage or damage to other nerves surrounding the shoulder. Proximal humeral fractures most commonly occur in older patients and are associated with osteoporosis.

The surgeon is challenged by the loss of normal anatomic relationships between the tuberosities and shaft that makes placement of the humeral head extremely difficult at its proper height and version. Some prosthetic systems do offer a jig, which may be of some assistance. In addition, the tuberosities and attached rotator cuff tendons must be repaired back to each other and the humeral shaft, usually with heavy sutures.

Postoperatively, rehabilitation of these patients proceeds in a fashion very similar to rehabilitation following repair of a massive rotator cuff tear. A study in 2007 comparing early (after 2 weeks) and late (after 6 weeks) mobilization of hemiarthroplasties for fractures demonstrated similar outcomes, although patients in the early mobilization group had a somewhat increased incidence of tuberosity displacement.[36] Functional outcome after hemiarthroplasty for fracture depends heavily on greater tuberosity healing, and thus active elevation of the arm is avoided for 6 weeks to protect the tuberosities, and passive stretching is used to regain flexibility. Post-traumatic inflammation and scarring more commonly lead to tightness of the shoulder following arthroplasty for fracture than in other diagnoses. A greater emphasis on stretching is required. Careful evaluation of the neurologic structures, especially the axillary nerve, is critical postoperatively because this structure cannot be adequately assessed before surgery because of pain and swelling.

The results of arthroplasty for acute fracture are by far superior to nonoperative management of these same fractures[37] but are generally inferior to the results in fractures that can be managed with open reduction and internal fixation.[11] Typically, pain relief is excellent in more than 80% of cases, although function is variable. The average patient regains active forward elevation of approximately 90° to 100° and regains the ability to perform only approximately 50% of their ADLs. Results are better in patients who are more than 65 years old, primarily because of lower demands.

Post-traumatic Arthritis

Post-traumatic glenohumeral joint arthritis is related to previous fractures or fracture-dislocations and is associated with extensive soft tissue scarring, bone loss, retraction of the tuberosities, bony malunion, and even nonunion. When previous attempts at open reduction and internal fixation were made, retained hardware is found and may complicate matters further. Nerve injuries may be associated with the initial trauma or subsequent surgery, and these patients have a higher risk of infection because of the previous operation. In addition, the rotator cuff may have been injured by the initial trauma as well.

In surgery, rotator cuff injuries, in the form both of scarring and tearing, must be addressed with attempts at mobilization and repair of the rotator cuff. Osteotomy of the tuberosities is avoid, if this is required, because results are clearly inferior when this procedure is performed.[38] The deltoid myofascial resting length must be restored by placement of the prosthesis at the proper height and version in the presence of altered anatomy. Modular prostheses currently in use have improved the surgeon's ability to modify the fit of the prosthesis to bony distortion of the proximal humerus following old fractures.

Postoperative rehabilitation must be individualized because this is a very heterogeneous group. Early PROM exercises are critical because this group has a greater tendency to post-operative stiffness. Instability following arthroplasty is of greatest risk in this patient group and must be prevented by modification of the rehabilitation program, depending on the areas of potential instability. These patients often require 1 full year of rehabilitation to maximize the results of surgery.

The results of arthroplasty for post-traumatic arthritis are inferior to those seen in acute trauma.[39] Active forward elevation has been reported to average approximately 60°, with external rotation of approximately 20°. Pain relief is also inferior to that observed for arthroplasty following early trauma.

REHABILITATION

The overall goals for postoperative rehabilitation following arthroplasty include pain relief and improvement in function. Specifically, physical therapy must focus on limiting postoperative contractures following arthroplasty and increasing the strength of the rotator cuff and deltoid muscles to maximize functional improvement. Early in the course of physical therapy, the subscapularis and any other repaired structure must be protected, and the patient's comfort must be maintained at reasonable levels. As time progresses, more emphasis on strengthening and functional improvement is critical. Careful communication with the surgeon and teamwork among the patient, therapist, and surgeon are critical to a successful outcome following shoulder arthroplasty.

Categories of Rehabilitation following Shoulder Arthroplasty

The steps of rehabilitation and overall goals following shoulder arthroplasty vary according to the diagnosis. Patients fall into three general categories for rehabilitation: (A) programs for patients with a good rotator cuff and deltoid: (B) programs for patients with a poor or repaired rotator cuff and deltoid; and (C) "limited goals" programs. Patients in category A generally include those with osteoarthritis, rheumatoid arthritis with a good cuff, arthritis of dislocation, or avascular necrosis. Patients in category B generally include those with rheumatoid arthritis with a repaired cuff, patients with acute fracture, and some patients with post-traumatic arthritis. Patients in the limited goals category C include patients with rheumatoid arthritis with an irreparable rotator cuff, patients with previously failed cuff surgery, those with cuff tear arthropathy, patients with neurologic problems, and those with previously failed shoulder arthroplasty.

The protocols given in Appendix 20-1 can serve as a guide in the progression of rehabilitation after shoulder arthroplasty for the various diagnoses outlined previously. Careful communication with the surgeon and patient is a prerequisite for safe and tolerable progression. The time lines specified are general recommendations and must be adjusted individually, based on feedback from the patient and demonstration of functional improvement.

Patients in the limited goals category are placed there by the surgeon, based on pathologic conditions encountered at the time of surgery. The goals in this patient group are reasonable pain relief and adequate function from "eyes to thighs."

Critical Points and Technique

Because of the numerous pathologic conditions encountered during shoulder arthroplasty, clear communication, either written or oral, between the therapist and the surgeon is critical. The therapist must know whether the rotator cuff was repaired during the surgical procedure because this will require 6 weeks of passive elevation, rather than the usual active-assisted exercises. If posterior instability is a concern, supine exercises may be dangerous. If the quality of the subscapularis was poor because of prior surgery, external rotation may require further limitations.

The first step toward achieving a cooperative relationship in postoperative therapy is for the surgeon and the therapist to gain the patient's trust and confidence. The session in which the arm is moved passively for the first time sets the stage for the rest of the program and must be accomplished with confidence and compassion. It is more important to gain the patient's trust than to achieve a specific goal of motion in the first session. Confidence on the part of the therapist comes from a clear understanding of that patient's particular pathologic condition and its implications on the postoperative rehabilitation program.

Arm elevation is most comfortably obtained in the plane of the scapula with the patient's back and scapula well supported, either in the supine or the sitting position. A more proximal and certainly firm grasp of the patient's arm allows better control by the therapist and results in better relaxation on the part of the patient (Fig. 20-5).

To externally rotate the patient's arm comfortably, the therapist first should make sure that the arm is not in extension because this will place further stress on the anterior suture line. If the patient is supine, bolstering under the elbow is helpful. Slight abduction (approximately 30°) is also beneficial for unlocking the greater tuberosity from underneath the acromion (Fig. 20-6).

The volume and intensity of daily exercises provided to the patient should be kept at a reasonable level. Patients who have undergone shoulder arthroplasty tend to be older and may have associated medical problems or arthritic processes involving other joints. Exercises can be performed in repetitions of 5 to 10 at a frequency of 2 to 3 times per day. As a group, these patients tend to be motivated and at times must be cautioned to avoid excessive stress on their replacement shoulder. Irritation of the rotator cuff can occur

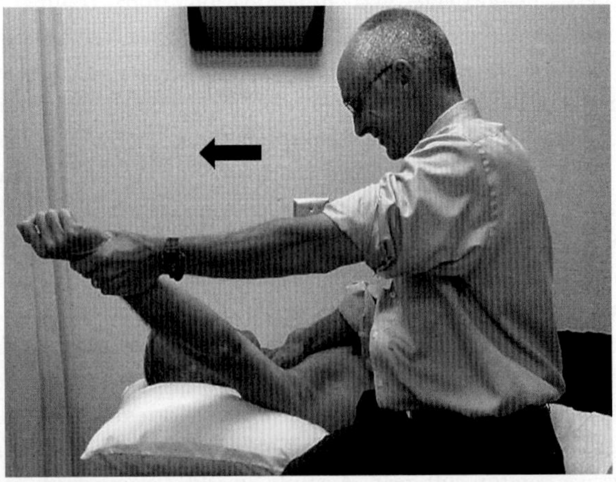

Figure 20-5 Passive forward elevation in the plane of the scapula with the assistance of a therapist or family member.

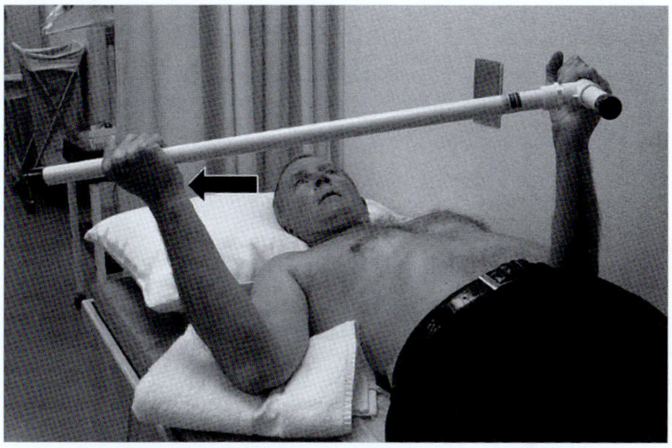

Figure 20-6 Passive external rotation of the shoulder by using a stick with the arm supported by a bolster.

at transitions in the exercise program, especially when initiating resistive exercises. The exercise program can be modified individually, based on response to exercises and levels of pain.

The progression to resistive exercises is allowed when muscle tendon units, such as the subscapularis, have safely healed to bone. These exercises are orchestrated to lead the patient gradually from light muscle reeducation to full activities. The usual program progresses from light isometrics (Fig. 20-7) to gravity-eliminated exercises (Fig. 20-8) and active-assisted ROM exercises (Figs. 20-9 and 20-10). At this point, the patient is allowed to begin eccentric lowering following active-assisted elevation (Fig. 20-11) and then active ROM exercises (Fig. 20-12). This is followed by light resistive exercises with elastic bands (Fig. 20-13) and dumbbells (Figs. 20-14 and 20-15; see also Fig. 20-12). Modified and then full activities follow.

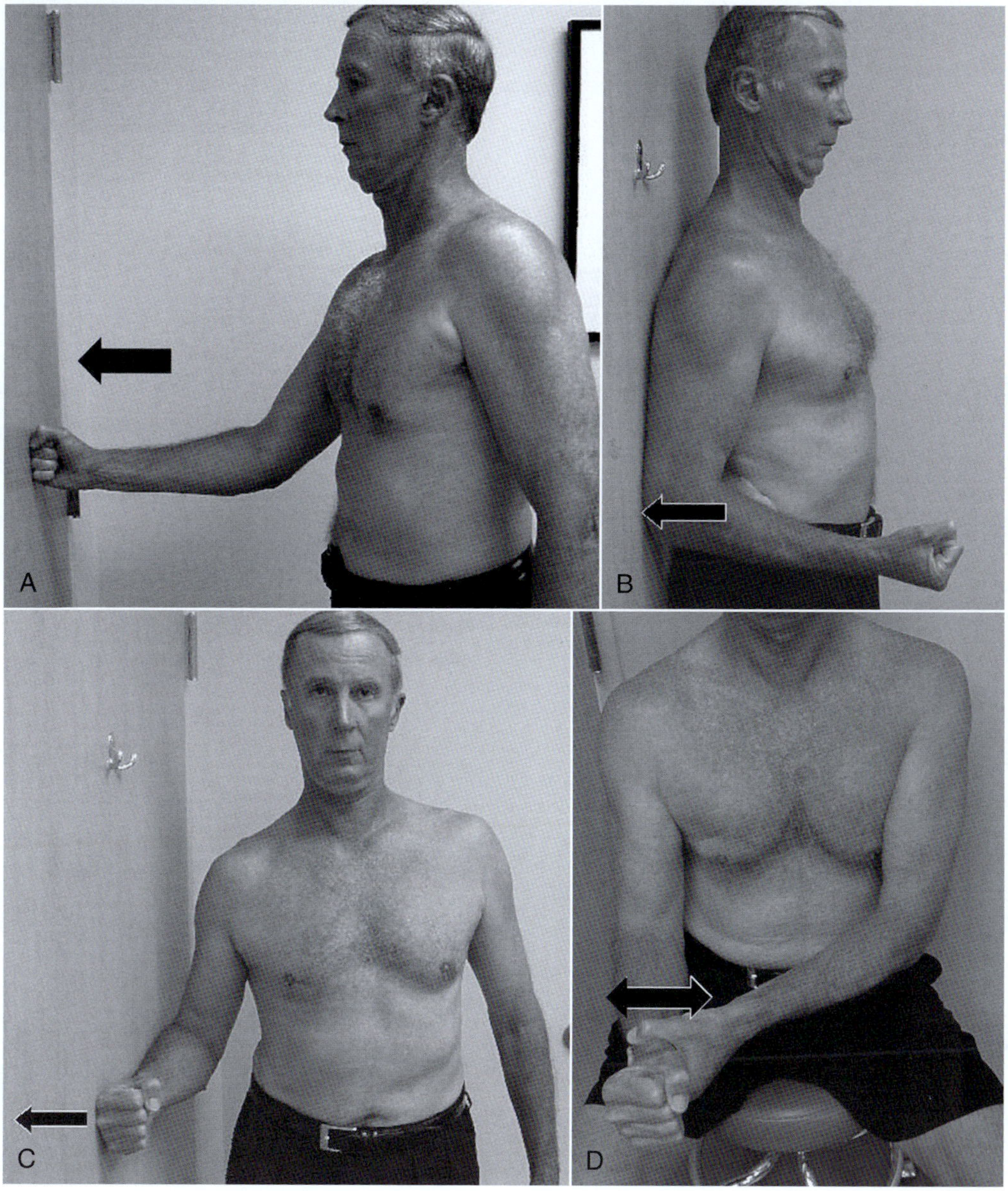

Figure 20-7 Five-way isometric exercises for the glenohumeral joint with the elbow fixed at 90°. **A,** Flexion. **B,** Extension. **C,** Abduction. **D,** Internal and external rotation.

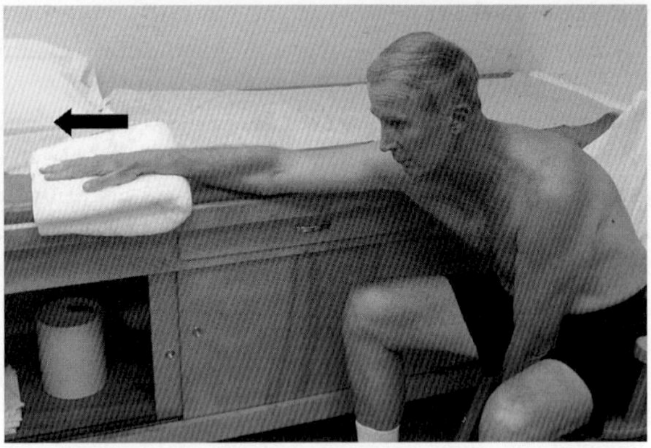

Figure 20-8 Gravity-eliminated elevation on a table top.

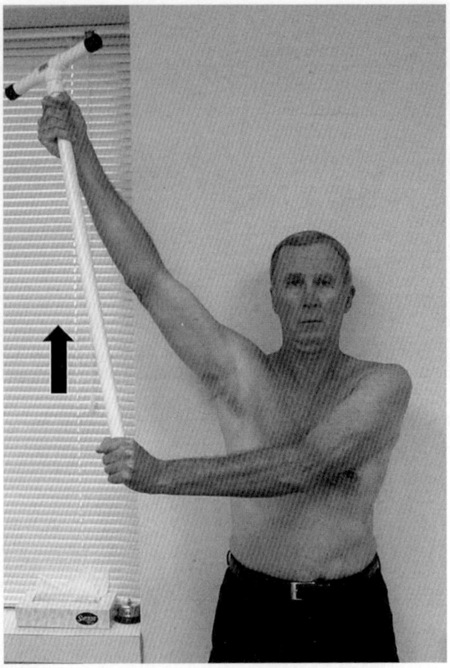

Figure 20-10 Active-assisted elevation with a stick in the plane of the scapula.

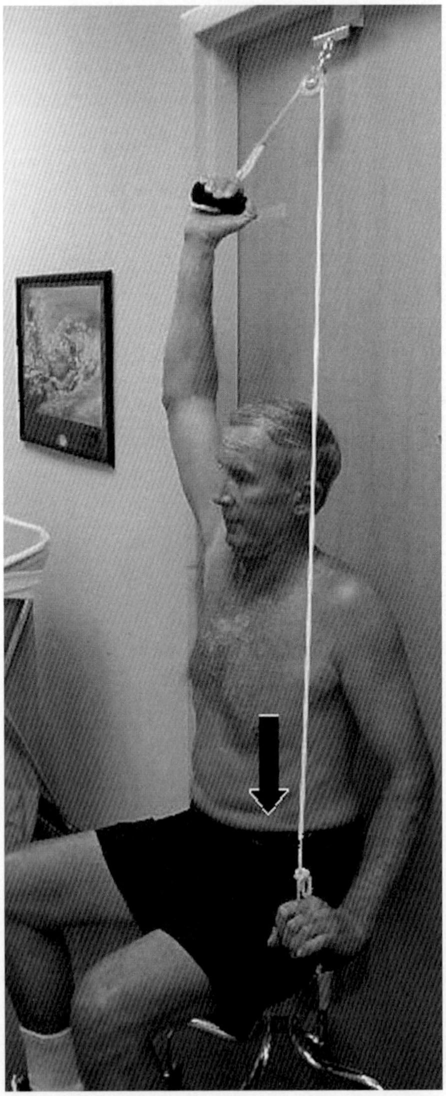

Figure 20-9 Active-assisted elevation of the arm in the plane of the scapula using a pulley system.

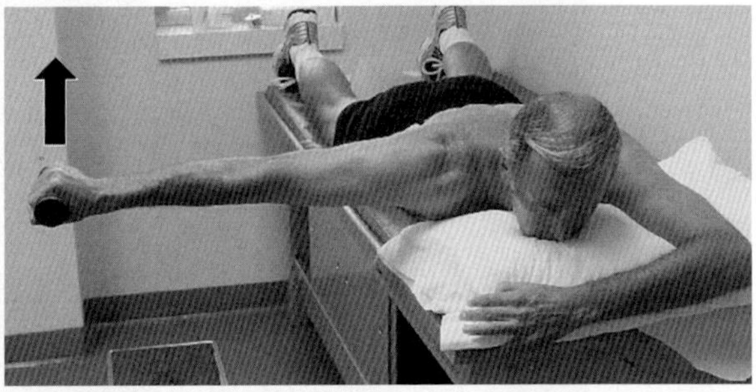

Figure 20-11 Prone horizontal abduction to strengthen the supraspinatus.

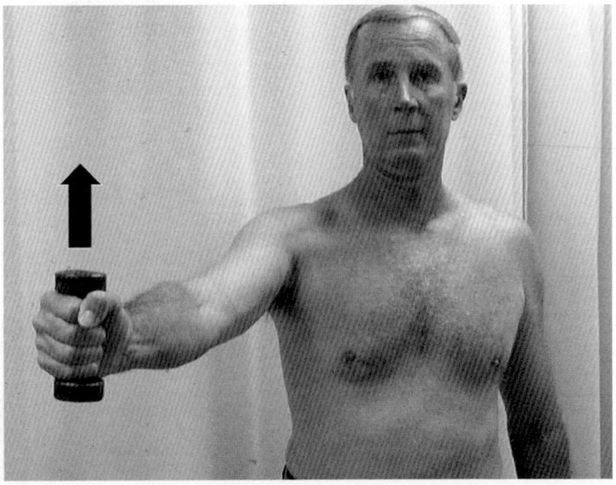

Figure 20-12 Active elevation of the arm in the plane of the scapula (scaption).

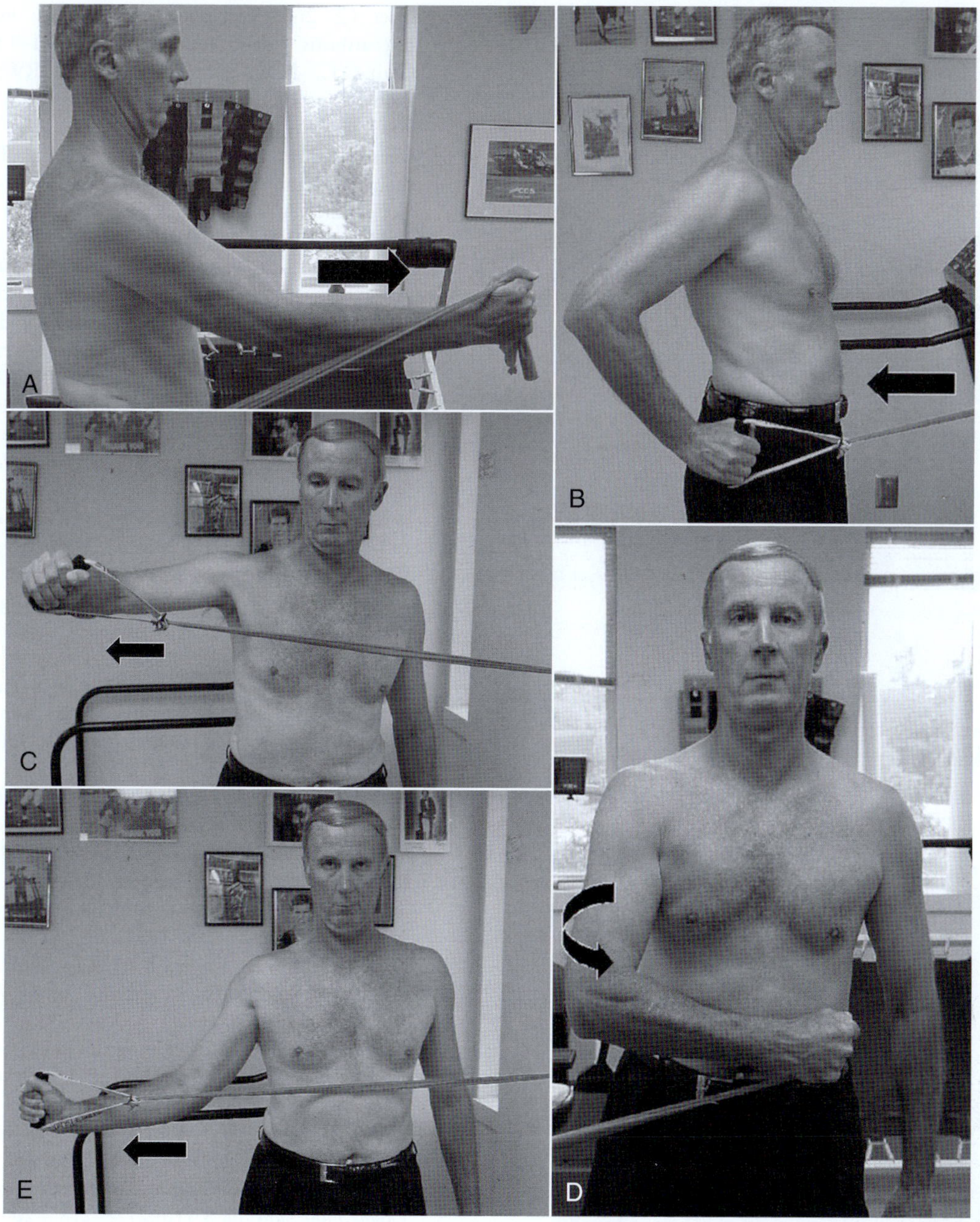

Figure 20-13 Thera-Band resistive exercises for the rotator cuff and deltoid. **A,** Flexion. **B,** Extension. **C,** Abduction. **D,** Internal rotation. **E,** External rotation.

Progression from one level to another is allowed when a patient can demonstrate the exercises comfortably and in a biomechanically correct fashion. Depending on the amount of atrophy and associated pathologic conditions in the shoulder, each patient progresses at a different rate.

SUMMARY

Successful outcome following shoulder arthroplasty requires meticulous surgical technique and a well-orchestrated and safe rehabilitation program. This chapter outlines the variety of pathologic conditions encountered in arthritic processes involving the shoulder and details special surgical techniques required with each diagnosis. Understanding the implications of these techniques on postoperative rehabilitation and the overall prognosis with each of the various diagnoses leading to glenohumeral joint arthritis will assist the therapist in organizing a safe rehabilitation program with realistic and reachable goals. Communication among the therapist, physician, and patient is critical to the successful management of these patients.

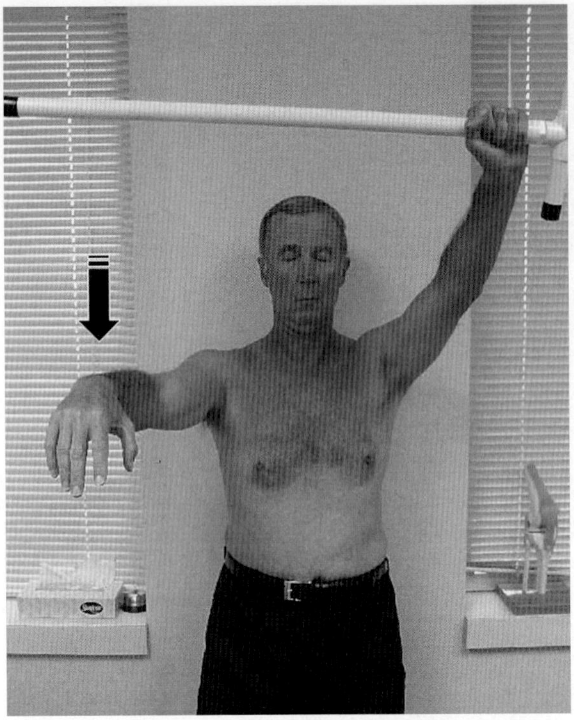

Figure 20-14 Passive elevation with a stick, followed by active eccentric lowering as tolerated.

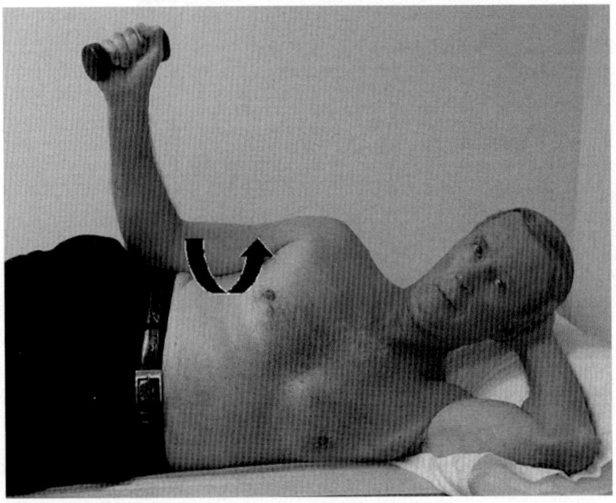

Figure 20-15 External rotation exercises with a dumbbell while the patient is lying on the contralateral side.

REFERENCES

1. Matsen FA 3rd: Early effectiveness of shoulder arthroplasty for patients who have primary glenohumeral degenerative joint disease, *J Bone Joint Surg Am* 78(2):260–264, 1996.
2. Pean JE, Bick EM: The classic: on prosthetic methods intended to repair bone fragments, *Clin Orthop Relat Res* 94:4–7, 1973.
3. Neer CS 2nd: Indications for replacement of the proximal humeral articulation, *Am J Surg* 89(4):901–907, 1955.
4. Neer CS 2nd: Replacement arthroplasty for glenohumeral osteoarthritis, *J Bone Joint Surg Am* 56(1):1–13, 1974.
5. Gerber C, Pennington SD, Nyffeler RW: Reverse total shoulder arthroplasty, *J Am Acad Orthop Surg* 17(5):284–295, 2009.
6. Matsen FA III, Boileau P, Walch G, et al: The reverse total shoulder arthroplasty, *Instr Course Lect* 57:167–174, 2008.
7. Godeneche A, Boileau P, Favard L, et al: Prosthetic replacement in the treatment of osteoarthritis of the shoulder: early results of 268 cases, *J Shoulder Elbow Surg* 11(1):11–18, 2002.
8. Arlet J, Ficat P, Gedeon A, et al: [Necrosis and ischemia of the femoral head in arteritis obliterans of the lower limbs (apropos of 5 cases)], *Rev Rhum Mal Osteoartic* 39(8):523–529, 1972.
9. Arntz CT, Jackins S, Matsen FA 3rd: Prosthetic replacement of the shoulder for the treatment of defects in the rotator cuff and the surface of the glenohumeral joint, *J Bone Joint Surg Am* 75 (4):485–491, 1993.
10. Williams GR Jr Rockwood CA Jr: Hemiarthroplasty in rotator cuff-deficient shoulders, *J Shoulder Elbow Surg* 5(5):362–367, 1996.
11. Solberg BD, Moon CN, Franco DP, et al: Surgical treatment of three and four-part proximal humeral fractures, *J Bone Joint Surg Am* 91(7):1689–1697, 2009.
12. Kontakis G, Koutras C, Tosounidis T, et al: Early management of proximal humeral fractures with hemiarthroplasty: a systematic review, *J Bone Joint Surg Br* 90(11):1407–1413, 2008.
13. Boileau P, Trojani C, Walch G, et al: Shoulder arthroplasty for the treatment of the sequelae of fractures of the proximal humerus, *J Shoulder Elbow Surg* 10(4):299–308, 2001.
14. Richards RR, An KN, Bigliani LU, et al: A standardized method to the assessment of shoulder function, *J Shoulder Elbow Surg* 3(6):347–352, 1994.
15. Kelly IG, Foster RS, Fisher WD: Neer total shoulder replacement in rheumatoid arthritis, *J Bone Joint Surg Br* 69 (5):723–726, 1987.
16. Norris TR, Iannotti JP: Functional outcome after shoulder arthroplasty for primary osteoarthritis: a multicenter study, *J Shoulder Elbow Surg* 11(2):130–135, 2002.
17. Lo IK, Litchfield RB, Griffin S, et al: Quality-of-life outcome following hemiarthroplasty or total shoulder arthroplasty in patients with osteoarthritis: a prospective, randomized trial, *J Bone Joint Surg Am* 87(10):2178–2185, 2005.
18. Bryant D, Litchfield R, Sandow M, et al: A comparison of pain, strength, range of motion, and functional outcomes after hemiarthroplasty and total shoulder arthroplasty in patients with osteoarthritis of the shoulder: a systematic review and meta-analysis, *J Bone Joint Surg Am* 87(9):1947–1956, 2005.
19. Athwal GS, Sperling JW, Rispoli DM, et al: Periprosthetic humeral fractures during shoulder arthroplasty, *J Bone Joint Surg Am* 91(3):594–603, 2009.
20. Sperling JW, Cofield RH, Rowland CM: Minimum fifteen-year follow-up of Neer hemiarthroplasty and total shoulder arthroplasty in patients aged fifty years or younger, *J Shoulder Elbow Surg* 13(6):604–613, 2004.
21. Sojbjerg JO, Frich LH, Johannsen HV, et al: Late results of total shoulder replacement in patients with rheumatoid arthritis, *Clin Orthop Relat Res* 366:39–45, 1999.
22. Neer CS 2nd: Degenerative lesions of the proximal humeral articular surface, *Clin Orthop Relat Res* 20:116–125, 1961.

23. Franklin JL, Barrett WP, Jackins SE, et al: Glenoid loosening in total shoulder arthroplasty: association with rotator cuff deficiency, *J Arthroplasty* 3(1):39–46, 1988.
24. Sperling JW, Cofield RH, Schleck CD, et al: Total shoulder arthroplasty versus hemiarthroplasty for rheumatoid arthritis of the shoulder: results of 303 consecutive cases, *J Shoulder Elbow Surg* 16(6):683–690, 2007.
25. Green A, Norris TR: Shoulder arthroplasty for advanced glenohumeral arthritis after anterior instability repair, *J Shoulder Elbow Surg* 10(6):539–545, 2001.
26. Bigliani LU, Weinstein DM, Glasgow MT, et al: Glenohumeral arthroplasty for arthritis after instability surgery, *J Shoulder Elbow Surg* 4(2):87–94, 1995.
27. Feeley BT, Fealy S, Dines DM, et al: Hemiarthroplasty and total shoulder arthroplasty for avascular necrosis of the humeral head, *J Shoulder Elbow Surg* 17(5):689–694, 2008.
28. Neer CS 2nd, Craig EV, Fukuda H: Cuff-tear arthropathy, *J Bone Joint Surg Am* 65(9):1232–1244, 1983.
29. Grammont PM, Baulot E: Delta shoulder prosthesis for rotator cuff rupture, *Orthopedics* 16(1):65–68, 1993.
30. Nyffeler RW, Werner CM, Gerber C: Biomechanical relevance of glenoid component positioning in the reverse Delta III total shoulder prosthesis, *J Shoulder Elbow Surg* 14(5):524–528, 2005.
31. Boileau P, Watkinson DJ, Hatzidakis AM, et al: Grammont reverse prosthesis: design, rationale, and biomechanics, *J Shoulder Elbow Surg* 14(1 Suppl):147S–161S, 2005.
32. Gerber C, Pennington SD, Lingenfelter EJ, et al: Reverse Delta-III total shoulder replacement combined with latissimus dorsi transfer: a preliminary report, *J Bone Joint Surg Am* 89 (5):940–947, 2007.
33. Boudreau S, Boudreau ED, Higgins LD, et al: Rehabilitation following reverse total shoulder arthroplasty, *J Orthop Sports Phys Ther* 37(12):734–743, 2007.
34. Neer CS 2nd: Displaced proximal humeral fractures. I. Classification and evaluation, *J Bone Joint Surg Am* 52 (6):1077–1089, 1970.
35. Neer CS 2nd: Displaced proximal humeral fractures. II. Treatment of three-part and four-part displacement, *J Bone Joint Surg Am* 52(6):1090–1103, 1970.
36. Agorastides I, Sinopidis C, El Meligy M, et al: Early versus late mobilization after hemiarthroplasty for proximal humeral fractures, *J Shoulder Elbow Surg* 16(3 Suppl):S33–S38, 2007.
37. Compito CA, Self EB, Bigliani LU: Arthroplasty and acute shoulder trauma: reasons for success and failure, *Clin Orthop Relat Res* 307:27–36, 1994.
38. Boileau P, Chuinard C, Le Huec JC, et al: Proximal humerus fracture sequelae: impact of a new radiographic classification on arthroplasty, *Clin Orthop Relat Res* 442:121–130, 2006.
39. Bosch U, Skutek M, Fremerey RW, et al: Outcome after primary and secondary hemiarthroplasty in elderly patients with fractures of the proximal humerus, *J Shoulder Elbow Surg* 7 (5):479–484, 1998.

APPENDIX 20-1. REHABILITATION PROGRAMS FOLLOWING TOTAL SHOULDER ARTHROPLASTY

CATEGORY A: POSTOPERATIVE REHABILITATION PROGRAM FOR TOTAL SHOULDER ARTHROPLASTY: GOOD ROTATOR CUFF AND DELTOID

Day 1

- Arm in sling at rest
- Out of bed as tolerated
- Elbow, wrist, and finger active exercises
- Passive external rotation with a stick to pain tolerance but less than 30°
- Pendulum exercises (Fig. 20-16)
- Light use of arm for eating

Days 2 to 3

- Family instructed in passive elevation exercises
- Passive elevation in the plane of the scapula
- Use of pulley by the patient begun when 120° of elevation reached and arm control adequate
- Instruction in ADL use
- Discharge from the hospital

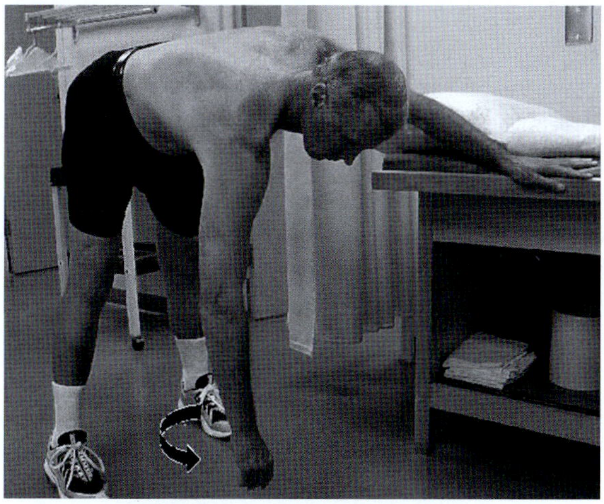

Figure 20-16 Pendulum exercises allow early passive motion following shoulder arthroplasty.

Home Program

Time Frame	Protection and Use	Modalities	Exercises
Weeks 1–2	Sling for outdoor use Patient may be more comfortable out of sling when indoors May bring hand to mouth for eating or washing May place hand pointing straight ahead as on armrest of chair May use hand for writing May begin gentle active use as tolerated	Cold pack Ultrasound to scapular muscles Transcutaneous electrical nerve stimulation (TENS) for pain if needed Advance to hot packs after sutures removed	Precaution: Avoid excessive resistance Gentle elbow ROM exercises Codman's pendulum exercises Full passive forward elevation as tolerated External rotation as tolerated Light isometrics for muscle reeducation Pulley exercises as tolerated No extension exercises Avoid scapular substitution May begin scapular stabilizing exercises (Fig. 20-17)
Weeks 2–4	Same	Same	Advance ROM as tolerated in elevation and external rotation Add overhead training as tolerated Supine elevation with a stick advancing to standing elevation with a stick Continue pulley No extension exercises No internal rotation up back
Weeks 4–6	Same	Same	Begin gravity-eliminated elevation on table top (Fig. 20-18) Begin wall stretches for full ROM (Fig. 20-19) May begin internal rotation and extension stretches
Weeks 6–12	Discontinue sling Advance use in ADLs as strength and pain allow	Same as needed	Add isometric exercises for strengthening of rotator cuff and deltoid Advance to resistive exercises as tolerated Avoid excessive resistance in internal rotation to protect subscapularis Advance passive strengthening exercises to full PROM (Figs. 20-20 and 20-21)
Weeks 12–16			May add isokinetics when patient obtains 85% of normal AROM and at least 4/5 strength for anterior deltoid and internal and external rotators Allow modified sports: short irons and putting in golf, and ground stroke in tennis
4+ Months			Allow progressive return to sports Progress stretching and strengthening

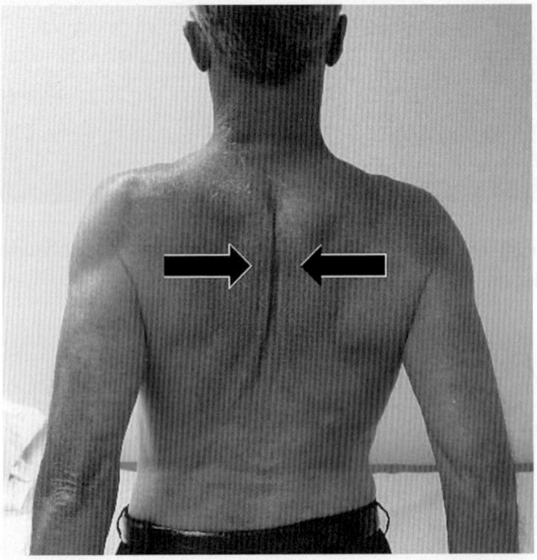

Figure 20-17 Scapular stabilizing exercises of retraction and elevation.

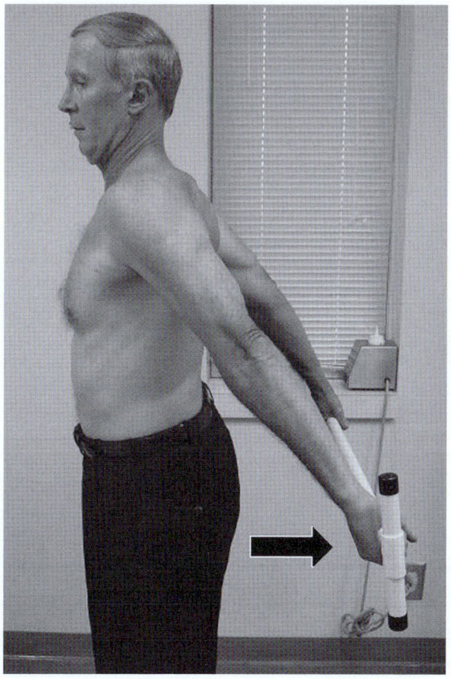

Figure 20-18 Extension exercises with a stick.

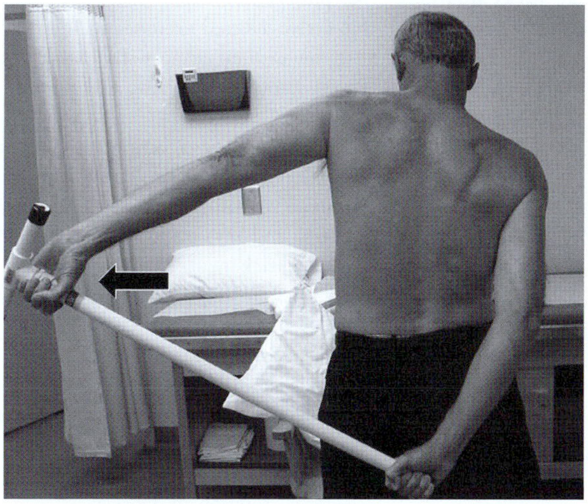

Figure 20-19 Internal rotation exercises using a stick.

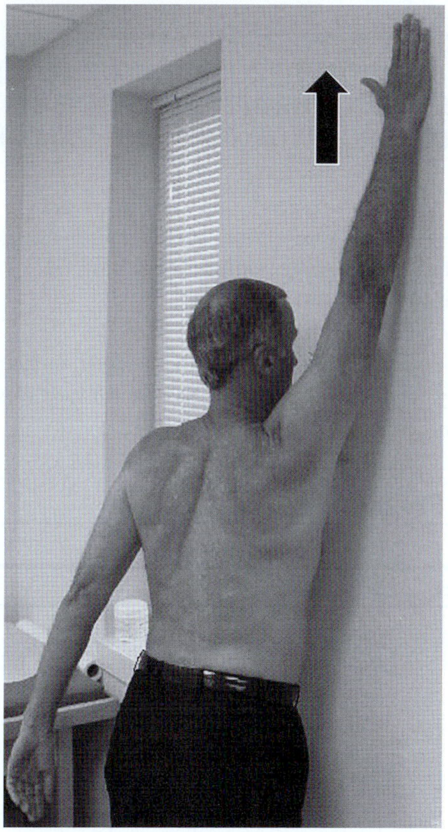

Figure 20-20 Wall slides for terminal elevation.

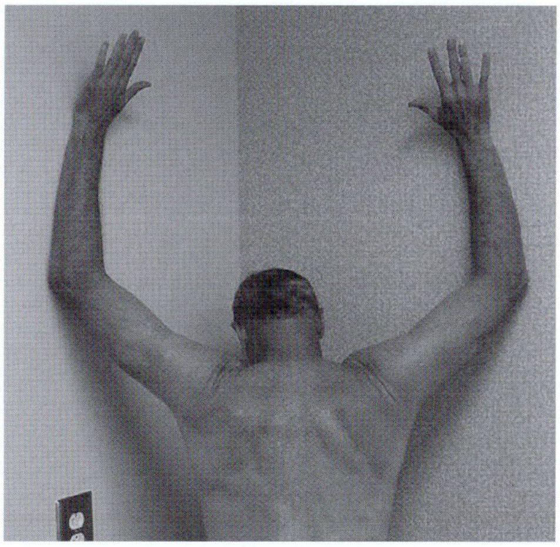

Figure 20-21 Corner or doorway stretch for terminal external rotation in abduction.

CATEGORY B: POSTOPERATIVE REHABILITATION PROGRAM FOR TOTAL SHOULDER ARTHROPLASTY: POOR OR REPAIRED ROTATOR CUFF AND DELTOID

Days 1 to 3

- Arm in sling or abduction pillow in hospital
- Out of bed ambulating
- Elbow, wrist, and finger AROM exercises
- Passive pendulum exercises with therapist to tolerance
- Family member instructed in passive forward elevation within limits set at surgery

Home Program

Time Frame	Protection and Use	Modalities	Exercises
Weeks 1–6	Wear sling outdoors and to sleep Patient may or may not have abduction pillow, and exercises may be performed from pillow May take arm out of sling indoors but should protect arm at all times; do not take shoulder below position it was in while in pillow Patient may bring hand to mouth for eating or washing while maintaining elbow at the side May place hand pointing straight ahead, as on armrest of chair No active elevation	Cold pack Ultrasound to scapular muscles TENS for pain if needed May advance to hot packs after sutures removed	Goal in ROM determined at time of surgery Passive elevation to limit set at surgery Passive external rotation to limit set at surgery Codman's pendulum exercises No pulleys No active-assisted exercises including supine arm elevation with a stick Begin scapular stabilizing exercises at week 4
Weeks 6–8	Discontinue sling or abduction pillow May begin active elevation as tolerated beginning with weight of the arm	Same	Goal: Full passive elevation and external rotation Begin active-assisted supine elevation with a stick and advance to standing elevation with a stick Start table or thigh-level slides before wall slides Begin internal rotation and extension exercises Light isometrics for muscle reeducation Begin pulley Advance to assisted wall slides and external rotation in doorway Begin passive elevation with active eccentric arm lowering
Weeks 8–10	Same	Same	Begin isometric exercises for strengthening of deltoid and rotator cuff as tolerated Begin terminal stretching for elevation and external rotation
Weeks 10–12	Same	Same	Advance to resistive exercises as tolerated with elastic bands or dumbbells Minimize pain and avoid recurrent impingement problems
12+ Weeks	Same	Same	Advance to isokinetic exercises Focus on correct scapulothoracic rhythm with AROM exercises

CATEGORY C: LIMITED GOALS PROGRAM

In hospital

- Arm in sling
- Elbow, wrist, and finger AROM exercises
- May or may not begin limited passive ROM exercises of the shoulder
- No use of arm with ADLs
- Pendulum exercises

Time Frame	Recommendations
Weeks 2–3	May begin limited passive elevation exercises with family member
Week 6	Gradual wean from sling Begin scapular stabilizing exercises to pain tolerance Begin passive external rotation to 20°
Week 12	Begin isometric strengthening Begin gravity-eliminated activities within pain tolerance
Month 4	Begin light elastic resistive exercises
Expected results	Active elevation to 120° Active external rotation to 30° Pain free use of arm below shoulder level

CATEGTORY D: REVERSE PROSTHESIS

Days 1 to 3 in Hospital

- Arm in sling or abduction pillow
- Out of bed ambulating
- Elbow, wrist, and finger AROM exercises
- Passive forward flexion in the scapular plane allowed to 90°
- Passive external rotation allowed to 30°

Home Program

Time Frame	Protection and Use	Exercises
Weeks 1–3	Wear sling at all times, except to flex and extend the elbow and during supervised therapy Avoid placing the arm in an adducted, internally rotated, and extended position (the position of dislocation for reverse prostheses) Patient may bring hand to mouth for eating or washing while maintaining elbow at their side No active elevation	Passive forward flexion to 90° and passive external rotation to 30° Deltoid and periscapular isometrics No pulleys No active-assisted exercises, including supine arm elevation with a stick
Weeks 3–6	Same	Passive forward flexion to 120° and passive external rotation to 45° Deltoid and periscapular isometrics
Weeks 6–12	Discontinue the sling Maintain dislocation precautions	Passive forward flexion to tolerance Begin passive internal rotation with the arm in 60° of abduction Begin activeassisted ROM, initially supine with the scapula stabilized
Weeks 10–12		Advance to AROM
12+ Weeks		Begin resistive exercises

Index

Note: Page numbers followed by *b* indicate boxes, *f* indicate figures and *t* indicate tables.

B

D

G

J

K

L

M

Q

R

S